2nd Edition

HARRISON'S™
CARDIOVASCULAR MEDICINE

Derived from Harrison's Principles of Internal Medicine, 18th Edition

Editors

DAN L. LONGO, MD

Professor of Medicine, Harvard Medical School;
Senior Physician, Brigham and Women's Hospital;
Deputy Editor, New England Journal of Medicine,
Boston, Massachusetts

DENNIS L. KASPER, MD

William Ellery Channing Professor of Medicine,
Professor of Microbiology and Molecular Genetics,
Harvard Medical School; Director, Channing Laboratory,
Department of Medicine, Brigham and Women's Hospital,
Boston, Massachusetts

J. LARRY JAMESON, MD, PhD

Robert G. Dunlop Professor of Medicine;
Dean, University of Pennsylvania School of Medicine;
Executive Vice-President of the University of Pennsylvania
for the Health System, Philadelphia, Pennsylvania

ANTHONY S. FAUCI, MD

Chief, Laboratory of Immunoregulation;
Director, National Institute of Alergy and Infectious Diseases,
National Institutes of Health,
Bethesda, Maryland

STEPHEN L. HAUSER, MD

Robert A. Fishman Distinguished Professor
and Chairman, Department of Neurology,
Univery of California, San Francisco,
San Francisco, California

JOSEPH LOSCALZO, MD, PhD

Hersey Professor of the Teory and Practice of Medicine,
Harvard Medical School; Chiman, Department of Medicine;
Physician-in-Chief, Brigham and Women's Hospital,
Boston, Massachusetts

2nd Edition

HARRISON'S™

CARDIOVASCULAR MEDICINE

EDITOR

Joseph Loscalzo, MD, PhD

Hersey Professor of the Theory and Practice of Medicine, Harvard Medical School;
Chairman, Department of Medicine; Physician-in-Chief, Brigham and Women's Hospital,
Boston, Massachusetts

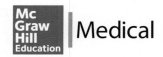

New York   Chicago   San Francisco   Lisbon   London   Madrid   Mexico City
Milan   New Delhi   San Juan   Seoul   Singapore   Sydney   Toronto

1 2 3 4 5 6 7 8 9 0   CTP/CTP   18 17 16 15 14 13

ISBN 978-0-07-181498-0
MHID 0-07-181498-1

This book was set in Bembo by Cenveo® Publisher Services. The editors were James F. Shanahan and Kim J. Davis. The production supervisor was Catherine H. Saggese. Project management was provided by Tania Andrabi, Cenveo Publisher Services. The cover design was by Thomas DePierro. Cover illustration, the coronary vessels of the heart, © MedicalRF.com/Corbis.

China Translation & Printing Services, Ltd. was the printer and binder.

Library of Congress Cataloging-in-Publication Data

Harrison's cardiovascular medicine / editor, Joseph Loscalzo. — 2nd ed.
    p. ; cm.
  Cardiovascular medicine
  Based on 18th edition of Harrison's principles of internal medicine.
  Includes bibliographical references and index.
  ISBN 978-0-07-181498-0 (pbk. : alk. paper) —
  ISBN 0-07-181498-1 (pbk. : alk. paper)
I. Loscalzo, Joseph.   II. Harrison, Tinsley Randolph, 1900-1978.   III. Harrison's principles of internal medicine.   IV. Title: Cardiovascular medicine.
  [DNLM: 1. Cardiovascular Diseases. WG 100]

616.1'2—dc23

2012040509

McGraw-Hill Education books are available at special quantity discounts to use as premiums and sales promotions, or for use in corporate training programs. To contact a representative please e-mail us at bulksales@mcgraw-hill.com.

CONTENTS

v

CONTRIBUTORS

Numbers in brackets refer to the chapter(s) written or cowritten by the contributor.

Jamil Aboulhosn, MD
Assistant Professor, Departments of Medicine and Pediatrics, David Geffen School of Medicine, University of California, Los Angeles, Los Angeles, California [19]

Elliott M. Antman, MD
Professor of Medicine, Harvard Medical School; Brigham and Women's Hospital, Boston, Massachusetts [33, 35]

Eric H. Awtry, MD
Assistant Professor of Medicine, Boston University School of Medicine; Inpatient Clinical Director, Section of Cardiology, Boston Medical Center, Boston, Massachusetts [23, 24]

Robert C. Basner, MD
Professor of Clinical Medicine, Division of Pulmonary, Allergy, and Critical Care Medicine, Columbia University College of Physicians and Surgeons, New York, New York [Appendix]

Deepak L. Bhatt, MD, MPH
Associate Professor of Medicine, Harvard Medical School; Chief of Cardiology, VA Boston Healthcare System; Director, Integrated Interventional Cardiovascular Program, Brigham and Women's Hospital and VA Boston Healthcare System; Senior Investigator, TIMI Study Group, Boston, Massachusetts [36, 44]

Eugene Braunwald, MD, MA (Hon), ScD (Hon) FRCP
Distinguished Hersey Professor of Medicine, Harvard Medical School; Founding Chairman, TIMI Study Group, Brigham and Women's Hospital, Boston, Massachusetts [7, 22, 34]

Cynthia D. Brown, MD
Assistant Professor of Medicine, Division of Pulmonary and Critical Care Medicine, University of Virginia, Charlottesville, Virginia [Review and Self-Assessment]

Christopher P. Cannon, MD
Associate Professor of Medicine, Harvard Medical School; Senior Investigator, TIMI Study Group, Brigham and Women's Hospital, Boston, Massachusetts [34]

Jonathan Carapetis, PhD, MBBS, FRACP, FAFPHM
Director, Menzies School of Health Research, Charles Darwin University, Darwin, Australia [26]

Agustin Castellanos, MD
Professor of Medicine, and Director, Clinical Electrophysiology, Division of Cardiology, University of Miami Miller School of Medicine, Miami, Florida [29]

Murali Chakinala, MD
Associate Professor of Medicine, Division of Pulmonary and Critical Care Medicine, Washington University School of Medicine, St. Louis, Missouri [17]

Panithaya Chareonthaitawee, MD
Associate Professor of Medicine, Mayo Clinic College of Medicine, Rochester, Minnesota [12, 42]

John S. Child, MD, FACC, FAHA, FASE
Streisand Professor of Medicine and Cardiology, Geffen School of Medicine, University of California, Los Angeles (UCLA); Director, Ahmanson-UCLA Adult Congenital Heart Disease Center; Director, UCLA Adult Noninvasive Cardiodiagnostics Laboratory, Ronald Reagan-UCLA Medical Center, Los Angeles, California [19]

Wilson S. Colucci, MD
Thomas J. Ryan Professor of Medicine, Boston University School of Medicine; Chief of Cardiovascular Medicine, Boston Medical Center, Boston, Massachusetts [23, 24]

Mark A. Creager, MD
Professor of Medicine, Harvard Medical School; Simon C. Fireman Scholar in Cardiovascular Medicine; Director, Vascular Center, Brigham and Women's Hospital, Boston, Massachusetts [38, 39]

Robert H. Eckel, MD
Professor of Medicine, Division of Endocrinology, Metabolism and Diabetes, Division of Cardiology; Professor of Physiology and Biophysics, Charles A. Boettcher, II Chair in Atherosclerosis, University of Colorado School of Medicine, Anschutz Medical Campus, Director Lipid Clinic, University of Colorado Hospital, Aurora, Colorado [32]

Andrew J. Einstein, MD, PhD
Assistant Professor of Clinical Medicine, Columbia University College of Physicians and Surgeons; Department of Medicine, Division of Cardiology, Department of Radiology, Columbia University Medical Center and New York-Presbyterian Hospital, New York, New York [Appendix]

Jonathan A. Epstein, MD, DTMH
William Wikoff Smith Professor of Medicine; Chairman, Department of Cell and Developmental Biology; Scientific Director, Cardiovascular Institute, University of Pennsylvania, Philadelphia, Pennsylvania [1]

David P. Faxon, MD
Senior Lecturer, Harvard Medical School; Vice Chair of Medicine for Strategic Planning, Department of Medicine, Brigham and Women's Hospital, Boston, Massachusetts [13, 36, 44]

J. Michael Gaziano, MD, MPH
Professor of Medicine, Harvard Medical School; Chief, Division of Aging, Brigham and Women's Hospital; Director, Massachusetts Veterans Epidemiology Center, Boston VA Healthcare System, Boston, Massachusetts [2]

Thomas A. Gaziano, MD, MSc
Assistant Professor, Harvard Medical School; Assistant Professor, Health Policy and Management, Center for Health Decision Sciences, Harvard School of Public Health; Associate Physician in Cardiovascular Medicine, Department of Cardiology, Brigham and Women's Hospital, Boston, Massachusetts [2]

Ary L. Goldberger, MD
Professor of Medicine, Harvard Medical School; Wyss Institute for Biologically Inspired Engineering, Harvard University; Beth Israel Deaconess Medical Center, Boston, Massachusetts [11, 41, 43]

Anna R. Hemnes, MD
Assistant Professor, Division of Allergy, Pulmonary, and Critical Care Medicine, Vanderbilt University Medical Center, Nashville, Tennessee [Review and Self-Assessment]

Helen H. Hobbs, MD
Professor of Internal Medicine and Molecular Genetics, University of Texas Southwestern Medical Center, Dallas, Texas; Investigator, Howard Hughes Medical Institute, Chevy Chase, Maryland [31]

Judith S. Hochman, MD
Harold Snyder Family Professor of Cardiology; Clinical Chief, Leon Charney Division of Cardiology; Co-Director, NYU-HHC Clinical and Translational Science Institute; Director, Cardiovascular Clinical Research Center, New York University School of Medicine, New York, New York [28]

Sharon A. Hunt, MD, FACC
Professor, Division of Cardiovascular Medicine, Stanford University, Palo Alto, California [18]

David H. Ingbar, MD
Professor of Medicine, Pediatrics, and Physiology; Director, Pulmonary Allergy, Critical Care and Sleep Division, University of Minnesota School of Medicine, Minneapolis, Minnesota [28]

Adolf W. Karchmer, MD
Professor of Medicine, Harvard Medical School; Division of Infectious Diseases, Beth Israel Deaconess Medical Center, Boston, Massachusetts [25]

Louis V. Kirchhoff, MD, MPH
Professor of Internal Medicine (Infectious Diseases) and Epidemiology, Department of Internal Medicine, The University of Iowa, Iowa City, Iowa [27]

Theodore A. Kotchen, MD
Professor Emeritus, Department of Medicine; Associate Dean for Clinical Research, Medical College of Wisconsin, Milwaukee, Wisconsin [37]

Alexander Kratz, MD, PhD, MPH
Associate Professor of Pathology and Cell Biology, Columbia University College of Physicians and Surgeons; Director, Core Laboratory, Columbia University Medical Center, New York, New York [Appendix]

Thomas H. Lee, MD, MSc
Professor of Medicine, Harvard Medical School; Network President, Partners Healthcare System, Boston, Massachusetts [4]

Jane A. Leopold, MD
Associate Professor of Medicine, Harvard Medical School; Brigham and Women's Hospital, Boston, Massachusetts [13, 44]

Peter Libby, MD
Mallinckrodt Professor of Medicine, Harvard Medical School; Chief, Cardiovascular Medicine, Brigham and Women's Hospital, Boston, Massachusetts [1, 30]

Joseph Loscalzo, MD, PhD
Hersey Professor of the Theory and Practice of Medicine, Harvard Medical School; Chairman, Department of Medicine; Physician-in-Chief, Brigham and Women's Hospital, Boston, Massachusetts [1, 3, 6–10, 20, 21, 33, 35, 38, 39]

Hari R. Mallidi, MD
Assistant Professor of Cardiothoracic Surgery; Director of Mechanical Circulatory Support, Stanford University Medical Center, Stanford, California [18]

Douglas L. Mann, MD
Lewin Chair and Chief, Cardiovascular Division; Professor of Medicine, Cell Biology and Physiology, Washington University School of Medicine, St. Louis, Missouri [17]

Francis Marchlinski, MD
Professor of Medicine; Director, Cardiac Electrophysiology, University of Pennsylvania Health System, Philadelphia, Pennsylvania [16]

Matthew Martinez, MD
Lehigh Valley Physician Group, Lehigh Valley Heart Specialists, Allentown, Pennsylvania [12, 42]

Robert J. Myerburg, MD
Professor, Departments of Medicine and Physiology, Division of Cardiology; AHA Chair in Cardiovascular Research, University of Miami Miller School of Medicine, Miami, Florida [29]

Rick A. Nishimura, MD, FACC, FACP
Judd and Mary Morris Leighton Professor of Cardiovascular Diseases; Professor of Medicine; Consultant, Division of Cardiovascular Diseases and Internal Medicine, Mayo Clinic College of Medicine, Rochester, Minnesota [12, 42]

Patrick T. O'Gara, MD
Professor of Medicine, Harvard Medical School; Director, Clinical Cardiology, Brigham and Women's Hospital, Boston, Massachusetts [9, 10, 20]

Michael A. Pesce, PhD
Professor Emeritus of Pathology and Cell Biology, Columbia University College of Physicians and Surgeons; Columbia University Medical Center, New York, New York [Appendix]

Daniel J. Rader, MD
Cooper-McClure Professor of Medicine and Pharmacology, University of Pennsylvania School of Medicine, Philadelphia, Pennsylvania [31]

Anis Rassi, Jr., MD, PhD, FACC, FACP, FAHA
Scientific Director, Anis Rassi Hospital, Goiânia, Brazil [27]

Stuart Rich, MD
Professor of Medicine, Department of Medicine, Section of Cardiology, University of Chicago, Chicago, Illinois [40]

Richard M. Schwartzstein, MD
Ellen and Melvin Gordon Professor of Medicine and Medical Education; Associate Chief, Division of Pulmonary, Critical Care, and Sleep Medicine, Beth Israel Deaconess Medical Center, Harvard Medical School, Boston, Massachusetts [5]

Andrew P. Selwyn, MD, MBCHB
Professor of Medicine, Harvard Medical School; Brigham and Women's Hospital, Boston, Massachusetts [33]

David D. Spragg, MD
Assistant Professor of Medicine, Johns Hopkins University, Baltimore, Maryland [14, 15]

Lynne Warner Stevenson, MD
Professor of Medicine, Harvard Medical School; Director, Heart Failure Program, Brigham and Women's Hospital, Boston, Massachusetts [21]

Gordon F. Tomaselli, MD
Michel Mirowski, MD Professor of Cardiology; Professor of Medicine and Cellular and Molecular Medicine; Chief, Division of Cardiology, Johns Hopkins University, Baltimore, Maryland [14, 15]

Charles M. Wiener, MD
Dean/CEO Perdana University Graduate School of Medicine, Selangor, Malaysia; Professor of Medicine and Physiology, Johns Hopkins University School of Medicine, Baltimore, Maryland [Review and Self-Assessment]

PREFACE

Harrison's Principles of Internal Medicine has been a respected information source for more than 60 years. Over time, the traditional textbook has evolved to meet the needs of internists, family physicians, nurses, and other health care providers. The growing list of *Harrison's* products now includes *Harrison's for the iPad, Harrison's Manual of Medicine,* and *Harrison's Online.* This book, *Harrison's Cardiovascular Medicine,* now in its second edition, is a compilation of chapters related to cardiovascular disorders.

Our readers consistently note the sophistication of the material in the specialty sections of *Harrison's.* Our goal was to bring this information to our audience in a more compact and usable form. Because the topic is more focused, it is possible to enhance the presentation of the material by enlarging the text and the tables. We have also included a Review and Self-Assessment section that includes questions and answers to provoke reflection and to provide additional teaching points.

Cardiovascular disease is the leading cause of death in the United States, and is rapidly becoming a major cause of death in the developing world. Advances in the therapy and prevention of cardiovascular diseases have clearly improved the lives of patients with these common, potentially devastating disorders; yet, the disease prevalence and the risk factor burden for disease (especially obesity in the United States and smoking worldwide) continue to increase globally. Cardiovascular medicine is, therefore, of crucial importance to the field of internal medicine.

Cardiovascular medicine is a large and growing subspecialty, and comprises a number of specific subfields, including coronary heart disease, congenital heart disease, valvular heart disease, cardiovascular imaging, electrophysiology, and interventional cardiology. Many of these areas involve novel technologies that facilitate diagnosis and therapy. The highly specialized nature of these disciplines within cardiology and the increasing specialization of cardiologists argue for the importance of a broad view of cardiovascular medicine by the internist in helping to guide the patient through illness and the decisions that arise in the course of its treatment.

The scientific underpinnings of cardiovascular medicine have also been evolving rapidly. The molecular pathogenesis and genetic basis for many diseases are now known and, with this knowledge, diagnostics and therapeutics are becoming increasingly individualized. Cardiovascular diseases are largely complex phenotypes, and this structural and physiological complexity recapitulates the complex molecular and genetic systems that underlie it. As knowledge about these complex systems expands, the opportunity for identifying unique therapeutic targets increases, holding great promise for definitive interventions in the future. Regenerative medicine is another area of cardiovascular medicine that is rapidly achieving translation. Recognition that the adult human heart can repair itself, albeit sparingly with typical injury, and that cardiac precursor (stem) cells reside within the myocardium to do this can be expanded, and can be used to repair if not regenerate a normal heart is an exciting advance in the field. These concepts represent a completely novel paradigm that will revolutionize the future of the subspecialty.

In view of the importance of cardiovascular medicine to the field of internal medicine, and the rapidity with which the scientific basis for the discipline is advancing, *Harrison's Cardiovascular Medicine* was developed. The purpose of this sectional is to provide the readers with a succinct overview of the field of cardiovascular medicine. To achieve this goal, *Harrison's Cardiovascular Medicine* comprises the key cardiovascular chapters contained in the eighteenth edition of *Harrison's Principles of Internal Medicine,* contributed by leading experts in the field. This sectional is designed not only for physicians-in-training on cardiology rotations, but also for practicing clinicians, other health care professionals, and medical students who seek to enrich and update their knowledge of this rapidly changing field. The editors trust that this book will increase both the readers' knowledge of the field, and their appreciation for its importance.

The first section of the book, "Introduction to Cardiovascular Disorders," provides a systems overview, beginning with the basic biology of the cardiovascular system, followed by epidemiology of cardiovascular disease, and approach to the patient. The integration of pathophysiology with clinical management is a hallmark of *Harrison's,* and can be found throughout each of the subsequent disease-oriented chapters. The book is divided into six main sections that reflect the scope of cardiovascular medicine: (I) Introduction to the Cardiovascular System; (II) Diagnosis of Cardiovascular Disorders; (III) Heart Rhythm Disturbances; (IV) Disorders of the Heart; (V) Disorders of the Vasculature; and (VI) Cardiovascular Atlases.

Our access to information through web-based journals and databases is remarkably efficient. Although these sources of information are invaluable, the daunting body of data creates an even greater need for synthesis by experts in the field. Thus, the preparation of these chapters is a special craft that requires the ability to distill core information from the ever-expanding knowledge base. The editors are, therefore, indebted to our authors, a group of internationally recognized authorities who are masters at providing a comprehensive overview while being able to distill a topic into a concise and interesting chapter. We are indebted to our colleagues at

McGraw-Hill. Jim Shanahan is a champion for *Harrison's* and these books were impeccably produced by Kim Davis. We hope you find this book useful in your effort to achieve continuous learning on behalf of your patients.

Joseph Loscalzo, MD, PhD

Review and self-assessment questions and answers were taken from Wiener CM, Brown CD, Hemnes AR (eds). *Harrison's Self-Assessment and Board Review*, 18th ed. New York, McGraw-Hill, 2012, ISBN 978-0-07-177195-5.

 The global icons call greater attention to key epidemiologic and clinical differences in the practice of medicine throughout the world.

 The genetic icons identify a clinical issue with an explicit genetic relationship.

SECTION I

INTRODUCTION TO CARDIOVASCULAR DISORDERS

CHAPTER 1

BASIC BIOLOGY OF THE CARDIOVASCULAR SYSTEM

Joseph Loscalzo ■ Peter Libby ■ Jonathan Epstein

THE BLOOD VESSEL

VASCULAR ULTRASTRUCTURE

Blood vessels participate in homeostasis on a moment-to-moment basis and contribute to the pathophysiology of diseases of virtually every organ system. Hence, an understanding of the fundamentals of vascular biology furnishes a foundation for understanding the normal function of all organ systems and many diseases. The smallest blood vessels—capillaries—consist of a monolayer of endothelial cells apposed to a basement membrane, adjacent to occasional smooth-muscle-like cells known as *pericytes* (**Fig. 1-1A**). Unlike larger vessels, pericytes do not invest the entire microvessel to form a continuous sheath. Veins and arteries typically have a trilaminar structure (**Fig. 1-1B–E**). The *intima* consists of a monolayer of endothelial cells continuous with those of the capillaries. The middle layer, or *tunica media*, consists of layers of smooth-muscle cells; in veins, the media can contain just a few layers of smooth-muscle cells (Fig. 1-1B). The outer layer, the *adventitia*, consists of looser extracellular matrix with occasional fibroblasts, mast cells, and nerve terminals. Larger arteries have their own vasculature, the *vasa vasorum*, which nourishes the outer aspects of the tunica media. The adventitia of many veins surpasses the intima in thickness.

The tone of muscular arterioles regulates blood pressure and flow through various arterial beds. These smaller arteries have a relatively thick tunica media in relation to the adventitia (Fig. 1-1C). Medium-size muscular arteries similarly contain a prominent tunica media (Fig. 1-1D); atherosclerosis commonly affects this type of muscular artery. The larger elastic arteries have a much more structured tunica media consisting of concentric bands of smooth-muscle cells, interspersed with strata of elastin-rich extracellular matrix sandwiched between layers of smooth-muscle cells (Fig. 1-1E). Larger arteries have a clearly demarcated internal elastic lamina that forms the barrier between the intima and the media. An external elastic lamina demarcates the media of arteries from the surrounding adventitia.

ORIGIN OF VASCULAR CELLS

The intima in human arteries often contains occasional resident smooth-muscle cells beneath the monolayer of vascular endothelial cells. The embryonic origin of smooth-muscle cells in various types of arteries differs. Some upper-body arterial smooth-muscle cells derive from the neural crest, whereas lower-body arteries generally recruit smooth-muscle cells from neighboring mesodermal structures during development. Derivatives of the proepicardial organ, which gives rise to the epicardial layer of the heart, contribute to the vascular smooth-muscle cells of the coronary arteries. Recent evidence suggests that bone marrow may give rise to both vascular endothelial cells and smooth-muscle cells, particularly under conditions of injury repair or vascular lesion formation. Indeed, the ability of bone marrow to repair an injured endothelial monolayer may contribute to maintenance of vascular health, whereas failure to do so may lead to arterial disease. The precise sources of endothelial and mesenchymal progenitor cells or their stem cell precursors remain the subject of active investigation.

VASCULAR CELL BIOLOGY
Endothelial cell

The key cell of the vascular intima, the endothelial cell, has manifold functions in health and disease. Most obviously, the endothelium forms the interface between

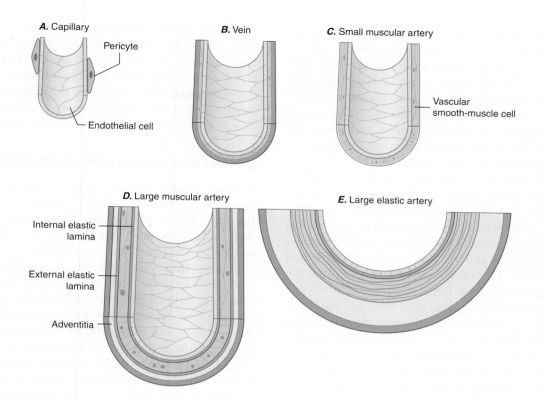

FIGURE 1-1

Schematics of the structures of various types of blood vessels. A. Capillaries consist of an endothelial tube in contact with a discontinuous population of pericytes. **B.** Veins typically have thin medias and thicker adventitias. **C.** A small muscular artery features a prominent tunica media. **D.** Larger muscular arteries have a prominent media with smooth-muscle cells embedded in a complex extracellular matrix. **E.** Larger elastic arteries have cylindrical layers of elastic tissue alternating with concentric rings of smooth-muscle cells.

tissues and the blood compartment. It therefore must regulate the entry of molecules and cells into tissues in a selective manner. The ability of endothelial cells to serve as a selectively permeable barrier fails in many vascular disorders, including atherosclerosis and hypertension. This dysregulation of permeability also occurs in pulmonary edema and other situations of "capillary leak."

The endothelium also participates in the local regulation of blood flow and vascular caliber. Endogenous substances produced by endothelial cells such as prostacyclin, endothelium-derived hyperpolarizing factor, nitric oxide (NO), and hydrogen peroxide (H_2O_2) provide tonic vasodilatory stimuli under physiologic conditions in vivo (Table 1-1). Impaired production or excess catabolism of NO impairs this endothelium-dependent vasodilator function and may contribute to excessive vasoconstriction in various pathologic situations. By contrast, endothelial cells also produce potent vasoconstrictor substances such as endothelin in a regulated fashion. Excessive production of reactive oxygen species, such as superoxide anion (O_2^-), by endothelial or smooth-muscle cells under pathologic conditions (e.g., excessive exposure to angiotensin II) can promote local oxidative stress and inactivate NO.

The endothelial monolayer contributes critically to inflammatory processes involved in normal host defenses and pathologic states. The normal endothelium resists prolonged contact with blood leukocytes; however, when activated by bacterial products such as endotoxin or proinflammatory cytokines released during infection or injury, endothelial cells express an array of leukocyte adhesion molecules that bind various classes of

TABLE 1-1

ENDOTHELIAL FUNCTIONS IN HEALTH AND DISEASE

HOMEOSTATIC PHENOTYPE	DYSFUNCTIONAL PHENOTYPE
Vasodilation	Impaired dilation, vasoconstriction
Antithrombotic, profibrinolytic	Prothrombotic, antifibrinolytic
Anti-inflammatory	Proinflammatory
Antiproliferative	Proproliferative
Antioxidant	Prooxidant
Permselectivity	Impaired barrier function

leukocytes. The endothelial cells appear to recruit selectively different classes of leukocytes in different pathologic conditions. The gamut of adhesion molecules and chemokines generated during acute bacterial infection tends to recruit granulocytes. In chronic inflammatory diseases such as tuberculosis and atherosclerosis, endothelial cells express adhesion molecules that favor the recruitment of mononuclear leukocytes that characteristically accumulate in these conditions.

The endothelium also dynamically regulates thrombosis and hemostasis. Nitric oxide, in addition to its vasodilatory properties, can limit platelet activation and aggregation. Like NO, prostacyclin produced by endothelial cells under normal conditions not only provides a vasodilatory stimulus but also antagonizes platelet activation and aggregation. Thrombomodulin expressed on the surface of endothelial cells binds thrombin at low concentrations and inhibits coagulation through activation of the protein C pathway, inactivating clotting factors Va and VIIIa and thus combating thrombus formation. The surface of endothelial cells contains heparan sulfate glycosaminoglycans that furnish an endogenous antithrombotic coating to the vasculature. Endothelial cells also participate actively in fibrinolysis and its regulation. They express receptors for plasminogen and plasminogen activators and produce tissue-type plasminogen activators. Through local generation of plasmin, the normal endothelial monolayer can promote the lysis of nascent thrombi.

When activated by inflammatory cytokines, bacterial endotoxin, or angiotensin II, for example, endothelial cells can produce substantial quantities of the major inhibitor of fibrinolysis, plasminogen activator inhibitor 1 (PAI-1). Thus, in pathologic circumstances, the endothelial cell may promote local thrombus accumulation rather than combat it. Inflammatory stimuli also induce the expression of the potent procoagulant tissue factor, a contributor to disseminated intravascular coagulation in sepsis.

Endothelial cells also participate in the pathophysiology of a number of immune-mediated diseases. Lysis of endothelial cells mediated by complement provides an example of immunologically mediated tissue injury. The presentation of foreign histocompatibility complex antigens by endothelial cells in solid-organ allografts can trigger immunologic rejection. In addition, immune-mediated endothelial injury may contribute in some patients with thrombotic thrombocytopenic purpura and patients with hemolytic-uremic syndrome. Thus, in addition to contributing to innate immune responses, endothelial cells participate actively in both humoral and cellular limbs of the immune response.

Endothelial cells regulate growth of the subjacent smooth-muscle cells as well. Heparan sulfate glycosaminoglycans elaborated by endothelial cells can hold smooth-muscle proliferation in check. In contrast, when exposed to various injurious stimuli, endothelial cells can elaborate growth factors and chemoattractants, such as platelet-derived growth factor, that can promote the migration and proliferation of vascular smooth-muscle cells. Dysregulated elaboration of these growth-stimulatory molecules may promote smooth-muscle accumulation in atherosclerotic lesions.

Clinical assessment of endothelial function

Various invasive and noninvasive approaches can be used to evaluate endothelial vasodilator function in humans. Either pharmacologic agonists or increased flow stimulates the endothelium to release acutely molecular effectors that alter underlying smooth-muscle cell tone. Invasively, infusion of the cholinergic agonists acetylcholine and methacholine stimulates the release of NO from normal endothelial cells. Changes in coronary diameter can be quantitatively measured in response to an intracoronary infusion of these short-lived, rapidly acting agents. Noninvasive assessment of endothelial function in the forearm circulation typically involves occlusion of brachial artery blood flow with a blood pressure cuff, which elicits reactive hyperemia after release; the resulting flow increase normally causes endothelium-dependent vasodilation, which is measured as the change in brachial artery blood flow and diameter by ultrasound (Fig. 1-2). This approach depends on shear stress–dependent changes in endothelial release of NO after restoration of blood flow, as well as the effect of adenosine released (transiently) from ischemic tissue in the forearm.

Typically, these invasive and noninvasive approaches detect inducible vasodilatory changes in vessel diameter of ~10%. In individuals with atherosclerosis or its risk factors (especially hypertension, hypercholesterolemia, diabetes mellitus, and smoking), such studies can detect endothelial dysfunction as defined by a smaller change in diameter and, in the extreme case, a so-called paradoxical vasoconstrictor response owing to the direct effect of cholinergic agonists on vascular smooth-muscle cell tone.

Vascular smooth-muscle cell

The vascular smooth-muscle cell, the major cell type of the media layer of blood vessels, also contributes actively to vascular pathobiology. Contraction and relaxation of smooth-muscle cells at the level of the muscular arteries controls blood pressure, and, hence, regional blood flow and the afterload experienced by the left ventricle (see later). The vasomotor tone of veins, which is governed by smooth-muscle cell tone, regulates the capacitance of the venous tree and influences the preload experienced by both ventricles. Smooth-muscle cells in the adult vessel seldom of contractile proteins and greater production of extracellular matrix macromolecules, can contribute to the development of arterial stenoses in atherosclerosis, arteriolar remodeling that can sustain and propagate hypertension, and the hyperplastic response of arteries injured by angioplasty or stent deployment. In the pulmonary circulation, smooth-muscle migration and proliferation contribute decisively to the pulmonary vascular disease that gradually occurs in response to sustained high-flow states such as left-to-right shunts. Such pulmonary vascular disease provides a major obstacle to the management of many patients with adult congenital heart disease. Elucidation of the signaling pathways that regulate the reversible transition of the vascular smooth-muscle cell phenotype remains an active focus of investigation. Among other mediators, microRNAs have emerged as powerful regulators of this transition, offering new targets for intervention.

The activated, phenotypically modulated smooth-muscle cells secrete the bulk of vascular extracellular matrix. Excessive production of collagen and glycosaminoglycans contributes to the remodeling and altered biology and biomechanics of arteries affected by hypertension or atherosclerosis. In larger elastic arteries, the elastin synthesized by smooth-muscle cells serves to maintain not only normal arterial structure but also hemodynamic function. The ability of the larger arteries, such as the aorta, to store the kinetic energy of systole promotes tissue perfusion during diastole. Arterial stiffness associated with aging or disease, as manifested by a widening pulse pressure, increases left ventricular afterload and portends a poor outcome.

Like endothelial cells, vascular smooth-muscle cells do not merely respond to vasomotor or inflammatory stimuli elaborated by other cell types but can themselves serve as a source of such stimuli. For example, when exposed to bacterial endotoxin or other proinflammatory stimuli, smooth-muscle cells can elaborate cytokines and other inflammatory mediators. Like endothelial cells, upon inflammatory activation, arterial smooth-muscle cells can produce prothrombotic mediators such as tissue factor, the antifibrinolytic protein PAI-1, and other molecules that modulate thrombosis and fibrinolysis. Smooth-muscle cells also elaborate autocrine growth factors that can amplify hyperplastic responses to arterial injury.

Vascular smooth-muscle cell function

Vascular smooth-muscle cells govern vessel tone. Those cells contract when stimulated by a rise in intracellular calcium concentration by calcium influx through the plasma membrane and by calcium release from intracellular stores (**Fig. 1-3**). In vascular smooth-muscle cells, voltage-dependent L-type calcium channels open with membrane depolarization, which is

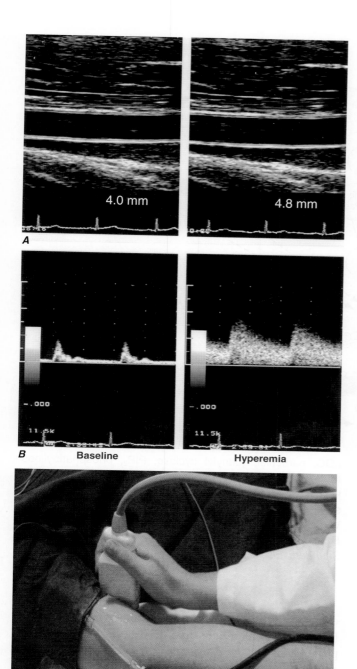

A

4.0 mm   4.8 mm

B   Baseline   Hyperemia

C

FIGURE 1-2

Assessment of endothelial function in vivo using blood pressure cuff-occlusion and release. Upon deflation of the cuff, changes in diameter (**A**) and blood flow (**B**) of the brachial artery are monitored with an ultrasound probe (**C**). (*Reproduced with permission of J. Vita, MD.*)

replicate. This homeostatic quiescence of smooth-muscle cells changes in conditions of arterial injury or inflammatory activation. Proliferation and migration of arterial smooth-muscle cells, which is associated with a change in phenotype characterized by lower content

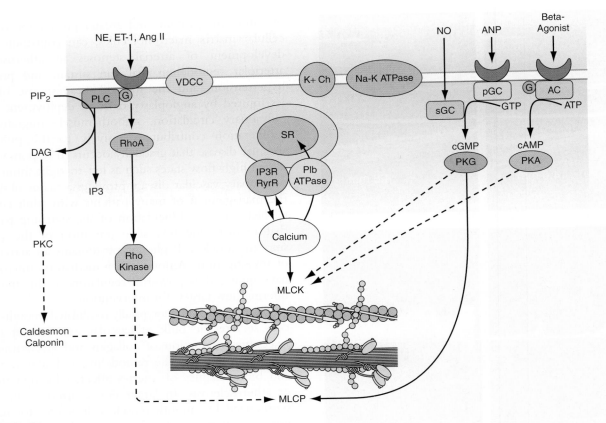

FIGURE 1-3

Regulation of vascular smooth-muscle cell calcium concentration and actomyosin ATPase-dependent contraction. AC, adenylyl cyclase; Ang II, angiotensin II; ANP, antrial natriuretic peptide; DAG, diacylglycerol; ET-1, endothelin-1; G, G-protein; IP₃, inositol 1,4,5-trisphosphate; MLCK, myosin light chain kinase; MLCP, myosin light chain phosphatase; NE, norepinephrine; NO, nitric oxide; pGC, particular guanylyl cyclase; PIP₂, phosphatidylinositol 4,5-bisphosphate; PKA, protein kinase A; PKC, protein kinase C; PKG, protein kinase G; PLC, phospholipase C; sGC, soluble guanylyl cyclase; SR, sarcoplasmic reticulum; VDCC, voltage-dependent calcium channel. *(Modified from B Berk, in Vascular Medicine, 3rd ed, p 23. Philadelphia, Saunders, Elsevier, 2006; with permission.)*

regulated by energy-dependent ion pumps such as the Na⁺,K⁺-ATPase pump and ion channels such as the Ca²⁺-sensitive K⁺ channel. Local changes in intracellular calcium concentration, termed *calcium sparks*, result from the influx of calcium through the voltage-dependent calcium channel and are caused by the coordinated activation of a cluster of ryanodine-sensitive calcium release channels in the sarcoplasmic reticulum (see later). Calcium sparks directly augment intracellular calcium concentration and indirectly increase intracellular calcium concentration by activating chloride channels. In addition, calcium sparks reduce smooth-muscle contractility by activating large-conductance calcium-sensitive K⁺ channels, hyperpolarizing the cell membrane and thereby limiting further voltage-dependent increases in intracellular calcium.

Biochemical agonists also increase intracellular calcium concentration, in this case by receptor-dependent activation of phospholipase C with hydrolysis of phosphatidylinositol 4,5-bisphosphate, resulting in generation of diacylglycerol (DAG) and inositol 1,4,5-trisphosphate (IP₃). These membrane lipid derivatives in turn activate protein kinase C and increase intracellular calcium concentration. In addition, IP₃ binds to specific receptors on the sarcoplasmic reticulum membrane to increase calcium efflux from this calcium storage pool into the cytoplasm.

Vascular smooth-muscle cell contraction is controlled principally by the phosphorylation of myosin light chain, which in the steady state depends on the balance between the actions of myosin light chain kinase and myosin light chain phosphatase. Calcium activates myosin light chain kinase through the formation of a calcium-calmodulin complex. Phosphorylation of myosin light chain by this kinase augments myosin ATPase activity and enhances contraction. Myosin light chain phosphatase dephosphorylates myosin light chain, reducing myosin ATPase activity and contractile force. Phosphorylation of the myosin-binding subunit (thr695) of myosin light chain phosphatase by Rho kinase inhibits phosphatase activity and induces calcium sensitization of the contractile apparatus. Rho kinase is itself activated by the small GTPase RhoA, which is stimulated by guanosine exchange factors and inhibited by GTPase-activating proteins.

Both cyclic AMP and cyclic GMP relax vascular smooth-muscle cells through complex mechanisms. β agonists, acting through their G-protein-coupled receptors activate adenylyl cyclase to convert ATP to cyclic AMP; NO and atrial natriuretic peptide acting directly and via a G-protein-coupled receptor, respectively, activate guanylyl cyclase to convert GTP to cyclic GMP. These agents in turn activate protein kinase A and protein kinase G, respectively, which inactivate myosin light chain kinase and decrease vascular smooth-muscle cell tone. In addition, protein kinase G can interact directly with the myosin-binding substrate subunit of myosin light chain phosphatase, increasing phosphatase activity and decreasing vascular tone. Finally, several mechanisms drive NO-dependent, protein kinase G–mediated reductions in vascular smooth-muscle cell calcium concentration, including phosphorylation-dependent inactivation of RhoA; decreased IP_3 formation; phosphorylation of the IP_3 receptor–associated cyclic GMP kinase substrate, with subsequent inhibition of IP_3 receptor function; phosphorylation of phospholamban, which increases calcium ATPase activity and sequestration of calcium in the sarcoplasmic reticulum; and protein kinase G–dependent stimulation of plasma membrane calcium ATPase activity, perhaps by activation of the Na^+,K^+-ATPase pump or hyperpolarization of the cell membrane by activation of calcium-dependent K^+ channels.

Control of vascular smooth-muscle cell tone

The tone of vascular smooth-muscle cells is governed by the autonomic nervous system and by the endothelium in tightly regulated control networks. Autonomic neurons enter the blood vessel medial layer from the adventitia and modulate vascular smooth-muscle cell tone in response to baroreceptors and chemoreceptors within the aortic arch and carotid bodies and in response to thermoreceptors in the skin. These regulatory components include rapidly acting reflex arcs modulated by central inputs that respond to sensory inputs (olfactory, visual, auditory, and tactile) as well as emotional stimuli. Three classes of nerves mediate autonomic regulation of vascular tone: *sympathetic*, whose principal neurotransmitters are epinephrine and norepinephrine; *parasympathetic*, whose principal neurotransmitter is acetylcholine; and *nonadrenergic/noncholinergic*, which include two subgroups—nitrergic, whose principal neurotransmitter is NO, and peptidergic, whose principal neurotransmitters are substance P, vasoactive intestinal peptide, calcitonin gene-related peptide, and ATP.

Each of these neurotransmitters acts through specific receptors on the vascular smooth-muscle cell to modulate intracellular calcium and, consequently, contractile tone. Norepinephrine activates α receptors, and epinephrine activates α and β receptors (adrenergic receptors); in most blood vessels, norepinephrine activates postjunctional α_1 receptors in large arteries and α_2 receptors in small arteries and arterioles, leading to vasoconstriction. Most blood vessels express β_2-adrenergic receptors on their vascular smooth-muscle cells and respond to β agonists by cyclic AMP–dependent relaxation. Acetylcholine released from parasympathetic neurons binds to muscarinic receptors (of which there are five subtypes, M_{1-5}) on vascular smooth-muscle cells to yield vasorelaxation. In addition, NO stimulates presynaptic neurons to release acetylcholine, which can stimulate the release of NO from the endothelium. Nitrergic neurons release NO produced by neuronal NO synthase, which causes vascular smooth-muscle cell relaxation via the cyclic GMP–dependent and –independent mechanisms described earlier. The peptidergic neurotransmitters all potently vasodilate, acting either directly or through endothelium-dependent NO release to decrease vascular smooth-muscle cell tone.

The endothelium modulates vascular smooth-muscle tone by the direct release of several effectors, including NO, prostacyclin, hydrogen sulfide, and endothelium-derived hyperpolarizing factor, all of which cause vasorelaxation, and endothelin, which causes vasoconstriction. The release of these endothelial effectors of vascular smooth-muscle cell tone is stimulated by mechanical (shear stress, cyclic strain, etc.) and biochemical mediators (purinergic agonists, muscarinic agonists, peptidergic agonists), with the biochemical mediators acting through endothelial receptors specific to each class. In addition to these local paracrine modulators of vascular smooth-muscle cell tone, circulating mediators can affect tone, including norepinephrine and epinephrine, vasopressin, angiotensin II, bradykinin, and the natriuretic peptides (ANP, BNP, CNP, and DNP), as discussed earlier.

VASCULAR REGENERATION

Growth of new blood vessels can occur in response to conditions such as chronic hypoxemia and tissue ischemia. Growth factors, including vascular endothelial growth factor (VEGF) and forms of fibroblast growth factor (FGF), activate a signaling cascade that stimulates endothelial proliferation and tube formation, defined as *angiogenesis*. The development of collateral vascular networks in the ischemic myocardium reflects this process and can result from selective activation of endothelial progenitor cells, which may reside in the blood vessel wall or home to the ischemic tissue

TABLE 1-2

GENETIC POLYMORPHISMS IN VASCULAR FUNCTION AND DISEASE RISK

GENE	POLYMORPHIC ALLELE	CLINICAL IMPLICATIONS
α-Adrenergic Receptors		
α_{1A}	Arg492Cys	None
α_{2B}	Glu9/G1712	Increased CHD events
α_{2C}	A2cDcl3232-325	Ethnic differences in risk of hypertension or heart failure
Angiotensin-converting enzyme (ACE)	Insertion/deletion polymorphism in intron 16	D allele or DD genotype-increased response to ACE inhibitors; inconsistent data for increased risk of atherosclerotic heart disease, and hypertension
Ang II type I receptor	1166A → C Ala-Cys	Increased response to Ang II and increased risk of pregnancy-associated hypertension
β-Adrenergic Receptors		
β_1	Ser49Gly	Increased HR and DCM risk
	Arg389Gly	Increased heart failure in blacks
β_2	Arg16Gly	Familial hypertension, increased obesity risk
	Glu27Gln	Hypertension in white type II diabetics
	Thr164Ile	Decreased agonist affinity and worse HF outcome
B2-Bradykinin receptor	Cys58Thr, Cys412Gly, Thr21Met	Increased risk of hypertension in some ethnic groups
Endothelial nitric oxide synthase (eNOS)	Nucleotide repeats in introns 4 and 13, Glu298Asp	Increased MI and venous thrombosis
	Thr785Cys	Early coronary artery disease

Abbreviations: CHD, coronary heart disease; HR, heart rate; DCM, dilated cardiomyopathy; HF, heart failure; MI, myocardial infarction.
Source: Derived from B Schaefer et al: Heart Dis 5:129, 2003.

subtended by an occluded or severely stenotic vessel from the bone marrow. True arteriogenesis, or the development of a new blood vessel that includes all three cell layers, normally does not occur in the cardiovascular system of adult mammals. The molecular mechanisms and progenitor cells that can recapitulate blood vessel development de novo are under rapidly advancing study.

VASCULAR PHARMACOGENOMICS

The last decade has witnessed considerable progress in efforts to define the genetic differences underlying individual variations in vascular pharmacologic responses. Many investigators have focused on receptors and enzymes associated with neurohumoral modulation of vascular function as well as hepatic enzymes that metabolize drugs that affect vascular tone. The genetic polymorphisms thus far associated with differences in vascular response often (but not invariably) relate to functional differences in the activity or expression of the receptor or enzyme of interest. Some of these polymorphisms appear to have different allele frequencies in specific ethnic groups. A summary of recently identified polymorphisms defining these vascular pharmacogenomic differences is provided in **Table 1-2**.

CELLULAR BASIS OF CARDIAC CONTRACTION

CARDIAC ULTRASTRUCTURE

About three-fourths of the ventricular mass is composed of cardiomyocytes, normally 60–140 μm in length and 17–25 μm in diameter **(Fig. 1-4A)**. Each cell contains multiple, rodlike cross-banded strands (myofibrils) that

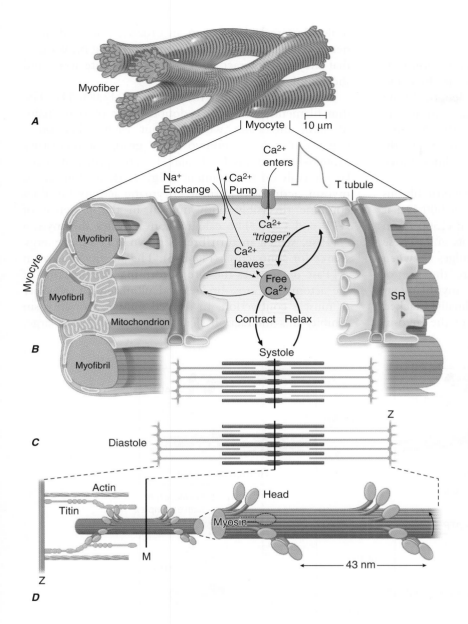

FIGURE 1-4

A shows the branching myocytes making up the cardiac myofibers. **B** illustrates the critical role played by the changing [Ca²⁺] in the myocardial cytosol. Ca²⁺ ions are schematically shown as entering through the calcium channel that opens in response to the wave of depolarization that travels along the sarcolemma. These Ca²⁺ ions "trigger" the release of more calcium from the sarcoplasmic reticulum (SR) and thereby initiate a contraction-relaxation cycle. Eventually, the small quantity of Ca²⁺ that has entered the cell leaves predominantly through an Na⁺/Ca²⁺ exchanger, with a lesser role for the sarcolemmal Ca²⁺ pump. The varying actin-myosin overlap is shown for (**B**) systole, when [Ca²⁺] is maximal, and (**C**) diastole, when [Ca²⁺] is minimal. **D**. The myosin heads, attached to the thick filaments, interact with the thin actin filaments. *(From LH Opie, Heart Physiology, reprinted with permission. Copyright LH Opie, 2004.)*

run the length of the cell and are composed of serially repeating structures, the sarcomeres. The cytoplasm between the myofibrils contains other cell constituents, including the single centrally located nucleus, numerous mitochondria, and the intracellular membrane system, the sarcoplasmic reticulum.

The *sarcomere*, the structural and functional unit of contraction, lies between adjacent Z lines, which are dark repeating bands that are apparent on transmission electron microscopy. The distance between Z lines varies with the degree of contraction or stretch of the muscle and ranges between 1.6 and 2.2 μm. Within the confines of the sarcomere are alternating light and dark bands, giving the myocardial fibers their striated appearance under the light microscope. At the center of the sarcomere is a dark band of constant length

(1.5 μm), the A band, which is flanked by two lighter bands, the I bands, which are of variable length. The sarcomere of heart muscle, like that of skeletal muscle, consists of two sets of interdigitating myofilaments. Thicker filaments, composed principally of the protein myosin, traverse the A band; they are about 10 nm (100 Å) in diameter, with tapered ends. Thinner filaments, composed primarily of actin, course from the Z lines through the I band into the A band; they are approximately 5 nm (50 Å) in diameter and 1.0 μm in length. Thus, thick and thin filaments overlap only within the (dark) A band, whereas the (light) I band contains only thin filaments. On electron-microscopic examination, bridges may be seen to extend between the thick and thin filaments within the A band; these are myosin heads bound to actin filaments.

THE CONTRACTILE PROCESS

The sliding filament model for muscle contraction rests on the fundamental observation that both the thick and the thin filaments are constant in overall length during both contraction and relaxation. With activation, the actin filaments are propelled farther into the A band. In the process, the A band remains constant in length, whereas the I band shortens and the Z lines move toward one another.

The *myosin* molecule is a complex, asymmetric fibrous protein with a molecular mass of about 500,000 Da; it has a rodlike portion that is about 150 nm (1500 Å) in length with a globular portion (head) at its end. These globular portions of myosin form the bridges between the myosin and actin molecules and are the site of ATPase activity. In forming the thick myofilament, which is composed of ~300 longitudinally stacked myosin molecules, the rodlike segments of the myosin molecules are laid down in an orderly, polarized manner, leaving the globular portions projecting outward so that they can interact with actin to generate force and shortening **(Fig. 1-4B)**.

Actin has a molecular mass of about 47,000 Da. The thin filament consists of a double helix of two chains of actin molecules wound about each other on a larger molecule, tropomyosin. A group of regulatory proteins—troponins C, I, and T—are spaced at regular intervals on this filament **(Fig. 1-5)**. In contrast to myosin, actin lacks intrinsic enzymatic activity but does combine reversibly with myosin in the presence of ATP and Ca^{2+}. The calcium ion activates the myosin ATPase, which in turn breaks down ATP, the energy source for contraction (Fig. 1-5). The activity of myosin ATPase determines the rate of forming and breaking of the actomyosin cross-bridges and ultimately the velocity of muscle contraction. In relaxed muscle, tropomyosin inhibits this interaction. *Titin* **(Fig. 1-4D)** is a large,

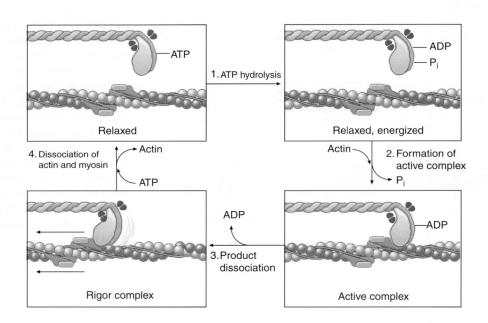

FIGURE 1-5

Four steps in cardiac muscle contraction and relaxation. In relaxed muscle **(upper left)**, ATP bound to the myosin cross-bridge dissociates the thick and thin filaments. **Step 1:** Hydrolysis of myosin-bound ATP by the ATPase site on the myosin head transfers the chemical energy of the nucleotide to the activated cross-bridge **(upper right)**. When cytosolic Ca^{2+} concentration is low, as in relaxed muscle, the reaction cannot proceed because tropomyosin and the troponin complex on the thin filament do not allow the active sites on actin to interact with the cross-bridges. Therefore, even though the cross-bridges are energized, they cannot interact with actin. **Step 2:** When Ca^{2+} binding to troponin C has exposed active sites on the thin filament, actin interacts with the myosin cross-bridges to form an active complex **(lower right)** in which the energy derived from ATP is retained in the actin-bound cross-bridge, whose orientation has not yet shifted. **Step 3:** The muscle contracts when ADP dissociates from the cross-bridge. This step leads to the formation of the low-energy rigor complex **(lower left)** in which the chemical energy derived from ATP hydrolysis has been expended to perform mechanical work (the "rowing" motion of the cross-bridge). **Step 4:** The muscle returns to its resting state, and the cycle ends when a new molecule of ATP binds to the rigor complex and dissociates the cross-bridge from the thin filament. This cycle continues until calcium is dissociated from troponin C in the thin filament, which causes the contractile proteins to return to the resting state with the cross-bridge in the energized state. ATP, adenosine triphosphate; ATPase, adenosine triphosphatase; ADP, adenosine diphosphate. (*From AM Katz: Heart failure: Cardiac function and dysfunction, in Atlas of Heart Diseases, 3rd ed, WS Colucci [ed]. Philadelphia, Current Medicine, 2002. Reprinted with permission.*)

flexible, myofibrillar protein that connects myosin to the Z line; its stretching contributes to the elasticity of the heart. Dystrophin is a long cytoskeletal protein that has an amino-terminal actin-binding domain and a carboxy-terminal domain that binds to the dystroglycan complex at adherens junctions on the cell membrane, thus tethering the sarcomere to the cell membrane at regions tightly coupled to adjacent contracting myocytes. Mutations in components of the dystrophin complex lead to muscular dystrophy and associated cardiomyopathy.

During activation of the cardiac myocyte, Ca^{2+} becomes attached to one of three components of the heterotrimer troponin C, which results in a conformational change in the regulatory protein tropomyosin; the latter, in turn, exposes the actin cross-bridge interaction sites (Fig. 1-5). Repetitive interaction between myosin heads and actin filaments is termed *cross-bridge cycling*, which results in sliding of the actin along the myosin filaments, ultimately causing muscle shortening and/or the development of tension. The splitting of ATP then dissociates the myosin cross-bridge from actin. In the presence of ATP (Fig. 1-5), linkages between actin and myosin filaments are made and broken cyclically as long as sufficient Ca^{2+} is present; these linkages cease when $[Ca^{2+}]$ falls below a critical level, and the troponin-tropomyosin complex once more prevents interactions between the myosin cross-bridges and actin filaments **(Fig. 1-6)**.

Intracytoplasmic Ca^{2+} is a principal determinant of the inotropic state of the heart. Most agents that stimulate myocardial contractility (positive inotropic stimuli), including the digitalis glycosides and β-adrenergic agonists, increase the $[Ca^{2+}]$ in the vicinity of the myofilaments, which in turn triggers cross-bridge cycling. Increased impulse traffic in the cardiac adrenergic nerves stimulates myocardial contractility as a consequence of the release of norepinephrine from cardiac adrenergic nerve endings. Norepinephrine activates myocardial β receptors and, through the G_s-stimulated guanine nucleotide-binding protein, activates the enzyme adenylyl cyclase, which leads to the formation of the intracellular second messenger cyclic AMP from ATP (Fig. 1-6). Cyclic AMP in turn activates protein kinase A (PKA), which phosphorylates the Ca^{2+} channel in the myocardial sarcolemma, thereby enhancing the influx of Ca^{2+} into the myocyte. Other functions of PKA are discussed later.

The *sarcoplasmic reticulum* (SR) **(Fig. 1-7)**, a complex network of anastomosing intracellular channels, invests the myofibrils. Its longitudinally disposed tubules closely invest the surfaces of individual sarcomeres but have no direct continuity with the outside of the cell. However, closely related to the SR, both structurally and functionally, are the transverse tubules, or T system, formed by tubelike invaginations of the sarcolemma that extend into the myocardial fiber along the Z lines, i.e., the ends of the sarcomeres.

CARDIAC ACTIVATION

In the inactive state, the cardiac cell is electrically polarized; i.e., the interior has a negative charge relative to the outside of the cell, with a transmembrane potential of −80 to −100 mV (Chap. 14). The sarcolemma, which in the resting state is largely impermeable to Na^+, has a Na^+- and K^+-stimulating pump energized by ATP that extrudes Na^+ from the cell; this pump plays a critical role in establishing the resting potential. Thus, intracellular $[K^+]$ is relatively high and $[Na^+]$ is far lower; conversely, extracellular $[Na^+]$ is high and $[K^+]$ is low. At the same time, in the resting state, extracellular $[Ca^{2+}]$ greatly exceeds free intracellular $[Ca^{2+}]$.

The action potential has four phases (Fig. 14-1*B*). During the plateau of the action potential (phase 2), there is a slow inward current through L-type Ca^{2+} channels in the sarcolemma (Fig. 1-7). The depolarizing current not only extends across the surface of the cell but penetrates deeply into the cell by way of the ramifying T tubular system. The absolute quantity of Ca^{2+} that crosses the sarcolemma and the T system is relatively small and by itself appears to be insufficient to bring about full activation of the contractile apparatus. However, this Ca^{2+} current triggers the release of much larger quantities of Ca^{2+} from the SR, a process termed *Ca^{2+}-induced Ca^{2+} release*. The latter is a major determinant of intracytoplasmic $[Ca^{2+}]$ and therefore of myocardial contractility.

Ca^{2+} is released from the SR through a Ca^{2+} release channel, a cardiac isoform of the ryanodine receptor (RyR2), which controls intracytoplasmic $[Ca^{2+}]$ and, as in vascular smooth-muscle cells, leads to the local changes in intracellular $[Ca^{2+}]$ called calcium sparks. A number of regulatory proteins, including *calstabin 2*, inhibit RyR2 and thereby the release of Ca^{2+} from the SR. PKA dissociates calstabin from the RyR2, enhancing Ca^{2+} release and thereby myocardial contractility. Excessive plasma catecholamine levels and cardiac sympathetic neuronal release of norepinephrine cause hyperphosphorylation of PKA, leading to calstabin 2–depleted RyR2. The latter depletes SR Ca^{2+} stores and thereby impairs cardiac contraction, leading to heart failure, and also triggers ventricular arrhythmias.

The Ca^{2+} released from the SR then diffuses toward the myofibrils, where, as already described, it combines with troponin C (Fig. 1-6). By repressing this inhibitor of contraction, Ca^{2+} activates the myofilaments to shorten. During repolarization, the activity of the Ca^{2+} pump in the SR, the SR Ca^{2+} ATPase (SERCA$_2$A), reaccumulates Ca^{2+} against a concentration gradient, and the Ca^{2+} is stored in the SR by its attachment to a protein, *calsequestrin*.

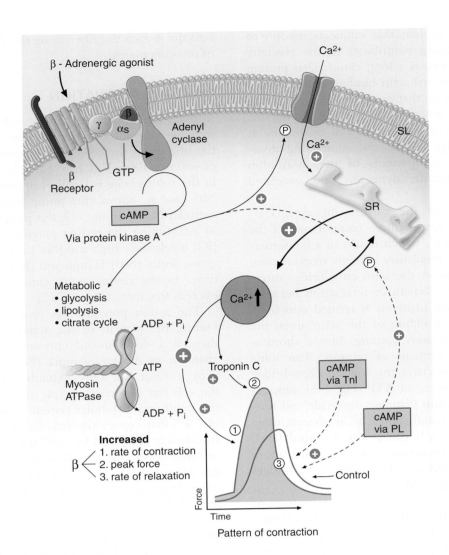

FIGURE 1-6

Signal systems involved in positive inotropic and lusitropic (enhanced relaxation) effects of β-adrenergic stimulation.
When the β-adrenergic agonist interacts with the β receptor, a series of G protein–mediated changes leads to activation of adenylyl cyclase and the formation of cyclic adenosine monophosphate (cAMP). The latter acts via protein kinase A to stimulate metabolism (**left**) and phosphorylate the Ca^{2+} channel protein (**right**). The result is an enhanced opening probability of the Ca^{2+} channel, thereby increasing the inward movement of Ca^{2+} ions through the sarcolemma (SL) of the T tubule. These Ca^{2+} ions release more calcium from the sarcoplasmic reticulum (SR) to increase cytosolic Ca^{2+} and activate troponin C. Ca^{2+} ions

also increase the rate of breakdown of adenosine triphosphate (ATP) to adenosine diphosphate (ADP) and inorganic phosphate (Pi). Enhanced myosin ATPase activity explains the increased rate of contraction, with increased activation of troponin C explaining increased peak force development. An increased rate of relaxation is explained by the fact that cAMP also activates the protein phospholamban, situated on the membrane of the SR, that controls the rate of uptake of calcium into the SR. The latter effect explains enhanced relaxation (lusitropic effect). P, phosphorylation; PL, phospholamban; TnI, troponin I. *(Modified from LH Opie, Heart Physiology, reprinted with permission. Copyright LH Opie, 2004.)*

This reaccumulation of Ca^{2+} is an energy (ATP)-requiring process that lowers the cytoplasmic $[Ca^{2+}]$ to a level that inhibits the actomyosin interaction responsible for contraction, and in this manner leads to myocardial relaxation. Also, there is an exchange of Ca^{2+} for Na^+ at the sarcolemma (Fig. 1-7), reducing the cytoplasmic $[Ca^{2+}]$. Cyclic AMP–dependent PKA phosphorylates the SR protein *phospholamban*; the latter, in turn, permits activation of the Ca^{2+} pump, thereby increasing the uptake of Ca^{2+} by the SR, accelerating

the rate of relaxation and providing larger quantities of Ca^{2+} in the SR for release by subsequent depolarization, thereby stimulating contraction.

Thus, the combination of the cell membrane, transverse tubules, and SR, with their ability to transmit the action potential and release and then reaccumulate Ca^{2+}, plays a fundamental role in the rhythmic contraction and relaxation of heart muscle. Genetic or pharmacologic alterations of any component, whatever its etiology, can disturb these functions.

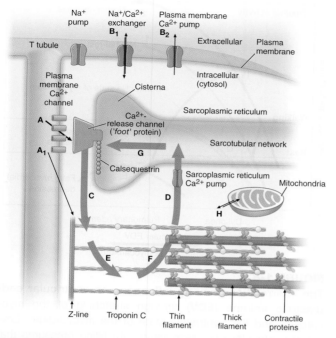

FIGURE 1-7

The Ca²⁺ fluxes and key structures involved in cardiac excitation-contraction coupling. The arrows denote the direction of Ca²⁺ fluxes. The thickness of each arrow indicates the magnitude of the calcium flux. Two Ca²⁺ cycles regulate excitation-contraction coupling and relaxation. The larger cycle is entirely intracellular and involves Ca²⁺ fluxes into and out of the sarcoplasmic reticulum, as well as Ca²⁺ binding to and release from troponin C. The smaller extracellular Ca²⁺ cycle occurs when this cation moves into and out of the cell. The action potential opens plasma membrane Ca²⁺ channels to allow passive entry of Ca²⁺ into the cell from the extracellular fluid (*arrow A*). Only a small portion of the Ca²⁺ that enters the cell directly activates the contractile proteins (*arrow A₁*). The extracellular cycle is completed when Ca²⁺ is actively transported back out to the extracellular fluid by way of two plasma membrane fluxes mediated by the sodium-calcium exchanger (*arrow B₁*) and the plasma membrane calcium pump (*arrow B₂*). In the intracellular Ca²⁺ cycle, passive Ca²⁺ release occurs through channels in the cisternae (*arrow C*) and initiates contraction; active Ca²⁺ uptake by the Ca²⁺ pump of the sarcotubular network (*arrow D*) relaxes the heart. Diffusion of Ca²⁺ within the sarcoplasmic reticulum (*arrow G*) returns this activator cation to the cisternae, where it is stored in a complex with calsequestrin and other calcium-binding proteins. Ca²⁺ released from the sarcoplasmic reticulum initiates systole when it binds to troponin C (*arrow E*). Lowering of cytosolic [Ca²⁺] by the sarcoplasmic reticulum (SR) causes this ion to dissociate from troponin (*arrow F*) and relaxes the heart. Ca²⁺ also may move between mitochondria and cytoplasm *(H)*. (Adapted from AM Katz: Physiology of the Heart, 4th ed. Philadelphia, Lippincott, Williams & Wilkins, 2005; with permission.)

CONTROL OF CARDIAC PERFORMANCE AND OUTPUT

The extent of shortening of heart muscle and, therefore, the stroke volume of the ventricle in the intact heart depend on three major influences: (1) the length of the muscle at the onset of contraction, i.e., the preload; (2) the tension that the muscle is called on to develop during contraction, i.e., the afterload; and (3) the contractility of the muscle, i.e., the extent and velocity of shortening at any given preload and afterload. The major determinants of preload, afterload, and contractility are shown in **Table 1-3**.

The role of muscle length (preload)

The preload determines the length of the sarcomeres at the onset of contraction. The length of the sarcomeres associated with the most forceful contraction is

TABLE 1-3

DETERMINANTS OF STROKE VOLUME
I. Ventricular Preload
A. Blood volume
B. Distribution of blood volume
1. Body position
2. Intrathoracic pressure
3. Intrapericardial pressure
4. Venous tone
5. Pumping action of skeletal muscles
C. Atrial contraction
II. Ventricular Afterload
A. Systemic vascular resistance
B. Elasticity of arterial tree
C. Arterial blood volume
D. Ventricular wall tension
1. Ventricular radius
2. Ventricular wall thickness
III. Myocardial Contractility[a]
A. Intramyocardial [Ca²⁺] ↑↓
B. Cardiac adrenergic nerve activity ↑↓[b]
C. Circulating catecholamines ↑↓[b]
D. Cardiac rate ↑↓[b]
E. Exogenous inotropic agents↑
F. Myocardial ischemia ↓
G. Myocardial cell death (necrosis, apoptosis, autophagy) ↓
H. Alterations of sarcomeric and cytoskeletal proteins ↓
1. Genetic
2. Hemodynamic overload
I. Myocardial fibrosis ↓
J. Chronic overexpression of neurohormones ↓
K. Ventricular remodeling ↓
L. Chronic and/or excessive myocardial hypertrophy ↓

[a]Arrows indicate directional effects of determinants of contractility.
[b]Contractility rises initially but later becomes depressed.

~2.2 μm. This length provides the optimum configuration for the interaction between the two sets of myofilaments. The length of the sarcomere also regulates the extent of activation of the contractile system, i.e., its sensitivity to Ca^{2+}. According to this concept, termed *length-dependent activation*, myofilament sensitivity to Ca^{2+} is also maximal at the optimal sarcomere length. The relation between the initial length of the muscle fibers and the developed force has prime importance for the function of heart muscle. This relationship forms the basis of Starling's law of the heart, which states that within limits, the force of ventricular contraction depends on the end-diastolic length of the cardiac muscle; in the intact heart, the latter relates closely to the ventricular end-diastolic volume.

Cardiac performance

The ventricular end-diastolic or "filling" pressure sometimes is used as a surrogate for the end-diastolic volume. In isolated heart and heart-lung preparations, the stroke volume varies directly with the end-diastolic fiber length (preload) and inversely with the arterial resistance (afterload), and as the heart fails—i.e., as its contractility declines—it delivers a progressively smaller stroke volume from a normal or even elevated end-diastolic volume. The relation between the ventricular end-diastolic pressure and the stroke work of the ventricle (the ventricular function curve) provides a useful definition of the level of contractility of the heart in the intact organism. An increase in contractility is accompanied by a shift of the ventricular function curve upward and to the left (greater stroke work at any level of ventricular end-diastolic pressure, or lower end-diastolic volume at any level of stroke work), whereas a shift downward and to the right characterizes depression of contractility (**Fig. 1–8**).

Ventricular afterload

In the intact heart, as in isolated cardiac muscle, the extent and velocity of shortening of ventricular muscle fibers at any level of preload and of myocardial contractility relate inversely to the afterload, i.e., the load that opposes shortening. In the intact heart, the afterload may be defined as the tension developed in the ventricular wall during ejection. Afterload is determined by the aortic pressure as well as by the volume and thickness of the ventricular cavity. Laplace's law states that the tension of the myocardial fiber is the product of the intracavitary ventricular pressure and ventricular radius divided by wall thickness. Therefore, at any particular level of aortic pressure, the afterload on a dilated left ventricle exceeds that on a normal-sized ventricle. Conversely, at the same aortic pressure and ventricular diastolic volume, the afterload on a hypertrophied ventricle is lower that of a normal chamber. The aortic

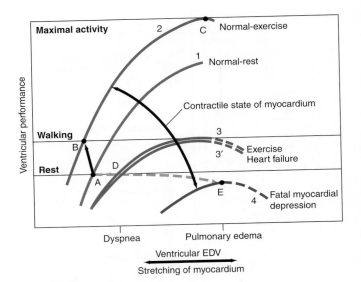

FIGURE 1-8

The interrelations among influences on ventricular end-diastolic volume (EDV) through stretching of the myocardium and the contractile state of the myocardium. Levels of ventricular EDV associated with filling pressures that result in dyspnea and pulmonary edema are shown on the abscissa. Levels of ventricular performance required when the subject is at rest, while walking, and during maximal activity are designated on the ordinate. The broken lines are the descending limbs of the ventricular-performance curves, which are rarely seen during life but show the level of ventricular performance if end-diastolic volume could be elevated to very high levels. For further explanation, see text. (*Modified from WS Colucci and E Braunwald: Pathophysiology of heart failure, in Braunwald's Heart Disease, 7th ed, DP Zipes et al [eds]. Philadelphia: Elsevier, 2005, pp 509–538.*)

pressure in turn depends on the peripheral vascular resistance, the physical characteristics of the arterial tree, and the volume of blood it contains at the onset of ejection.

Ventricular afterload critically regulates cardiovascular performance (**Fig. 1–9**). As already noted, elevations in both preload and contractility increase myocardial fiber shortening, whereas increases in afterload reduce it. The extent of myocardial fiber shortening and left ventricular size determine stroke volume. An increase in arterial pressure induced by vasoconstriction, for example, augments afterload, which opposes myocardial fiber shortening, reducing stroke volume.

When myocardial contractility becomes impaired and the ventricle dilates, afterload rises (Laplace's law) and limits cardiac output. Increased afterload also may result from neural and humoral stimuli that occur in response to a fall in cardiac output. This increased afterload may reduce cardiac output further, thereby increasing ventricular volume and initiating a vicious circle, especially in patients with ischemic heart disease and limited myocardial O_2 supply. Treatment with vasodilators has the

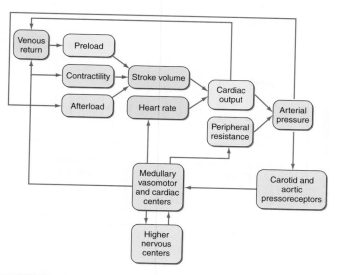

FIGURE 1-9

Interactions in the intact circulation of preload, contractility, and afterload in producing stroke volume. Stroke volume combined with heart rate determines cardiac output, which, when combined with peripheral vascular resistance, determines arterial pressure for tissue perfusion. The characteristics of the arterial system also contribute to afterload, an increase which reduces stroke volume. The interaction of these components with carotid and aortic arch baroreceptors provides a feedback mechanism to higher medullary and vasomotor cardiac centers and to higher levels in the central nervous system to effect a modulating influence on heart rate, peripheral vascular resistance, venous return, and contractility. (*From MR Starling: Physiology of myocardial contraction, in Atlas of Heart Failure: Cardiac Function and Dysfunction, 3rd ed, WS Colucci and E Braunwald [eds]. Philadelphia: Current Medicine, 2002, pp 19–35.*)

opposite effect; when afterload is reduced, cardiac output rises (Chap. 17).

Under normal circumstances, the various influences acting on cardiac performance enumerated earlier interact in a complex fashion to maintain cardiac output at a level appropriate to the requirements of the metabolizing tissues (Fig. 1-9); interference with a single mechanism may not influence the cardiac output. For example, a moderate reduction of blood volume or the loss of the atrial contribution to ventricular contraction ordinarily can be sustained without a reduction in the cardiac output at rest. Under these circumstances, other factors, such as increases in the frequency of adrenergic nerve impulses to the heart, heart rate, and venous tone, will serve as compensatory mechanisms and sustain cardiac output in a normal individual.

Exercise

The integrated response to exercise illustrates the interactions among the three determinants of stroke volume:

preload, afterload, and contractility (Fig. 1-8). Hyperventilation, the pumping action of the exercising muscles, and venoconstriction during exercise all augment venous return and hence ventricular filling and preload (Table 1-3). Simultaneously, the increase in the adrenergic nerve impulse traffic to the myocardium, the increased concentration of circulating catecholamines, and the tachycardia that occur during exercise combine to augment the contractility of the myocardium (Fig. 1-8, curves 1 and 2) and together elevate stroke volume and stroke work, without a change in or even a reduction of end-diastolic pressure and volume (Fig. 1-8, points A and B). Vasodilation occurs in the exercising muscles, thus tending to limit the increase in arterial pressure that otherwise would occur as cardiac output rises to levels as high as five times greater than basal levels during maximal exercise. This vasodilation ultimately allows the achievement of a greatly elevated cardiac output during exercise at an arterial pressure only moderately higher than in the resting state.

ASSESSMENT OF CARDIAC FUNCTION

Several techniques can define impaired cardiac function in clinical practice. The cardiac output and stroke volume may be depressed in the presence of heart failure, but not uncommonly, these variables are within normal limits in this condition. A somewhat more sensitive index of cardiac function is the ejection fraction, i.e., the ratio of stroke volume to end-diastolic volume (normal value = 67 ± 8%), which is frequently depressed in systolic heart failure even when the stroke volume itself is normal. Alternatively, abnormally elevated ventricular end-diastolic volume (normal value = 75 ± 20 mL/m^2) or end-systolic volume (normal value = 25 ± 7 mL/m^2) signifies impairment of left ventricular systolic function.

Noninvasive techniques, particularly echocardiography as well as radionuclide scintigraphy and cardiac magnetic resonance imaging (MRI) (Chap. 12), have great value in the clinical assessment of myocardial function. They provide measurements of end-diastolic and end-systolic volumes, ejection fraction, and systolic shortening rate, and they allow assessment of ventricular filling (see later) as well as regional contraction and relaxation. The latter measurements are particularly important in ischemic heart disease, as myocardial infarction causes regional myocardial damage.

A limitation of measurements of cardiac output, ejection fraction, and ventricular volumes in assessing cardiac function is that ventricular loading conditions strongly influence these variables. Thus, a depressed ejection fraction and lowered cardiac output may be observed in patients with normal ventricular function but reduced preload, as occurs in hypovolemia, or with increased afterload, as occurs in acutely elevated arterial pressure.

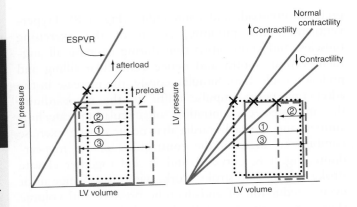

FIGURE 1-10

The responses of the left ventricle to increased afterload, increased preload, and increased and reduced contractility are shown in the pressure-volume plane. **Left.** Effects of increases in preload and afterload on the pressure-volume loop. Since there has been no change in contractility, ESPVR (the end-systolic pressure-volume relation) is unchanged. With an increase in afterload, stroke volume falls (1 → 2); with an increase in preload, stroke volume rises (1 → 3). **Right.** With increased myocardial contractility and constant LV end-diastolic volume, the ESPVR moves to the left of the normal line (lower end-systolic volume at any end-systolic pressure) and stroke volume rises (1 → 3). With reduced myocardial contractility, the ESPVR moves to the right; end-systolic volume is increased, and stroke volume falls (1 → 2).

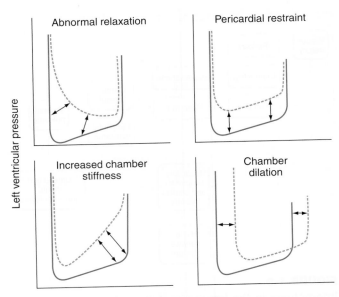

FIGURE 1-11

Mechanisms that cause diastolic dysfunction reflected in the pressure-volume relation. The bottom half of the pressure-volume loop is depicted. Solid lines represent normal subjects; broken lines represent patients with diastolic dysfunction. *(From JD Carroll et al: The differential effects of positive inotropic and vasodilator therapy on diastolic properties in patients with congestive cardiomyopathy. Circulation 74:815, 1986; with permission.)*

The end-systolic left ventricular pressure–volume relationship is a particularly useful index of ventricular performance since it does not depend on preload and afterload **(Fig. 1-10)**. At any level of myocardial contractility, left ventricular end-systolic volume varies inversely with end-systolic pressure; as contractility declines, end-systolic volume (at any level of end-systolic pressure) rises.

DIASTOLIC FUNCTION

Ventricular filling is influenced by the extent and speed of myocardial relaxation, which in turn depends on the rate of uptake of Ca^{2+} by the SR; the latter may be enhanced by adrenergic activation and reduced by ischemia, which reduces the ATP available for pumping Ca^{2+} into the SR (see earlier). The stiffness of the ventricular wall also may impede filling. Ventricular stiffness increases with hypertrophy and conditions that infiltrate the ventricle, such as amyloid, or is caused by an extrinsic constraint (e.g., pericardial compression) **(Fig. 1-11)**.

Ventricular filling can be assessed by continuously measuring the velocity of flow across the mitral valve, using Doppler ultrasound. Normally, the velocity of inflow is more rapid in early diastole than during atrial systole; with mild to moderately impaired relaxation, the rate of early diastolic filling declines, whereas the rate of presystolic filling rises. With further impairment of filling, the pattern is "pseudo-normalized," and early ventricular filling becomes more rapid as left atrial pressure upstream to the stiff left ventricle rises.

CARDIAC METABOLISM

The heart requires a continuous supply of energy (in the form of ATP) not only to perform its mechanical pumping functions, but also to regulate intracellular and transsarcolemmal ionic movements and concentration gradients. Among its pumping functions, the development of tension, the frequency of contraction, and the level of myocardial contractility are the principal determinants of the heart's substantial energy needs, making its O_2 requirements approximately 15% of that of the entire organism.

Most ATP production depends on the oxidation of substrate (glucose and free fatty acids [FFAs]). Myocardial FFAs are derived from circulating FFAs, which result principally from lipolysis in adipose tissue, whereas the myocyte's glucose derives from plasma as well as from the cell's breakdown of its glycogen stores (glycogenolysis). These two principal sources of acetyl coenzyme A in cardiac muscle vary reciprocally. Glucose is broken down in the cytoplasm into a three-carbon product, pyruvate, which passes into the mitochondria, where it is metabolized to the two-carbon fragment, acetyl-Co-A, and undergoes oxidation. FFAs are converted to acyl-CoA in the cytoplasm and acetyl-CoA in the mitochondria. Acetyl-CoA enters the citric acid (Krebs) cycle to produce ATP by oxidative phosphorylation within the mitochondria; ATP then enters the cytoplasm from the mitochondrial compartment. Intracellular ADP, resulting from the breakdown of ATP, enhances mitochondrial ATP production.

In the fasted, resting state, circulating FFA concentrations and their myocardial uptake are high, and they furnish most of the heart's acetyl-CoA (~70%). In the fed state, with elevations of blood glucose and insulin, glucose oxidation increases and FFA oxidation subsides. Increased cardiac work, the administration of inotropic agents, hypoxia, and mild ischemia all enhance myocardial glucose uptake, glucose production resulting from glycogenolysis, and glucose metabolism to pyruvate (glycolysis). By contrast, β-adrenergic stimulation, as occurs during stress, raises the circulating levels and metabolism of FFAs in favor of glucose. Severe ischemia inhibits the cytoplasmic enzyme pyruvate dehydrogenase, and despite both glycogen and glucose breakdown, glucose is metabolized only to lactic acid (anaerobic glycolysis), which does not enter the citric acid cycle. Anaerobic glycolysis produces much less ATP than does aerobic glucose metabolism, in which glucose is metabolized to pyruvate and subsequently oxidized to CO_2. High concentrations of circulating FFAs, which can occur when adrenergic stimulation is superimposed on severe ischemia, reduce oxidative phosphorylation and also cause ATP wastage; the myocardial content of ATP declines and impairs myocardial contraction. In addition, products of FFA breakdown can exert toxic effects on cardiac cell membranes and may be arrhythmogenic.

Myocardial energy is stored as creatine phosphate (CP), which is in equilibrium with ATP, the immediate source of energy. In states of reduced energy availability, the CP stores decline first. Cardiac hypertrophy, fibrosis, tachycardia, increased wall tension resulting from ventricular dilation, and increased intracytoplasmic $[Ca^{2+}]$ all contribute to increased myocardial energy needs. When coupled with reduced coronary flow reserve, as occurs with obstruction of coronary arteries or abnormalities of the coronary microcirculation, an imbalance in myocardial ATP production relative to demand may occur, and the resulting ischemia can worsen or cause heart failure.

Developmental biology of the cardiovascular system

The heart is the first organ to form during embryogenesis (**Fig. 1-12**) and must accomplish the simultaneous challenges of circulating blood, nutrients, and oxygen to the other forming organs while continuing to grow and undergo complex morphogenetic changes. Early progenitors of the heart arise within very early crescent-shaped fields of lateral splanchnic mesoderm under the influence of multiple signals, including those derived from neural ectoderm long before neural tube closure. Early cardiac precursors express regulatory transcription factors that play reiterated roles in cardiac development, such as NKX2-5 and GATA4; these mutations are responsible for some forms of inherited congenital heart disease. Early cardiac precursors form two bilateral heart tubes, each composed of a single cell layer of endocardium surrounded by a single layer of myocardial precursors. Subsequently, a single midline heart tube is formed by the medial migration and midline fusion of these bilateral structures. The caudal, inflow region of the heart tube adopts a more rostral final position and represents the atrial anlagen, whereas the rostral, outflow portion of the tube forms the truncus arteriosus, which divides to produce the aorta and the proximal pulmonary artery. Between these extremes lie the structural precursors of the ventricles.

The linear heart tube undergoes an asymmetric looping process (the first gross evidence of left-right asymmetry in the developing embryo), which positions the portion of the heart tube destined to become the left ventricle to the left of the more rostral precursors of the right ventricle and outflow tract. Looping is coordinated with chamber specification and ballooning of various regions of the heart tube to produce the presumptive atria and ventricles.

Relatively recent work has demonstrated that significant portions of the right ventricle are formed by cells that are added to the developing heart after looping has occurred. These cells, which are derived from what is called the second heart field, derive from progenitors in the ventral pharynx and express markers that allow for their identification, including islet-1. Different embryologic origins of cells within the right and left ventricles may help explain why some forms of congenital and adult heart diseases affect these regions of the heart to varying degrees.

After looping and chamber formation, a series of septation events divide the left and right sides of the heart, separate the atria from the ventricles, and form the aorta and pulmonary artery from the truncus arteriosus. Cardiac valves form between the atria and the ventricles and between the ventricles and the outflow vessels. Early in development, the single layer of myocardial cells secretes an extracellular matrix rich in hyaluronic acid. This extracellular matrix, termed "cardiac jelly," accumulates within the endocardial cushions, precursors of the cardiac valves. Signals from overlying myocardial cells, including members of the transforming growth factor β family, trigger migration, invasion, and phenotypic changes of underlying endocardial cells, which undergo an epithelial-mesenchymal transformation and

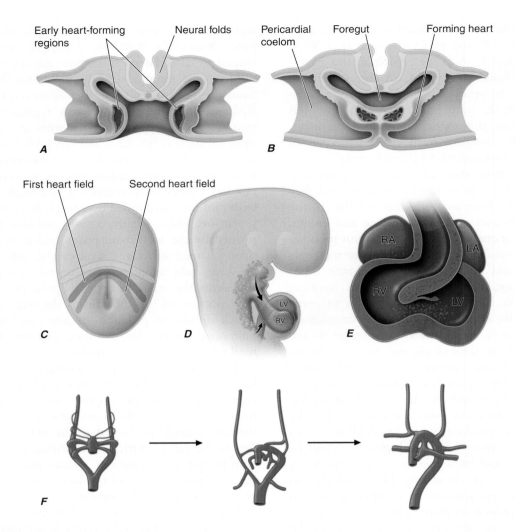

FIGURE 1-12

A. Schematic depiction of a transverse section through an early embryo depicts the bilateral regions where early heart tubes form. **B.** The bilateral heart tubes subsequently migrate to the midline and fuse to form the linear heart tube. **C.** At the early cardiac crescent stage of embryonic development, cardiac precursors include a primary heart field fated to form the linear heart tube and a second heart field fated to add myocardium to the inflow and outflow poles of the

heart. **D.** Second heart field cells populate the pharyngeal region before subsequently migrating to the maturing heart. **E.** Large portions of the right ventricle and outflow tract and some cells within the atria derive from the second heart field. **F.** The aortic arch arteries form as symmetric sets of vessels that then remodel under the influence of the neural crest to form the asymmetric mature vasculature.

invade the cardiac jelly to cellularize the endocardial cushions. Mesenchymal components proliferate and remodel to form the mature valve leaflets.

The great vessels form as a series of bilaterally symmetric aortic arch arteries that undergo asymmetric remodeling events to form the mature vasculature. The immigration of neural crest cells that arise in the dorsal neural tube orchestrates this process. These cells are required for aortic arch remodeling and septation of the truncus arteriosus. They develop into smooth-muscle cells within the tunica media of the aortic arch, the ductus arteriosus, and the carotid arteries. Smooth-muscle cells within the descending aorta arise from a different

embryologic source, the lateral plate mesoderm. Neural crest cells are sensitive to both vitamin A and folic acid, and congenital heart disease involving abnormal remodeling of the aortic arch arteries has been associated with maternal deficiencies of these vitamins. Genetic syndromes associated with aortic arch defects can be associated with other abnormalities of neural crest craniofacial derivatives, including the palate.

Coronary artery formation requires yet another cell population that initiates extrinsic to the embryonic heart fields. Epicardial cells arise in the proepicardial organ, a derivative of the septum transversum, which also contributes to the fibrous portion of the diaphragm and to the liver. Proepicardial cells contribute to the smooth-muscle cells of the coronary arteries and are required for their proper patterning. Other cell types within the heart, including fibroblasts and potentially some myocardial cells, also can arise from the proepicardium.

The cardiac conduction system, which functions both to generate and to propagate electrical impulses, develops primarily from multipotential cardiac precursors. The conduction system is composed of slow (proximal) components, such as the sinoatrial (SA) and atrioventricular (AV) nodes, as well as fast (distal) components, including the His bundle, bundle branches, and Purkinje fibers. The AV node primarily serves to delay the electrical impulse between atria and ventricles (manifesting decremental conduction), whereas the distal conduction system rapidly delivers the impulse throughout the ventricles. Significant recent attention has been focused on the embryologic origins of various components of the specialized conduction network. Precursors within the sinus venosus give rise to the SA node, whereas those within the AV canal mature into heterogeneous cell types that compose the AV node. Myocardial cells transdifferentiate into Purkinje fibers to form the distal conduction system. Fast and slow conducting cell types within the nodes and bundles are characterized by expression of distinct gap junction proteins, including connexins, and ion channels that characterize unique cell fates and electrical properties of the tissues. Developmental defects in conduction system morphogenesis and lineage determination can lead to various electrophysiologic disorders, including congenital heart block and preexcitation syndromes such as Wolff-Parkinson-White syndrome (Chap. 16).

Studies of cardiac stem and progenitor cells suggest that progressive lineage restriction results in the gradual and stepwise determination of mature cell fates within the heart, with early precursors capable of adopting endothelial, smooth-muscle, or cardiac phenotypes, and subsequent further specialization into atrial, ventricular, and specialized conduction cell types.

REGENERATING CARDIAC TISSUE

Until very recently, adult mammalian myocardial cells were viewed as fully differentiated and without regenerative potential. Evidence currently supports the existence of limited endogenous regenerative potential of mature cardiac myocytes, resident cardiac progenitors, and/or bone marrow–derived stem cells. Considerable current effort is being devoted to evaluating the utility of cells from these sources to enhance the regenerative potential of the heart. The success of such approaches would offer the exciting possibility of reconstructing an infarcted or failing ventricle.

CHAPTER 2

EPIDEMIOLOGY OF CARDIOVASCULAR DISEASE

Thomas A. Gaziano ■ **J. Michael Gaziano**

Cardiovascular disease (CVD) is now the most common cause of death worldwide. Before 1900, infectious diseases and malnutrition were the most common causes and CVD was responsible for less than 10% of all deaths. Today, CVD accounts for approximately 30% of deaths worldwide, including nearly 40% in high-income countries and about 28% in low- and middle-income countries.

THE EPIDEMIOLOGIC TRANSITION

The global rise in CVD is the result of an unprecedented transformation in the causes of morbidity and mortality during the twentieth and twenty-first centuries. Known as the epidemiologic transition, this shift is driven by industrialization, urbanization, and associated lifestyle changes and is taking place in every part of the world among all races, ethnic groups, and cultures. The transition is divided into four basic stages: pestilence and famine, receding pandemics, degenerative and human-made diseases, and delayed degenerative diseases. A fifth stage, characterized by an epidemic of inactivity and obesity, may be emerging in some countries **(Table 2-1)**.

Malnutrition, infectious diseases, and high infant and child mortality rates that are offset by high fertility mark the *age of pestilence and famine*. Tuberculosis, dysentery, cholera, and influenza are often fatal, resulting in a mean life expectancy of about 30 years. Cardiovascular disease, which accounts for less than 10% of deaths, takes the form of rheumatic heart disease and cardiomyopathies due to infection and malnutrition. Approximately 10% of the world's population remains in the age of pestilence and famine.

Per capita income and life expectancy increase during the *age of receding pandemics* as the emergence of public health systems, cleaner water supplies, and improved nutrition combine to drive down deaths from infectious disease and malnutrition. Infant and childhood mortality rates also decline, but deaths due to CVD increase to between 10% and 35% of all deaths. Rheumatic valvular disease, hypertension, coronary heart disease (CHD), and stroke are the predominant forms of CVD. Almost 40% of the world's population is currently in this stage.

The *age of degenerative and human-made diseases* is distinguished by mortality from noncommunicable diseases—primarily CVD—surpassing mortality from malnutrition and infectious diseases. Caloric intake, particularly from animal fat, increases. Coronary heart disease and stroke are prevalent, and 35–65% of all deaths can be traced to CVD. Typically, the rate of CHD deaths exceeds that of stroke by a ratio of 2:1 to 3:1. During this period, average life expectancy surpasses 50 years. Roughly 35% of the world's population falls into this category.

In the *age of delayed degenerative diseases*, CVD and cancer remain the major causes of morbidity and mortality, with CVD accounting for 40% of all deaths. However, age-adjusted CVD mortality declines, aided by preventive strategies such as smoking cessation programs and effective blood pressure control, acute hospital management, and technological advances such as the availability of bypass surgery. CHD, stroke, and congestive heart failure are the primary forms of CVD. About 15% of the world's population is now in the age of delayed degenerative diseases or is exiting this age and moving into the fifth stage of the epidemiologic transition.

In the industrialized world, physical activity continues to decline while total caloric intake increases. The resulting epidemic of overweight and obesity may signal the start of the *age of inactivity and obesity*. Rates of

TABLE 2-1

FIVE STAGES OF THE EPIDEMIOLOGIC TRANSITION

STAGE	DESCRIPTION	DEATHS RELATED TO CVD, %	PREDOMINANT CVD TYPE
Pestilence and famine	Predominance of malnutrition and infectious diseases as causes of death; high rates of infant and child mortality; low mean life expectancy	<10	Rheumatic heart disease, cardiomyopathies caused by infection and malnutrition
Receding pandemics	Improvements in nutrition and public health lead to decrease in rates of deaths related to malnutrition and infection; precipitous decline in infant and child mortality rates	10–35	Rheumatic valvular disease, hypertension, CHD, and stroke (predominantly hemorrhagic)
Degenerative and human-made diseases	Increased fat and caloric intake and decrease in physical activity lead to emergence of hypertension and atherosclerosis; with increase in life expectancy, mortality from chronic, noncommunicable diseases exceeds mortality from malnutrition and infectious disease	35–65	CHD and stroke (ischemic and hemorrhagic)
Delayed degenerative diseases	CVD and cancer are the major causes of morbidity and mortality; better treatment and prevention efforts help avoid deaths among those with disease and delay primary events; age-adjusted CVD morality rate declines; CVD affecting older and older individuals	40–50	CHD, stroke, and congestive heart failure
Inactivity and obesity	Overweight and obesity increase at alarming rate; diabetes and hypertension increase; decline in smoking rates levels off; a minority of the population meets physical activity recommendations	Possible reversal of age-adjusted declines in mortality	CHD, stroke, and congestive heart failure, peripheral vascular disease

Abbreviations: CHD, coronary heart disease; CVD, cardiovascular disease.
Source: Adapted from AR Omran: Milbank Mem Fund Q 49:509, 1971; and SJ Olshansky, AB Ault: Milbank Q 64:355, 1986.

type 2 diabetes mellitus, hypertension, and lipid abnormalities are on the rise, trends that are particularly evident in children. If these risk factor trends continue, age-adjusted CVD mortality rates could increase in the coming years.

THE EPIDEMIOLOGIC TRANSITION IN THE UNITED STATES

The United States, like other high-income countries, has proceeded through four stages of the epidemiologic transition. Recent trends, however, suggest that the rates of decline of some chronic and degenerative diseases have slowed. Because of the large amount of available data, the United States serves as a useful reference point for comparisons.

The age of pestilence and famine (before 1900)

The American colonies were born into pestilence and famine, with half the Pilgrims who arrived in 1620 dying of infection and malnutrition by the following spring. At the end of the 1800s, the U.S. economy was still largely agrarian, with more than 60% of the population living in rural settings. By 1900, average life expectancy had increased to about 50 years. However, tuberculosis, pneumonia, and other infectious diseases still accounted for more deaths than any other cause. CVD accounted for less than 10% of all deaths.

The age of receding pandemics (1900–1930)

By 1900, a public health infrastructure was in place: Forty states had health departments, many larger towns had major public works efforts to improve the water supply and sewage systems, municipal use of chlorine to disinfect water was widespread, pasteurization and other improvements in food handling were introduced, and the educational quality of health care personnel improved. Those changes led to dramatic declines in infectious disease mortality rates. However, the continued shift from a rural, agriculture-based economy to an urban, industrial economy had a number of consequences on risk behaviors and factors for CVD. Owing to a lack of refrigerated transport from farms to urban centers, consumption of fresh fruits and vegetables declined and consumption of meat and grains increased, resulting in diets that were higher in animal fat and processed carbohydrates. In addition, the availability of factory-rolled cigarettes made tobacco more accessible and affordable for the mass population. Age-adjusted CVD mortality rates rose from 300 per 100,000 people in 1900 to approximately 390 per 100,000 during this period, driven by rapidly rising CHD rates.

The age of degenerative and human-made diseases (1930–1965)

During this period, deaths from infectious diseases fell to fewer than 50 per 100,000 per year and life expectancy increased to almost 70 years. At the same time, the country became increasingly urbanized and industrialized, precipitating a number of important lifestyle changes. By 1955, 55% of adult men were smoking, and fat consumption accounted for approximately 40% of total calories. Lower activity levels, high-fat diets, and increased smoking pushed CVD death rates to peak levels.

The age of delayed degenerative diseases (1965–2000)

Substantial declines in age-adjusted CVD mortality rates began in the mid-1960s. In the 1970s and 1980s, age-adjusted CHD mortality rates fell approximately 2% per year and stroke rates fell 3% per year. A main characteristic of this phase is the steadily rising age at which a first CVD event occurs. Two significant advances have been credited with the decline in CVD mortality rates: new therapeutic approaches and the implementation of prevention measures. Treatments once considered advanced, such as angioplasty, bypass surgery, and implantation of defibrillators, are now considered the standard of care. Treatments for hypertension and elevated cholesterol along with the widespread use of aspirin have also contributed significantly to reducing deaths from CVD. In addition, Americans have been exposed to public health campaigns promoting lifestyle modifications effective at reducing the prevalence of smoking, hypertension, and dyslipidemia.

Is the United States entering the fifth age?

The decline in the age-adjusted CVD death rate of 3% per year through the 1970s and 1980s tapered off in the 1990s to 2%. However, CVD death rates declined by 3–5% per year during the first decade of the new millennium. In 2000, the age-adjusted CVD death rate was 341 per 100,000. By 2006, it had fallen to 263 per 100,000. Competing trends appear to be in play. On the one hand, the well-recognized increase in the prevalence of diabetes and obesity, a slowing in the rate of decline of smoking, and a leveling off in the rate of detection and treatment for hypertension are in the negative column. On the other hand, cholesterol levels continue to decline in the face of increased statin use.

CURRENT WORLDWIDE VARIATIONS

An epidemiologic transition much like that which occurred in the United States is occurring throughout the world, but unique regional features have modified aspects of the transition in various parts of the world. In terms of economic development, the world can be divided into two broad categories, (1) high-income countries and (2) low- and middle-income countries, which can be further subdivided into six distinct economic/geographic regions. Currently, 85% of the world's population lives in low- and middle-income countries, and it is those countries which are driving the rates of change in the global burden of CVD (Fig. 2-1). Three million CVD deaths occurred in high-income countries in 2001, compared with 13 million in the rest of the world.

High-income countries

Approximately 940 million people live in high-income countries, where CHD is the dominant form of CVD, with rates that tend to be twofold to fivefold higher than stroke rates. The rates of CVD in Canada, New Zealand, Australia, and Western Europe tend to be similar to those in the United States; however, among the countries of Western Europe, the absolute rates vary threefold with a clear north/south gradient. The highest CVD death rates are in the northern countries, such as Finland, Ireland, and Scotland, and the lowest rates are in the Mediterranean countries of France, Spain, and Italy. Japan is unique among the high-income countries: stroke rates increased dramatically, but CHD rates did not rise as sharply over the last century. This difference may stem in part from genetic factors, but it is more likely that the fish- and plant-based low-fat diet and resulting low cholesterol levels have played a larger role. Importantly, Japanese dietary habits are undergoing substantial changes, reflected in an increase in cholesterol levels.

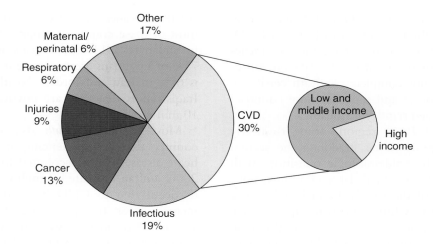

FIGURE 2-1

CVD data compared with other causes of death. CVD: cardiovascular disease. *(Based on data from CD Mathers et al: Deaths and Disease Burden by Cause: Global Burden of* *Disease Estimates for 2001 by World Bank Country Groups. Disease Control Priorities Working Paper 18. April 2004, revised January 2005.)*

Low- and middle-income countries

The World Bank groups the low- and middle-income countries (gross national income per capita less than US $9200) into six geographic regions: East Asia and the Pacific, (Eastern) Europe and Central Asia, Latin America and the Caribbean, Middle East and North Africa, South Asia, and Sub-Saharan Africa. Although communicable diseases continue to be a major cause of death, CVD has emerged as a significant health concern in

low- and middle-income countries. In most, an urban/rural gradient has emerged for CHD, stroke, and hypertension, with higher rates in urban centers.

Although CVD rates are rapidly rising, there are vast differences among the regions and countries and even within individual countries **(Fig. 2-2)**. Many factors contribute to this heterogeneity. First, the regions are in various stages of the epidemiologic transition. Second, vast differences in lifestyle and behavioral risk

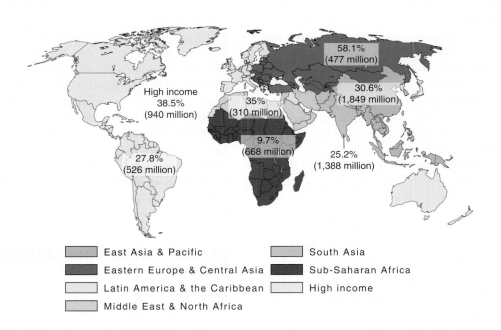

FIGURE 2-2

CVD death as a percentage of total deaths and total population in seven economic regions of the world defined by the World Bank. *(Based on data from CD Mathers et al: Deaths and* *Disease Burden by Cause: Global Burden of Disease Estimates for 2001 by World Bank Country Groups. Disease Control Priorities Working Paper 18. April 2004, revised January 2005.)*

factors exist. Third, racial and ethnic differences may lead to altered susceptibilities to various forms of CVD. In addition, it should be noted that for most countries in these regions, accurate countrywide data on cause-specific mortality are not complete, as death certificate completion is not routine and most of those countries do not have a centralized registry for deaths.

The *East Asia and Pacific* region, home to nearly 2 billion people, appears to be straddling the second and third phases of the epidemiologic transition, with China, Indonesia, and Sri Lanka's large combined population driving most of the trends. Overall, CVD is a major cause of death in China, but as in Japan, stroke (particularly hemorrhagic) causes more deaths than does CHD, at a ratio of about 3:1. However, age-adjusted CHD mortality increased 40% from 1984 to 1999, suggesting further epidemiologic transition. China also appears to have a geographic gradient like that of Western Europe, with higher CVD rates in northern China than in southern China by a factor of 6. Other countries, such as Vietnam and Cambodia, are just emerging from the pestilence and famine era.

The *Eastern Europe and Central Asia* region is firmly at the peak of the third phase, with the highest death rates (58%) due to CVD in the world, nearly double the rate of high-income countries. More troubling is that nearly 35% of deaths from CHD occur among working-age adults, which is three times the rate in the United States. In Russia, increased CVD rates have contributed to falling life expectancy, particularly for men, whose life expectancy dropped from 71.6 in 1986 to 59 years today. In Poland, by contrast, the age-adjusted mortality rate decreased by approximately 30% for men during the 1990s and slightly more among women. Slovenia, Hungary, the Czech Republic, and Slovakia have had similar declines.

In general, *Latin America* appears to be in the third phase of the epidemiologic transition, although as in other low- and middle-income regions, there is vast regional heterogeneity, with some areas in the second phase of the transition and some in the fourth. Today, approximately 28% of all deaths in this region are attributable to CVD, with CHD rates (35%) higher than stroke rates (29%). As in Eastern Europe, some countries—Mexico, Costa Rica, and Venezuela—continued an overall increase in age-adjusted CHD mortality of 3–10% between 1970 and 2002, whereas in others—Argentina, Brazil, Chile, and Columbia—rates appear to have declined by as much as 2% per year over the same period. The *Middle East and North Africa* region appears to be entering the third phase of the epidemiologic transition, with increasing life expectancy overall and CVD death rates just below those of developed nations. CHD is responsible for 17% of all deaths, and stroke for 7%. The traditional high-fiber diet, low in fat and cholesterol, has changed rapidly. Over the

last few decades, daily fat consumption has increased in most of these countries, ranging from a 13.6% increase in Sudan to a 143.3% increase in Saudi Arabia. Over 75% of Egyptians are overweight or obese, and the rate is 67% in Iraq and Jordan. Nearly 60% of Syrians and Iraqis report that they are physically inactive (less than 10 min per day).

Most people in *South Asia* live in rural India, a country that is experiencing an alarming increase in heart disease. CVD accounted for 32% of all deaths in 2000, and an estimated 2 million deaths were expected to occur due to CHD by 2010, representing a 30% increase over the preceding decade. The transition appears to be in the Western style, with CHD as the dominant form of CVD. In 1960, CHD represented 4% of all CVD deaths in India, whereas in 1990 the proportion was >50%. This is somewhat unexpected because stroke tends to be a more dominant factor early in the epidemiologic transition. This finding may reflect inaccuracies in cause-specific mortality estimates or possibly an underlying genetic component. It has been suggested that Indians have exaggerated insulin insensitivity in response to the Western lifestyle pattern that may differentially increase rates of CHD over stroke. The South Asia region has the highest overall prevalence of diabetes in the low-income regions, with rates as high as 14% in urban centers. In certain rural areas, the prevalence of CVD and its risk factors is approaching urban rates. Nonetheless, rheumatic heart disease continues to be a major cause of morbidity and mortality.

For the most part, *Sub-Saharan Africa* remains in the first phase of the epidemiologic transition, with CVD rates half those in developed nations. Life expectancy has decreased by an average of 5 years since the early 1990s largely because of HIV/AIDS and other chronic diseases, according to the World Bank; life expectancies are the lowest in the world. Still, CVD accounts for 46% of noncommunicable deaths and is the leading cause of death among adults >age 35. As more HIV/AIDS patients receive antiretroviral treatment, managing CVD risk factors such as dyslipidemia in this population requires more attention. However, hypertension continues to be the major public health concern and has resulted in stroke being the dominant form of CVD. Rheumatic heart disease is still an important cause of CVD mortality and morbidity.

GLOBAL TRENDS IN CARDIOVASCULAR DISEASE

In 1990, CVD accounted for 28% of the world's 50.4 million deaths and 9.7% of the 1.4 billion lost disability-adjusted life years (DALYs), and by 2001, CVD was responsible for 29% of all deaths and 14% of the 1.5 billion lost DALYs. By 2030, when the population is expected to reach 8.2 billion, 33% of all deaths

TABLE 2-2

ESTIMATED MORBIDITY RELATED TO HEART DISEASE: 2010-2030		
DEATHS	**BY 2010**	**BY 2030**
CVD deaths: annual number of all deaths	18.1 million	24.2 million
CVD deaths: percentage of all deaths	30.8%	32.5%
CHD deaths: percentage of all male deaths	13.1%	14.9%
CHD deaths: percentage of all female deaths	13.6%	13.1%
Stroke deaths: percentage of all male deaths	9.2%	10.4%
Stroke deaths: percentage of all female deaths	11.5%	11.8%

Abbreviations: CVD, cardiovascular disease; CHD, coronary heart disease.
Source: Adapted from J Mackay, G Mensah: *Atlas of Heart Disease and Stroke.* Geneva, World Health Organization, 2004.

will be the result of CVD (**Table 2–2**). Of these, 14.9% of deaths in men and 13.1% of deaths in women will be due to CHD. Stroke will be responsible for 10.4% of all male deaths and 11.8% of all female deaths.

In the *high-income countries*, population growth will be fueled by emigration from the low- and middle-income countries, but the populations of high-income countries will shrink as a proportion of the world's population. The modest decline in CVD death rates that began in the high-income countries in the latter third of the twentieth century will continue, but the rate of decline appears to be slowing. However, these countries are expected to see an increase in the prevalence of CVD, as well as the absolute number of deaths as the population ages.

Significant proportions of the population living in *low- and middle-income countries* have entered the third phase of the epidemiologic transition, and some are entering the fourth stage. Changing demographics play a significant role in future predictions for CVD throughout the world. For example, between 1990 and 2001, the population of Eastern Europe and Central Asia grew by 1 million people per year, whereas South Asia added 25 million people each year.

CVD rates will also have an economic impact. Even assuming no increase in CVD risk factors, most countries, but especially India and South Africa, will see a large number of people between 35 and 64 die of CVD over the next 30 years as well as an increasing level of morbidity among middle-aged people related to heart disease and stroke. In China, it is estimated that there

will be 9 million deaths from CVD in 2030—up from 2.4 million in 2002—with half occurring in individuals between 35 and 64 years old.

REGIONAL TRENDS IN RISK FACTORS

As indicated earlier, the global variation in CVD rates is related to temporal and regional variations in known risk behaviors and factors. Ecological analyses of major CVD risk factors and mortality demonstrate high correlations between expected and observed mortality rates for the three main risk factors—smoking, serum cholesterol, and hypertension—and suggest that many of the regional variations are based on differences in conventional risk factors.

BEHAVIORAL RISK FACTORS

Tobacco

Every year, more than 5.5 trillion cigarettes are produced, enough to provide every person on the planet with 1000 cigarettes. Worldwide, 1.3 billion people smoked in 2003, a number that is projected to increase to 1.6 billion by 2030. Tobacco currently causes about 5 million deaths—9% of all deaths—annually. Approximately 1.6 million are CVD-related. If current smoking patterns continue, by 2030 the global burden of disease attributable to tobacco will reach 10 million deaths annually. A unique feature of the low- and middle-income countries is easy access to smoking during the early stages of the epidemiologic transition due to the availability of relatively inexpensive tobacco products. In South Asia, the prominence of locally produced forms of tobacco other than manufactured cigarettes makes control of consumption more challenging.

Diet

Total caloric intake per capita increases as countries develop. With regard to cardiovascular disease, a key element of dietary change is an increase in intake of saturated animal fats and hydrogenated vegetable fats, which contain atherogenic trans-fatty acids, along with a decrease in intake of plant-based foods and an increase in simple carbohydrates. Fat contributes less than 20% of calories in rural China and India, less than 30% in Japan, and well above 30% in the United States. Caloric contributions from fat appear to be falling in the high-income countries. In the United States, between 1971 and 2000, the percentage of calories derived from saturated fat decreased from 13% to 11%.

Physical inactivity

The increased mechanization that accompanies the economic transition leads to a shift from physically demanding agriculture-based work to largely sedentary industry- and office-based work. In the United States, approximately one-quarter of the population does not participate in any leisure-time physical activity and only 22% report engaging in sustained physical activity for at least 30 min on 5 or more days per week (the current recommendation). In contrast, in countries such as China, physical activity is still integral to everyday life. Approximately 90% of the urban population walks or rides a bicycle to work, shopping, or school daily.

METABOLIC RISK FACTORS

Lipid levels

Worldwide, high cholesterol levels are estimated to cause 56% of ischemic heart disease and 18% of strokes, amounting to 4.4 million deaths annually. As countries move through the epidemiologic transition, mean population plasma cholesterol levels tend to rise. Social and individual changes that accompany urbanization clearly play a role because plasma cholesterol levels tend to be higher among urban residents than among rural residents. This shift is driven largely by greater consumption of dietary fats—primarily from animal products and processed vegetable oils—and decreased physical activity. In the high-income countries, in general, mean population cholesterol levels are falling, whereas wide variation is seen in the low- and middle-income countries.

Hypertension

Elevated blood pressure is an early indicator of the epidemiologic transition. Worldwide, approximately 62% of strokes and 49% of cases of ischemic heart disease are attributable to suboptimal (>115 mmHg systolic) blood pressure, which is believed to account for more than 7 million deaths annually. Remarkably, nearly half of this burden occurs among those with systolic blood pressure <140 mmHg, even as this level is used at the arbitrary threshold for defining hypertension in many national guidelines. Rising mean population blood pressure is apparent as populations industrialize and move from rural to urban settings. Among urban-dwelling men and women in India, for example, the prevalence of hypertension is 25.5% and 29.0%, respectively, whereas it is 14.0% and 10.8%, respectively, in rural communities. One major concern in low- and middle-income countries is the high rate of undetected, and therefore untreated, hypertension. This may explain, at least in part, the higher stroke rates in these countries in relation to CHD rates during the early stages of the transition. The high rates of hypertension, especially undiagnosed hypertension, throughout Asia probably contribute to the high prevalence of hemorrhagic stroke in the region.

Obesity

Although clearly associated with increased risk of CHD, much of the risk posed by obesity may be mediated by other CVD risk factors, including hypertension, diabetes mellitus, and lipid profile imbalances. In the mid-1980s, the World Health Organization's MONICA Project sampled 48 populations for cardiovascular risk factors. In all but one male population (China) and in most of the female populations, between 50% and 75% of adults age 35–64 years were overweight or obese. In addition, the prevalence of extreme obesity (BMI >40 kg/m^2) more than tripled, increasing from 1.3% to 4.9%. In many of the low- and middle-income countries, obesity appears to coexist with undernutrition and malnutrition. Obesity is increasing throughout the world, particularly in developing countries, where the trajectories are steeper than those experienced in the developed countries. According to the latest World Health Organization (WHO) data, this is equivalent to about 1.3 billion overweight adults in the world. A survey undertaken in 1998 found that as many as 58% of African women living in South Africa might have been overweight or obese.

Diabetes mellitus

As a consequence of, or in addition to, increasing body mass index and decreasing levels of physical activity, worldwide rates of diabetes—predominantly type 2 diabetes—are on the rise. In 2003, 194 million adults, or 5% of the world's population, had diabetes. By 2025, this number is predicted to increase 72 percent to 333 million. By 2025, the number of people with type 2 diabetes is projected to double in three of the six low- and middle-income regions: the Middle East and North Africa, South Asia, and Sub-Saharan Africa. There appear to be clear genetic susceptibilities to diabetes mellitus in various racial and ethnic groups. For example, migration studies suggest that South Asians and Indians tend to be at higher risk than are people of European ancestry.

SUMMARY

Although CVD rates are declining in the high-income countries, they are increasing in virtually every other region of the world. The consequences of this preventable epidemic will be substantial on many levels: individual mortality and morbidity rates, family suffering, and staggering economic costs.

Three complementary strategies can be used to lessen the impact. First, the overall burden of CVD risk factors can be lowered through population-wide public health measures such as national campaigns against cigarette smoking, unhealthy diets, and physical inactivity. Second, it is important to identify higher-risk subgroups of the population that stand to benefit the most from specific, low-cost prevention interventions, including screening for and treatment of hypertension and elevated cholesterol. Simple, low-cost interventions, such as the "polypill," a regimen of aspirin, a statin, and an anithypertensive agent, also need to be explored. Third, resources should be allocated to acute as well as secondary prevention interventions. For countries with limited resources, a critical first step in developing a comprehensive plan is better assessment of cause-specific mortality and morbidity, as well as the prevalence of the major preventable risk factors.

In the meantime, the high-income countries must continue to bear the burden of research and development aimed at prevention and treatment, being mindful of the economic limitations of many countries. The concept of the epidemiologic transition provides insight into methods to alter the course of the CVD epidemic. The efficient transfer of low-cost preventive and therapeutic strategies could alter the natural course of this epidemic and thereby reduce the excess global burden of preventable CVD.

CHAPTER 3

APPROACH TO THE PATIENT WITH POSSIBLE CARDIOVASCULAR DISEASE

Joseph Loscalzo

THE MAGNITUDE OF THE PROBLEM

Cardiovascular diseases comprise the most prevalent serious disorders in industrialized nations and are a rapidly growing problem in developing nations (Chap. 2). Age-adjusted death rates for coronary heart disease have declined by two-thirds in the last four decades in the United States, reflecting the identification and reduction of risk factors as well as improved treatments and interventions for the management of coronary artery disease, arrhythmias, and heart failure. Nonetheless, cardiovascular diseases remain the most common causes of death, responsible for 35% of all deaths, almost 1 million deaths each year. Approximately one-fourth of these deaths are sudden. In addition, cardiovascular diseases are highly prevalent, diagnosed in 80 million adults, or ~35% of the adult population. The growing prevalence of obesity, type 2 diabetes mellitus, and metabolic syndrome (Chap. 32), which are important risk factors for atherosclerosis, now threatens to reverse the progress that has been made in the age-adjusted reduction in the mortality rate of coronary heart disease.

For many years cardiovascular disease was considered to be more common in men than in women. In fact, the percentage of all deaths secondary to cardiovascular disease is higher among women (43%) than among men (37%). In addition, although the absolute number of deaths secondary to cardiovascular disease has declined over the past decades in men, this number has actually risen in women. Inflammation, obesity, type 2 diabetes mellitus, and the metabolic syndrome appear to play more prominent roles in the development of coronary atherosclerosis in women than in men. Coronary artery disease (CAD) is more frequently associated with dysfunction of the coronary microcirculation in women than in men. Exercise electrocardiography has a lower diagnostic accuracy in the prediction of epicardial obstruction in women than in men.

CARDIAC SYMPTOMS

The symptoms caused by heart disease result most commonly from myocardial ischemia, disturbance of the contraction and/or relaxation of the myocardium, obstruction to blood flow, or an abnormal cardiac rhythm or rate. Ischemia, which is caused by an imbalance between the heart's oxygen supply and demand, is manifest most frequently as chest discomfort (Chap. 4), whereas reduction of the pumping ability of the heart commonly leads to fatigue and elevated intravascular pressure upstream of the failing ventricle. The latter results in abnormal fluid accumulation, with peripheral edema (Chap. 7) or pulmonary congestion and dyspnea (Chap. 5). Obstruction to blood flow, as occurs in valvular stenosis, can cause symptoms resembling those of myocardial failure (Chap. 17). Cardiac arrhythmias often develop suddenly, and the resulting symptoms and signs—palpitations (Chap. 8), dyspnea, hypotension, and syncope—generally occur abruptly and may disappear as rapidly as they develop.

Although dyspnea, chest discomfort, edema, and syncope are cardinal manifestations of cardiac disease, they occur in other conditions as well. Thus, dyspnea is observed in disorders as diverse as pulmonary disease, marked obesity, and anxiety (Chap. 5). Similarly, chest discomfort may result from a variety of noncardiac and cardiac causes other than myocardial ischemia (Chap. 4). Edema, an important finding in untreated or inadequately treated heart failure, also may occur with primary renal disease and in hepatic cirrhosis (Chap. 7). Syncope occurs not only with serious cardiac arrhythmias but in a number of neurologic conditions as well. Whether heart disease is responsible for these symptoms frequently can be determined by carrying out a careful clinical examination (Chap. 9), supplemented by noninvasive testing using electrocardiography at rest and during exercise (Chap. 11), echocardiography, roentgenography, and other forms of myocardial imaging (Chap. 12).

Myocardial or coronary function that may be adequate at rest may be insufficient during exertion. Thus, dyspnea and/or chest discomfort that appear during activity are characteristic of patients with heart disease, whereas the opposite pattern, i.e., the appearance of these symptoms at rest and their remission during exertion, is rarely observed in such patients. It is important, therefore, to question the patient carefully about the relation of symptoms to exertion.

Many patients with cardiovascular disease may be asymptomatic both at rest and during exertion but may present with an abnormal physical finding such as a heart murmur, elevated arterial pressure, or an abnormality of the electrocardiogram (ECG) or the cardiac silhouette on the chest roentgenogram or other imaging test. It is important to assess the global risk of CAD in asymptomatic individuals, using a combination of clinical assessment and measurement of cholesterol and its fractions, as well as other biomarkers, such as C-reactive protein, in some patients (Chap. 30). Since the first clinical manifestation of CAD may be catastrophic—sudden cardiac death, acute myocardial infarction, or stroke in previous asymptomatic persons—it is mandatory to identify those at high risk of such events and institute further testing and preventive measures.

DIAGNOSIS

As outlined by the New York Heart Association (NYHA), the elements of a complete cardiac diagnosis include the systematic consideration of the following:

1. *The underlying etiology.* Is the disease congenital, hypertensive, ischemic, or inflammatory in origin?
2. *The anatomical abnormalities.* Which chambers are involved? Are they hypertrophied, dilated, or both? Which valves are affected? Are they regurgitant and/or stenotic? Is there pericardial involvement? Has there been a myocardial infarction?
3. *The physiological disturbances.* Is an arrhythmia present? Is there evidence of congestive heart failure or myocardial ischemia?
4. *Functional disability.* How strenuous is the physical activity required to elicit symptoms? The classification provided by the NYHA has been found to be useful in describing functional disability (Table 3-1).

TABLE 3-1

NEW YORK HEART ASSOCIATION FUNCTIONAL CLASSIFICATION	

Class I
  No limitation of physical activity
  No symptoms with ordinary exertion
Class II
  Slight limitation of physical activity
  Ordinary activity causes symptoms
	Class III
	  Marked limitation of physical activity
	  Less than ordinary activity causes symptoms
	  Asymptomatic at rest
	Class IV
	  Inability to carry out any physical activity without discomfort
	  Symptoms at rest

Source: Modified from The Criteria Committee of the New York Heart Association: *Nomenclature and Criteria for Diagnosis*, 9th ed. Boston, Little, Brown, 1994.

One example may serve to illustrate the importance of establishing a complete diagnosis. In a patient who presents with exertional chest discomfort, the identification of myocardial ischemia as the etiology is of great clinical importance. However, the simple recognition of ischemia is insufficient to formulate a therapeutic strategy or prognosis until the underlying anatomical abnormalities responsible for the myocardial ischemia, e.g., coronary atherosclerosis or aortic stenosis, are identified and a judgment is made about whether other physiologic disturbances that cause an imbalance between myocardial oxygen supply and demand, such as severe anemia, thyrotoxicosis, or supraventricular tachycardia, play contributory roles. Finally, the severity of the disability should govern the extent and tempo of the workup and strongly influence the therapeutic strategy that is selected.

The establishment of a correct and complete cardiac diagnosis usually commences with the history and physical examination (Chap. 9). Indeed, the clinical examination remains the basis for the diagnosis of a wide variety of disorders. The clinical examination may then be supplemented by five types of laboratory tests: (1) ECG (Chap. 11), (2) noninvasive imaging examinations (chest roentgenogram, echocardiogram, radionuclide imaging, computed tomographic imaging, and magnetic resonance imaging (Chap. 12), (3) blood tests to assess risk (e.g., lipid determinations, C-reactive protein [Chap. 30]) or cardiac function (e.g., brain natriuretic peptide [BNP] [Chap. 17]), (4) occasionally specialized invasive examinations (i.e., cardiac catheterization and coronary arteriography [Chap. 13]), and (5) genetic tests to identify monogenic cardiac diseases (e.g., hypertrophic cardiomyopathy [Chap. 21], Marfan syndrome, and abnormalities of cardiac ion channels that lead to prolongation of the QT interval and an increase in the risk of sudden death [Chap. 16]). These tests are becoming more widely available.

FAMILY HISTORY

In eliciting the history of a patient with known or suspected cardiovascular disease, particular attention should be directed to the family history. Familial clustering is common in many forms of heart disease. Mendelian transmission of single-gene defects may occur, as in hypertrophic cardiomyopathy (Chap. 21), Marfan syndrome, and sudden death associated with a prolonged QT syndrome (Chap. 16). Premature coronary disease and essential hypertension, type 2 diabetes mellitus, and hyperlipidemia (the most important risk factors for coronary artery disease) are usually polygenic disorders. Although familial transmission may be less obvious than in the monogenic disorders, it is helpful in assessing risk and prognosis in polygenic disorders. Familial clustering of cardiovascular diseases not only may occur on a genetic basis but also may be related to familial dietary or behavior patterns such as excessive ingestion of salt or calories and cigarette smoking.

ASSESSMENT OF FUNCTIONAL IMPAIRMENT

When an attempt is made to determine the severity of functional impairment in a patient with heart disease, it is helpful to ascertain the level of activity and the rate at which it is performed before symptoms develop. Thus, it is not sufficient to state that the patient complains of dyspnea. The breathlessness that occurs after running up two long flights of stairs denotes far less functional impairment than do similar symptoms that occur after taking a few steps on level ground. Also, the degree of customary physical activity at work and during recreation should be considered. The development of two-flight dyspnea in a well-conditioned marathon runner may be far more significant than the development of one-flight dyspnea in a previously sedentary person. The history should include a detailed consideration of the patient's therapeutic regimen. For example, the persistence or development of edema, breathlessness, and other manifestations of heart failure in a patient who is receiving optimal doses of diuretics and other therapies for heart failure (Chap. 17) is far graver than are similar manifestations in the absence of treatment. Similarly, the presence of angina pectoris despite treatment with optimal doses of multiple antianginal drugs (Chap. 33) is more serious than it is in a patient on no therapy. In an effort to determine the progression of symptoms, and thus the severity of the underlying illness, it may be useful to ascertain what, if any, specific tasks the patient could have carried out 6 months or 1 year earlier that he or she cannot carry out at present.

ELECTROCARDIOGRAM

(See also Chap. 11) Although an ECG usually should be recorded in patients with known or suspected heart disease, with the exception of the identification of arrhythmias, conduction abnormalities, ventricular hypertrophy, and acute myocardial infarction, it generally does not establish a specific diagnosis. The range of normal electrocardiographic findings is wide, and the tracing can be affected significantly by many noncardiac factors, such as age, body habitus, and serum electrolyte concentrations. In general, electrocardiographic changes should be interpreted in the context of other abnormal cardiovascular findings.

ASSESSMENT OF THE PATIENT WITH A HEART MURMUR

(Fig. 3–1) The cause of a heart murmur can often be readily elucidated from a systematic evaluation of its major attributes: timing, duration, intensity, quality, frequency, configuration, location, and radiation when considered in the light of the history, general physical examination, and other features of the cardiac examination, as described in Chap. 9.

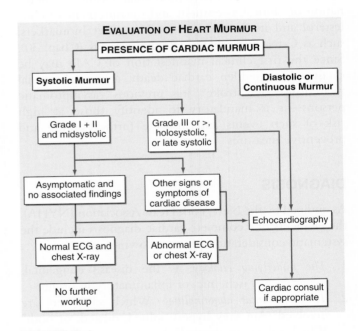

FIGURE 3-1

An alternative "echocardiography first" approach to the evaluation of a heart murmur that also uses the results of the electrocardiogram (ECG) and chest x-ray in asymptomatic patients with soft midsystolic murmurs and no other physical findings. This algorithm is useful for patients over age 40 years in whom the prevalence of coronary artery disease and aortic stenosis increases as the cause of systolic murmur. (*From RA O'Rourke, in Primary Cardiology, 2nd ed, E Braunwald, L Goldman [eds]. Philadelphia, Saunders, 2003.*)

The majority of heart murmurs are midsystolic and soft (grades I–II/VI). When such a murmur occurs in an asymptomatic child or young adult *without* other evidence of heart disease on clinical examination, it is usually benign and echocardiography generally is not required. By contrast, two-dimensional and Doppler echocardiography (Chap. 12) are indicated in patients with loud systolic murmurs (grades ≥III/VI), especially those that are holosystolic or late systolic, and in most patients with diastolic or continuous murmurs.

NATURAL HISTORY

Cardiovascular disorders often present acutely, as in a previously asymptomatic person who develops an acute myocardial infarction (Chap. 35), or a previously asymptomatic patient with hypertrophic cardiomyopathy (Chap. 21), or with a prolonged QT interval (Chap. 16) whose first clinical manifestation is syncope or even sudden death. However, the alert physician may recognize the patient at risk for these complications long before they occur and often can take measures to prevent their occurrence. For example, a patient with acute myocardial infarction will often have had risk factors for atherosclerosis for many years. Had these risk factors been recognized, their elimination or reduction might have delayed or even prevented the infarction. Similarly, a patient with hypertrophic cardiomyopathy may have had a heart murmur for years and a family history of this disorder. These findings could have led to an echocardiographic examination, recognition of the condition, and appropriate therapy long before the occurrence of a serious acute manifestation.

Patients with valvular heart disease or idiopathic dilated cardiomyopathy, by contrast, may have a prolonged course of gradually increasing dyspnea and other manifestations of chronic heart failure that is punctuated by episodes of acute deterioration only late in the course of the disease. Understanding the natural history of various cardiac disorders is essential for applying appropriate diagnostic and therapeutic measures to each stage of the condition, as well as for providing the patient and family with the likely prognosis.

PITFALLS IN CARDIOVASCULAR MEDICINE

Increasing subspecialization in internal medicine and the perfection of advanced diagnostic techniques in cardiology can lead to several undesirable consequences. Examples include the following:

1. Failure by the *noncardiologist* to recognize important cardiac manifestations of systemic illnesses. For example,

the presence of mitral stenosis, patent foramen ovale, and/or transient atrial arrhythmia should be considered in a patient with stroke, or the presence of pulmonary hypertension and cor pulmonale should be considered in a patient with scleroderma or Raynaud's syndrome. A cardiovascular examination should be carried out to identify and estimate the severity of the cardiovascular involvement that accompanies many noncardiac disorders.

2. Failure by the *cardiologist* to recognize underlying systemic disorders in patients with heart disease. For example, hyperthyroidism should be considered in an elderly patient with atrial fibrillation and unexplained heart failure, and Lyme disease should be considered in a patient with an unexplained fluctuating atrioventricular block. A cardiovascular abnormality may provide the clue critical to the recognition of some systemic disorders. For instance, an unexplained pericardial effusion may provide an early clue to the diagnosis of tuberculosis or a neoplasm.

3. Overreliance on and overutilization of laboratory tests, particularly invasive techniques, for the evaluation of the cardiovascular system. Cardiac catheterization and coronary arteriography (Chap. 13) provide precise diagnostic information that may be crucial in developing a therapeutic plan in patients with known or suspected CAD. Although a great deal of attention has been directed to these examinations, it is important to recognize that they serve to *supplement*, not *supplant*, a careful examination carried out with clinical and noninvasive techniques. A coronary arteriogram should not be performed in lieu of a careful history in patients with chest pain suspected of having ischemic heart disease. Although coronary arteriography may establish whether the coronary arteries are obstructed and to what extent, the results of the procedure by themselves often do not provide a definitive answer to the question of whether a patient's complaint of chest discomfort is attributable to coronary atherosclerosis and whether or not revascularization is indicated.

Despite the value of invasive tests in certain circumstances, they entail some small risk to the patient, involve discomfort and substantial cost, and place a strain on medical facilities. Therefore, they should be carried out only if the results can be expected to modify the patient's management.

DISEASE PREVENTION AND MANAGEMENT

The prevention of heart disease, especially of CAD, is one of the most important tasks of primary care health givers as well as cardiologists. Prevention begins with risk assessment, followed by attention to lifestyle, such as achieving optimal weight, physical activity, smoking cessation, and then aggressive treatment of all abnormal risk factors, such as hypertension, hyperlipidemia, and diabetes mellitus.

After a complete diagnosis has been established in patients with known heart disease, a number of management options are usually available. Several examples may be used to demonstrate some of the principles of cardiovascular therapeutics:

1. In the absence of evidence of heart disease, the patient should be clearly informed of this assessment and *not* be asked to return at intervals for repeated examinations. If there is no evidence of disease, such continued attention may lead to the patient's developing inappropriate concern about the possibility of heart disease.

2. If there is no evidence of cardiovascular disease but the patient has one or more risk factors for the development of ischemic heart disease (Chap. 33), a plan for their reduction should be developed and the patient should be retested at intervals to assess compliance and efficacy in risk reduction.

3. Asymptomatic or mildly symptomatic patients with valvular heart disease that is anatomically severe should be evaluated periodically, every 6 to 12 months, by clinical and noninvasive examinations. Early signs of deterioration of ventricular function may signify the need for surgical treatment before the development of disabling symptoms, irreversible myocardial damage, and excessive risk of surgical treatment (Chap. 20).

4. In patients with CAD (Chap. 33), available practice guidelines should be considered in the decision on the form of treatment (medical, percutaneous coronary intervention, or surgical revascularization). Mechanical revascularization may be employed too frequently in the United States and too infrequently in Eastern Europe and developing nations. The mere presence of angina pectoris and/or the demonstration of critical coronary arterial narrowing at angiography should not reflexively evoke a decision to treat the patient by revascularization. Instead, these interventions should be limited to patients with CAD whose angina has not responded adequately to medical treatment or in whom revascularization has been shown to improve the natural history (e.g., acute coronary syndrome or multivessel CAD with left ventricular dysfunction).

ACKNOWLEDGMENT

Dr. Eugene Braunwald authored this chapter for the previous edition of Harrison's Principles of Internal Medicine. Some of the material from the 17th edition has been carried forward.

SECTION II

DIAGNOSIS OF CARDIOVASCULAR DISORDERS

CHAPTER 4

CHEST DISCOMFORT

Thomas H. Lee

Chest discomfort is a common challenge for clinicians in the office or emergency department. The differential diagnosis includes conditions affecting organs throughout the thorax and abdomen, with prognostic implications that vary from benign to life threatening (Table 4-1). Failure to recognize potentially serious conditions such as acute ischemic heart disease, aortic dissection, tension pneumothorax, or pulmonary embolism can lead to serious complications, including death. Conversely, overly conservative management of low-risk patients leads to unnecessary hospital admissions, tests, procedures, and anxiety.

CAUSES OF CHEST DISCOMFORT

Myocardial ischemia and injury

Myocardial ischemia occurs when the oxygen supply to the heart is insufficient to meet metabolic needs. This mismatch can result from a decrease in oxygen supply, a rise in demand, or both. The most common underlying cause of myocardial ischemia is obstruction of coronary arteries by atherosclerosis; in the presence of such obstruction, transient ischemic episodes are usually precipitated by an increase in oxygen demand as a result of physical exertion. However, ischemia can also result from psychological stress, fever, or large meals or from compromised oxygen delivery due to anemia, hypoxia, or hypotension. Ventricular hypertrophy due to valvular heart disease, hypertrophic cardiomyopathy, or hypertension can predispose the myocardium to ischemia because of impaired penetration of blood flow from epicardial coronary arteries to the endocardium.

Angina pectoris

(See also Chap. 33) The chest discomfort of myocardial ischemia is a visceral discomfort that is usually described as a heaviness, pressure, or squeezing (Table 4-2). Other common adjectives for anginal pain are burning and aching. Some patients deny any

TABLE 4-1

DIAGNOSES AMONG CHEST PAIN PATIENTS WITHOUT MYOCARDIAL INFARCTION

DIAGNOSIS	PERCENT

Gastroesophageal disease[a]
  Gastroesophageal reflux
  Esophageal motility disorders
  Peptic ulcer
  Gallstones
	42

Ischemic heart disease	31
Chest wall syndromes	28
Pericarditis	4
Pleuritis/pneumonia	2
Pulmonary embolism	2
Lung cancer	1.5
Aortic aneurysm	1
Aortic stenosis	1
Herpes zoster	1

[a]In order of frequency.
Source: P Fruergaard et al: Eur Heart J 17:1028, 1996.

"pain" but may admit to dyspnea or a vague sense of anxiety. The word "sharp" is sometimes used by patients to describe intensity rather than quality.

The location of angina pectoris is usually retrosternal; most patients do not localize the pain to any small area. The discomfort may radiate to the neck, jaw, teeth, arms, or shoulders, reflecting the common origin in the posterior horn of the spinal cord of sensory neurons supplying the heart and these areas. Some patients present with aching in sites of radiated pain as their only symptoms of ischemia. Occasional patients report epigastric distress with ischemic episodes. Less common is radiation to below the umbilicus or to the back.

Stable angina pectoris usually develops gradually with exertion, emotional excitement, or after heavy meals.

TABLE 4-2

TYPICAL CLINICAL FEATURES OF MAJOR CAUSES OF ACUTE CHEST DISCOMFORT

CONDITION	DURATION	QUALITY	LOCATION	ASSOCIATED FEATURES
Angina	More than 2 and less than 10 min	Pressure, tightness, squeezing, heaviness, burning	Retrosternal, often with radiation to or isolated discomfort in neck, jaw, shoulders, or arms—frequently on left	Precipitated by exertion, exposure to cold, psychologic stress S_4 gallop or mitral regurgitation murmur during pain
Unstable angina	10–20 min	Similar to angina but often more severe	Similar to angina	Similar to angina, but occurs with low levels of exertion or even at rest
Acute myocardial infarction	Variable; often more than 30 min	Similar to angina but often more severe	Similar to angina	Unrelieved by nitroglycerin May be associated with evidence of heart failure or arrhythmia
Aortic stenosis	Recurrent episodes as described for angina	As described for angina	As described for angina	Late-peaking systolic murmur radiating to carotid arteries
Pericarditis	Hours to days; may be episodic	Sharp	Retrosternal or toward cardiac apex; may radiate to left shoulder	May be relieved by sitting up and leaning forward Pericardial friction rub
Aortic dissection	Abrupt onset of unrelenting pain	Tearing or ripping sensation; knifelike	Anterior chest, often radiating to back, between shoulder blades	Associated with hypertension and/or underlying connective tissue disorder, e.g., Marfan syndrome Murmur of aortic insufficiency, pericardial rub, pericardial tamponade, or loss of peripheral pulses
Pulmonary embolism	Abrupt onset; several minutes to a few hours	Pleuritic	Often lateral, on the side of the embolism	Dyspnea, tachypnea, tachycardia, and hypotension
Pulmonary hypertension	Variable	Pressure	Substernal	Dyspnea, signs of increased venous pressure including edema and jugular venous distention
Pneumonia or pleuritis	Variable	Pleuritic	Unilateral, often localized	Dyspnea, cough, fever, rales, occasional rub
Spontaneous pneumothorax	Sudden onset; several hours	Pleuritic	Lateral to side of pneumothorax	Dyspnea, decreased breath sounds on side of pneumothorax
Esophageal reflux	10–60 min	Burning	Substernal, epigastric	Worsened by postprandial recumbency Relieved by antacids
Esophageal spasm	2–30 min	Pressure, tightness, burning	Retrosternal	Can closely mimic angina
Peptic ulcer	Prolonged	Burning	Epigastric, substernal	Relieved with food or antacids
Gallbladder disease	Prolonged	Burning, pressure	Epigastric, right upper quadrant, substernal	May follow meal
Musculoskeletal disease	Variable	Aching	Variable	Aggravated by movement May be reproduced by localized pressure on examination
Herpes zoster	Variable	Sharp or burning	Dermatomal distribution	Vesicular rash in area of discomfort
Emotional and psychiatric conditions	Variable; may be fleeting	Variable	Variable; may be retrosternal	Situational factors may precipitate symptoms Anxiety or depression often detectable with careful history

Rest or treatment with sublingual nitroglycerin typically leads to relief within several minutes. In contrast, pain that is fleeting (lasting only a few seconds) is rarely ischemic in origin. Similarly, pain that lasts for several hours is unlikely to represent angina, particularly if the patient's electrocardiogram (ECG) does not show evidence of ischemia.

Anginal episodes can be precipitated by any physiologic or psychological stress that induces tachycardia. Most myocardial perfusion occurs during diastole, when there is minimal pressure opposing coronary artery flow from within the left ventricle. Since tachycardia decreases the percentage of the time in which the heart is in diastole, it decreases myocardial perfusion.

Unstable angina and myocardial infarction

(See also Chaps. 34 and 35) Patients with these acute ischemic syndromes usually complain of symptoms similar in quality to angina pectoris, but more prolonged and severe. The onset of these syndromes may occur with the patient at rest, or awakened from sleep, and sublingual nitroglycerin may lead to transient or no relief. Accompanying symptoms may include diaphoresis, dyspnea, nausea, and light-headedness.

The physical examination may be completely normal in patients with chest discomfort due to ischemic heart disease. Careful auscultation during ischemic episodes may reveal a third or fourth heart sound, reflecting myocardial systolic or diastolic dysfunction. A transient murmur of mitral regurgitation suggests ischemic papillary muscle dysfunction. Severe episodes of ischemia can lead to pulmonary congestion and even pulmonary edema.

Other cardiac causes

Myocardial ischemia caused by hypertrophic cardiomyopathy or aortic stenosis leads to angina pectoris similar to that caused by coronary atherosclerosis. In such cases, a loud systolic murmur or other findings usually suggest that abnormalities other than coronary atherosclerosis may be contributing to the patient's symptoms. Some patients with chest pain and normal coronary angiograms have functional abnormalities of the coronary circulation, ranging from coronary spasm visible on coronary angiography to abnormal vasodilator responses and heightened vasoconstrictor responses. The term "cardiac syndrome X" is used to describe patients with angina-like chest pain and ischemic-appearing ST-segment depression during stress despite normal coronary arteriograms. Some data indicate that many such patients have limited changes in coronary flow in response to pacing stress or coronary vasodilators.

Pericarditis

(See also Chap. 22) The pain in pericarditis is believed to be due to inflammation of the adjacent parietal pleura, since most of the pericardium is believed to be insensitive to pain. Thus, infectious pericarditis, which usually involves adjoining pleural surfaces, tends to be associated with pain, while conditions that cause only local inflammation (e.g., myocardial infarction or uremia) and cardiac tamponade tend to result in mild or no chest pain.

The adjacent parietal pleura receives its sensory supply from several sources, so the pain of pericarditis can be experienced in areas ranging from the shoulder and neck to the abdomen and back. Most typically, the pain is retrosternal and is aggravated by coughing, deep breaths, or changes in position—all of which lead to movements of pleural surfaces. The pain is often worse in the supine position and relieved by sitting upright and leaning forward. Less common is a steady aching discomfort that mimics acute myocardial infarction.

Diseases of the aorta

(See also Chap. 38) *Aortic dissection* is a potentially catastrophic condition that is due to spread of a subintimal hematoma within the wall of the aorta. The hematoma may begin with a tear in the intima of the aorta or with rupture of the vasa vasorum within the aortic media. This syndrome can occur with trauma to the aorta, including motor vehicle accidents or medical procedures in which catheters or intraaortic balloon pumps damage the intima of the aorta. Nontraumatic aortic dissections are rare in the absence of hypertension and/or conditions associated with deterioration of the elastic or muscular components of the media within the aorta's wall. Cystic medial degeneration is a feature of several inherited connective tissue diseases, including Marfan and Ehlers-Danlos syndromes. About half of all aortic dissections in women under 40 years of age occur during pregnancy.

Almost all patients with acute dissections present with severe chest pain, although some patients with chronic dissections are identified without associated symptoms. Unlike the pain of ischemic heart disease, symptoms of aortic dissection tend to reach peak severity immediately, often causing the patient to collapse from its intensity. The classic teaching is that the adjectives used to describe the pain reflect the process occurring within the wall of the aorta—"ripping" and "tearing"—but more recent data suggest that the most common presenting complaint is sudden onset of severe, sharp pain. The location often correlates with the site and extent of the dissection. Thus, dissections that begin in the ascending aorta and extend to the descending aorta tend to cause pain in the front of the chest that extends into the back, between the shoulder blades.

Physical findings may also reflect extension of the aortic dissection that compromises flow into arteries branching off the aorta. Thus, loss of a pulse in one or both arms, cerebrovascular accident, or paraplegia can all be catastrophic consequences of aortic dissection. Hematomas that extend proximally and undermine the coronary arteries or aortic valve apparatus may lead to acute myocardial infarction or acute aortic insufficiency. Rupture of the hematoma into the pericardial space leads to pericardial tamponade.

Another abnormality of the aorta that can cause chest pain is a *thoracic aortic aneurysm*. Aortic aneurysms are frequently asymptomatic but can cause chest pain and other symptoms by compressing adjacent structures. This pain tends to be steady, deep, and sometimes severe.

Pulmonary embolism

Chest pain due to pulmonary embolism is believed to be due to distention of the pulmonary artery or infarction of a segment of the lung adjacent to the pleura. Massive pulmonary emboli may lead to substernal pain that is suggestive of acute myocardial infarction. More commonly, smaller emboli lead to focal pulmonary infarctions that cause pain that is lateral and pleuritic. Associated symptoms include dyspnea and, occasionally, hemoptysis. Tachycardia is usually present. Although not always present, certain characteristic ECG changes can support the diagnosis.

Pneumothorax

Sudden onset of pleuritic chest pain and respiratory distress should lead to consideration of spontaneous pneumothorax, as well as pulmonary embolism. Such events may occur without a precipitating event in persons without lung disease, or as a consequence of underlying lung disorders.

Pneumonia or pleuritis

Lung diseases that damage and cause inflammation of the pleura of the lung usually cause a sharp, knifelike pain that is aggravated by inspiration or coughing.

Gastrointestinal conditions

Esophageal pain from acid reflux from the stomach, spasm, obstruction, or injury can be difficult to differentiate from myocardial syndromes. Acid reflux typically causes a deep burning discomfort that may be exacerbated by alcohol, aspirin, or some foods; this discomfort is often relieved by antacid or other acid-reducing therapies. Acid reflux tends to be exacerbated by lying down and may be worse in early morning when the stomach is empty of food that might otherwise absorb gastric acid.

Esophageal spasm may occur in the presence or absence of acid reflux and leads to a squeezing pain indistinguishable from angina. Prompt relief of esophageal spasm is often provided by antianginal therapies such as sublingual nifedipine, further promoting confusion between these syndromes. Chest pain can also result from injury to the esophagus, such as a Mallory-Weiss tear caused by severe vomiting.

Chest pain can result from diseases of the gastrointestinal tract below the diaphragm, including *peptic ulcer disease*, *biliary disease*, and *pancreatitis*. These conditions usually cause abdominal pain as well as chest discomfort; symptoms are not likely to be associated with exertion. The pain of ulcer disease typically occurs 60 to 90 min after meals, when postprandial acid production is no longer neutralized by food in the stomach. Cholecystitis usually causes a pain that is described as aching, occurring an hour or more after meals.

Neuromusculoskeletal conditions

Cervical disk disease can cause chest pain by compression of nerve roots. Pain in a dermatomal distribution can also be caused by *intercostal muscle cramps* or by *herpes zoster*. Chest pain symptoms due to herpes zoster may occur before skin lesions are apparent.

Costochondral and *chondrosternal syndromes* are the most common causes of anterior chest musculoskeletal pain. Only occasionally are physical signs of costochondritis such as swelling, redness, and warmth (Tietze's syndrome) present. The pain of such syndromes is usually fleeting and sharp, but some patients experience a dull ache that lasts for hours. Direct pressure on the chondrosternal and costochondral junctions may reproduce the pain from these and other musculoskeletal syndromes. Arthritis of the shoulder and spine and bursitis may also cause chest pain. Some patients who have these conditions and myocardial ischemia blur and confuse symptoms of these syndromes.

Emotional and psychiatric conditions

As many as 10% of patients who present to emergency departments with acute chest discomfort have panic disorder or other emotional conditions. The symptoms in these populations are highly variable, but frequently the discomfort is described as visceral tightness or aching that lasts more than 30 min. Some patients offer other atypical descriptions, such as pain that is fleeting, sharp, and/or localized to a small region. The ECG in patients with emotional conditions may be difficult to interpret if hyperventilation causes ST-T-wave abnormalities. A careful history may elicit clues of depression, prior panic attacks, somatization, agoraphobia, or other phobias.

APPROACH TO THE PATIENT | Chest Discomfort

The evaluation of the patient with chest discomfort must accommodate two goals—determining the diagnosis and assessing the safety of the immediate management plan. The latter issue is often dominant when the patient has acute chest discomfort, such as patients seen in the emergency department. In such settings, the clinician must focus first on identifying patients who require aggressive interventions to diagnose or manage potentially life-threatening conditions, including acute ischemic heart disease, acute aortic dissection, pulmonary embolism, and tension pneumothorax. If such conditions are unlikely, the clinician must address questions such as the safety of discharge to home, admission to a noncoronary care unit facility, or immediate exercise testing. Table 4-3 displays a sequence of questions that can be used in the evaluation of the patient with chest discomfort, with the diagnostic entities that are most important for consideration at each stage of the evaluation.

TABLE 4-3

CONSIDERATIONS IN THE ASSESSMENT OF THE PATIENT WITH CHEST DISCOMFORT

1. Could the chest discomfort be due to an acute, potentially life-threatening condition that warrants immediate hospitalization and aggressive evaluation?

Acute ischemic heart disease	Pulmonary embolism
Aortic dissection	Spontaneous pneumothorax

2. If not, could the discomfort be due to a chronic condition likely to lead to serious complications?

Stable angina

Aortic stenosis

Pulmonary hypertension

3. If not, could the discomfort be due to an acute condition that warrants specific treatment?

Pericarditis
Pneumonia/pleuritis
Herpes zoster

4. If not, could the discomfort be due to another treatable chronic condition?

Esophageal reflux	Cervical disk disease
Esophageal spasm	Arthritis of the shoulder or spine
Peptic ulcer disease	Costochondritis
Gallbladder disease	Other musculoskeletal disorders
Other gastrointestinal conditions	Anxiety state

ACUTE CHEST DISCOMFORT In patients with acute chest discomfort, the clinician must first assess the patient's respiratory and hemodynamic status. If either is compromised, initial management should focus on stabilizing the patient before the diagnostic evaluation is pursued. If, however, the patient does not require emergent interventions, then a focused history, physical examination, and laboratory evaluation should be performed to assess the patient's risk of life-threatening conditions.

Clinicians who are seeing patients in the office setting should not assume that they do not have acute ischemic heart disease, even if the prevalence may be lower. Malpractice litigation related to myocardial infarctions that were missed during office evaluations is becoming increasingly common, and ECGs were not performed in many such cases. The prevalence of high-risk patients seen in office settings may be increasing due to congestion in emergency departments.

In either setting, the *history* should include questions about the quality and location of the chest discomfort (Table 4-2). The patient should also be asked about the nature of onset of the pain and its duration. Myocardial ischemia is usually associated with a gradual intensification of symptoms over a period of minutes. Pain that is fleeting or that lasts hours without being associated with electrocardiographic changes is not likely to be ischemic in origin. Although the presence of risk factors for coronary artery disease may heighten concern for this diagnosis, the absence of such risk factors does not lower the risk for myocardial ischemia enough to be used to justify a decision to discharge a patient.

Wide radiation of chest pain increases probability that pain is due to myocardial infarction. Radiation of chest pain to the left arm is common with acute ischemic heart disease, but radiation to the right arm is also highly consistent with this diagnosis. Figure 4-1 shows estimates derived from several studies of the impact of various clinical features from the history on the probability that a patient has an acute myocardial infarction.

Right shoulder pain is also common with acute cholecystitis, but this syndrome is usually accompanied by pain that is located in the abdomen rather than the chest. Chest pain that radiates between the scapulae raises the question of aortic dissection.

The *physical examination* should include evaluation of blood pressure in both arms and of pulses in both legs. Poor perfusion of a limb may be due to an aortic dissection that has compromised flow to an artery branching from the aorta. Chest auscultation may reveal diminished breath sounds; a pleural rub; or evidence of pneumothorax, pulmonary embolism, pneumonia, or pleurisy. Tension pneumothorax may lead to a shift in the trachea from the midline, away from the side of the pneumothorax. The cardiac examination should seek

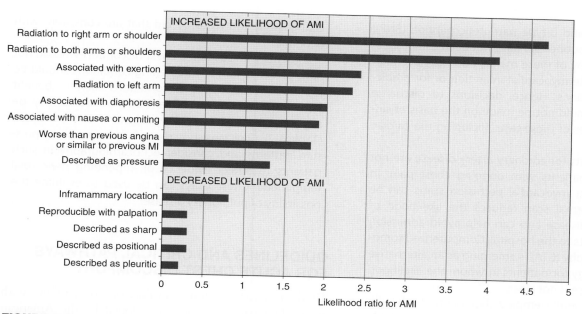

FIGURE 4-1
Impact of chest pain characteristics on odds of acute myocardial infarction (AMI). (*Figure prepared from data in CJ Swap, JT Nagurney: JAMA 294:2623, 2005.*)

pericardial rubs, systolic and diastolic murmurs, and third or fourth heart sounds. Pressure on the chest wall may reproduce symptoms in patients with musculoskeletal causes of chest pain; it is important that the clinician ask the patient if the chest pain syndrome is being completely reproduced before drawing too much reassurance that more serious underlying conditions are not present.

An *ECG* is an essential test for adults with chest discomfort that is not due to an obvious traumatic cause. In such patients, the presence of electrocardiographic changes consistent with ischemia or infarction (Chap. 11) is associated with high risks of acute myocardial infarction or unstable angina (Table 4-4); such patients should be admitted to a unit with electrocardiographic monitoring and the capacity to respond to a cardiac arrest. The absence of such changes does not exclude acute ischemic heart disease, but the risk of life-threatening complications is low for patients with normal electrocardiograms or only nonspecific ST-T-wave changes. If these patients are not considered appropriate for immediate discharge, they are often candidates for early or immediate exercise testing.

Markers of myocardial injury are often obtained in the emergency department evaluation of acute chest discomfort. In recent years, the cardiac troponins (I and T) have superceded creatine kinase (CK) and CK-MB as the markers of choice for detecting myocardial injury. Some data support the use of other markers, such as

TABLE 4-4

PREVALENCE OF ACUTE ISCHEMIC HEART DISEASE SYNDROMES AMONG SUBSETS OF EMERGENCY DEPARTMENT PATIENTS WITH CHEST PAIN

FINDING	PREVALENCE MYOCARDIAL INFARCTION, %	UNSTABLE ANGINA, %
ST elevation (≥1 mm) or Q waves on ECG not known to be old	79	12
Ischemia or strain on ECG not known to be old (ST depression ≥1 mm or ischemic T waves)	20	41
None of the preceding ECG changes but a prior history of angina or myocardial infarction (history of heart attack or nitroglycerin use)	4	51
None of the preceding ECG changes and no prior history of angina or myocardial infarction (history of heart attack or nitroglycerin use)	2	14

Abbreviation: ECG, electrocardiogram.
Source: Unpublished data from Brigham and Women's Hospital Chest Pain Study, 1997–1999.

myeloperoxidase and B-type natriuretic peptide (BNP), but their roles in routine care have not been established. Single values of any of these markers do not have high sensitivity for acute myocardial infarction or for prediction of complications. Hence, decisions to discharge patients home should not be made on the basis of single negative values of these tests, including the cardiac troponins.

Provocative tests for coronary artery disease are not appropriate for patients with ongoing chest pain. In such patients, rest myocardial perfusion scans can be considered; a normal scan reduces the likelihood of coronary artery disease and can help avoid admission of low-risk patients to the hospital. Computerized tomographic angiography (CTA) is emerging as an alternative diagnostic strategy for patients in whom the likelihood of coronary disease is not clear.

Clinicians frequently employ therapeutic trials with sublingual nitroglycerin or antacids or, in the stable patient seen in the office setting, a proton pump inhibitor. A common error is to assume that a response to any of these interventions clarifies the diagnosis. While such information is often helpful, the patient's response may be due to the placebo effect. Hence, myocardial ischemia should never be considered excluded solely because of a response to antacid therapy. Similarly, failure of nitroglycerin to relieve pain does not exclude the diagnosis of coronary disease.

If the patient's history or examination is consistent with aortic dissection, imaging studies to evaluate the aorta must be pursued promptly because of the high risk of catastrophic complications with this condition. Appropriate tests include a chest CT scan with contrast, MRI, or transesophageal echocardiography. Current data indicate that elevated D-dimer levels should raise clinicians' suspicion of aortic dissection.

Acute pulmonary embolism should be considered in patients with respiratory symptoms, pleuritic chest pain, hemoptysis, or a history of venous thromboembolism or coagulation abnormalities. Initial tests usually include CT angiography or a lung scan, which are sometimes combined with lower extremity venous ultrasound or D-dimer testing.

If patients with acute chest discomfort show no evidence of life-threatening conditions, the clinician should then focus on serious chronic conditions with the potential to cause major complications, the most common of which is stable angina. Early use of exercise electrocardiography, stress echocardiography, or stress perfusion imaging for such patients, whether in the office or the emergency department, is now an accepted management strategy for low-risk patients. Exercise testing is not appropriate, however, for patients who (1) report pain that is believed to be ischemic occurring at rest or (2) have electrocardiographic changes not known to be old that are consistent with ischemia.

Patients with sustained chest discomfort who do not have evidence for life-threatening conditions should be evaluated for evidence of conditions likely to benefit from acute treatment (Table 4-3). Pericarditis may be suggested by the history, physical examination, and ECG (Table 4-2). Clinicians should carefully assess blood pressure patterns and consider echocardiography in such patients to detect evidence of impending pericardial tamponade. Chest x-rays can be used to evaluate the possibility of pulmonary disease.

GUIDELINES AND CRITICAL PATHWAYS FOR ACUTE CHEST DISCOMFORT

Guidelines for the initial evaluation for patients with acute chest pain have been developed by the American College of Cardiology, American Heart Association, and other organizations. These guidelines recommend performance of an ECG for virtually all patients with chest pain who do not have an obvious noncardiac cause of their pain, and performance of a chest x-ray for patients with signs or symptoms consistent with congestive heart failure, valvular heart disease, pericardial disease, or aortic dissection or aneurysm.

The American College of Cardiology/American Heart Association guidelines on exercise testing support its use in low-risk patients presenting to the emergency department, as well as in selected intermediate-risk patients. However, these guidelines emphasize that exercise tests should be performed only after patients have been screened for high-risk features or other indicators for hospital admission.

Many medical centers have adopted critical pathways and other forms of guidelines to increase efficiency and to expedite the treatment of patients with high-risk acute ischemic heart disease syndromes. These guidelines emphasize the following strategies:

- Rapid identification and treatment of patients for whom emergent reperfusion therapy, either via percutaneous coronary interventions or thrombolytic agents, is likely to lead to improved outcomes.
- Triage to non-coronary care unit monitored facilities such as intermediate-care units or chest pain units of patients with a low risk for complications, such as patients without new ischemic changes on their ECGs and without ongoing chest pain. Such patients can usually be safely observed in non-coronary care unit settings, undergo early exercise testing, or be discharged home. Risk stratification can be assisted through use of prospectively validated multivariate algorithms that have been published for acute ischemic heart disease and its complications.

- Shortening lengths of stay in the coronary care unit and hospital. Recommendations regarding the minimum length of stay in a monitored bed for a patient who has no further symptoms have decreased in recent years to 12 h or less if exercise testing or other risk stratification technologies are available.

Nonacute chest discomfort

The management of patients who do not require admission to the hospital or who no longer require inpatient observation should seek to identify the cause of the symptoms and the likelihood of major complications. Noninvasive tests for coronary disease serve both to diagnose this condition and to identify patients with high-risk forms of coronary disease who may benefit from revascularization. Gastrointestinal causes of chest pain can be evaluated via endoscopy or radiology studies, or with trials of medical therapy. Emotional and psychiatric conditions warrant appropriate evaluation and treatment; randomized trial data indicate that cognitive therapy and group interventions lead to decreases in symptoms for such patients.

CHAPTER 5

DYSPNEA

Richard M. Schwartzstein

DYSPNEA

The American Thoracic Society defines *dyspnea* as a "subjective experience of breathing discomfort that consists of qualitatively distinct sensations that vary in intensity. The experience derives from interactions among multiple physiological, psychological, social, and environmental factors and may induce secondary physiological and behavioral responses." Dyspnea, a symptom, must be distinguished from the signs of increased work of breathing.

MECHANISMS OF DYSPNEA

Respiratory sensations are the consequence of interactions between the *efferent*, or outgoing, motor output from the brain to the ventilatory muscles (feed-forward) and the *afferent*, or incoming, sensory input from receptors throughout the body (feedback), as well as the integrative processing of this information that we infer must be occurring in the brain (Fig. 5-1). In contrast to painful sensations, which can often be attributed to the stimulation of a single nerve ending, dyspnea sensations are more commonly viewed as holistic, more akin to hunger or thirst. A given disease state may lead to dyspnea by one or more mechanisms, some of which may be operative under some circumstances, e.g., exercise, but not others, e.g., a change in position.

Motor efferents

Disorders of the ventilatory pump, most commonly increase airway resistance or stiffness (decreased compliance) of the respiratory system, are associated with increased work of breathing or a sense of an increased effort to breathe. When the muscles are weak or fatigued, greater effort is required, even though the mechanics of the system are normal. The increased neural output from the motor cortex is sensed via a

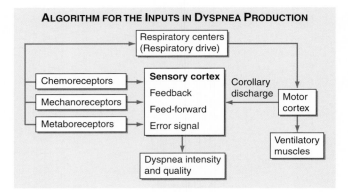

ALGORITHM FOR THE INPUTS IN DYSPNEA PRODUCTION

FIGURE 5-1

Hypothetical model for integration of sensory inputs in the production of dyspnea. Afferent information from the receptors throughout the respiratory system projects directly to the sensory cortex to contribute to primary qualitative sensory experiences and provide feedback on the action of the ventilatory pump. Afferents also project to the areas of the brain responsible for control of ventilation. The motor cortex, responding to input from the control centers, sends neural messages to the ventilatory muscles and a corollary discharge to the sensory cortex (feed-forward with respect to the instructions sent to the muscles). If the feed-forward and feedback messages do not match, an error signal is generated and the intensity of dyspnea increases. *(Adapted from MA Gillette, RM Schwartzstein: Mechanisms of dyspnea, in Supportive Care in Respiratory Disease, SH Ahmedzai and MF Muer [eds]. Oxford, UK, Oxford University Press, 2005.)*

corollary discharge, a neural signal that is sent to the sensory cortex at the same time that motor output is directed to the ventilatory muscles.

Sensory afferents

Chemoreceptors in the carotid bodies and medulla are activated by hypoxemia, acute hypercapnia, and acidemia. Stimulation of these receptors, as well as others that lead to an increase in ventilation, produce a sensation of air hunger. Mechanoreceptors in the lungs, when stimulated by bronchospasm, lead to a sensation of chest tightness. J-receptors, sensitive to interstitial edema, and pulmonary vascular receptors, activated by acute changes in pulmonary artery pressure, appear to contribute to air hunger. Hyperinflation is associated with the sensation of increased work of breathing and an inability to get a deep breath or of an unsatisfying breath. Metaboreceptors, located in skeletal muscle, are believed to be activated by changes in the local biochemical milieu of the tissue active during exercise and, when stimulated, contribute to the breathing discomfort.

Integration: Efferent-reafferent mismatch

A discrepancy or mismatch between the feed-forward message to the ventilatory muscles and the feedback from receptors that monitor the response of the ventilatory pump increases the intensity of dyspnea. This is particularly important when there is a mechanical derangement of the ventilatory pump, such as in asthma or chronic obstructive pulmonary disease (COPD).

Anxiety

Acute anxiety may increase the severity of dyspnea either by altering the interpretation of sensory data or by leading to patterns of breathing that heighten physiologic abnormalities in the respiratory system. In patients with expiratory flow limitation, for example, the increased respiratory rate that accompanies acute anxiety leads to hyperinflation, increased work and effort of breathing, and a sense of an unsatisfying breath.

ASSESSING DYSPNEA
Quality of sensation

As with pain, dyspnea assessment begins with a determination of the quality of the discomfort (Table 5-1). Dyspnea questionnaires, or lists of phrases commonly used by patients, assist those who have difficulty describing their breathing sensations.

Sensory intensity

A modified Borg scale or visual analogue scale can be utilized to measure dyspnea at rest, immediately following exercise, or on recall of a reproducible physical task, e.g., climbing the stairs at home. An alternative approach is to inquire about the activities a patient can do, i.e., to gain a sense of the patient's disability. The Baseline Dyspnea Index and the Chronic Respiratory Disease Questionnaire are commonly used tools for this purpose.

TABLE 5-1

ASSOCIATION OF QUALITATIVE DESCRIPTORS AND PATHOPHYSIOLOGIC MECHANISMS OF SHORTNESS OF BREATH

DESCRIPTOR	PATHOPHYSIOLOGY
Chest tightness or constriction	Bronchoconstriction, interstitial edema (asthma, myocardial ischemia)
Increased work or effort of breathing	Airway obstruction, neuromuscular disease (COPD, moderate to severe asthma, myopathy, kyphoscoliosis)
Air hunger, need to breathe, urge to breathe	Increased drive to breathe (CHF, pulmonary embolism, moderate to severe airflow obstruction)
Cannot get a deep breath, unsatisfying breath	Hyperinflation (asthma, COPD) and restricted tidal volume (pulmonary fibrosis, chest wall restriction)
Heavy breathing, rapid breathing, breathing more	Deconditioning

Abbreviations: CHF, congestive heart failure; COPD, chronic obstructive pulmonary disease.
Source: From RM Schwartzstein: The language of dyspnea, in *Dyspnea: Mechanisms, Measurement, and Management*, DA Mahler and DE O'Donnell (eds). New York, Marcel Dekker, 2005 and RM Schwartzstein, D Feller-Kopman: Shortness of breath, in *Primary Cardiology*, 2nd ed, E Braunwald and L Goldman (eds). Philadelphia, WB Saunders, 2003.

Affective dimension

For a sensation to be reported as a symptom, it must be perceived as unpleasant and interpreted as abnormal. Laboratory studies have demonstrated that air hunger evokes a stronger affective response than does increased effort or work of breathing. Some therapies for dyspnea, such as pulmonary rehabilitation, may reduce breathing discomfort, in part, by altering this dimension.

DIFFERENTIAL DIAGNOSIS

Dyspnea is the consequence of deviations from normal function in the cardiopulmonary systems. These deviations produce breathlessness as a consequence of increased drive to breathe; increased effort or work of breathing; and/or stimulation of receptors in the heart, lungs, or vascular system. Most diseases of the respiratory system are associated with alterations in the mechanical properties of the lungs and/or chest wall, frequently as a consequence of disease of the airways or lung parenchyma. In contrast, disorders of the cardiovascular system more commonly lead to dyspnea by causing gas exchange abnormalities or stimulating pulmonary and/or vascular receptors (Table 5-2).

TABLE 5-2

MECHANISMS OF DYSPNEA IN COMMON DISEASES

DISEASE	↑ WORK OF BREATHING	↑ DRIVE TO BREATHE	HYPOXEMIA[a]	ACUTE HYPERCAPNIA[a]	STIMULATION OF PULMONARY RECEPTORS	STIMULATION OF VASCULAR RECEPTORS	METABORECEPTORS
COPD	•		•	•			
Asthma	•	•	•	•	•		
ILD	•	•	•	•	•		
PVD		•	•				
CPE	•	•	•		•	•	•
NCPE	•	•	•		•		
Anemia							•
Decond							•

[a]Hypoxemia and hypercapnia are not always present in these conditions. When hypoxemia is present, dyspnea usually persists, albeit at a reduced intensity, with correction of hypoxemia by the administration of supplemental oxygen.
Abbreviations: COPD, chronic obstructive pulmonary disease; CPE, cardiogenic pulmonary edema; Decond, deconditioning; ILD, interstitial lung disease; NCPE, noncardiogenic pulmonary edema; PVD, pulmonary vascular disease.

Respiratory system dyspnea

Diseases of the airways

Asthma and COPD, the most common obstructive lung diseases, are characterized by expiratory airflow obstruction, which typically leads to dynamic hyperinflation of the lungs and chest wall. Patients with moderate to severe disease have increased resistive and elastic loads (a term that relates to the stiffness of the system) on the ventilatory muscles and increased work of breathing. Patients with acute bronchoconstriction also complain of a sense of tightness, which can exist even when lung function is still within the normal range. These patients commonly hyperventilate. Both the chest tightness and hyperventilation are probably due to stimulation of pulmonary receptors. Both asthma and COPD may lead to hypoxemia and hypercapnia from ventilation-perfusion (V̇/Q) mismatch (and diffusion limitation during exercise with emphysema); hypoxemia is much more common than hypercapnia as a consequence of the different ways in which oxygen and carbon dioxide bind to hemoglobin.

Diseases of the chest wall

Conditions that stiffen the chest wall, such as kyphoscoliosis, or that weaken ventilatory muscles, such as myasthenia gravis or the Guillain-Barré syndrome, are also associated with an increased effort to breathe. Large pleural effusions may contribute to dyspnea, both by increasing the work of breathing and by stimulating pulmonary receptors if there is associated atelectasis.

Diseases of the lung parenchyma

Interstitial lung diseases, which may arise from infections, occupational exposures, or autoimmune disorders, are associated with increased stiffness (decreased compliance) of the lungs and increased work of breathing. In addition, V̇/Q mismatch, and destruction and/or thickening of the alveolar-capillary interface may lead to hypoxemia and an increased drive to breathe. Stimulation of pulmonary receptors may further enhance the hyperventilation characteristic of mild to moderate interstitial disease.

Cardiovascular system dyspnea

Diseases of the left heart

Diseases of the myocardium resulting from coronary artery disease and nonischemic cardiomyopathies result in a greater left-ventricular end-diastolic volume and an elevation of the left-ventricular end-diastolic, as well as pulmonary capillary pressures. These elevated pressures lead to interstitial edema and stimulation of pulmonary receptors, thereby causing dyspnea; hypoxemia due to V̇/Q mismatch may also contribute to breathlessness. Diastolic dysfunction, characterized by a very stiff left ventricle, may lead to severe dyspnea with relatively mild degrees of physical activity, particularly if it is associated with mitral regurgitation.

Diseases of the pulmonary vasculature

Pulmonary thromboembolic disease and primary diseases of the pulmonary circulation (primary pulmonary hypertension, pulmonary vasculitis) cause dyspnea via increased pulmonary-artery pressure and stimulation of pulmonary receptors. Hyperventilation is common, and hypoxemia may be present. However, in most cases, use of supplemental oxygen has minimal effect on the severity of dyspnea and hyperventilation.

Diseases of the pericardium

Constrictive pericarditis and cardiac tamponade are both associated with increased intracardiac and pulmonary vascular pressures, which are the likely cause of dyspnea in these conditions. To the extent that cardiac output is limited, at rest or with exercise, stimulation of metaboreceptors and chemoreceptors (if lactic acidosis develops) contribute as well.

Dyspnea with normal respiratory and cardiovascular systems

Mild to moderate anemia is associated with breathing discomfort during exercise. This is thought to be related to stimulation of metaboreceptors; oxygen saturation is normal in patients with anemia. The breathlessness associated with obesity is probably due to multiple mechanisms, including high cardiac output and impaired ventilatory pump function (decreased compliance of the chest wall). Cardiovascular deconditioning (poor fitness) is characterized by the early development of anaerobic metabolism and the stimulation of chemoreceptors and metaboreceptors.

APPROACH TO THE PATIENT   Dyspnea

(Fig. 5-2) In obtaining a *history*, the patient should be asked to describe in his/her own words what the discomfort feels like, as well as the effect of position, infections, and environmental stimuli on the dyspnea. Orthopnea is a common indicator of congestive heart failure (CHF), mechanical impairment of the diaphragm associated with obesity, or asthma triggered by esophageal reflux. Nocturnal dyspnea suggests CHF or asthma. Acute, intermittent episodes of dyspnea are more likely to reflect episodes of myocardial ischemia, bronchospasm, or pulmonary embolism, while chronic persistent dyspnea is typical of COPD, interstitial lung disease, and chronic thromboembolic disease. Risk factors for occupational lung disease and for coronary artery disease should be elicited. Left atrial myxoma or hepatopulmonary syndrome should be considered when the patient complains of *platypnea*, defined as dyspnea in the upright position with relief in the supine position.

The *physical examination* should begin during the interview of the patient. Inability of the patient to speak in full sentences before stopping to get a deep breath suggests a condition that leads to stimulation of the controller or an impairment of the ventilatory pump with reduced vital capacity. Evidence for increased work of breathing (supraclavicular retractions, use of accessory muscles of ventilation, and the tripod position, characterized by sitting with one's hands braced on the knees) is indicative of increased airway resistance or stiff lungs and chest wall. When measuring the vital signs, one should accurately assess the respiratory rate and measure the pulsus paradoxus (Chap. 22); if it is >10 mmHg, consider the presence of COPD or acute asthma. During the general examination, signs of anemia (pale conjunctivae), cyanosis, and cirrhosis (spider angiomata, gynecomastia) should be sought. Examination of the chest should focus on symmetry of movement; percussion (dullness indicative of pleural effusion, hyperresonance a sign of emphysema); and auscultation (wheezes, rales, rhonchi, prolonged expiratory phase, diminished breath sounds, which are clues to disorders of the airways, and interstitial edema or fibrosis). The cardiac examination should focus on signs of elevated right heart pressures (jugular venous distention, edema, accentuated pulmonic component to the second heart sound); left ventricular dysfunction (S3 and S4 gallops); and valvular disease (murmurs). When examining the abdomen with the patient in the supine position, it should be noted whether there is paradoxical movement of the abdomen (inward motion during inspiration), a sign of diaphragmatic weakness; rounding of the abdomen during exhalation is suggestive of pulmonary edema. Clubbing of the digits may be an indication of interstitial pulmonary fibrosis, and the presence of joint swelling or deformation as well as changes consistent with Raynaud's disease may be indicative of a collagen-vascular process that can be associated with pulmonary disease.

Patients with exertional dyspnea should be asked to walk under observation in order to reproduce the symptoms. The patient should be examined for new findings that were not present at rest and for oxygen saturation.

Following the history and physical examination, a *chest radiograph* should be obtained. The lung volumes should be assessed (hyperinflation indicates obstructive lung disease; low lung volumes suggest interstitial edema or fibrosis, diaphragmatic dysfunction, or impaired chest wall motion). The pulmonary parenchyma should be examined for evidence of interstitial disease and emphysema. Prominent pulmonary vasculature in the upper zones indicates pulmonary venous hypertension, while enlarged central pulmonary arteries suggest pulmonary artery hypertension. An enlarged cardiac silhouette suggests a dilated cardiomyopathy or valvular disease. Bilateral pleural effusions are typical of CHF and some forms of collagen vascular disease. Unilateral effusions raise the specter of carcinoma and pulmonary embolism but may also occur in heart failure. *Computed tomography* (CT) *of the chest* is generally reserved for further evaluation of the lung parenchyma (interstitial lung disease) and possible pulmonary embolism.

Laboratory studies should include an electrocardiogram to look for evidence of ventricular hypertrophy and prior myocardial infarction. Echocardiography is indicated in patients in

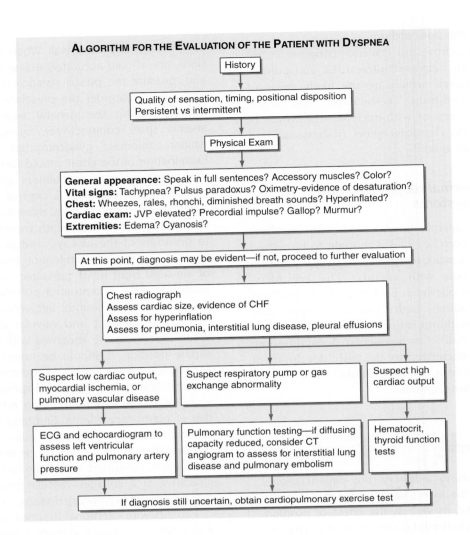

ALGORITHM FOR THE EVALUATION OF THE PATIENT WITH DYSPNEA

History

↓

Quality of sensation, timing, positional disposition
Persistent vs intermittent

↓

Physical Exam

↓

General appearance: Speak in full sentences? Accessory muscles? Color?
Vital signs: Tachypnea? Pulsus paradoxus? Oximetry-evidence of desaturation?
Chest: Wheezes, rales, rhonchi, diminished breath sounds? Hyperinflated?
Cardiac exam: JVP elevated? Precordial impulse? Gallop? Murmur?
Extremities: Edema? Cyanosis?

↓

At this point, diagnosis may be evident—if not, proceed to further evaluation

↓

Chest radiograph
Assess cardiac size, evidence of CHF
Assess for hyperinflation
Assess for pneumonia, interstitial lung disease, pleural effusions

Suspect low cardiac output, myocardial ischemia, or pulmonary vascular disease	Suspect respiratory pump or gas exchange abnormality	Suspect high cardiac output
ECG and echocardiogram to assess left ventricular function and pulmonary artery pressure	Pulmonary function testing—if diffusing capacity reduced, consider CT angiogram to assess for interstitial lung disease and pulmonary embolism	Hematocrit, thyroid function tests

If diagnosis still uncertain, obtain cardiopulmonary exercise test

FIGURE 5-2

An algorithm for the evaluation of the patient with dyspnea. JVP, jugular venous pulse; CHF, congestive heart failure; ECG, electrocardiogram; CT, computed tomography. (*Adapted from RM Schwartzstein: The language of dyspnea, in Dyspnea: Mechanisms, Measurement, and Management,* *DA Mahler and DE O'Donnell [eds]. New York, Marcel Dekker, 2005 and RM Schwartzstein, D Feller-Kopman: Shortness of breath, in Primary Cardiology, 2nd ed, E Braunwald and L Goldman [eds]. Philadelphia, WB Saunders, 2003.)*

whom systolic dysfunction, pulmonary hypertension, or valvular heart disease is suspected. Bronchoprovocation testing is useful in patients with intermittent symptoms suggestive of asthma but normal physical examination and lung function; up to one-third of patients with the clinical diagnosis of asthma do not have reactive airways disease when formally tested.

DISTINGUISHING CARDIOVASCULAR FROM RESPIRATORY SYSTEM DYSPNEA

If a patient has evidence of both pulmonary and cardiac disease, a cardiopulmonary exercise test should be carried out to determine which system is responsible for the exercise limitation. If, at peak exercise, the patient achieves predicted maximal ventilation, demonstrates an increase in dead space or hypoxemia, or develops bronchospasm, the respiratory system is probably the cause of

the problem. Alternatively, if the heart rate is >85% of the predicted maximum, if anaerobic threshold occurs early, if the blood pressure becomes excessively high or decreases during exercise, if the O_2 pulse (O_2 consumption/heart rate, an indicator of stroke volume) falls, or if there are ischemic changes on the electrocardiogram, an abnormality of the cardiovascular system is likely the explanation for the breathing discomfort.

TREATMENT Dyspnea

The first goal is to correct the underlying problem responsible for the symptom. If this is not possible, one attempts to lessen the intensity of the symptom and its effect on the patient's quality of life. Supplemental

O$_2$ should be administered if the resting O$_2$ saturation is ≤89% or if the patient's saturation drops to these levels with activity. For patients with COPD, pulmonary rehabilitation programs have demonstrated positive effects on dyspnea, exercise capacity, and rates of hospitalization. Studies of anxiolytics and antidepressants have not demonstrated consistent benefit. Experimental interventions—e.g., cold air on the face, chest-wall vibration, and inhaled furosemide—to modulate the afferent information from receptors throughout the respiratory system are being studied.

PULMONARY EDEMA

MECHANISMS OF FLUID ACCUMULATION

The extent to which fluid accumulates in the interstitium of the lung depends on the balance of hydrostatic and oncotic forces within the pulmonary capillaries and in the surrounding tissue. Hydrostatic pressure favors movement of fluid from the capillary into the interstitium. The oncotic pressure, which is determined by the protein concentration in the blood, favors movement of fluid into the vessel. Albumin, the primary protein in the plasma, may be low in conditions such as cirrhosis and nephrotic syndrome. While hypoalbuminemia favors movement of fluid into the tissue for any given hydrostatic pressure in the capillary, it is usually not sufficient by itself to cause interstitial edema. In a healthy individual, the tight junctions of the capillary endothelium are impermeable to proteins, and the lymphatics in the tissue carry away the small amounts of protein that may leak out; together, these factors result in an oncotic force that maintains fluid in the capillary. Disruption of the endothelial barrier, however, allows protein to escape the capillary bed and enhances the movement of fluid into the tissue of the lung.

Cardiogenic pulmonary edema

(See also Chap. 28) Cardiac abnormalities that lead to an increase in pulmonary venous pressure shift the balance of forces between the capillary and the interstitium. Hydrostatic pressure is increased and fluid exits the capillary at an increased rate, resulting in interstitial and, in more severe cases, alveolar edema. The development of pleural effusions may further compromise respiratory system function and contribute to breathing discomfort.

Early signs of pulmonary edema include exertional dyspnea and orthopnea. Chest radiographs show peribronchial thickening, prominent vascular markings in the upper lung zones, and Kerley B lines. As the pulmonary edema worsens, alveoli fill with fluid; the chest radiograph shows patchy alveolar filling, typically in a perihilar distribution, which then progresses to diffuse alveolar infiltrates. Increasing airway edema is associated with rhonchi and wheezes.

Noncardiogenic pulmonary edema

In noncardiogenic pulmonary edema, lung water increases due to damage of the pulmonary capillary lining with leakage of proteins and other macromolecules into the tissue; fluid follows the protein as oncotic forces are shifted from the vessel to the surrounding lung tissue. This process is associated with dysfunction of the surfactant lining the alveoli, increased surface forces, and a propensity for the alveoli to collapse at low lung volumes. Physiologically, noncardiogenic pulmonary edema is characterized by intrapulmonary shunt with hypoxemia and decreased pulmonary compliance. Pathologically, hyaline membranes are evident in the alveoli, and inflammation leading to pulmonary fibrosis may be seen. Clinically, the picture ranges from mild dyspnea to respiratory failure. Auscultation of the lungs may be relatively normal despite chest radiographs that show diffuse alveolar infiltrates. CT scans demonstrate that the distribution of alveolar edema is more heterogeneous than was once thought. Although normal intracardiac pressures are considered by many to be part of the definition of noncardiogenic pulmonary edema, the pathology of the process, as described earlier, is distinctly different, and one can observe a combination of cardiogenic and noncardiogenic pulmonary edema in some patients.

It is useful to categorize the causes of noncardiogenic pulmonary edema in terms of whether the injury to the lung is likely to result from direct, indirect, or pulmonary vascular causes (Table 5-3). Direct injuries are mediated via the airways (e.g., aspiration) or as the consequence of blunt chest trauma. Indirect injury is the consequence of mediators that reach the lung via the bloodstream. The third category includes conditions that may be the consequence of acute changes in pulmonary vascular pressures, possibly the result of sudden autonomic discharge in the case of neurogenic and high-altitude pulmonary edema, or sudden swings of pleural pressure, as well as transient damage to the pulmonary capillaries in the case of reexpansion pulmonary edema.

Distinguishing cardiogenic from noncardiogenic pulmonary edema

The *history* is essential for assessing the likelihood of underlying cardiac disease as well as for identification of one of the conditions associated with noncardiogenic pulmonary edema. The *physical examination* in cardiogenic pulmonary edema is notable for evidence of

TABLE 5-3

COMMON CAUSES OF NONCARDIOGENIC PULMONARY EDEMA

Direct Injury to Lung

Chest trauma, pulmonary contusion
Aspiration
Smoke inhalation
Pneumonia
Oxygen toxicity
Pulmonary embolism, reperfusion

Hematogenous Injury to Lung

Sepsis
Pancreatitis
Nonthoracic trauma
Leukoagglutination reactions
Multiple transfusions
Intravenous drug use, e.g., heroin
Cardiopulmonary bypass

Possible Lung Injury Plus Elevated Hydrostatic Pressures

High-altitude pulmonary edema
Neurogenic pulmonary edema
Reexpansion pulmonary edema

increased intracardiac pressures (S3 gallop, elevated jugular venous pulse, peripheral edema), and rales and/or wheezes on auscultation of the chest. In contrast, the physical examination in noncardiogenic pulmonary edema is dominated by the findings of the precipitating condition; pulmonary findings may be relatively normal in the early stages. The *chest radiograph* in cardiogenic pulmonary edema typically shows an enlarged cardiac silhouette, vascular redistribution, interstitial thickening, and perihilar alveolar infiltrates; pleural effusions are common. In noncardiogenic pulmonary edema, heart size is normal, alveolar infiltrates are distributed more uniformly throughout the lungs, and pleural effusions are uncommon. Finally, the *hypoxemia* of cardiogenic pulmonary edema is due largely to $\dot{V}/\dot{Q}$ mismatch and responds to the administration of supplemental oxygen. In contrast, hypoxemia in noncardiogenic pulmonary edema is due primarily to intrapulmonary shunting and typically persists despite high concentrations of inhaled O_2.

CHAPTER 6
HYPOXIA AND CYANOSIS

Joseph Loscalzo

HYPOXIA

The fundamental purpose of the cardiorespiratory system is to deliver O_2 and nutrients to cells and to remove CO_2 and other metabolic products from them. Proper maintenance of this function depends not only on intact cardiovascular and respiratory systems but also on an adequate number of red blood cells and hemoglobin and a supply of inspired gas containing adequate O_2.

RESPONSES TO HYPOXIA

Decreased O_2 availability to cells results in an inhibition of oxidative phosphorylation and increased anaerobic glycolysis. This switch from aerobic to anaerobic metabolism, the Pasteur effect, maintains some, albeit reduced, adenosine 5'-triphosphate (ATP) production. In severe hypoxia, when ATP production is inadequate to meet the energy requirements of ionic and osmotic equilibrium, cell membrane depolarization leads to uncontrolled Ca^{2+} influx and activation of Ca^{2+}-dependent phospholipases and proteases. These events, in turn, cause cell swelling and, ultimately, cell death.

The adaptations to hypoxia are mediated, in part, by the upregulation of genes encoding a variety of proteins, including glycolytic enzymes such as phosphoglycerate kinase and phosphofructokinase, as well as the glucose transporters Glut-1 and Glut-2; and by growth factors, such as vascular endothelial growth factor (VEGF) and erythropoietin, which enhance erythrocyte production. The hypoxia-induced increase in expression of these key proteins is governed by the hypoxia-sensitive transcription factor, hypoxia-inducible factor-1 (HIF-1).

During hypoxia, systemic arterioles dilate, at least in part, by opening of K_{ATP} channels in vascular smooth-muscle cells due to the hypoxia-induced reduction in ATP concentration. By contrast, in pulmonary vascular smooth-muscle cells, inhibition of K^+ channels causes depolarization which, in turn, activates voltage-gated Ca^{2+} channels raising the cytosolic $[Ca^{2+}]$ and causing smooth-muscle cell contraction. Hypoxia-induced pulmonary arterial constriction shunts blood away from poorly ventilated portions toward better ventilated portions of the lung; however, it also increases pulmonary vascular resistance and right ventricular afterload.

Effects on the central nervous system

Changes in the central nervous system (CNS), particularly the higher centers, are especially important consequences of hypoxia. Acute hypoxia causes impaired judgment, motor incoordination, and a clinical picture resembling acute alcohol intoxication. High-altitude illness is characterized by headache secondary to cerebral vasodilation, gastrointestinal symptoms, dizziness, insomnia, fatigue, or somnolence. Pulmonary arterial and sometimes venous constriction cause capillary leakage and high-altitude pulmonary edema (HAPE) (Chap. 5), which intensifies hypoxia, further promoting vasoconstriction. Rarely, high-altitude cerebral edema (HACE) develops, which is manifest by severe headache and papilledema and can cause coma. As hypoxia becomes more severe, the regulatory centers of the brainstem are affected, and death usually results from respiratory failure.

CAUSES OF HYPOXIA
Respiratory hypoxia

When hypoxia occurs from respiratory failure, PaO_2 declines, and when respiratory failure is persistent, the hemoglobin-oxygen (Hb-O_2) dissociation curve is displaced to the right, with greater quantities of O_2 released at any level of tissue PO_2. Arterial hypoxemia, i.e., a reduction of O_2 saturation of arterial blood (SaO_2), and consequent cyanosis are likely to be more marked when such depression of PaO_2 results from pulmonary disease than when the depression occurs as the result of a decline in the fraction of oxygen in inspired air (FIO_2). In this latter situation, $PaCO_2$ falls secondary to anoxia-induced hyperventilation and the Hb-O_2 dissociation curve is displaced to the left, limiting the decline in SaO_2 at any level of PaO_2.

The most common cause of respiratory hypoxia is *ventilation-perfusion mismatch* resulting from perfusion of poorly ventilated alveoli. Respiratory hypoxemia may also be caused by *hypoventilation*, in which case it is then associated with an elevation of $PaCO_2$. These two forms of respiratory hypoxia are usually correctable by inspiring 100% O_2 for several minutes. A third cause of respiratory hypoxia is shunting of blood across the lung from the pulmonary arterial to the venous bed (*intrapulmonary right-to-left shunting*) by perfusion of nonventilated portions of the lung, as in pulmonary atelectasis or through pulmonary arteriovenous connections. The low PaO_2 in this situation is only partially corrected by an FIO_2 of 100%.

Hypoxia secondary to high altitude

As one ascends rapidly to 3000 m (~10,000 ft), the reduction of the O_2 content of inspired air (FIO_2) leads to a decrease in alveolar PO_2 to approximately 60 mmHg, and a condition termed *high-altitude illness* develops (see earlier). At higher altitudes, arterial saturation declines rapidly and symptoms become more serious; and at 5000 m, unacclimated individuals usually cease to be able to function normally owing to the changes in CNS function described earlier.

Hypoxia secondary to right-to-left extrapulmonary shunting

From a physiologic viewpoint, this cause of hypoxia resembles intrapulmonary right-to-left shunting but is caused by congenital cardiac malformations, such as tetralogy of Fallot, transposition of the great arteries, and Eisenmenger's syndrome (Chap. 19). As in pulmonary right-to-left shunting, the PaO_2 cannot be restored to normal with inspiration of 100% O_2.

Anemic hypoxia

A reduction in hemoglobin concentration of the blood is accompanied by a corresponding decline in the O_2-carrying capacity of the blood. Although the PaO_2 is normal in anemic hypoxia, the absolute quantity of O_2 transported per unit volume of blood is diminished. As the anemic blood passes through the capillaries and the usual quantity of O_2 is removed from it, the PO_2 and saturation in the venous blood decline to a greater extent than normal.

Carbon monoxide (CO) intoxication

Hemoglobin that binds with CO (carboxyhemoglobin, COHb) is unavailable for O_2 transport. In addition, the presence of COHb shifts the Hb-O_2 dissociation curve to the left so that O_2 is unloaded only at lower tensions, contributing further to tissue hypoxia.

Circulatory hypoxia

As in anemic hypoxia, the PaO_2 is usually normal, but venous and tissue PO_2 values are reduced as a consequence of reduced tissue perfusion and greater tissue O_2 extraction. This pathophysiology leads to an increased arterial-mixed venous O_2 difference (a-v-O_2 difference), or gradient. Generalized circulatory hypoxia occurs in heart failure (Chap. 17) and in most forms of shock.

Specific organ hypoxia

Localized circulatory hypoxia may occur as a result of decreased perfusion secondary to arterial obstruction, as in localized atherosclerosis in any vascular bed, or as a consequence of vasoconstriction, as observed in Raynaud's phenomenon (Chap. 39). Localized hypoxia may also result from venous obstruction and the resultant expansion of interstitial fluid causing arteriolar compression and, thereby, reduction of arterial inflow. Edema, which increases the distance through which O_2 must diffuse before it reaches cells, can also cause localized hypoxia. In an attempt to maintain adequate perfusion to more vital organs in patients with reduced cardiac output secondary to heart failure or hypovolemic shock, vasoconstriction may reduce perfusion in the limbs and skin, causing hypoxia of these regions.

Increased O_2 requirements

If the O_2 consumption of tissues is elevated without a corresponding increase in perfusion, tissue hypoxia ensues and the PO_2 in venous blood declines. Ordinarily, the clinical picture of patients with hypoxia due to an elevated metabolic rate, as in fever or thyrotoxicosis, is quite different from that in other types of hypoxia: the skin is warm and flushed owing to increased cutaneous blood flow that dissipates the excessive heat produced, and cyanosis is usually absent.

Exercise is a classic example of increased tissue O_2 requirements. These increased demands are normally met by several mechanisms operating simultaneously: (1) increase in the cardiac output and ventilation and, thus, O_2 delivery to the tissues; (2) a preferential shift in blood flow to the exercising muscles by changing vascular resistances in the circulatory beds of exercising tissues, directly and/or reflexly; (3) an increase in O_2 extraction from the delivered blood and a widening of the arteriovenous O_2 difference; and (4) a reduction in the pH of the tissues and capillary blood, shifting the $Hb-O_2$ curve to the right, and unloading more O_2 from hemoglobin. If the capacity of these mechanisms is exceeded, then hypoxia, especially of the exercising muscles, will result.

Improper oxygen utilization

Cyanide and several other similarly acting poisons cause cellular hypoxia. The tissues are unable to utilize O_2, and, as a consequence, the venous blood tends to have a high O_2 tension. This condition has been termed *histotoxic hypoxia*.

ADAPTATION TO HYPOXIA

An important component of the respiratory response to hypoxia originates in special chemosensitive cells in the carotid and aortic bodies and in the respiratory center in the brainstem. The stimulation of these cells by hypoxia increases ventilation, with a loss of CO_2, and can lead to respiratory alkalosis. When combined with the metabolic acidosis resulting from the production of lactic acid, the serum bicarbonate level declines.

With the reduction of PaO_2, cerebrovascular resistance decreases and cerebral blood flow increases in an attempt to maintain O_2 delivery to the brain. However, when the reduction of PaO_2 is accompanied by hyperventilation and a reduction of $PaCO_2$, cerebrovascular resistance rises, cerebral blood flow falls, and tissue hypoxia intensifies.

The diffuse, systemic vasodilation that occurs in generalized hypoxia increases the cardiac output. In patients with underlying heart disease, the requirements of peripheral tissues for an increase of cardiac output with hypoxia may precipitate congestive heart failure. In patients with ischemic heart disease, a reduced PaO_2 may intensify myocardial ischemia and further impair left ventricular function.

One of the important compensatory mechanisms for chronic hypoxia is an increase in the hemoglobin concentration and in the number of red blood cells in the circulating blood, i.e., the development of polycythemia secondary to erythropoietin production. In persons with chronic hypoxemia secondary to prolonged residence at a high altitude (>13,000 ft, 4200 m), a condition termed *chronic mountain sickness* develops. This disorder is characterized by a blunted respiratory drive, reduced ventilation, erythrocytosis, cyanosis, weakness, right ventricular enlargement secondary to pulmonary hypertension, and even stupor.

CYANOSIS

Cyanosis refers to a bluish color of the skin and mucous membranes resulting from an increased quantity of reduced hemoglobin (i.e., deoxygenated hemoglobin) or of hemoglobin derivatives (e.g., methemoglobin or sulfhemoglobin) in the small blood vessels of those tissues. It is usually most marked in the lips, nail beds, ears, and malar eminences. Cyanosis, especially if developed recently, is more commonly detected by a family member than the patient. The florid skin characteristic of polycythemia vera must be distinguished from the true cyanosis discussed here. A cherry-colored flush, rather than cyanosis, is caused by COHb.

The degree of cyanosis is modified by the color of the cutaneous pigment and the thickness of the skin, as well as by the state of the cutaneous capillaries. The accurate clinical detection of the presence and degree of cyanosis is difficult, as proved by oximetric studies. In some instances, central cyanosis can be detected reliably when the SaO_2 has fallen to 85%; in others, particularly in dark-skinned persons, it may not be detected until it has declined to 75%. In the latter case, examination of the mucous membranes in the oral cavity and the conjunctivae rather than examination of the skin is more helpful in the detection of cyanosis.

The increase in the quantity of reduced hemoglobin in the mucocutaneous vessels that produces cyanosis may be brought about either by an increase in the quantity of venous blood as a result of dilation of the venules and venous ends of the capillaries or by a reduction in the SaO_2 in the capillary blood. In general, cyanosis becomes apparent when the concentration of reduced hemoglobin in capillary blood exceeds 40 g/L (4 g/dL).

It is the *absolute*, rather than the *relative*, quantity of reduced hemoglobin that is important in producing cyanosis. Thus, in a patient with severe anemia, the *relative* quantity of reduced hemoglobin in the venous blood may be very large when considered in relation to the total quantity of hemoglobin in the blood. However, since the concentration of the latter is markedly reduced, the *absolute* quantity of reduced hemoglobin may still be small, and, therefore, patients with severe anemia and even *marked* arterial desaturation may not display cyanosis. Conversely, the higher the total hemoglobin content, the greater the tendency toward cyanosis; thus, patients with marked polycythemia tend to be cyanotic at higher levels of SaO_2 than patients with normal hematocrit values. Likewise, local passive congestion, which causes an increase in the total quantity of reduced hemoglobin in the vessels in a given area, may cause cyanosis. Cyanosis is also observed when nonfunctional hemoglobin, such as methemoglobin or sulfhemoglobin, is present in blood.

Cyanosis may be subdivided into central and peripheral types. In *central* cyanosis, the SaO_2 is reduced or an abnormal hemoglobin derivative is present, and the mucous membranes and skin are both affected. *Peripheral* cyanosis is due to a slowing of blood flow and abnormally great extraction of O_2 from normally saturated arterial blood; it results from vasoconstriction and diminished peripheral blood flow, such as occurs in cold exposure, shock, congestive failure, and peripheral vascular disease. Often in these conditions, the mucous membranes of the oral cavity or those beneath the tongue may be spared. Clinical differentiation between central and peripheral cyanosis may not always be simple, and in conditions such as cardiogenic shock with pulmonary edema there may be a mixture of both types.

DIFFERENTIAL DIAGNOSIS

Central cyanosis

(Table 6-1) Decreased SaO_2 results from a marked reduction in the PaO_2. This reduction may be brought about by a decline in the FIO_2 without sufficient compensatory alveolar hyperventilation to maintain alveolar PO_2. Cyanosis usually becomes manifest in an ascent to an altitude of 4000 m (13,000 ft).

Seriously *impaired pulmonary function*, through perfusion of unventilated or poorly ventilated areas of the lung or alveolar hypoventilation, is a common cause of central cyanosis. This condition may occur acutely, as in extensive pneumonia or pulmonary edema, or chronically, with chronic pulmonary diseases (e.g., emphysema). In the latter situation, secondary polycythemia is generally present and clubbing of the fingers (see later) may occur. Another cause of reduced SaO_2 is *shunting of systemic venous blood into the arterial circuit*. Certain forms of congenital heart disease are associated with cyanosis on this basis (see earlier and Chap. 19).

Pulmonary arteriovenous fistulae may be congenital or acquired, solitary or multiple, microscopic or massive. The severity of cyanosis produced by these fistulae depends on their size and number. They occur with some frequency in hereditary hemorrhagic telangiectasia. SaO_2 reduction and cyanosis may also occur in some patients with cirrhosis, presumably as a consequence of pulmonary arteriovenous fistulae or portal vein–pulmonary vein anastomoses.

In patients with cardiac or pulmonary right-to-left shunts, the presence and severity of cyanosis depend on the size of the shunt relative to the systemic flow as well as on the Hb-O_2 saturation of the venous blood. With increased extraction of O_2 from the blood by the exercising muscles, the venous blood returning to the right side of the heart is more unsaturated than at rest, and shunting of this blood intensifies the cyanosis. Secondary polycythemia occurs frequently in patients in this setting and contributes to the cyanosis.

Cyanosis can be caused by small quantities of circulating methemoglobin (Hb Fe^{3+}) and by even smaller quantities of sulfhemoglobin; both of these hemoglobin derivatives are unable to bind oxygen. Although they are uncommon causes of cyanosis, these abnormal hemoglobin species should be sought by spectroscopy when cyanosis is not readily explained by malfunction of the circulatory or respiratory systems. Generally, digital clubbing does not occur with them.

Peripheral cyanosis

Probably the most common cause of peripheral cyanosis is the normal vasoconstriction resulting from exposure to cold air or water. When cardiac output is reduced, cutaneous vasoconstriction occurs as a compensatory mechanism so that blood is diverted from the skin to more vital areas such as the CNS and heart, and cyanosis of the extremities may result even though the arterial blood is normally saturated.

Arterial obstruction to an extremity, as with an embolus, or arteriolar constriction, as in cold-induced vasospasm (Raynaud's phenomenon) (Chap. 39), generally results in pallor and coldness, and there may be associated cyanosis. Venous obstruction, as in thrombophlebitis or deep venous thrombosis, dilates the subpapillary venous plexuses and thereby intensifies cyanosis.

TABLE 6-1

CAUSES OF CYANOSIS
Central Cyanosis
Decreased arterial oxygen saturation
Decreased atmospheric pressure—high altitude
Impaired pulmonary function
Alveolar hypoventilation
Uneven relationships between pulmonary ventilation and perfusion (perfusion of hypoventilated alveoli)
Impaired oxygen diffusion
Anatomic shunts
Certain types of congenital heart disease
Pulmonary arteriovenous fistulas
Multiple small intrapulmonary shunts
Hemoglobin with low affinity for oxygen
Hemoglobin abnormalities
Methemoglobinemia—hereditary, acquired
Sulfhemoglobinemia—acquired
Carboxyhemoglobinemia (not true cyanosis)
Peripheral Cyanosis
Reduced cardiac output
Cold exposure
Redistribution of blood flow from extremities
Arterial obstruction
Venous obstruction

APPROACH TO THE PATIENT | Cyanosis

Certain features are important in arriving at the cause of cyanosis:

1. It is important to ascertain the time of onset of cyanosis. Cyanosis present since birth or infancy is usually due to congenital heart disease.

2. Central and peripheral cyanosis must be differentiated. Evidence of disorders of the respiratory or cardiovascular systems are helpful. Massage or gentle warming of a cyanotic extremity will increase peripheral blood flow and abolish peripheral, but not central, cyanosis.

3. The presence or absence of clubbing of the digits (see next section) should be ascertained. The combination of cyanosis and clubbing is frequent in patients with congenital heart disease and right-to-left shunting and is seen occasionally in patients with pulmonary disease, such as lung abscess or pulmonary arteriovenous fistulae. In contrast, peripheral cyanosis or acutely developing central cyanosis is *not* associated with clubbed digits.

4. PaO_2 and SaO_2 should be determined, and, in patients with cyanosis in whom the mechanism is obscure, spectroscopic examination of the blood performed to look for abnormal types of hemoglobin (critical in the differential diagnosis of cyanosis).

CLUBBING

The selective bulbous enlargement of the distal segments of the fingers and toes due to proliferation of connective tissue, particularly on the dorsal surface, is termed *clubbing*; there is also increased sponginess of the soft tissue at the base of the clubbed nail. Clubbing may be hereditary, idiopathic, or acquired and associated with a variety of disorders, including cyanotic congenital heart disease (see earlier), infective endocarditis, and a variety of pulmonary conditions (among them primary and metastatic lung cancer, bronchiectasis, asbestosis, sarcoidosis, lung abscess, cystic fibrosis, tuberculosis, and mesothelioma), as well as with some gastrointestinal diseases (including inflammatory bowel disease and hepatic cirrhosis). In some instances, it is occupational, e.g., in jackhammer operators.

Clubbing in patients with primary and metastatic lung cancer, mesothelioma, bronchiectasis, or hepatic cirrhosis may be associated with *hypertrophic osteoarthropathy*. In this condition, the subperiosteal formation of new bone in the distal diaphyses of the long bones of the extremities causes pain and symmetric arthritis-like changes in the shoulders, knees, ankles, wrists, and elbows. The diagnosis of hypertrophic osteoarthropathy may be confirmed by bone radiograph or MRI. Although the mechanism of clubbing is unclear, it appears to be secondary to humoral substances that cause dilation of the vessels of the distal digits as well as growth factors released from unfragmented platelet precursors in the digital circulation.

ACKNOWLEDGMENT

Dr. Eugene Braunwald authored this chapter in the previous edition of Harrison's Principles of Internal Medicine. Some of the material from the 17th edition has been carried forward.

CHAPTER 7

EDEMA

Eugene Braunwald ■ Joseph Loscalzo

Edema is defined as a clinically apparent increase in the interstitial fluid volume, which may expand by several liters before the abnormality is evident. Therefore, a weight gain of several kilograms usually precedes overt manifestations of edema, and a similar weight loss from diuresis can be induced in a slightly edematous patient before "dry weight" is achieved. *Anasarca* refers to gross, generalized edema. *Ascites* and *hydrothorax* refer to accumulation of excess fluid in the peritoneal and pleural cavities, respectively, and are considered special forms of edema.

Depending on its cause and mechanism, edema may be localized or have a generalized distribution. Edema is recognized in its generalized form by puffiness of the face, which is most readily apparent in the periorbital areas, and by the persistence of an indentation of the skin after pressure; this is known as "pitting" edema. In its more subtle form, edema may be detected by noting that after the stethoscope is removed from the chest wall, the rim of the bell leaves an indentation on the skin of the chest for a few minutes. When the ring on a finger fits more snugly than in the past or when a patient complains of difficulty putting on shoes, particularly in the evening, edema may be present.

PATHOGENESIS

About one-third of total-body water is confined to the extracellular space. Approximately 75% of the latter is interstitial fluid, and the remainder is in the plasma compartment.

Starling forces

The forces that regulate the disposition of fluid between these two components of the extracellular compartment frequently are referred to as the *Starling forces*. The hydrostatic pressure within the vascular system and the colloid oncotic pressure in the interstitial fluid tend to promote movement of fluid from the vascular to the extravascular space. By contrast, the colloid oncotic pressure contributed by plasma proteins and the hydrostatic pressure within the interstitial fluid promote the movement of fluid into the vascular compartment.

As a consequence of these forces, there is movement of water and diffusible solutes from the vascular space at the arteriolar end of the capillaries. Fluid is returned from the interstitial space into the vascular system at the venous end of the capillaries and by way of the lymphatics. Unless these channels are obstructed, lymph flow rises with increases in net movement of fluid from the vascular compartment to the interstitium. These flows are usually balanced so that there is a steady state in the sizes of the intravascular and interstitial compartments, yet a large exchange between them occurs. However, if either the hydrostatic or the oncotic pressure gradient is altered significantly, a further net movement of fluid between the two components of the extracellular space will take place. The development of edema then depends on one or more alterations in the Starling forces so that there is increased flow of fluid from the vascular system into the interstitium or into a body cavity.

Edema due to an increase in capillary pressure may result from an elevation of venous pressure caused by obstruction to venous and/or lymphatic drainage. An increase in capillary pressure may be generalized, as occurs in congestive heart failure (see later). The Starling forces also may be imbalanced when the colloid oncotic pressure of the plasma is reduced owing to any factor that may induce hypoalbuminemia, such as severe malnutrition, liver disease, loss of protein into the urine or into the gastrointestinal tract, or a severe catabolic state. Edema may be localized to one extremity when venous pressure is elevated due to unilateral thrombophlebitis (see later).

Capillary damage

Edema may also result from damage to the capillary endothelium, which increases its permeability and permits the transfer of proteins into the interstitial compartment. Injury to the capillary wall can result from drugs, viral or bacterial agents, and thermal or mechanical trauma. Increased capillary permeability also may be a consequence of a hypersensitivity reaction and is characteristic of immune injury. Damage to the capillary endothelium is presumably responsible for inflammatory edema, which is usually nonpitting, localized, and accompanied by other signs of inflammation—i.e., erythema, heat, and tenderness.

Reduction of effective arterial volume

In many forms of edema, the effective arterial blood volume, a parameter that represents the filling of the arterial tree, is reduced. Underfilling of the arterial tree may be caused by a reduction of cardiac output and/or systemic vascular resistance. As a consequence of underfilling, a series of physiologic responses designed to restore the effective arterial volume to normal are set into motion. A key element of these responses is the retention of salt and, therefore, of water, ultimately leading to edema.

Renal factors and the renin-angiotensin-aldosterone (RAA) system

In the final analysis, renal retention of Na$^+$ is central to the development of generalized edema (Fig. 7-1). The diminished renal blood flow characteristic of states in which the effective arterial blood volume is reduced is translated by the renal juxtaglomerular cells (specialized myoepithelial cells surrounding the afferent arteriole) into a signal for increased renin release. Renin is an enzyme with a molecular mass of about 40,000 Da that acts on its substrate, angiotensinogen, an α_2-globulin synthesized by the liver, to release angiotensin I, a decapeptide, which in turn is converted to angiotensin II (AII), an octapeptide. AII has generalized vasoconstrictor properties; it is especially active on the renal efferent arterioles. This action reduces the hydrostatic pressure in the peritubular capillaries, whereas the increased filtration fraction raises the colloid osmotic pressure in these vessels, thereby enhancing salt and water reabsorption in the proximal tubule as well as in the ascending limb of the loop of Henle.

The renin-angiotensin-aldosterone (RAA) system has long been recognized as a hormonal system; however, it also operates locally. Intrarenally produced AII contributes to glomerular efferent arteriolar constriction, and this "tubuloglomerular feedback" causes salt and water

retention and thereby contributes to the formation of edema.

AII that enters the systemic circulation stimulates the production of aldosterone by the zona glomerulosa of the adrenal cortex. Aldosterone in turn enhances Na$^+$ reabsorption (and K$^+$ excretion) by the collecting tubule. In patients with heart failure, not only is aldosterone secretion elevated but the biologic half-life of aldosterone is prolonged, which increases further the plasma level of the hormone. A depression of hepatic blood flow, especially during exercise, is responsible for reduced hepatic catabolism of aldosterone.

Increased quantities of aldosterone are secreted in heart failure and in other edematous states, and blockade of the action of aldosterone by spironolactone or eplerenone (aldosterone antagonists) or by amiloride (a blocker of epithelial Na$^+$ channels) often induces a moderate diuresis in edematous states. Yet persistently augmented levels of aldosterone (or other mineralocorticoids) alone do not always promote accumulation of edema, as witnessed by the lack of significant fluid retention in most instances of primary aldosteronism. Furthermore, although normal individuals retain some NaCl and water with the administration of potent mineralocorticoids, such as deoxycorticosterone acetate and fludrocortisone, this accumulation is self-limiting despite continued exposure to the steroid, a phenomenon known as *mineralocorticoid escape*. The failure of normal individuals who receive large doses of mineralocorticoids to accumulate large quantities of extracellular fluid and develop edema is probably a consequence of an increase in glomerular filtration rate (pressure natriuresis) and the action of natriuretic substance(s) (see later). The continued secretion of aldosterone may be more important in the accumulation of fluid in edematous states because patients with edema secondary to heart failure, nephrotic syndrome, and hepatic cirrhosis are generally unable to repair the deficit in effective arterial blood volume. As a consequence, they do not develop pressure natriuresis.

Arginine vasopressin (AVP)

The secretion of AVP occurs in response to increased intracellular osmolar concentration, and, by stimulating V$_2$ receptors, AVP increases the reabsorption of free water in the renal distal tubule and collecting duct, thereby increasing total-body water. Circulating AVP is elevated in many patients with heart failure secondary to a nonosmotic stimulus associated with decreased effective arterial volume. Such patients fail to show the normal reduction of AVP with a reduction of osmolality, contributing to edema formation and hyponatremia.

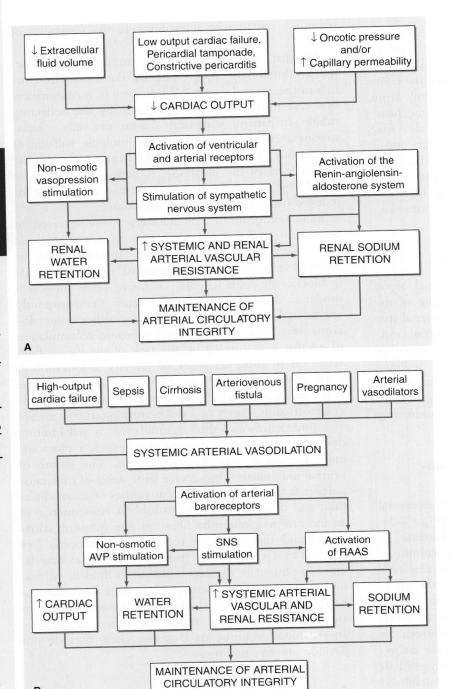

FIGURE 7-1

Clinical conditions in which a decrease in cardiac output (*A*) and systemic arterial vasodilation (*B*) cause arterial underfilling with resulting neurohumoral activation and renal sodium and water retention. In addition to activating the neurohumoral axis, adrenergic stimulation causes renal vasoconstriction and enhances sodium and fluid transport by the proximal tubule epithelium. SNS, sympathetic nervous system; RAAS, renin-angiotensin aldosterone system. (*Reprinted from RW Schrier: Ann Intern Med 113:155, 1990.*)

Endothelin

This potent peptide vasoconstrictor is released by endothelial cells. Its concentration is elevated in heart failure and contributes to renal vasoconstriction, Na^+ retention, and edema in heart failure.

Natriuretic peptides

Atrial distention and/or a Na^+ load cause release into the circulation of atrial natriuretic peptide (ANP),

a polypeptide; a high–molecular-weight precursor of ANP is stored in secretory granules within atrial myocytes. Release of ANP causes (1) excretion of sodium and water by augmenting glomerular filtration rate, inhibiting sodium reabsorption in the proximal tubule, and inhibiting release of renin and aldosterone and (2) arteriolar and venous dilation by antagonizing the vasoconstrictor actions of AII, AVP, and sympathetic stimulation. Thus, ANP has the capacity to oppose Na^+ retention and arterial pressure elevation in hypervolemic states.

The closely related brain natriuretic peptide (BNP) is stored primarily in ventricular myocardium and is released when ventricular diastolic pressure rises. Its actions are similar to those of ANP, and both BNP and ANP bind to the natriuretic receptor-A, which is found in the myocardium. Yet another natriuretic peptide, C-type (CNP), is of endothelial and renal origin. CNP binds preferentially to the natriuretic peptide receptor-B, which is expressed principally in veins. Circulating levels of ANP and BNP are elevated in congestive heart failure and in cirrhosis with ascites, but obviously not sufficiently to prevent edema formation. In addition, in edematous states there is abnormal resistance to the actions of natriuretic peptides.

CLINICAL CAUSES OF EDEMA

Obstruction of venous (and lymphatic) drainage of a limb

In this condition, the hydrostatic pressure in the capillary bed upstream (proximal) to the obstruction increases so that an abnormal quantity of fluid is transferred from the vascular to the interstitial space. Since the alternative route (i.e., the lymphatic channels) also may be obstructed or maximally filled, an increased volume of interstitial fluid in the limb develops (i.e., there is trapping of fluid in the interstitium of the extremity). The displacement of fluid into a limb may occur at the expense of the blood volume in the remainder of the body, thereby reducing effective arterial blood volume and leading to the retention of NaCl and H_2O until the deficit in plasma volume has been corrected.

Congestive heart failure

(See also Chap. 17) In this disorder the impaired systolic emptying of the ventricle(s) and/or the impairment of ventricular relaxation promotes an accumulation of blood in the venous circulation at the expense of the effective arterial volume, and the aforementioned sequence of events (Fig. 7-1) is initiated. In mild heart failure, a small increment of total blood volume may repair the deficit of arterial volume and establish a new steady state. Through the operation of Starling's law of the heart, an increase in ventricular diastolic volume promotes a more forceful contraction and may thereby maintain the cardiac output. However, if the cardiac disorder is more severe, fluid retention continues, and the increment in blood volume accumulates in the venous circulation, raising venous pressure and causing edema.

Incomplete ventricular emptying (systolic heart failure) and/or inadequate ventricular relaxation (diastolic heart failure) both lead to an elevation of ventricular diastolic pressure. If the impairment of cardiac function primarily involves the right ventricle, pressures in the systemic veins and capillaries rise, augmenting the transudation of fluid into the interstitial space and enhancing the likelihood of peripheral edema. The elevated systemic venous pressure is transmitted to the thoracic duct with consequent reduction of lymph drainage, further increasing the accumulation of edema. If the impairment of cardiac function involves the left ventricle primarily, pulmonary venous and capillary pressures rise. Pulmonary artery pressure rises, and this in turn interferes with the emptying of the right ventricle, leading to an elevation of right ventricular diastolic and central and systemic venous pressures, enhancing the likelihood of the formation of peripheral edema. The elevation of pulmonary capillary pressure may cause pulmonary edema, which impairs gas exchange. The resulting hypoxemia may impair cardiac function further, sometimes causing a vicious circle.

Nephrotic syndrome and other hypoalbuminemic states

The primary alteration in this disorder is a diminished colloid oncotic pressure due to losses of large quantities of protein into the urine. With severe hypoalbuminemia and the consequent reduced colloid osmotic pressure, the NaCl and H_2O that are retained cannot be restrained within the vascular compartment, and total and effective arterial blood volumes decline. This process initiates the edema-forming sequence of events described earlier, including activation of the RAA system. Impaired renal function contributes further to the formation of edema. A similar sequence of events occurs in other conditions that lead to *severe* hypoalbuminemia, including (1) severe nutritional deficiency states, (2) severe, chronic liver disease (see later), and (3) protein-losing enteropathy.

Cirrhosis

This condition is characterized in part by hepatic venous outflow blockade, which in turn expands the splanchnic blood volume and increases hepatic lymph formation. Intrahepatic hypertension acts as a stimulus for renal Na^+ retention and a reduction of effective arterial blood volume. These alterations frequently are complicated by hypoalbuminemia secondary to reduced hepatic synthesis, as well as systemic vasodilation. These effects reduce the effective arterial blood volume further, leading to activation of the RAA system, renal sympathetic nerves, and other NaCl- and H_2O-retaining mechanisms. The concentration of circulating aldosterone often is elevated by the failure of the liver to metabolize this hormone. Initially, the excess interstitial fluid is localized preferentially proximal (upstream) to the congested portal venous system

TABLE 7-1

DRUGS ASSOCIATED WITH EDEMA FORMATION

Nonsteroidal anti-inflammatory drugs
Antihypertensive agents
   Direct arterial/arteriolar vasodilators
      Hydralazine
      Clonidine
      Methyldopa
      Guanethidine
      Minoxidil
   Calcium channel antagonists
   α-Adrenergic antagonists
   Thiazolidinediones
Steroid hormones
   Glucocorticoids
   Anabolic steroids
   Estrogens
   Progestins
Cyclosporine
Growth hormone
Immunotherapies
   Interleukin 2
   OKT3 monoclonal antibody

Source: From GM Chertow: Approach to the patient with edema, in *Primary Cardiology*, 2nd ed, E Braunwald, L Goldman (eds). Philadelphia, Saunders 2003.

and obstructed hepatic lymphatics, i.e., in the peritoneal cavity (ascites). In later stages, particularly when there is severe hypoalbuminemia, peripheral edema may develop. The excess production of prostaglandins (PGE_2 and PGI_2) in cirrhosis attenuates renal Na^+ retention. When the synthesis of these substances is inhibited by nonsteroidal anti-inflammatory drugs (NSAIDs), renal function deteriorates and Na^+ retention increases.

Drug-induced edema

A large number of widely used drugs can cause edema (**Table 7-1**). Mechanisms include renal vasoconstriction (NSAIDs and cyclosporine), arteriolar dilation (vasodilators), augmented renal Na^+ reabsorption (steroid hormones), and capillary damage (interleukin 2).

DIFFERENTIAL DIAGNOSIS

Localized edema

(See also Chap. 39) Localized edema due to venous or lymphatic obstruction may be caused by thrombophlebitis, chronic lymphangitis, resection of regional lymph nodes, filariasis, etc. Lymphedema is particularly intractable because restriction of lymphatic flow results in increased protein concentration in the interstitial fluid, a circumstance that aggravates retention of fluid.

GENERALIZED EDEMA

The differences among the major causes of generalized edema are shown in **Table 7-2**.

A majority of patients with generalized edema develop cardiac, renal, hepatic, or nutritional disorders. Consequently, the differential diagnosis of generalized edema should be directed toward identifying or excluding these several conditions.

Edema of heart failure

(See also Chap. 17) The presence of heart disease, as manifested by cardiac enlargement and a gallop rhythm, together with evidence of cardiac failure, such as dyspnea, basilar rales, venous distention, and hepatomegaly, usually indicates that edema results from heart failure. Noninvasive tests such as echocardiography may be helpful in establishing the diagnosis of heart disease. The edema of heart failure typically occurs in the dependent portions of the body.

Edema of acute glomerulonephritis and other forms of renal failure

The edema that occurs during the acute phases of glomerulonephritis is characteristically associated with hematuria, proteinuria, and hypertension. Although some evidence supports the view that the fluid retention is due to increased capillary permeability, in most instances, the edema results from primary retention of NaCl and H_2O by the kidneys owing to renal insufficiency. This state differs from congestive heart failure in that it is characterized by a normal (or sometimes even increased) cardiac output and a normal arterial–mixed venous oxygen difference. Patients with edema due to renal failure commonly have evidence of arterial hypertension as well as pulmonary congestion on chest roentgenogram even without cardiac enlargement, but they may not develop orthopnea. Patients with *chronic* renal failure may also develop edema due to primary renal retention of NaCl and H_2O.

Edema of the nephrotic syndrome

Marked proteinuria (>3.5 g/d), hypoalbuminemia (<35 g/L), and, in some instances, hypercholesterolemia are present. This syndrome may occur during the course of a variety of kidney diseases, which include glomerulonephritis, diabetic glomerulosclerosis, and hypersensitivity reactions. A history of previous renal disease may or may not be elicited.

Edema of cirrhosis

Ascites and biochemical and clinical evidence of hepatic disease (collateral venous channels, jaundice, and spider

TABLE 7-2

59

CHAPTER 7 Edema

PRINCIPAL CAUSES OF GENERALIZED EDEMA: HISTORY, PHYSICAL EXAMINATION, AND LABORATORY FINDINGS

ORGAN SYSTEM	HISTORY	PHYSICAL EXAMINATION	LABORATORY FINDINGS
Cardiac	Dyspnea with exertion prominent—often associated with orthopnea—or paroxysmal nocturnal dyspnea	Elevated jugular venous pressure, ventricular (S_3) gallop; occasionally with displaced or dyskinetic apical pulse; peripheral cyanosis, cool extremities, small pulse pressure when severe	Elevated urea nitrogen-to-creatinine ratio common; elevated uric acid; serum sodium often diminished; liver enzymes occasionally elevated with hepatic congestion
Hepatic	Dyspnea uncommon, except if associated with significant degree of ascites; most often a history of ethanol abuse	Frequently associated with ascites; jugular venous pressure normal or low; blood pressure lower than in renal or cardiac disease; one or more additional signs of chronic liver disease (jaundice, palmar erythema, Dupuytren's contracture, spider angiomata, male gynecomastia; asterixis and other signs of encephalopathy) may be present	If severe, reductions in serum albumin, cholesterol, other hepatic proteins (transferrin, fibrinogen); liver enzymes elevated, depending on the cause and acuity of liver injury; tendency toward hypokalemia, respiratory alkalosis; macrocytosis from folate deficiency
Renal (CRF)	Usually chronic: may be associated with uremic signs and symptoms, including decreased appetite, altered (metallic or fishy) taste, altered sleep pattern, difficulty concentrating, restless legs or myoclonus; dyspnea can be present, but generally less prominent than in heart failure	Elevated blood pressure; hypertensive retinopathy; nitrogenous fetor; pericardial friction rub in advanced cases with uremia	Albuminuria, hypoalbuminemia; sometimes, elevation of serum creatinine and urea nitrogen; hyperkalemia, metabolic acidosis, hyperphosphatemia, hypocalcemia, anemia (usually normocytic)
Renal (NS)	Childhood diabetes mellitus; plasma cell dyscrasias	Periorbital edema; hypertension	Proteinuria (3.5 g/d); hypoalbuminemia; hypercholesterolemia; microscopic hematuria

Abbreviations: CRF, chronic renal failure; NS, nephrotic syndrome.
Source: Modified from GM Chertow: Approach to the patient with edema, in *Primary Cardiology*, 2nd ed, E Braunwald, L Goldman (eds). Philadelphia, Saunders 2003.

angiomata) characterize edema of hepatic origin. The ascites is frequently refractory to treatment because it collects as a result of a combination of obstruction of hepatic lymphatic drainage, portal hypertension, and hypoalbuminemia. A sizable accumulation of ascitic fluid may increase intraabdominal pressure and impede venous return from the lower extremities; hence, it tends to promote accumulation of edema in this region as well.

Edema of nutritional origin

A diet grossly deficient in protein over a prolonged period may produce hypoproteinemia and edema. The latter may be intensified by the development of beriberi heart disease, which also is of nutritional origin, in which multiple peripheral arteriovenous fistulas result in reduced effective systemic perfusion and effective arterial blood volume, thereby enhancing edema formation. Edema may actually become intensified when famished subjects are first provided with an adequate diet. The ingestion of more food may increase the quantity of NaCl ingested, which is then retained along with H_2O. So-called refeeding edema also may be linked to increased release of insulin, which directly increases tubular Na^+ reabsorption. In addition to hypoalbuminemia, hypokalemia and caloric deficits may be involved in the edema of starvation.

Other causes of edema

These causes include hypothyroidism (myxedema) and hyperthyroidism (pretibial myxedema secondary to Graves' disease), the edema in which is typically non-pitting and due to deposition of hyaluronic acid and, in Graves' disease, lymphocytic infiltration and inflammation; exogenous hyperadrenocortism; pregnancy; and administration of estrogens and vasodilators, particularly dihydropyridines such as nifedipine.

DISTRIBUTION OF EDEMA

The distribution of edema is an important guide to its cause. Thus, edema limited to one leg or to one or both arms is usually the result of venous and/or lymphatic obstruction. Edema resulting from hypoproteinemia characteristically is generalized, but it is especially evident in the very soft tissues of the eyelids and face and tends to be most pronounced in the morning because of the recumbent posture assumed during the night. Less common causes of facial edema include trichinosis, allergic reactions, and myxedema. Edema associated with heart failure, by contrast, tends to be more extensive in the legs and to be accentuated in the evening, a feature also determined largely by posture. When patients with heart failure have been confined to bed, edema may be most prominent in the presacral region. Paralysis reduces lymphatic and venous drainage on the affected side and may be responsible for unilateral edema.

ADDITIONAL FACTORS IN DIAGNOSIS

The color, thickness, and sensitivity of the skin are significant. Local tenderness and warmth suggest inflammation. Local cyanosis may signify venous obstruction. In individuals who have had repeated episodes of prolonged edema, the skin over the involved areas may be thickened, indurated, and often red.

Estimation of the venous pressure is of importance in evaluating edema. Ordinarily, a significant generalized increase in venous pressure can be recognized by the level at which cervical veins collapse (Chap. 9). In patients with obstruction of the superior vena cava, edema is confined to the face, neck, and upper extremities, in which the venous pressure is elevated compared with that in the lower extremities. Severe heart failure may cause ascites that may be distinguished from the ascites caused by hepatic cirrhosis by the jugular venous pressure, which is usually elevated in heart failure and normal in cirrhosis.

Determination of the concentration of serum albumin aids importantly in identifying those patients in whom edema is due, at least in part, to diminished intravascular colloid oncotic pressure. The presence of proteinuria also affords useful clues. The absence of proteinuria excludes nephrotic syndrome but cannot exclude nonproteinuric causes of renal failure. Slight to moderate proteinuria is the rule in patients with heart failure.

APPROACH TO THE
PATIENT   Edema

An important first question is whether the edema is localized or generalized. If it is localized, the local phenomena that may be responsible should be considered. If the edema is generalized, one should first determine if there is serious hypoalbuminemia, e.g., serum albumin <25 g/L. If so, the history, physical examination, urinalysis, and other laboratory data will help evaluate the question of cirrhosis, severe malnutrition, or the nephrotic syndrome as the underlying disorder. If hypoalbuminemia is not present, one should determine if there is evidence of congestive heart failure severe enough to promote generalized edema. Finally, one should determine whether the patient has an adequate urine output or if there is significant oliguria or anuria.

CHAPTER 8
PALPITATIONS

Joseph Loscalzo

Palpitations are extremely common among patients who present to their internist and can best be defined as an intermittent "thumping," "pounding," or "fluttering" sensation in the chest. This sensation can be either intermittent or sustained and either regular or irregular. Most patients interpret palpitations as an unusual awareness of the heartbeat, and become especially concerned when they sense that they have had "skipped" or "missing" heartbeats. Palpitations are often noted when the patient is quietly resting, during which time other stimuli are minimal. Palpitations that are positional generally reflect a structural process within (e.g., atrial myxoma) or adjacent to (e.g., mediastinal mass) the heart.

Palpitations are brought about by cardiac (43%), psychiatric (31%), miscellaneous (10%), and unknown (16%) causes, according to one large series. Among the cardiovascular causes are premature atrial and ventricular contractions, supraventricular and ventricular arrhythmias, mitral valve prolapse (with or without associated arrhythmias), aortic insufficiency, atrial myxoma, and pulmonary embolism. Intermittent palpitations are commonly caused by premature atrial or ventricular contractions: the postextrasystolic beat is sensed by the patient owing to the increase in ventricular end–diastolic dimension following the pause in the cardiac cycle and the increased strength of contraction (postextrasystolic potentiation) of that beat. Regular, sustained palpitations can be caused by regular supraventricular and ventricular tachycardias. Irregular, sustained palpitations can be caused by atrial fibrillation. It is important to note that most arrhythmias are not associated with palpitations. In those that are, it is often useful either to ask the patient to "tap out" the rhythm of the palpitations or to take his/her pulse while experiencing palpitations. In general, hyperdynamic cardiovascular states caused by catecholaminergic stimulation from exercise, stress, or pheochromocytoma can lead to palpitations. Palpitations are common among athletes, especially older endurance athletes. In addition, the enlarged ventricle of aortic regurgitation and accompanying hyperdynamic precordium frequently lead to the sensation of palpitations. Other factors that enhance the strength of myocardial contraction, including tobacco, caffeine, aminophylline, atropine, thyroxine, cocaine, and amphetamines, can cause palpitations.

Psychiatric causes of palpitations include panic attacks or disorders, anxiety states, and somatization, alone or in combination. Patients with psychiatric causes for palpitations more commonly report a longer duration of the sensation (>15 min) and other accompanying symptoms than do patients with other causes. Among the miscellaneous causes of palpitations included are thyrotoxicosis, drugs (see earlier) and ethanol, spontaneous skeletal muscle contractions of the chest wall, pheochromocytoma, and systemic mastocytosis.

APPROACH TO THE PATIENT | **Palpitations**

The principal goal in assessing patients with palpitations is to determine if the symptom is caused by a life-threatening arrhythmia. Patients with preexisting coronary artery disease (CAD) or risk factors for CAD are at greatest risk for ventricular arrhythmias as a cause for palpitations. In addition, the association of palpitations with other symptoms suggesting hemodynamic compromise, including syncope or lightheadedness, supports this diagnosis. Palpitations caused by sustained tachyarrhythmias in patients with CAD can be accompanied by angina pectoris or dyspnea, and in patients with ventricular dysfunction (systolic or diastolic), aortic stenosis, hypertrophic cardiomyopathy, or mitral stenosis, with or without CAD, can be accompanied by dyspnea from increased left atrial and pulmonary venous pressure.

Key features of the physical examination that will help confirm or refute the presence of an arrhythmia as a cause for the palpitations and its adverse hemodynamic consequences include measurement of the vital signs, assessment of the jugular venous pressure and pulse, and auscultation of the chest and precordium. A resting electrocardiogram can be used to document the arrhythmia. If exertion is known to induce the arrhythmia and accompanying palpitations, exercise electrocardiography can be used to make the diagnosis. If the arrhythmia is sufficiently infrequent, other methods must be used, including continuous electrocardiographic (Holter) monitoring; telephonic monitoring, through which the patient can transmit an electrocardiographic tracing during a sensed episode; loop recordings (external or implantable), which can capture the electrocardiographic event for later review; and mobile cardiac outpatient telemetry. Recent data suggest that Holter monitoring is of limited clinical utility, while the implantable loop recorder and mobile cardiac outpatient telemetry are safe and possibly more cost-effective in the assessment of patients with recurrent, unexplained palpitations.

Most patients with palpitations do not have serious arrhythmias or underlying structural heart disease. Occasional benign atrial or ventricular premature contractions can often be managed with beta-blocker therapy if sufficiently troubling to the patient. Palpitations incited by alcohol, tobacco, or illicit drugs need to be managed by abstention, while those caused by pharmacologic agents should be addressed by considering alternate therapies when appropriate or possible. Psychiatric causes of palpitations may benefit from cognitive or pharmacotherapies. The physician should note that palpitations are at the very least bothersome and, on occasion, frightening to the patient. Once serious causes for the symptom have been excluded, the patient should be reassured that the palpitations will not adversely affect prognosis.

CHAPTER 9

PHYSICAL EXAMINATION OF THE CARDIOVASCULAR SYSTEM

Patrick T. O'Gara ■ Joseph Loscalzo

The approach to a patient with known or suspected cardiovascular disease begins with the time-honored traditions of a directed history and a targeted physical examination. The scope of these activities depends on the clinical context at the time of presentation, ranging from an elective ambulatory follow-up visit to a more focused emergency department encounter. There has been a gradual decline in physical examination skills over the last two decades at every level, from student to faculty specialist, a development of great concern to both clinicians and medical educators. Classic cardiac findings are recognized by only a minority of internal medicine and family practice residents. Despite popular perceptions, clinical performance does not improve predictably as a function of experience; instead, the acquisition of new examination skills may become more difficult for a busy individual practitioner. Less time is now devoted to mentored cardiovascular examinations during the training of students and residents. One widely recognized outcome of these trends is the progressive overutilization of noninvasive imaging studies to establish the presence and severity of cardiovascular disease even when the examination findings imply a low pretest probability of significant pathology. Educational techniques to improve bedside skills include repetition, patient-centered teaching conferences, and visual display feedback of auscultatory events with Doppler echocardiographic imaging.

The evidence base that links the findings from the history and physical examination to the presence, severity, and prognosis of cardiovascular disease has been established most rigorously for coronary artery disease, heart failure, and valvular heart disease. For example, observations regarding heart rate, blood pressure, signs of pulmonary congestion, and the presence of mitral regurgitation (MR) contribute importantly to bedside

risk assessment in patients with acute coronary syndromes. Observations from the physical examination in this setting can inform clinical decision making before the results of cardiac biomarkers testing are known. The prognosis of patients with systolic heart failure can be predicted on the basis of the jugular venous pressure (JVP) and the presence or absence of a third heart sound (S_3). Accurate characterization of cardiac murmurs provides important insight into the natural history of many valvular and congenital heart lesions. Finally, the important role played by the physical examination in enhancing the clinician-patient relationship cannot be overestimated.

THE GENERAL PHYSICAL EXAMINATION

Any examination begins with an assessment of the general appearance of the patient, with notation of age, posture, demeanor, and overall health status. Is the patient in pain or resting quietly, dyspneic or diaphoretic? Does the patient choose to avoid certain body positions to reduce or eliminate pain, as might be the case with suspected acute pericarditis? Are there clues indicating that dyspnea may have a pulmonary cause, such as a barrel chest deformity with an increased anterior-posterior diameter, tachypnea, and pursed-lip breathing? Skin pallor, cyanosis, and jaundice can be appreciated readily and provide additional clues. A chronically ill-appearing emaciated patient may suggest the presence of long-standing heart failure or another systemic disorder, such as a malignancy. Various genetic syndromes, often with cardiovascular involvement, can also be recognized easily, such as trisomy 21, Marfan syndrome, and Holt-Oram syndrome. Height and weight should be measured routinely, and both body mass index and body surface area should be calculated. Knowledge of the waist circumference and the waist-to-hip ratio can be used to predict long-term cardiovascular risk. Mental status, level of alertness, and mood should be assessed continuously during the interview and examination.

Skin

Central cyanosis occurs with significant right-to-left shunting at the level of the heart or lungs, allowing deoxygenated blood to reach the systemic circulation. Peripheral cyanosis or acrocyanosis, in contrast, is usually related to reduced extremity blood flow due to small vessel constriction, as seen in patients with severe heart failure, shock, or peripheral vascular disease; it can be aggravated by the use of β-adrenergic blockers with unopposed α-mediated constriction. Differential cyanosis refers to isolated cyanosis affecting the lower but not the upper extremities in a patient with a large patent ductus arteriosus (PDA) and secondary pulmonary hypertension with right-to-left shunting at the great vessel level. Hereditary telangiectasias on the lips, tongue, and mucous membranes, as part of the Osler-Weber-Rendu syndrome (hereditary hemorrhagic telangiectasia), resemble spider nevi and can be a source of right-to-left shunting when also present in the lung. Malar telangiectasias also are seen in patients with advanced mitral stenosis and scleroderma. An unusually tan or bronze discoloration of the skin may suggest hemochromatosis as the cause of the associated systolic heart failure. Jaundice, which may be visible first in the sclerae, has a broad differential diagnosis but in the appropriate setting can be consistent with advanced right heart failure and congestive hepatomegaly or late-term "cardiac cirrhosis." Cutaneous ecchymoses are seen frequently among patients taking vitamin K antagonists or antiplatelet agents such as aspirin and thienopyridines. Various lipid disorders sometimes are associated with subcutaneous xanthomas, particularly along the tendon sheaths or over the extensor surfaces of the extremities. Severe hypertriglyceridemia can be associated with eruptive xanthomatosis and lipemia retinalis. Palmar crease xanthomas are specific for type III hyperlipoproteinemia. Pseudoxanthoma elasticum, a disease associated with premature atherosclerosis, is manifested by a leathery, cobblestoned appearance of the skin in the axilla and neck creases and by angioid streaks on funduscopic examination. Extensive lentiginoses have been described in a variety of development delay–cardiovascular syndromes, including Carney syndrome, which includes multiple atrial myxomas. Cutaneous manifestations of sarcoidosis such as lupus pernio and erythema nodosum may suggest this disease as a cause of an associated dilated cardiomyopathy, especially with heart block, intraventricular conduction delay, or ventricular tachycardia.

Head and neck

Dentition and oral hygiene should be assessed in every patient both as a source of potential infection and as an index of general health. A high-arched palate is a feature of Marfan syndrome and other connective tissue disease syndromes. Bifid uvula has been described in patients with Loeys-Dietz syndrome, and orange tonsils are characteristic of Tangier disease. The ocular manifestations of hyperthyroidism have been well described. Many patients with congenital heart disease have associated hypertelorism, low-set ears, or micrognathia. Blue sclerae are a feature of osteogenesis imperfecta. An arcus senilis pattern lacks specificity as an index of coronary heart disease risk. The funduscopic examination is an often underutilized method by which to assess the microvasculature, especially among patients with established atherosclerosis, hypertension, or diabetes mellitus. A mydriatic agent may be necessary for optimal visualization. A funduscopic examination should be performed routinely in the assessment of patients with suspected endocarditis and those with a history of acute visual change. Branch retinal artery occlusion or visualization of a Hollenhorst plaque can narrow the differential diagnosis rapidly in the appropriate setting. Relapsing polychondritis may manifest as an inflamed pinna or, in its later stages, as a saddle-nose deformity because of destruction of nasal cartilage; Wegener's granulomatosis can also lead to a saddle-nose deformity.

Chest

Midline sternotomy, left posterolateral thoracotomy, or infraclavicular scars at the site of pacemaker/defibrillator generator implantation should not be overlooked and may provide the first clue regarding an underlying cardiovascular disorder in patients unable to provide a relevant history. A prominent venous collateral pattern may suggest subclavian or vena caval obstruction. If the head and neck appear dusky and slightly cyanotic and the venous pressure is grossly elevated without visible pulsations, a diagnosis of superior vena cava syndrome should be entertained. Thoracic cage abnormalities have been well described among patients with connective tissue disease syndromes. They include pectus carinatum ("pigeon chest") and pectus excavatum ("funnel chest"). Obstructive lung disease is suggested by a barrel chest deformity, especially with tachypnea, pursed-lip breathing, and use of accessory muscles. The characteristically severe kyphosis and compensatory lumbar, pelvic, and knee flexion of ankylosing spondylitis should prompt careful auscultation for a murmur of aortic regurgitation (AR). Straight back syndrome refers to the loss of the normal kyphosis of the thoracic spine and has been described in patients with mitral valve prolapse (MVP) and its variants. In some patients with cyanotic congenital heart disease, the chest wall appears to be asymmetric, with anterior displacement of the left hemithorax. The respiratory rate and pattern should be noted during spontaneous breathing, with additional attention to depth, audible wheezing, and stridor. Lung examination can reveal adventitious sounds indicative of pulmonary edema, pneumonia, or pleuritis.

Abdomen

In some patients with advanced obstructive lung disease, the point of maximal cardiac impulse may be in the epigastrium. The liver is frequently enlarged and tender in patients with chronic heart failure. Systolic pulsations over the liver signify severe tricuspid regurgitation (TR). Splenomegaly may be a feature of infective endocarditis, particularly when symptoms have persisted for weeks or months. Ascites is a nonspecific finding but may be present with advanced chronic right heart failure, constrictive pericarditis, hepatic cirrhosis, or an intraperitoneal malignancy. The finding of an elevated JVP implies a cardiovascular etiology. In nonobese patients, the aorta typically is palpated between the epigastrium and the umbilicus. The sensitivity of palpation for the detection of an abdominal aortic aneurysm (pulsatile and expansile mass) decreases as a function of body size. Because palpation alone is not sufficiently accurate to establish this diagnosis, a screening ultrasound examination is advised. The presence of an arterial bruit over the abdomen suggests high-grade atherosclerotic disease, though precise localization is difficult.

Extremities

The temperature and color of the extremities, the presence of clubbing, arachnodactyly, and pertinent nail findings can be surmised quickly during the examination. Clubbing implies the presence of central right-to-left shunting, although it has also been described in patients with endocarditis. Its appearance can range from cyanosis and softening of the root of the nail bed, to the classic loss of the normal angle between the base of the nail and the skin, to the skeletal and periosteal bony changes of hypertrophic osteoarthropathy, which is seen rarely in patients with advanced lung or liver disease. Patients with the Holt-Oram syndrome have an unopposable, "fingerized" thumb, whereas patients with Marfan syndrome may have arachnodactyly and a positive "wrist" (overlapping of the thumb and fifth finger around the wrist) or "thumb" (protrusion of the thumb beyond the ulnar aspect of the hand when the fingers are clenched over the thumb in a fist) sign. The Janeway lesions of endocarditis are nontender, slightly raised hemorrhages on the palms and soles, whereas Osler's nodes are tender, raised nodules on the pads of

the fingers or toes. Splinter hemorrhages are classically identified as linear petechiae in the midposition of the nail bed and should be distinguished from the more common traumatic petechiae, which are seen closer to the distal edge.

Lower extremity or presacral edema in the setting of an elevated JVP defines volume overload and may be a feature of chronic heart failure or constrictive pericarditis. Lower extremity edema in the absence of jugular venous hypertension may be due to lymphatic or venous obstruction or, more commonly, to venous insufficiency, as further suggested by the appearance of varicosities, venous ulcers (typically medial in location), and brownish cutaneous discoloration from hemosiderin deposition (eburnation). Pitting edema can also be seen in patients who use dihydropyridine calcium channel blockers. A Homan's sign (posterior calf pain on active dorsiflexion of the foot against resistance) is neither specific nor sensitive for deep venous thrombosis. Muscular atrophy or the absence of hair along an extremity is consistent with severe arterial insufficiency or a primary neuromuscular disorder.

CARDIOVASCULAR EXAMINATION

Jugular venous pressure and waveform

Jugular venous pressure is the single most important bedside measurement from which to estimate the volume status. The internal jugular vein is preferred because the external jugular vein is valved and not directly in line with the superior vena cava and right atrium. Nevertheless, the external jugular vein has been used to discriminate between high and low central venous pressure (CVP) when tested among medical students, residents, and attending physicians. Precise estimation of the central venous or right atrial pressure from bedside assessment of the jugular venous waveform has proved difficult. Venous pressure traditionally has been measured as the vertical distance between the top of the jugular venous pulsation and the sternal inflection point (angle of Louis). A distance >4.5 cm at 30° elevation is considered abnormal. However, the actual distance between the mid-right atrium and the angle of Louis varies considerably as a function of both body size and the patient angle at which the assessment is made (30°, 45°, or 60°). The use of the sternal angle as a reference point leads to systematic underestimation of CVP, and this method should be used less for semiquantification than to distinguish a normal from an abnormally elevated CVP. The use of the clavicle may provide an easier reference for standardization. Venous pulsations above this level in the sitting position are clearly abnormal, as the distance between the clavicle and the right atrium is at least 10 cm. The patient should always be placed in the sitting position, with the legs dangling below the bedside, when an elevated pressure is suspected in the semisupine position. It should also be noted that bedside estimates of CVP are made in centimeters of water but must be converted to millimeters of mercury to provide correlation with accepted hemodynamic norms (1.36 cmH$_2$O = 1.0 mmHg).

The venous waveform sometimes can be difficult to distinguish from the carotid pulse, especially during casual inspection. Nevertheless, the venous waveform has several characteristic features, and its individual components can be appreciated in most patients (Fig. 9-1). In patients in sinus rhythm, the venous waveform is typically biphasic, whereas the carotid upstroke is monophasic.

The venous waveform is divided into several distinct peaks. The *a* wave reflects right atrial presystolic contraction and occurs just after the electrocardiographic P wave, preceding the first heart sound (S$_1$). A prominent *a* wave is seen in patients with reduced right ventricular compliance; a cannon *a* wave occurs with atrioventricular (AV) dissociation and right atrial contraction against a closed tricuspid valve. In a patient with a wide complex tachycardia, the appreciation of cannon *a* waves in the jugular venous waveform identifies the rhythm as ventricular in origin. The *a* wave is not present with atrial fibrillation. The *x* descent defines the fall in right atrial pressure after inscription of the *a* wave. The *c* wave interrupts this *x* descent and is followed by a further descent. The *v* wave represents atrial filling (atrial diastole) and occurs during ventricular systole. The height of the *v* wave is determined by right atrial compliance as well as the volume of blood returning to the right atrium either antegrade from the cavae or retrograde through an incompetent tricuspid valve. In patients with TR, the *v* wave is accentuated and the subsequent fall in pressure (*y* descent) is rapid. With progressive degrees of TR, the *v* wave merges with the *c* wave, and the right atrial and jugular vein waveforms become "ventricularized." The *y* descent, which follows the peak of the *v* wave, can become prolonged or blunted with obstruction to right ventricular inflow, as may occur with tricuspid stenosis (TS) or pericardial tamponade. Normally, the venous pressure should fall by at least 3 mmHg with inspiration. Kussmaul's sign is defined by either a rise or a lack of fall of the JVP with inspiration and is classically associated with constrictive pericarditis, although it has been reported in patients with restrictive cardiomyopathy, massive pulmonary embolism, right ventricular infarction, and advanced left ventricular systolic heart failure.

Venous hypertension sometimes can be elicited by performance of the abdominojugular reflex or with passive leg elevation. When these signs are positive, a volume-overloaded state with limited compliance of an overly distended or constricted venous system is present. The abdominojugular reflex is elicited with firm

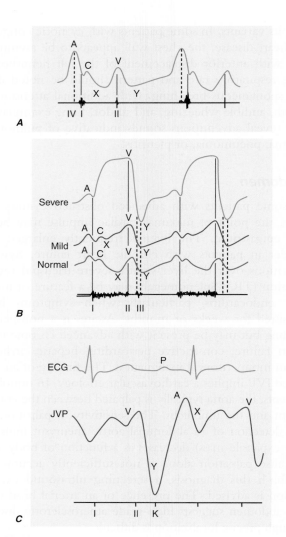

FIGURE 9-1

A. **Jugular venous pulse wave tracing** (*top*) with heart sounds (*bottom*). The A wave represents right atrial presystolic contraction and occurs just after the electrocardiographic P wave and just before the first heart sound (I). In this example, the A wave is accentuated and larger than normal due to decreased right ventricular compliance, as also suggested by the right-sided S$_4$ (IV). The C wave may reflect the carotid pulsation in the neck and/or an early systolic increase in right atrial pressure as the right ventricle pushes the closed tricuspid valve into the right atrium. The x descent follows the A wave just as atrial pressure continues to fall. The V wave represents atrial filling during ventricular systole and peaks at the second heart sound (II). The y descent corresponds to the fall in right atrial pressure after tricuspid valve opening. *B.* Jugular venous waveforms in mild (*middle*) and severe (*top*) tricuspid regurgitation, compared with normal, with phonocardiographic representation of the corresponding heart sounds below. With increasing degrees of tricuspid regurgitation, the waveform becomes "ventricularized." *C.* ECG (*top*), jugular venous waveform (*middle*), and heart sounds (*bottom*) in pericardial constriction. Note the prominent and rapid y descent, corresponding in timing to the pericardial knock (K). (*From J Abrams: Synopsis of Cardiac Physical Diagnosis, 2nd ed. Boston, Butterworth Heinemann, 2001, pp 25–35.*)

and consistent pressure over the upper portion of the abdomen, preferably over the right upper quadrant, for at least 10 s. A positive response is defined by a sustained rise of more than 3 cm in JVP for at least 15 s after release of the hand. Patients must be coached to refrain from breath holding or a Valsalva-like maneuver during the procedure. The abdominojugular reflex is useful in predicting a pulmonary artery wedge pressure in excess of 15 mmHg in patients with heart failure.

Although the JVP estimates right ventricular filling pressure, it has a predictable relationship with the pulmonary artery wedge pressure. In a large study of patients with advanced heart failure, the presence of a right atrial pressure >10 mmHg (as predicted on bedside examination) had a positive value of 88% for the prediction of a pulmonary artery wedge pressure of >22 mmHg. In addition, an elevated JVP has prognostic significance in patients with both symptomatic heart failure and asymptomatic left ventricular systolic dysfunction. The presence of an elevated JVP is associated with a higher risk of subsequent hospitalization for heart failure, death from heart failure, or both.

Assessment of blood pressure

Measurement of blood pressure usually is delegated to a medical assistant but should be repeated by the clinician. Accurate measurement depends on body position, arm size, time of measurement, place of measurement, device, device size, technique, and examiner. In general, physician-recorded blood pressures are higher than nurse-recorded pressures. Blood pressure is best measured in the seated position with the arm at the level of the heart, using an appropriately sized cuff, after 5–10 min of relaxation. When it is measured in the supine position, the arm should be raised to bring it to the level of the mid-right atrium. The length and width of the blood pressure cuff bladder should be 80% and 40% of the arm's circumference, respectively. A common source of error in practice is to use an inappropriately small cuff, resulting in marked overestimation of true blood pressure, or an inappropriately large cuff, resulting in underestimation of true blood pressure. The cuff should be inflated to 30 mmHg above the expected systolic pressure and the pressure released at a rate of 2–3 mmHg/s. Systolic and diastolic pressures are defined by the first and fifth Korotkoff sounds, respectively. Very low (even 0 mmHg) diastolic blood pressures may be recorded in patients with chronic, severe AR or a large arteriovenous fistula because of enhanced diastolic "runoff." In these instances, both the phase IV and phase V Korotkoff sounds should be recorded. Blood pressure is best assessed at the brachial artery level, though it can be measured at the radial, popliteal, or pedal pulse level. In general, systolic pressure increases and diastolic pressure decreases when measured in more distal arteries.

Blood pressure should be measured in both arms, and the difference should be less than 10 mmHg. A blood pressure differential that exceeds this threshold may be associated with atherosclerotic or inflammatory subclavian artery disease, supravalvular aortic stenosis, aortic coarctation, or aortic dissection. Systolic leg pressures are usually as much as 20 mmHg higher than systolic arm pressures. Greater leg–arm pressure differences are seen in patients with chronic severe AR as well as patients with extensive and calcified lower extremity peripheral arterial disease. The ankle-brachial index (lower pressure in the dorsalis pedis or posterior tibial artery divided by the higher of the two brachial artery pressures) is a powerful predictor of long-term cardiovascular mortality.

The blood pressure measured in an office or hospital setting may not accurately reflect the pressure in other venues. "White coat hypertension" is defined by at least three separate clinic-based measurements >140/90 mmHg and at least two non-clinic-based measurements <140/90 mmHg in the absence of any evidence of target organ damage. Individuals with white coat hypertension may not benefit from drug therapy, although they may be more likely to develop sustained hypertension over time. Masked hypertension should be suspected when normal or even low blood pressures are recorded in patients with advanced atherosclerotic disease, especially when evidence of target organ damage is present or bruits are audible.

Orthostatic hypotension is defined by a fall in systolic pressure >20 mmHg or in diastolic pressure >10 mmHg in response to assumption of the upright posture from a supine position within 3 min. There may also be a lack of a compensatory tachycardia, an abnormal response that suggests autonomic insufficiency, as may be seen in patients with diabetes or Parkinson's disease. Orthostatic hypotension is a common cause of postural lightheadedness/syncope and should be assessed routinely in patients for whom this diagnosis might pertain. It can be exacerbated by advanced age, dehydration, certain medications, food, deconditioning, and ambient temperature.

Arterial pulse

The carotid artery pulse occurs just after the ascending aortic pulse. The aortic pulse is best appreciated in the epigastrium, just above the level of the umbilicus. Peripheral arterial pulses that should be assessed routinely include the subclavian, brachial, radial, ulnar, femoral, popliteal, dorsalis pedis, and posterior tibial. In patients in whom the diagnosis of either temporal arteritis or polymyalgia rheumatica is suspected, the temporal arteries also should be examined. Although one of the two pedal pulses may not be palpable in up to 10% of normal subjects, the pair should be symmetric. The integrity of the arcuate system of the hand is assessed by Allen's test, which is performed routinely before instrumentation of the radial artery. The pulses should be examined for their symmetry, volume, timing, contour, amplitude, and duration. If necessary, simultaneous auscultation of the heart can help identify a delay in the arrival of an arterial pulse. Simultaneous palpation of the radial and femoral pulses may reveal a femoral delay in a patient with hypertension and suspected aortic coarctation. The carotid upstrokes should never be examined simultaneously or before listening for a bruit. Light pressure should always be used to avoid precipitation of carotid hypersensitivity syndrome and syncope in a susceptible elderly individual. The arterial pulse usually becomes more rapid and spiking as a function of its distance from the heart, a phenomenon that reflects the muscular status of the more peripheral arteries and the summation of the incident and reflected waves. In general, the character and contour of the arterial pulse depend on the stroke volume, ejection velocity, vascular compliance, and systemic vascular resistance. The pulse examination can be misleading in patients with reduced cardiac output and in those with stiffened arteries from aging, chronic hypertension, or peripheral arterial disease.

The character of the pulse is best appreciated at the carotid level (**Fig. 9-2**). A weak and delayed pulse (*pulsus parvus et tardus*) defines severe aortic stenosis (AS). Some patients with AS may also have a slow, notched, or interrupted upstroke (anacrotic pulse) with a thrill or shudder. With chronic severe AR, by contrast, the carotid upstroke has a sharp rise and rapid fall-off (Corrigan's or water-hammer pulse). Some patients with advanced AR may have a bifid or bisferiens pulse, in which two systolic peaks can be appreciated. A bifid pulse is also described in patients with hypertrophic obstructive cardiomyopathy (HOCM), with inscription of percussion and tidal waves. A bifid pulse is easily appreciated in patients on intraaortic balloon counterpulsation (IABP), in whom the second pulse is diastolic in timing.

Pulsus paradoxus refers to a fall in systolic pressure >10 mmHg with inspiration that is seen in patients with pericardial tamponade but also is described in those with massive pulmonary embolism, hemorrhagic shock, severe obstructive lung disease, and tension pneumothorax. Pulsus paradoxus is measured by noting the difference between the systolic pressure at which the Korotkoff sounds are first heard (during expiration) and the systolic pressure at which the Korotkoff sounds are heard with each heartbeat, independent of the respiratory phase. Between these two pressures, the Korotkoff sounds are heard only intermittently and during expiration. The cuff pressure must be decreased slowly to appreciate the finding. It can be difficult to measure pulsus paradoxus in patients with tachycardia, atrial

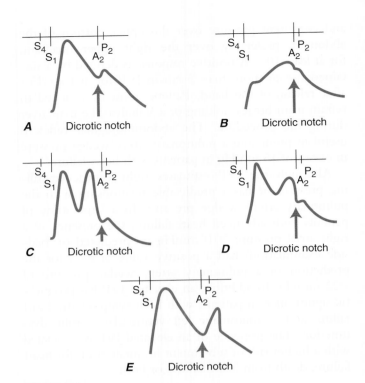

FIGURE 9-2

Schematic diagrams of the configurational changes in carotid pulse and their differential diagnoses. Heart sounds are also illustrated. **A**. Normal. S_4, fourth heart sound; S_1, first heart sound; A_2 aortic component of second heart sound; P_2 pulmonic component of second heart sound. **B**. Aortic stenosis. Anacrotic pulse with slow upstroke to a reduced peak. **C**. Bisferiens pulse with two peaks in systole. This pulse is rarely appreciated in patients with severe aortic regurgitation. **D**. Bisferiens pulse in hypertrophic obstructive cardiomyopathy. There is a rapid upstroke to the first peak (percussion wave) and a slower rise to the second peak (tidal wave). **E**. Dicrotic pulse with peaks in systole and diastole. This waveform may be seen in patients with sepsis or during intraaortic balloon counterpulsation with inflation just after the dicrotic notch. (*From K Chatterjee, W Parmley [eds]: Cardiology: An Illustrated Text/Reference. Philadelphia, JB Lippincott, 1991.*)

fibrillation, or tachypnea. A pulsus paradoxus may be palpable at the brachial artery or femoral artery level when the pressure difference exceeds 15 mmHg. This inspiratory fall in systolic pressure is an exaggerated consequence of interventricular dependence.

Pulsus alternans, in contrast, is defined by beat-to-beat variability of pulse amplitude. It is present only when every other phase I Korotkoff sound is audible as the cuff pressure is lowered slowly, typically in a patient with a regular heart rhythm and independent of the respiratory cycle. Pulsus alternans is seen in patients with severe left ventricular systolic heart failure and is thought to be due to cyclic changes in intracellular calcium and action potential duration. Interestingly, when pulsus alternans is associated with electrocardiographic T-wave alternans, the risk for an arrhythmic event appears to be increased.

Ascending aortic aneurysms can rarely be appreciated as a pulsatile mass in the right parasternal. Appreciation of a prominent abdominal aortic pulse should prompt noninvasive imaging for better characterization. Femoral and/or popliteal artery aneurysms should be sought in patients with abdominal aortic aneurysm disease.

The level of a claudication-producing arterial obstruction can often be identified on physical examination (Fig. 9-3). For example, in a patient with calf claudication, a decrease in pulse amplitude between the common femoral and popliteal arteries will localize the obstruction to the level of the superficial femoral artery, although inflow obstruction above the level of the common femoral artery may coexist. Auscultation for carotid, subclavian, abdominal aortic, and femoral artery bruits should be routine. However, the correlation between the presence of a bruit and the degree of vascular obstruction is poor. A cervical bruit is a weak indicator of the degree of carotid artery stenosis; the absence of a bruit does not exclude the presence of significant luminal obstruction. If a bruit extends into diastole or if a thrill is present, the obstruction is generally severe. Other causes of arterial bruits include an arteriovenous fistula with enhanced flow.

The likelihood of significant lower extremity peripheral arterial disease increases with typical symptoms of claudication, cool skin, abnormalities on pulse examination, or the presence of a vascular bruit. Abnormal pulse oximetry (a >2% difference between finger and toe oxygen saturation) can be used to detect lower extremity peripheral arterial disease and is comparable in its performance characteristics to the ankle-brachial index.

Inspection and palpation of the heart

The left ventricular apex beat may be visible in the midclavicular line at the fifth intercostal space in thin-chested adults. Visible pulsations anywhere other than this expected location are abnormal. The left anterior

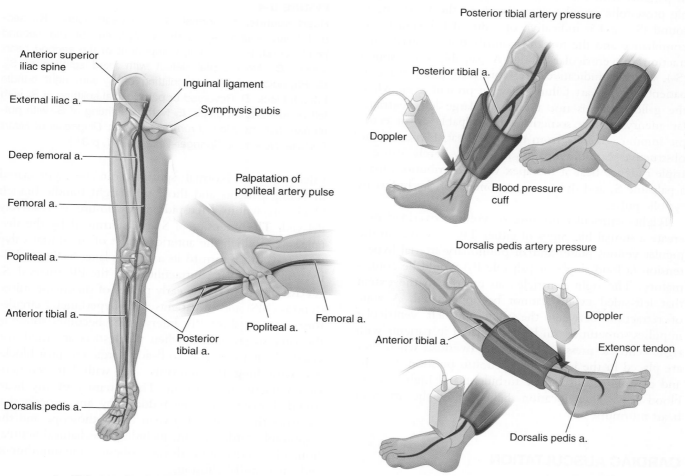

A   Major arteries of the lower limb

B   Measurement of ankle systolic pressure

FIGURE 9-3

A. Anatomy of the major arteries of the leg. *B*. Measurement of the ankle systolic pressure. (*From NA Khan et al: JAMA 295: 536–546, 2006.*)

chest wall may heave in patients with an enlarged or hyperdynamic left or right ventricle. As noted previously, a visible right upper parasternal pulsation may be suggestive of ascending aortic aneurysm disease. In thin, tall patients and patients with advanced obstructive lung disease and flattened diaphragms, the cardiac impulse may be visible in the epigastrium and should be distinguished from a pulsatile liver edge.

Palpation of the heart begins with the patient in the supine position at 30° and can be enhanced by placing the patient in the left lateral decubitus position. The normal left ventricular impulse is less than 2 cm in diameter and moves quickly away from the fingers; it is better appreciated at end expiration, with the heart closer to the anterior chest wall. Characteristics such as size, amplitude, and rate of force development should be noted.

Enlargement of the left ventricular cavity is manifested by a leftward and downward displacement of an enlarged apex beat. A sustained apex beat is a sign of pressure overload, such as that which may be present in patients with AS or chronic hypertension. A palpable presystolic impulse corresponds to the fourth heart sound (S_4) and is indicative of reduced left ventricular compliance and the forceful contribution of atrial contraction to ventricular filling. A palpable third sound (S_3), which is indicative of a rapid early filling wave in patients with heart failure, may be present even when the gallop itself is not audible. A large left ventricular aneurysm may sometimes be palpable as an ectopic impulse, discrete from the apex beat. Hypertrophic obstructive cardiomyopathy may very rarely cause a triple cadence beat at the apex with contributions from a palpable S_4 and the two components of the bisferiens systolic pulse.

Right ventricular pressure or volume overload may create a sternal lift. Signs of either TR (*cv* waves in the jugular venous pulse) and/or pulmonary arterial hypertension (a loud single or palpable P_2) would be confirmatory. The right ventricle can enlarge to the extent that left-sided events cannot be appreciated. A zone of retraction between the right and left ventricular impulses sometimes can be appreciated in patients with right ventricle pressure or volume overload when they are placed in the left lateral decubitus position. Systolic and diastolic thrills signify turbulent and high-velocity blood flow. Their locations help identify the origin of heart murmurs.

CARDIAC AUSCULTATION

Heart sounds

Ventricular systole is defined by the interval between the first (S_1) and second (S_2) heart sounds (Fig. 9-4). The first heart sound (S_1) includes mitral and tricuspid

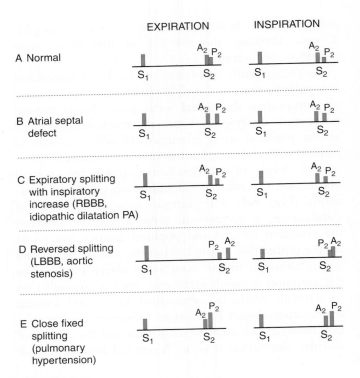

FIGURE 9-4

Heart sounds. *A*. Normal. S_1, first heart sound; S_2, second heart sound; A_2, aortic component of the second heart sound; P_2, pulmonic component of the second heart sound. ***B*.** Atrial septal defect with fixed splitting of S_2. ***C*.** Physiologic but wide splitting of S_2 with right bundle branch block. ***D*.** Reversed or paradoxical splitting of S_2 with left bundle branch block. ***E*.** Narrow splitting of S_2 with pulmonary hypertension. (*From NO Fowler: Diagnosis of Heart Disease. New York, Springer-Verlag, 1991, p 31.*)

valve closure. Normal splitting can be appreciated in young patients and those with right bundle branch block, in whom tricuspid valve closure is relatively delayed. The intensity of S_1 is determined by the distance over which the anterior leaflet of the mitral valve must travel to return to its annular plane, leaflet mobility, left ventricular contractility, and the PR interval. S_1 is classically loud in the early phases of rheumatic mitral stenosis (MS) and in patients with hyperkinetic circulatory states or short PR intervals. S_1 becomes softer in the later stages of MS when the leaflets are rigid and calcified, after exposure to β-adrenergic receptor blockers, with long PR intervals, and with left ventricular contractile dysfunction. The intensity of any heart sound, however, can be reduced by any process that increases the distance between the stethoscope and the responsible cardiac event, including mechanical ventilation, obstructive lung disease, obesity, pneumothorax, and a pericardial effusion.

Aortic and pulmonic valve closure constitutes the second heart sound (S_2). With normal or physiologic splitting, the A_2–P_2 interval increases with inspiration and narrows during expiration. This physiologic interval will widen with right bundle branch block because of the further delay in pulmonic valve closure and in patients with severe MR because of the premature closure of the aortic valve. An unusually narrowly split or even a singular S_2 is a feature of pulmonary arterial hypertension. Fixed splitting of S_2, in which the A_2–P_2 interval is wide and does not change during the respiratory cycle, occurs in patients with a secundum atrial septal defect. Reversed or paradoxical splitting refers to a pathologic delay in aortic valve closure, such as that which occurs in patients with left bundle branch block, right ventricular apical pacing, severe AS, HOCM, and acute myocardial ischemia. With reversed or paradoxical splitting, the individual components of S_2 are audible at end expiration, and their interval narrows with inspiration, the opposite of what would be expected under normal physiologic conditions. P_2 is considered loud when its intensity exceeds that of A_2 at the base, when it can be palpated in the area of the proximal pulmonary artery (second left interspace), or when both components of S_2 can be appreciated at the lower left sternal border or apex. The intensity of A_2 and P_2 decreases with aortic and pulmonic stenosis, respectively. In these conditions, a single S_2 may result.

Systolic sounds

An ejection sound is a high-pitched early systolic sound that corresponds in timing to the upstroke of the carotid pulse. It usually is associated with congenital bicuspid aortic or pulmonic valve disease; however, ejection sounds are also sometimes audible in patients with isolated aortic or pulmonary root dilation and normal semilunar valves. The ejection sound that accompanies bicuspid aortic valve disease becomes softer and then inaudible as the valve calcifies and becomes more rigid. The ejection sound that accompanies pulmonic stenosis (PS) moves closer to the first heart sound as the severity of the stenosis increases. In addition, the pulmonic ejection sound is the only right-sided acoustic event that decreases in intensity with inspiration. Ejection sounds are often heard more easily at the lower left sternal border than they are at the base. Nonejection sounds (clicks), which occur after the onset of the carotid upstroke, are related to mitral valve prolapse and may be single or multiple. The nonejection click may introduce a murmur. This click-murmur complex will move away from the first heart sound with maneuvers that increase ventricular preload, such as squatting. On standing, the click and murmur move closer to S_1.

Diastolic sounds

The high-pitched opening snap (OS) of MS occurs after a very short interval after the second heart sound. The A_2–OS interval is inversely proportional to the height of the left atrial–left ventricular diastolic pressure gradient. The intensity of both S_1 and the OS of MS decreases with progressive calcification and rigidity of the anterior mitral leaflets. The pericardial knock (PK) is also high pitched and occurs slightly later than the opening snap, corresponding in timing to the abrupt cessation of ventricular expansion after tricuspid valve opening and to an exaggerated y descent seen in the jugular venous waveform in patients with constrictive pericarditis. A tumor plop is a lower-pitched sound that rarely can be heard in patients with atrial myxoma. It may be appreciated only in certain positions and arises from the diastolic prolapse of the tumor across the mitral valve.

The third heart sound (S_3) occurs during the rapid filling phase of ventricular diastole. It can be a normal finding in children, adolescents, and young adults; however, in older patients it signifies heart failure. A left-sided S_3 is a low-pitched sound best heard over the left ventricular (LV) apex. A right-sided S_3 is usually better heard over the lower left sternal border and becomes louder with inspiration. A left-sided S_3 in patients with chronic heart failure is predictive of cardiovascular morbidity and mortality. Interestingly, an S_3 is equally prevalent among heart failure patients with and without LV systolic dysfunction.

The fourth heart sound (S_4) occurs during the atrial filling phase of ventricular diastole and indicates left ventricular presystolic expansion. An S_4 is more common among patients who derive significant benefit from the atrial contribution to ventricular filling, such as those with chronic left ventricular hypertrophy or active myocardial ischemia. An S_4 is not present with atrial fibrillation.

Cardiac murmurs

Heart murmurs result from audible vibrations that are caused by increased turbulence and are defined by their timing within the cardiac cycle. Not all murmurs are indicative of structural heart disease, and the accurate identification of a benign or functional systolic murmur often can obviate the need for additional testing in healthy subjects. The duration, frequency, configuration, and intensity of a heart murmur are dictated by the magnitude, variability, and duration of the responsible pressure difference between two cardiac chambers, the two ventricles, or the ventricles and their respective great arteries. The intensity of a heart murmur is graded on a scale of 1 to 6; a thrill is present with murmurs of grade 4 or greater intensity. Other attributes of the murmur that aid in its accurate identification include its location, radiation, and response to bedside maneuvers. Although clinicians can detect and correctly identify heart murmurs with only fair reliability, a careful and complete bedside examination usually can identify individuals with valvular heart disease for whom transthoracic echocardiography and clinical follow-up are indicated and exclude subjects for whom no further evaluation is necessary.

Systolic murmurs can be early, mid-, late, or holosystolic in timing (Fig. 9–5). Acute severe MR results in a decrescendo early systolic murmur, the characteristics of which are related to the progressive attenuation of the left ventricular to left atrial pressure gradient during systole because of the steep and rapid rise in left atrial pressure in this clinical context. Severe MR associated with posterior leaflet prolapse or flail radiates anteriorly and to the base, where it can be confused with the murmur of aortic stenosis. MR that is due to anterior leaflet involvement radiates posteriorly and to the axilla. With acute TR in patients with normal pulmonary arterty (PA) pressures, an early systolic murmur that may increase in intensity with inspiration may be heard at the left lower sternal border, with regurgitant *cv* waves visible in the jugular venous pulse.

A midsystolic murmur begins after S_1 and ends before S_2; it is typically crescendo-decrescendo in configuration. Aortic stenosis is the most common cause of a midsystolic murmur in an adult. It is often difficult to estimate the severity of the valve lesion on the basis of the physical examination findings, especially in older hypertensive patients with stiffened carotid arteries or patients with low cardiac output in whom the intensity of the systolic heart murmur is misleadingly soft. Examination findings consistent with severe AS would include parvus et tardus carotid upstrokes, a late-peaking grade 3 or greater midsystolic murmur, a soft A_2, a sustained LV apical impulse, and an S_4. It is sometimes difficult to distinguish aortic sclerosis from more advanced degrees of valve stenosis. The former is defined by focal thickening and calcification of the aortic valve leaflets that is not severe enough to result in obstruction. These valve changes are associated with a Doppler jet velocity across the aortic valve of 2.5 m/s or less. Patients with aortic sclerosis can have grade 2 or 3 midsystolic murmurs identical in their acoustic characteristics to the murmurs heard in patients with more advanced degrees of AS. Other causes of a midsystolic heart murmur include pulmonic valve stenosis (with or without an ejection sound), HOCM, increased pulmonary blood flow in patients with a large atrial septal defect and left-to-right shunting, and several states associated with accelerated blood flow in the absence of structural heart disease, such as fever, thyrotoxicosis, pregnancy, anemia, and normal adolescence.

The murmur of hypertrophic obstructive cardiomyopathy has features of both obstruction to left ventricular outflow and MR, as would be expected from knowledge of the pathophysiology of this condition. The systolic murmur of HOCM usually can be distinguished from other causes on the basis of its response to bedside maneuvers, including Valsalva, passive leg raising, and standing/squatting. In general, maneuvers that decrease left ventricular preload (or increase left ventricular contractility) will cause the murmur to intensify, whereas maneuvers that increase left ventricular preload or afterload will cause a decrease in the intensity of the murmur. Accordingly, the systolic murmur of HOCM becomes louder during the strain phase of the Valsalva maneuver and after standing quickly from a squatting position. The murmur becomes softer with passive leg raising and when squatting. The murmur of AS is typically loudest in the second right interspace with radiation into the carotids, whereas the murmur of HOCM is best heard between the lower left sternal border and the apex. The murmur of PS is best heard in the second left interspace. The midsystolic murmur associated with enhanced pulmonic blood flow in the setting of a large atrial septal defect (ASD) is usually loudest at the mid-left sternal border.

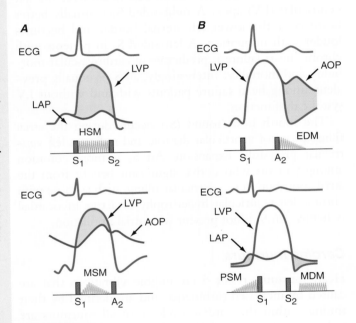

FIGURE 9-5

A. Top. Graphic representation of the systolic pressure difference (green shaded area) between left ventricle and left atrium with phonocardiographic recording of a holosystolic murmur (HSM) indicative of mitral regurgitation. ECG, electrocardiogram; LVP, left ventricular pressure; LAP, left atrial pressure; S_1, first heart sound; S_2 second heart sound. *Bottom.* Graphic representation of the systolic pressure gradient (green shaded area) between left ventricle and aorta in patient with aortic stenosis. A mid-systolic murmur (MSM) with a crescendo-decrescendo configuration is recorded. AOP, aortic pressure. *B. Top.* Graphic representation of the diastolic pressure difference between the aorta and left ventricle (blue shaded area) in a patient with aortic regurgitation, resulting in a decrescendo, early diastolic murmur (EDM) beginning with A_2. *Bottom.* Graphic representation of the diastolic left atrial–left ventricular gradient (blue areas) in a patient with mitral stenosis with a mid-diastolic murmur (MDM) and late presystolic murmurs (PSM).

A late systolic murmur, heard best at the apex, indicates MVP. As previously noted, the murmur may or may not be introduced by a nonejection click. Differential radiation of the murmur, as previously described, may help identify the specific leaflet involved by the myxomatous process. The click-murmur complex behaves in a manner directionally similar to that demonstrated by the murmur of HOCM during the Valsalva and stand/squat maneuvers (Fig. 9-6). The murmur of MVP can be identified by the accompanying nonejection click.

Holosystolic murmurs are plateau in configuration and reflect a continuous and wide pressure gradient between the left ventricle and left atrium with chronic MR, the left ventricle and right ventricle with a ventricular septal defect (VSD), and the right ventricle and right atrium with TR. In contrast to acute MR, in chronic MR the left atrium is enlarged and its compliance is normal or increased to the extent that there is little if any further increase in left atrial pressure from any increase in regurgitant volume. The murmur of MR is best heard over the cardiac apex. The intensity of the murmur increases with maneuvers that increase left ventricular afterload, such as sustained hand grip. The murmur of a VSD (without significant pulmonary hypertension) is holosystolic and loudest at the mid-left sternal border, where a thrill is usually present.

The murmur of TR is loudest at the lower left sternal border, increases in intensity with inspiration (Carvallo's sign), and is accompanied by visible *cv* waves in the jugular venous waveform and, on occasion, by pulsatile hepatomegaly.

Diastolic murmurs

In contrast to some systolic murmurs, diastolic heart murmurs always signify structural heart disease (Fig. 9-5). The murmur associated with acute, severe AR is relatively soft and of short duration because of the rapid rise in left ventricular diastolic pressure and the progressive diminution of the aortic–left ventricular diastolic pressure gradient. In contrast, the murmur of chronic severe AR is classically heard as a decrescendo, blowing diastolic murmur along the left sternal border in patients with primary valve pathology and sometimes along the right sternal border in patients with primary aortic root pathology. With chronic AR, the pulse pressure is wide and the arterial pulses are bounding in character. These signs of significant diastolic run-off are absent in the acute phase. The murmur of pulmonic regurgitation (PR) is also heard along the left sternal border. It is most commonly due to pulmonary hypertension and enlargement of the annulus of the pulmonic valve. S$_2$ is single and loud and may be palpable. There is a right

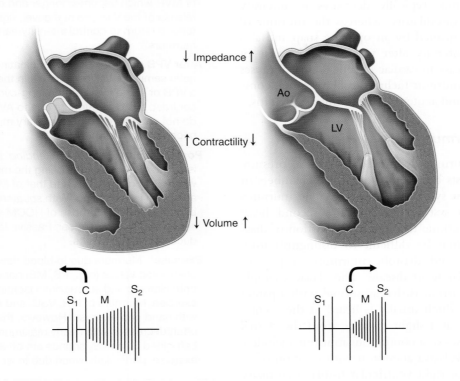

FIGURE 9-6

Behavior of the click (C) and murmur (M) of mitral valve prolapse with changes in loading (volume, impedance) and contractility. S$_1$, first heart sound; S$_2$, second heart sound. With standing (left side of figure), volume and impedance decrease, as a result of which the click and murmur move closer to S$_1$. With squatting (right), the click and murmur move away from S$_1$ owing to the increases in left ventricular volume and impedance (afterload). (*Adapted from RA O'Rourke, MH Crawford: Curr Prob Cardiol 1:9, 1976.*)

ventricular/parasternal lift that is indicative of chronic right ventricular pressure overload. A less impressive murmur of PR is present after repair of tetralogy of Fallot or pulmonic valve atresia. In this postoperative setting, the murmur is softer and lower pitched and the severity of the accompanying pulmonic regurgitation can be underestimated significantly.

Mitral stenosis is the classic cause of a mid- to late diastolic murmur, which is best heard over the apex in the left lateral decubitus position and is low-pitched or rumbling and is introduced by an OS in the early stages of the rheumatic disease process. Presystolic accentuation refers to an increase in the intensity of the murmur just before the first heart sound and occurs in patients with sinus rhythm. It is absent in patients with atrial fibrillation. The auscultatory findings in patients with rheumatic tricuspid stenosis typically are obscured by left-sided events, though they are similar in nature to those described in patients with MS. "Functional" mitral or tricuspid stenosis refers to the generation of mid-diastolic murmurs that are created by increased and accelerated transvalvular diastolic flow, even in the absence of valvular obstruction, in the setting of severe MR, severe TR, or a large ASD with left-to-right shunting. The Austin Flint murmur of chronic severe AR is a low-pitched mid- to late apical diastolic murmur that sometimes can be confused with MS. The Austin Flint murmur typically decreases in intensity after exposure to vasodilators, whereas the murmur of MS may be accompanied by an opening snap and also may increase in intensity after vasodilators because of the associated increase in cardiac output. Unusual causes of a mid-diastolic murmur include atrial myxoma, complete heart block, and acute rheumatic mitral valvulitis.

Continuous murmur

A continuous murmur is predicated on a pressure gradient that persists between two cardiac chambers or blood vessels across systole and diastole. The murmurs typically begin in systole, envelop the second heart sound (S_2), and continue through some portion of diastole. They can often be difficult to distinguish from individual systolic and diastolic murmurs in patients with mixed valvular heart disease. The classic example of a continuous murmur is that associated with a patent ductus arteriosus, which usually is heard in the second or third interspace at a slight distance from the sternal border. Other causes of a continuous murmur include a ruptured sinus of Valsalva aneurysm with creation of an aortic–right atrial or right ventricular fistula, a coronary or great vessel arteriovenous fistula, and an arteriovenous fistula constructed to provide dialysis access. There are two types of benign continuous murmurs. The cervical venous hum is heard in children or adolescents in the supraclavicular fossa. It can be obliterated with firm pressure applied to the diaphragm of the stethoscope, especially when the subject turns his or her head toward the examiner. The mammary souffle of pregnancy relates to enhanced arterial blood flow through engorged breasts. The diastolic component of the murmur can be obliterated with firm pressure over the stethoscope.

Dynamic auscultation

Diagnostic accuracy can be enhanced by the performance of simple bedside maneuvers to identify heart murmurs and characterize their significance (Table 9-1). Except for the pulmonic ejection sound, right-sided events increase in intensity with inspiration and decrease with expiration; left-sided events behave oppositely (100% sensitivity, 88% specificity). As previously noted, the intensity

TABLE 9-1

EFFECTS OF PHYSIOLOGIC AND PHARMACOLOGIC INTERVENTIONS ON THE INTENSITY OF HEART MURMURS AND SOUNDS

Respiration Right-sided murmurs and sounds generally increase with inspiration, except for the PES. Left-sided murmurs and sounds are usually louder during expiration.

Valsalva maneuver Most murmurs decrease in length and intensity. Two exceptions are the systolic murmur of HOCM, which usually becomes much louder, and that of MVP, which becomes longer and often louder. After release of the Valsalva maneuver, right-sided murmurs tend to return to control intensity earlier than do left-sided murmurs.

After VPB or AF Murmurs originating at normal or stenotic semilunar valves increase in the cardiac cycle after a VPB or in the cycle after a long-cycle length in AF. By contrast, systolic murmurs due to AV valve regurgitation do not change, diminish (papillary muscle dysfunction), or become shorter (MVP).

Positional changes With *standing*, most murmurs diminish, with two exceptions being the murmur of HOCM, which becomes louder, and that of MVP, which lengthens and often is intensified. With *squatting*, most murmurs become louder, but those of HOCM and MVP usually soften and may disappear. Passive leg raising usually produces the same results.

Exercise Murmurs due to blood flow across normal or obstructed valves (e.g., PS, MS) become louder with both isotonic and submaximal isometric (hand grip) exercise. Murmurs of MR, VSD, and AR also increase with hand grip exercise. However, the murmur of HOCM often decreases with nearly maximum hand grip exercise. Left-sided S_4 and S_3 sounds are often accentuated by exercise, particularly when due to ischemic heart disease.

Abbreviations: AF, atrial fibrillation; AR, aortic regurgitation; HOCM, hypertrophic obstructive cardiomyopathy; MR, mitral regurgitation; MS, mitral stenosis; MVP, mitral valve prolapse; PES, pulmonic ejection sound; PR, pulmonic regurgitation; PS, pulmonic stenosis; TR, tricuspid regurgitation; TS, tricuspid stenosis; VPB, ventricular premature beat; VSD, ventricular septal defect.

of the murmurs associated with MR, VSD, and AR will increase in response to maneuvers that increase LV afterload, such as hand grip and vasopressors. The intensity of these murmurs will decrease after exposure to vasodilating agents. Squatting is associated with an abrupt increase in LV preload and afterload, whereas rapid standing results in a sudden decrease in preload. In patients with MVP, the click and murmur move away from the first heart sound with squatting because of the delay in onset of leaflet prolapse at higher ventricular volumes. With rapid standing, however, the click and murmur move closer to the first heart sound as prolapse occurs earlier in systole at a smaller chamber dimension. The murmur of HOCM behaves similarly, becoming softer and shorter with squatting (95% sensitivity, 85% specificity) and longer and louder on rapid standing (95% sensitivity, 84% specificity). A change in the intensity of a systolic murmur in the first beat after a premature beat or in the beat after a long cycle length in patients with atrial fibrillation suggests valvular AS rather than MR, particularly in an older patient in whom the murmur of the AS may be well transmitted to the apex (Gallavardin effect). Of note, however, the systolic murmur of HOCM also increases in intensity in the beat after a premature beat. This increase in intensity of any LV outflow murmur in the beat after a premature beat relates to the combined effects of enhanced LV filling (from the longer diastolic period) and postextrasystolic potentiation of LV contractile function. In either instance, forward flow will accelerate, causing an increase in the gradient across the LV outflow tract (dynamic or fixed) and a louder systolic murmur. In contrast, the intensity of the murmur of MR does not change in a postpremature beat, as there is relatively little change in the nearly constant LV to left atrial pressure gradient or further alteration in mitral valve flow. Bedside exercise can sometimes be performed to increase cardiac output and, secondarily, the intensity of both systolic and diastolic heart murmurs. Most left-sided heart murmurs decrease in intensity and duration during the strain phase of the Valsalva maneuver. The murmurs associated with MVP and HOCM are the two notable exceptions. The Valsalva maneuver also can be used to assess the integrity of the heart and vasculature in the setting of advanced heart failure.

Prosthetic heart valves

The first clue that prosthetic valve dysfunction may contribute to recurrent symptoms is frequently a change in the quality of the heart sounds or the appearance of a new murmur. The heart sounds with a bioprosthetic valve resemble those generated by native valves. A mitral bioprosthesis usually is associated with a grade 2 or 3 mid-systolic murmur along the left sternal border (created by turbulence across the valve struts as they project into the LV outflow tract) as well as by a soft mid-diastolic murmur that occurs with normal LV filling. This diastolic murmur often can be heard only in the left lateral decubitus position and after exercise. A high-pitched or holosystolic apical murmur is indicative of paravalvular leak or bioprosthetic regurgitation, for which additional imaging is indicated. Clinical deterioration can occur rapidly after the first expression of bioprosthetic failure. A tissue valve in the aortic position is always associated with a grade 2 to 3 mid-systolic murmur at the base or just below the suprasternal notch. A diastolic murmur of AR is abnormal in any circumstances. Mechanical valve dysfunction may first be suggested by a decrease in the intensity of either the opening or the closing sound. A high-pitched apical systolic murmur in patients with a mechanical mitral prosthesis and a diastolic decrescendo murmur in patients with a mechanical aortic prosthesis indicate paravalvular regurgitation. Patients with prosthetic valve thrombosis may present clinically with signs of shock, muffled heart sounds, and soft murmurs.

Pericardial disease

A pericardial friction rub is nearly 100% specific for the diagnosis of acute pericarditis, though the sensitivity of this finding is not nearly as high, as the rub may come and go over the course of an acute illness or be very difficult to elicit. The rub is heard as a leathery or scratchy three-component or two-component sound, though it may be monophasic. Classically, the three components are ventricular systole, rapid early diastolic filling, and late presystolic filling after atrial contraction in patients in sinus rhythm. It is necessary to listen to the heart in several positions. Additional clues may be present from the history and 12-lead electrocardiogram. The rub typically disappears as the volume of any pericardial effusion increases. Pericardial tamponade can be diagnosed with a sensitivity of 98%, a specificity of 83%, and a positive likelihood ratio of 5.9 (95% confidence intervals 2.4 to 14) by a pulsus paradoxus that exceeds 12 mmHg in a patient with a large pericardial effusion.

The findings on physical examination are integrated with the symptoms previously elicited with a careful history to construct an appropriate differential diagnosis and proceed with indicated imaging and laboratory assessment. The physical examination is an irreplaceable component of the diagnostic algorithm and in selected patients can inform prognosis. Educational efforts to improve clinician competence eventually may result in cost saving, particularly if the indications for imaging can be influenced by the examination findings.

CHAPTER 10

APPROACH TO THE PATIENT WITH A HEART MURMUR

Patrick T. O'Gara ■ Joseph Loscalzo

INTRODUCTION

The differential diagnosis of a heart murmur begins with a careful assessment of its major attributes and responses to bedside maneuvers. The history, clinical context, and associated physical examination findings provide additional clues by which the significance of a heart murmur is established. Accurate bedside identification of a heart murmur can inform decisions regarding the indications for noninvasive testing and the need for referral to a cardiovascular specialist. Preliminary discussions can be held with the patient regarding antibiotic or rheumatic fever prophylaxis, the need to restrict various forms of physical activity, and the potential role for family screening.

Heart murmurs are caused by audible vibrations that are due to increased turbulence from accelerated blood flow through normal or abnormal orifices, flow through a narrowed or irregular orifice into a dilated vessel or chamber, or backward flow through an incompetent valve, ventricular septal defect, or patent ductus arteriosus. They traditionally are defined in terms of their timing within the cardiac cycle (**Fig. 10-1**). *Systolic murmurs* begin with or after the first heart sound (S_1) and terminate at or before the component (A_2 or P_2) of the second heart sound (S_2) that corresponds to their site of origin (left or right, respectively). *Diastolic murmurs* begin with or after the associated component of S_2 and end at or before the subsequent S_1. *Continuous murmurs* are not confined to either phase of the cardiac cycle but instead begin in early systole and proceed through S_2 into all or part of diastole. The accurate timing of heart murmurs is the first step in their identification. The distinction between S_1 and S_2 and, therefore, systole and diastole is usually a straightforward process but can be difficult in the setting of a tachyarrhythmia, in which case the heart sounds can be distinguished by simultaneous palpation of the carotid upstroke, which should closely follow S_1.

Duration

The duration of a heart murmur depends on the length of time over which a pressure difference exists between two cardiac chambers, the left ventricle and the aorta, the right ventricle and the pulmonary artery, or the great vessels. The magnitude and variability of this pressure difference, coupled with the geometry and compliance of the involved chambers or vessels, dictate the velocity of flow; the degree of turbulence; and the resulting frequency, configuration, and intensity of the murmur. The diastolic murmur of chronic aortic regurgitation (AR) is a blowing, high-frequency event, whereas the murmur of mitral stenosis (MS), indicative of the left atrial–left ventricular diastolic pressure gradient, is a low-frequency event, heard as a rumbling sound with the bell of the stethoscope. The frequency components of a heart murmur may vary at different sites of auscultation. The coarse systolic murmur of aortic stenosis (AS) may sound higher pitched and more acoustically pure at the apex, a phenomenon eponymously referred to as the *Gallavardin effect*. Some murmurs may have a distinct or unusual quality, such as the "honking" sound appreciated in some patients with mitral regurgitation (MR) due to mitral valve prolapse (MVP).

The configuration of a heart murmur may be described as crescendo, decrescendo, crescendo-decrescendo, or plateau. The decrescendo configuration of the murmur of chronic AR (**Fig. 10-1E**) can be understood in terms of the progressive decline in the diastolic pressure gradient between the aorta and the left ventricle. The crescendo-decrescendo configuration of the murmur of AS reflects the changes in the systolic pressure gradient between the

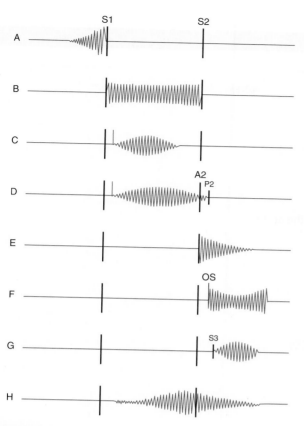

FIGURE 10-1

Diagram depicting principal heart murmurs. A. Presystolic murmur of mitral or tricuspid stenosis. **B.** Holosystolic (pansystolic) murmur of mitral or tricuspid regurgitation or of ventricular septal defect. **C.** Aortic ejection murmur beginning with an ejection click and fading before the second heart sound. **D.** Systolic murmur in pulmonic stenosis spilling through the aortic second sound, pulmonic valve closure being delayed. **E.** Aortic or pulmonary diastolic murmur. **F.** Long diastolic murmur of mitral stenosis after the opening snap (OS). **G.** Short mid-diastolic inflow murmur after a third heart sound. **H.** Continuous murmur of patent ductus arteriosus. *(Adapted from P Wood, Diseases of the Heart and Circulation, London, Eyre & Spottiswood, 1968. Permission granted courtesy of Antony and Julie Wood.)*

left ventricle and the aorta as ejection occurs, whereas the plateau configuration of the murmur of chronic MR **(Fig. 10-1B)** is consistent with the large and nearly constant pressure difference between the left ventricle and the left atrium.

Intensity

The intensity of a heart murmur is graded on a scale of 1–6 (or I–VI). A grade 1 murmur is very soft and is heard only with great effort. A grade 2 murmur is easily heard but not particularly loud. A grade 3 murmur is loud but is not accompanied by a palpable thrill over the site of maximal intensity. A grade 4 murmur is very loud and is

accompanied by a thrill. A grade 5 murmur is loud enough to be heard with only the edge of the stethoscope touching the chest, whereas a grade 6 murmur is loud enough to be heard with the stethoscope slightly off the chest. Murmurs of grade 3 or greater intensity usually signify important structural heart disease and indicate high blood flow velocity at the site of murmur production. Small ventricular septal defects (VSDs), for example, are accompanied by loud, usually grade 4 or greater, systolic murmurs as blood is ejected at high velocity from the left ventricle to the right ventricle. Low-velocity events, such as left-to-right shunting across an atrial septal defect (ASD), are usually silent. The intensity of a heart murmur also may be diminished by any process that increases the distance between the intracardiac source and the stethoscope on the chest wall, such as obesity, obstructive lung disease, and a large pericardial effusion. The intensity of a murmur also may be misleadingly soft when cardiac output is reduced significantly or when the pressure gradient between the involved cardiac structures is low.

Location and radiation

Recognition of the location and radiation of the murmur helps facilitate its accurate identification **(Fig. 10-2)**. Adventitious sounds, such as a systolic click or diastolic snap, or abnormalities of S₁ or S₂ may provide additional clues. Careful attention to the characteristics of the murmur and other heart sounds during the respiratory cycle and the performance of simple bedside maneuvers complete the auscultatory examination. These features, along with recommendations for further testing, are discussed later in the context of specific systolic, diastolic, and continuous heart murmurs **(Table 10-1)**.

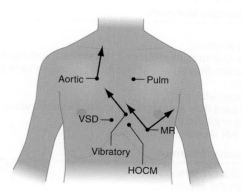

FIGURE 10-2

Maximal intensity and radiation of six isolated systolic murmurs. HOCM, hypertrophic obstructive cardiomyopathy; MR, mitral regurgitation; Pulm, pulmonary stenosis; Aortic, aortic stenosis; VSD, ventricular septal defect. *(From JB Barlow, Perspectives on the Mitral Valve. Philadelphia, FA Davis, 1987, p 140.)*

TABLE 10-1

PRINCIPAL CAUSES OF HEART MURMURS

Systolic Murmurs

Early systolic
  Mitral
    Acute MR
  VSD
    Muscular
    Nonrestrictive with pulmonary hypertension
  Tricuspid
    TR with normal pulmonary artery pressure
Mid-systolic
  Aortic
    Obstructive
      Supravalvular—supravalvular aortic stenosis, coarctation of the aorta
      Valvular—AS and aortic sclerosis
      Subvalvular—discrete, tunnel or HOCM
    Increased flow, hyperkinetic states, AR, complete heart block
    Dilation of ascending aorta, atheroma, aortitis
  Pulmonary
    Obstructive
      Supravalvular—pulmonary artery stenosis
      Valvular–pulmonic valve stenosis
      Subvalvular–infundibular stenosis (dynamic)
    Increased flow, hyperkinetic states, left-to-right shunt (e.g., ASD)
    Dilation of pulmonary artery
Late systolic
  Mitral
    MVP, acute myocardial ischemia
  Tricuspid
    TVP
Holosystolic
  Atrioventricular valve regurgitation (MR, TR)
  Left-to-right shunt at ventricular level (VSD)

Early Diastolic Murmurs

Aortic regurgitation
  Valvular: congenital (bicuspid valve), rheumatic deformity, endocarditis, prolapse, trauma, post-valvulotomy
  Dilation of valve ring: aortic dissection, annulo-aortic ectasia, cystic medial degeneration, hypertension, ankylosing spondylitis
  Widening of commissures: syphilis
Pulmonic regurgitation
  Valvular: post-valvulotomy, endocarditis, rheumatic fever, carcinoid
  Dilation of valve ring: pulmonary hypertension; Marfan syndrome
  Congenital: isolated or associated with tetralogy of Fallot, VSD, pulmonic stenosis

Mid-Diastolic Murmurs

Mitral
  Mitral stenosis
  Carey-Coombs murmur (mid-diastolic apical murmur in acute rheumatic fever)
  Increased flow across nonstenotic mitral valve (e.g., MR, VSD, PDA, high-output states, and complete heart block)
Tricuspid
  Tricuspid stenosis
  Increased flow across nonstenotic tricuspid valve (e.g., TR, ASD, and anomalous pulmonary venous return)
Left and right atrial tumors (myxoma)
Severe AR (Austin Flint murmur)

Continuous Murmurs

Patent ductus arteriosus
Coronary AV fistula
Ruptured sinus of Valsalva aneurysm
Aortic septal defect
Cervical venous hum
Anomalous left coronary artery

Proximal coronary artery stenosis
Mammary souffle of pregnancy
Pulmonary artery branch stenosis
Bronchial collateral circulation
Small (restrictive) ASD with MS
Intercostal AV fistula

Abbreviations: AR, aortic regurgitation; AS, aortic stenosis; ASD, atrial septal defect; AV, arteriovenous; HOCM, hypertrophic obstructive cardiomyopathy; MR, mitral regurgitation; MS, mitral stenosis; MVP, mitral valve prolapse; PDA, patent ductus arteriosus; TR, tricuspid regurgitation; TVP, tricuspid valve prolapse; VSD, ventricular septal defect.
Source: E Braunwald, JK Perloff, in D Zipes et al (eds): *Braunwald's Heart Disease*, 7th ed. Philadelphia, Elsevier, 2005; PJ Norton, RA O'Rourke, in E Braunwald, L Goldman (eds): *Primary Cardiology*, 2nd ed. Philadelphia, Elsevier, 2003.

SYSTOLIC HEART MURMURS

Early systolic murmurs

Early systolic murmurs begin with S_1 and extend for a variable period, ending well before S_2. Their causes are relatively few in number. *Acute, severe MR* into a normal-sized, relatively noncompliant left atrium results in an early, decrescendo systolic murmur best heard at or just medial to the apical impulse. These characteristics reflect the progressive attenuation of the pressure gradient between the left ventricle and the left atrium during systole owing to the rapid rise in left atrial pressure caused by the sudden volume load into an unprepared chamber and contrast sharply with the auscultatory features of chronic MR. Clinical settings in which acute, severe MR occur include (1) papillary muscle rupture complicating acute myocardial infarction (MI) (Chap. 35), (2) rupture of chordae tendineae in the setting of myxomatous mitral valve disease (MVP, Chap. 20), (3) infective endocarditis (Chap. 25), and (4) blunt chest wall trauma.

Acute, severe MR from papillary muscle rupture usually accompanies an inferior, posterior, or lateral MI and occurs 2–7 days after presentation. It often is signaled by chest pain, hypotension, and pulmonary edema, but a murmur may be absent in up to 50% of cases. The posteromedial papillary muscle is involved 6 to 10 times more frequently than the anterolateral papillary muscle. The murmur is to be distinguished from that associated with post-MI ventricular septal rupture, which is accompanied by a systolic thrill at the left sternal border in nearly all patients and is holosystolic in duration. A new heart murmur after an MI is an indication for transthoracic echocardiography (TTE) (Chap. 12), which allows bedside delineation of its etiology and pathophysiologic significance. The distinction between acute MR and ventricular septal rupture also can be achieved with right heart catheterization, sequential determination of oxygen saturations, and analysis of the pressure waveforms (tall v wave in the pulmonary artery wedge pressure in MR). Post-MI mechanical complications of this nature mandate aggressive medical stabilization and prompt referral for surgical repair.

Spontaneous chordal rupture can complicate the course of myxomatous mitral valve disease (MVP) and result in new-onset or "acute on chronic" severe MR. MVP may occur as an isolated phenomenon, or the lesion may be part of a more generalized connective tissue disorder as seen, for example, in patients with Marfan syndrome. Acute, severe MR as a consequence of infective endocarditis results from destruction of leaflet tissue, chordal rupture, or both. Blunt chest wall trauma is usually self-evident but may be disarmingly trivial; it can result in papillary muscle contusion and rupture, chordal detachment, or leaflet avulsion. TTE is indicated in all cases of suspected acute, severe MR to define its mechanism and severity, delineate left ventricular size and systolic function, and provide an assessment of suitability for primary valve repair.

A congenital, small muscular VSD (Chap. 19) may be associated with an early systolic murmur. The defect closes progressively during septal contraction, and thus, the murmur is confined to early systole. It is localized to the left sternal border (Fig. 10-2) and is usually of grade 4 or 5 intensity. Signs of pulmonary hypertension or left ventricular volume overload are absent. Anatomically large and uncorrected VSDs, which usually involve the membranous portion of the septum, may lead to pulmonary hypertension. The murmur associated with the left-to-right shunt, which earlier may have been holosystolic, becomes limited to the first portion of systole as the elevated pulmonary vascular resistance leads to an abrupt rise in right ventricular pressure and an attenuation of the interventricular pressure gradient during the remainder of the cardiac cycle. In such instances, signs of pulmonary hypertension (right ventricular lift, loud and single or closely split S_2) may predominate. The murmur is best heard along the left sternal border but is softer. Suspicion of a VSD is an indication for TTE.

Tricuspid regurgitation (TR) with normal pulmonary artery pressures, as may occur with infective endocarditis, may produce an early systolic murmur. The murmur is soft (grade 1 or 2), is best heard at the lower left sternal border, and may increase in intensity with inspiration (Carvallo's sign). Regurgitant "*c–v*" waves may be visible in the jugular venous pulse. TR in this setting is not associated with signs of right heart failure.

Mid-systolic murmurs

Mid-systolic murmurs begin at a short interval after S_1, end before S_2 **(Fig. 10-1C)**, and are usually crescendo-decrescendo in configuration. Aortic stenosis is the most common cause of a mid-systolic murmur in an adult. The murmur of AS is usually loudest to the right of the sternum in the second intercostal space (aortic area, Fig. 10-2) and radiates into the carotids. Transmission of the mid-systolic murmur to the apex, where it becomes higher pitched, is common (Gallavardin effect; see earlier).

Differentiation of this apical systolic murmur from MR can be difficult. The murmur of AS will increase in intensity, or become louder, in the beat after a premature beat, whereas the murmur of MR will have constant intensity from beat to beat. The intensity of the AS murmur also varies directly with the cardiac output. With a normal cardiac output, a systolic thrill and a grade 4 or higher murmur suggest severe AS. The murmur is softer in the setting of heart failure and low cardiac output. Other auscultatory findings of severe AS include a soft or absent A_2, paradoxical splitting of S_2, an apical S_4, and a late-peaking systolic murmur. In children, adolescents, and young adults with congenital valvular AS, an early ejection sound (click) is usually audible, more often along the left sternal border than at the base. Its presence signifies a flexible, noncalcified bicuspid valve (or one of its variants) and localizes the left ventricular outflow obstruction to the valvular (rather than sub- or supravalvular) level.

Assessment of the volume and rate of rise of the carotid pulse can provide additional information. A small and delayed upstroke (*parvus et tardus*) is consistent with severe AS. The carotid pulse examination is less discriminatory, however, in older patients with stiffened arteries. The electrocardiogram (ECG) shows signs of left ventricular hypertrophy (LVH) as the severity of the stenosis increases. TTE is indicated to assess the anatomic features of the aortic valve, the severity of the stenosis, left ventricular size, wall thickness and function, and the size and contour of the aortic root and proximal ascending aorta.

The obstructive form of hypertrophic cardiomyopathy (HOCM) is associated with a mid-systolic murmur that is usually loudest along the left sternal border or between the left lower sternal border and the apex (Chap. 21, Fig. 10-2). The murmur is produced by both dynamic left ventricular outflow tract obstruction and MR, and thus, its configuration is a hybrid between ejection and regurgitant phenomena. The intensity of the murmur may vary from beat to beat and after provocative maneuvers but usually does not exceed grade 3. The murmur classically will increase in intensity with maneuvers that result in increasing degrees of outflow tract obstruction, such as a reduction in preload or afterload (Valsalva, standing, vasodilators), or with an augmentation of contractility (inotropic stimulation). Maneuvers that increase preload (squatting, passive leg raising, volume administration) or afterload (squatting, vasopressors) or that reduce contractility (β-adrenoreceptor blockers) decrease the intensity of the murmur. In rare patients, there may be reversed splitting of S_2. A sustained left ventricular apical impulse and an S_4 may be appreciated. In contrast to AS, the carotid upstroke is rapid and of normal volume. Rarely, it is bisferiens or bifid in contour (see Fig. 9-2D) due to mid-systolic closure of the aortic valve. LVH is present on the ECG, and the diagnosis is confirmed by TTE. Although the systolic murmur associated with MVP behaves similarly to that due to HOCM in response to the Valsalva maneuver and to standing/squatting (**Fig. 10-3**), these two lesions can be distinguished on the basis of their associated findings, such as the presence of LVH in HOCM or a nonejection click in MVP.

The mid-systolic, crescendo-decrescendo murmur of congenital pulmonic stenosis (PS, Chap. 19) is best appreciated in the second and third left intercostal spaces (pulmonic area) (Figs. 10-2 and **10-4**). The duration of the murmur lengthens and the intensity of P_2 diminishes with increasing degrees of valvular stenosis (**Fig. 10-1D**). An early ejection sound, the

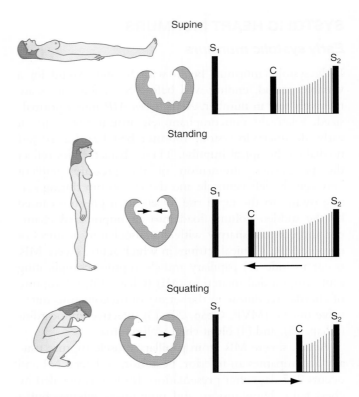

FIGURE 10-3

A mid-systolic nonejection sound (C) occurs in mitral valve prolapse and is followed by a late systolic murmur that crescendos to the second heart sound (S_2). Standing decreases venous return; the heart becomes smaller; C moves closer to the first heart sound (S_1), and the mitral regurgitant murmur has an earlier onset. With prompt squatting, venous return increases; the heart becomes larger; C moves toward S_2, and the duration of the murmur shortens. *(From JA Shaver, JJ Leonard, DF Leon, Examination of the Heart, Part IV, Auscultation of the Heart. Dallas, American Heart Association, 1990, p 13. Copyright, American Heart Association.)*

intensity of which decreases with inspiration, is heard in younger patients. A parasternal lift and ECG evidence of right ventricular hypertrophy indicate severe pressure overload. If obtained, the chest x-ray may show poststenotic dilation of the main pulmonary artery. TTE is recommended for complete characterization.

Significant left-to-right intracardiac shunting due to an ASD (Chap. 19) leads to an increase in pulmonary blood flow and a grade 2–3 mid-systolic murmur at the middle to upper left sternal border attributed to increased flow rates across the pulmonic valve with fixed splitting of S_2. Ostium secundum ASDs are the most common cause of these shunts in adults. Features suggestive of a primum ASD include the coexistence of MR due to a cleft anterior mitral valve leaflet and left axis deviation of the QRS complex on the ECG. With sinus venosus ASDs, the left-to-right shunt is usually not large enough to result in a systolic murmur, although the ECG may show abnormalities of sinus node function. A grade 2 or 3 mid-systolic murmur

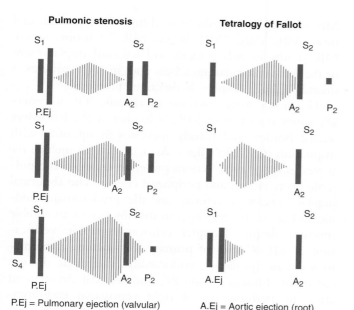

Pulmonic stenosis

S₁   S₂

P.Ej   A₂   P₂

S₁   S₂

P.Ej   A₂   P₂

S₁   S₂

S₄

P.Ej   A₂   P₂

Tetralogy of Fallot

S₁   S₂

A₂   P₂

S₁   S₂

A₂

S₁   S₂

A.Ej   A₂

P.Ej = Pulmonary ejection (valvular)   A.Ej = Aortic ejection (root)

FIGURE 10-4

Left. In valvular pulmonic stenosis with intact ventricular septum, right ventricular systolic ejection becomes progressively longer, with increasing obstruction to flow. As a result, the murmur becomes longer and louder, enveloping the aortic component of the second heart sound (A₂). The pulmonic component (P₂) occurs later, and splitting becomes wider but more difficult to hear because A₂ is lost in the murmur and P₂ becomes progressively fainter and lower pitched. As the pulmonic gradient increases, isometric contraction shortens until the pulmonic valve ejection sound fuses with the first heart sound (S₁). In severe pulmonic stenosis with concentric hypertrophy and decreasing right ventricular compliance, a fourth heart sound appears. ***Right.*** In tetralogy of Fallot with increasing obstruction at the pulmonic infundibular area, an increasing amount of right ventricular blood is shunted across the silent ventricular septal defect and flow across the obstructed outflow tract decreases. Therefore, with increasing obstruction the murmur becomes shorter, earlier, and fainter. P₂ is absent in severe tetralogy of Fallot. A large aortic root receives almost all cardiac output from both ventricular chambers, and the aorta dilates and is accompanied by a root ejection sound that does not vary with respiration. *(From JA Shaver, JJ Leonard, DF Leon, Examination of the Heart, Part IV, Auscultation of the Heart. Dallas, American Heart Association, 1990, p 45. Copyright, American Heart Association.)*

may also be heard best at the upper left sternal border in patients with idiopathic dilation of the pulmonary artery; a pulmonary ejection sound is also present in these patients. TTE is indicated to evaluate a grade 2 or 3 mid-systolic murmur when there are other signs of cardiac disease.

An isolated grade 1 or 2 mid-systolic murmur, heard in the absence of symptoms or signs of heart disease, is most often a benign finding for which no further evaluation, including TTE, is necessary. The most common example of a murmur of this type in an older adult

patient is the crescendo-decrescendo murmur of aortic valve sclerosis, heard at the second right interspace (Fig. 10-2). Aortic sclerosis is defined as focal thickening and calcification of the aortic valve to a degree that does not interfere with leaflet opening. The carotid upstrokes are normal, and electrocardiographic LVH is not present. A grade 1 or 2 mid-systolic murmur often can be heard at the left sternal border with pregnancy, hyperthyroidism, or anemia, physiologic states that are associated with accelerated blood flow. *Still's murmur* refers to a benign grade 2, vibratory mid-systolic murmur at the lower left sternal border in normal children and adolescents (Fig. 10-2).

Late systolic murmurs

A late systolic murmur that is best heard at the left ventricular apex is usually due to MVP (Chap. 20). Often, this murmur is introduced by one or more nonejection clicks. The radiation of the murmur can help identify the specific mitral leaflet involved in the process of prolapse or flail. The term *flail* refers to the movement made by an unsupported portion of the leaflet after loss of its chordal attachment(s). With posterior leaflet prolapse or flail, the resultant jet of MR is directed anteriorly and medially, as a result of which the murmur radiates to the base of the heart and masquerades as AS. Anterior leaflet prolapse or flail results in a posteriorly directed MR jet that radiates to the axilla or left infrascapular region. Leaflet flail is associated with a murmur of grade 3 or 4 intensity that can be heard throughout the precordium in thin-chested patients. The presence of an S₃ or a short, rumbling mid-diastolic murmur due to enhanced flow signifies severe MR.

Bedside maneuvers that decrease left ventricular preload, such as standing, will cause the click and murmur of MVP to move closer to the first heart sound, as leaflet prolapse occurs earlier in systole. Standing also causes the murmur to become louder and longer. With squatting, left ventricular preload and afterload are increased abruptly, leading to an increase in left ventricular volume, and the click and murmur move away from the first heart sound as leaflet prolapse is delayed; the murmur becomes softer and shorter in duration (Fig. 10-3). As noted earlier, these responses to standing and squatting are directionally similar to those observed in patients with HOCM.

A late, apical systolic murmur indicative of MR may be heard transiently in the setting of acute myocardial ischemia; it is due to apical tethering and malcoaptation of the leaflets in response to structural and functional changes of the ventricle and mitral annulus. The intensity of the murmur varies as a function of left ventricular afterload and will increase in the setting of hypertension. TTE is recommended for assessment of late systolic murmurs.

Holosystolic murmurs

(Figs. 10-1*B* and **10-5**) Holosystolic murmurs begin with S_1 and continue through systole to S_2. They are usually indicative of chronic mitral or tricuspid valve regurgitation or a VSD and warrant TTE for further characterization. The holosystolic murmur of chronic MR is best heard at the left ventricular apex and radiates to the axilla (Fig. 10-2); it is usually high pitched and plateau in configuration because of the wide difference between left ventricular and left atrial pressure throughout systole. In contrast to acute MR, left atrial compliance is normal or even increased in chronic MR. As a result, there is only a small increase in left atrial pressure for any increase in regurgitant volume.

Several conditions are associated with chronic MR and an apical holosystolic murmur, including rheumatic scarring of the leaflets, mitral annular calcification, postinfarction left ventricular remodeling, and severe left ventricular chamber enlargement. The circumference of the mitral annulus increases as the left ventricle enlarges and leads to failure of leaflet coaptation with central MR in patients with dilated cardiomyopathy (Chap. 21). The severity of the MR is worsened by any contribution from apical displacement of the papillary muscles and leaflet tethering (remodeling). Because the mitral annulus is contiguous with the left atrial endocardium, gradual enlargement of the left atrium from chronic MR will result in further stretching of the annulus and more MR; thus, "MR begets MR." Chronic severe MR results in enlargement and leftward displacement of the left ventricular apex beat and, in some patients, a diastolic filling complex, as described previously.

The holosystolic murmur of chronic TR is generally softer than that of MR, is loudest at the left lower sternal border, and usually increases in intensity with inspiration (Carvallo's sign). Associated signs include *c-v* waves in the jugular venous pulse, an enlarged and pulsatile liver, ascites, and peripheral edema. The abnormal jugular venous waveforms are the predominant finding and are seen very often in the absence of an audible murmur despite Doppler echocardiographic verification of TR. Causes of primary TR include myxomatous disease (prolapse), endocarditis, rheumatic disease, carcinoid, Ebstein's anomaly, and chordal detachment after the performance of right ventricular endomyocardial biopsy. TR is more commonly a passive process that results secondarily from chronic elevations of pulmonary artery and right ventricular pressures, leading to right ventricular enlargement, annular dilation, papillary muscle displacement, and failure of leaflet coaptation.

The holosystolic murmur of a VSD is loudest at the mid- to lower left sternal border (Fig. 10-2) and radiates widely. A thrill is present at the site of maximal intensity in the majority of patients. There is no change in the intensity of the murmur with inspiration.

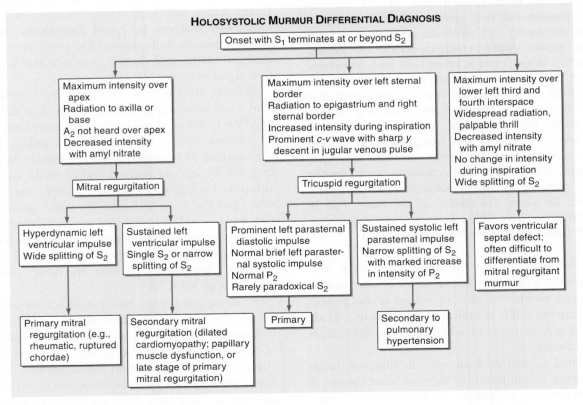

FIGURE 10-5
Differential diagnosis of a holosystolic murmur.

The intensity of the murmur varies as a function of the anatomic size of the defect. Small, restrictive VSDs, as exemplified by the *maladie de Roger*, create a very loud murmur due to the significant and sustained systolic pressure gradient between the left and right ventricles. With large defects, the ventricular pressures tend to equalize, shunt flow is balanced, and a murmur is not appreciated. The distinction between post-MI ventricular septal rupture and MR has been reviewed previously.

DIASTOLIC HEART MURMURS

Early diastolic murmurs

(Fig. 10-1E) Chronic AR results in a high-pitched, blowing, decrescendo, early to mid-diastolic murmur that begins after the aortic component of S_2 (A_2) and is best heard at the second right interspace (Fig. 10-6). The murmur may be soft and difficult to hear unless auscultation is performed with the patient leaning forward at end expiration. This maneuver brings the aortic root closer to the anterior chest wall. Radiation of the murmur may provide a clue to the cause of the AR. With primary valve disease, such as that due to congenital bicuspid disease, prolapse, or endocarditis, the diastolic murmur tends to radiate along the left sternal border, where it is often louder than appreciated in the second right interspace. When AR is caused by aortic root disease, the diastolic murmur may radiate along the right sternal border. Diseases of the aortic root cause dilation or distortion of the aortic annulus and failure of leaflet coaptation. Causes include Marfan

syndrome with aneurysm formation, annulo-aortic ectasia, ankylosing spondylitis, and aortic dissection.

Chronic, severe AR also may produce a lower-pitched mid- to late, grade 1 or 2 diastolic murmur at the apex (Austin Flint murmur), which is thought to reflect turbulence at the mitral inflow area from the admixture of regurgitant (aortic) and forward (mitral) blood flow (Fig. 10-1G). This lower-pitched, apical diastolic murmur can be distinguished from that due to MS by the absence of an opening snap and the response of the murmur to a vasodilator challenge. Lowering afterload with an agent such as amyl nitrite will decrease the duration and magnitude of the aortic–left ventricular diastolic pressure gradient, and thus, the Austin Flint murmur of severe AR will become shorter and softer. The intensity of the diastolic murmur of mitral stenosis (Fig. 10-6) may either remain constant or increase with afterload reduction because of the reflex increase in cardiac output and mitral valve flow.

Although AS and AR may coexist, a grade 2 or 3 crescendo-decrescendo mid-systolic murmur frequently is heard at the base of the heart in patients with isolated, severe AR and is due to an increased volume and rate of systolic flow. Accurate bedside identification of coexistent AS can be difficult unless the carotid pulse examination is abnormal or the mid-systolic murmur is of grade 4 or greater intensity. In the absence of heart failure, chronic severe AR is accompanied by several peripheral signs of significant diastolic run-off, including a wide pulse pressure, a "water-hammer" carotid upstroke (Corrigan's pulse), and Quincke's pulsations of

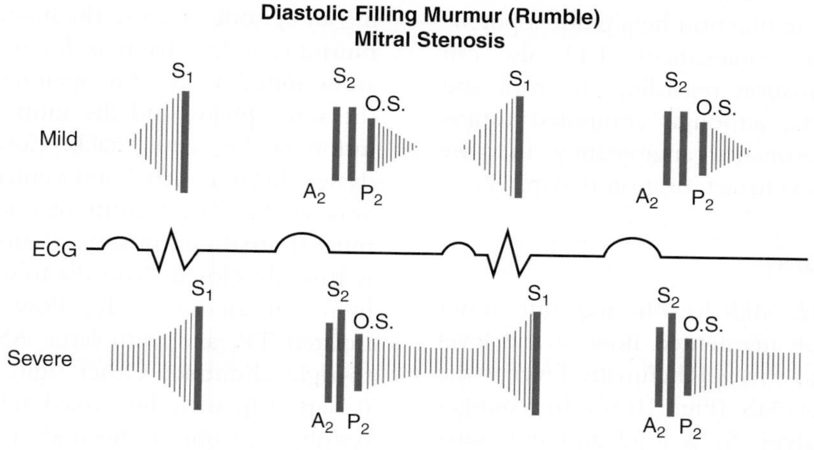

Diastolic Filling Murmur (Rumble)
Mitral Stenosis

FIGURE 10-6

Diastolic filling murmur (rumble) in mitral stenosis. In mild mitral stenosis, the diastolic gradient across the valve is limited to the phases of rapid ventricular filling in early diastole and presystole. The rumble may occur during either or both periods. As the stenotic process becomes severe, a large pressure gradient exists across the valve during the entire diastolic filling period, and the rumble persists throughout diastole. As the left atrial pressure becomes greater, the

interval between A_2 (or P_2) and the opening snap (O.S.) shortens. In severe mitral stenosis, secondary pulmonary hypertension develops and results in a loud P_2 and the splitting interval usually narrows. ECG, electrocardiogram. *(From JA Shaver, JJ Leonard, DF Leon, Examination of the Heart, Part IV, Auscultation of the Heart. Dallas, American Heart Association, 1990, p 55. Copyright, American Heart Association.)*

the nail beds. The diastolic murmur of *acute, severe AR* is notably shorter in duration and lower pitched than the murmur of chronic AR. It can be very difficult to appreciate in the presence of a rapid heart rate. These attributes reflect the abrupt rate of rise of diastolic pressure within the unprepared and noncompliant left ventricle and the correspondingly rapid decline in the aortic–left ventricular diastolic pressure gradient. Left ventricular diastolic pressure may increase sufficiently to result in premature closure of the mitral valve and a soft first heart sound. Peripheral signs of significant diastolic run-off are not present.

Pulmonic regurgitation (PR) results in a decrescendo, early to mid-diastolic murmur (*Graham Steell murmur*) that begins after the pulmonic component of S_2 (P_2), is best heard at the second left interspace, and radiates along the left sternal border. The intensity of the murmur may increase with inspiration. PR is most commonly due to dilation of the valve annulus from chronic elevation of the pulmonary artery pressure. Signs of pulmonary hypertension, including a right ventricular lift and a loud single or narrowly split S_2, are present. These features also help distinguish PR from AR as the cause of a decrescendo diastolic murmur heard along the left sternal border. PR in the absence of pulmonary hypertension can occur with endocarditis or a congenitally deformed valve. It is usually present after repair of tetralogy of Fallot in childhood. When pulmonary hypertension is not present, the diastolic murmur is softer and lower pitched than the classic Graham Steell murmur, and the severity of the PR can be difficult to appreciate.

TTE is indicated for the further evaluation of a patient with an early to mid-diastolic murmur. Longitudinal assessment of the severity of the valve lesion and ventricular size and systolic function help guide a potential decision for surgical management. TTE also can provide anatomic information regarding the root and proximal ascending aorta, although computed tomographic or magnetic resonance angiography may be indicated for more precise characterization (Chap. 12).

Mid-diastolic murmurs

(Figs. 10-1*G* and **10-1*H***) Mid-diastolic murmurs result from obstruction and/or augmented flow at the level of the mitral or tricuspid valve. Rheumatic fever is the most common cause of MS (Fig. 10-6). In younger patients with pliable valves, S_1 is loud and the murmur begins after an opening snap, which is a high-pitched sound that occurs shortly after S_2. The interval between the pulmonic component of the second heart sound (P_2) and the opening snap is inversely related to the magnitude of the left atrial–left ventricular pressure gradient. The murmur of MS is low pitched and thus is best heard with the bell of the stethoscope. It is loudest at the left ventricular apex and often is appreciated only when the patient is turned in the left lateral

decubitus position. It is usually of grade 1 or 2 intensity but may be absent when the cardiac output is severely reduced despite significant obstruction. The intensity of the murmur increases during maneuvers that increase cardiac output and mitral valve flow, such as exercise. The duration of the murmur reflects the length of time over which left atrial pressure exceeds left ventricular diastolic pressure. An increase in the intensity of the murmur just before S_1, a phenomenon known as *presystolic accentuation* (Figs. 10-1*A* and 10-6), occurs in patients in sinus rhythm and is due to a late increase in transmitral flow with atrial contraction. Presystolic accentuation does not occur in patients with atrial fibrillation.

The mid-diastolic murmur associated with tricuspid stenosis is best heard at the lower left sternal border and increases in intensity with inspiration. A prolonged γ descent may be visible in the jugular venous waveform. This murmur is very difficult to hear and often is obscured by left-sided acoustical events.

There are several other causes of mid-diastolic murmurs. Large left atrial myxomas may prolapse across the mitral valve and cause variable degrees of obstruction to left ventricular inflow (Chap. 23). The murmur associated with an atrial myxoma may change in duration and intensity with changes in body position. An opening snap is not present, and there is no presystolic accentuation. Augmented mitral diastolic flow can occur with isolated severe MR or with a large left-to-right shunt at the ventricular or great vessel level and produce a soft, rapid filling sound (S_3) followed by a short, low-pitched mid-diastolic apical murmur. The Austin Flint murmur of severe, chronic AR has already been described.

A short, mid-diastolic murmur is rarely heard during an episode of acute rheumatic fever (Carey-Coombs murmur) and probably is due to flow through an edematous mitral valve. An opening snap is not present in the acute phase, and the murmur dissipates with resolution of the acute attack. Complete heart block with dyssynchronous atrial and ventricular activation may be associated with intermittent mid- to late diastolic murmurs if atrial contraction occurs when the mitral valve is partially closed. Mid-diastolic murmurs indicative of increased tricuspid valve flow can occur with severe, isolated TR and with large ASDs and significant left-to-right shunting. Other signs of an ASD are present (Chap. 19), including fixed splitting of S_2 and a mid-systolic murmur at the mid- to upper left sternal border. TTE is indicated for evaluation of a patient with a mid- to late diastolic murmur. Findings specific to the diseases discussed earlier will help guide management.

CONTINUOUS MURMURS

(Figs. 10-1*H* and **10-7***) Continuous murmurs begin in systole, peak near the second heart sound, and continue into all or part of diastole. Their presence throughout

Continuous Murmur vs. To-Fro Murmur

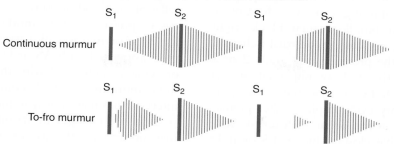

FIGURE 10-7

Comparison of the continuous murmur and the to-fro murmur. During abnormal communication between high-pressure and low-pressure systems, a large pressure gradient exists throughout the cardiac cycle, producing a continuous murmur. A classic example is patent ductus arteriosus. At times, this type of murmur can be confused with a to-fro murmur, which is a combination of systolic ejection murmur and a murmur of semilunar valve incompetence. A classic example of a to-fro murmur is aortic stenosis and regurgitation. A continuous murmur crescendos to around the second heart sound (S_2), whereas a to-fro murmur has two components. The mid-systolic ejection component decrescendos and disappears as it approaches S_2. (*From JA Shaver, JJ Leonard, DF Leon, Examination of the Heart, Part IV, Auscultation of the Heart. Dallas, American Heart Association, 1990, p 55. Copyright, American Heart Association.*)

the cardiac cycle implies a pressure gradient between two chambers or vessels during both systole and diastole. The continuous murmur associated with a patent ductus arteriosus is best heard at the upper left sternal border. Large, uncorrected shunts may lead to pulmonary hypertension, attenuation or obliteration of the diastolic component of the murmur, reversal of shunt flow, and differential cyanosis of the lower extremities. A ruptured sinus of Valsalva aneurysm creates a continuous murmur of abrupt onset at the upper right sternal border. Rupture typically occurs into a right heart chamber, and the murmur is indicative of a continuous pressure difference between the aorta and either the right ventricle or the right atrium. A continuous murmur also may be audible along the left sternal border with a coronary arteriovenous fistula and at the site of an arteriovenous fistula used for hemodialysis access. Enhanced flow through enlarged intercostal collateral arteries in patients with aortic coarctation may produce a continuous murmur along the course of one or more ribs. A cervical bruit with both systolic and diastolic components (a to-fro murmur, Fig. 10-7) usually indicates a high-grade carotid artery stenosis.

Not all continuous murmurs are pathologic. A continuous venous hum can be heard in healthy children and young adults, especially during pregnancy; it is best appreciated in the right supraclavicular fossa and can be obliterated by pressure over the right internal jugular vein or by having the patient turn his or her head toward the examiner. The continuous mammary souffle of pregnancy is created by enhanced arterial flow through engorged breasts and usually appears during the late third trimester or early puerperium. The murmur is louder in systole. Firm pressure with the diaphragm of the stethoscope can eliminate the diastolic portion of the murmur.

DYNAMIC AUSCULTATION

(Tables 10-2 and 9-1) Careful attention to the behavior of heart murmurs during simple maneuvers that alter cardiac hemodynamics can provide important clues to their cause and significance.

Respiration

Auscultation should be performed during quiet respiration or with a modest increase in inspiratory effort, as more forceful movement of the chest tends to obscure the heart sounds. Left-sided murmurs may be best heard at end expiration, when lung volumes are minimized and the heart and great vessels are brought closer to the chest wall. This phenomenon is characteristic of the murmur of AR. Murmurs of right-sided origin, such as tricuspid or pulmonic regurgitation, increase in intensity during inspiration. The intensity of left-sided murmurs either remains constant or decreases with inspiration.

Bedside assessment also should evaluate the behavior of S_2 with respiration and the dynamic relationship

TABLE 10-2

DYNAMIC AUSCULTATION: BEDSIDE MANEUVERS THAT CAN BE USED TO CHANGE THE INTENSITY OF CARDIAC MURMURS (SEE TEXT)

1. Respiration
2. Isometric exercise (hand grip)
3. Transient arterial occlusion
4. Pharmacologic manipulation of preload and/or afterload
5. Valsalva maneuver
6. Rapid standing/squatting
7. Passive leg raising
8. Post-premature beat

between the aortic and pulmonic components (Fig. 10-8). Reversed splitting can be a feature of severe AS, HOCM, left bundle branch block, right ventricular apical pacing, or acute myocardial ischemia. Fixed splitting of S$_2$ in the presence of a grade 2 or 3 mid-systolic murmur at the mid- or upper left sternal border indicates an ASD. Physiologic but wide splitting during the respiratory cycle implies either premature aortic valve closure, as can occur with severe MR, or delayed pulmonic valve closure due to PS or right bundle branch block.

Alterations of systemic vascular resistance

Murmurs can change characteristics after maneuvers that alter systemic vascular resistance and left ventricular afterload. The systolic murmurs of MR and VSD

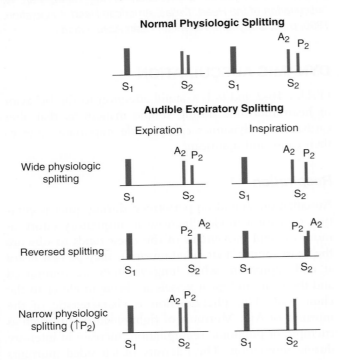

Normal Physiologic Splitting

Audible Expiratory Splitting

FIGURE 10-8

Top. Normal physiologic splitting. During expiration, the aortic (A$_2$) and pulmonic (P$_2$) components of the second heart sound are separated by <30 ms and are appreciated as a single sound. During inspiration, the splitting interval widens, and A$_2$ and P$_2$ are clearly separated into two distinct sounds. **Bottom.** Audible expiratory splitting. Wide physiologic splitting is caused by a delay in P$_2$. Reversed splitting is caused by a delay in A$_2$, resulting in paradoxical movement; i.e., with inspiration P$_2$ moves toward A$_2$, and the splitting interval narrows. Narrow physiologic splitting occurs in pulmonary hypertension, and both A$_2$ and P$_2$ are heard during expiration at a narrow splitting interval because of the increased intensity and high-frequency composition of P$_2$. *(From JA Shaver, JJ Leonard, DF Leon, Examination of the Heart, Part IV, Auscultation of the Heart. Dallas, American Heart Association, 1990, p 17. Copyright, American Heart Association.)*

become louder during sustained hand grip, simultaneous inflation of blood pressure cuffs on both upper extremities to pressures 20–40 mmHg above systolic pressure for 20 s, or infusion of a vasopressor agent. The murmurs associated with AS or HOCM will become softer or remain unchanged with these maneuvers. The diastolic murmur of AR becomes louder in response to interventions that raise systemic vascular resistance.

Opposite changes in systolic and diastolic murmurs may occur with the use of pharmacologic agents that lower systemic vascular resistance. Inhaled amyl nitrite is now rarely used for this purpose but can help distinguish the murmur of AS or HOCM from that of either MR or VSD, if necessary. The former two murmurs increase in intensity, whereas the latter two become softer after exposure to amyl nitrite. As noted previously, the Austin Flint murmur of severe AR becomes softer, but the mid-diastolic rumble of MS becomes louder, in response to the abrupt lowering of systemic vascular resistance with amyl nitrite.

Changes in venous return

The Valsalva maneuver results in an increase in intrathoracic pressure, followed by a decrease in venous return, ventricular filling, and cardiac output. The majority of murmurs decrease in intensity during the strain phase of the maneuver. Two notable exceptions are the murmurs associated with MVP and obstructive HOCM, both of which become louder during the Valsalva maneuver. The murmur of MVP may also become longer as leaflet prolapse occurs earlier in systole at smaller ventricular volumes. These murmurs behave in a similar and parallel fashion with standing. Both the click and the murmur of MVP move closer in timing to S$_1$ on rapid standing from a squatting position (Fig. 10-3). The increase in the intensity of the murmur of HOCM is predicated on the augmentation of the dynamic left ventricular outflow tract gradient that occurs with reduced ventricular filling. Squatting results in abrupt increases in both venous return (preload) and left ventricular afterload that increases ventricular volume, changes that predictably cause a decrease in the intensity and duration of the murmurs associated with MVP and HOCM; the click and murmur of MVP move away from S$_1$ with squatting. Passive leg raising can be used to increase venous return in patients who are unable to squat and stand. This maneuver may lead to a decrease in the intensity of the murmur associated with HOCM but has less effect in patients with MVP.

Post-premature ventricular contraction

A change in the intensity of a systolic murmur in the first beat after a premature beat, or in the beat after a long cycle length in patients with atrial fibrillation, can help distinguish AS from MR, particularly in an older patient in whom the murmur of AS is well transmitted to the apex. Systolic murmurs due to left ventricular outflow obstruction, including that due to AS, increase in intensity in the beat after a premature beat because of the combined effects of enhanced left ventricular filling and postextrasystolic potentiation of contractile function. Forward flow accelerates, causing an increase in the gradient and a louder murmur. The intensity of the murmur of MR does not change in the post-premature beat as there is relatively little further increase in mitral valve flow or change in the left ventricular–left atrial gradient.

THE CLINICAL CONTEXT

Additional clues to the etiology and importance of a heart murmur can be gleaned from the history and other physical examination findings. Symptoms suggestive of cardiovascular, neurologic, or pulmonary disease help focus the differential diagnosis, as do findings relevant to the jugular venous pressure and waveforms, the arterial pulses, other heart sounds, the lungs, the abdomen, the skin, and the extremities. In many instances, laboratory studies, an ECG, and/or a chest x-ray may have been obtained earlier and may contain valuable information. A patient with suspected infective endocarditis, for example, may have a murmur in the setting of fever, chills, anorexia, fatigue, dyspnea, splenomegaly, petechiae, and positive blood cultures. A new systolic murmur in a patient with a marked fall in blood pressure after a recent MI suggests myocardial rupture.

By contrast, an isolated grade 1 or 2 mid-systolic murmur at the left sternal border in a healthy, active, and asymptomatic young adult is most likely a benign finding for which no further evaluation is indicated. The context in which the murmur is appreciated often dictates the need for further testing.

ECHOCARDIOGRAPHY

(See **Fig. 10-9**, Chaps. 9 and 12) Echocardiography with color flow and spectral Doppler is a valuable tool for the assessment of cardiac murmurs. Information regarding valve structure and function, chamber size, wall thickness, ventricular function, estimated pulmonary artery pressures, intracardiac shunt flow, pulmonary and hepatic vein flow, and aortic flow can be ascertained readily. It is important to note that Doppler signals of trace or mild valvular regurgitation of no clinical consequence can be detected with structurally normal tricuspid, pulmonic, and mitral valves. Such signals are not likely to generate enough turbulence to create an audible murmur.

Echocardiography is indicated for the evaluation of patients with early, late, or holosystolic murmurs and patients with grade 3 or louder mid-systolic murmurs. Patients with grade 1 or 2 mid-systolic murmurs but other symptoms or signs of cardiovascular disease, including those from ECG or chest x-ray, should also undergo echocardiography. Echocardiography is indicated for the evaluation of any patient with a diastolic murmur and for patients with continuous murmurs not due to a venous hum or mammary souffle.

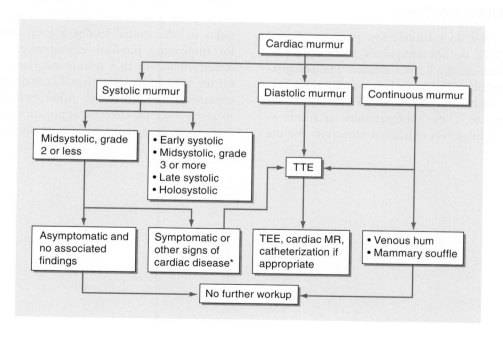

FIGURE 10-9

Strategy for evaluating heart murmurs. *If an electrocardiogram or chest x-ray has been obtained and is abnormal, echocardiography is indicated. TTE, transthoracic echocardiography; TEE, transesophageal echocardiography; MR, magnetic resonance. *(Adapted from RO Bonow et al: J Am Coll Cardiol 32:1486, 1998.)*

Echocardiography also should be considered when there is a clinical need to verify normal cardiac structure and function in a patient whose symptoms and signs are probably noncardiac in origin. The performance of serial echocardiography to follow the course of asymptomatic individuals with valvular heart disease is a central feature of their longitudinal assessment and provides valuable information that may have an impact on decisions regarding the timing of surgery. Routine echocardiography is *not* recommended for asymptomatic patients with a grade 1 or 2 mid-systolic murmur without other signs of heart disease. For this category of patients, referral to a cardiovascular specialist should be considered if there is doubt about the significance of the murmur after the initial examination.

The selective use of echocardiography outlined earlier has not been subjected to rigorous analysis of its cost-effectiveness. At least one study has suggested that initial referral of pediatric patients with heart murmurs to a specialist results in modest cost savings. For some clinicians, handheld or miniaturized cardiac ultrasound devices have replaced the stethoscope. Although several reports attest to the improved sensitivity of such devices for the detection of valvular heart disease, accuracy is highly operator-dependent, and incremental cost considerations have not been addressed adequately. The use of electronic or digital stethoscopes with spectral display capabilities has also been proposed as a method to improve the characterization of heart murmurs and the mentored teaching of cardiac auscultation.

OTHER CARDIAC TESTING

(Chap. 12, Fig. 10-9) In relatively few patients, clinical assessment and TTE do not adequately characterize the origin and significance of a heart murmur. Transesophageal echocardiography (TEE) can be considered for further evaluation, especially when the TTE windows are limited by body size, chest configuration, or intrathoracic pathology. TEE offers enhanced sensitivity for the detection of a wide range of structural cardiac disorders. Electrocardiographically gated cardiac magnetic resonance (CMR) imaging, although limited in its ability to display valvular morphology, can provide quantitative information regarding valvular function, stenosis severity, regurgitant fraction, regurgitant volume, shunt flow, chamber and great vessel size, ventricular function, and myocardial perfusion. CMR has greater capability than cardiac computed tomography (CCT) in this regard and has largely supplanted the need for cardiac catheterization and invasive hemodynamic assessment when there is a discrepancy between the clinical and echocardiographic findings. Invasive coronary angiography is performed routinely in most adult patients before valve surgery, especially when there is a suspicion of coronary artery disease predicated on symptoms, risk factors, and/or age. The use of computed tomography coronary angiography (CCTA) to exclude coronary artery disease in young patients with a low pretest probability of disease before valve surgery is under active investigation.

INTEGRATED APPROACH

The accurate identification of a heart murmur begins with a systematic approach to cardiac auscultation. Characterization of its major attributes, as reviewed earlier, allows the examiner to construct a preliminary differential diagnosis, which is then refined by integration of information available from the history, associated cardiac findings, the general physical examination, and the clinical context. The need for and urgency of further testing follow sequentially. Correlation of the findings on auscultation with the noninvasive data provides an educational feedback loop and an opportunity for improving physical examination skills. Cost constraints mandate that noninvasive imaging be justified on the basis of its incremental contribution to diagnosis, treatment, and outcome. Additional study is required to assess the cost-effective application of newer imaging technology in patients with heart murmurs.

CHAPTER 11
ELECTROCARDIOGRAPHY

Ary L. Goldberger

An electrocardiogram (ECG or EKG) is a graphic recording of electric potentials generated by the heart. The signals are detected by means of metal electrodes attached to the extremities and chest wall and then are amplified and recorded by the electrocardiograph. ECG *leads* actually display the instantaneous *differences* in potential between the electrodes.

The clinical utility of the ECG derives from its immediate availability as a noninvasive, inexpensive, and highly versatile test. In addition to its use in detecting arrhythmias, conduction disturbances, and myocardial ischemia, electrocardiography may reveal other findings related to life-threatening metabolic disturbances (e.g., hyperkalemia) or increased susceptibility to sudden cardiac death (e.g., QT prolongation syndromes).

ELECTROPHYSIOLOGY

(See also Chaps. 15 and 16) Depolarization of the heart is the initiating event for cardiac contraction. The electric currents that spread through the heart are produced by three components: cardiac pacemaker cells, specialized conduction tissue, and the heart muscle itself. The ECG, however, records only the depolarization (stimulation) and repolarization (recovery) potentials generated by the atrial and ventricular myocardium.

The depolarization stimulus for the normal heartbeat originates in the *sinoatrial* (SA) *node* (**Fig. 11-1**), or *sinus node*, a collection of *pacemaker cells*. These cells fire spontaneously; that is, they exhibit *automaticity*. The first phase of cardiac electrical activation is the spread of the depolarization wave through the right and left atria, followed by atrial contraction. Next, the impulse stimulates pacemaker and specialized conduction tissues in the atrioventricular (AV) nodal and His-bundle areas; together, these two regions constitute the AV junction. The bundle of His bifurcates into two main branches, the right and left bundles, which rapidly

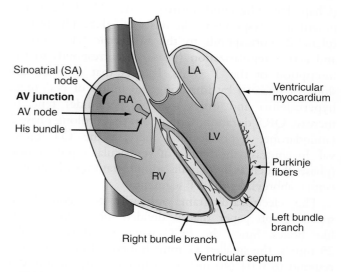

FIGURE 11-1
Schematic of the cardiac conduction system.

transmit depolarization wave fronts to the right and left ventricular myocardium by way of Purkinje fibers. The main left bundle bifurcates into two primary subdivisions: a left anterior fascicle and a left posterior fascicle. The depolarization wave fronts then spread through the ventricular wall, from endocardium to epicardium, triggering ventricular contraction.

Since the cardiac depolarization and repolarization waves have direction and magnitude, they can be represented by vectors. Vector analysis illustrates a central concept of electrocardiography: The ECG records the complex spatial and temporal summation of electrical potentials from multiple myocardial fibers conducted to the surface of the body. This principle accounts for inherent limitations in both ECG *sensitivity* (activity from certain cardiac regions may be canceled out or may be too weak to be recorded) and *specificity* (the same vectorial sum can result from either a selective gain or a loss of forces in opposite directions).

ECG WAVEFORMS AND INTERVALS

The ECG waveforms are labeled alphabetically, beginning with the P wave, which represents atrial depolarization (Fig. 11-2). The QRS complex represents ventricular depolarization, and the ST-T-U complex (ST segment, T wave, and U wave) represents ventricular repolarization. The J point is the junction between the end of the QRS complex and the beginning of the ST segment. Atrial repolarization is usually too low in amplitude to be detected, but it may become apparent in conditions such as acute pericarditis and atrial infarction.

The QRS-T waveforms of the surface ECG correspond in a general way with the different phases of simultaneously obtained ventricular *action potentials*, the intracellular recordings from single myocardial fibers (Chap. 15). The rapid upstroke (phase 0) of the action potential corresponds to the onset of QRS. The plateau (phase 2) corresponds to the isoelectric ST segment, and active repolarization (phase 3) corresponds to the inscription of the T wave. Factors that decrease the slope of phase 0 by impairing the influx of Na^+ (e.g., hyperkalemia and drugs such as flecainide) tend to increase QRS duration. Conditions that prolong phase 2 (amiodarone, hypocalcemia) increase the QT interval. In contrast, shortening of ventricular repolarization (phase 2), such as by digitalis administration or hypercalcemia, abbreviates the ST segment.

The electrocardiogram ordinarily is recorded on special graph paper that is divided into 1-mm² gridlike boxes. Since the ECG paper speed is generally 25 mm/s, the smallest (1 mm) horizontal divisions correspond to 0.04 (40 ms), with heavier lines at intervals of 0.20 s (200 ms). Vertically, the ECG graph measures the amplitude of a specific wave or deflection (1 mV = 10 mm with standard calibration; the voltage criteria for hypertrophy mentioned below are given in millimeters).

There are four major ECG intervals: R-R, PR, QRS, and QT (Fig. 11-2). The heart rate (beats per minute) can be computed readily from the interbeat (R-R) interval by dividing the number of large (0.20 s) time units between consecutive R waves into 300 or the number of small (0.04 s) units into 1500. The PR interval measures the time (normally 120–200 ms) between atrial and ventricular depolarization, which includes the physiologic delay imposed by stimulation of cells in the AV junction area. The QRS interval (normally 100–110 ms or less) reflects the duration of ventricular depolarization. The QT interval includes both ventricular depolarization and repolarization times and varies inversely with the heart rate. A rate-related ("corrected") QT interval, QT_c, can be calculated as $QT/\sqrt{R\text{-}R}$ and normally is ≤0.44 s. (Some references give QT_c upper normal limits as 0.43 s in men and 0.45 s in women. Also, a number of different formulas have been proposed, without consensus, for calculating the QT_c.)

The QRS complex is subdivided into specific deflections or waves. If the initial QRS deflection in a particular lead is negative, it is termed a Q *wave*; the first positive deflection is termed an R *wave*. A negative deflection after an R wave is an S *wave*. Subsequent positive or negative waves are labeled R′ and S′, respectively. Lowercase letters (qrs) are used for waves of relatively small amplitude. An entirely negative QRS complex is termed a QS *wave*.

ECG LEADS

The 12 conventional ECG leads record the difference in potential between electrodes placed on the surface of the body. These leads are divided into two groups: six limb (extremity) leads and six chest (precordial) leads. The limb leads record potentials transmitted onto the *frontal plane* (Fig. 11-3A), and the chest leads record potentials transmitted onto the *horizontal plane* (Fig. 11-3B).

The spatial orientation and polarity of the six frontal plane leads is represented on the hexaxial diagram (Fig. 11-4). The six chest leads (Fig. 11-5) are unipolar recordings obtained by electrodes in the following positions: lead V_1, fourth intercostal space, just to the right of the sternum; lead V_2, fourth intercostal space, just to the left of the sternum; lead V_3, midway between V_2 and V_4; lead V_4, midclavicular line, fifth intercostal space; lead V_5, anterior axillary line, same level as V_4; and lead V_6, midaxillary line, same level as V_4 and V_5.

Together, the frontal and horizontal plane electrodes provide a three-dimensional representation of cardiac electrical activity. Each lead can be likened to a different video camera angle "looking" at the same events—atrial and ventricular depolarization and repolarization—from different spatial orientations. The conventional 12-lead ECG can be supplemented with additional leads in

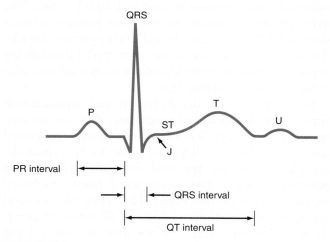

FIGURE 11-2

Basic ECG waveforms and intervals. Not shown is the R-R interval, the time between consecutive QRS complexes.

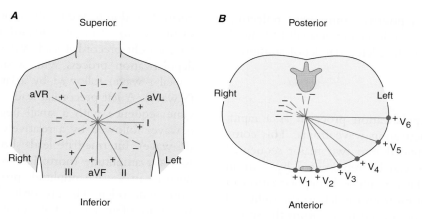

FIGURE 11-3

The six frontal plane (*A*) and six horizontal plane (*B*) leads provide a three-dimensional representation of cardiac electrical activity.

special circumstances. For example, right precordial leads V_3R, V_4R, etc., are useful in detecting evidence of acute right ventricular ischemia. Bedside monitors and ambulatory ECG (Holter) recordings usually employ only one or two modified leads. Intracardiac electrocardiography and electrophysiologic testing are discussed in Chaps. 15 and 16.

The ECG leads are configured so that a positive (upright) deflection is recorded in a lead if a wave of depolarization spreads toward the positive pole of that lead, and a negative deflection is recorded if the wave spreads toward the negative pole. If the mean orientation

of the depolarization vector is at right angles to a particular lead axis, a biphasic (equally positive and negative) deflection will be recorded.

GENESIS OF THE NORMAL ECG

P WAVE

The normal atrial depolarization vector is oriented downward and toward the subject's left, reflecting the spread of depolarization from the sinus node to the right and then the left atrial myocardium. Since this vector points toward the positive pole of lead II and toward the negative pole of lead aVR, the normal P wave will be positive in lead II and negative in lead aVR. By contrast, activation of the atria from an ectopic pacemaker in the lower part of either atrium or in the AV junction region may produce retrograde P waves (negative in lead II, positive in lead aVR). The normal P wave in lead V_1

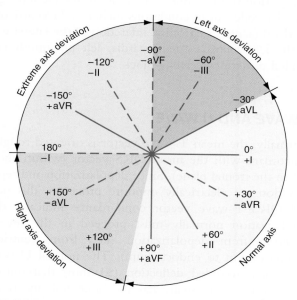

FIGURE 11-4

The frontal plane (limb or extremity) leads are represented on a hexaxial diagram. Each ECG lead has a specific spatial orientation and polarity. The positive pole of each lead axis (*solid line*) and the negative pole (*hatched line*) are designated by their angular position relative to the positive pole of lead I (0°). The mean electrical axis of the QRS complex is measured with respect to this display.

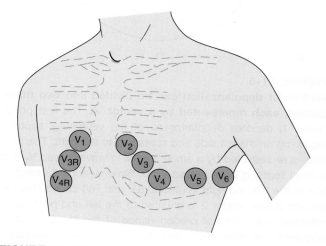

FIGURE 11-5

The horizontal plane (chest or precordial) leads are obtained with electrodes in the locations shown.

may be biphasic with a positive component reflecting right atrial depolarization, followed by a small (<1 mm²) negative component reflecting left atrial depolarization.

QRS COMPLEX

Normal ventricular depolarization proceeds as a rapid, continuous spread of activation wave fronts. This complex process can be divided into two major sequential phases, and each phase can be represented by a mean vector (Fig. 11-6). The first phase is depolarization of the interventricular septum from the left to the right and anteriorly (vector 1). The second results from the simultaneous depolarization of the right and left ventricles; it

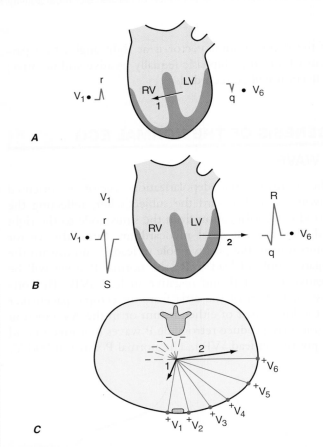

FIGURE 11-6

Ventricular depolarization can be divided into two major phases, each represented by a vector. A. The first phase (*arrow 1*) denotes depolarization of the ventricular septum, beginning on the left side and spreading to the right. This process is represented by a small "septal" r wave in lead V₁ and a small septal q wave in lead V₆. **B.** Simultaneous depolarization of the left and right ventricles (LV and RV) constitutes the second phase. Vector 2 is oriented to the left and posteriorly, reflecting the electrical predominance of the LV. **C.** Vectors (*arrows*) representing these two phases are shown in reference to the horizontal plane leads. (*After AL Goldberger: Clinical Electrocardiography: A Simplified Approach, 8th ed. Philadelphia, Elsevier/Saunders, 2013.*)

normally is dominated by the more massive left ventricle, so that vector 2 points leftward and posteriorly. Therefore, a right precordial lead (V₁) will record this biphasic depolarization process with a small positive deflection (septal r wave) followed by a larger negative deflection (S wave). A left precordial lead, e.g., V₆, will record the same sequence with a small negative deflection (septal q wave) followed by a relatively tall positive deflection (R wave). Intermediate leads show a relative increase in R-wave amplitude (normal R-wave progression) and a decrease in S-wave amplitude progressing across the chest from right to left. The precordial lead where the R and S waves are of approximately equal amplitude is referred to as the *transition zone* (usually V₃ or V₄) (Fig. 11-7).

The QRS pattern in the extremity leads may vary considerably from one normal subject to another depending on the *electrical axis* of the QRS, which describes the mean orientation of the QRS vector with reference to the six frontal plane leads. Normally, the QRS axis ranges from −30° to +100° (Fig. 11-4). An axis more negative than −30° is referred to as *left axis deviation*, and an axis more positive than +100° is referred to as *right axis deviation*. Left axis deviation may occur as a normal variant but is more commonly associated with left ventricular hypertrophy, a block in the anterior fascicle of the left bundle system (left anterior fascicular block or hemiblock), or inferior myocardial infarction. Right axis deviation also may occur as a normal variant (particularly in children and young adults), as a spurious finding due to reversal of the left and right arm electrodes, or in conditions such as right ventricular overload (acute or chronic), infarction of the lateral wall of the left ventricle, dextrocardia, left pneumothorax, and left posterior fascicular block.

T WAVE AND U WAVE

Normally, the mean T-wave vector is oriented roughly concordant with the mean QRS vector (within about 45° in the frontal plane). Since depolarization and repolarization are electrically opposite processes, this normal QRS–T-wave vector concordance indicates that repolarization normally must proceed in the reverse direction from depolarization (i.e., from ventricular epicardium to endocardium). The normal U wave is a small, rounded deflection (≤1 mm) that follows the T wave and usually has the same polarity as the T wave. An abnormal increase in U-wave amplitude is most commonly due to drugs (e.g., dofetilide, amiodarone, sotalol, quinidine, procainamide, disopyramide) or to hypokalemia. Very prominent U waves are a marker of increased susceptibility to the *torsades de pointes* type of ventricular tachycardia (Chap. 16). Inversion of the U wave in the precordial leads is abnormal and may be a subtle sign of ischemia.

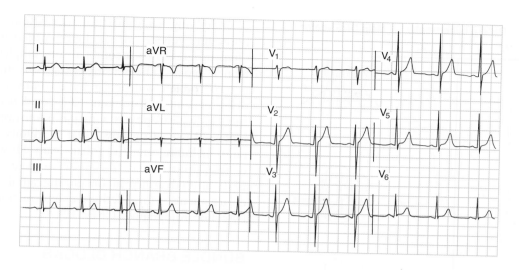

FIGURE 11-7

Normal electrocardiogram from a healthy subject. Sinus rhythm is present with a heart rate of 75 beats per minute. PR interval is 0.16 s; QRS interval (duration) is 0.08 s; QT interval is 0.36 s; QT_c is 0.40 s; the mean QRS axis is about +70°. The precordial leads show normal R-wave progression with the transition zone (R wave = S wave) in lead V_3.

MAJOR ECG ABNORMALITIES

CARDIAC ENLARGEMENT AND HYPERTROPHY

Right atrial overload (acute or chronic) may lead to an increase in P-wave amplitude (≥2.5 mm) **(Fig. 11-8)**. Left atrial overload typically produces a biphasic P wave in V_1 with a broad negative component or a broad (≥120 ms), often notched P wave in one or more limb leads (Fig. 11-8). This pattern may also occur with left atrial conduction delays in the absence of actual atrial enlargement, leading to the more general designation of *left atrial abnormality.*

Right ventricular hypertrophy due to a pressure load (as from pulmonic valve stenosis or pulmonary artery hypertension) is characterized by a relatively tall R wave in lead V_1 (R ≥ S wave), usually with right axis deviation **(Fig. 11-9)**; alternatively, there may be a qR pattern in V_1 or V_3R. ST depression and T-wave inversion in the right-to-midprecordial leads are also often present. This pattern, formerly called right ventricular "strain," is attributed to repolarization abnormalities in acutely or chronically overloaded muscle. Prominent S waves may occur in the left lateral precordial leads. Right ventricular hypertrophy due to ostium secundum–type atrial septal defects, with the accompanying right ventricular volume overload, is commonly associated with an incomplete or complete right bundle branch block pattern with a rightward QRS axis.

Acute cor pulmonale due to pulmonary embolism, for example, may be associated with a normal ECG or a variety of abnormalities. Sinus tachycardia is the most common arrhythmia, although other tachyarrhythmias, such as atrial fibrillation or flutter, may occur. The QRS axis may shift to the right, sometimes in concert with the so-called $S_1Q_3T_3$ pattern (prominence of the S wave in lead I and the Q wave in lead III, with T-wave inversion in lead III). Acute right ventricular dilation also may be associated with slow R-wave progression and ST-T abnormalities in V_1 to V_4 simulating acute anterior infarction. A right ventricular conduction disturbance may appear.

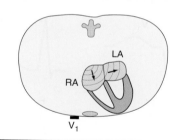

FIGURE 11-8

Right atrial (RA) overload may cause tall, peaked P waves in the limb or precordial leads. Left atrial (LA) abnormality may cause broad, often notched P waves in the limb leads and a biphasic P wave in lead V_1 with a prominent negative component representing delayed depolarization of the LA. (*After MK Park, WG Guntheroth: How to Read Pediatric ECGs, 4th ed. St. Louis, Mosby/Elsevier, 2006.*)

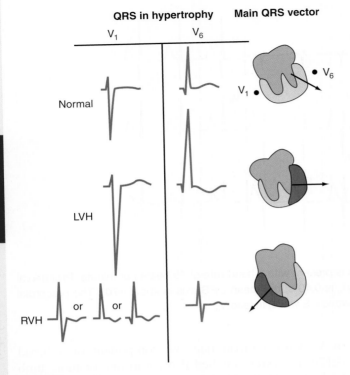

QRS in hypertrophy   **Main QRS vector**

FIGURE 11-9

Left ventricular hypertrophy (LVH) increases the amplitude of electrical forces directed to the left and posteriorly. In addition, repolarization abnormalities may cause ST-segment depression and T-wave inversion in leads with a prominent R wave. Right ventricular hypertrophy (RVH) may shift the QRS vector to the right; this effect usually is associated with an R, RS, or qR complex in lead V_1. T-wave inversions may be present in right precordial leads.

Chronic cor pulmonale due to obstructive lung disease (Chap. 17) usually does not produce the classic ECG patterns of right ventricular hypertrophy noted earlier. Instead of tall right precordial R waves, chronic lung disease more typically is associated with small R waves in right-to-midprecordial leads (slow R-wave progression) due in part to downward displacement of the diaphragm and the heart. Low-voltage complexes are commonly present, owing to hyperaeration of the lungs.

A number of different voltage criteria for *left ventricular hypertrophy* (Fig. 11-9) have been proposed on the basis of the presence of tall left precordial R waves and deep right precordial S waves (e.g., SV_1 + [RV_5 or RV_6] >35 mm). Repolarization abnormalities (ST depression with T-wave inversions, formerly called the left ventricular "strain" pattern) also may appear in leads with prominent R waves. However, prominent precordial voltages may occur as a normal variant, especially in athletic or young individuals. Left ventricular hypertrophy may increase limb lead voltage with or without increased precordial voltage (e.g., RaVL + SV_3 >20 mm in women and >28 mm in men). The presence of left atrial abnormality increases the likelihood

of underlying left ventricular hypertrophy in cases with borderline voltage criteria. Left ventricular hypertrophy often progresses to incomplete or complete left bundle branch block. The sensitivity of conventional voltage criteria for left ventricular hypertrophy is decreased in obese persons and smokers. ECG evidence for left ventricular hypertrophy is a major noninvasive marker of increased risk of cardiovascular morbidity and mortality rates, including sudden cardiac death. However, because of false-positive and false-negative diagnoses, the ECG is of limited utility in diagnosing atrial or ventricular enlargement. More definitive information is provided by echocardiography (Chap. 12).

BUNDLE BRANCH BLOCKS

Intrinsic impairment of conduction in either the right or the left bundle system (intraventricular conduction disturbances) leads to prolongation of the QRS interval. With complete bundle branch blocks, the QRS interval is ≥120 ms in duration; with incomplete blocks, the QRS interval is between 100 and 120 ms. The QRS vector usually is oriented in the direction of the myocardial region where depolarization is delayed (Fig. 11-10). Thus, with right bundle branch block, the terminal QRS vector is oriented to the right and anteriorly (rSR′ in V_1 and qRS in V_6, typically). Left bundle branch block alters both early and later phases of ventricular depolarization. The major QRS vector

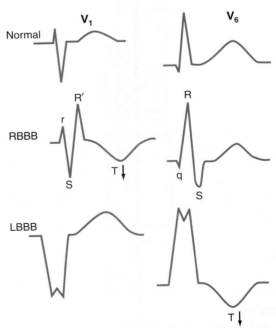

FIGURE 11-10

Comparison of typical QRS-T patterns in right bundle branch block (RBBB) and left bundle branch block (LBBB) with the normal pattern in leads V_1 and V_6. Note the secondary T-wave inversions (*arrows*) in leads with an rSR′ complex with RBBB and in leads with a wide R wave with LBBB.

is directed to the left and posteriorly. In addition, the normal early left-to-right pattern of septal activation is disrupted such that septal depolarization proceeds from right to left as well. As a result, left bundle branch block generates wide, predominantly negative (QS) complexes in lead V_1 and entirely positive (R) complexes in lead V_6. A pattern identical to that of left bundle branch block, preceded by a sharp spike, is seen in most cases of electronic right ventricular pacing because of the relative delay in left ventricular activation.

Bundle branch block may occur in a variety of conditions. In subjects without structural heart disease, right bundle branch block is seen more commonly than left bundle branch block. Right bundle branch block also occurs with heart disease, both congenital (e.g., atrial septal defect) and acquired (e.g., valvular, ischemic). Left bundle branch block is often a marker of one of four underlying conditions associated with increased risk of cardiovascular morbidity and mortality rates: coronary heart disease (frequently with impaired left ventricular function), hypertensive heart disease, aortic valve disease, and cardiomyopathy. Bundle branch blocks may be chronic or intermittent. A bundle branch block may be rate-related; for example, it often occurs when the heart rate exceeds some critical value.

Bundle branch blocks and depolarization abnormalities secondary to artificial pacemakers not only affect ventricular depolarization (QRS) but also are characteristically associated with secondary repolarization (ST-T) abnormalities. With bundle branch blocks, the T wave is typically opposite in polarity to the last deflection of the QRS (Fig. 11-10). This discordance of the QRS–T-wave vectors is caused by the altered sequence of repolarization that occurs secondary to altered depolarization. In contrast, primary repolarization abnormalities are independent of QRS changes and are related instead to actual alterations in the electrical properties of the myocardial fibers themselves (e.g., in the resting membrane potential or action potential duration), not just to changes in the sequence of repolarization. Ischemia, electrolyte imbalance, and drugs such as digitalis all cause such primary ST–T-wave changes. Primary and secondary T-wave changes may coexist. For example, T-wave inversions in the right precordial leads with left bundle branch block or in the left precordial leads with right bundle branch block may be important markers of underlying ischemia or other abnormalities. A distinctive abnormality simulating right bundle branch block with ST-segment elevations in the right chest leads is seen with the Brugada pattern (Chap. 16).

Partial blocks (fascicular or "hemiblocks") in the left bundle system (left anterior or posterior fascicular blocks) generally do not prolong the QRS duration substantially but instead are associated with shifts in the frontal plane QRS axis (leftward or rightward, respectively). More complex combinations of fascicular

and bundle branch blocks may occur that involve the left and right bundle system. Examples of bifascicular block include right bundle branch block and left posterior fascicular block, right bundle branch block with left anterior fascicular block, and complete left bundle branch block. Chronic bifascicular block in an asymptomatic individual is associated with a relatively low risk of progression to high-degree AV heart block. In contrast, new bifascicular block with acute anterior myocardial infarction carries a much greater risk of complete heart block. Alternation of right and left bundle branch block is a sign of trifascicular disease. However, the presence of a prolonged PR interval and bifascicular block does not necessarily indicate trifascicular involvement, since this combination may arise with AV node disease and bifascicular block. Intraventricular conduction delays also can be caused by extrinsic (toxic) factors that slow ventricular conduction, particularly hyperkalemia or drugs (e.g., class 1 antiarrhythmic agents, tricyclic antidepressants, phenothiazines).

Prolongation of QRS duration does not necessarily indicate a conduction delay but may be due to preexcitation of the ventricles via a bypass tract, as in Wolff-Parkinson-White (WPW) patterns (Chap. 16) and related variants. The diagnostic triad of WPW consists of a wide QRS complex associated with a relatively short PR interval and slurring of the initial part of the QRS (delta wave), with the latter effect being due to aberrant activation of ventricular myocardium. The presence of a bypass tract predisposes to reentrant supraventricular tachyarrhythmias.

MYOCARDIAL ISCHEMIA AND INFARCTION

(See also Chap. 35) The ECG is a cornerstone in the diagnosis of acute and chronic ischemic heart disease. The findings depend on several key factors: the nature of the process (reversible [i.e., ischemia] versus irreversible [i.e., infarction]), the duration (acute versus chronic), the extent (transmural versus subendocardial), and localization (anterior versus inferoposterior), as well as the presence of other underlying abnormalities (ventricular hypertrophy, conduction defects).

Ischemia exerts complex time-dependent effects on the electrical properties of myocardial cells. Severe, acute ischemia lowers the resting membrane potential and shortens the duration of the action potential. Such changes cause a voltage gradient between normal and ischemic zones. As a consequence, current flows between those regions. These currents of injury are represented on the surface ECG by deviation of the ST segment (Fig. 11-11). When the acute ischemia is transmural, the ST vector usually is shifted in the direction of the outer (epicardial) layers, producing ST elevations and sometimes, in the earliest stages of ischemia, tall, positive so-called hyperacute T waves over the

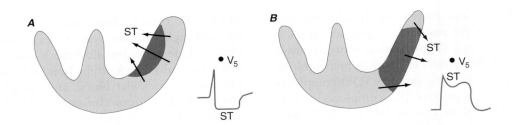

FIGURE 11-11

Acute ischemia causes a current of injury. With predominant subendocardial ischemia (**A**), the resultant ST vector will be directed toward the inner layer of the affected ventricle and the ventricular cavity. Overlying leads therefore will record ST depression. With ischemia involving the outer ventricular layer (**B**) (transmural or epicardial injury), the ST vector will be directed outward. Overlying leads will record ST elevation.

ischemic zone. With ischemia confined primarily to the *subendocardium*, the ST vector typically shifts toward the subendocardium and ventricular cavity, so that overlying (e.g., anterior precordial) leads show ST-segment depression (with ST elevation in lead aVR). Multiple factors affect the amplitude of acute ischemic ST deviations. Profound ST elevation or depression in multiple leads usually indicates very severe ischemia. From a clinical viewpoint, the division of acute myocardial infarction into ST-segment elevation and non-ST elevation types is useful since the efficacy of acute reperfusion therapy is limited to the former group.

The ECG leads are usually more helpful in localizing regions of ST elevation than non-ST elevation ischemia. For example, acute transmural anterior (including apical and lateral) wall ischemia is reflected by ST elevations or increased T-wave positivity in one or more of the precordial leads (V_1–V_6) and leads I and aVL. Inferior wall ischemia produces changes in leads II, III, and aVF. "Posterior" wall ischemia (usually associated with lateral or inferior involvement) may be indirectly recognized by *reciprocal* ST depressions in leads V_1 to V_3 (thus constituting an ST elevation "equivalent" acute coronary syndrome). Right ventricular ischemia usually produces ST elevations in right-sided chest leads (Fig. 11-5). When ischemic ST elevations occur as the earliest sign of acute infarction, they typically are followed within a period ranging from hours to days by evolving T-wave inversions and often by Q waves occurring in the same lead distribution. Reversible transmural ischemia, for example, due to coronary vasospasm (Prinzmetal's variant angina and probably the Tako-Tsubo "stress" cardiomyopathy syndrome), may cause transient ST-segment elevations without development of Q waves, as may very early reperfusion in acute coronary syndromes. Depending on the severity and duration of ischemia, the ST elevations may resolve completely in minutes or be followed by T-wave inversions that persist for hours or even days. Patients with ischemic chest pain who present with deep T-wave inversions in multiple precordial leads (e.g., V_1–V_4) with or without cardiac enzyme elevations typically have severe obstruction in the left anterior descending coronary artery system (Fig. 11-12). In contrast, patients whose baseline ECG already shows abnormal T-wave inversions may develop T-wave normalization (pseudonormalization) during episodes of acute transmural ischemia.

With infarction, depolarization (QRS) changes often accompany repolarization (ST-T) abnormalities. Necrosis of sufficient myocardial tissue may lead to decreased R-wave amplitude or abnormal Q waves (even in the absence of transmurality) in the anterior or inferior leads (Fig. 11-13). Previously, abnormal Q waves were considered markers of transmural myocardial infarction, whereas subendocardial infarcts were thought not to produce Q waves. However, careful ECG-pathology correlative studies have indicated that transmural infarcts may occur without Q waves and that subendocardial (nontransmural) infarcts sometimes may be associated with Q waves. Therefore, infarcts are more appropriately classified as "Q-wave" or "non-Q-wave."

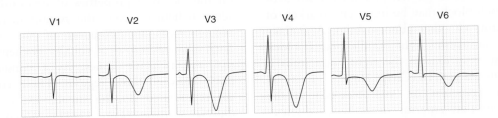

FIGURE 11-12

Severe anterior wall ischemia (with or without infarction) may cause prominent T-wave inversions in the precordial leads. This pattern (sometimes referred to as Wellens T waves) is usually associated with a high-grade stenosis of the left anterior descending coronary artery.

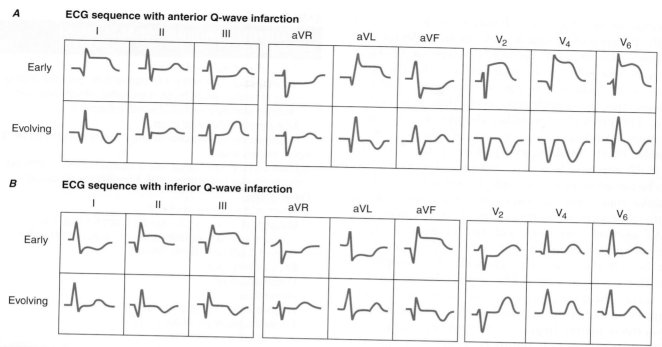

A ECG sequence with anterior Q-wave infarction

B ECG sequence with inferior Q-wave infarction

FIGURE 11-13

Sequence of depolarization and repolarization changes with (**A**) acute anterior and (**B**) acute inferior wall Q-wave infarctions. With anterior infarcts, ST elevation in leads I and aVL and the precordial leads may be accompanied by reciprocal ST depressions in leads II, III, and aVF. Conversely, acute inferior (or posterolateral) infarcts may be associated with reciprocal ST depressions in leads V₁ to V₃. *(After AL Goldberger: Clinical Electrocardiography: A Simplified Approach, 8th ed. Philadelphia, Elsevier/Saunders, 2013.)*

The major acute ECG changes in syndromes of ischemic heart disease are summarized schematically in Fig. 11-14. Loss of depolarization forces due to posterior or lateral infarction may cause reciprocal increases in R-wave amplitude in leads V_1 and V_2 without diagnostic Q waves in any of the conventional leads. Atrial infarction may be associated with PR-segment deviations due to an atrial current of injury, changes in P-wave morphology, or atrial arrhythmias.

In the weeks and months after infarction, these ECG changes may persist or begin to resolve. Complete normalization of the ECG after Q-wave infarction is uncommon but may occur, particularly with smaller infarcts. In contrast, ST-segment elevations that persist for several weeks or more after a Q-wave infarct usually correlate with a severe underlying wall motion disorder (akinetic or dyskinetic zone), although not necessarily a frank ventricular aneurysm. ECG changes due to ischemia may occur spontaneously or may be provoked by various exercise protocols (stress electrocardiography; Chap. 33).

The ECG has important limitations in both sensitivity and specificity in the diagnosis of ischemic heart disease. Although a single normal ECG does not exclude ischemia or even acute infarction, a normal ECG *throughout* the course of an acute infarct is distinctly uncommon. Prolonged chest pain without diagnostic ECG changes therefore should always prompt a careful search for other noncoronary causes of chest pain (Chap. 4). Furthermore, the diagnostic changes of acute or evolving ischemia are often masked by the presence of left bundle branch block, electronic ventricular pacemaker patterns, and Wolff-Parkinson-White preexcitation. However, clinicians

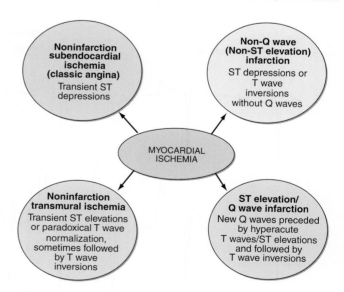

FIGURE 11-14

Variability of ECG patterns with acute myocardial ischemia. The ECG also may be normal or nonspecifically abnormal. Furthermore, these categorizations are not mutually exclusive. *(After AL Goldberger: Clinical Electrocardiography: A Simplified Approach, 7th ed. St. Louis, Mosby/Elsevier, 2006.)*

continue to overdiagnose ischemia or infarction based on the presence of ST-segment elevations or depressions; T-wave inversions; tall, positive T waves; or Q waves *not* related to ischemic heart disease (pseudoinfarct patterns). For example, ST-segment elevations simulating ischemia may occur with acute pericarditis or myocarditis, as a normal variant (including the typical "early repolarization" pattern), or in a variety of other conditions (Table 11-1). Similarly, tall, positive T waves do not invariably represent hyperacute ischemic changes but may also be caused by normal variants, hyperkalemia, cerebrovascular injury, and left ventricular volume overload due to mitral or aortic regurgitation, among other causes.

ST-segment elevations and tall, positive T waves are common findings in leads V_1 and V_2 in left bundle branch block or left ventricular hypertrophy in the absence of ischemia. The differential diagnosis of Q waves includes physiologic or positional variants, ventricular hypertrophy, acute or chronic noncoronary myocardial injury, hypertrophic cardiomyopathy, and ventricular conduction disorders. Digoxin, ventricular hypertrophy, hypokalemia, and a variety of other factors may cause ST-segment depression mimicking subendocardial ischemia. Prominent T-wave inversion may occur with ventricular hypertrophy, cardiomyopathies, myocarditis, and cerebrovascular injury (particularly intracranial bleeds), among many other conditions.

METABOLIC FACTORS AND DRUG EFFECTS

A variety of metabolic and pharmacologic agents alter the ECG and, in particular, cause changes in repolarization

TABLE 11-1

DIFFERENTIAL DIAGNOSIS OF ST-SEGMENT ELEVATIONS

Ischemia/myocardial infarction
  Noninfarction, transmural ischemia (Prinzmetal's angina, and probably Tako-Tsubo syndrome, which may also exactly simulate classical acute infarction)
  Acute myocardial infarction
  Postmyocardial infarction (ventricular aneurysm pattern)
Acute pericarditis
Normal variants (including "early repolarization" patterns)
Left ventricular hypertrophy/left bundle branch block[a]
Other (rarer)
  Acute pulmonary embolism[a]
  Brugada patterns (right bundle branch block–like pattern with ST elevations in right precordial leads)[a]
  Class 1C antiarrhythmic drugs[a]
  DC cardioversion
  Hypercalcemia[a]
  Hyperkalemia[a]
  Hypothermia (J [Osborn] waves)
  Nonischemic myocardial injury
    Myocarditis
    Tumor invading left ventricle
    Trauma to ventricles

[a]Usually localized to V_1–V_2 or V_3.
Source: Modified from AL Goldberger: *Clinical Electrocardiography: A Simplified Approach*, 8th ed. Philadelphia, Elsevier/Saunders, 2013.

(ST-T-U) and sometimes QRS prolongation. Certain life-threatening electrolyte disturbances may be diagnosed initially and monitored from the ECG. *Hyperkalemia* produces a sequence of changes (Fig. 11-15), usually beginning with narrowing and peaking (tenting) of the T waves. Further elevation of extracellular K⁺ leads to

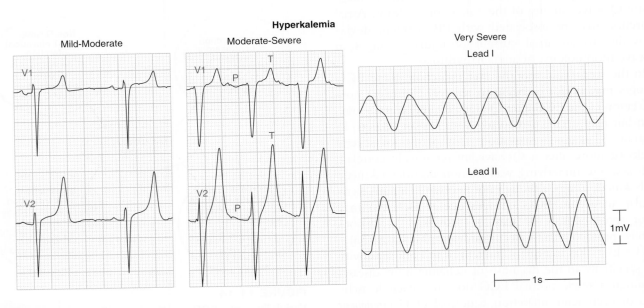

Hyperkalemia

Mild-Moderate   Moderate-Severe   Very Severe

FIGURE 11-15
The earliest ECG change with hyperkalemia is usually peaking ("tenting") of the T waves. With further increases in the serum potassium concentration, the QRS complexes widen, the P waves decrease in amplitude and may disappear, and finally a sine-wave pattern leads to asystole unless emergency therapy is given. (*After AL Goldberger: Clinical Electrocardiography: A Simplified Approach, 8th ed. Philadelphia, Elsevier/Saunders, 2013.*)

AV conduction disturbances, diminution in P-wave amplitude, and widening of the QRS interval. Severe hyperkalemia eventually causes cardiac arrest with a slow sinusoidal type of mechanism ("sine-wave" pattern) followed by asystole. *Hypokalemia* **(Fig. 11-16)** prolongs ventricular repolarization, often with prominent U waves. Prolongation of the QT interval is also seen with drugs that increase the duration of the ventricular action potential: class 1A antiarrhythmic agents and related drugs (e.g., quinidine, disopyramide, procainamide, tricyclic antidepressants, phenothiazines) and class III agents (e.g., amiodarone [Fig. 11-16], dofetilide, dronedarone, sotalol, ibutilide). Marked QT prolongation, sometimes with deep, wide T-wave inversions, may occur with intracranial bleeds, particularly subarachnoid hemorrhage ("CVA T-wave" pattern) (Fig. 11-16). Systemic *hypothermia* also prolongs repolarization, usually with a distinctive convex elevation of the J point (Osborn wave). *Hypocalcemia* typically prolongs the QT interval (ST portion), whereas *hypercalcemia* shortens it **(Fig. 11-17)**. Digitalis glycosides also shorten the QT interval, often with a characteristic "scooping" of the ST–T-wave complex (*digitalis effect*).

Many other factors are associated with ECG changes, particularly alterations in ventricular repolarization. T-wave flattening, minimal T-wave inversions, or slight ST-segment depression ("nonspecific ST–T-wave changes") may occur with a variety of electrolyte and acid-base disturbances, a variety of infectious processes, central nervous system disorders, endocrine abnormalities, many drugs, ischemia, hypoxia, and virtually any type of cardiopulmonary abnormality. Although subtle ST–T-wave changes may be markers of ischemia,

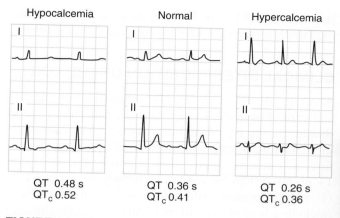

FIGURE 11-17
Prolongation of the Q-T interval (ST-segment portion) is typical of hypocalcemia. Hypercalcemia may cause abbreviation of the ST segment and shortening of the QT interval.

transient nonspecific repolarization changes may also occur after a meal or with postural (orthostatic) change, hyperventilation, or exercise in healthy individuals.

ELECTRICAL ALTERNANS

Electrical alternans—a beat-to-beat alternation in one or more components of the ECG signal—is a common type of nonlinear cardiovascular response to a variety of hemodynamic and electrophysiologic perturbations. Total electrical alternans (P-QRS-T) with sinus tachycardia is a relatively specific sign of pericardial effusion, usually with cardiac tamponade. The mechanism relates to a periodic swinging motion of the heart in the effusion at a frequency exactly one-half the heart rate.

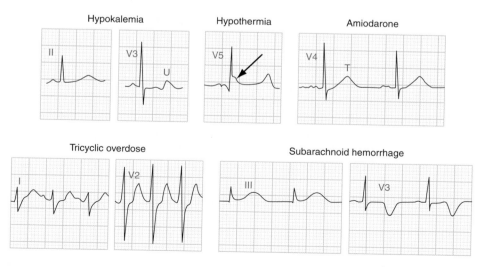

FIGURE 11-16

A variety of metabolic derangements, drug effects, and other factors may prolong ventricular repolarization with QT prolongation or prominent U waves. Prominent repolarization prolongation, particularly if due to hypokalemia, inherited "channelopathies," or certain pharmacologic agents, indicates increased susceptibility to *torsades des pointes*–type ventricular tachycardia (Chap. 16). Marked systemic hypothermia is associated with a distinctive convex "hump" at the J point (Osborn wave, *arrow*) due to altered ventricular action potential characteristics. Note QRS and QT prolongation along with sinus tachycardia in the case of tricyclic antidepressant overdose.

Repolarization (ST-T or U wave) alternans is a sign of electrical instability and may precede ventricular tachyarrhythmias.

CLINICAL INTERPRETATION OF THE ECG

Accurate analysis of ECGs requires thoroughness and care. The patient's age, gender, and clinical status should always be taken into account. Many mistakes in ECG interpretation are errors of omission. Therefore, a systematic approach is essential. The following 14 points should be analyzed carefully in every ECG: (1) standardization (calibration) and technical features (including lead placement and artifacts), (2) rhythm, (3) heart rate, (4) PR interval/AV conduction, (5) QRS interval, (6) QT/QT_c interval, (7) mean QRS electrical axis, (8) P waves, (9) QRS voltages, (10) precordial R-wave progression, (11) abnormal Q waves, (12) ST segments, (13) T waves, and (14) U waves.

Only after analyzing all these points should the interpretation be formulated. Where appropriate, important clinical correlates or inferences should be mentioned.

For example, sinus tachycardia with QRS and QT-(U) prolongation, especially in the context of changes in mental status, suggests tricyclic antidepressant overdose (Fig. 11-16). The triad of peaked T waves (hyperkalemia), a long QT due to ST-segment lengthening (hypocalcemia), and left ventricular hypertrophy (systemic hypertension) suggests chronic renal failure. Comparison with any previous ECGs is invaluable. The diagnosis and management of specific cardiac arrhythmias and conduction disturbances are discussed in Chaps. 15 and 16.

COMPUTERIZED ELECTROCARDIOGRAPHY

Computerized ECG systems are widely used for immediate retrieval of thousands of ECG records. Computer interpretation of ECGs still has major limitations. Incomplete or inaccurate readings are most likely with arrhythmias and complex abnormalities. Therefore, computerized interpretation (including measurements of basic ECG intervals) should not be accepted without careful clinician review.

CHAPTER 12

NONINVASIVE CARDIAC IMAGING: ECHOCARDIOGRAPHY, NUCLEAR CARDIOLOGY, AND MRI/CT IMAGING

Rick A. Nishimura ■ Panithaya Chareonthaitawee ■ Matthew Martinez

Cardiovascular imaging plays an essential role in the practice of cardiology. Two-dimensional (2D) echocardiography is able to visualize the heart directly in real time using ultrasound, providing instantaneous assessment of the myocardium, cardiac chambers, valves, pericardium, and great vessels. Doppler echocardiography measures the velocity of moving red blood cells and has become a noninvasive alternative to cardiac catheterization for assessment of hemodynamics. Transesophageal echocardiography (TEE) provides a unique window for high-resolution imaging of posterior structures of the heart, particularly the left atrium, mitral valve, and aorta. Nuclear cardiology uses radioactive tracers to provide assessment of myocardial perfusion and metabolism, along with ventricular function, and is applied primarily to the evaluation of patients with ischemic heart disease. Cardiac MRI and CT can delineate cardiac structure and function with high resolution. They are particularly useful in the examination of cardiac masses, the pericardium, the great vessels, and ventricular function and perfusion. Gadolinium enhancement during cardiac MRI adds information on myocardial perfusion. Detection of coronary calcification by CT as well as direct visualization of coronary arteries by CT angiography (CTA) may be useful in selected patients with suspected coronary artery disease (CAD). This chapter provides an overview of the basic concepts of these cardiac imaging modalities as well as the clinical indications for each procedure.

ECHOCARDIOGRAPHY

TWO-DIMENSIONAL ECHOCARDIOGRAPHY

Basic principles

2D echocardiography uses the principle of ultrasound reflection off cardiac structures to produce images of the heart (Table 12-1). For a transthoracic echocardiogram (TTE), the imaging is performed with a handheld transducer placed directly on the chest wall. In selected patients, a TEE may be performed, in which an ultrasound transducer is mounted on the tip of an endoscope placed in the esophagus and directed toward the cardiac structures.

Current echocardiographic machines are portable and can be wheeled directly to the patient's bedside. Thus, a major advantage of echocardiography over other imaging modalities is the ability to obtain instantaneous images of the cardiac structures for immediate

TABLE 12-1

CLINICAL USES OF ECHOCARDIOGRAPHY

Two-Dimensional Echocardiography	Doppler Echocardiography
Cardiac chambers	Valve stenosis
Chamber size	Gradient
Left ventricular	Valve area
hypertrophy	Valve regurgitation
Regional wall motion	Semiquantitation
abnormalities	Intracardiac pressures
Valve	Volumetric flow
Morphology and motion	Diastolic filling
Pericardium	Intracardiac shunts
Effusion	**Transesophageal**
Tamponade	**Echocardiography**
Masses	Inadequate transthoracic
Great vessels	images
Stress Echocardiography	Aortic disease
Two-dimensional	Infective endocarditis
Myocardial ischemia	Source of embolism
Viable myocardium	Valve prosthesis
Doppler	Intraoperative
Valve disease	

interpretation. Thus, echocardiography has become an ideal imaging modality for cardiac emergencies. A limitation of TTE is the inability to obtain high-quality images in all patients, especially those with a thick chest wall or severe lung disease, as ultrasound waves are poorly transmitted through lung parenchyma. Technology such as harmonic imaging and IV contrast agents (which traverse the pulmonary circulation) can be used to enhance endocardial borders in patients with poor acoustic windows.

Chamber size and function

2D echocardiography is an ideal imaging modality for assessing left ventricular (LV) size and function (Fig. 12-1). A qualitative assessment of the ventricular cavity and systolic function can be made directly from the 2D image by experienced observers. 2D echocardiography is useful in the diagnosis of LV hypertrophy and is the imaging modality of choice for the diagnosis of hypertrophic cardiomyopathy. Other chamber sizes are assessed by visual analysis, including the left atrium and right-sided chambers.

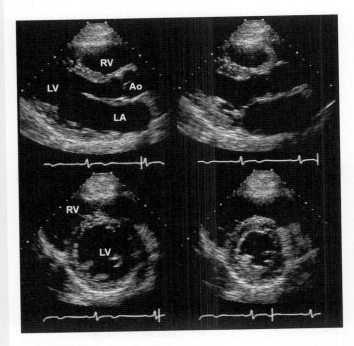

FIGURE 12-1
Two-dimensional echocardiographic still-frame images from a normal patient with a normal heart. *Upper:* Parasternal long-axis view during systole and diastole (*left*) and systole (*right*). During systole, there is thickening of the myocardium and reduction in the size of the left ventricle (LV). The valve leaflets are thin and open widely. *Lower:* Parasternal short-axis view during diastole (left) and systole (right) demonstrating a decrease in the left ventricular cavity size during systole as well as an increase in wall thickness. LA, left atrium; RV, right ventricle; Ao, aorta.

Valve abnormalities

2D echocardiography is the "gold standard" for imaging valve morphology and motion. Leaflet thickness and mobility, valve calcification, and the appearance of subvalvular and supravalvular structures can be assessed. Valve stenosis is reliably diagnosed by the thickening and decreased mobility of the valve. 2D echocardiography is also the gold standard for the diagnosis of mitral stenosis, which produces typical tethering and diastolic doming, and the severity of the stenosis can be ascertained from a direct planimetry measurement of the mitral valve orifice. The presence and often the etiology of stenosis of the semilunar valves can be made by 2D echocardiography (Fig. 12-2), but evaluation of the severity of the stenosis requires Doppler echocardiography (discussed later). The diagnosis of valvular regurgitation must be made by Doppler echocardiography, but 2D echocardiography is valuable for determining the etiology of the regurgitation, as well as its effects on ventricular dimensions, shape, and function.

Pericardial disease

2D echocardiography is the imaging modality of choice for the detection of pericardial effusion, which is easily visualized as a black echolucent ovoid structure surrounding the heart (Fig. 12-3). In the hemodynamically unstable patient with pericardial tamponade, typical echo findings include a dilated inferior vena cava, right atrial collapse, and then right ventricular collapse. Echocardiographically guided pericardiocentesis has now become a standard of care.

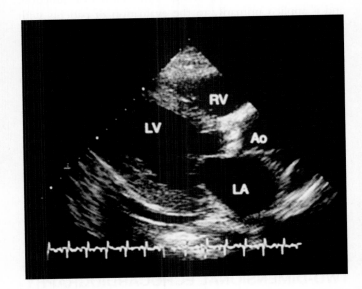

FIGURE 12-2
Two-dimensional echocardiographic still-frame images from a patient with aortic stenosis. Parasternal long-axis view shows a heavily calcified aortic valve. RV, right ventricle; LV, left ventricle; Ao, aorta; LA, left atrium.

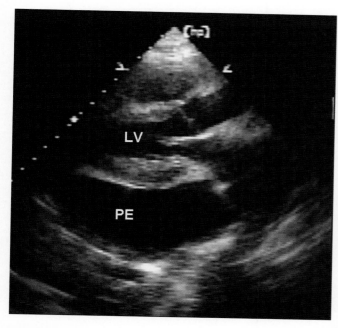

FIGURE 12-3

Two-dimensional echocardiographic still-frame image of a patient with a pericardial effusion. Pericardial effusion (PE) is shown as a black echo-free space surrounding the heart. LV, left ventricle.

Intracardiac masses

Intracardiac masses can be visualized on 2D echocardiography, provided that image quality is adequate. Solid masses appear as echo-dense structures, which can be located inside the cardiac chambers or infiltrating into the myocardium or pericardium. LV thrombus appears as an echo-dense structure, usually in the apical region associated with regional wall motion abnormalities. The appearance and mobility of the thrombus are predictive of embolic events. Vegetations appear as mobile linear echo densities attached to valve leaflets. Atrial myxoma can be diagnosed by the appearance of a

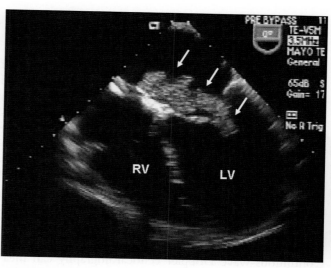

FIGURE 12-4

Transesophageal still-frame echocardiographic images of a patient with a left atrial myxoma. There is a large echo-dense mass in the left atrium, attached to the atrial septum. The mass moves across the mitral valve in diastole. LV, left ventricle; RV, right ventricle.

well-circumscribed mobile mass with attachments to the atrial septum (**Fig. 12-4**). The high-resolution images provided by TEE may be required for further delineation of myocardial masses, especially those <1 cm in diameter.

Aortic disease

2D echocardiography can provide extremely useful information on diseases of the aorta. The proximal ascending aorta, the arch, and the distal descending aorta can usually be visualized via the transthoracic approach. The definitive diagnosis of a suspected aortic dissection usually requires a TEE, which can rapidly provide high-resolution images of the proximal ascending and descending thoracic aorta (**Fig. 12-5**).

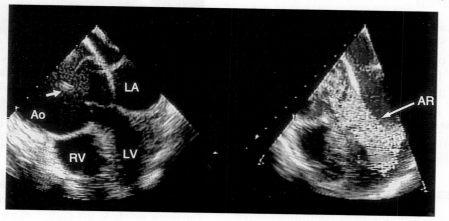

FIGURE 12-5

Transesophageal still-frame echocardiographic view of a patient with a dilated aorta, aortic dissection, and severe aortic regurgitation. The arrow points to the intimal flap that is seen in the dilated ascending aorta. **Left:** The long-axis apex-down view of the black-and-white two-dimensional image in diastole. **Right:** Color-flow imaging that demonstrates a large mosaic jet of aortic regurgitation. Ao, aorta; RV, right ventricle; AR, aortic regurgitation.

DOPPLER ECHOCARDIOGRAPHY

Basic principles

Doppler echocardiography uses ultrasound reflecting off moving red blood cells to measure the velocity of blood flow across valves, within cardiac chambers, and through the great vessels. Normal and abnormal blood flow patterns can be assessed noninvasively. Color-flow Doppler imaging displays the blood velocities in real time superimposed upon a 2D echocardiographic image. The different colors indicate the direction of blood flow (red toward and blue away from the transducer), with green superimposed when there is turbulent flow. Pulsed-wave Doppler measures the blood flow velocity in a specific location on the 2D echocardiographic image. Continuous-wave Doppler echocardiography can measure high velocities of blood flow directed along the line of the Doppler beam, such as occur in the presence of valve stenosis, valve regurgitation, or intracardiac shunts. These high velocities can be used to determine intracardiac pressure gradients by a modified Bernoulli equation:

$$\text{Pressure change} = 4 \text{ times (velocity)}^2$$

Tissue Doppler echocardiography measures the velocity of myocardial motion. Myocardial velocities can be used to determine myocardial strain rate, which is a quantitative measure of regional myocardial contraction and relaxation.

Valve gradients

In the presence of valvular stenosis, there is an increase in the velocity of blood flow across the stenotic valve. A continuous-wave Doppler can be used to determine the pressure gradient across the valve (Fig. 12-6). A valve area can also be calculated from the Doppler velocities.

Valvular regurgitation

Valvular regurgitation is diagnosed by Doppler echocardiography when there is abnormal retrograde flow across the valve. Color-flow imaging is the Doppler method used most frequently to detect valve regurgitation by visualization of a high-velocity turbulent jet in the chamber proximal to the regurgitant valve (Fig. 12-7). The size and extent of the color-flow jet into the receiving cardiac chamber provide a semiquantitative estimate of the severity of regurgitation.

Intracardiac pressures

These can be calculated from the peak continuous-wave Doppler signal of a regurgitant lesion, which reflects the pressure gradient between two cardiac chambers. This approach is commonly applied to a tricuspid regurgitant jet, from which the systolic pressure gradient between

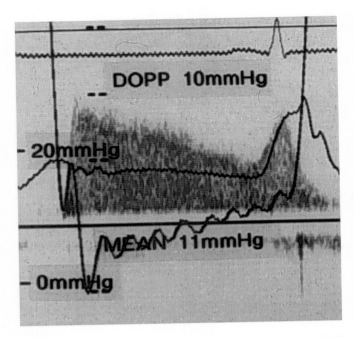

FIGURE 12-6
Continuous-wave Doppler of mitral valve velocities in a patient with mitral stenosis. The mean gradient calculated from Doppler (DOPP) of 10 mmHg is similar to the mean gradient of 11 mmHg from simultaneous cardiac catheterization in this patient.

the right atrium and right ventricle can be calculated, yielding an accurate measurement of pulmonary artery systolic pressure (Fig. 12-8).

Cardiac output

Volume flow rates (or stroke volume and cardiac output) can be reliably measured noninvasively by Doppler echocardiography. Flow is calculated as the product

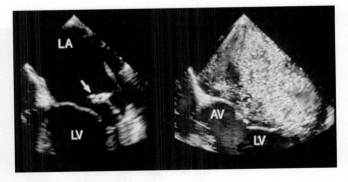

FIGURE 12-7
Left: Transesophageal echocardiographic view of a patient with severe mitral regurgitation due to a flail posterior leaflet. The arrow points to the portion of the posterior leaflet that is unsupported and moves into the left atrium during systole. *Right:* Color-flow imaging demonstrating a large mosaic jet of mitral regurgitation during systole. LA, left atrium; LV, left ventricle; AV, aortic valve.

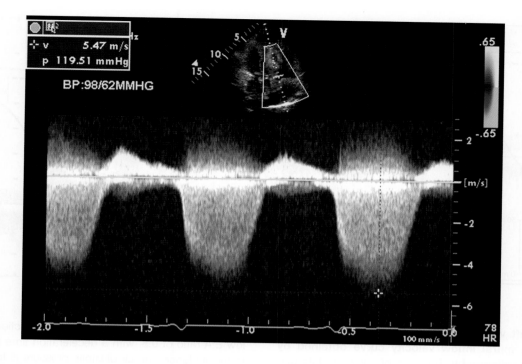

FIGURE 12-8

Continuous-wave Doppler of tricuspid regurgitation in a patient with pulmonary hypertension. There is an increase in the velocity to 5.4 m/s. Using the modified Bernoulli equation, the peak pressure gradient between the right ventricle and right atrium during systole is 116 mmHg. Assuming a right atrial pressure of 10 mmHg, the right ventricular systolic pressure is 126 mmHg. In the absence of right ventricular outflow tract obstruction, this indicates there is severe pulmonary hypertension with a pulmonary artery systolic pressure of 126 mmHg.

of the cross-sectional area of the vessel or chamber through which blood moves and the velocity of blood flow as assessed by Doppler.

Diastolic filling

Doppler echocardiography allows noninvasive evaluation of ventricular diastolic filling. The transmitral velocity curves reflect the relative pressure gradients between the left atrium and ventricle throughout diastole and are influenced by the rate of ventricular relaxation, the driving force across the valve, and the compliance of the ventricle. In the early phase of diastolic dysfunction there is primarily an impairment of LV relaxation, with reduced early transmitral flow and a compensatory increase in flow during atrial contraction (Fig. 12-9). As disease progresses and ventricular compliance declines, left atrial pressure rises, resulting in a higher early transmitral velocity and shortening of the deceleration of flow in early diastole. Analysis of Doppler tissue velocities of annular motion and myocardial strain provides further information concerning the diastolic properties of the heart.

Congenital heart disease

2D and Doppler echocardiography have been useful in the evaluation of patients with congenital heart disease.

Congenital stenotic or regurgitant valve lesions can be assessed. The detection of intracardiac shunts is possible by 2D and Doppler echocardiography. Patency of surgical shunts and conduits can also be evaluated.

STRESS ECHOCARDIOGRAPHY

2D and Doppler echocardiography are usually performed with the patient in the resting state. Further information can be obtained by reimaging during either exercise or pharmacologic stress. The primary indications for stress echocardiography are to confirm the suspicion of ischemic heart disease and determine the extent of ischemia.

A decrease in systolic contraction of an ischemic area (segment) of myocardium, termed a regional wall motion abnormality, occurs before symptoms or electrocardiographic changes (Fig. 12-10). New regional wall motion abnormalities, a decline in ejection fraction, and an increase in end-systolic volume with stress are all indicators of myocardial ischemia. Exercise stress testing is usually done with exercise protocols using either upright treadmill or bicycle exercise. In patients who are not able to exercise, pharmacologic testing can be performed by infusion of dobutamine to increase myocardial oxygen demand. Dobutamine echocardiography has also been used to assess myocardial viability in patients

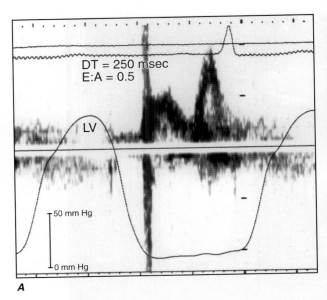

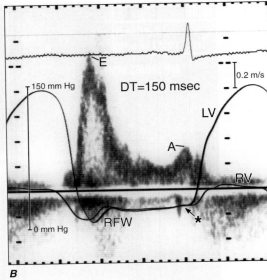

A

B

FIGURE 12-9

High-fidelity left ventricular (LV) pressure curves super-imposed on a mitral inflow velocity curve obtained by Doppler echocardiography. The ratio of early and late diastolic flows is termed the E:A ratio. The deceleration time (DT) measures the rate of decline of early velocity and reflects the effective operative compliance of the left ventricle. **Left:** In early stages of diastolic dysfunction, there is an abnormality of relaxation. There is a decrease in the early diastolic filling and an increase with filling at atrial contraction, resulting in a low E:A ratio of 0.5, with a deceleration time (DT) of 250 ms. In this instance, the LV diastolic pressure is low at 6 mmHg. **Right:** As diastolic dysfunction progresses, there is a restriction to filling, in which there is a high early diastolic velocity and low velocity at atrial contraction resulting in a high E:A ratio of 3.0, with DT of 150 ms. In this instance, the LV diastolic pressure is markedly elevated to 34 mmHg.

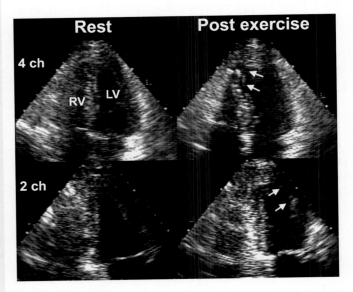

FIGURE 12-10

Systolic still-frame two-dimensional echocardiographic images of a patient undergoing a stress echocardiogram. During rest (**left**), there is contraction of all segments of the myocardium. During exercise (**right**), there are regional wall motion abnormalities in the anterior and anteroapical segments (**arrows**). 4 ch = four-chamber view, 2 ch = two-chamber views, LV = left ventricle, RV = right ventricle.

with poor systolic function and concomitant CAD; when used for this purpose, dobutamine is administered at lower doses than standard pharmacologic stress doses.

Doppler echocardiography can be used at rest and during exercise in patients with valvular heart disease to determine the hemodynamic response of valve gradients and pulmonary pressures (**Fig. 12–11**). In patients with low-output, low-gradient aortic stenosis, the response of the gradient to dobutamine stimulation is of diagnostic and therapeutic value.

TRANSESOPHAGEAL ECHOCARDIOGRAPHY

When limited information is obtained from a TTE due to poor imaging windows, TEE can be useful. Diseases of the aorta, such as aortic dissection, can be readily diagnosed by TEE. Defining the source of embolism is a common indication for TEE, as abnormalities such as atrial thrombi, patent foramen ovale, and aortic plaques can be detected. Other masses, particularly those in the atria, can be visualized. The presence of vegetations for the diagnosis of infective endocarditis and its complications can be assessed by TEE. This technique has been used before cardioversion in patients with atrial fibrillation to rule out a thrombus in the left atrium or left atrial appendage.

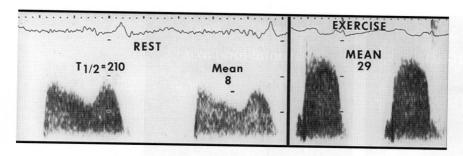

FIGURE 12-11
Continuous-wave Doppler echocardiogram across the mitral valve of a patient with mitral stenosis. In the resting state (***left***), there is a mean gradient of 8 mmHg. During exercise (***right***), the mean gradient rises to 29 mmHg, indicating a hemodynamically significant mitral stenosis.

NUCLEAR CARDIOLOGY

BASIC PRINCIPLES OF NUCLEAR CARDIOLOGY

Nuclear (or radionuclide) imaging requires intravenous administration of radiopharmaceuticals (isotopes or tracers). Once injected, the isotope traces physiologic processes and undergoes uptake in specific organs. During this process, radiation is emitted in the form of photons, generally gamma rays, generated during radioactive decay when the nucleus of an isotope changes from one energy level to a lower one. A special camera detects these photons and creates images via a computer interface. The two most commonly used technologies in clinical nuclear cardiology are single-photon emission computed tomography (SPECT) and positron emission tomography (PET). These technologies differ in instrumentation, acquisition, resolution, and nuclides used.

CLINICAL APPLICATIONS

Assessment of myocardial perfusion and coronary artery disease

Nuclear myocardial perfusion imaging (MPI) using SPECT and more recently PET has an established role in the evaluation and management of patients with known or suspected coronary artery disease (CAD). Both SPECT and PET MRI require the injection of

isotopes at rest and during stress to produce images of regional myocardial uptake proportional to regional blood flow. Normally, myocardial blood flow can be increased up to fivefold above the resting state to meet the increased myocardial oxygen demand during stress. In the presence of a fixed coronary stenosis, the inability to increase myocardial perfusion in the territory supplied by the stenosis creates a flow differential and inhomogeneous myocardial tracer uptake. In patients unable to exercise, pharmacologic agents are used to increase blood flow and create similar inhomogeneities.

The most commonly used SPECT perfusion tracers are thallium-201 (^{201}Tl) and technetium-99m (^{99m}Tc) labeled isonitriles. ^{99m}Tc isonitriles have higher photon energies and shorter physical half-lives than ^{201}Tl, permitting injection of higher doses with less radiation exposure while concurrently producing higher-quality images. The FDA-approved PET tracers are rubidium-82 (^{82}Rb) and ^{13}N ammonia (^{13}NH$_3$) for high-dose administration and shorter imaging protocols.

Both SPECT and PET myocardial perfusion images are commonly interpreted by visual analysis, which may be supplemented with quantitative software. Normal myocardial perfusion images demonstrate uniform tracer uptake throughout the LV myocardium (**Fig. 12-12**). In contrast, regions with reduced myocardial blood flow demonstrate varying degrees of reduced tracer uptake (**Fig. 12-13**), which can be graded on a semiquantitative scale. Reduced tracer uptake in a myocardial region

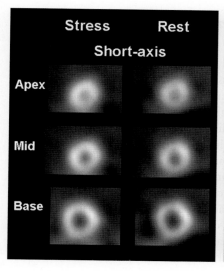

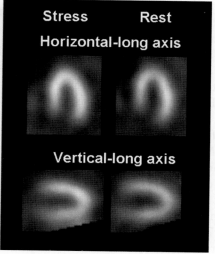

FIGURE 12-12
Exercise technetium-99m sestamibi images in a 65-year-old man with atypical angina. Images are shown in three standard views; stress (***left***) and rest (***right***) in each panel. There is uniform tracer uptake throughout the left ventricular myocardium at rest and peak stress in all three views.

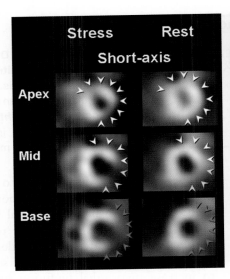
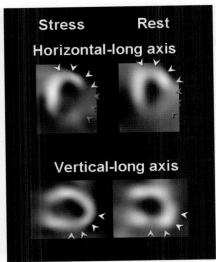

FIGURE 12-13

Exercise technetium-99m sestamibi and rest thallium-201 images in a 72-year-old woman with typical angina. Images are shown in three standard views, with stress (*left*) and rest (*right*) in each panel. Stress images demonstrate reduced tracer uptake in the apical, mid-anterior, mid-lateral, and mid-inferior regions (*white arrowheads*) with normal or near-normal tracer uptake in the corresponding regions on the rest images (*white arrowheads*), signifying a reversible defect consistent with ischemia. The lack of complete normalization (or reversibility) of tracer uptake on the rest images at the mid-inferior and mid-lateral regions represents associated infarction in that area (*yellow arrowheads*). On both stress and rest images, the basal inferior and basal lateral regions exhibit severely reduced tracer uptake, signifying a fixed defect consistent with infarction (*red arrowheads*). Subsequent invasive coronary angiography demonstrated severe stenosis of the mid-left anterior descending coronary artery and occlusion of the left circumflex coronary artery with collaterals.

on both resting and stress images is called a fixed defect and is consistent with infarction. Reduced tracer uptake on the stress image with relatively preserved or improved uptake on the rest image is called a reversible defect and indicates ischemia. PET has the ability to quantify myocardial blood flow and flow reserve in absolute terms.

For the diagnosis of angiographically significant CAD, SPECT using ^{201}Tl and ^{99m}Tc isonitriles and either exercise or pharmacologic stress has an average sensitivity of 87% and specificity of 73%. In comparison, PET MPI has higher accuracy (average sensitivity 90%; specificity of 89%). The robust methods for attenuation correction with PET improve the specificity, particularly in obese populations and women, while the superior resolution and higher extraction fraction of PET tracers increase the sensitivity **(Fig. 12-14)**. PET has not been as widely used as SPECT due to decreased availability and less local experience, but PET scanners are becoming more widely available **(Table 12-2)**.

Both SPECT and PET MPI have powerful prognostic value. In patients with normal SPECT MPI results, the annual rate of cardiac death or myocardial infarction is generally very low (<0.7%). Annual death/event rates increase with the extent and severity of imaging abnormalities and are generally about 3% in those with mild to moderate abnormalities and about 7% in those with severe abnormalities; rates are higher in specific populations such as diabetics and those with high-risk exercise treadmill results. High-risk SPECT MPI findings include severe resting or poststress LV systolic dysfunction, large or multiple stress-induced defects, or a large fixed defect with LV dilation or increased ^{201}Tl lung uptake. The incremental prognostic value of SPECT MPI has been established in many clinical settings, including populations with known CAD, prior myocardial infarction and/or revascularization, and acute chest pain in the emergency department.

Assessment of myocardial metabolism and viability

PET has traditionally been regarded as the gold standard technique for the assessment of myocardial viability. The positron-emitting tracer F-18 fluorodeoxyglucose (FDG) assesses myocardial glucose metabolism and is an indicator of myocardial viability. Because uptake is heterogeneous in normal myocardium in the fasting state, oral glucose loading or a combination of insulin and glucose infusions is used to enhance myocardial uptake. With reduced myocardial blood flow and ischemia, substrate utilization switches from fatty acids and lactate toward glucose, leading to enhanced myocardial FDG uptake. This pattern of enhanced FDG uptake in regions of decreased perfusion (termed flow/metabolism "mismatch") identifies areas

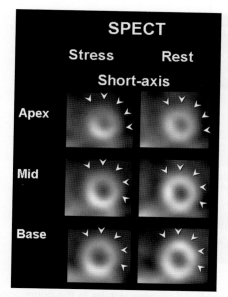

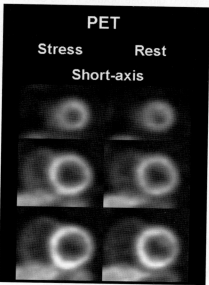

FIGURE 12-14

SPECT and PET images in a 67-year-old woman with atypical angina. Images are shown in short-axis views, with stress (***top***) and rest (***bottom***) in each panel. Shifting breast position between the rest and stress SPECT acquisitions produced an apparent reversible apical, anterior, and anterolateral attenuation artifact (*arrowheads*) resembling ischemia. With PET and its built-in attenuation correction in the same patient, the defect was not present. SPECT, single-photon emission computed tomography; PET, positron emission tomography.

of ischemic or hibernating myocardium that are likely to improve in function after revascularization (**Fig. 12-15**). This mismatch has a sensitivity and specificity of 92% and 63%, respectively, for regional contractile recovery after revascularization. The SPECT radiopharmaceuticals, ^{201}Tl and ^{99m}Tc isonitriles, require an intact (viable) cell membrane for uptake and also provide an assessment of myocardial viability in addition to perfusion. However, PET identifies ischemic or hibernating myocardium in 10–20%

TABLE 12-2

RELATIVE ADVANTAGES AND DISADVANTAGES OF SPECT AND PET

SPECT

Thallium-201

Lower radiopharmaceutical cost
Measurement of increased pulmonary uptake
Less hepatobiliary and bowel uptake
Detection of resting ischemia (hibernating myocardium)
Longer physical half-life of tracers (limiting dose administration)
Lower energy level

Technetium-99m isonitriles
Better image quality
Ventricular function assessment (gated SPECT)
Shorter imaging time
Shorter imaging protocols (patient/scheduling convenience)
Acute imaging in myocardial infarction and unstable angina
Superior quantification

PET
Robust attenuation correction
Short physical half-life of tracers
Best image quality (particularly in obese patients and women)
Shorter imaging time (particularly for rubidium-82)
Very short imaging protocols (particularly for rubidium-82)
More complex imaging protocols (particularly viability assessment)
Detection of viability
Absolute quantification
High diagnostic accuracy
Limited prognostic studies
N-13 ammonia requires on-site cyclotron
Rubidium-82 generally requires costly commercial generator
Lower radiation exposure, particularly for N-13 ammonia

High Risk Perfusion Imaging Features
Severe resting or exercise LV systolic dysfunction (EF<35%)
Stress-induced large perfusion defect (especially if anterior)
Stress-induced multiple perfusion defects of moderate size
Large, fixed perfusion defect with LV dilatation
Transient (poststress) LV dilatation
Increased lung uptake (thallium)

Abbreviatons: EF, ejection fraction; LV, left ventricle; PET, positron emission tomography; SPECT, single–photon emission computed tomography.

of regions otherwise classified as fibrotic (infarcted) by SPECT perfusion tracers. Patients with ischemic heart failure, who have viable myocardium identified by PET or SPECT and undergo revascularization, have a better survival than those who do not have viable myocardium or do not undergo revascularization.

Assessment of ventricular function

In addition to perfusion and metabolic information, LV systolic function and volumes are now routinely obtained with gated SPECT and PET acquisitions, as long as the heart rate is relatively constant. An automated technique determines the endocardial borders of the LV cavity, and a geometric model is used to calculate the LVEF and

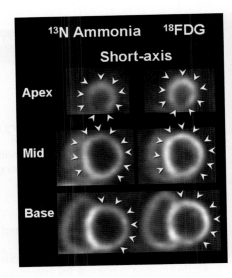
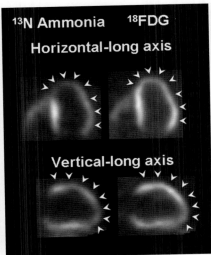

FIGURE 12-15

PET viability study in a 63-year-old woman with heart failure, severe LV systolic dysfunction, and severe coronary artery disease. Images are shown in three standard views, with perfusion (*left*) and glucose metabolism (*right*) in each panel. The N-13 ammonia images show a very large apical, septal, anterior, and lateral perfusion defect (*arrowheads*), but F-18 fluorodeoxyglucose (18FDG) images demonstrate relatively preserved glucose uptake in the corresponding segments (*arrowheads*). This PET perfusion-metabolism mismatch is consistent with hibernating myocardium. The patient underwent coronary artery bypass grafting surgery with improvement in left ventricular systolic function (ejection fraction increased from 26% pre- to 45% postoperatively). All regions identified as viable recovered contractile function after revascularization.

volumes with a high level of reproducibility. Regional wall motion can also be assessed by visual examination. The combined variables of perfusion and function are more effective in risk stratification than either alone.

Another established but less widely available nuclear technique for assessing LV function and volumes is equilibrium radionuclide angiography RNA, also known as multiple-gated blood pool acquisition (MUGA). This technique involves imaging of ^{99m}Tc-labeled albumin or red cells that are uniformly distributed throughout the blood volume. LV volumes throughout the cardiac cycle are calculated from a time-activity curve generated using regions of interest.

Innovations in hybrid imaging technology, especially PET/CT and SPECT/CT, are occurring rapidly and contribute to their emerging role in the combined assessments of anatomy and physiology in patients with suspected or known CAD. The diagnostic literature is evolving for these hybrid technologies but radiation exposure is a concern and large-scale clinical trials are still needed to validate their clinical applications, determine their prognostic value, and address their cost-effectiveness and appropriateness.

MRI AND CT IMAGING

MAGNETIC RESONANCE IMAGING

Basic principles

MRI is a technique based on the magnetic properties of hydrogen nuclei. In the presence of a large magnetic field, nuclear spin transitions from the ground state to excited states can be induced by an electric field, and as the nuclei relax and return to their ground state, they release energy in the form of electromagnetic radiation that is detected and processed into an image. Although the large vascular vessels can be visualized on MRI without contrast agents, gadolinium is frequently employed as a contrast agent to produce magnetic resonance angiograms (MRAs). Contrast agents also provide enhanced soft tissue contrast as well as the opportunity to obtain rapid angiographic images during the first pass of contrast through the vascular system.

Cardiac MRI is challenging because of the rapid motion of the heart and coronary arteries. However, both static and cine images can usually now be obtained using electrocardiographic triggering, often within short breath holds of 10–15 s. Cine images can be acquired in any plane with excellent blood-myocardial contrast. These images can be used to quantify accurately ejection fraction, end-systolic and end-diastolic volumes, and cardiac mass with high accuracy, reliability, and reproducibility, and without the need for ionizing radiation.

Clinical utility

The multiplanar capabilities of MRI, coupled with excellent contrast and spatial resolution, provide superb images of the myocardium and great vessels. MRI is of great value in defining anatomic relationships in patients with complex congenital heart disease (**Fig. 12-16**) and cardiomyopathies (**Fig. 12-17**). Cardiac masses can be characterized and distinguished from thrombus

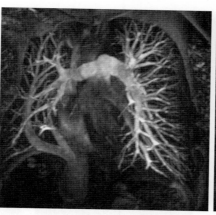
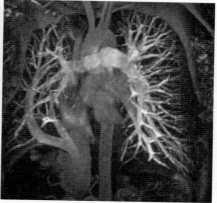

FIGURE 12-16

MRA scan of a patient with partial anomalous pulmonary venous drainage of the right lung into the inferior vena cava (scimitar syndrome). MRA is able to define the abnormal anatomic relationships of cardiac structures and great vessels in patients with congenital heart disease.

(Fig. 12–18). In addition to defining their relationship to normal anatomic structures, MRI can determine whether a mediastinal or pulmonary mass has invaded the pericardium or heart. The entire pericardium can be visualized in multiple planes, and MRI has proved useful in characterizing pericardial effusions, pericardial thickening, and inflammation. Specialized pulse sequences can measure the velocity of blood in each pixel of the image, so that flow across valves and within blood vessels may be determined with accuracy, thereby aiding in the evaluation of valvular disease and intracardiac shunts.

MRA is a standard technique for imaging the aorta and large vessels of the chest and abdomen, with results essentially identical to conventional angiography. MRA of the coronary arteries is a much more difficult challenge, both because of the small size of these vessels and because of their rapid and complex motion during the cardiac cycle; thus, coronary MRA is not yet a reliable clinical technique.

MRI is now an accepted technology for the evaluation of patients with suspected or known coronary disease. Ventricular function and wall motion can be assessed at rest and during infusion of inotropic agents.

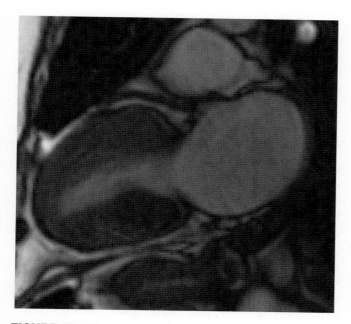

FIGURE 12-17

MRI scan of a patient with hypertrophic cardiomyopathy, showing the severe increase in left ventricular wall thickness. Cardiac MRI is an ideal imaging modality for diagnosing cardiomyopathies.

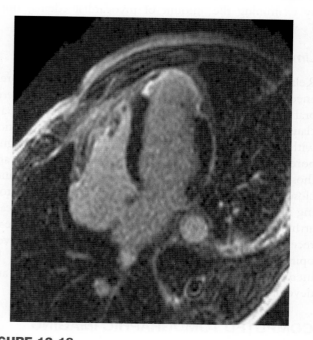

FIGURE 12-18

MRI scan with delayed gadolinium enhancement in a patient with a large anteroapical infarction. The gadolinium (white area) accumulated in the extracellular space in the presence of cell death from myocardial infarction.

Assessment of myocardial perfusion can be performed by injecting a bolus of gadolinium contrast and then continuously scanning the heart as the gadolinium passes through the cardiac chambers and into the myocardium. Relative perfusion deficits are reflected as regions of low signal intensity within the myocardium. Pharmacologic stress (typically achieved with vasodilators) can be applied during perfusion imaging to detect physiologically significant coronary artery lesions. Myocardial perfusion imaging with cardiac MRI is more sensitive than SPECT imaging for detecting subendocardial ischemia due to its enhanced spatial resolution.

Myocardial viability and infarction may be determined by imaging the heart 10–20 min after gadolinium injection, known as delayed enhancement magnetic resonance imaging. In normal myocardium, gadolinium cannot penetrate the membranes of the densely packed myocytes. Abnormal myocardial tissue accumulates excess gadolinium following intravenous injection, as ruptured myocyte membranes allow gadolinium to passively diffuse into intracellular space. In chronic infarction, the tissue concentration of gadolinium is increased due to an expansion of the intracellular space from collagenous scar (Fig. 12-18). Thus, delayed enhancement is indicative of nonviable or infarcted myocardium, the subendocardial versus transmural extent of which is accurately assessed by the high spatial resolution of MRI. The presence and pattern of gadolinium enhancement not only is useful for determining viability but also has prognostic value in the patient with an ischemic cardiomyopathy. "Myocardium at risk" following myocardial infarction can be assessed by examining the amount of myocardial edema, using T_2-weighted sequences (Fig. 12–19).

Limitations of MRI

Relative contraindications to MRI include the presence of pacemakers, internal defibrillators, or cerebral aneurysm clips. A small percentage of patients are claustrophobic and unable to tolerate the examination within the relatively confined quarters of the magnet bore. Examination of clinically unstable patients and those undergoing stress testing is problematic, since close hemodynamic and electrocardiographic monitoring is difficult. Image quality in patients with significant arrhythmias is often limited. Patients with renal disease receiving gadolinium contrast may be at risk of developing nephrogenic systemic fibrosis, characterized by increased tissue deposition of collagen in the skin and development of fibrosis in skin and other organs.

COMPUTED TOMOGRAPHIC IMAGING

Basic principles

CT is a fast, simple, noninvasive technique that provides images of the myocardium and great vessels with excellent spatial resolution and good soft tissue contrast.

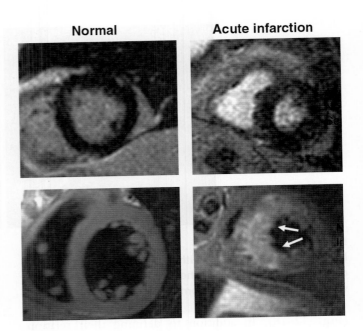

Normal   **Acute infarction**

FIGURE 12-19

Left: Normal delayed enhancement and "edema"-sensitive images. **Top (*left*):** Delayed enhancement image illustrating normal black myocardium without infarction/fibrosis. **Bottom (*left*):** A triple inversion recovery sequence that is T2-weighted demonstrating normal homogenous-appearing gray myocardium. *Right:* A patient postmyocardial infarction and early revascularization without evidence of an infarction and an edematous myocardium in the septum. **Top (*right*):** Delayed enhanced with normal black myocardium without infarction or fibrosis. **Bottom (*right*):** A triple inversion recovery sequence illustrating edema in the septum without infarction. This is the area of "salvaged" myocardium.

The development of electron-beam CT and multidetector-row CT have led to improved temporal resolution and routine imaging of the beating heart. Motion-free high-spatial-resolution images are now possible with multidetector CT technology ($\geq$64 channel) that allows imaging of the coronary arteries.

Clinical applications

Cardiac CT has important clinical applications. Pericardial calcification is easily detected by CT (Fig. 12-20). CT is useful in characterizing cardiac masses, particularly those containing fat or calcium. The ability to detect small amounts of fat with high spatial resolution makes CT an attractive technique for imaging patients with suspected arrhythmogenic right ventricular dysplasia. Cine images can be used to evaluate wall motion and to determine ejection fraction, end-diastolic and end-systolic volumes, and cardiac mass.

CT angiography (CTA) has demonstrated accuracy similar to MRA in imaging the aorta and great vessels, and CTA is the examination of choice in the evaluation of patients with suspected pulmonary embolus. CTA is an excellent imaging modality for the diagnosis of aortic

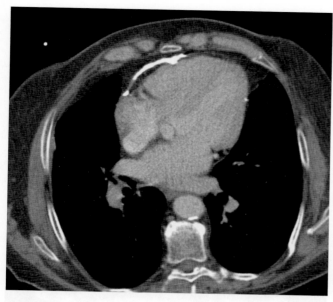

FIGURE 12-20
CT scan showing pericardial calcification, seen as a white linear density anterior to the myocardium.

dissection or penetrating ulcers. Complete visualization of the entire aorta and its branches is possible by CTA using a single contrast medial bolus injection.

Coronary calcification

Calcium in the coronary arteries occurs in athero-sclerosis and is absent in the normal coronary artery **(Fig. 12-21)**. CT is very sensitive for the detection of coronary artery calcification, and the absence of coronary calcification excludes significant epicardial coronary disease. The quantity of coronary calcification (coronary calcium score) is related to the severity of CAD and prognosis. However, the utility of CT calcification score in clinical practice in the asymptomatic patient is limited to those with a moderate risk of coronary heart disease in whom the result will change management.

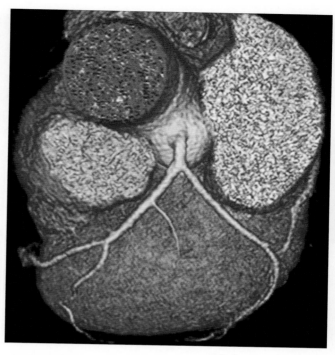

FIGURE 12-22
Three-dimensional volume rendered image of a contrast-enhanced CT angiogram demonstrating a normal left main coronary artery arising from the aorta and its two branches, the left anterior descending artery (***left***) and the circumflex artery (***right***).

Contrast-enhanced CT angiography

With the high temporal and spatial resolution of multislice spiral CT, accurate assessment of luminal narrowing in the major branches of the coronary arteries is possible in selected patients. Studies at experienced centers have shown a sensitivity and specificity of >90% for detecting coronary artery lesions as compared to cardiac catheterization. The highest accuracy has been noted in the left main and the proximal portions of the left-sided coronary arteries with decreased sensitivities in the more distal segments and in the more rapidly moving right coronary artery **(Fig. 12-22)**.

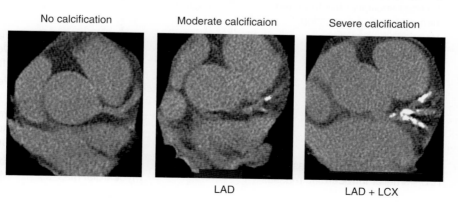

No calcification　　　Moderate calcificaion　　　Severe calcification

LAD　　　　　　LAD + LCX

FIGURE 12-21
CT scans of three patients showing the ability to detect coronary calcification. ***Left:*** Normal coronary arteries without calcification. ***Middle:*** Calcification in the left anterior

artery (LAD). ***Right:*** Severe calcification in the LAD and circumflex (CX) arteries.

The concept of "noninvasive coronary angiography" has generated great interest in CTA. However, as with any imaging modalities, CTA has technical limitations requiring proper patient selection and preparation. The integration of CTA into clinical practice requires knowledge of pretest diagnostic and prognostic data and the incremental information that will alter management. The well-accepted indication for coronary CTA is in the evaluation of suspected coronary artery anomalies for which CTA not only confirms the diagnosis but also shows the course of the arteries related to the great vessels (Fig. 12-23). For patients with chest pain syndromes, CTA is best used to rule out significant coronary disease, given its high negative predictive value. Thus, it is the patient with an intermediate pretest probability of CAD who cannot exercise or has uninterpretable or equivocal results on prior testing who would be best suited for CTA. The benefit of CTA in other groups of patients is still unclear.

Limitations of CT

Limitations of CT include its dependence on ionizing radiation (in contrast to MRI) and the need for iodinated contrast. Techniques to lower radiation doses continue to evolve, as the radiation doses for coronary CTA generally exceed those delivered during standard diagnostic cardiac catheterization. Fast or irregular heart rhythms and body motion limit the accuracy of CTA. Heavy calcification and artifacts from stents preclude accurate assessment of the severity of a stenosis.

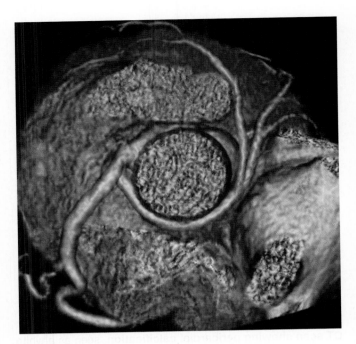

FIGURE 12-23

Three-dimensional volume rendered image of a contrast-enhanced CT angiogram illustrating an anomalous left coronary artery arising from the right coronary artery and traveling posterior to the aorta.

SELECTION OF IMAGING TESTS (TABLE 12-3)

BASIC PREMISE

The choice of the optimal imaging modality for a particular patient should be based upon the major problem

TABLE 12-3

SELECTION OF IMAGING TESTS

	ECHO	NUCLEAR	CT[a]	MRI[b]
LV size/function	Initial modality of choice Low cost, portable Provides ancillary structural and hemodynamic information	Available from gated SPECT or PET imaging	Best resolution Highest cost	Best resolution Highest cost
Valve disease	Initial modality of choice Valve motion Doppler hemodynamics			Visualize valve motion Delineate abnormal flow
Pericardial disease	Pericardial effusion Doppler hemodynamics		Pericardial thickening	Pericardial thickening
Aortic disease	TEE rapid diagnosis[c] Acute dissection		Image entire aorta Acute aneurysm Aortic dissection	Image entire aorta Aortic aneurysm Chronic dissection
Cardiac masses	TTE—large intracardiac masses TEE—smaller intracardiac masses[c]		Extracardiac masses Myocardial masses	Extracardiac masses Myocardial masses

[a]Contrast required.
[b]Relative contraindication: pacemakers, metallic objects, claustrophobic.
[c]When not seen on TTE.
Abbreviations: Echo, echocardiography; PET, positron emission tomography; SPECT, single-photon emission computed tomography; TEE, transesophageal echocardiography; TTE, transthoracic echocardiogram.

being addressed, other concomitant clinical questions, as well as the local expertise and equipment available in an institution. The clinical urgency and costs of each test also need to be considered. To ensure the effective use of cardiovascular imaging tools, Appropriateness Criteria have been developed by the national societies to examine the incremental clinical benefit of imaging modalities.

COMMON CLINICAL QUESTIONS

Left ventricular size and function

2D echocardiography is the primary imaging modality obtained for assessment of LV cavity size, systolic function, and wall thickness. Echocardiography can also provide concomitant information on valve function, pulmonary artery pressures, and diastolic filling, which are valuable in the patient presenting with possible heart failure. The disadvantage is poor endocardial resolution in some patients and the lack of reproducible quantitative measurements.

Equilibrium radionuclide angiography can provide an accurate quantitative measurement of LV volumes and function but is not widely available and cannot be used in patients with irregular rhythms. Gated SPECT and PET measure LV systolic function and volumes as a part of myocardial perfusion and/or viability imaging but also require relatively regular rhythm. Both MRI and CT scanning provide the highest quality resolution of the endocardial border and, thus, are the most accurate of all modalities. However, they are of higher cost, lack portability, and do not provide concomitant hemodynamic information as echocardiography does.

Valvular heart disease

2D and Doppler echocardiography provide both anatomic and hemodynamic information regarding valve disease, and are the first test of choice. MRI can also visualize valve motion and determine abnormal flow velocities across valves, but there is less validation of quantitative hemodynamic measurements in comparison to echocardiography.

Pericardial disease

Echocardiography is the first imaging modality of choice in patients with suspected pericardial effusion and tamponade owing to its rapid image display and portability. For patients with suspected constrictive pericarditis, either MRI or CT scanning is the imaging modality that best delineates pericardial thickness. Hemodynamic analysis of the enhancement of ventricular interaction that occurs in pericardial constriction can be assessed by Doppler echocardiography.

Aortic disease

Both CT scanning and MRI are the imaging modalities of choice for the evaluation of the stable patient with suspected aortic aneurysm or aortic dissection. In the acutely ill patient with suspected aortic dissection, either TEE or CT scanning is a reliable imaging modality.

Cardiac masses

2D TTE is the first test to rule out an intracardiac mass; masses >1.0 cm in diameter are usually well visualized. Intracardiac masses of smaller size may be visualized by TEE. CT scanning and MRI are optimal for evaluating masses extrinsic to the heart or involving the myocardium.

CHOOSING THE APPROPRIATE IMAGING TEST FOR THE EVALUATION OF KNOWN OR SUSPECTED CAD

The choice of an initial test should be based on the evaluation of the patient's resting electrocardiogram, the ability to perform exercise, the clinical features, the patient's body habitus, and the available local expertise and technology (Fig. 12-24). For the standard assessment of CAD, the exercise electrocardiographic test should be the initial consideration in patients with an interpretable electrocardiogram who are able to exercise. If there are resting electrocardiographic abnormalities, or if the patient has had prior coronary revascularization, an imaging modality (either nuclear imaging or echocardiography) should be used for initial evaluation. Imaging tests can add prognostic information to a standard exercise electrocardiographic test and, thus, are especially useful when the initial results fall into an intermediate risk category. Pharmacologic stress testing with imaging should be used in patients who are unable to exercise. The utility of CT coronary angiography is evolving.

While the patient is often best evaluated with the imaging modality for which most experience and expertise are available, there are additional considerations and certain situations where one imaging modality has an advantage over another. Echocardiography provides structural information. Therefore, if there is a question of concomitant valve disease, pericardial disease, or aortic disease, stress echocardiography should be considered. In patients with previous infarction and/or LV systolic dysfunction on the basis of CAD, nuclear imaging, particularly PET, or MRI, is the preferred modality as it also establishes viability. In general, nuclear imaging is more sensitive and less specific than echocardiography for the detection of myocardial ischemia and viability.

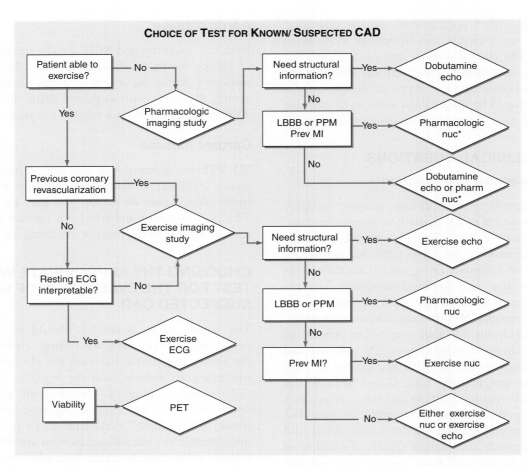

CHOICE OF TEST FOR KNOWN/ SUSPECTED CAD

FIGURE 12-24

Flow diagram showing selection of initial stress test in a patient with chest pain. Patients who are able to exercise, without previous revascularization, and with an interpretable resting ECG can be tested with an exercise ECG. The appropriate imaging study for other patients depends on multiple factors (see text). LBBB, left bundle branch block; Prev MI-Reg ischemia, previous MI with a need to detect regional ischemia; nuc, SPECT nuclear imaging study; Pharm, pharmacologic. *Consider PET if morbidly obese or female with large/dense breasts.

CHAPTER 13

DIAGNOSTIC CARDIAC CATHETERIZATION AND CORONARY ANGIOGRAPHY

Jane A. Leopold ■ David P. Faxon

Diagnostic cardiac catheterization and coronary angiography are considered the gold standard in the assessment of the anatomy and physiology of the heart and its associated vasculature. In 1929, Forssmann demonstrated the feasibility of cardiac catheterization in humans when he passed a urological catheter from a vein in his arm to his right atrium and documented the catheter's position in the heart by x-ray. In the 1940s, Cournand and Richards applied this technique to patients with cardiovascular disease to evaluate cardiac function. These three physicians were awarded the Nobel Prize in 1956. In 1958, Sones inadvertently performed the first selective coronary angiography when a catheter in the left ventricle slipped back across the aortic valve, engaged the right coronary artery, and power-injected 40 mL of contrast down the vessel. The resulting angiogram provided superb anatomic detail of the artery, and the patient suffered no adverse effects. Sones went on to develop selective coronary catheters, which were modified further by Judkins, who developed preformed catheters and allowed coronary artery angiography to gain widespread use as a diagnostic tool. In the United States, cardiac catheterization is the second most common operative procedure, with nearly 3 million procedures performed annually.

CARDIAC CATHETERIZATION

INDICATIONS, RISKS, AND PREPROCEDURE MANAGEMENT

Cardiac catheterization and coronary angiography are indicated to evaluate the extent and severity of cardiac disease in symptomatic patients and to determine if medical, surgical, or catheter-based interventions are warranted (Table 13-1). They are also used to exclude severe disease in symptomatic patients with equivocal findings on noninvasive studies and in patients with chest-pain syndromes of unclear etiology for whom a definitive diagnosis is necessary for management. Cardiac catheterization is not mandatory prior to cardiac surgery in some younger patients who have congenital or valvular heart disease that is well defined by noninvasive imaging and who do not have symptoms or risk factors that suggest concomitant coronary artery disease.

The risks associated with elective cardiac catheterization are relatively low, with a reported risk of 0.05% for myocardial infarction, 0.07% for stroke, and 0.08–0.14% for death. These risks increase substantially if the catheterization is performed emergently, during acute myocardial infarction, or in hemodynamically unstable patients. Additional risks of the procedure include tachy- or bradyarrhythmias that require countershock or pharmacologic therapy, acute renal failure leading to transient or permanent dialysis, vascular complications that necessitate surgical repair, and significant access-site bleeding. Of these risks, vascular access-site bleeding is the most common complication, occurring in 1.5–2.0% of patients, with major bleeding events associated with a worse short- and long-term outcome.

In patients who understand and accept the risks associated with cardiac catheterization, there are no absolute contraindications when the procedure is performed in anticipation of a life-saving intervention. Relative contraindications do, however, exist; these include decompensated congestive heart failure; acute renal failure; severe chronic renal insufficiency, unless dialysis is planned; bacteremia; acute stroke; active gastrointestinal bleeding; severe, uncorrected electrolyte abnormalities; a history of an anaphylactic/anaphylactoid reaction to iodinated contrast agents; and a history of allergy/bronchospasm to aspirin in patients for whom progression to a percutaneous coronary intervention is likely.

Contrast allergy and contrast-induced renal failure merit further consideration, because these adverse

TABLE 13-1

INDICATIONS FOR CARDIAC CATHETERIZATION AND CORONARY ANGIOGRAPHY

CORONARY ARTERY DISEASE

Asymptomatic or Symptomatic

High risk for adverse outcome based on noninvasive testing

Sudden cardiac death

Sustained (>30 s) monomorphic ventricular tachycardia

Nonsustained (<30 s) polymorphic ventricular tachycardia

Symptomatic

Canadian Cardiology Society class III or IV angina on medical therapy

Unstable angina—high or intermediate risk

Chest-pain syndrome of unclear etiology and equivocal findings on noninvasive tests

Acute Myocardial Infarction

Reperfusion with primary percutaneous coronary intervention

Persistent or recurrent ischemia

Severe pulmonary edema

Cardiogenic shock or hemodynamic instability

Mechanical complications—mitral regurgitation, ventricular septal defect

VALVULAR HEART DISEASE

Suspected valve disease in symptomatic patients—dyspnea, angina, heart failure, syncope

Infective endocarditis with coronary embolization

Asymptomatic patients with aortic regurgitation and cardiac enlargement or ↓ ejection fraction

Prevalve surgery in older patients with coronary artery disease risk factors

CONGESTIVE HEART FAILURE

New onset with angina or suspected undiagnosed coronary artery disease

CONGENITAL HEART DISEASE

Prior to surgical correction, when symptoms or noninvasive testing suggests coronary disease

Suspicion for congenital coronary anomalies

Forms of congenital heart disease associated with coronary anomalies

PERICARDIAL DISEASE

Symptomatic patients with suspected cardiac tamponade or constrictive pericarditis

CARDIAC TRANSPLANTATION

Preoperative and postsurgical evaluation

OTHER CONDITIONS

Hypertrophic cardiomyopathy with angina

Diseases of the aorta when knowledge of coronary artery involvement is necessary for management

Source: Adapted from American College of Cardiology/American Heart Association Ad Hoc Task Force on Practice Guidelines: ACC/AHA Guidelines for Coronary Angiography. Circulation 1999;99:2345–2357.

events may occur in otherwise healthy individuals and prophylactic measures exist to reduce risk. Allergic reactions to contrast agents occur in <5% of cases with severe anaphylactoid (clinically indistinguishable from anaphylaxis, but not mediated by an IgE mechanism) reactions occurring in 0.1–0.2% of patients. Mild reactions manifest as nausea, vomiting, and urticaria, while severe anaphylactoid reactions lead to hypotensive shock, pulmonary edema, and cardiorespiratory arrest. Patients with a history of significant contrast allergy should be premedicated with corticosteroids and antihistamines (H_1- and H_2-blockers) and studies performed with nonionic, low-osmolar contrast agents that have a lower reported rate of allergic reactions.

Contrast-induced nephropathy, defined as an increase in creatinine >0.5 mg/dL or 25% above baseline that occurs 48–72 h after contrast administration, occurs in ~2–7% of patients with rates of 20–30% reported in high-risk patients, including those with diabetes mellitus, congestive heart failure, chronic kidney disease, anemia, and older age. Dialysis is required in 0.3–0.7% of patients and is associated with a five-fold increase in in-hospital mortality. For all patients, adequate intravascular volume expansion with intravenous 0.9% saline (1.0–1.5 mL/kg per hour) for 3–12 h before and continued 6–24 h after the procedure limits the risk of contrast-induced nephropathy. In patients with chronic kidney disease, additional pretreatment with *N*-acetylcysteine (Mucomist, 600 mg bid orally before and two days after catheterization) also decreases risk. Diabetic patients treated with metformin should stop the drug 48 h prior to the procedure to limit the associated risk of lactic acidosis. Other strategies to decrease risk include the administration of sodium bicarbonate, although there is conflicting data regarding its efficacy; use of low- or iso-osmolar contrast agents; and limiting the volume of contrast to <100 mL per procedure.

Cardiac catheterization is performed after the patient has fasted for 6 h and has received IV conscious sedation to remain awake but sedated during the procedure. All patients with suspected coronary artery disease are pretreated with 325 mg aspirin. In patients in whom the procedure is likely to progress to a percutaneous coronary intervention, a clopidogrel 600-mg loading dose followed by 75 mg daily should be started. Warfarin is held starting 48 h prior to the catheterization to allow the international normalized ratio (INR) to fall to <2.0 and limit access-site bleeding complications. Cardiac catheterization is a sterile procedure, so antibiotic prophylaxis is not required.

TECHNIQUE

Cardiac catheterization and coronary angiography provide a detailed hemodynamic and anatomic assessment of the heart and coronary arteries. The selection of procedures is dependent upon the patient's symptoms and clinical condition, with some direction provided by noninvasive studies.

Vascular access

Cardiac catheterization procedures are performed using a percutaneous technique to enter the femoral artery and vein as the preferred access sites for left and right heart catheterization, respectively. A flexible sheath is inserted into the vessel over a guidewire, allowing diagnostic catheters to be introduced into the vessel and advanced toward the heart using fluoroscopic guidance. The brachial or radial artery may also be used as an arterial access site in patients with peripheral arterial disease that involves the abdominal aorta, iliac, or femoral vessels; severe iliac-artery tortuosity; morbid obesity; or preference for early postprocedure ambulation. Use of radial-artery access is gaining popularity owing to a lower rate of access-site bleeding complications. A normal Allen's test confirming dual blood supply to the hand from the radial and ulnar arteries is a prerequisite to access this site. The internal jugular vein serves as an alternate access site to the right heart when the patient has an inferior vena cava filter in place or requires prolonged hemodynamic monitoring.

Right heart catheterization

This procedure measures pressures in the right heart. Right heart catheterization is no longer a routine part of diagnostic cardiac catheterization, but it is reasonable in patients with unexplained dyspnea, valvular heart disease, pericardial disease, right and/or left ventricular dysfunction, congenital heart disease, and suspected intracardiac shunts. Right heart catheterization uses a balloon-tipped flotation catheter that is inserted into the femoral or jugular vein. Using fluoroscopic guidance, the catheter is advanced sequentially to the right atrium, right ventricle, pulmonary artery, and pulmonary wedge position (as a surrogate for left atrial pressure); in each cardiac chamber, pressure is measured and blood samples are obtained for oxygen-saturation analysis to screen for intracardiac shunts.

Left heart catheterization

This procedure measures pressures in the left heart as a determinant of left ventricular performance. With the aid of fluoroscopy, a catheter is guided to the ascending aorta and across the aortic valve into the left ventricle to provide a direct measure of left ventricular pressure. In patients with a tilting-disc prosthetic aortic valve, crossing the valve with a catheter is contraindicated and the left heart may be accessed from the right atrium using a needle-tipped catheter to puncture the atrial septum at the fossa ovalis. Once the catheter crosses from the right to the left atrium, it can be advanced across the mitral valve to the left ventricle. This technique is also used for mitral valvuloplasty. Heparin is given for prolonged procedures to limit the risk of stroke from embolism of clots that may form on the catheter.

HEMODYNAMICS

A comprehensive hemodynamic assessment involves obtaining pressure measurements in the right and left heart and peripheral arterial system and determining the cardiac output (Table 13-2). The shape and magnitude of the pressure waveforms provide important diagnostic information; an example of normal pressure tracings is shown in Fig. 13-1. In the absence of valvular heart disease, the atria and ventricles are "one chamber" during diastole when the tricuspid and mitral valves are open while in systole, when the pulmonary and aortic valves are open, the ventricles and their respective outflow tracts are considered "one chamber." These concepts form the basis by which hemodynamic measurements are used to assess valvular stenosis. When aortic stenosis is present, there is a systolic pressure gradient between the left ventricle and the aorta; when mitral stenosis is present, there is a diastolic pressure gradient between the pulmonary capillary wedge

TABLE 13-2

NORMAL VALUES FOR HEMODYNAMIC MEASUREMENTS	
Pressures (mmHg)	
Right atrium	
Mean	0–5
a wave	1–7
v wave	1–7
Right ventricle	
Peak systolic/end diastolic	17–32/1–7
Pulmonary artery	
Peak systolic/end diastolic	17–32/1–7
Mean	9–19
Pulmonary capillary wedge (mean)	4–12
Left atrium	
Mean	4–12
a wave	4–15
v wave	4–15
Left ventricle	
Peak systolic/end diastolic	90–140/5–12
Aorta	
Peak systolic/end diastolic	90–140/60–90
Mean	70–105
Resistances ([dyn-s]/cm^5)	
Systemic vascular resistance	900–1400
Pulmonary vascular resistance	40–120
Oxygen Consumption Index ([L-min]/m^2)	115–140
Arteriovenous oxygen difference (vol %)	3.5–4.8
Cardiac index ([L-min]/m^2)]	2.8–4.2

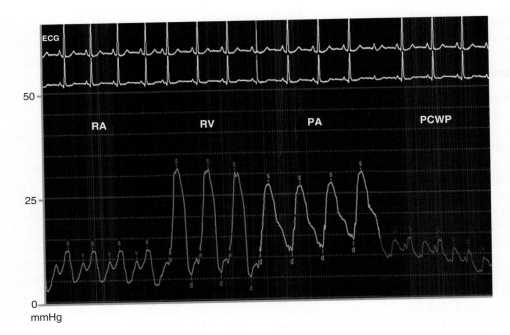

FIGURE 13-1

Normal hemodynamic waveforms recorded during right heart catheterization. Atrial pressure tracings have a characteristic "*a*" wave that reflects atrial contraction and a "*v*" wave that reflects pressure changes in the atrium during ventricular systole. Ventricular pressure tracings have a low

pressure diastolic filling period and a sharp rise in pressure that occurs during ventricular systole. RA, right atrium; RV, right ventricle; PA, pulmonary artery; PCWP, pulmonary capillary wedge pessure; s, systole; d, diastole.

(left atrial) pressure and the left ventricle (**Fig. 13-2**). Hemodynamic measurements also discriminate between aortic stenosis and hypertrophic obstructive cardiomyopathy where the asymmetrically hypertrophied septum

creates a dynamic intraventricular pressure gradient during ventricular systole. The magnitude of this obstruction is measured using an end-hole catheter positioned at the left ventricular apex that is pulled back while

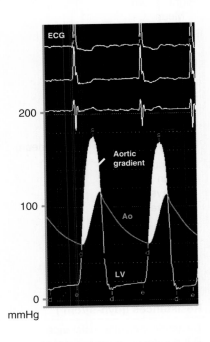

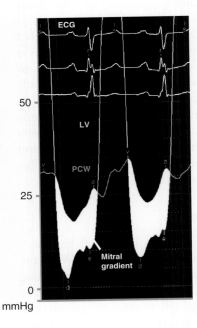

FIGURE 13-2

Severe aortic and mitral stenosis. Simultaneous recording of left ventricular (LV) and aortic (Ao) pressure tracings demonstrate a 62-mmHg mean systolic gradient (shaded area) that corresponds to an aortic valve area of 0.6 cm² (left). Simultaneous recording of LV and pulmonary capillary wedge

(PCW) pressure tracings reveal a 14-mmHg mean diastolic gradient (shaded area) that is consistent with critical mitral stenosis (mitral valve area = 0.5 cm²). s, systole; d, diastole; e, end diastole.

recording pressure; once the catheter has passed the septal obstruction and is positioned in the apex of the left ventricle, a gradient can be measured between the left ventricular apex and the aorta. Hypertrophic obstructive cardiomyopathy is confirmed by the Brockenbrough-Braunwald sign: following a premature ventricular contraction, there is an increase in the left ventricular–aorta pressure gradient with a simultaneous decrease in the aortic pulse pressure. These findings are absent in aortic stenosis.

Regurgitant valvular lesions increase volume (and pressure) in the "receiving" cardiac chamber. In severe mitral and tricuspid regurgitation, the increase in blood flow to the atria takes place during ventricular systole, leading to an increase in the v wave (two times greater than the mean pressure). Severe aortic regurgitation leads to a decrease in aortic diastolic pressure with a concomitant rise in left ventricular end-diastolic pressure, resulting in equalization of pressures between the two chambers at end diastole.

Hemodynamic measurements are also used to differentiate between cardiac tamponade, constrictive pericarditis, and restrictive cardiomyopathy. In cardiac tamponade, right atrial pressure is increased with a decreased "y" descent, indicative of impaired right atrial emptying in diastole, and there is diastolic equalization of pressures in all cardiac chambers. In constrictive pericarditis, right atrial pressure is elevated with a prominent "y" descent, indicating rapid filling of the right ventricle during early diastole. A diastolic dip and plateau or "square root sign," in the ventricular waveforms due to an abrupt halt in ventricular filling during diastole; right ventricular and pulmonary artery pressures are elevated; and discordant pressure changes in the right and left ventricles with inspiration (right ventricular systolic pressure increases while left ventricular systolic pressure decreases) are observed. The latter hemodynamic phenomenon is the most specific for constriction. Restrictive cardiomyopathy may be distinguished from constrictive pericarditis by a marked increase in right ventricular and pulmonary artery systolic pressures (usually >60 mmHg), a separation of the left and right ventricular diastolic pressures by >5 mmHg (at baseline or with acute volume loading), and concordant changes in left and right ventricular diastolic filling pressures with inspiration (both increase).

Cardiac output

Cardiac output is measured by the Fick method or the thermodilution technique or calculated from left ventricular angiography. Typically, the Fick method and thermodilution technique are both performed during cardiac catheterization, although the Fick method is considered more reliable in the presence of tricuspid regurgitation and in low-output states. The Fick method uses oxygen as the indicator substance and is based on the principle that the amount of a substance taken up or released by an organ (oxygen consumption) is equal to the product of its blood flow (cardiac output) and the difference in the concentration of the substance in the arterial and venous circulation (arterial-venous oxygen difference). Thus, the formula for calculating the Fick cardiac output is:

Cardiac output (L/min) = (oxygen consumption [mL/min])/(arterial-venous oxygen difference [mL/L])

Oxygen consumption is estimated as 125 mL oxygen/minute × body surface area, and the arterial-venous oxygen difference is determined by first calculating the oxygen-carrying capacity of blood (hemoglobin [g/100 mL] × 1.36 [mL oxygen/g hemoglobin] × 10) and multiplying this product by the fractional oxygen saturation. The thermodilution method measures a substance that is injected into and adequately mixes with blood. In contemporary practice, thermodilution cardiac outputs are measured using temperature as the indicator. Measurements are made with a thermistor-tipped catheter that detects temperature deviations in the pulmonary artery after the injection of 10 mL of room-temperature normal saline into the right atrium. Cardiac output may also be calculated from the left ventriculogram by first determining left ventricular volumes in end diastole and end systole using the area-length method. Cardiac output is equal to the heart rate × stroke volume, which is the difference between the end-diastolic volume and the end-systolic volume.

Vascular resistance

Resistance across the systemic and pulmonary circulations is calculated by extrapolating from Ohm's law of electrical resistance and is equal to the mean pressure gradient divided by the mean flow (cardiac output). Therefore, systemic vascular resistance is ([mean aortic pressure − mean right atrial pressure]/cardiac output) multiplied by 80 to convert the resistance from Wood units to dyn-s-cm^{-5}. Similarly, the pulmonary vascular resistance is ([mean pulmonary artery − mean pulmonary capillary wedge pressure]/cardiac output) × 80. Pulmonary vascular resistance is lowered by oxygen, nitroprusside, calcium channel blockers, prostacyclin infusions, and inhaled nitric oxide; these therapies may be administered during catheterization to determine if increased pulmonary vascular resistance is fixed or reversible.

Valve area

Hemodynamic data may also be used to calculate the valve area using the Gorlin formula that equates the area to the flow across the valve divided by the pressure gradient between the cardiac chambers surrounding the valve. The formula for the assessment of valve area is: Area = (cardiac output [cm^3/min]/[systolic ejection period or diastolic filling period][heart rate])/44.3 C × square root of the pressure gradient, where C = 1 for aortic valve and 0.85 for the mitral valve. A valve area of <1.0 cm^2 and a mean gradient of greater than 40 mmHg indicate severe aortic stenosis, while a valve area of <1.5 cm^2 and a mean gradient >5–10 mmHg is consistent with moderate-to-severe mitral stenosis; in symptomatic patients with a mitral valve area >1.5 cm^2, a mean gradient >15 mmHg, pulmonary artery pressure >60 mmHg, or a pulmonary artery wedge pressure >25 mmHg after exercise is also considered significant and may warrant intervention. The modified Hakki formula has also been used to estimate aortic valve area. This formula calculates the valve area as the cardiac output (L/min) divided by the square root of the pressure gradient. Aortic valve area calculations based on the Gorlin formula are flow-dependent and, therefore, for patients with low cardiac outputs, it is imperative to determine if a decreased valve area actually reflects a fixed stenosis or is overestimated by a low cardiac output and stroke volume that is insufficient to open the valve leaflets fully. In these instances, cautious hemodynamic manipulation using dobutamine to increase the cardiac output and recalculation of the aortic valve area may be necessary.

Intracardiac shunts

In patients with congenital heart disease, detection, localization, and quantification of the intracardiac shunt should be evaluated. A shunt should be suspected when there is unexplained arterial desaturation or increased oxygen saturation of venous blood. A "step up" or increase in oxygen content indicates the presence of a left-to-right shunt while a "step down" indicates a right-to-left shunt. The shunt is localized by detecting a difference in oxygen saturation levels of 5–7% between adjacent cardiac chambers. The severity of the shunt is determined by the ratio of pulmonary blood flow (Q_p) to the systemic blood flow (Q_s), or $Q_p/Q_s =$ ([systemic arterial oxygen content − mixed venous oxygen content]/pulmonary vein oxygen content − pulmonary artery oxygen content). For an atrial septal defect, a shunt ratio of 1.5 is considered significant and factored with other clinical variables to determine the need for intervention. When a congenital ventricular septal defect is present, a shunt ratio of ≥ 2.0 with evidence of left ventricular volume overload is a class I indication for surgical correction.

VENTRICULOGRAPHY AND AORTOGRAPHY

Ventriculography to assess left ventricular function may be performed during cardiac catheterization. A pigtail catheter is advanced retrograde across the aortic valve into the left ventricle and 30–45 mL of contrast is power-injected to visualize the left ventricular chamber during the cardiac cycle. The ventriculogram is usually performed in the right anterior oblique projection to examine wall motion and mitral valve function. Normal wall motion is observed as symmetric contraction of all segments; hypokinetic segments have decreased contraction, akinetic segments do not contract, and dyskinetic segments appear to bulge paradoxically during systole (Fig. 13-3). Ventriculography may also reveal

DIASTOLE   SYSTOLE

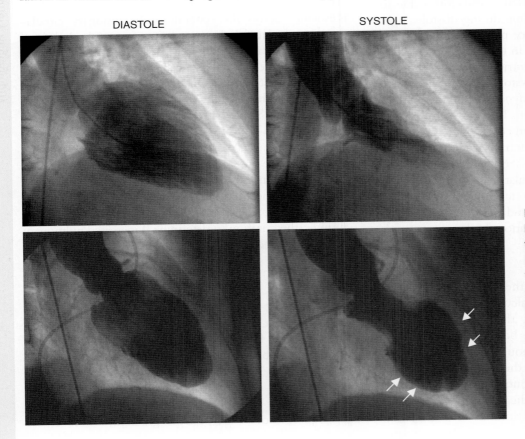

FIGURE 13-3

Left ventriculogram at end diastole (left) and end systole (right). In patients with normal left ventricular function, the ventriculogram reveals symmetric contraction of all walls (top). Patients with coronary artery disease may have wall motion abnormalities on ventriculography as seen in this 60-year-old male following a large anterior myocardial infarction. In systole, the anterior, apical, and inferior walls are akinetic (white arrows) (bottom).

a left ventricular aneurysm, pseudoaneurysm, or diverticulum and can be used to assess mitral valve prolapse and the severity of mitral regurgitation. The degree of mitral regurgitation is estimated by comparing the density of contrast opacification of the left atrium with that of the left ventricle. Minimal contrast reflux into the left atrium is considered 1+ mitral regurgitation while contrast density in the left atrium that is greater than that in the left ventricle with reflux of contrast into the pulmonary veins within three beats defines 4+ mitral regurgitation.

Aortography in the cardiac catheterization laboratory visualizes abnormalities of the ascending aorta, including aneurysmal dilation and involvement of the great vessels, as well as dissection with compression of the true lumen by an intimal flap that separates the true and false lumina. Aortography can also be used to identify patent saphenous vein grafts that elude selective cannulation, identify shunts that involve the aorta such as a patent ductus arteriosus, and provide a qualitative assessment of aortic regurgitation using a 1+ − 4+ scale similar to that used for mitral regurgitation.

CORONARY ANGIOGRAPHY

Selective coronary angiography is almost always performed during cardiac catheterization and is used to define the coronary anatomy and determine the extent of epicardial coronary artery and coronary artery bypass graft disease. Specially shaped coronary catheters are used to engage the left and right coronary ostia. Hand

injection of radiopaque contrast agents create a coronary "luminogram" that is recorded on a radiographic images (cine angiography). Because the coronary arteries are three-dimensional objects that are in motion with the cardiac cycle, angiograms of the vessels using several different orthogonal projections are taken to best visualize the vessels without overlap or foreshortening.

The normal coronary anatomy is highly variable between individuals, but, in general, there are two coronary ostia and three major coronary vessels—the left anterior descending, the left circumflex, and the right coronary arteries with the left anterior descending and left circumflex arteries arising from the left main coronary artery (Fig. 13-4). When the right coronary artery is the origin of the A-V nodal branch, the posterior descending artery, and the posterior lateral vessels, the circulation is defined as right dominant; this is found in ~85% of individuals. When these branches arise from the left circumflex artery as occurs in ~5% of individuals, the circulation is defined as left dominant. The remaining ~10% of patients have a codominant circulation with vessels arising from both the right and left coronary circulation. In some patients, a ramus intermedius branch arises directly from the left main coronary artery; this finding is a normal variant. Coronary artery anomalies occur in 1–2% of patients, with separate ostia for the left anterior descending and left circumflex arteries being the most common (0.41%).

Coronary angiography visualizes coronary artery stenoses as luminal narrowings on the cine angiogram. The degree of narrowing is referred to as the percent stenosis and is determined visually by comparing the most severely diseased segment with a proximal or distal

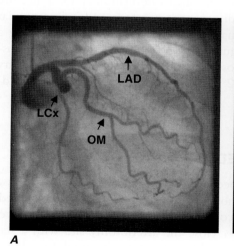 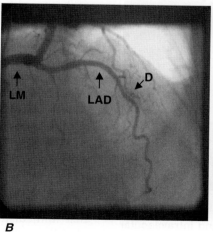 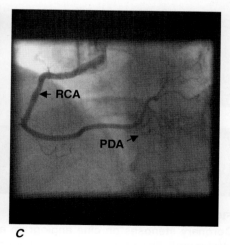

FIGURE 13-4

Normal coronary artery anatomy. A. Coronary angiogram showing the left circumflex (LCx) artery and its obtuse marginal (OM) branches. The left anterior descending artery (LAD) is also seen but may be foreshortened in this view. **B.** The LAD and its diagonal (D) branches are best seen in cranial views. In this angiogram, the left main (LM) coronary artery is also seen. **C.** The right coronary artery gives off the posterior descending artery (PDA) so this is a right-dominant circulation.

"normal segment" mg; a stenosis >50% is considered significant **(Fig. 13–5)**. Online quantitative coronary angiography can provide a more accurate assessment of the percent stenosis and lessen the tendency to overestimate lesion severity visually. The presence of a myocardial bridge, which most commonly involves the left anterior descending artery, may be mistaken for a significant stenosis; this occurs when a portion of the vessel dips below the epicardial surface into the myocardium and is subject to compressive forces during ventricular systole. The key to differentiating a myocardial bridge from a fixed stenosis is that the "stenosed" part of the vessel returns to normal during diastole. Coronary calcification is also seen during angiography prior to the injection of contrast agents. Collateral blood vessels may be seen traversing from one vessel to the distal vasculature of a severely stenosed or totally occluded vessel. Thrombolysis in myocardial infarction (TIMI) flow grade, a measure of the relative duration of time that it takes for contrast to opacify the coronary artery fully, may provide an additional clue to the degree of lesion severity, and the presence of TIMI grade 1 or 2 flow suggests that a significant coronary artery stenosis is present.

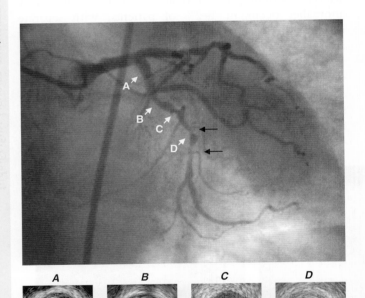

FIGURE 13-5

Coronary stenoses on cine angiogram and intravascular ultrasound. Significant stenoses in the coronary artery are seen as narrowings (black arrows) of the vessel. Intravascular ultrasound shows a normal segment of artery (**A**), areas with eccentric plaque (**B, C**), and near total obliteration of the lumen at the site of the significant stenosis (**D**). Note that the intravascular ultrasound catheter is present in the images as a black circle.

INTRAVASCULAR ULTRASOUND, FRACTIONAL FLOW RESERVE, AND CORONARY FLOW RESERVE

During coronary angiography, intermediate stenoses (40–70%), indeterminate findings, or anatomic findings that are incongruous with the patient's symptoms may require further interrogation. In these cases, intravascular ultrasound provides a more accurate anatomic assessment of the coronary artery and the degree of coronary atherosclerosis (Fig. 13-5). Intravascular ultrasound is performed using a small flexible catheter with a 40-mHz transducer at its tip that is advanced into the coronary artery over a guidewire. Data from intravascular ultrasound studies may be used to image atherosclerotic plaque precisely, determine luminal cross-sectional area, and measure vessel size; it is also used during or following percutaneous coronary intervention to assess the stenosis and determine the adequacy of stent placement. Measurement of the fractional flow reserve provides a functional assessment of the stenosis. The fractional flow reserve is the ratio of the pressure in the coronary artery distal to the stenosis divided by the pressure in the artery proximal to the stenosis at maximal vasodilation. Fractional flow reserve is measured using a coronary pressure–sensor guidewire at rest and at maximal hyperemia following the injection of adenosine. A fractional flow reserve of <0.75 indicates a hemodynamically significant stenosis that would benefit from intervention. Measurement of coronary flow reserve is another technique to assess the functional severity of a stenosis, although this technique is used with less frequency than fractional flow reserve. The coronary flow reserve is the maximal coronary blood flow increase above resting conditions during maximal vasodilation and is a measure of both epicardial coronary artery and microvascular function. Coronary flow reserve is determined using a Doppler flow guidewire before and after the administration of adenosine to induce hyperemia. A coronary flow reserve <2:1 after maximal hyperemia is considered abnormal.

POSTPROCEDURE CARE

Once the procedure is completed, vascular access sheaths are removed. If the femoral approach is used, direct manual compression or vascular closure devices that immediately close the arteriotomy site with a staple/clip, collagen plug, or suture are used to achieve hemostasis. These devices decrease the length of bed rest (from 6 h to 2–4 h) and improve patient satisfaction but have not been shown definitively to be superior to manual compression with respect to access-site complications. When cardiac catheterization is performed as an elective outpatient procedure, the patient completes postprocedure bed rest in a monitored setting and is discharged home with instructions to liberalize fluids because contrast agents promote an osmotic diuresis, to avoid strenuous activity, and to observe the vascular access site for signs of complications. Overnight hospitalization may be required for high-risk patients with significant comorbidities, patients with complications occurring during the catheterization, or in patients who have undergone a percutaneous coronary intervention. Hypotension early after the procedure may be due to inadequate fluid replacement or retroperitoneal bleeding from the access site.

SECTION III

HEART RHYTHM
DISTURBANCES

SECTION III

CHAPTER 14
PRINCIPLES OF ELECTROPHYSIOLOGY

David D. Spragg ■ Gordon F. Tomaselli

HISTORY AND INTRODUCTION

The field of cardiac electrophysiology was ushered in with the development of the electrocardiogram (ECG) by Einthoven at the turn of the twentieth century. The recording of cellular membrane currents revealed that the body surface ECG is the timed sum of the cellular action potentials in the atria and ventricles. In the late 1960s, the development of intracavitary recording, in particular the ability to record His bundle electrograms with programmed stimulation of the heart, marked the beginning of contemporary clinical electrophysiology. Adoption of radio frequency technology to ablate cardiac tissue in the early 1990s heralded the birth of interventional cardiac electrophysiology.

The clinical problem of sudden death caused by ventricular arrhythmias, most commonly in the setting of coronary obstruction, was recognized as early as the late nineteenth century. The problem was vexing and led to the development of pharmacologic and nonpharmacologic therapies, including transthoracic defibrillators, cardiac massage, and, most recently, implantable defibrillators. Over time the limitations of antiarrhythmic drug therapy have been highlighted repeatedly in clinical trials, and now ablation and devices are first-line therapy for a number of cardiac arrhythmias.

In the last two decades, the genetic basis of a number of heritable arrhythmias has been elucidated, revealing important insights into the mechanisms not only of these rare arrhythmias but also of similar rhythm disturbances observed in more common forms of heart disease.

DESCRIPTIVE PHYSIOLOGY

The normal cardiac impulse is generated by pacemaker cells in the sinoatrial node situated at the junction of the right atrium and the superior vena cava (see Fig. 11-1).

This impulse is transmitted slowly through nodal tissue to the anatomically complex atria, where it is conducted more rapidly to the atrioventricular node (AVN), inscribing the P wave of the ECG (see Fig. 11-2). There is a perceptible delay in conduction through the anatomically and functionally heterogeneous AVN. The time needed for activation of the atria and the AVN delay is represented as the PR interval of the ECG. The AVN is the only electrical connection between the atria and the ventricles in the normal heart. The electrical impulse emerges from the AVN and is transmitted to the His-Purkinje system, specifically the common bundle of His, then the left and right bundle branches, and then to the Purkinje network, facilitating activation of ventricular muscle. In normal circumstances, the ventricles are activated rapidly in a well-defined fashion that is determined by the course of the Purkinje network, and this inscribes the QRS complex (see Fig. 11-2). Recovery of electrical excitability occurs more slowly and is governed by the time of activation and duration of regional action potentials. The relative brevity of epicardial action potentials in the ventricle results in repolarization that occurs first on the epicardial surface and then proceeds to the endocardium, which inscribes a T wave normally of the same polarity as the QRS complex. The duration of activation and recovery is determined by the action potential duration represented on the body surface ECG by the QT interval (see Fig. 11-2).

Cardiac myocytes exhibit a characteristically long action potential (200–400 ms) compared with neurons and skeletal muscle cells (1–5 ms). The action potential profile is sculpted by the orchestrated activity of multiple distinctive time- and voltage-dependent ionic currents (Fig. 14-1A). The currents in turn are carried by transmembrane proteins that passively conduct ions down their electrochemical gradients through selective pores (ion channels), actively transport ions against their

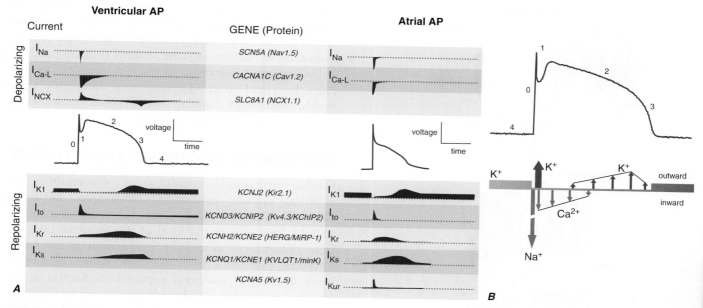

FIGURE 14-1

A. Cellular atrial and ventricular action potentials. Phases 0–4 are the rapid upstroke, early repolarization, plateau, late repolarization, and diastole, respectively. The ionic currents and their respective genes are shown above and below the action potentials. The currents that underlie the action potentials vary in atrial and ventricular myocytes. **B.** A ventricular action potential with a schematic of the ionic currents flowing during the phases of the action potential. Potassium current (I_{K1}) is the principal current during phase 4 and determines

the resting membrane potential of the myocyte. Sodium current generates the upstroke of the action potential (phase 0); activation of I_{to} with inactivation of the Na current inscribes early repolarization (phase 1). The plateau (phase 2) is generated by a balance of repolarizing potassium currents and depolarizing calcium current. Inactivation of the calcium current with persistent activation of potassium currents (predominantly I_{Kr} and I_{Ks}) causes phase 3 repolarization.

electrochemical gradient (pumps, transporters), or electrogenically exchange ionic species (exchangers).

Action potentials in the heart are regionally distinct. The regional variability in cardiac action potentials is a result of differences in the number and types of ion channel proteins expressed by different cell types in the heart. Further, unique sets of ionic currents are active in pacemaking and muscle cells, and the relative contributions of these currents may vary in the same cell type in different regions of the heart (Fig. 14-1*A*).

Ion channels are complex, multisubunit transmembrane glycoproteins that open and close in response to a number of biologic stimuli, including a change in membrane voltage, ligand binding (directly to the channel or to a G protein–coupled receptor), and mechanical deformation (**Fig. 14-2**). Other ion motive exchangers and transporters contribute importantly to cellular excitability in the heart. Ion pumps establish and maintain the ionic gradients across the cell membrane that serve as the driving force for current flow through ion channels. Transporters or exchangers that do not move ions in an electrically neutral manner (e.g., the sodium-calcium exchanger transports three Na$^+$ for one Ca^{2+}) are termed *electrogenic* and contribute directly to the action potential profile.

The most abundant superfamily of ion channels expressed in the heart is voltage gated. Several structural themes are common to all voltage-dependent ion channels. First, the architecture is modular, consisting either of four homologous subunits (e.g., K channels) or of four internally homologous domains (e.g., Na and Ca channels). Second, the proteins fold around a central pore lined by amino acids that exhibit exquisite conservation within a given channel family of like selectivity (e.g., jellyfish, eel, fruit fly, and human Na channels have very similar P segments). Third, the general strategy for activation gating (opening and closing in response to changes in membrane voltage) is highly conserved: the fourth transmembrane segment (S4), studded with positively charged residues, lies within the membrane field and moves in response to depolarization, opening the channel. Fourth, most ion channel complexes include not only the pore-forming proteins (α subunits) but also auxiliary subunits (e.g., β subunits) that modify channel function (Fig. 14-2).

Na and Ca channels are the primary carriers of depolarizing current in both the atria and the ventricles; inactivation of these currents and activation of repolarizing K currents hyperpolarize the heart cells, reestablishing the negative resting membrane potential (**Fig. 14-1***B*). The *plateau phase* is a time when

K channels

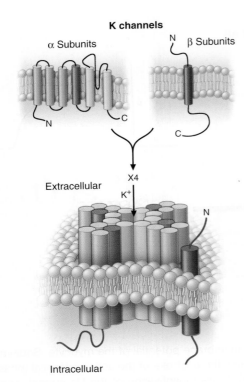

Na channels

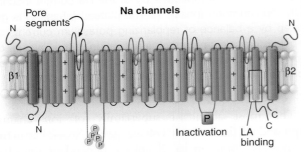

Ca channels

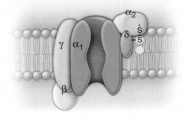

FIGURE 14-2

Topology and subunit composition of the voltage-dependent ion channels. Potassium channels are formed by the tetramerization of α or pore-forming subunits and one or more β subunits; only single β subunits are shown for clarity. Sodium and calcium channels are composed of α subunits with four homologous domains and one or more ancillary subunits. In all channel types the loop of protein between the fifth and sixth membrane-spanning repeat in each subunit or domain forms the ion-selective pore. In the case of the sodium channel, the channel is a target for phosphorylation, the linker between the third and fourth homologous domain is critical to inactivation, and the sixth membrane-spanning repeat in the fourth domain is important in local anesthetic antiarrhythmic drug binding.

little current is flowing, and relatively minor changes in depolarizing or repolarizing currents can have profound effects on the shape and duration of the action profile. Mutations in subunits of these channel proteins produce arrhythmogenic alterations in the action potentials that cause long and short QT syndrome, idiopathic ventricular fibrillation, familial atrial fibrillation, and some forms of conduction system disease.

MECHANISMS OF CARDIAC ARRHYTHMIAS

Cardiac arrhythmias result from abnormalities of electrical impulse generation, conduction, or both. Bradyarrhythmias typically arise from disturbances in impulse formation at the level of the sinoatrial node or from disturbances in impulse propagation at any level, including exit block from the sinus node, conduction block in the AV node, and impaired conduction in the His-Purkinje system. Tachyarrhythmias can be classified according to mechanism, including enhanced automaticity (spontaneous depolarization of atrial, junctional, or ventricular pacemakers), reentry (circus propagation of a depolarizing wavefront), or triggered arrhythmias (initiated by afterdepolarizations) occurring during or immediately after cardiac repolarization, during phase 3 or 4 of the action potential. A variety of mapping and pacing maneuvers typically performed during invasive electrophysiologic testing can often determine the underlying mechanism of a tachyarrhythmia **(Table 14-1)**.

Alterations in impulse initiation: Automaticity

Spontaneous (phase 4) diastolic depolarization underlies the property of automaticity (pacemaking) characteristic of cells in the sinoatrial (SA) and atrioventricular (AV) nodes, His-Purkinje system, coronary sinus, and pulmonary veins. Phase 4 depolarization results from the concerted action of a number of ionic currents, including K^+ currents, Ca^{2+} currents, electrogenic Na, K-ATPase, the Na-Ca exchanger, and the so-called funny, or pacemaker, current (I_f); however, the relative importance of these currents remains controversial.

The rate of phase 4 depolarization and, therefore, the firing rates of pacemaker cells are dynamically regulated. Prominent among the factors that modulate phase 4 is autonomic nervous system tone. The negative chronotropic effect of activation of the parasympathetic nervous system is a result of the release of acetylcholine that binds to muscarinic receptors, releasing G protein βγ subunits that activate a potassium current (I_{KACh}) in nodal and atrial cells. The resulting increase in K^+ conductance opposes membrane depolarization, slowing the rate of rise of phase 4 of the action potential. Conversely, augmentation of sympathetic nervous system tone increases myocardial catecholamine concentrations, which activate both α– and β–adrenergic receptors.

TABLE 14-1

ARRHYTHMIA MECHANISMS

ELECTROPHYSIOLOGIC PROPERTY	MOLECULAR COMPONENTS	MECHANISM	PROTOTYPIC ARRHYTHMIAS
Cellular			
Impulse Initiation			
Automaticity	I_f, I_{Ca-L}, I_{Ca-T}, I_K, I_{K1}	Suppression/acceleration of phase 4	Sinus bradycardia, sinus tachycardia
Triggered automaticity	Calcium overload, I_{TI}	DADs	Digitalis toxicity, reperfusion VT
	I_{Ca-L}, I_K, I_{Na}	EADs	Torsades des pointes, congenital and acquired
Excitation	I_{Na}	Suppression of phase 0	Ischemic VF
	I_{K-ATP}	AP shortening, inexcitability	AV block
	I_{Ca-L}	Suppression	
Repolarization	I_{Na}, I_{Ca-L}, I_K, I_{K1}, Ca^{2+} homeostasis	AP prolongation, EADs, DADs	Polymorphic VT (HF, LVH)
	I_{Ca-L}, K channels, Ca^{2+} homeostasis	AP shortening	Atrial fibrillation
Multicellular			
Cellular Coupling	Connexins (Cx43), I_{Na}, I_{K-ATP}	Decreased coupling	Ischemic VT/VF
Tissue Structure	Extracellular matrix, collagen	Excitable gap and functional reentry	Monomorphic VT, atrial fibrillation

Abbreviations: AP, action potential; AV, atrioventricular; DADs, delayed afterdepolarizations; EADs, early afterdepolarizations; HF, heart failure; LVH, left ventricular hypertrophy; VF, ventricular fibrillation; VT, ventricular tachyarrhythmia.

The effect of β_1-adrenergic stimulation predominates in pacemaking cells, augmenting both L-type Ca current (I_{Ca-L}) and I_f, thus increasing the slope of phase 4. Enhanced sympathetic nervous system activity can dramatically increase the rate of firing of SA nodal cells, producing sinus tachycardia with rates >200 beats/min. By contrast, the increased rate of firing of Purkinje cells is more limited, rarely producing ventricular tachyarrhythmias >120 beats/min.

Normal automaticity may be affected by a number other factors associated with heart disease. Hypokalemia and ischemia may reduce the activity of Na, K-ATPase, thereby reducing the background repolarizing current and enhancing phase 4 diastolic depolarization. The end result would be an increase in the spontaneous firing rate of pacemaking cells. Modest increases in extracellular potassium may render the maximum diastolic potential more positive, thereby also increasing the firing rate of pacemaking cells. A more significant increase in $[K^+]_o$, however, renders the heart inexcitable by depolarizing the membrane potential.

Normal or enhanced automaticity of subsidiary latent pacemakers produces escape rhythms in the setting of failure of more dominant pacemakers. Suppression of a pacemaker cell by a faster rhythm leads to an increased intracellular Na^+ load ($[Na^+]_i$), and extrusion of Na^+ from the cell by Na, K-ATPase produces an increased background repolarizing current that slows phase 4 diastolic depolarization. At slower rates, $[Na^+]_i$ is decreased, as is the activity of the Na, K-ATPase, resulting in

progressively more rapid diastolic depolarization and warm-up of the tachycardia rate. Overdrive suppression and warm-up are characteristic of, but may not be observed in, all automatic tachycardias. Abnormal conduction into tissue with enhanced automaticity (*entrance block*) may blunt or eliminate the phenomena of overdrive suppression and warm-up of automatic tissue.

Abnormal automaticity may underlie atrial tachycardia, accelerated idioventricular rhythms, and ventricular tachycardia, particularly that associated with ischemia and reperfusion. It has also been suggested that injury currents at the borders of ischemic myocardium may depolarize adjacent nonischemic tissue, predisposing to automatic ventricular tachycardia.

Afterdepolarizations and triggered automaticity

Triggered automaticity or activity refers to impulse initiation that is dependent on afterdepolarizations (Fig. 14-3). Afterdepolarizations are membrane voltage oscillations that occur during (early afterdepolarizations, EADs) or after (delayed afterdepolarizations, DADs) an action potential.

The cellular feature common to the induction of DADs is the presence of an increased Ca^{2+} load in the cytosol and sarcoplasmic reticulum. Digitalis glycoside toxicity, catecholamines, and ischemia all can enhance Ca^{2+} loading sufficiently to produce DADs. Accumulation of lysophospholipids in ischemic myocardium with consequent Na^+ and Ca^{2+} overload has been suggested as a mechanism

CHAPTER 14 Principles of Electrophysiology

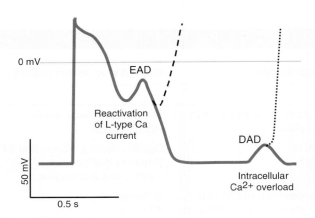

FIGURE 14-3

Schematic action potentials with early afterdepolarizations (EADs) and delayed afterdepolarizations (DADs). Afterdepolarizations are spontaneous depolarizations in cardiac myocytes. EADs occur before the end of the action potential (phases 2 and 3), interrupting repolarization. DADs occur during phase 4 of the action potential after completion of repolarization. The cellular mechanisms of EADs and DADs differ (see text).

for DADs and triggered automaticity. Cells from damaged areas or cells that survive a myocardial infarction may display spontaneous release of calcium from the sarcoplasmic reticulum, and this may generate "waves" of intracellular calcium elevation and arrhythmias.

EADs occur during the action potential and interrupt the orderly repolarization of the myocyte. Traditionally, EADs have been thought to arise from action potential prolongation and reactivation of depolarizing currents, but more recent experimental evidence suggests a previously unappreciated interrelationship between intracellular calcium loading and EADs. Cytosolic calcium may increase when action potentials are prolonged. This, in turn, appears to enhance L-type Ca current, further prolonging action potential duration as well as providing the inward current driving EADs. Intracellular calcium loading by action potential prolongation may also enhance the likelihood of DADs. The interrelationship among intracellular $[Ca^{2+}]$, EADs, and DADs may be one explanation for the susceptibility of hearts that are calcium loaded (e.g., in ischemia or congestive heart failure) to develop arrhythmias, particularly on exposure to action potential–prolonging drugs.

EAD-triggered arrhythmias exhibit rate dependence. In general, the amplitude of an EAD is augmented at slow rates when action potentials are longer. Indeed, a fundamental condition that underlies the development of EADs is action potential and QT prolongation. Hypokalemia, hypomagnesemia, bradycardia, and, most commonly, drugs can predispose to the generation of EADs, invariably in the context of prolonging the action potential. Antiarrhythmics with class IA and III action (see later) produce action potential and QT prolongation intended to be therapeutic but frequently causing arrhythmias.

Noncardiac drugs such as phenothiazines, nonsedating antihistamines, and some antibiotics can also prolong the action potential duration and predispose to EAD-mediated triggered arrhythmias. Decreased $[K^+]_o$ paradoxically may decrease membrane potassium currents (particularly the delayed rectifier current, I_{Kr}) in the ventricular myocyte, explaining why hypokalemia causes action potential prolongation and EADs. In fact, potassium infusions in patients with the congenital long QT syndrome (LQTS) and in those with drug-induced acquired QT prolongation shorten the QT interval.

EAD-mediated triggered activity probably underlies initiation of the characteristic polymorphic ventricular tachycardia, torsades des pointes, seen in patients with congenital and acquired forms of LQTS. Structural heart disease such as cardiac hypertrophy and failure may also delay ventricular repolarization (so-called electrical remodeling) and predispose to arrhythmias related to abnormalities of repolarization. The abnormalities of repolarization in hypertrophy and heart failure are often magnified by concomitant drug therapy or electrolyte disturbances.

Abnormal impulse conduction: Reentry

The most common arrhythmia mechanism is reentry. Fundamentally, reentry is defined as circulation of an activation wave around an inexcitable obstacle. Thus, the requirements for reentry are two electrophysiologically dissimilar pathways for impulse propagation around an inexcitable region such that unidirectional block occurs in one of the pathways and a region of excitable tissue exists at the head of the propagating wavefront **(Fig. 14-4)**. Structural and electrophysiologic properties

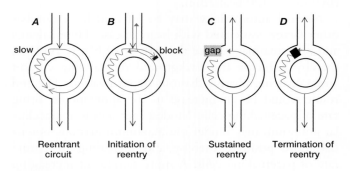

FIGURE 14-4

Schematic diagram of reentry. A. The circuit contains two limbs, one with slow conduction. **B.** A premature impulse blocks in the fast pathway and conducts over the slow pathway, allowing the fast pathway to recover so that the activation wave can reenter the fast pathway from the retrograde direction. **C.** During sustained reentry utilizing such a circuit, a gap (excitable gap) exists between the activating head of the wave and the recovering tail. **D.** One mechanism of termination of reentry occurs when the conduction and recovery characteristics of the circuit change and the activating head of the wave collides with the tail, extinguishing the tachycardia.

of the heart may contribute to the development of the inexcitable obstacle and that of unidirectional block. The complex geometry of muscle bundles in the heart and spatial heterogeneity of cellular coupling or other active membrane properties (i.e., ionic currents) appear to be critical.

A key feature in classifying reentrant arrhythmias, particularly for therapy, is the presence and size of an excitable gap. An excitable gap exists when the tachycardia circuit is longer than the tachycardia wavelength (λ = conduction velocity $\times$ refractory period, representing the size of the circuit that can sustain reentry), allowing appropriately timed stimuli to reset propagation in the circuit. Reentrant arrhythmias may exist in the heart in the absence of an excitable gap and with a tachycardia wavelength nearly the same size as the path length. In this case, the wavefront propagates through partially refractory tissue with no anatomic obstacle and no fully excitable gap; this is referred to as *leading circle reentry*, a form of functional reentry (reentry that depends on functional properties of the tissue). Unlike excitable gap reentry, there is no fixed anatomic circuit in leading circle reentry, and it may therefore not be possible to disrupt the tachycardia with pacing or destruction of a part of the circuit. Furthermore, the circuit in leading circle reentry tends to be less stable than that in excitable gap reentrant arrhythmias, with large variations in cycle length and a predilection to termination.

Anatomically determined, excitable gap reentry can explain several clinically important tachycardias, such as AV reentry, atrial flutter, bundle branch reentry ventricular tachycardia, and ventricular tachycardia in scarred myocardium. There is strong evidence to suggest that other, less organized arrhythmias, such as atrial and ventricular fibrillation, are associated with more complex activation of the heart and are due to functional reentry.

Structural heart disease is associated with changes in conduction and refractoriness that increase the risk of reentrant arrhythmias. Chronically ischemic myocardium exhibits a downregulation of the gap junction channel protein (connexin 43) that carries intercellular ionic current. The border zones of infarcted and failing ventricular myocardium exhibit not only functional alterations of ionic currents but also remodeling of tissue and altered distribution of gap junctions. The changes in gap junction channel expression and distribution, in combination with macroscopic tissue alterations, support a role for slowed conduction in reentrant arrhythmias that complicate chronic coronary artery disease (CAD). Aged human atrial myocardium exhibits altered conduction, manifest as highly fractionated atrial electrograms, producing an ideal substrate for the reentry that may underlie the very common development of atrial fibrillation in the elderly.

APPROACH TO THE PATIENT: Cardiac Arrhythmias

The evaluation of patients with suspected cardiac arrhythmias is highly individualized; however, two key features—the history and ECG—are pivotal in directing the diagnostic workup and therapy. Patients with cardiac arrhythmias exhibit a wide spectrum of clinical presentations that range from asymptomatic ECG abnormalities to survival from cardiac arrest. In general, the more severe the presenting symptoms are, the more aggressive the evaluation and treatment are. Loss of consciousness that is believed to be of cardiac origin typically mandates an exhaustive search for the etiology and often requires invasive, device-based therapy. The presence of structural heart disease and prior myocardial infarction dictates a change in the approach to the management of syncope or ventricular arrhythmias. The presence of a family history of serious ventricular arrhythmias or premature sudden death will influence the evaluation of presumed heritable arrhythmias.

The physical examination is focused on determining whether there is cardiopulmonary disease that is associated with specific cardiac arrhythmias. The absence of significant cardiopulmonary disease often, but not always, suggests benignity of the rhythm disturbance. In contrast, palpitations, syncope, or near syncope in the setting of significant heart or lung disease have more ominous implications. In addition, the physical examination may reveal the presence of a persistent arrhythmia such as atrial fibrillation.

The judicious use of noninvasive diagnostic tests is an important element in the evaluation of patients with arrhythmias, and there is no test more important than the ECG, particularly if recorded at the time of symptoms. Uncommon but diagnostically important signatures of electrophysiologic disturbances may be unearthed on the resting ECG, such as delta waves in Wolff-Parkinson-White (WPW) syndrome, prolongation or shortening of the QT interval, right precordial ST-segment abnormalities in Brugada syndrome, and epsilon waves in arrhythmogenic right ventricular dysplasia. Variants of body surface ECG recording can provide important information about arrhythmia substrates and triggers. Holter monitoring and event recording, either continuous or intermittent, record the body surface ECG over longer periods, enhancing the possibility of observing the cardiac rhythm during symptoms. Implantable long-term monitors and commercial ambulatory ECG monitoring services permit prolonged telemetric monitoring both for diagnosis and to assess the efficacy of therapy.

Long-term recordings permit the assessment of the time-varying behavior of the heart rhythm. Heart rate variability (HRV) and QT interval variability (QTV) provide noninvasive methods to assess autonomic nervous system influence on the heart. A decrease in HRV has been associated with increased sympathetic nervous system tone and increased mortality rates in patients after myocardial infarction. Signal-averaged electrocardiography (SAECG) uses signal-averaging techniques to amplify small potentials in the body surface ECG that are associated with slow conduction in the myocardium. The presence of these small potentials, referred to as *late potentials* because of their timing with respect to the QRS complex, and prolongation of the filtered (or averaged) QRS duration are indicative of slowed conduction in the ventricle and have been associated with an increased risk of ventricular arrhythmias after myocardial infarction. Exercise electrocardiography is important in determining the presence of myocardial demand ischemia; more recently, analysis of the morphology of the QT interval with exercise has been used to assess the risk of serious ventricular arrhythmias. Microscopic alterations in the T wave (T wave alternans, TWA) at low heart rates may identify patients at risk for ventricular arrhythmias. Cardiac imaging plays an important role in the detection and characterization of myocardial structural abnormalities that may render the heart more susceptible to arrhythmia. Ventricular tachyarrhythmias, for instance, occur more frequently in patients with ventricular systolic dysfunction and chamber dilation, in hypertrophic cardiomyopathy, and in the setting of infiltrative diseases such as sarcoidosis. Supraventricular arrhythmias may be associated with particular congenital conditions, including AV reentry in the setting of Ebstein's anomaly. Echocardiography is a frequently employed imaging technique to screen for disorders of cardiac structure and function. Increasingly, magnetic resonance (MR) imaging of the myocardium is being used to screen for scar burden, fibrofatty infiltration of the myocardium as seen in arrhythmogenic right ventricular cardiomyopathy, and other structural changes that affect arrhythmia susceptibility.

Head-up tilt (HUT) testing is useful in the evaluation of some patients with syncope. The physiologic response to HUT is incompletely understood; however, redistribution of blood volume and increased ventricular contractility occur consistently. Exaggerated activation of a central reflex in response to HUT produces a stereotypic response of an initial increase in heart rate, then a drop in blood pressure followed by a reduction in heart rate characteristic of neurally mediated hypotension. Other responses to HUT may be observed in patients with orthostatic hypotension and autonomic insufficiency. HUT is used most often in patients with recurrent syncope, although it may be useful in patients with single syncopal episodes with associated injury, particularly in the absence of structural heart disease. In patients with structural heart disease, HUT may be indicated in those with syncope, in whom other causes (e.g., asystole, ventricular tachyarrhythmias) have been excluded. HUT has been suggested as a useful tool in the diagnosis of and therapy for recurrent idiopathic vertigo, chronic fatigue syndrome, recurrent transient ischemic attacks, and repeated falls of unknown etiology in the elderly. Importantly, HUT is relatively contraindicated in the presence of severe CAD with proximal coronary stenoses, known severe cerebrovascular disease, severe mitral stenosis, and obstruction to left ventricular outflow (e.g., aortic stenosis). The method of HUT is variable, but the angle of tilt and the duration of upright posture are central to the diagnostic utility of the test. Pharmacologic provocation of orthostatic stress with isoproterenol, nitrates, adenosine, and edrophonium has been used to shorten the test and enhance specificity.

Electrophysiologic testing is central to the understanding and treatment of many cardiac arrhythmias. Indeed, most frequently, electrophysiologic testing is interventional, providing both diagnosis and therapy. The components of the electrophysiologic test are baseline measurements of conduction under resting and stressed (rate or pharmacologic) conditions and maneuvers, both pacing and pharmacologic, to induce arrhythmias. A number of sophisticated electrical mapping and catheter-guidance techniques have been developed to facilitate catheter-based therapeutics in the electrophysiology laboratory.

TREATMENT **Cardiac Arrhythmias**

Antiarrhythmic Drug Therapy The interaction of antiarrhythmic drugs with cardiac tissues and the resulting electrophysiologic changes are complex. An incomplete understanding of the effects of these drugs has produced serious missteps that have had adverse effects on patient outcomes and the development of newer pharmacologic agents. Currently, antiarrhythmic drugs have been relegated to an ancillary role in the treatment of most cardiac arrhythmias.

There are several explanations for the complexity of antiarrhythmic drug action: the structural similarity of target ion channels; regional differences in the levels of expression of channels and transporters, which change with disease; time and voltage dependence of drug action; and the effect of these drugs on targets other than ion channels. Because of the limitations of any scheme to classify antiarrhythmic agents, a shorthand that is useful in describing the major mechanisms of action is of some utility. Such a classification scheme was proposed in 1970 by Vaughan-Williams and later modified by Singh and Harrison. The classes of antiarrhythmic action are class I, local anesthetic effect due to blockade of Na^+ current; class II, interference with the action of catecholamines at the β-adrenergic receptor; class III, delay of repolarization due to inhibition of K^+ current or activation of depolarizing current; class IV, interference with calcium conductance (Table 14-2). The limitations of the Vaughan-Williams classification scheme include multiple actions of most drugs, overwhelming consideration of antagonism as a mechanism of action, and the fact that several agents have none of the four classes of action in the scheme.

Catheter Ablation The use of catheter ablation is based on the principle that there is a critical anatomic region of impulse generation or propagation that is required for the initiation and maintenance of cardiac arrhythmias. Destruction of such a critical region results in the elimination of the arrhythmia. The use of radio frequency (RF) energy in clinical medicine is nearly a century old. The first catheter ablation using a DC energy source was performed in the early 1980s by Scheinman and colleagues. By the early 1990s, RF had been adapted for use in catheter-based ablation in the heart (Fig. 14-5).

The RF frequency band (300–30,000 kHz) is used to generate energy for several biomedical applications, including coagulation and cauterization of tissues. Energy of this frequency will not stimulate skeletal muscle or the heart and heats tissue by a resistive mechanism, with the intensity of heating and tissue destruction being proportional to the delivered power. Alternative, less frequently used energy sources for catheter ablation of cardiac arrhythmias include microwaves (915 MHz or 2450 MHz), lasers, ultrasound, and freezing (cryoablation). Of these alternative ablation techniques, cryoablation is being used clinically with the most frequency, especially ablation in the region of the AV node. At temperatures just below 32°C, membrane ion transport is disrupted, producing depolarization of cells, decreased action potential amplitude and duration, and slowed conduction velocity (resulting in local conduction block)—all of which are reversible if the tissue is rewarmed in a timely fashion. Tissue cooling can be used for mapping and ablation. Cryomapping can be used to confirm the location of a desired ablation target, such as an accessory pathway in WPW syndrome, or can be used to determine the safety of ablation around the AV node by monitoring AV conduction during cooling. Another advantage of cryoablation is that once the catheter tip cools below freezing, it adheres to the tissue, increasing catheter stability independent of the rhythm or pacing.

Device Therapy Bradyarrhythmias due either to primary sinus node dysfunction or to atrioventricular conduction defects are readily treated through implantation

TABLE 14-2

ANTIARRHYTHMIC DRUG ACTIONS

DRUG	CLASS ACTIONS				MISCELLANEOUS ACTION
	I	II	III	IV	
Quinidine	++		++		α-Adrenergic blockade
Procainamide	++		++		Ganglionic blockade
Flecainide	+++		+		
Propafenone	++	+			
Sotalol		++	+++		
Dofetilide			+++		
Amiodarone	++	++	+++	+	α-Adrenergic blockade
Ibutilide			+++		Na^+ channel activator

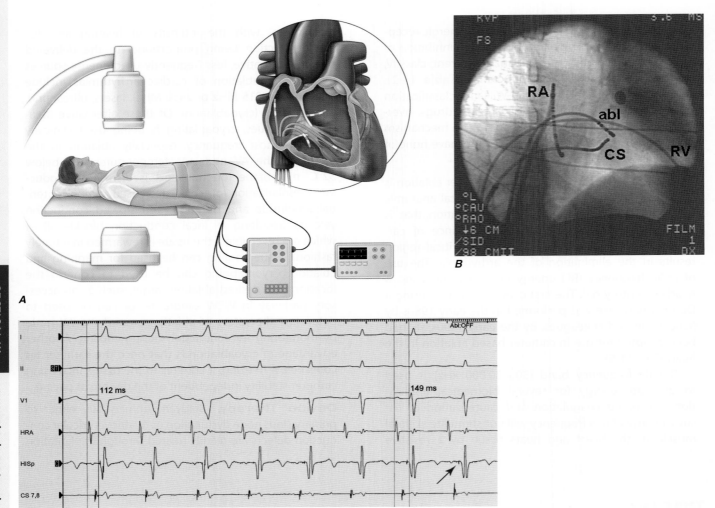

FIGURE 14-5

Catheter ablation of cardiac arrhythmias. A. A schematic of the catheter system and generator in a patient undergoing radio frequency catheter ablation (RFCA); the circuit involves the catheter in the heart and a dispersive patch placed on the body surface (usually the back). The inset shows a diagram of the heart with a catheter located at the AV valve ring for ablation of an accessory pathway. **B.** A right anterior oblique fluoroscopic image of the catheter position for ablation of a left-sided accessory pathway. A catheter is placed in the atrial side of the mitral valve ring (abl) via a transseptal puncture. Other catheters are placed in the coronary sinus, in the right atrium (RA), and in the right ventricular (RV) apex to record local electrical activation. **C.** Body surface ECG recordings (I, II, V₁) and endocardial electrograms (HRA, high right atrium; HISp, proximal His bundle electrogram; CS 7,8, recordings from poles 7 and 8 of a decapolar catheter placed in the coronary sinus) during RFCA of a left-sided accessory pathway in a patient with Wolff-Parkinson-White syndrome. The QRS narrows at the fourth complex; the arrow shows the His bundle electrogram, which becomes apparent with elimination of ventricular preexcitation over the accessory pathway.

of a permanent pacemaker. Clinical indications for pacemaker implantation often depend on the presence either of symptomatic bradycardia or of an unreliable endogenous escape rhythm and are more fully reviewed in Chap. 15.

Ventricular tachyarrhythmias, particularly those occurring in the context of progressive structural heart diseases such as ischemic cardiomyopathy or arrhythmogenic right ventricular cardiomyopathy, may recur despite therapy with antiarrhythmic drugs or catheter ablation.

In appropriate candidates, implantation of an internal cardioverter-defibrillator (ICD) may reduce mortality rates from sudden cardiac death. In a subset of patients with congestive heart failure (CHF) and ventricular mechanical dyssynchrony, ICD or pacemaker platforms can be used to provide cardiac resynchronization therapy, typically through implantation of a left ventricular pacing lead. In patients with dyssynchronous CHF, such therapy has been shown to improve both morbidity and mortality rates.

CHAPTER 15

THE BRADYARRHYTHMIAS

David D. Spragg ■ Gordon F. Tomaselli

Electrical activation of the heart normally originates in the sinoatrial (SA) node, the predominant pacemaker. Other subsidiary pacemakers in the atrioventricular (AV) node, specialized conducting system, and muscle may initiate electrical activation if the SA node is dysfunctional or suppressed. Typically, subsidiary pacemakers discharge at a slower rate and, in the absence of an appropriate increase in stroke volume, may result in tissue hypoperfusion.

Spontaneous activation and contraction of the heart are a consequence of the specialized pacemaking tissue in these anatomic locales. As described in Chap. 14, action potentials in the heart are regionally heterogeneous. The action potentials in cells isolated from nodal tissue are distinct from those recorded from atrial and ventricular myocytes (Fig. 15-1). The complement of ionic currents present in nodal cells results in a less negative resting membrane potential compared with atrial or ventricular myocytes. Electrical diastole in nodal cells is characterized by slow diastolic depolarization (phase 4), which generates an action potential as the membrane voltage reaches threshold. The action potential upstrokes (phase 0) are slow compared with atrial or ventricular myocytes, being mediated by calcium rather than sodium current. Cells with properties of SA and AV nodal tissue are electrically connected to the remainder of the myocardium by cells with an electrophysiologic phenotype between that of nodal cells and that of atrial or ventricular myocytes. Cells in the SA node exhibit the most rapid phase 4 depolarization and thus are the dominant pacemakers in a normal heart.

Bradycardia results from a failure of either impulse initiation or impulse conduction. Failure of impulse initiation may be caused by depressed automaticity resulting from a slowing or failure of phase 4 diastolic depolarization (Fig. 15-2), which may result from disease or exposure to drugs. Prominently, the autonomic nervous system modulates the rate of phase 4 diastolic depolarization and thus the firing rate of both primary (SA node) and subsidiary pacemakers. Failure of conduction of an impulse from nodal tissue to atrial or ventricular myocardium may produce bradycardia as a result of exit block. Conditions that alter the activation and connectivity of cells (e.g., fibrosis) in the heart may result in failure of impulse conduction.

SA node dysfunction and AV conduction block are the most common causes of pathologic bradycardia. SA node dysfunction may be difficult to distinguish from physiologic sinus bradycardia, particularly in the young. SA node dysfunction increases in frequency between the fifth and sixth decades of life and should be considered in patients with fatigue, exercise intolerance, or syncope and sinus bradycardia. Transient AV block is common in the young and probably is a result of the high vagal tone found in up to 10% of young adults. Acquired and persistent failure of AV conduction is decidedly rare in healthy adult populations, with an estimated incidence of ~200/million population per year.

Permanent pacemaking is the only reliable therapy for symptomatic bradycardia in the absence of extrinsic and reversible etiologies such as increased vagal tone, hypoxia, hypothermia, and drugs (Table 15-1). Approximately 50% of the 150,000 permanent pacemakers implanted in the United States and 20–30% of the 150,000 of those in Europe were implanted for SA node disease.

SA NODE DISEASE

Structure and physiology of the SA node

The SA node is composed of a cluster of small fusiform cells in the sulcus terminalis on the epicardial surface of the heart at the right atrial–superior vena caval junction, where they envelop the SA nodal artery. The SA node is structurally heterogeneous, but the central prototypic nodal cells have fewer distinct myofibrils than does the surrounding atrial myocardium, no intercalated

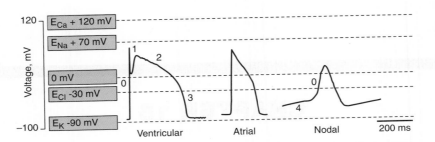

FIGURE 15-1

Action potential profiles recorded in cells isolated from sinoatrial or atrioventricular nodal tissue compared with those of cells from atrial or ventricular myocardium. Nodal cell action potentials exhibit more depolarized resting membrane potentials, slower phase 0 upstrokes, and phase 4 diastolic depolarization.

disks visible on light microscopy, a poorly developed sarcoplasmic reticulum, and no T-tubules. Cells in the peripheral regions of the SA node are transitional in both structure and function. The SA nodal artery arises from the right coronary artery in 55–60% and the left circumflex artery in 40–45% of persons. The SA node is richly innervated by sympathetic and parasympathetic nerves and ganglia.

Irregular and slow propagation of impulses from the SA node can be explained by the electrophysiology of nodal cells and the structure of the SA node itself. The action potentials of SA nodal cells are characterized by a relatively depolarized membrane potential (Fig. 15-1) of −40 to −60 mV, slow phase 0 upstroke, and relatively rapid phase 4 diastolic depolarization compared with the action potentials recorded in cardiac muscle

cells. The relative absence of inward rectifier potassium current (I_{K1}) accounts for the depolarized membrane

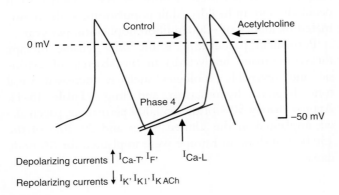

FIGURE 15-2

Schematics of nodal action potentials and the currents that contribute to phase 4 depolarization. Relative increases in depolarizing L- (I_{Ca-L}) and T- (I_{Ca-T}) type calcium and pacemaker currents (I_f) along with a reduction in repolarizing inward rectifier (I_{K1}) and delayed rectifier (I_K) potassium currents result in depolarization. Activation of ACh-gated (I_{KACh}) potassium current and beta blockade slow the rate of phase 4 and decrease the pacing rate. (*Modified from J Jalife et al: Basic Cardiac Electrophysiology for the Clinician, Blackwell Publishing, 1999.*)

TABLE 15-1
ETIOLOGIES OF SA NODE DYSFUNCTION

EXTRINSIC	INTRINSIC
Autonomic	Sick-sinus syndrome (SSS)
Carotid sinus hypersensitivity	Coronary artery disease (chronic and acute MI)
Vasovagal (cardioinhibitory) stimulation	Inflammatory
Drugs	Pericarditis
Beta blockers	Myocarditis (including viral)
Calcium channel blockers	Rheumatic heart disease
Digoxin	Collagen vascular diseases
Antiarrhythmics (class I and III)	Lyme disease
Adenosine	Senile amyloidosis
Clonidine (other sympatholytics)	Congenital heart disease
Lithium carbonate	TGA/Mustard and Fontan repairs
Cimetidine	Iatrogenic
Amitriptyline	Radiation therapy
Phenothiazines	Postsurgical
Narcotics (methadone)	Chest trauma
Pentamidine	Familial
Hypothyroidism	AD SSS, OMIM #163800 (15q24-25)
Sleep apnea	AR SSS, OMIM #608567 (3p21)
Hypoxia	SA node disease with myopia, OMIM 182190
Endotracheal suctioning (vagal maneuvers)	Kearns-Sayre syndrome, OMIM #530000
Hypothermia	Myotonic dystrophy
Increased intracranial pressure	Type 1, OMIM #160900 (19q13.2-13.3)
	Type 2, OMIM #602668 (3q13.3-q24)
	Friedreich's ataxia, OMIM #229300 (9q13, 9p23-p11)

Abbreviations: AD, autosomal dominant; AR, autosomal recessive; MI, myocardial infarction; OMIM, Online Mendelian Inheritance in Man (database); TGA, transposition of the great arteries.

potential; the slow upstroke of phase 0 results from the absence of available fast sodium current (I_{Na}) and is mediated by L-type calcium current (I_{Ca-L}); and phase 4 depolarization is a result of the aggregate activity of a number of ionic currents. Prominently, both L- and T-type (I_{Ca-T}) calcium currents, the pacemaker current (so-called funny current, or I_f) formed by the tetramerization of hyperpolarization-activated cyclic nucleotide-gated channels, and the electrogenic sodium-calcium exchanger provide depolarizing current that is antagonized by delayed rectifier (I_{Kr}) and acetylcholine-gated (I_{KACh}) potassium currents. I_{Ca-L}, I_{Ca-T}, and I_f are modulated by β–adrenergic stimulation and I_{KACh} by vagal stimulation, explaining the exquisite sensitivity of diastolic depolarization to autonomic nervous system activity. The slow conduction within the SA node is explained by the absence of I_{Na} and poor electrical coupling of cells in the node, resulting from sizable amounts of interstitial tissue and a low abundance of gap junctions. The poor coupling allows for graded electrophysiologic properties within the node, with the peripheral transitional cells being silenced by electrotonic coupling to atrial myocardium.

Etiology of SA nodal disease

SA nodal dysfunction has been classified as intrinsic or extrinsic. The distinction is important because extrinsic dysfunction is often reversible and generally should be corrected before pacemaker therapy is considered (Table 15-1). The most common causes of extrinsic SA node dysfunction are drugs and autonomic nervous system influences that suppress automaticity and/or compromise conduction. Other extrinsic causes include hypothyroidism, sleep apnea, and conditions likely to occur in critically ill patients such as hypothermia, hypoxia, increased intracranial pressure (Cushing's response), and endotracheal suctioning via activation of the vagus nerve.

Intrinsic sinus node dysfunction is degenerative and often is characterized pathologically by fibrous replacement of the SA node or its connections to the atrium. Acute and chronic coronary artery disease (CAD) may be associated with SA node dysfunction, although in the setting of acute myocardial infarction (MI; typically inferior), the vabnormalities are transient. Inflammatory processes may alter SA node function, ultimately producing replacement fibrosis. Pericarditis, myocarditis, and rheumatic heart disease have been associated with SA nodal disease with sinus bradycardia, sinus arrest, and exit block. Carditis associated with systemic lupus erythematosus (SLE), rheumatoid arthritis (RA), and mixed connective tissue disorders (MCTDs) may also affect SA node structure and function. Senile amyloidosis is an infiltrative disorder in patients typically in the ninth decade of life; deposition of amyloid protein

in the atrial myocardium can impair SA node function. Some SA node disease is iatrogenic and results from direct injury to the SA node during cardiothoracic surgery.

Rare heritable forms of sinus node disease have been described, and several have been characterized genetically. Autosomal dominant sinus node dysfunction in conjunction with supraventricular tachycardia (i.e., tachycardia-bradycardia variant of sick-sinus syndrome [SSS]) has been linked to mutations in the pacemaker current (I_f) subunit gene *HCN4* on chromosome 15. An autosomal recessive form of SSS with the prominent feature of atrial inexcitability and absence of P waves on the electrocardiogram (ECG) is caused by mutations in the cardiac sodium channel gene, *SCN5A*, on chromosome 3. SSS associated with myopia has been described but not genetically characterized. There are several neuromuscular diseases, including Kearns-Sayre syndrome (ophthalmoplegia, pigmentary degeneration of the retina, and cardiomyopathy) and myotonic dystrophy, that have a predilection for the conducting system and SA node.

SSS in both the young and the elderly is associated with an increase in fibrous tissue in the SA node. The onset of SSS may be hastened by coexisting disease, such as CAD, diabetes mellitus, hypertension, and valvular diseases and cardiomyopathies.

Clinical features of SA node disease

SA node dysfunction may be completely asymptomatic and manifest as an ECG anomaly such as sinus bradycardia; sinus arrest and exit block; or alternating supraventricular tachycardia, usually atrial fibrillation, and bradycardia. Symptoms associated with SA node dysfunction, in particular tachycardia-bradycardia syndrome, may be related to both slow and fast heart rates. For example, tachycardia may be associated with palpitations, angina pectoris, and heart failure, and bradycardia may be associated with hypotension, syncope, presyncope, fatigue, and weakness. In the setting of SSS, overdrive suppression of the SA node may result in prolonged pauses and syncope upon termination of the tachycardia. In many cases, symptoms associated with SA node dysfunction result from concomitant cardiovascular disease. A significant minority of patients with SSS develop signs and symptoms of heart failure that may be related to slow or fast heart rates.

One-third to one-half of patients with SA node dysfunction develop supraventricular tachycardia, usually atrial fibrillation or atrial flutter. The incidence of persistent atrial fibrillation in patients with SA node dysfunction increases with advanced age, hypertension, diabetes mellitus, left ventricular dilation, valvular heart disease, and ventricular pacing. Remarkably, some symptomatic patients may experience an improvement

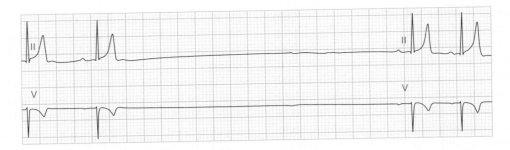

FIGURE 15-3

Sinus slowing and pauses on the ECG. The ECG is recorded during sleep in a young patient without heart disease. The heart rate before the pause is slow, and the PR interval is prolonged, consistent with an increase in vagal tone. The P waves have a morphology consistent with sinus rhythm. The recording is from a two-lead telemetry system in which the tracing labeled II mimics frontal lead II and V represents Modified Central Lead 1, which mimics lead V1 of the standard 12-lead ECG.

in symptoms with the development of atrial fibrillation, presumably from an increase in their average heart rate. Patients with the tachycardia-bradycardia variant of SSS, similar to patients with atrial fibrillation, are at risk for thromboembolism, and *those at greatest risk*, including patients ≥65 years and patients with a prior history of stroke, valvular heart disease, left ventricular dysfunction, or atrial enlargement, should be treated with anticoagulants. Up to one-quarter of patients with SA node disease will have concurrent AV conduction disease, although only a minority will require specific therapy for high-grade AV block.

The natural history of SA node dysfunction is one of varying intensity of symptoms even in patients who present with syncope. Symptoms related to SA node dysfunction may be significant, but overall mortality usually is not compromised in the absence of other significant comorbid conditions. These features of the natural history need to be taken into account in considering therapy for these patients.

Electrocardiography of SA node disease

The electrocardiographic manifestations of SA node dysfunction include sinus bradycardia, sinus pauses, sinus arrest, sinus exit block, tachycardia (in SSS), and chronotropic incompetence. It is often difficult to distinguish pathologic from physiologic sinus bradycardia.

By definition, sinus bradycardia is a rhythm driven by the SA node with a rate of <60 beats/min; sinus bradycardia is very common and typically benign. Resting heart rates <60 beats/min are very common in young healthy individuals and physically conditioned subjects. A sinus rate of <40 beats/min in the awake state in the absence of physical conditioning generally is considered abnormal. Sinus pauses and sinus arrest result from failure of the SA node to discharge, producing a pause without P waves visible on the ECG (**Fig. 15-3**). Sinus pauses of up to 3 s are common in awake athletes, and pauses of this duration or longer may be observed in asymptomatic elderly subjects. Intermittent failure of conduction from the SA node produces sinus exit block. The severity of sinus exit block may vary in a manner similar to that of AV block (see later). Prolongation of conduction from the sinus node will not be apparent on the ECG; second-degree SA block will produce intermittent conduction from the SA node and a regularly irregular atrial rhythm.

Type I second-degree SA block results from progressive prolongation of SA node conduction with intermittent failure of the impulses originating in the sinus node to conduct to the surrounding atrial tissue. Second-degree SA block appears on the ECG as an intermittent absence of P waves (**Fig. 15-4**). In type II second-degree SA block, there is no change in SA node conduction before the pause. Complete

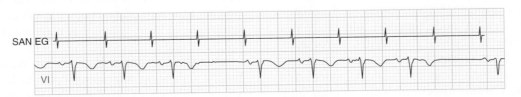

FIGURE 15-4

Mobitz type I SA nodal exit block. A theoretical SA node electrogram (SAN EG) is shown. Note that there is grouped beating producing a regularly irregular heart rhythm. The SA node EG rate is constant with progressive delay in exit from the node and activation of the atria, inscribing the P wave. This produces subtly decreasing P-P intervals before the pause, and the pause is less than twice the cycle length of the last sinus interval.

or third-degree SA block results in no P waves on the ECG. Tachycardia-bradycardia syndrome is manifest as alternating sinus bradycardia and atrial tachyarrhythmias. Although atrial tachycardia, atrial flutter, and atrial fibrillation may be observed, the latter is the most common tachycardia. Chronotropic incompetence is the inability to increase the heart rate in response to exercise or other stress appropriately and is defined in greater detail later.

Diagnostic testing

SA node dysfunction is most commonly a clinical or electrocardiographic diagnosis. Sinus bradycardia or pauses on the resting ECG are rarely sufficient to diagnose SA node disease, and longer-term recording and symptom correlation generally are required. Symptoms in the absence of sinus bradyarrhythmias may be sufficient to exclude a diagnosis of SA node dysfunction.

Electrocardiographic recording plays a central role in the diagnosis and management of SA node dysfunction. Despite the limitations of the resting ECG, longer-term recording employing Holter or event monitors may permit correlation of symptoms with the cardiac rhythm. Many contemporary event monitors may be automatically triggered to record the ECG when certain programmed heart rate criteria are met. Implantable ECG monitors permit long-term recording (12–18 months) in particularly challenging patients.

Failure to increase the heart rate with exercise is referred to as *chronotropic incompetence*. This is alternatively defined as failure to reach 85% of predicted maximal heart rate at peak exercise or failure to achieve a heart rate >100 beats/min with exercise or a maximal heart rate with exercise less than two standard deviations below that of an age-matched control population. Exercise testing may be useful in discriminating chronotropic incompetence from resting bradycardia and may aid in the identification of the mechanism of exercise intolerance.

Autonomic nervous system testing is useful in diagnosing carotid sinus hypersensitivity; pauses >3 s are consistent with the diagnosis but may be present in asymptomatic elderly subjects. Determining the intrinsic heart rate (IHR) may distinguish SA node dysfunction from slow heart rates that result from high vagal tone. The normal IHR after administration of 0.2 mg/kg propranolol and 0.04 mg/kg atropine is 117.2 − (0.53 × age) in beats/min; a low IHR is indicative of SA disease.

Electrophysiologic testing may play a role in the assessment of patients with presumed SA node dysfunction and in the evaluation of syncope, particularly in the setting of structural heart disease. In this circumstance, electrophysiologic testing is used to rule out more malignant etiologies of syncope, such as ventricular tachyarrhythmias and AV conduction block. There are several ways to assess SA node function invasively. They include the sinus node recovery time (SNRT), defined as the longest pause after cessation of overdrive pacing of the right atrium near the SA node (normal: <1500 ms or, corrected for sinus cycle length, <550 ms), and the sinoatrial conduction time (SACT), defined as one-half the difference between the intrinsic sinus cycle length and a noncompensatory pause after a premature atrial stimulus (normal <125 ms). The combination of an abnormal SNRT, an abnormal SACT, and a low IHR is a sensitive and specific indicator of intrinsic SA node disease.

TREATMENT Sinoatrial Node Dysfunction

Since SA node dysfunction is not associated with increased mortality rates, the aim of therapy is alleviation of symptoms. Exclusion of extrinsic causes of SA node dysfunction and correlation of the cardiac rhythm with symptoms is an essential part of patient management. Pacemaker implantation is the primary therapeutic intervention in patients with symptomatic SA node dysfunction. Pharmacologic considerations are important in the evaluation and management of patients with SA nodal disease. A number of drugs modulate SA node function and are extrinsic causes of dysfunction (Table 15-1). Beta blockers and calcium channel blockers increase SNRT in patients with SA node dysfunction, and antiarrhythmic drugs with class I and III action may promote SA node exit block. In general, such agents should be discontinued before decisions regarding the need for permanent pacing in patients with SA node disease are made. Chronic pharmacologic therapy for sinus bradyarrhythmias is limited. Some pharmacologic agents may improve SA node function; digitalis, for example, has been shown to shorten SNRT in patients with SA node dysfunction. Isoproterenol or atropine administered IV may increase the sinus rate acutely. Theophylline has been used both acutely and chronically to increase heart rate but has liabilities when used in patients with tachycardia-bradycardia syndrome, increasing the frequency of supraventricular tachyarrhythmias, and in patients with structural heart disease, increasing the risk of potentially serious ventricular arrhythmias. At the current time, there is only a single randomized study of therapy for SA node dysfunction. In patients with resting heart rates <50 and >30 beats/min on a Holter monitor, patients who received dual-chamber pacemakers experienced significantly fewer syncopal episodes and had symptomatic improvement compared with patients randomized to theophylline or no treatment.

In certain circumstances, sinus bradycardia requires no specific treatment or only temporary rate support. Sinus bradycardia is common in patients with acute inferior or posterior MI and can be exacerbated by vagal activation induced by pain or the use of drugs such as morphine. Ischemia of the SA nodal artery probably occurs in acute coronary syndromes more typically with involvement with the right coronary artery, and even with infarction, the effect on SA node function most often is transient.

Sinus bradycardia is a prominent feature of carotid sinus hypersensitivity and neurally mediated hypotension associated with vasovagal syncope that responds to pacemaker therapy. Carotid hypersensitivity with recurrent syncope or presyncope associated with a predominant cardioinhibitory component responds to pacemaker implantation. Several randomized trials have investigated the efficacy of permanent pacing in patients with drug-refractory vasovagal syncope, with mixed results. Although initial trials suggested that patients undergoing pacemaker implantation have fewer recurrences and a longer time to recurrence of symptoms, at least one follow-up study did not confirm these results.

The details of pacing modes and indications for pacing in SA node dysfunction are discussed below.

ATRIOVENTRICULAR CONDUCTION DISEASE

Structure and physiology of the AV node

The AV conduction axis is structurally complex, involving the atria and ventricles as well as the AV node. Unlike the SA node, the AV node is a subendocardial structure originating in the transitional zone, which is composed of aggregates of cells in the posterior-inferior right atrium. Superior, medial, and posterior transitional atrionodal bundles converge on the compact AV node. The compact AV node ($\sim$1 $\times$ 3 $\times$ 5 mm) is situated at the apex of the triangle of Koch, which is defined by the coronary sinus ostium posteriorly, the septal tricuspid valve annulus anteriorly, and the tendon of Todaro superiorly. The compact AV node continues as the penetrating AV bundle where it immediately traverses the central fibrous body and is in close proximity to the aortic, mitral, and tricuspid valve annuli; thus, it is subject to injury in the setting of valvular heart disease or its surgical treatment. The penetrating AV bundle continues through the annulus fibrosis and emerges along the ventricular septum adjacent to the membranous septum as the bundle of His. The right bundle branch (RBB) emerges from the distal AV bundle in a band that traverses the right ventricle (moderator band). In contrast, the left bundle branch (LBB) is a broad subendocardial sheet of tissue on the septal left ventricle. The Purkinje fiber network emerges from the RBB and LBB and extensively ramifies on the endocardial surfaces of the right and left ventricles, respectively.

The blood supply to the penetrating AV bundle is from the AV nodal artery and first septal perforator of the left anterior descending coronary artery. The bundle branches also have a dual blood supply from the septal perforators of the left anterior descending coronary artery and branches of the posterior descending coronary artery. The AV node is highly innervated with postganglionic sympathetic and parasympathetic nerves. The bundle of His and distal conducting system are minimally influenced by autonomic tone.

The cells that constitute the AV node complex are heterogeneous with a range of action potential profiles. In the transitional zones, the cells have an electrical phenotype between those of atrial myocytes and cells of the compact node (Fig. 15-1). Atrionodal transitional connections may exhibit *decremental conduction*, defined as slowing of conduction with increasingly rapid rates of stimulation. Fast and slow AV nodal pathways have been described, but it is controversial whether these two types of pathway are anatomically distinct or represent functional heterogeneities in different regions of the AV nodal complex. Myocytes that constitute the compact node are depolarized (resting membrane potential $\sim$−60 mV) and exhibit action potentials with low amplitudes, slow upstrokes of phase 0 (<10 V/s), and phase 4 diastolic depolarization; high-input resistance; and relative insensitivity to external [K+]. The action potential phenotype is explained by the complement of ionic currents expressed. AV nodal cells lack I_{K1} and I_{Na}; I_{Ca-L} is responsible for phase 0; and phase 4 depolarization reflects the composite activity of the depolarizing currents I_f, I_{Ca-L}, I_{Ca-T}, and I_{NCX} and the repolarizing currents I_{Kr} and I_{KACh}. Electrical coupling between cells in the AV node is tenuous due to the relatively sparse expression of gap junction channels (predominantly connexin-40) and increased extracellular volume.

The His bundle and the bundle branches are insulated from ventricular myocardium. The most rapid conduction in the heart is observed in these tissues. The action potentials exhibit very rapid upstrokes (phase 0), prolonged plateaus (phase 2), and modest automaticity (phase 4 depolarization). Gap junctions, composed largely of connexin-40, are abundant, but bundles are poorly connected transversely to ventricular myocardium.

Etiology of AV conduction disease

Conduction block from the atrium to the ventricle can occur for a variety of reasons in a number of clinical situations, and AV conduction block may be classified in a number of ways. The etiologies may be functional or structural, in part analogous to extrinsic and intrinsic causes of SA nodal dysfunction. The block may be classified by its severity from first to third degree or complete AV block or by the location of block within the AV conduction system. **Table 15-2** summarizes the etiologies of AV conduction block. Those which are functional (autonomic, metabolic/endocrine, and drug related) tend to be reversible. Most other etiologies produce structural changes, typically fibrosis, in segments of the AV conduction axis that are generally permanent. Heightened vagal tone during sleep or in well-conditioned individuals can be associated with all grades of AV block. Carotid sinus hypersensitivity, vasovagal syncope, and cough and micturition syncope may be associated with SA node slowing and AV conduction block. Transient metabolic and endocrinologic disturbances as well as a number of pharmacologic agents also may produce reversible AV conduction block.

Several infectious diseases have a predilection for the conducting system. Lyme disease may involve the heart in up to 50% of cases; 10% of patients with Lyme carditis develop AV conduction block, which is generally reversible but may require temporary pacing support. Chagas' disease, which is common in Latin America, and syphilis may produce more persistent AV conduction disturbances. Some autoimmune and infiltrative diseases may produce AV conduction block, including SLE, RA, MCTD, scleroderma, amyloidosis (primary and secondary), sarcoidosis, and hemochromatosis; rare malignancies also may impair AV conduction.

Idiopathic progressive fibrosis of the conduction system is one of the more common and degenerative causes of AV conduction block. Aging is associated with degenerative changes in the summit of the ventricular septum, central fibrous body, and aortic and mitral annuli and has been described as "sclerosis of the left cardiac skeleton." The process typically begins in the fourth decade of life and may be accelerated by atherosclerosis, hypertension, and diabetes mellitus. Accelerated forms of progressive familial heart block have been identified in families with mutations in the cardiac sodium channel gene (*SCN5A*) and other loci that have been mapped to chromosomes 1 and 19.

AV conduction block has been associated with heritable neuromuscular diseases, including the nucleotide repeat disease myotonic dystrophy, the mitochondrial myopathy Kearns-Sayre syndrome, and several of the monogenic muscular dystrophies. Congenital AV block may be observed in complex congenital cardiac anomalies (Chap. 19), such as transposition of the great arteries, ostium primum atrial septal defects (ASDs), ventricular septal defects (VSDs), endocardial cushion defects, and some single-ventricle defects. Congenital AV block in the setting of a structurally normal heart has been seen in children born to mothers with SLE. Iatrogenic AV block may occur during mitral or aortic valve surgery, rarely in the setting of thoracic radiation, and as a

TABLE 15-2

ETIOLOGIES OF ATRIOVENTRICULAR BLOCK

Autonomic

Carotid sinus hypersensitivity	Vasovagal

Metabolic/Endocrine

Hyperkalemia	Hypothyroidism
Hypermagnesemia	Adrenal insufficiency

Drug-Related

Beta blockers	Adenosine
Calcium channel blockers	Antiarrhythmics (class I and III)
Digitalis	Lithium

Infectious

Endocarditis	Tuberculosis
Lyme disease	Diphtheria
Chagas' disease	Toxoplasmosis
Syphilis	

Heritable/Congenital

Congenital heart disease Maternal SLE	Facioscapulohumeral MD, OMIM #158900 (4q35)
Kearns-Sayre syndrome, OMIM #530000	Emery-Dreifuss MD, OMIM #310300 (Xq28)
Myotonic dystrophy Type 1, OMIM #160900 (19q13.2-13.3)	Progressive familial heart block, OMIM #113900 (19q13.2-q13.3, 3p21)
Type 2, OMIM #602668 (3q13.3-q24)	

Inflammatory

SLE	MCTD
Rheumatoid arthritis	Scleroderma

Infiltrative

Amyloidosis	Hemochromatosis
Sarcoidosis	

Neoplastic/Traumatic

Lymphoma	Radiation
Mesothelioma	Catheter ablation
Melanoma	

Degenerative

Lev disease	Lenègre disease

Coronary Artery Disease

Acute MI

Abbreviations: MCTD, mixed connective tissue disease; MI, myocardial infarction; OMIM, Online Mendelian Inheritance in Man (database); SLE, systemic lupus erythematosus.

consequence of catheter ablation. AV block is a decidedly rare complication of the surgical repair of VSDs or ASDs but may complicate repairs of transposition of the great arteries.

CAD may produce transient or persistent AV block. In the setting of coronary spasm, ischemia, particularly in the right coronary artery distribution, may produce

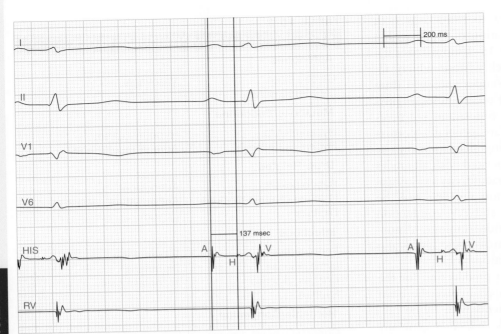

FIGURE 15-5

First-degree AV block with slowing of conduction in the AV node as indicated by the prolonged atrial-to-His bundle electrogram (AH) interval, in this case 157 ms. The His bundle-to-earliest ventricular activation on the surface ECG (HV) interval is normal. The normal HV interval suggests normal conduction below the AV node to the ventricle. I and V1 are surface ECG leads, HIS is the recording of the endocavitary electrogram at the His bundle position. A, H, and V are labels for the atrial, His bundle, and right ventricular electrograms, respectively.

transient AV block. In acute MI, AV block transiently develops in 10–25% of patients; most commonly this is first- or second-degree AV block, but complete heart block (CHB) may also occur. Second-degree and higher-grade AV block tends to occur more often in inferior than in anterior acute MI; however, the level of block in inferior MI tends to be in the AV node with more stable, narrow escape rhythms. In contrast, acute anterior MI is associated with block in the distal AV nodal complex, His bundle, or bundle branches and results in wide complex, unstable escape rhythms and a worse prognosis with high mortality rates.

Electrocardiography and electrophysiology of AV conduction block

Atrioventricular conduction block typically is diagnosed electrocardiographically, which characterizes the severity of the conduction disturbance and allows one to draw inferences about the location of the block. AV conduction block manifests as slow conduction in its mildest forms and failure to conduct, either intermittent or persistently, in more severe varieties. First-degree AV

block (PR interval >200 ms) is a slowing of conduction through the AV junction (**Fig. 15-5**). The site of delay is typically in the AV node but may be in the atria, bundle of His, or His-Purkinje system. A wide QRS is suggestive of delay in the distal conduction system, whereas a narrow QRS suggests delay in the AV node proper or, less commonly, in the bundle of His. In second-degree AV block there is an intermittent failure of electrical impulse conduction from atrium to ventricle. Second-degree AV block is subclassified as Mobitz type I (Wenckebach) or Mobitz type II. The periodic failure of conduction in Mobitz type I block is characterized by a progressively lengthening PR interval, shortening of the RR interval, and a pause that is less than two times the immediately preceding RR interval on the ECG. The ECG complex after the pause exhibits a shorter PR interval than that immediately preceding the pause (**Fig. 15-6**). This ECG pattern most often arises because of decremental conduction of electrical impulses in the AV node.

It is important to distinguish type I from type II second-degree AV nodal block because the latter has more serious prognostic implications. Type II

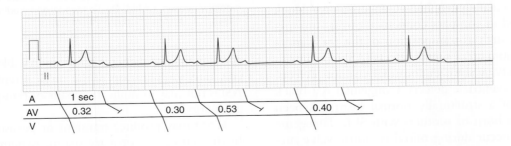

FIGURE 15-6

Mobitz type I second-degree AV block. The PR interval prolongs before the pause, as shown in the ladder diagram.

The ECG pattern results from slowing of conduction in the AV node.

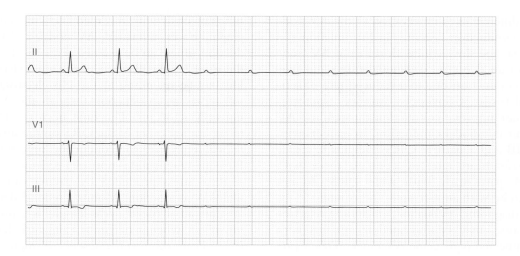

FIGURE 15-7

Paroxysmal AV block. Multiple nonconducted P waves after a period of sinus bradycardia with a normal PR interval. This implies significant conduction system disease, requiring permanent pacemaker implantation.

second-degree AV block is characterized by intermittent failure of conduction of the P wave without changes in the preceding PR or RR intervals. When AV block is 2:1, it may be difficult to distinguish type I from type II block. Type II second-degree AV block typically occurs in the distal or infra-His conduction system, is often associated with intraventricular conduction delays (e.g., bundle branch block), and is more likely to proceed to higher grades of AV block than is type I second-degree AV block. Second-degree AV block (particularly type II) may be associated with a series of nonconducted P waves, referred to as *paroxysmal AV block* **(Fig. 15–7)**, and implies significant conduction system disease and is an indication for permanent pacing. Complete failure of conduction from atrium to ventricle is referred to as complete or third-degree AV block. AV block that is intermediate between second degree and third degree is referred to as high-grade AV block and, as with CHB, implies advanced AV conduction system disease. In both cases, the block is most often distal to the AV node,

and the duration of the QRS complex can be helpful in determining the level of the block. In the absence of a preexisting bundle branch block, a wide QRS escape rhythm **(Fig. 15-8B)** implies a block in the distal His or bundle branches; in contrast, a narrow QRS rhythm implies a block in the AV node or proximal His and an escape rhythm originating in the AV junction **(Fig. 15-8A)**. Narrow QRS escape rhythms are typically faster and more stable than wide QRS escape rhythms and originate more proximally in the AV conduction system.

Diagnostic testing

Diagnostic testing in the evaluation of AV block is aimed at determining the level of conduction block, particularly in asymptomatic patients, since the prognosis and therapy depend on whether the block is in or below the AV node. Vagal maneuvers, carotid sinus massage, exercise, and administration of drugs such as atropine and isoproterenol may be diagnostically informative.

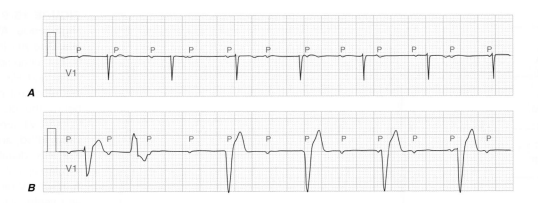

FIGURE 15-8

High-grade AV block. A. Multiple nonconducted P waves with a regular narrow complex QRS escape rhythm probably emanating from the AV junction. **B.** A wide complex QRS escape and a single premature ventricular contraction. In both cases, there is no consistent temporal relationship between the P waves and QRS complexes.

Owing to the differences in innervation of the AV node and infranodal conduction system, vagal stimulation and carotid sinus massage slow conduction in the AV node but have less of an effect on infranodal tissue and may even improve conduction due to a reduced rate of activation of distal tissues. Conversely, atropine, isoproterenol, and exercise improve conduction through the AV node and impair infranodal conduction. In patients with congenital CHB and a narrow QRS complex, exercise typically increases heart rate; by contrast, those with acquired CHB, particularly with wide QRS, do not respond to exercise with an increase in heart rate.

Additional diagnostic evaluation, including electrophysiologic testing, may be indicated in patients with syncope and suspected high-grade AV block. This is particularly relevant if noninvasive testing does not reveal the cause of syncope or if the patient has structural heart disease with ventricular tachyarrhythmias as a cause of symptoms. Electrophysiologic testing provides more precise information regarding the location of AV conduction block and permits studies of AV conduction under conditions of pharmacologic stress and exercise. Recording of the His bundle electrogram by a catheter positioned at the superior margin of the tricuspid valve annulus provides information about conduction at all levels of the AV conduction axis. A properly recorded His bundle electrogram reveals local atrial activity, the His electrogram, and local ventricular activation; when it is monitored simultaneously with recorded body surface electrocardiographic traces, intraatrial, AV nodal, and infranodal conduction times can be assessed (Fig. 15-5). The time from the most rapid deflection of the atrial electrogram in the His bundle recording to the His electrogram (*AH interval*) represents conduction through the AV node and is normally <130 ms. The time from the His electrogram to the earliest onset of the QRS on the surface ECG (*HV interval*) represents the conduction time through the His-Purkinje system and is normally ≤55 ms.

Rate stress produced by pacing can unveil abnormal AV conduction. Mobitz I second-degree AV block at short atrial paced cycle lengths is a normal response. However, when it occurs at atrial cycle lengths >500 ms (<120 beats/min) in the absence of high vagal tone, it is abnormal. Typically, type I second-degree AV block is associated with prolongation of the AH interval, representing conduction slowing and block in the AV node. AH prolongation occasionally is due to the effect of drugs (beta blockers, calcium channel blockers, digitalis) or increased vagal tone. Atropine can be used to reverse high vagal tone; however, if AH prolongation and AV block at long pacing cycle lengths persist, intrinsic AV node disease is likely. Type II second-degree block is typically infranodal, often in the His-Purkinje system. Block below the node with prolongation of the HV interval or a His bundle electrogram with no ventricular activation (**Fig. 15-9**) is abnormal unless it is elicited

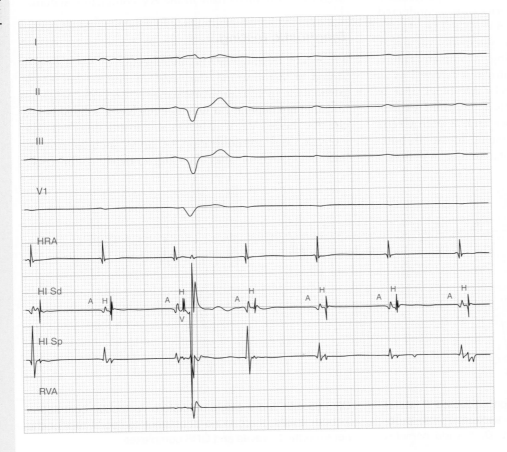

FIGURE 15-9

High-grade AV block below the His. The AH interval is normal and is not changing before the block. Atrial and His bundle electrograms are recorded consistent with block below the distal AV junction. I, II, III, and V1 are surface ECG leads. HISp, HISd, and RVA are the proximal HIS, distal HIS, and right ventricular apical electrical recordings. A, H, and V represent the atrial, His, and ventricular electrograms on the His bundle recording. (*Tracing courtesy of Dr. Joseph Marine; with permission.*)

at fast pacing rates or short coupling intervals with extra stimulation. It is often difficult to determine the type of second–degree AV block when 2:1 conduction is present; however, the finding of a His bundle electrogram after every atrial electrogram indicates that block is occurring in the distal conduction system.

Intracardiac recording at electrophysiologic study that reveals prolongation of conduction through the His-Purkinje system (i.e., long HV interval) is associated with an increased risk of progression to higher grades of block and is generally an indication for pacing. In the setting of bundle branch block, the HV interval may reveal the condition of the unblocked bundle and the prognosis for developing more advanced AV conduction block. Prolongation of the HV interval in patients with asymptomatic bundle branch block is associated with an increased risk of developing higher-grade AV block. The risk increases with greater prolongation of the HV interval such that in patients with an HV interval >100 ms, the annual incidence of complete AV block approaches 10%, indicating a need for pacing. In patients with acquired CHB, even if intermittent, there is little role for electrophysiologic testing, and pacemaker implantation is almost always indicated.

| TREATMENT | Management of AV Conduction Block |

Temporary or permanent artificial pacing is the most reliable treatment for patients with symptomatic AV conduction system disease. However, exclusion of reversible causes of AV block and the need for temporary heart rate support based on the hemodynamic condition of the patient are essential considerations in each patient. Correction of electrolyte derangements and ischemia, inhibition of excessive vagal tone, and withholding of drugs with AV nodal blocking properties may increase the heart rate. Adjunctive pharmacologic treatment with atropine or isoproterenol may be useful if the block is in the AV node. Since most pharmacologic treatment may take some time to initiate and become effective, temporary pacing may be necessary. The most expeditious technique is the use of transcutaneous pacing, where pacing patches are placed anteriorly over the cardiac apex (cathode) and posteriorly between the spine and the scapula or above the right nipple (anode). Acutely, transcutaneous pacing is highly effective, but its duration is limited by patient discomfort and longer-term failure to capture the ventricle owing to changes in lead impedance. If a patient requires more than a few minutes of pacemaker support, transvenous temporary pacing should be instituted. Temporary pacing leads can be placed from the jugular or subclavian venous system and advanced to the right ventricle, permitting stable temporary pacing for many days, if necessary. In most circumstances, in the absence of prompt resolution, conduction block distal to the AV node requires permanent pacemaking.

PERMANENT PACEMAKERS

Nomenclature and Complications

The main therapeutic intervention in SA node dysfunction and AV conduction block is permanent pacing. Since the first implementation of permanent pacing in the 1950s, many advances in technology have resulted in miniaturization, increased longevity of pulse generators, improvement in leads, and increased functionality. To better understand pacemaker therapy for bradycardias, it is important to be familiar with the fundamentals of pacemaking. Pacemaker modes and function are named using a five-letter code. The first letter indicates the chamber(s) that is paced (O, none; A, atrium; V, ventricle; D, dual; S, single), the second is the chamber(s) in which sensing occurs (O, none; A, atrium; V, ventricle; D, dual; S, single), the third is the response to a sensed event (O, none; I, inhibition; T, triggered; D, inhibition + triggered), the fourth refers to the programmability or rate response (R, rate responsive), and the fifth refers to the existence of antitachycardia functions if present (O, none; P, antitachycardia pacing; S, shock; D, pace + shock). Almost all modern pacemakers are multiprogrammable and have the capability for rate responsiveness using one of several rate sensors: activity or motion, minute ventilation, or QT interval. The most commonly programmed modes of implanted single- and dual-chamber pacemakers are VVIR and DDDR, respectively, although multiple modes can be programmed in modern pacemakers.

Although pacemakers are highly reliable, they are subject to a number of complications related to implantation and electronic function. In adults, permanent pacemakers are most commonly implanted with access to the heart by way of the subclavian–superior vena cava venous system. Rare, but possible, acute complications of transvenous pacemaker implantation include infection, hematoma, pneumothorax, cardiac perforation, diaphragmatic/phrenic nerve stimulation, and lead dislodgment. Limitations of chronic pacemaker therapy include infection, erosion, lead failure, and abnormalities resulting from inappropriate programming or interaction with the patient's native electrical cardiac function. Rotation of the pacemaker pulse generator in its subcutaneous pocket, either intentionally or inadvertently, often referred to as "twiddler's syndrome," can wrap the leads around the generator and produce dislodgment with failure to sense or pace the heart. The small size and light weight of contemporary pacemakers make this a rare complication.

Complications stemming from chronic cardiac pacing also result from disturbances in atrioventricular synchrony and/or left ventricular mechanical synchrony. Pacing modes that interrupt or fail to restore atrioventricular synchrony may lead to a constellation of signs and symptoms, collectively referred to as pacemaker syndrome, that include neck pulsation, fatigue, palpitations, cough, confusion, exertional dyspnea, dizziness, syncope, elevation in jugular venous pressure, canon A waves, and stigmata of congestive heart failure, including edema, rales, and a third heart sound. Right ventricular apical pacing can induce dyssynchronous activation of the left ventricle, leading to compromised left ventricular (LV) systolic function, mitral valve regurgitation, and the previously mentioned stigmata of congestive heart failure. Maintenance of AV synchrony can minimize the sequelae of pacemaker syndrome. Selection of pacing modes that minimize unnecessary ventricular pacing or implantation of a device capable of right and left ventricular pacing (biventricular pacing) can help minimize the deleterious consequences of pacing-induced mechanical dyssynchrony at the ventricular level.

Pacemaker Therapy in SA Node Dysfunction Pacing in SA nodal disease is indicated to alleviate symptoms of bradycardia. Consensus guidelines published by the American Heart Association (AHA)/American College of Cardiology/Heart Rhythm Society (ACC/HRS) outline the indications for the use of pacemakers and categorize them by class based on levels of evidence. Class I conditions are those for which there is evidence or consensus of opinion that therapy is useful and effective. In class II conditions there is conflicting evidence or a divergence of opinion about the efficacy of a procedure or treatment; in class IIa conditions the weight of evidence or opinion favors treatment, and in class IIb conditions efficacy is less well established by the evidence or opinion of experts. In class III conditions, the evidence or weight of opinion indicates that the therapy is not efficacious or useful and may be harmful.

Class I indications for pacing in SA node dysfunction include documented symptomatic bradycardia, sinus node dysfunction–associated long-term drug therapy for which there is no alternative, and symptomatic chronotropic incompetence. Class IIa indications include those outlined previously in which sinus node dysfunction is suspected but not documented and for syncope of unexplained origin in the presence of major abnormalities of SA node dysfunction. Mildly symptomatic individuals with heart rates consistently <40 beats/min constitute a class IIb indication for pacing. Pacing is not indicated in patients with SA node dysfunction who do not have symptoms and in those in whom bradycardia is associated with the use of nonessential drugs (Table 15-3).

There is some controversy about the mode of pacing that should be employed in SA node disease. A number

TABLE 15-3

SUMMARY OF GUIDELINES FOR PACEMAKER IMPLANTATION IN SA NODE DYSFUNCTION
Class I
1. SA node dysfunction with symptomatic bradycardia or sinus pauses
2. Symptomatic SA node dysfunction as a result of essential long-term drug therapy with no acceptable alternatives
3. Symptomatic chronotropic incompetence
4. Atrial fibrillation with bradycardia and pauses >5s
Class IIa
1. SA node dysfunction with heart rates <40 beats/min without a clear and consistent relationship between bradycardia and symptoms
2. SA node dysfunction with heart rates <40 beats/min on an essential long-term drug therapy with no acceptable alternatives, without a clear and consistent relationship between bradycardia and symptoms
3. Syncope of unknown origin when major abnormalities of SA node dysfunction are discovered or provoked by electrophysiologic testing
Class IIb
1. Mildly symptomatic patients with waking chronic heart rates <40 beats/min
Class III
1. SA node dysfunction in asymptomatic patients, even those with heart rates <40 beats/min
2. SA node dysfunction in which symptoms suggestive of bradycardia are not associated with a slow heart rate
3. SA node dysfunction with symptomatic bradycardia due to nonessential drug therapy

Source: Modified from AE Epstein et al: J Am Coll Cardiol 51:e1, 2008 and G Gregoratos et al: J Am Coll Cardiol 40:703, 2002.

of randomized, single-blind trials of pacing mode have been performed. There are no trials that demonstrate an improvement in mortality rate with AV synchronous pacing compared with single-chamber pacing in SA node disease. In some of these studies, the incidence of atrial fibrillation and thromboembolic events was reduced with AV synchronous pacing. In trials of patients with dual-chamber pacemakers designed to compare single-chamber with dual-chamber pacing by crossover design, the need for AV synchronous pacing due to pacemaker syndrome was common. Pacing modes that preserve AV synchrony appear to be associated with a reduction in the incidence of atrial fibrillation and improved quality of life. Because of the low but finite incidence of AV conduction disease, patients with SA node dysfunction usually undergo dual-chamber pacemaker implantation.

Pacemaker Therapy in Carotid Sinus Hypersensitivity and Vasovagal Syncope Carotid sinus hypersensitivity, if accompanied by a significant cardioinhibitory component, responds well to pacing. In this circumstance, pacing is required only intermittently and single-chamber ventricular pacing is often sufficient. The mechanism of vasovagal syncope is incompletely understood but appears to involve activation of cardiac mechanoreceptors with consequent activation of neural centers that mediate vagal activation and withdrawal of sympathetic nervous system tone. Several randomized clinical trials have been performed in patients with drug-refractory vasovagal syncope, with some studies suggesting reduction in the frequency and the time to recurrent syncope in patients who were paced compared with those who were not. A recent follow-up study to one of those initial trials, however, found less convincing results, casting some doubt on the utility of pacing for vagally mediated syncope.

Pacemakers in AV Conduction Disease

There are no randomized trials that evaluate the efficacy of pacing in patients with AV block, as there are no reliable therapeutic alternatives for AV block and untreated high-grade AV block is potentially lethal. The consensus guidelines for pacing in acquired AV conduction block in adults provide a general outline for situations in which pacing is indicated (Table 15-4). Pacemaker implantation should be performed in any patient with symptomatic bradycardia and irreversible second- or third-degree AV block, regardless of the cause or level of block in the conducting system. Symptoms may include those directly related to bradycardia and low cardiac output or to worsening heart failure, angina, or intolerance to an essential medication. Pacing in patients with asymptomatic AV block should be individualized; situations in which pacing should be considered are patients with acquired CHB, particularly in the setting of cardiac enlargement; left ventricular dysfunction; and waking heart rates ≤40 beats/min. Patients who have asymptomatic second-degree AV block of either type should be considered for pacing if the block is demonstrated to be intra- or infra-His or is associated with a wide QRS complex. Pacing may be indicated in asymptomatic patients in special circumstances, in patients with profound first-degree AV block and left ventricular dysfunction in whom a shorter AV interval produces hemodynamic improvement, and in the setting of milder forms of AV conduction delay (first-degree AV block, intraventricular conduction delay) in patients with neuromuscular diseases that have a predilection for the conduction system, such as myotonic dystrophy and other muscular dystrophies, and Kearns-Sayre syndrome.

Pacemaker Therapy in Myocardial Infarction

Atrioventricular block in acute MI is often transient, particularly in inferior infarction. The circumstances in which pacing is indicated in acute MI are persistent second- or third-degree AV block, particularly

TABLE 15-4

GUIDELINE SUMMARY FOR PACEMAKER IMPLANTATION IN ACQUIRED AV BLOCK

Class I

1. Third-degree or high-grade AV block at any anatomic level associated with:
   a. Symptomatic bradycardia
   b. Essential drug therapy that produces symptomatic bradycardia
   c. Periods of asystole >3 s or any escape rate <40 beats/min while awake
   d. Postoperative AV block not expected to resolve
   e. Catheter ablation of the AV junction
   f. Neuromuscular diseases such as myotonic dystrophy, Kearns-Sayre syndrome, Erb dystrophy, and peroneal muscular atrophy, regardless of the presence of symptoms
2. Second-degree AV block with symptomatic bradycardia
3. Type II second-degree AV block with a wide QRS complex with or without symptoms
4. Exercise-induced second- or third-degree AV block in the absence of ischemia
5. Atrial fibrillation with bradycardia and pauses >5s

Class IIa

1. Asymptomatic third-degree AV block regardless of level
2. Asymptomatic type II second-degree AV block with a narrow QRS complex
3. Asymptomatic type II second-degree AV block with block within or below the His at electrophysiologic study
4. First- or second-degree AV block with symptoms similar to pacemaker syndrome

Class IIb

1. Marked first-degree AV block (PR interval >300 ms) in patients with LV dysfunction in whom shortening the AV delay would improve hemodynamics
2. Neuromuscular diseases such as myotonic dystrophy, Kearns-Sayre syndrome, Erb dystrophy, and peroneal muscular atrophy with any degree of AV block regardless of the presence of symptoms

Class III

1. Asymptomatic first-degree AV block
2. Asymptomatic type I second-degree AV block at the AV node level
3. AV block that is expected to resolve or is unlikely to recur (Lyme disease, drug toxicity)

Source: Modified from AE Epstein et al: J Am Coll Cardiol 51:e1, 2008 and G Gregoratos et al: J Am Coll Cardiol 40:703, 2002.

if symptomatic, and transient second- or third-degree AV block associated with bundle branch block (Table 15-5). Pacing is generally not indicated in the setting of transient AV block in the absence of intraventricular conduction delays or in the presence of fascicular block or first-degree AV block that develops in the setting of preexisting bundle branch block. Fascicular blocks that develop in acute MI in the absence of other

TABLE 15-5

GUIDELINE SUMMARY FOR PACEMAKER IMPLANTATION IN AV CONDUCTION BLOCK IN ACUTE MYOCARDIAL INFARCTION (AMI)

Class I
1. Persistent second-degree AV block in the His-Purkinje system with bilateral bundle branch block or third-degree block within or below the His after AMI
2. Transient advanced (second- or third-degree) infranodal AV block and associated bundle branch block. If the site of block is uncertain, an electrophysiologic study may be necessary
3. Persistent and symptomatic second- or third-degree AV block

Class IIb
1. Persistent second- or third-degree AV block at the AV node level

Class III
1. Transient AV block in the absence of intraventricular conduction defects
2. Transient AV block in the presence of isolated left anterior fascicular block
3. Acquired left anterior fascicular block in the absence of AV block
4. Persistent first-degree AV block in the presence of bundle branch block that is old or age-indeterminate

Source: Modified from AE Epstein et al: J Am Coll Cardiol 51:e1, 2008 and G Gregoratos et al: J Am Coll Cardiol 40:703, 2002.

TABLE 15-6

INDICATIONS FOR PACEMAKER IMPLANTATION IN CHRONIC BIFASCICULAR AND TRIFASCICULAR BLOCK

Class I
1. Intermittent third-degree AV block
2. Type II second-degree AV block
3. Alternating bundle branch block

Class IIa
1. Syncope not demonstrated to be due to AV block when other likely causes (e.g., ventricular tachycardia) have been excluded
2. Incidental finding at electrophysiologic study of a markedly prolonged HV interval (>100 ms) in asymptomatic patients
3. Incidental finding at electrophysiologic study of pacing-induced infra-His block that is not physiologic

Class IIb
1. Neuromuscular diseases such as myotonic dystrophy, Kearns-Sayre syndrome, Erb dystrophy, and peroneal muscular atrophy with any degree of fascicular block regardless of the presence of symptoms, because there may be unpredictable progression of AV conduction disease

Class III
1. Fascicular block without AV block or symptoms
2. Fascicular block with first-degree AV block without symptoms

Source: Modified from AE Epstein et al: J Am Coll Cardiol 51:e1, 2008 and G Gregoratos et al: J Am Coll Cardiol 40:703, 2002.

forms of AV block also do not require pacing (Table 15-5 and Table 15-6).

Pacemaker Therapy in Bifascicular and Trifascicular Block Distal forms of AV conduction block may require pacemaker implantation in certain clinical settings. Patients with bifascicular or trifascicular block and symptoms, particularly syncope that is not attributable to other causes, should undergo pacemaker implantation. Pacemaking is indicated in asymptomatic patients with bifascicular or trifascicular block who experience intermittent third-degree, type II second-degree AV block or alternating bundle branch block. In patients with fascicular block who are undergoing electrophysiologic study, a markedly prolonged HV interval or block below the His at long cycle lengths also may constitute an indication for permanent pacing. Patients with fascicular block and the neuromuscular diseases

previously described should also undergo pacemaker implantation (Table 15-6).

Selection of Pacing Mode In general, a pacing mode that maintains AV synchrony reduces complications of pacing such as pacemaker syndrome and pacemaker-mediated tachycardia. This is particularly true in younger patients; the importance of dual-chamber pacing in the elderly, however, is not well established. Several studies have failed to demonstrate a difference in mortality rate in older patients with AV block treated with a single-(VVI) compared with a dual-(DDD) chamber pacing mode. In some of the studies that randomized pacing mode, the risk of chronic atrial fibrillation and stroke risk decreased with physiologic pacing. In patients with sinus rhythm and AV block, the very modest increase in risk with dual-chamber pacemaker implantation appears to be justified to avoid the possible complications of single-chamber pacing.

CHAPTER 16

THE TACHYARRHYTHMIAS

Francis Marchlinski

The term *tachyarrhythmias* typically refers to nonsustained and sustained forms of tachycardia originating from myocardial foci or reentrant circuits. The standard definition of tachycardia is a rhythm that produces a ventricular rate >100 beats per minute. This definition has some limitations in that atrial rates can exceed 100 beats per minute despite a slow ventricular rate. Furthermore, ventricular rates may exceed the baseline sinus rate and be <100 beats per minute but still represent an important "tachycardia" response, as is observed with accelerated ventricular rhythms. Premature complexes (depolarizations) are considered under the category of tachyarrhythmias because they may cause arrhythmia-related symptoms and/or serve as triggering events for more sustained forms of tachycardia.

SYMPTOMS DUE TO TACHYARRHYTHMIAS

Tachyarrhythmias classically produce symptoms of palpitations or racing of the pulse. With premature beats, skipping of the pulse or a pause may be experienced, and patients may even sense slowing of the heart rate or dizziness. A more dramatic irregularity of the pulse is experienced with chaotic rapid rhythms or tachyarrhythmias that originate in the atrium and conduct variably to the ventricles. With rapid tachyarrhythmias, hemodynamic compromise can occur, as can dizziness or syncope due to a decrease in cardiac output or breathlessness due to a marked increase in cardiac filling pressures. Occasionally, chest discomfort may be experienced that mimics symptoms of myocardial ischemia. The underlying cardiac condition typically dictates the severity of symptoms at any specific heart rate. Even patients with normal systolic left ventricular (LV) function may experience severe symptoms if diastolic compliance due to hypertrophy or valvular obstruction is present and a tachycardia develops. Hemodynamic collapse with the development of ventricular fibrillation (VF) can lead to sudden cardiac death (SCD) (Chap. 29).

DIAGNOSTIC TESTS IN EVALUATING TACHYARRHYTHMIAS

In patients who present with nonlife-threatening symptoms such as palpitations or dizziness, electrocardiographic (ECG) confirmation of an arrhythmia with the development of recurrent symptoms is essential. A 24-h Holter monitor should be considered only for patients with daily symptoms. For intermittent symptoms that are of prolonged duration, a patient-activated event monitor can be used to obtain the ECG information without the need for continuous ECG lead attachment and recordings. A patient-activated monitor with a continuously recorded memory loop ("loop recorder") can be used to document short-lived episodes and the onset of the arrhythmia. This is the preferred monitoring technique for symptomatic patients with less frequent arrhythmia events, but it requires continuous ECG recording. A monitor that automatically triggers to record a fast rhythm can be used to detect asymptomatic arrhythmias. Patients with infrequent, severe symptoms that cannot be identified by intermittent ECG monitoring may receive an implanted loop ECG monitor that provides more extended periods of monitoring and automatic arrhythmia detection (Fig. 16-1).

In patients who present with more severe symptoms, such as syncope, outpatient monitoring may be insufficient. In patients with structural heart disease and syncope in whom there is suspicion of ventricular tachycardia (VT), hospitalization and diagnostic electrophysiologic testing are warranted, with strong consideration of an implantable cardioverter/defibrillator (ICD) device. The 12-lead ECG recorded in sinus rhythm should be assessed carefully in patients without structural heart disease for evidence of ST-segment elevation in leads V_1 and V_2 consistent with Brugada syndrome, QT interval changes consistent with long or short QT syndromes, or a short PR interval and delta wave

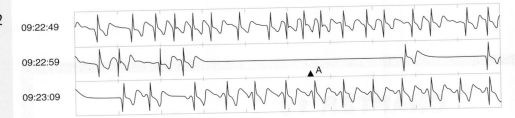

09:22:49

09:22:59

▲A

09:23:09

FIGURE 16-1

Spontaneous termination of atrial fibrillation at the time of a syncopal episode identified from implantable loop ECG recording.

consistent with Wolff-Parkinson-White (WPW) syndrome. These ECG patterns identify a possible arrhythmogenic substrate that may cause intermittent life-threatening symptoms and warrant further evaluation and therapy. The individual syndromes are discussed in detail later in this chapter.

Monitoring for asymptomatic tachyarrhythmias is indicated in several specific situations. In patients with a suspected tachycardia-induced cardiomyopathy marked by chamber dilation and depression in systolic function, the demonstration of arrhythmia control is essential. Monitoring for asymptomatic ventricular premature complexes (VPCs) and nonsustained VT can be helpful in stratifying the risk of SCD in patients with depressed LV function after myocardial infarction (MI). Finally, in patients with asymptomatic atrial fibrillation (AF), anticoagulation treatment strategies depend on an accurate assessment of the presence of this arrhythmia. The duration of monitoring for asymptomatic arrhythmias may have to be extended to optimize detection capabilities.

A 12-lead ECG recording during the tachycardia can be an important diagnostic tool in identifying the mechanism and origin of a tachycardia to a degree not afforded by one- or two-lead ECG recordings. A 12-lead ECG of the tachyarrhythmia should be recorded and incorporated as a permanent part of the medical record whenever possible. For patients whose arrhythmias are provoked by exercise, an exercise test may provide an opportunity to obtain 12-lead ECG recordings of the arrhythmia and may obviate the need for more extended periods of monitoring.

Many paroxysmal supraventricular tachyarrhythmias are not associated with a significant risk of structural heart disease, and an evaluation for the presence of ischemic heart disease and cardiac function is required infrequently unless dictated by the severity or characteristics of the symptoms. However, in patients with focal or macroreentrant atrial tachycardias (ATs), atrial flutter (AFL), or AF, an evaluation of cardiac chamber size and function and of valve function is warranted. In patients with VT, an echocardiographic assessment of LV and right ventricular (RV) size and function should be the norm. Ventricular tachycardia that occurs in the setting of depressed LV function should raise the suspicion of advanced coronary artery disease (CAD). Ventricular tachycardia in the setting of isolated RV dilation should raise concern about the diagnosis of arrhythmogenic RV cardiomyopathy. Polymorphic VT in the absence of QT prolongation should always raise concern for a potentially unstable ischemic process that may need to be corrected to effect VT control.

MECHANISMS OF TACHYARRHYTHMIAS

Tachycardias are due to abnormalities of impulse formation and/or abnormalities of impulse propagation (Fig. 16-2).

Abnormalities in impulse formation

An increase in automaticity normally causes an increase in sinus rate and sinus tachycardia (Fig. 16-2A). Abnormal automaticity is due to an increase in the slope of phase 4 depolarization or a reduced threshold for action potential depolarization in myocardium other than the sinus node. Abnormal automaticity is thought to be responsible for most atrial premature complexes (APCs) and VPCs and some ATs. Pacing does not provoke automatic rhythms. Less commonly, abnormal impulse formation is due to triggered activity. Triggered activity is related to cellular afterdepolarizations that occur at the end of the action potential, during phase 3, and are referred to as *early afterdepolarizations;* when they occur after the action potential, during phase 4, they are referred to as *late afterdepolarizations.* Afterdepolarizations are attributable to an increase in intracellular calcium accumulation. If sufficient afterdepolarization amplitude is achieved, repeated myocardial depolarization and a tachycardic response can occur. Early afterdepolarizations may be responsible for the VPCs that trigger the polymorphic ventricular arrhythmia known as *torsades des pointes* (TDP). Late afterdepolarizations are thought to be responsible for atrial, junctional, and fascicular tachyarrhythmias caused by digoxin toxicity and also appear to be the basis for catecholamine-sensitive VT originating in the outflow tract. In contrast to automatic tachycardias, those due to triggered activity (Fig. 16-2B) frequently can be provoked with pacing maneuvers.

Abnormalities in impulse propagation

Reentry is due to inhomogeneities in myocardial conduction and/or recovery properties. The presence of a

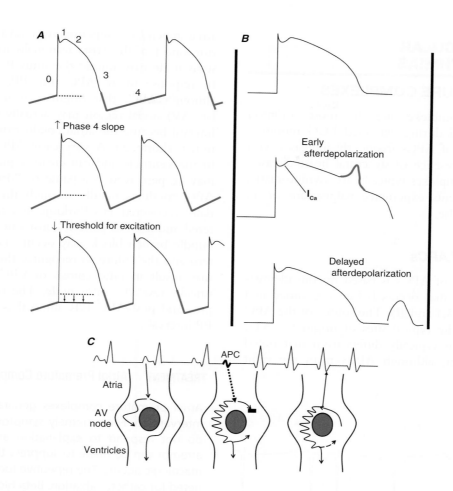

FIGURE 16-2

Schematic representation of the different mechanisms for arrhythmias. A. Abnormal automaticity due to an increased slope of phase 4 of the action potential or a decrease in the threshold for phase 0. **B.** Triggered activity due to early afterdepolarizations (EADs) during phase 3 of the action potential due to alteration of plateau currents or delayed afterdepolarizations (DADs) during phase 4 of the action potential due to intracellular calcium accumulation.

C. Reentry with basic requirements of two pathways that have heterogeneous electrophysiologic properties which allows conduction to block in one pathway and propagate slowly in the other, allowing for sufficient delay so that the blocked site has time for recovery to allow for reentry or circus movement tachycardia. Shown is a typical schema for reentry in the AV node. AV, atrioventricular; APC, atrial premature complex.

unidirectional block with slow conduction to allow for retrograde recovery of the blocked myocardium allows the formation of a circuit that, if perpetuated, can sustain a tachycardia (**Fig. 16-2C**). These inhomogeneities are somewhat inherent but are minimized in normal myocardial activation/recovery. The inhomogeneities can be exaggerated by the presence of extra pathways, as occurs with the WPW syndrome; generalized genetically determined myocardial ion channel abnormalities, as occur with long QT syndrome (LQTS); or the interruption of normal myocardial patterns of activation due to the development of fibrosis.

Reentry appears to be the basis for most abnormal sustained supraventricular tachycardias (SVTs) and VTs. In general, reentry can be anatomically driven (fixed) based on the presence of "extra" pathways, natural anatomic barriers of conduction such as the crista terminalis,

the vertical crest on the interior wall of the right atrium that separates the nontrabeculated posterior right atrium from the rest of the trabeculated right atrium located lateral to the structure, and/or extensive fibrosis created by underlying myocardial disease. This form of reentry seems to be more stable and results in a tachycardia that has a uniform (often monomorphic), repetitive appearance. Other forms of reentry appear to be more functional and are more dependent on dynamic changes in electrophysiologic properties of the myocardium. These tachycardias tend to be more unstable and may result in tachycardias that have a polymorphic appearance. Two classic examples of reentry that are primarily functional are VF due to acute myocardial ischemia and polymorphic VT in patients with a genetically determined ion channel abnormality such as Brugada syndrome, LQTS, or catecholaminergic polymorphic VT.

SUPRAVENTRICULAR TACHYARRHYTHMIAS

ATRIAL PREMATURE COMPLEXES

Atrial premature complexes are the most common arrhythmia identified during extended ECG monitoring. The incidence of APCs frequently increases with age and with the presence of structural heart diseases. Atrial premature complexes typically are asymptomatic, although some patients experience palpitations or an irregularity of the pulse.

ECG diagnosis of APCs

The ECG diagnosis of APCs is based on the identification of a P wave that occurs before the anticipated sinus beat (Fig. 16-3*A* and *B*). The source of the APC appears to parallel the typical sites of origin for ATs. The P-wave contour typically differs from that noted during sinus rhythm, although APCs from the right

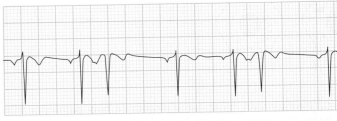

A

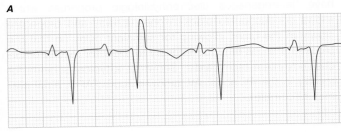

B

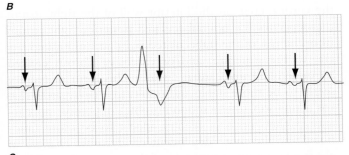

C

FIGURE 16-3

Atrial and ventricular premature complexes (APCs, VPCs). The APC resets the sinus node, and no compensatory pause is present **A.** even when conducted aberrantly in the ventricles with a bundle branch block-type QRS pattern **B.** VPCs tend not to reset the sinus activity (*arrows*) and will demonstrate a full compensatory pause **C.**

atrial appendage, superior vena cava (SVC), and superior aspect of the crista terminalis in the region of the sinus node may mimic the sinus P-wave morphology. In response to an APC, the PR interval lengthens, although APCs that originate near the atrioventricular (AV) nodal region may actually have a shorter PR interval because the atrial conduction time to the junction is shortened. A very early APC may not conduct to the ventricle and can create a pulse irregularity that may be perceived as a pause or "dropped beat." If the APC conducts rapidly through the AV node, a partially recovered His-Purkinje system will be encountered and a QRS pattern consistent with a right or left bundle branch block may occur. This wide QRS pattern and the failure to recognize the preceding P wave may result in misdiagnosis of VPCs. APCs characteristically reset the sinus node. The resulting sum of the pre- and post-APC RR interval is less than two sinus PP intervals.

TREATMENT	Atrial Premature Complexes

Atrial premature complexes generally do not require intervention. For extremely symptomatic patients who do not respond to explanation and reassurance, an attempt can be made to suppress the APCs with pharmacologic agents. The repetitive focus can even be targeted for catheter ablation. Beta blockers may be tried. Of note, these agents may uncommonly exacerbate symptoms if AV block occurs with the APC and irregularity of the pulse consequently becomes more profound. The use of class IC antiarrhythmic agents may eliminate the APCs but should be avoided if structural heart disease is present.

JUNCTIONAL PREMATURE COMPLEXES

Junctional premature complexes are extremely uncommon. The complexes originate from the AV node and His bundle region and may produce retrograde atrial activation with the P wave distorting the initial or terminal portions of the QRS complex, producing pseudo Q or S waves in leads II, III, and aVF. Extrasystoles originating in the bundle of His that do not conduct to the ventricle and also block the atria can produce unexplained surface ECG PR prolongation that does not follow a typical Wenckebach periodicity (i.e., gradual PR prolongation culminating in atrial activity that fails to conduct to the ventricles). Intracardiac recordings frequently can identify a His depolarization, thus identifying the origin of the complex to the AV junction. Symptomatic patients typically may be treated with beta blockers or, if there is no structural heart disease, class IC antiarrhythmic agents.

SINUS TACHYCARDIA

Physiologic sinus tachycardia represents a normal or appropriate response to physiologic stress, such as that which occurs with exercise, anxiety, or fever. Pathologic conditions such as thyrotoxicosis, anemia, and hypotension also may produce sinus tachycardia. It is important to distinguish sinus tachycardia from other SVTs. Sinus tachycardia will produce a P-wave contour consistent with its origin from the sinus node located in the superior-lateral and posterior aspect of the right atrium. The P wave is upright in leads II, III, and aVF and negative in lead aVR. The P-wave morphology in lead V_1 characteristically has a biphasic, positive/negative contour. Onset of sinus tachycardia is gradual, and in response to carotid sinus pressure there may be some modest and transient slowing but no abrupt termination. Importantly, the diagnosis should not be based on the PR interval or the presence of a P wave before every QRS complex. The PR interval and the presence of 1:1 AV conduction properties are determined by AV nodal and His-Purkinje conduction; therefore, the PR interval can be dramatically prolonged while sinus tachycardia remains the atrial mechanism.

TREATMENT Physiologic Sinus Tachycardia

Treatment of physiologic sinus tachycardia is directed at the underlying condition causing the tachycardia response. Uncommonly, beta blockers are used to minimize the tachycardia response if it is determined to be potentially harmful, as may occur in a patient with ischemic heart disease and rate-related anginal symptoms.

Inappropriate sinus tachycardia represents an uncommon but important medical condition in which the heart rate increases either spontaneously or out of proportion to the degree of physiologic stress/exercise. Dizziness and even frank syncope often accompany the sinus tachycardia and symptoms of palpitations. The syndrome can be quite disabling. Associated symptoms of chest pain, headaches, and gastrointestinal upset are common. In many patients, the syndrome occurs after a viral illness and may resolve spontaneously over the course of 3–12 months, suggesting a postviral dysautonomia.

Excluding the diagnosis of an automatic AT that originates in the region of the sinus node can be difficult and may require invasive electrophysiologic evaluation. Frequently, patients are misdiagnosed as having an anxiety disorder with physiologic sinus tachycardia.

TREATMENT Inappropriate Sinus Tachycardia

For symptomatic patients, maintaining an increased state of hydration, salt loading, and careful titration of beta blockers to the maximum tolerated dose, administered in divided doses, frequently minimize symptoms. For severely symptomatic patients who are intolerant of or unresponsive to beta blockers, catheter ablation directed at modifying the sinus node may be effective. Because of the high recurrence rate after ablation and the frequent need for atrial pacing therapy, this intervention remains second-line treatment.

ATRIAL FIBRILLATION

(Fig. 16-4) Atrial fibrillation is the most common sustained arrhythmia. It is marked by disorganized, rapid, and irregular atrial activation. The ventricular response to the rapid atrial activation is also irregular. In an untreated patient, the ventricular rate also tends to be rapid and is entirely dependent on the conduction properties of the AV junction. Although typically the rate will vary between 120 and 160 beats per minute, in some patients it can be >200 beats per minute. In other patients, because of heightened vagal tone or intrinsic AV nodal conduction properties, the ventricular response is <100 beats per minute and occasionally even profoundly slow. The mechanism for AF initiation and maintenance, although still debated, appears to be a complex interaction between drivers responsible for the initiation and the complex anatomic atrial substrate that promotes the maintenance of multiple wavelets of (micro)reentry. The drivers appear to originate predominantly from the atrialized musculature that enters the pulmonary veins and represent either focal abnormal automaticity or triggered firing that is somewhat modulated by autonomic influences. Sustained forms of microreentry as drivers also have been documented around the orifice of pulmonary veins; nonpulmonary vein drivers also have been demonstrated. The role these drivers play in maintaining the tachycardias may be significant and may explain the success of pulmonary vein isolation procedures in eliminating more chronic or persistent forms of AF.

Although AF is common in the adult population, it is extremely unusual in children unless structural heart disease is present or there is another arrhythmia that precipitates the AF, such as paroxysmal SVT in patients with WPW syndrome. The incidence of AF increases with age such that >5% of the adult population over 70 will experience the arrhythmia. As many patients are asymptomatic with AF, it is anticipated that the overall incidence, particularly that noted in the elderly, may be more than double the previously reported rates. Occasionally, AF appears to have a well-defined

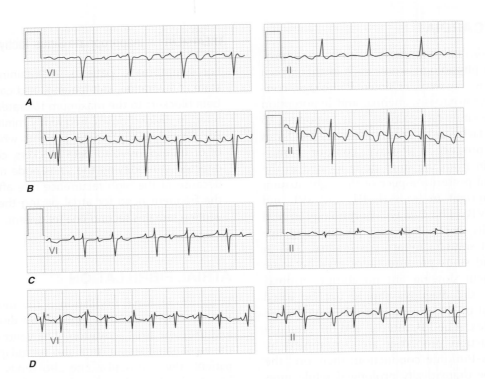

FIGURE 16-4

Supraventricular tachycardias with irregular ventricular rates. Atrial fibrillation (**A**), atrial flutter (**B**), atrial tachycardia (**C**), and multifocal atrial tachycardia (MAT; **D**) are shown. The characteristics of the atrial activity with respect to the morphology and rate provide the clues to the diagnosis. The variable ventricular response to the atrial flutter and the atrial tachycardia suggest a Wenckebach-type periodicity.

etiology, such as acute hyperthyroidism, an acute vagotonic episode, or acute alcohol intoxication. Acute AF is particularly common during the acute or early recovery phase of major vascular, abdominal, and thoracic surgery, in which case autonomic fluxes and/or direct mechanical irritation potentiate the arrhythmia. AF also may be triggered by other supraventricular tachycardias, such as AV nodal reentrant tachycardia (AVNRT), and elimination of these arrhythmias may prevent AF recurrence.

AF has clinical importance related to (1) the loss of atrial contractility, (2) the inappropriate fast ventricular response, and (3) the loss of atrial appendage contractility and emptying leading to the risk of clot formation and subsequent thromboembolic events.

Symptoms from AF vary dramatically. Many patients are asymptomatic and have no apparent hemodynamic consequences from the development of AF. Other patients experience only minor palpitations or sense irregularity of the pulse. Many patients, however, experience severe palpitations. The hemodynamic effect in patients can be quite dramatic, depending on the need for normal atrial contractility and the ventricular response. Hypotension, pulmonary congestion, and anginal symptoms may be severe in some patients. In patients with LV diastolic dysfunction that occurs with hypertension, hypertrophic cardiomyopathy, or obstructive aortic valvular disease, symptoms may be even more dramatic, especially if the ventricular rate does not permit adequate ventricular filling. Exercise intolerance and easy fatigability are the hallmarks of poor rate control with exertion. Occasionally, the only manifestation of AF is severe dizziness or syncope associated with the pause that occurs upon termination of AF before sinus rhythm resumes (Fig. 16-1).

The ECG in AF is characterized by the lack of organized atrial activity and the irregularly irregular ventricular response. Occasionally, one needs to record from multiple ECG leads simultaneously to identify the chaotic continuous atrial activation. Lead V_1 frequently shows the appearance of organized atrial activity that mimics AFL. This occurs because the crista terminalis serves as an effective anatomic barrier to electrical conduction, and the activation of the lateral right atrium may be represented by a more uniform activation wave front that originates over the roof of the right atrium. ECG assessment of the PP interval (<200 ms) and the chaotic P-wave morphology in the remaining ECG leads will confirm the presence of AF.

Evaluation of a patient with AF should include a search for a reversible cause of the arrhythmia, such as hyperthyroidism or anemia. An echocardiogram should be performed to determine whether there is structural heart disease. Persistent or labile hypertension should be identified and treated.

Treatment for AF must take into account the clinical situation in which the arrhythmia is encountered, the chronicity of the AF, the status of the patient's level of anticoagulation, risk factors for stroke, the patient's symptoms, the hemodynamic impact of the AF, and the ventricular rate.

ACUTE RATE CONTROL In the absence of hemodynamic compromise that might warrant emergent cardioversion to terminate the AF, the initial goals of therapy are to (1) establish control of the ventricular rate and (2) address anticoagulation status and begin IV heparin treatment if the duration of AF is >12 h and risk factors for stroke with AF are present (Table 16-1). Ventricular rate control for acute AF is best established with beta blockers and/or the calcium channel blocking agents verapamil and diltiazem. The route of administration and dose will be dictated by the ventricular rate and clinical status. Digoxin may add to the rate-controlling benefit of the other agents but is uncommonly used as a stand-alone agent, especially in acute AF.

Anticoagulation is of particular importance in patients who have known risk factors for stroke associated with AF. Factors associated with the highest risk of stroke include a history of stroke, transient ischemic attack (TIA) or systemic embolism, and the presence of rheumatic mitral stenosis. Other identified risk factors include age >65 years, history of congestive heart failure (CHF), diabetes mellitus, hypertension, LV dysfunction, and evidence of marked left atrial enlargement (>5.0 cm). Chronic anticoagulation with warfarin targeted to achieve an international normalized ratio (INR) between 2.0 and 3.0 is recommended in patients with persistent or frequent and long-lived paroxysmal AF and risk factors. If patients have not been adequately anticoagulated and the AF is more than 24–48 h in duration, a transesophageal echocardiogram (TEE) can be performed to exclude the presence of a left atrial thrombus that might dislodge with the attempted restoration of sinus rhythm with either nonpharmacologic or pharmacologic therapy. Anticoagulation must be instituted coincident with the TEE and maintained for at least

1 month after restoration of sinus rhythm if the duration of AF has been prolonged or is unknown. Heparin is maintained routinely until the INR is 1.8 with the administration of warfarin after the TEE. For patients who do not warrant early cardioversion of AF, anticoagulation should be maintained for at least 3 weeks with the INR confirmed to be >1.8 on at least two separate occasions before attempts at cardioversion.

Termination of AF acutely may be warranted on the basis of clinical parameters and/or hemodynamic status. Confirmation of appropriate anticoagulation status as described earlier in the chapter must be documented unless symptoms and clinical status warrant emergent intervention. Direct current transthoracic cardioversion during short-acting anesthesia is a reliable way to terminate AF. Conversion rates using a 200-J biphasic shock delivered synchronously with the QRS complex typically are >90%. Pharmacologic therapy to terminate AF is less reliable. Oral and/or IV administration of amiodarone or procainamide has only modest success. The acute IV administration of ibutilide appears to be somewhat more effective and may be used in selected patients to facilitate termination with direct current (DC) cardioversion (Tables 16-2 and 16-3).

Pharmacologic therapy to maintain sinus rhythm can be instituted once sinus rhythm has been established or in anticipation of cardioversion to attempt to maintain sinus rhythm (Table 16-3). A single episode of AF may not warrant any intervention or only a short course of beta blocker therapy. To prevent recurrent AF unresponsive to beta blockade, a trial of antiarrhythmic therapy may be warranted, particularly if the AF is associated with rapid rates and/or significant symptoms. The selection of antiarrhythmic agents should be dictated primarily by the presence or absence of CAD, depressed LV function not attributable to a reversible tachycardia-induced cardiomyopathy, and/or severe hypertension with evidence of marked LV hypertrophy. The presence of any significant structural heart disease typically narrows treatment to the use of sotalol, amiodarone, dofetilide, or dronedarone. Severely depressed LV function with heart failure symptoms precludes the use of dronedarone and may limit sotalol therapy. Owing to the risk of QT prolongation and polymorphic VT, sotalol and dofetilide have to be initiated in the hospital in most cases.

In patients without evidence of structural heart disease or hypertensive heart disease without evidence of severe hypertrophy, the use of the class IC antiarrhythmic agents flecainide or propafenone appears to be well tolerated and does not have significant proarrhythmia risk. It is important to recognize that no drug is uniformly effective, and arrhythmia recurrence should be anticipated in over one-half of the patients during

TABLE 16-1

RISK FACTORS FOR STROKE IN ATRIAL FIBRILLATION	
History of stroke or transient ischemic attack	Age >75 years
Mitral stenosis	Congestive heart failure
Hypertension	Left ventricular dysfunction
Diabetes mellitus	Marked left atrial enlargement (>5.0 cm)
	Spontaneous echo contrast

TABLE 16-2

COMMONLY USED ANTIARRHYTHMIC AGENTS—INTRAVENOUS DOSE RANGE/PRIMARY INDICATION				
DRUG	**LOADING**	**MAINTENANCE**	**PRIMARY INDICATION**	**CLASS**[a]
Adenosine	6–18 mg (rapid bolus)	N/A	Terminate reentrant SVT involving AV node	—
Amiodarone	15 mg/min for 10 min, 1 mg/min for 6 h	0.5–1 mg/min	AF, AFL, SVT, VT/VF	III
Digoxin	0.25 mg q2h until 1 mg total	0.125–0.25 mg/d	AF/AFL rate control	—
Diltiazem	0.25 mg/kg over 3–5 min (max 20 mg)	5–15 mg/h	SVT, AF/AFL rate control	IV
Esmolol	500 µg/kg over 1 min	50 µg/kg per min	AF/AFL rate control	II
Ibutilide	1 mg over 10 min if over 60 kg	N/A	Terminate AF/AFL	III
Lidocaine	1–3 mg/kg at 20–50 mg/min	1–4 mg/min	VT	IB
Metoprolol	5 mg over 3–5 min × 3 doses	1.25–5 mg q6h	SVT, AF rate control; exercise-induced VT; long QT	II
Procainamide	15 mg/kg over 60 min	1–4 mg/min	Convert/prevent AF/VT	IA
Quinidine	6–10 mg/kg at 0.3–0.5 mg/kg per min	N/A	Convert/prevent AF/VT	IA
Verapamil	5–10 mg over 3–5 min	2.5–10 mg/h	SVT, AF rate control	IV

[a]Classification of antiarrhythmic drugs: Class I—agents that primarily block inward sodium current; class IA agents also prolong action potential duration; class II—antisympathetic agents; class III—agents that primarily prolong action potential duration; class IV—calcium channel-blocking agents.
Abbreviations: AF, atrial fibrillation; AFL, atrial flutter; AV, atrioventricular; SVT, supraventricular tachycardia; VF, ventricular fibrillation; VT, ventricular tachycardia.

long-term follow-up regardless of the type and number of agents tried. It is also important to recognize that although the maintenance of sinus rhythm has been associated with improved long-term survival, the survival outcome of patients randomized to the pharmacologic maintenance of sinus rhythm was not superior to that of patients treated with rate control and anticoagulation in the AFFIRM and RACE trials. The AFFIRM and RACE trials compared outcome with respect to survival and thromboembolic events in patients with AF and risk factors for stroke using the two treatment strategies. It is believed that the poor outcome related to pharmacologic therapy used to maintain sinus rhythm was primarily due to the common inefficacy of such drug therapy and an increased incidence of asymptomatic AF. Many of the drugs used for rhythm control, including sotalol, amiodarone, propafenone, dronedarone, and flecainide, enhance slowing of AV nodal conduction. The absence of symptoms frequently leads to stopping anticoagulant therapy, and asymptomatic AF without anticoagulation increases stroke risk. Any consideration for stopping anticoagulation therefore must be accompanied by a prolonged period of ECG monitoring to document asymptomatic AF. It is also recommended that patients participate in monitoring by learning to take their pulse on a twice-daily basis and reliably identify its regularity if discontinuing anticoagulant therapy is contemplated seriously.

It is clear that to reduce the risk of drug-induced complications in treating AF, a thorough understanding of the drug planned to be used is critical—its dosing, metabolism, and common side effects and important drug-drug interactions. This information has been summarized in Tables 16-2, 16-3, **16-4**, and **16-5** and serves as a starting point for a more complete review. In using antiarrhythmic agents that slow atrial conduction, strong consideration should be given to adding a beta blocker or a calcium channel blocker (verapamil or diltiazem) to the treatment regimen. This should help avoid a rapid ventricular response if AF is converted to "slow" AFL with the drug therapy (**Fig. 16-5**).

CHRONIC RATE CONTROL This is an option in patients who are asymptomatic or symptomatic due to the resulting tachycardia. Rate control is frequently difficult to achieve in patients who have paroxysmal AF. In patients with more persistent forms of AF, rate control with beta blockers, the calcium channel blockers diltiazem and verapamil, and/or digoxin frequently can be achieved. Using the drugs in combination may avoid some of the common side effects seen with high-dose monotherapy. An effort should be made to document the adequacy of rate control to reduce the risk of a tachycardia-induced cardiomyopathy. Heart rates >80 beats/min at rest or 100 beats/min with very modest physical activity are indications that rate control may

TABLE 16-3

COMMONLY USED ANTIARRHYTHMIC AGENTS: CHRONIC ORAL DOSING/PRIMARY INDICATIONS

DRUG	DOSING ORAL, MG, MAINTENANCE	HALF-LIFE, H	PRIMARY ROUTE(S) OF METABOLISM/ELIMINATION	MOST COMMON INDICATION	CLASS[a]
Acebutolol	200–400 q12h	6–7	Renal/hepatic	AF rate control/SVT Long QT/RVOT VT	II
Amiodarone	100–400 qd	40–55 d	Hepatic	AF/VT prevention	III[b]
Atenolol	25–100 per d	6–9	Renal	AF rate control/SVT Long QT/RVOT VT	II
Digoxin	0.125–0.5 qd	38–48	Renal	AF rate control	—
Diltiazem	30–60 q6h	3–4.5	Hepatic	AF rate control/SVT	IV
Disopyramide	100–300 q6–8h	4–10	Renal 50%/hepatic	AF/SVT prevention	Ia
Dofetilide	0.125–0.5 q12h	10	Renal	AF prevention	III
Dronedarone	400 q12 hr	13–19	Hepatic	AF prevention	IIIb
Flecainide	50–200 q12h	7–22	Hepatic 75%/renal	AF/SVT/VT prevention	Ic ✓
Metoprolol	25–100 q6h	3–8	Hepatic	AF rate control/SVT Long QT/RVOT VT	II
Mexiletine	150–300 q8–12h	10–14	Hepatic	VT prevention	Ib
Moricizine	100–400 q8h	3–13	Hepatic 60%/renal	AF prevention	Ic
Nadolol	40–240 per d	10–24	Renal	Same as metoprolol	II
Procainamide	250–500 q3–6h	3–5	Hepatic/renal	AF/SVT/VT prevention	Ia
Propafenone	150–300 q8h	2–8	Hepatic	AF/SVT/VT prevention	Ic ✓
Quinidine	300–600 q6h	6–8	Hepatic 75%/renal	AF/SVT/VT prevention	Ia
Sotalol	80–160 q12h	12	Renal	AF/VT prevention	III
Verapamil	80–120 q6–8h	4.5–12	Hepatic/renal	AF rate control/RVOT VT Idiopathic LV VT	IV

[a]Classification of antiarrhythmic drugs: Class I—agents that primarily block inward sodium current; class II—antisympathetic agents; class III—agents that primarily prolong action potential duration; class IV—calcium channel-blocking agents.
[b]Amiodarone and dronedarone both are grouped in class III, but both also have class I, II, and IV properties.
Abbreviations: AF, atrial fibrillation; LV, left ventricular; RVOT, right ventricular outflow tract; SVT, supraventricular tachycardia; VT, ventricular tachycardia.

be inadequate in persistent AF. Extended periods of ECG monitoring and assessment of heart rate with exercise should be considered.

In patients with symptoms resulting from inadequate rate control with pharmacologic therapy or worsening LV function due to the persistent tachycardia, ablative therapy to attempt to eliminate atrial fibrillation, or an AV junction ablation can be performed. The AV junction ablation must be coupled with the implantation of an activity sensor pacemaker to maintain a physiologic range of heart rates. Recent evidence that RV pacing can occasionally modestly depress LV function should be taken into consideration in identifying which patients are appropriate candidates for the "ablate and pace" treatment strategy. Occasionally, biventricular pacing may be used to minimize the degree of dyssynchronization that can occur with RV apical pacing alone. Rate control treatment options must be coupled with chronic anticoagulation therapy in all cases. Trials evaluating the

elimination of embolic risk by elimination or isolation of the left atrial appendage or by endovascular insertion of a left atrial appendage-occluding device may provide other treatment options that can eliminate the need for chronic anticoagulation.

CATHETER AND SURGICAL ABLATIVE THERAPY TO PREVENT RECURRENT AF

Although the optimum ablation strategy has not been defined, most ablation strategies incorporate techniques that isolate the atrial muscle sleeves entering the pulmonary veins; these muscle sleeves have been identified as the source of the majority of triggers responsible for the initiation of AF. Ablation therapy is currently considered an alternative to additional pharmacologic therapy trials in patients with recurrent symptomatic AF or AF associated with poor rate control who have failed an initial attempt at rhythm control with pharmacologic management. Ablative therapy appears superior to additional

TABLE 16-4

COMMON NONARRHYTHMIC TOXICITY OF MOST FREQUENTLY USED ANTIARRHYTHMIC AGENTS

DRUG	COMMON NONARRHYTHMIC TOXICITY
Amiodarone	Tremor, peripheral neuropathy, pulmonary inflammation, hypo- and hyperthyroidism, photosensitivity
Adenosine	Cough, flushing
Digoxin	Anorexia, nausea, vomiting, visual changes
Disopyramide	Anticholinergic effects, decreased myocardial contractility
Dofetilide	Nausea
Dronedarone	Gastrointestinal intolerance, exacerbation of heart failure
Flecainide	Dizziness, nausea, headache, decreased myocardial contractility
Ibutilide	Nausea
Lidocaine	Dizziness, confusion, delirium, seizures, coma
Mexiletine	Ataxia, tremor, gait disturbances, rash, nausea
Moricizine	Mood changes, tremor, loss of mental clarity, nausea
Procainamide	Lupus erythematosus-like syndrome (more common in slow acetylators), anorexia, nausea, neutropenia
Propafenone	Taste disturbance, dyspepsia, nausea, vomiting
Quinidine	Diarrhea, nausea, vomiting, cinchonism, thrombocytopenia
Sotalol	Hypotension, bronchospasm

TABLE 16-5

PROARRHYTHMIC MANIFESTATIONS OF MOST FREQUENTLY USED ANTIARRHYTHMIC AGENTS

DRUG	COMMON PROARRHYTHMIC TOXICITY
Amiodarone	Sinus bradycardia, AV block, increase in defibrillation threshold Rare: long QT and torsades des pointes, 1:1 ventricular conduction with atrial flutter
Adenosine	All arrhythmias potentiated by profound pauses, atrial fibrillation
Digoxin	High-grade AV block, fascicular tachycardia, accelerated junctional rhythm, atrial tachycardia
Disopyramide	Long QT and torsades des pointes, 1:1 ventricular response to atrial flutter; increased risk of some ventricular tachycardias in patients with structural heart disease
Dofetilide	Long QT and torsades des pointes
Dronedarone	Bradyarrhythmias and AV block, long QT and torsades des pointes
Flecainide	1:1 Ventricular response to atrial flutter; increased risk of some ventricular tachycardias in patients with structural heart disease; sinus bradycardia
Ibutilide	Long QT and torsades des pointes
Procainamide	Long QT and torsades des pointes, 1:1 ventricular response to atrial flutter; increased risk of some ventricular tachycardias in patients with structural heart disease
Propafenone	1:1 Ventricular response to atrial flutter; increased risk of some ventricular tachycardias in patients with structural heart disease; sinus bradycardia
Quinidine	Long QT and torsades des pointes, 1:1 ventricular response to atrial flutter; increased risk of some ventricular tachycardias in patients with structural heart disease
Sotalol	Long QT and torsades des pointes, sinus bradycardia

Abbreviation: AV, atrioventricular.

pharmacologic treatment aimed at rhythm control in this setting. Elimination of AF in 50–80% of patients with a catheter-based ablation procedure should be anticipated, depending on the chronicity of the AF, with additional patients becoming responsive to previously ineffective medications.

Catheter ablative therapy also holds promise in patients with more persistent forms of AF and even those with severe atrial dilation. Its confirmed efficacy suggests an important alternative to His bundle ablation and pacemaker insertion in many patients. Serious risks related to the left atrial ablation procedure, albeit low (overall 2–4%), include pulmonary vein stenosis, atrioesophageal fistula, systemic embolic events, perforation/tamponade, and phrenic nerve injury.

Surgical ablation of AF is typically performed at the time of other cardiac valve or coronary artery surgery and, less commonly, as a stand-alone procedure.

The surgical Cox-Maze procedure is designed to interrupt all macroreentrant circuits that might potentially develop in the atria, thereby precluding the ability of the atria to fibrillate. In an attempt to simplify the operation, the multiple incisions of the traditional Cox-Maze procedure have been replaced with linear lines of ablation and pulmonary vein isolation using a variety of energy sources.

Severity of AF symptoms and difficulties in rate and/or rhythm control with pharmacologic therapy frequently dictate the optimum AF treatment strategy. Similar to the approach with pharmacologic rhythm control, a cautious approach to eliminating anticoagulant therapy is recommended after catheter or surgical ablation. Careful ECG monitoring for asymptomatic AF, particularly in patients with multiple risk factors for stroke, should be considered until guidelines are firmly established. If the left atrial appendage has been removed surgically, the threshold for stopping anticoagulation may be lowered. Antiarrhythmic therapy typically can be discontinued after catheter or surgical ablation of AF. However, in selected patients, satisfactory AF control may require maintenance of previously ineffective drug therapy after the ablation intervention.

ATRIAL FLUTTER AND MACROREENTRANT ATRIAL TACHYCARDIAS

Macroreentrant arrhythmias involving the atrial myocardium are referred to collectively as AFL. The terms *AFL* and *macroreentrant AT* frequently are used interchangeably, with both denoting a nonfocal source of an atrial arrhythmia. The typical or most common AFL circuit rotates in a clockwise or counterclockwise direction in the right atrium around the tricuspid valve annulus. The posterior boundary of the right AFL circuit is defined by the crista terminalis, the eustachian ridge, and the inferior and superior vena cavae. Counterclockwise right AFL represents ~80% of all AFL with superiorly directed activation of the interatrial septum, which produces the saw-toothed appearance of the P waves in ECG leads II, III, and aVF. Clockwise rotation of the same right atrial circuit produces predominantly positive P waves in leads II, III, and aVF (Fig. 16-4). Macroreentrant left AFL also may develop, albeit much less commonly. This type of arrhythmia may be the sequela of surgical or catheter-based ablation procedures that create large anatomic barriers or promote slowing of conduction in the left atrium, especially around the mitral valve annulus or partially disconnected pulmonary veins. Atypical AFL or macroreentrant AT can also develop around incisions created during surgery for valvular or congenital heart disease or in and/or around large areas of atrial fibrosis.

Classic or typical right AFL has an atrial rate of 260–300 beats per minute with a ventricular response that tends to be 2:1, or typically 130–150 beats per minute. In the setting of severe atrial conduction disease and or antiarrhythmic drug therapy, the atrial rate can slow to <200 beats per minute. In this setting, a 1:1 rapid ventricular response may occur, particularly with exertion, and produce adverse hemodynamic effects (Fig. 16-5). Atypical AFL or macroreentrant AT related to prior surgical incisions and atrial fibrosis demonstrates less predictability in terms of the atrial rate and is more

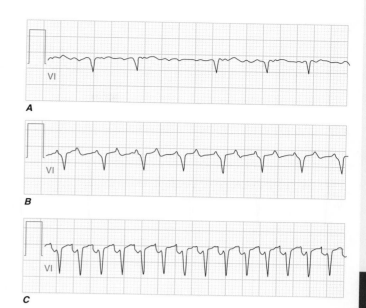

FIGURE 16-5
Atrial fibrillation. A. Transitions to "slow" atrial flutter during antiarrhythmic drug therapy. **B.** A rapid ventricular response with 1:1 atrioventricular conduction occurred with exercise, leading to **C.** symptoms of dizziness.

likely to demonstrate slower rates that overlap with those identified with focal atrial tachycardias.

Because lead V_1 is frequently monitored in a hospitalized patient, coarse AF may be misdiagnosed as AFL. This occurs because in both typical right AFL and coarse AF the crista terminalis in the right atrium may serve as an effective anatomic barrier. The free wall of the right atrium, whose electrical depolarization is best reflected on the body surface by lead V_1, may demonstrate a uniform wave front of atrial activation in both conditions. The timing of atrial activation is much more rapid in AF and always demonstrates variable atrial intervals with some intervals between defined P waves <200 ms (Fig. 16-6). A review of the other ECG leads demonstrates the disorganized atrial depolarization that is characteristic of AF. Frequently, an individual patient may alternate between AF and AFL or, less commonly, may manifest AF in one atrium and AFL in the other, making the distinction more difficult.

TREATMENT   Atrial Flutter

Because of the anticipated rapid regular ventricular rate associated with AFL and the failure to respond to pharmacologic therapy directed at slowing the ventricular rate, patients frequently are treated with DC cardioversion. The organized atrial flutter activity frequently can be terminated with low-energy external cardioversion of 50–100 J. The risk of thromboembolic events associated with typical AFL is high, and anticoagulation

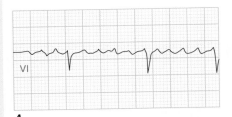
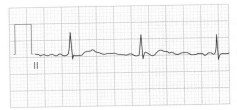

A

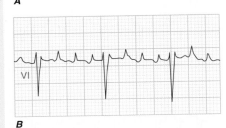
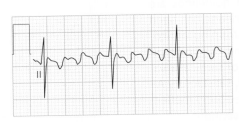

B

FIGURE 16-6
Atrial flutter/atrial fibrillation. Coarse atrial fibrillation (**A**) contrasted with organized atrial flutter (**B**).

must be managed similarly to what was described for patients with AF.

Asymptomatic patients with AFL may develop heart failure symptoms with tachycardia-induced severe LV dysfunction. In all patients, an effort should be made to control the ventricular rate pharmacologically or restore sinus rhythm. Rate control with calcium antagonists (diltiazem or verapamil), beta blockers, and/or digoxin may be difficult. Even higher-grade AV slowing, such as a 4:1 AV response, may be only transient and is easily overcome with activity or emotional stress. Owing to the typically faster ventricular rate, AFL tends to be poorly tolerated in comparison to AF.

In selected patients with high anesthetic risk, an attempt at pharmacologic cardioversion with procainamide, amiodarone, or ibutilide is appropriate. Antiarrhythmic drug therapy may also enhance the efficacy of DC cardioversion and the maintenance of sinus rhythm after cardioversion. Recurrence rates of AFL with pharmacologic attempts at rhythm control exceed 80% by 1 year.

Patients who manifest recurrent AFL appear to be effectively treated with catheter ablative therapy. For typical right AFL, an isthmus ablation line from the tricuspid annulus to the opening of the inferior vena cava can permanently eliminate flutter, with an anticipated success rate of >90% in most experienced centers. In patients with macroreentrant atrial tachycardia or AFL involving prior surgical incisions or catheter ablation or in areas of atrial fibrosis, detailed mapping of the arrhythmia circuit is required to design the best ablation strategy to interrupt the circuit. In selected patients with AF and typical right AFL, pharmacologic therapy may help prevent the AF but not the AFL. In this type of patient, hybrid therapy with antiarrhythmic agents coupled with a right atrial isthmus ablation may produce AF and AFL control.

MULTIFOCAL ATRIAL TACHYCARDIA

Multifocal AT (MAT) is the signature tachycardia of patients with significant pulmonary disease. The atrial rhythm is characterized by at least three distinct P-wave morphologies and often at least three different PR intervals, and the associated atrial and ventricular rates are typically between 100 and 150 beats per minute. The presence of an isoelectric baseline distinguishes this arrhythmia from AF (Fig. 16-4). The absence of any intervening sinus rhythm distinguishes MAT from normal sinus rhythm with frequent multifocal APCs, although this distinction may be moot as these processes define an electrophysiologic continuum.

| TREATMENT | Multifocal Atrial Tachycardia |

Therapy for MAT should be directed at improving the underlying medical condition, which is typically, although not invariably, chronic obstructive or restrictive lung disease. Treatment with the calcium channel blocker verapamil also may provide some benefit. The judicious use of flecainide or propafenone may also decrease atrial arrhythmias. Patients should be screened for the presence of significant ventricular dysfunction or CAD before these agents are started. Low-dose amiodarone therapy may also control the arrhythmia and minimize the risk of pulmonary toxicity noted with the drug.

FOCAL ATRIAL TACHYCARDIAS The two general mechanisms for focal ATs can be distinguished by observations made at AT initiation and in response to adenosine. *Automatic ATs* start with a "warm-up" period over the first 3–10 complexes and, similarly, slow in rate before termination. They may respond to adenosine not only with evidence of AV block but also with gradual slowing of the atrial rhythm and termination.

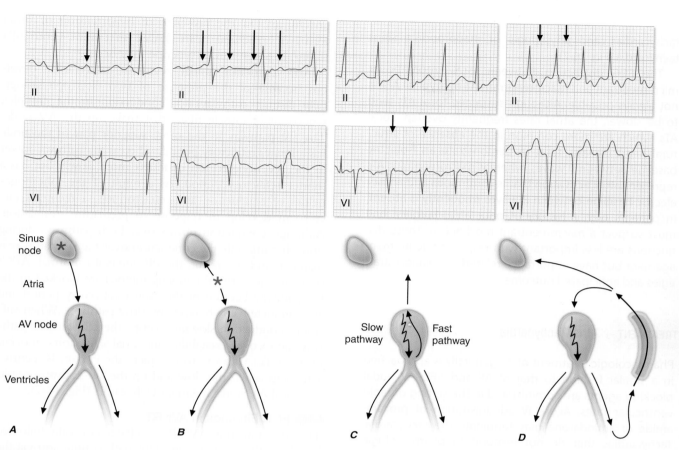

FIGURE 16-7

Pattern of atrial and ventricular activation and characteristic relationship of P-wave and QRS complex as recorded in leads II and V₁ during regular supraventricular tachycardias.

A. Sinus tachycardia. **B.** Atrial tachycardia from top of the atria. **C.** Atrioventricular nodal reentry. **D.** Accessory pathway–mediated orthodromic supraventricular tachycardia.

The initiation of automatic ATs frequently can be provoked by isoproterenol infusion. The first P wave of the tachycardia has the same morphology as the remaining waves. Some of the ATs may be triggered or provoked by burst atrial pacing but are not reliably initiated by programmed atrial stimulation.

In contrast, evidence supporting a focal reentrant AT includes the initiation of the tachycardia with programmed atrial stimulation or spontaneous premature beats. The P wave initiating the tachycardia will characteristically have a different morphology than the P wave during the sustained AT. In response to adenosine, reentrant ATs will demonstrate AV block but typically do not slow and/or terminate. Most focal ATs in the absence of structural heart disease originate from specific anatomic locations. These anatomic locations appear to be associated with anatomic ridges, such as the crista terminalis, the valve annuli, and the limbus of the fossa ovalis. ATs also appear to originate from the muscular sleeves associated with the cardiac thoracic veins, i.e., the SVC, the coronary sinus, and the pulmonary veins. As was indicated, repetitive firing of these foci also appears to serve as the triggering mechanism for AF in most patients.

It is important to distinguish focal ATs from reentrant tachycardias that incorporate the AV node in the circuit (**Fig. 16-7**). The primary distinction is related to the persistence of the AT in the presence of AV block that occurs spontaneously or is created by carotid sinus massage or the administration of adenosine (Fig. 16-4). Atrial activity drives the ventricles in AT and all changes in the PP interval accompanied by correlative changes in the RR intervals; in addition, the V–A relationship changes when the atrial rate changes. The P wave in AT is characteristically distinct from the sinus P-wave morphology, and unless there is significant AV nodal conduction delay, the PR interval is shorter than the measured RP interval when there is a 1:1 relationship between atria and ventricles (Fig. 16-7).

The P wave for ATs depends on the anatomic site of origin. In addition to attempting to create an AV block to establish the diagnosis of AT, analysis of the P-wave morphology on the 12-lead ECG may help exclude AV nodal reentry, AV bypass tract–mediated reentrant tachycardias, and physiologic or inappropriate sinus tachycardia (Fig. 16-7).

The ECG distinction between focal automatic or microreentrant and macroreentrant AT or atypical AFL is not always possible. Although sustained focal ATs tend to be slower, the atrial rates frequently overlap. Focal ATs, which are more common in the absence of structural heart disease, tend to demonstrate an isoelectric baseline between P waves, whereas macroreentrant ATs represent atrial activation that is continuous and an isoelectric baseline between P waves frequently is absent. In patients with a history of prior atrial surgery, one must suspect a macroreentrant mechanism. These distinctions are less important with respect to acute management but have importance related to ablation strategies and anticipated outcome.

TREATMENT   Atrial Tachycardia

Pharmacologic treatment of AT generally is approached in a similar fashion to that of AF and AFL. AV nodal blocking agents are administered in the setting of rapid ventricular rates. Acute IV administration of procainamide or amiodarone may terminate the tachycardia. Tachycardias that do not respond to pharmacologic therapy may be terminated with electrical cardioversion. Typically, anticoagulation before treatment is not needed unless there is evidence of severe atrial dilatation, >5 cm left atrial diameter with a high risk of AF, and/or a history of coincident paroxysmal AF. Most focal ATs are readily amenable to catheter ablative therapy. In patients who fail to respond to medical therapy or who are reluctant to take chronic drug therapy, this option should be considered, with an anticipated 90% cure rate. A parahisian location for the AT and/or a focus that is located in the left atrium may modestly increase the risk related to the procedure, and for this reason, every effort should be made to determine the likely origin of the AT based on an analysis of the P-wave morphology on 12-lead ECG before the procedure.

AV NODAL TACHYCARDIAS
AV nodal reentrant tachycardia

Atrioventricular nodal reentrant tachycardia is the most common paroxysmal regular SVT. It is more commonly observed in women than in men and is typically manifest in the second to fourth decades of life. In general, because AVNRT tends to occur in the absence of structural heart disease, it is usually well tolerated. Neck pulsations are usually felt because of the simultaneous atrial and ventricular contraction, and a "frog sign" can be identified on physical examination during the

arrhythmia. In the presence of hypertension or other forms of structural heart disease that limit ventricular filling, hypotension or syncope may occur.

Atrioventricular nodal reentrant tachycardia develops because of the presence of two electrophysiologically distinct pathways for conduction in the complex syncytium of muscle fibers that make up the AV node. The fast pathway in the more superior part of the node has a longer refractory period, whereas the pathway lower in the AV node region conducts more slowly but has a shorter refractory period. As a result of the inhomogeneities of conduction and refractoriness, a reentrant circuit can develop in response to premature stimulation. Although conduction occurs over both pathways during sinus rhythm, only the conduction over the fast pathway is manifest, and as a result, the PR interval is normal. APCs occurring at a critical coupling interval are blocked in the fast pathway because of the longer refractory period and are conducted slowly over the slow pathway. When sufficient conduction slowing occurs, the blocked fast pathway can recover excitability and atrial activation can occur over the fast pathway to complete the circuit. Repetitive activation down the slow and up the fast pathway results in typical AV nodal reentrant tachycardia (Fig. 16-7).

ECG Findings in AVNRT

The APC initiating AVNRT is characteristically followed by a long PR interval consistent with conduction via the slow pathway. AVNRT is manifest typically as a narrow QRS complex tachycardia at rates that range from 120 to 250 beats/min. The QRS-P wave pattern associated with typical AVNRT is quite characteristic, with simultaneous activation of the atria and ventricles from the reentrant AV nodal circuit. The P wave frequently is buried inside the QRS complex and either will not be visible or will distort the initial or terminal portion of the QRS complex (Fig. 16-7). Because atrial activation originates in the region of the AV node, a negative deflection will be generated by retrograde atrial depolarization when recording ECG leads II, III, or aVF.

Occasionally, AVNRT occurs with activation in the reverse direction, conducting down the fast pathway and returning up the slow pathway. This form of AVNRT occurs much less commonly and produces a prolonged RP interval during the tachycardia with a negative P wave in leads II, III, and aVF. This atypical form of AVNRT is more easily precipitated by ventricular stimulation.

TREATMENT   Atrioventricular Nodal Reentrant Tachycardia

ACUTE TREATMENT   Treatment is directed at altering conduction within the AV node. Vagal stimulation, such as that which occurs with the Valsalva maneuver or carotid sinus massage, can slow conduction in the AV node sufficiently to terminate AVNRT. In patients in whom physical maneuvers do not terminate the tachyarrhythmia, the administration of adenosine, 6–12 mg IV, frequently does so. Intravenous beta blockade or calcium channel therapy should be considered as second-line treatment. If hemodynamic compromise is present, R-wave synchronous DC cardioversion using 100–200 J can terminate the tachyarrhythmia.

PREVENTION Prevention may be achieved with drugs that slow conduction in the antegrade slow pathway, such as digitalis, beta blockers, and calcium channel blockers. In patients who have a history of exercise-precipitated AVNRT, the use of beta blockers frequently eliminates symptoms. In patients who do not respond to drug therapy directed at the antegrade slow pathway, treatment with class IA or IC agents directed at altering conduction of the fast pathway may be considered.

Catheter ablation, directed at elimination or modification of slow pathway conduction, is very effective in permanently eliminating AVNRT. Patients with recurrent AVNRT that produces significant symptoms or heart rates >200 beats/min and patients reluctant to take chronic drug therapy should be considered for ablative therapy. Catheter ablation can cure AV nodal reentry in >95% of patients with a single procedure. The risk of AV block requiring a permanent pacemaker is ~1% with the ablation procedure.

AV junctional tachycardias

These can also occur in the setting of enhanced normal automaticity, abnormal automaticity, or triggered activity. These tachycardias may or may not be associated with retrograde conduction to the atria, and the P waves may appear dissociated or produce intermittent conduction and early activation of the junction. These arrhythmias may occur as a manifestation of increased adrenergic tone or drug effect in patients with sinus node dysfunction or after surgical or catheter ablation. The arrhythmia may also be a manifestation of digoxin toxicity. The most common manifestation of digoxin intoxication is the sudden regularization of the response to AF. A junctional tachycardia due to digoxin toxicity typically does not manifest retrograde conduction. Sinus activity may appear dissociated or result in intermittent capture beats with a long PR interval. If the rate is >50 beats per minute and <100 beats per minute, the term *accelerated junctional rhythm* applies. Occasionally, automatic rhythms are mimicked by AVNRT that fails to conduct to the atrium. The triggering events associated with the onset of the tachycardia may provide a clue to the appropriate diagnosis. Initiation of the tachycardia without an atrial premature beat with a gradual acceleration in rate suggests an automatic focus.

TREATMENT Atrioventricular Junctional Tachycardias

Treatment of automatic/triggered junctional tachycardias is directed at decreasing adrenergic stimulation and reversing digoxin toxicity, if present. Digoxin therapy can be withheld if toxicity is suspected, and the administration of digoxin-specific antibody fragments can rapidly reverse digoxin toxicity if the tachycardia is producing significant symptoms and rapid termination is indicated. Junctional tachycardia due to abnormal automaticity can be treated pharmacologically with beta blockers. A trial of class IA or IC drugs may also be attempted. For incessant automatic junctional tachycardia, focal catheter ablation can be performed but is associated with an increased risk of AV block.

TACHYCARDIAS ASSOCIATED WITH ACCESSORY AV PATHWAYS

Tachycardias that involve accessory pathways (APs) between atria and ventricles commonly manifest a normal QRS complex with a short or long RP interval. They must be considered in the differential diagnosis of other narrow-complex tachycardias. Importantly, most tachycardias associated with APs involve a large macroreentrant circuit that includes the ventricles (Fig. 16-7). Thus, identifying these arrhythmias as "supraventricular" is actually a misnomer, and they deserve separate consideration.

Accessory pathways are typically capable of conducting rapidly in both an antegrade and a retrograde direction. In the absence of an AP, the sinus impulse normally activates the ventricles via the AV node and His-Purkinje system, resulting in a PR interval of 120–200 ms. When an antegradely conducting AP is present, the sinus impulse bypasses the AV node and can activate the ventricles rapidly, resulting in ventricular preexcitation. The resulting PR interval is shorter than anticipated. In addition, because the initial ventricular activation is due to muscle-to-muscle conduction, as opposed to rapid spread of activation via the His-Purkinje system, the initial portion of the QRS complex is slurred, creating the characteristic "delta wave." The remaining portion of the QRS complex in sinus rhythm is created by a fusion of the ventricular activation wave front originating from the Purkinje network and the continued spread of activation from the site of insertion of the AP (Fig. 16-8). Evidence of ventricular preexcitation includes evidence in sinus rhythm of a short PR interval and a delta wave.

The most common AP connects the left atrium to the left ventricle, followed by posterior septal, right free wall, and anterior septal APs. APs typically insert from the atrium into the adjacent ventricular myocardium. However, occasionally pathways, particularly those originating from the right atrium, can have a ventricular

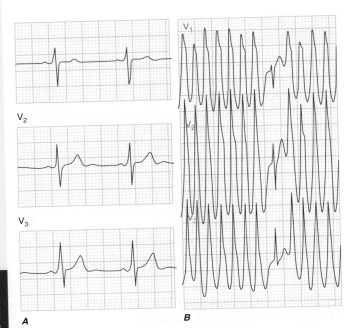

FIGURE 16-8

A. Sinus rhythm tracing of leads V₁–V₃ showing evidence of Wolff-Parkinson-White syndrome with short PR interval and delta wave. **B.** During atrial fibrillation, rapid conduction to the ventricles is observed producing a wide QRS complex tachycardia with marked irregularity of the ventricular response and morphology of the QRS complex.

insertion at a site distant from the AV groove in the fascicles. These pathways conduct more slowly and are referred to as *atriofascicular accessory pathways*. Atriofascicular APs are unique in their tendency to demonstrate decremental antegrade conduction.

Other accessory pathway connections from the AV node to the fascicles may exist. These pathways are referred to as *Mahaim fibers* and typically manifest a normal PR interval with a delta wave.

Patients with manifest preexcitation and WPW syndrome are typically subject to both macroreentrant tachycardias and a rapid response to AF (Fig. 16-8). The most common macroreentrant tachycardia associated with WPW syndrome is referred to as *orthodromic AV reentry*. Ventricular activation occurs via the AV node and the His-Purkinje system. Conduction then returns or reenters the atria via retrograde conduction over the AP. The reentrant circuit develops because of the inhomogeneity in conduction and refractoriness in the AP and the normal AV node.

Characteristically, the AP has more rapid conduction but a longer refractory period than that of the AV node. Typical APs do not show evidence of antegrade decremental conduction. An APC can block in the AP and conduct sufficiently slowly or with decrement via the AV node to allow for retrograde recovery of activation of the AP and, in turn, of the atria (Fig. 16-7). This retrograde activation of the atria via the AP is referred

to as an *echo beat*. If the pattern repeats itself, a tachycardia develops. Uncommonly, the reentrant circuit can be reversed so that the impulse reaches the ventricle via the AP and conducts retrogradely through to the atria via the His-Purkinje system and the AV node; this is referred to as *antidromic AV reentry* and/or *preexcitation macroreentry*, with the entire activation of the ventricle originating from the site of insertion of the AP. Although it is uncommon, it is important to recognize antidromic SVT. The ECG pattern during the tachycardia mimics VT originating from the site of ventricular insertion of the AP. The presence of manifest preexcitation in sinus rhythm provides a valuable clue to the diagnosis.

The second most common and potentially more serious arrhythmia associated with WPW syndrome is rapidly conducting AF. Nearly 50% of patients with evidence of APs are predisposed to episodes of AF. In patients who have rapid antegrade conduction from the atria to the ventricles over the AP, the AP can conduct rapidly in response to AF, resulting in a faster ventricular rate than would occur normally via the AV node. The rapid ventricular rates can result in hemodynamic compromise and even precipitate VF. The QRS pattern during AF in patients with manifest preexcitation can appear quite bizarre and change on a beat-to-beat basis due to the variability in the degree of fusion from activation over the AV node (Fig. 16-8).

Concealed APs

In ~50% of patients with APs, there is no antegrade conduction over the AP; however, retrograde conduction is preserved. As a result, the AP is not manifest in sinus rhythm and is manifest only during the sustained tachycardia. The presence of a concealed AP is suggested by the timing and pattern of atrial activation during the tachycardia: the P wave typically follows ventricular activation with a short RP wave interval (Fig. 16-7). Because many APs connect the left ventricle to the left atrium, the pattern of atrial activation during the tachycardia frequently produces negative P waves in leads I and aVL. The tachycardia circuit and therefore its ECG manifestation during orthodromic tachycardia are identical both in patients with overt preexcitation in sinus rhythm and in those with concealed APs. Patients with concealed APs, although prone to episodes of AF, are not at risk for developing a rapid ventricular response to the AF.

Occasionally, APs conduct extremely slowly in a retrograde fashion, resulting in longer retrograde conduction and the development of a long RP interval during the tachycardia (*long RP tachycardia*). Because of the presence of this dramatically slowed conduction, additional conduction slowing created by premature atrial complexes is not required for tachycardia to ensue.

These patients are more prone to frequent episodes of tachycardia and can present with "incessant" tachycardias and tachycardia-induced LV cardiomyopathy. The correct diagnosis of a long RP tachycardia may be suggested by the pattern of initiation and the P-wave morphology. Frequently, however, an electrophysiologic evaluation is required to establish the diagnosis.

TREATMENT	Accessory Pathway–Mediated Tachycardias

Acute treatment of AP-mediated macroreentrant orthodromic tachycardias is similar to that for AV nodal reentry and is directed at altering conduction in the AV node. Vagal stimulation with the Valsalva maneuver and carotid sinus pressure may create sufficient AV nodal slowing to terminate the AVRT. Intravenous administration of adenosine, 6–12 mg, is first-line pharmacologic therapy; IV, the calcium channel blockers verapamil and diltiazem or beta blockers may also be effective. In patients who manifest preexcitation and AF, therapy should be aimed at preventing a rapid ventricular response. In life-threatening situations, DC cardioversion should be used to terminate the AF. In nonlife-threatening situations, procainamide at a dose of 15 mg/kg administered IV over 20–30 min will slow the ventricular response and may organize and terminate AF. Ibutilide can also be used to facilitate termination of AF. During AF there may be rapid conduction over the AV node as well as the AP. Caution should be used in attempting to slow AV nodal conduction with the use of digoxin or verapamil; when administered IV, these drugs may actually result in an acute increase in rate over the AP, placing the patient at risk for development of VF. Digoxin appears to shorten the refractory period of the AP directly and thus increases the ventricular rate. Verapamil appears to shorten the refractory period indirectly by causing vasodilation and a reflex increase in sympathetic tone.

Chronic oral administration of beta blockers and/or verapamil or diltiazem may be used to prevent recurrent supraventricular reentrant tachycardias associated with APs. In patients with evidence of AF and a rapid ventricular response and in those with recurrences of SVT on AV nodal blocking drugs, strong consideration should be given to the administration of a class IA or IC antiarrhythmic drug such as quinidine, flecainide, or propafenone because these drugs slow conduction and increase refractoriness in the AP.

Patients with a history of recurrent symptomatic SVT episodes, incessant SVT, and heart rates >200 beats/min with SVT should be given strong consideration for undergoing catheter ablation. Patients who have demonstrated rapid antegrade conduction over their AP or the potential for rapid conduction should also be considered for catheter ablation. Catheter ablation therapy has been demonstrated to be successful in >95% of patients with documented WPW syndrome and appears effective regardless of age. The risk of catheter ablative therapy is low and is dictated primarily by the location of the AP. Ablation of parahisian APs is associated with a risk of heart block, and ablation in the left atrium is associated with a small but definite risk of thromboembolic phenomenon. These risks must be weighed against the potential serious complications associated with hemodynamic compromise, the risk of VF, and the severity of the patient's symptoms with AP-mediated tachycardias.

Patients who demonstrate evidence of ventricular preexcitation in the absence of any prior arrhythmia history merit special consideration. The first arrhythmia manifestation can be a rapid SVT or, albeit of low risk (<1%), a life-threatening rapid response to AF. Patients who demonstrate intermittent preexcitation during ECG monitoring or an abrupt loss of AP conduction during exercise testing are at low risk of a life-threatening rapid response to AF. All other patients should be advised of their risks and therapeutic options in advance of a documented arrhythmia event.

VENTRICULAR TACHYARRHYTHMIAS

VENTRICULAR PREMATURE COMPLEXES

The origin of premature beats in the ventricle at sites remote from the Purkinje network produces slow ventricular activation and a wide QRS complex that is typically >140 ms in duration. Ventricular premature complexes are common and increase with age and the presence of structural heart disease. VPCs can occur with a certain degree of periodicity that has become incorporated into the lexicon of electrocardiography. Ventricular premature complexes may occur in patterns of *bigeminy*, in which every sinus beat is followed by a VPC, or *trigeminy*, in which two sinus beats are followed by a VPC. VPCs may have different morphologies and are thus referred to as *multiformed*. Two successive VPCs are termed *pairs* or *couplets*. Three or more consecutive VPCs are termed *VT* when the rate is >100 beats per minute. If the repetitive VPCs terminate spontaneously and are more than three beats in duration, the arrhythmia is referred to as *nonsustained VT*.

APCs with aberrant ventricular conduction may also create a wide and early QRS complex. The premature P wave can occasionally be difficult to discern when it falls on the preceding T wave, and other clues must be used to make the diagnosis. The QRS pattern for a VPC does not appear to follow a typical right or left bundle branch block pattern as the QRS morphology is associated with aberrant atrial conduction and can be quite bizarre. On occasion, VPCs can arise from the Purkinje network of the ventricles, in which case the QRS pattern mimics aberration. The 12-lead ECG recording of the VPC may be required to identify subtle morphologic clues regarding the QRS complex to confirm its ventricular origin. Most commonly, VPCs are associated with a "fully compensatory pause" (i.e., the duration between the last QRS before the PVC and the next QRS complex is equal to twice the sinus rate [Fig. 16-3]). The VPC typically does not conduct to the atrium. If the VPC does conduct to the atrium, it may not be sufficiently early to reset the sinus node. As a result, sinus activity will occur and the antegrade wave front from the sinus node may encounter some delay in the AV node or His-Purkinje system from the blocked VPC wave front, or it may collide with the retrograde atrial wave front. Sinus activity will continue undisturbed, resulting in a delay to the next QRS complex (Fig. 16-3). Occasionally, the VPC can occur early enough and conduct retrograde to the atrium to reset the sinus node; the pause that results will be less than compensatory. VPCs that fail to influence the oncoming sinus impulse are termed *interpolated VPCs*. A ventricular focus that fires repetitively at a fixed interval may produce variably coupled VPCs, depending on the sinus rate. This type of focus is referred to as a *parasystolic focus* because its firing does not appear to be modulated by sinus activity and the conducted QRS complex. The ventricular ectopy will occur at a characteristic fixed integer or multiple of these intervals. The variability in coupling relative to the underlying QRS complex and a fixed interval between complexes of ventricular origin provide the diagnostic information necessary to identify a parasystolic focus.

TREATMENT Ventricular Premature Complexes

The threshold for treatment of VPCs is high, and the treatment is directed primarily at eliminating severe symptoms associated with palpitations. VPCs of sufficient frequency can cause a reversible cardiomyopathy. Depressed LV function in the setting of ventricular bigeminy and/or frequent nonsustained VT should raise the possibility of a cardiomyopathy that is reversible with control of the ventricular arrhythmia. In the absence of structural heart disease, VPCs do not appear to have prognostic significance. In patients with structural heart disease, frequent VPCs and runs of nonsustained VT have prognostic significance and may portend an increased risk of SCD. However, no study has documented that elimination of VPCs with antiarrhythmic drug therapy reduces the risk of arrhythmic death in patients with severe structural heart disease. In fact,

drug therapies that slow myocardial conduction and/or enhance dispersion of refractoriness can actually increase the risk of life-threatening arrhythmias (drug-induced QT prolongation and TDP) despite being effective at eliminating VPCs.

ACCELERATED IDIOVENTRICULAR RHYTHM (AIVR)

AIVR refers to a ventricular rhythm that is characterized by three or more complexes at a rate >40 beats per minute and <120 beats per minute. The arrhythmia mechanism causing AIVR is thought to be due to abnormal automaticity. By definition, there is an overlap between AIVR and "slow" VT; both rhythms can manifest rates between 90 and 120 beats per minute. Because AIVR tends to be a benign rhythm with different therapeutic implications, it is worthwhile to attempt to distinguish it from "slow" VT. AIVR has a characteristic gradual onset and offset and more variability in cycle length. It is typically a brief, self-limiting arrhythmia. AIVR can be seen in the absence of any structural heart disease, but it is frequently present in the setting of acute myocardial infarction (MI), cocaine intoxication, acute myocarditis, digoxin intoxication, and postoperative cardiac surgery. Sustained forms of AIVR can exist, particularly in the setting of acute MI and postoperatively. In the setting of sustained AIVR, hemodynamic compromise can occur because of the loss of AV synchrony. Patients with RV infarction associated with proximal right coronary artery occlusion are most susceptible to associated bradyarrhythmias and the hemodynamic consequences of AIVR. In these patients, acceleration of the atrial rate either by the cautious administration of atropine or by atrial pacing may be an important treatment consideration.

VENTRICULAR TACHYCARDIA

VT originates below the bundle of His at a rate >100 beats per minute; most VT patients have rates >120 beats per minute. Sustained VT at rates <120 beats per minute and even <100 beats per minute can be observed, particularly in association with the administration of antiarrhythmic agents that can slow the rate. Because of the overlap in rates with AIVR, the arrhythmia ECG characteristics and the clinical circumstance sometimes can be used to distinguish the two forms of tachycardia. Slow sustained VT is less likely to show a marked warm-up in rate and the marked cycle-length oscillations seen with AIVR, and it is more likely to occur in the setting of chronic infarction or cardiomyopathy and less likely with acute infarction or myocarditis. Obviously, significant overlap may exist. Typically, slow VT will be initiated with programmed stimulation and is found to represent a large macroreentrant circuit in chronically diseased myocardium capable of supporting markedly slow conduction.

The QRS complex during VT may be uniform (monomorphic) or may vary from beat to beat (polymorphic). Polymorphic VT in patients who demonstrate a long QT interval during their baseline rhythm typically is referred to as *torsades des pointes*. The polymorphic VT associated with QT prolongation dramatically oscillates around the baseline on most of the monitored ECG leads, mimicking the "turning of the points" stitching pattern (**Fig. 16-9**).

Monomorphic VT suggests a stable tachycardia focus in the absence of structural heart disease or a fixed anatomic abnormality that can create the substrate for a stable reentrant VT circuit when structural disease is present. Monomorphic VT tends to be a reproducible and recurrent phenomenon and may be initiated with pacing and programmed ventricular stimulation. In contrast, polymorphic VT suggests a more dynamic and/or unstable process and, by its very nature, is less reproducible. Polymorphic VT may be produced by acute ischemia, myocarditis, or dynamic changes in the QT interval and enhanced dispersion of ventricular refractoriness. Polymorphic VTs are not reliably initiated with pacing or programmed stimulation.

A time duration of 30 s frequently is used to distinguish sustained from nonsustained VT. Hemodynamically unstable VT that requires termination before 30 s or VT that is terminated by therapy from an implantable defibrillator is also typically classified as sustained. Ventricular flutter appears as a sine wave on the ECG and has a rate of >250 beats per minute. A rapid rate coupled with the sine wave nature of the arrhythmia makes it impossible to identify a discrete QRS morphology. When antiarrhythmic drugs are being administered, a sine wave appearance of the QRS complex can be observed, even at rates as low as 200 beats per minute. VF is characterized by completely disorganized ventricular activation on the surface ECG. Polymorphic

ventricular arrhythmias, ventricular flutter, and VF always produce hemodynamic collapse if allowed to continue. The hemodynamic stability of a unimorphic VT depends on the presence and severity of the underlying structural heart disease, the location of the site of origin of the arrhythmia, and the heart rate.

It is important to distinguish monomorphic VT from SVT with aberrant ventricular conduction due to right or left bundle branch block.

Importantly, the sinus or baseline 12-lead ECG tracing can provide important clues that help establish the correct diagnosis of a wide complex tachycardia. The presence of an aberrant QRS pattern that matches exactly that of the wide complex rhythm strongly supports the diagnosis of SVT. A right or left bundle branch block QRS pattern that does not match the QRS and/or that is wider in duration than the QRS during the wide complex tachycardia supports the diagnosis of VT. Most patients with VT have structural heart disease and show evidence of a prior Q wave MI during sinus rhythm. Important exceptions to this rule are discussed. Finally, the presence of a preexcited QRS pattern on the 12-lead ECG in sinus rhythm suggests that the wide complex rhythm represents an atrial arrhythmia, such as AFL or a focal AT, with rapid conduction over an AP or antidromic macroreentrant tachycardia (Fig. 16-8). If the arrhythmia is irregular with changing QRS complexes, the diagnosis of AF with ventricular preexcitation should be considered.

With the exception of some idiopathic outflow tract tachycardias, most VTs do not respond to vagal stimulation provoked by carotid sinus massage, the Valsalva maneuver, or adenosine administration. The IV administration of verapamil and/or adenosine is not recommended as a diagnostic test. Verapamil has been associated with hemodynamic collapse when administered to patients with structural heart disease and VT.

Patients with VT frequently demonstrate AV dissociation. Findings on physical examination of intermittent cannon *a* waves and variability of the first heart sound are consistent with AV dissociation. The presence of AV dissociation is characteristically marked by the presence of sinus capture or fusion beats. The presence of 1:1 ventriculoatrial conduction does not preclude a diagnosis of VT.

Additional characteristics of the 12-lead ECG during the tachycardia that suggest VT include (1) the presence of a QRS duration >140 ms in the absence of drug therapy, (2) a superior and rightward QRS frontal plane axis, (3) a bizarre QRS complex that does not mimic the characteristic QRS pattern associated with left or right bundle branch block, and (4) slurring of the initial portion of the QRS (Fig. 16-10). Table 16-6 provides a useful summary of ECG criteria that have evolved based on the described characteristics of VT.

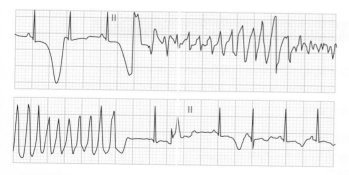

FIGURE 16-9

Sinus rhythm with long QT interval and the polymorphic ventricular arrhythmia torsades des pointes. Dramatic T wave alternans are present in sinus rhythm.

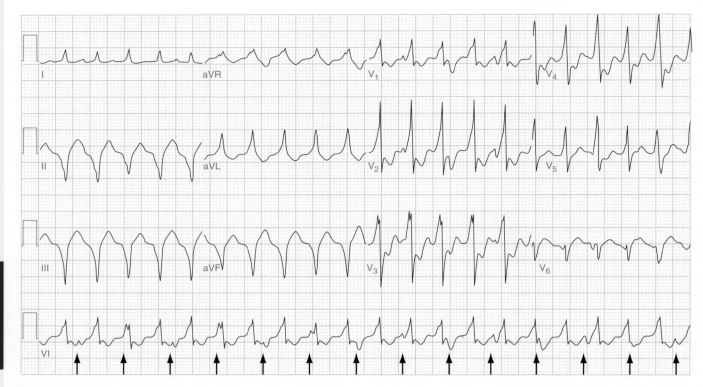

FIGURE 16-10

Ventricular tachycardia. ECG showing AV dissociation (arrows mark P waves), wide QRS >200 ms, superior frontal plane axis, slurring of the initial portion of the QRS, and large S wave in V₆—all clues to the diagnosis of ventricular tachycardia.

TREATMENT   Ventricular Tachycardia/Fibrillation

Sustained polymorphic VT, ventricular flutter, and VF all lead to immediate hemodynamic collapse. Emergency asynchronous defibrillation is therefore required, with at least 200-J monophasic or 100-J biphasic shock. The shock should be delivered asynchronously to avoid delays related to sensing of the QRS complex. If the arrhythmia persists, repeated shocks with the maximum energy output of the defibrillator are essential to optimize the chance of successful resuscitation. Intravenous lidocaine and/or amiodarone should be administered but should not delay repeated attempts at defibrillation.

For any monomorphic wide complex rhythm that results in hemodynamic compromise, a prompt R-wave synchronous shock is required. Conscious sedation should be provided if the hemodynamic status permits. For patients with a well-tolerated wide complex tachycardia, the appropriate diagnosis should be established on the basis of strict ECG criteria (Table 16-6). Pharmacologic treatment to terminate monomorphic VT is not

TABLE 16-6

ECG CLUES SUPPORTING THE DIAGNOSIS OF VENTRICULAR TACHYCARDIA
AV dissociation (atrial capture, fusion beats)
QRS duration >140 ms for RBBB type V₁ morphology; V₁ >160 ms for LBBB type V₁ morphology
Frontal plane axis −90° to 180°

Delayed activation during initial phase of the QRS complex
    LBBB pattern—R wave in V₁, V₂ >40 ms
    RBBB pattern—onset of R wave to nadir of S >100 ms

Bizarre QRS pattern that does not mimic typical RBBB or LBBB QRS complex
    Concordance of QRS complex in all precordial leads
    RS or dominant S in V₆ for RBBB VT
    Q wave in V₆ with LBBB QRS pattern
    Monophasic R or biphasic qR or R/S in V₁ with RBBB pattern

Abbreviations: AV, atrioventricular; RBBB/LBBB, right/left bundle branch block.

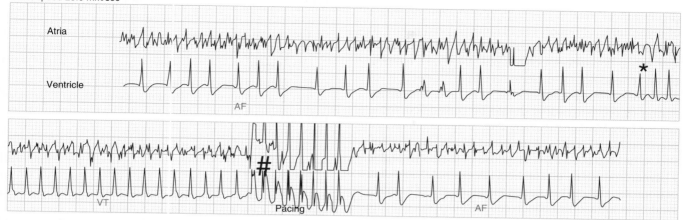

Chart speed 25.0 mm/sec

Atria

Ventricle

AF

*

VT

#

Pacing

AF

FIGURE 16-11

Ventricular tachycardia (VT) (*) during atrial fibrillation stopped by pacing (#) from an implantable cardioverter defibrillator (ICD) from recording stored by ICD. The atrial electrogram shows characteristic fibrillatory waves through the tracing. The ventricular electrogram shows an irregularly irregular response consistent with atrial fibrillation at the beginning of the tracing. The ventricular electrogram suddenly changes in morphology (*) and becomes regular, consistent with the diagnosis of VT. Pacing transiently accelerates the rate and interrupts the rapid VT. The patient was unaware of the life-threatening event.

typically successful (<30%). Intravenous procainamide, lidocaine, or amiodarone can be utilized. If the arrhythmia persists, synchronous R-wave cardioversion after the administration of conscious sedation is appropriate. Selected patients with focal outflow tract tachycardias who demonstrate triggered or automatic VT may respond to IV beta blocker administration. Idiopathic LV septal VT appears to respond uniquely to IV verapamil administration.

VT in patients with structural heart disease is now almost always treated with the implantation of an ICD to manage anticipated VT recurrence. The ICD can provide rapid pacing and shock therapy to treat most VTs effectively (Fig. 16-11).

Prevention of VT remains important, and >50% of patients with a history of VT and an ICD may need to be treated with adjunctive antiarrhythmic drug therapy to prevent VT recurrences or to manage atrial arrhythmias. Because of the presence of an ICD, there is more flexibility with respect to the selection of antiarrhythmic drug therapy. The use of sotalol or amiodarone represents first-line therapy for patients with a history of structural heart disease and life-threatening monomorphic or polymorphic VT not due to long QT syndrome. Importantly, sotalol has been associated with a decrease in the defibrillation threshold, which reflects the amount of energy necessary to terminate VF. Amiodarone may be better tolerated in patients with a more marginal hemodynamic status and systolic blood pressure. The risk of end-organ toxicity from amiodarone must be weighed against the ease of use and general efficacy. Antiarrhythmic drug therapy with agents such as quinidine, procainamide, and propafenone, which might not normally be used in patients with structural heart disease because of the risk of proarrhythmia, may be considered in patients with an ICD and recurrent VT.

Catheter ablative therapy for VT in patients without structural heart disease results in cure rates >90%. In patients with structural heart disease, catheter ablation that includes a strategy for eliminating unmappable/rapid VT and one that incorporates endocardial as well as epicardial mapping and ablation should be employed. In most patients, catheter ablation can reduce or eliminate the requirement for toxic drug therapy and should be considered in any patient with recurrent VT. The utilization of ablative therapy to reduce the incidence of ICD shocks for VT in patients who receive the ICD as part of primary prevention for VT is being actively investigated.

MANAGEMENT OF VT STORM Repeated VT episodes requiring external cardioversion/defibrillation or repeated appropriate ICD shock therapy are referred to as *VT storm*. Although a definition of more than two episodes in 24 h is used, most patients with VT storm will experience many more episodes. In the extreme form of VT storm, the tachycardia becomes incessant and the baseline rhythm cannot be restored for any extended period. In patients with recurrent polymorphic VT in the absence of the long QT interval, one should have a high suspicion of active ischemic disease or fulminant myocarditis. Intravenous lidocaine or amiodarone administration should be coupled with prompt assessment of the status of the coronary anatomy. Endomyocardial biopsy, if indicated by clinical circumstances, may be used to confirm the diagnosis of myocarditis, although the diagnostic yield is low. In patients who demonstrate QT prolongation and recurrent pause-dependent polymorphic VT (TDP), removal of an offending QT-prolonging drug, correction of potassium or magnesium deficiencies, and emergency pacing to prevent pauses should be considered. Intravenous beta blockade therapy should be considered for polymorphic VT storm. A targeted treatment strategy should be employed if the diagnosis of the polymorphic VT syndrome can be established. For example, quinidine or isoproterenol can be used in the treatment of Brugada syndrome. Intraaortic balloon counterpulsation or acute coronary angioplasty may be needed to stop recurrent polymorphic VT precipitated by acute ischemia. In selected patients with a repeating VPC trigger for their polymorphic VT, the VPC can be targeted for ablation to prevent recurrent VT.

In patients with recurrent monomorphic VT, acute IV administration of lidocaine, procainamide, or amiodarone can prevent recurrences. The use of such therapy is empirical, and a clinical response is not certain. Procainamide and amiodarone are more likely to slow the tachycardia and make it hemodynamically tolerated. Unfortunately, antiarrhythmic drugs, especially those that slow conduction (e.g., amiodarone, procainamide), can also facilitate recurrent VT or even result in incessant VT. VT catheter ablation can eliminate frequent recurrent or incessant VT and frequent ICD shocks. Such therapy should be deployed earlier in the course of arrhythmia events to prevent adverse consequences of recurrent VT episodes and adverse effects from antiarrhythmic drugs.

UNIQUE VT SYNDROMES

Although most ventricular arrhythmias occur in the setting of CAD with prior MI, a significant number of patients develop VT in other settings. A brief discussion of each unique VT syndrome is warranted. Information that illustrates a unique pathogenesis and enhances the ability to make the correct diagnosis and institute appropriate therapy will be highlighted.

Idiopathic outflow tract VT

VT in the absence of structural heart disease is referred to as *idiopathic VT*. There are two major varieties of these VTs. Outflow tachycardias originate in the RV and LV outflow tract regions. Approximately 80% of outflow tract VTs originate in the RV and ~20% in the LV outflow tract regions. Outflow tract VTs appear to originate from anatomic sites that form an arc that begins just above the tricuspid valve and extends along the roof of the outflow tract region to include the free wall and septal aspect of the right ventricle just beneath the pulmonic valve, the aortic valve region, and then the anterior/superior margin of the mitral valve annulus. These arrhythmias appear more commonly in women. Importantly, these ventricular arrhythmias are *rarely* associated with SCD unless manifest by very short coupled premature complexes that trigger VF. Patients manifest symptoms of palpitations with exercise, stress, and caffeine ingestion. In women, the arrhythmia is more commonly associated with hormonal triggers and can frequently be timed to the premenstrual period, gestation, and menopause. Uncommonly, the VPCs and VTs can be of sufficient frequency and duration to cause a tachycardia-induced cardiomyopathy.

The pathogenesis of outflow tract VT remains unknown, and there is no definite anatomic abnormality identified with these VTs. Vagal maneuvers, adenosine, and beta blockers tend to terminate the VTs, whereas catecholamine infusion, exercise, and stress tend to potentiate the outflow tract VTs. Based on these observations, the mechanism of the arrhythmia is most likely calcium-dependent triggered activity. Preliminary data suggest that at least in some patients, a somatic mutation of the inhibitory G protein ($G\alpha_{i2}$) may serve as the genetic basis for the VT. In contrast to VT in patients with CAD, outflow tract VTs are uncommonly initiated with programmed stimulation but are able to be initiated by rapid-burst atrial or ventricular pacing, particularly when coupled with the infusion of isoproterenol.

Outflow tract VT typically produces large monophasic R waves in the inferior frontal plane leads II, III, and aVF, and typically occurs as nonsustained bursts of VT and/or frequent premature beats. Cycle length oscillations during the tachycardia are common. Since most VT originates in the RV outflow tract, the VT typically has a left bundle branch block (LBBB) pattern in lead V_1 (negative QRS vector) **(Fig. 16-12)**. Outflow tract VTs, originating in the left ventricle, particularly those associated with an origin from the mitral valve annulus, have a right bundle branch block (RBBB) pattern in lead V_1 (positive QRS vector).

TREATMENT	Idiopathic Outflow Tract Ventricular Tachycardia

Acute medical therapy for idiopathic outflow tract VT is rarely required because the VT is hemodynamically tolerated and is typically nonsustained. Intravenous beta blockers frequently terminate the tachycardia. Chronic therapy with beta or calcium channel blockers frequently prevents recurrent episodes of the tachycardia. The arrhythmia also appears to respond to treatment with class IA or IC agents or with sotalol. Catheter ablative

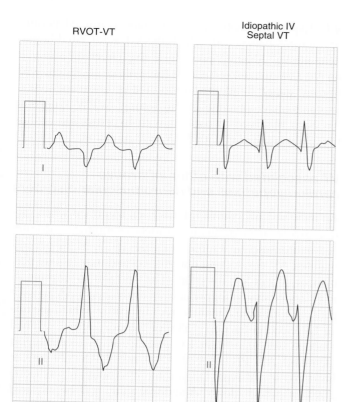
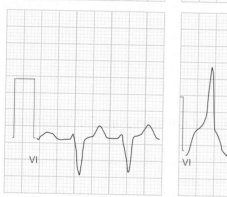
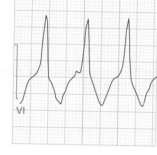

FIGURE 16-12

Common idiopathic ventricular tachycardia (VT) ECG patterns. Right ventricular outflow tract (RVOT) VT with typical left bundle QRS pattern in V₁ and inferiorly directed frontal plane axis, and left ventricular septal VT from the inferior septum with a narrow QRS RBBB pattern in V₁ and superior and leftward front plane QRS axis.

therapy has been utilized successfully to eliminate the tachycardia with success rates >90%. Because of the absence of structural heart disease and the focal nature of these arrhythmias, the 12-lead ECG pattern during VT can help localize the site of origin of the arrhythmia and help facilitate catheter ablation. Efficacy of therapy is assessed with treadmill testing and/or ECG monitoring, and electrophysiologic study is performed only when the diagnosis is in question or to perform catheter ablation.

Idiopathic LV septal/fascicular VT

The second most common idiopathic VT is linked anatomically to the Purkinje system in the left ventricle. The arrhythmia mechanism appears to be macroreentry involving calcium-dependent slow response fibers that are part of the Purkinje network, although automatic tachycardias have also been observed. A 12-lead ECG morphology of the VT shows a narrow RBBB pattern and a superior leftward axis or an inferior rightward axis, depending on whether the VT originates from the posterior or anterior fascicles (Fig. 16-12). Idiopathic LV septal VT is unique in its suppression with verapamil. Beta blockers also have been used with some success as primary or effective adjunctive therapy. Catheter ablation is very effective therapy for VT resistant to drug therapy or in patients reluctant to take daily therapy, with anticipated successful elimination of VT in >90% of patients.

VT associated with LV dilated cardiomyopathy

Monomorphic and polymorphic VTs may occur in patients with nonischemic dilated cardiomyopathy (Chap. 21). Although the myopathic process may be diffuse, there appears to be a predilection for the development of fibrosis around the mitral and aortic valvular regions. Most uniform sustained VT can be mapped to these regions of fibrosis. Drug therapy is usually ineffective in preventing VT, and empirical trials of sotalol or amiodarone are usually initiated only for recurrent VT episodes after ICD implantation. VT associated with nonischemic dilated cardiomyopathy appears to be less amenable to catheter ablative therapy from the endocardium; frequently, the VT originates from epicardial areas of fibrosis and catheter access to the epicardium can be gained via a percutaneous pericardial puncture to improve the outcome of ablation techniques. In patients with a history of depressed myocardial dysfunction due to a nonischemic cardiomyopathy with an LV ejection fraction <30%, data now support the implantation of a prophylactic ICD device to reduce the risk of SCD from the first VT/VF episode effectively.

Bundle branch reentrant VT

Monomorphic VT in patients with idiopathic nonischemic cardiomyopathy or valvular cardiomyopathy is frequently due to a large macroreentrant circuit involving the various elements of the His-Purkinje network. The arrhythmia usually occurs in the presence of underlying disease of the His-Purkinje system. In sinus rhythm, an incomplete left bundle block is typically present and the time it takes to traverse the His-Purkinje network is delayed; this slow conduction serves as the substrate for reentry. Characteristically, the VT circuit rotates in an antegrade direction down the right bundle and retrograde up the left posterior or anterior fascicles and left bundle branch. As a result, bundle branch reentrant VT typically has a QRS morphology with a left bundle branch block type of pattern and a leftward superior axis (Fig. 16–13). The circuit for bundle branch (LBB) reentrant VT can occasionally rotate in the opposite direction, antegrade through the left bundle and retrograde through the right bundle, in which case an RBBB pattern during VT will be manifest.

It is important to recognize bundle branch reentrant VT because it is readily amenable to ablative therapy that targets a component of the His-Purkinje system, typically the right bundle, to block the VT circuit. Less commonly, bundle branch reentry may occur in the absence of structural heart disease or in the setting of CAD. The use of adjunctive ICD therapy is dictated by the ability to eliminate the VT successfully and the severity of the LV dysfunction.

VT associated with hypertrophic cardiomyopathy

(See also Chap. 21) VT and VF have also been associated with hypertrophic cardiomyopathy. In patients with hypertrophic cardiomyopathy and a history of sustained VT/VF, unexplained syncope, a strong family history of SCD, LV septal thickness >30 mm, or nonsustained spontaneous VT, the risk of SCD is high and ICD implantation is usually indicated. Amiodarone, sotalol, and beta blockers have been used to control recurrent

VT. Experience with ablative therapy is limited because of the infrequency with which the VT is tolerated hemodynamically. Ablation procedures that target the substrate for VT/VF and ablate areas of low voltage consistent with fibrosis, which frequently are located in apical aneurysms, appear to have promise in this setting. WPW syndrome has been observed in patients with hypertrophic cardiomyopathy associated with *PRKAG2* mutations.

VT associated with other infiltrative cardiomyopathies and neuromuscular disorders

An increased arrhythmia risk has been identified when cardiac involvement occurs in a variety of infiltrative diseases and neuromuscular disorders (Table 16–7). Many patients manifest AV conduction disturbances and may require permanent pacemaker insertion. The decision to implant an ICD device should follow current established guidelines for patients with nonischemic cardiomyopathy, which include an LV ejection fraction <35% or a history of unexplained syncope with significant LV dysfunction. A recent report identified AF, PR interval >240 ms, QRS 120 ms, or heart block and type 1 myotonic dystrophy as predicting a risk of sudden death. Additional study will be required to determine if patients with lesser degrees of LV dysfunction or other more diffuse myopathic disease processes also have identifiable risk and warrant primary ICD implantation. A potential proarrhythmic risk of antiarrhythmic drug therapy should be acknowledged, and drug therapy should be reserved for symptomatic arrhythmias and limited to amiodarone or sotalol if an ICD is not present.

Arrhythmogenic RV cardiomyopathy/dysplasia (ARVCM/D)

(See also Chap. 21) ARVCM/D due to a genetically determined dysplastic process or after a suspected viral myocarditis is also associated with VT/VF. The sporadic nonfamilial/nondysplastic form of RV cardiomyopathy

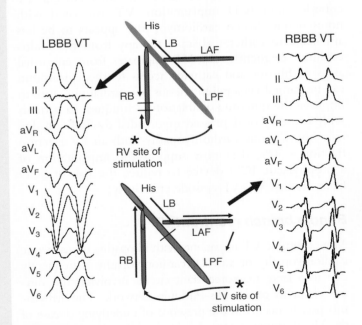

FIGURE 16-13
Bundle branch reentrant ventricular tachycardia (VT) showing typical QRS morphologies when VT is initiated with stimulation from the right ventricle (left bundle branch block [LBBB] VT pattern) or left ventricle (right bundle branch block [RBBB] VT pattern) and schema for circuit involving the His-Purkinje network.

TABLE 16-7

INFILTRATIVE/INFLAMMATORY AND NEUROMUSCULAR DISORDERS ASSOCIATED WITH AN INCREASED VENTRICULAR ARRHYTHMIA RISK	
Sarcoidosis[a]	Emery-Dreyfuss muscular dystrophy[a]
Chagas' disease[a]	Limb-girdle muscular dystrophy[a]
Amyloidosis[a]	Duchenne muscular dystrophy
Fabry disease	Becker muscular dystrophy
Hemochromatosis	Kearn-Sayre syndrome[a]
Myotonic muscular dystrophy[a]	Friedreich's ataxia

[a]High frequency of ventricular arrhythmias noted.

appears to be more common; however, this may vary with ethnicity. In patients predisposed to VT, there appears to be a predominance of perivalvular fibrosis involving mostly the free wall of the right ventricle in proximity to the tricuspid and pulmonic valves. The surface ECG leads that reflect RV activation, including V_1–V_3, may show terminal notching of the QRS complex and inverted T waves in sinus rhythm. When the terminal notching is distinct and appears separated from the QRS complex, it is referred to as an *epsilon wave* (**Fig. 16-14**). Epsilon waves are consistent with markedly delayed ventricular activation in the region of the RV free wall near the base of the tricuspid and pulmonic valves in areas of extensive fibrosis.

In patients with ARVCM/D, echocardiography demonstrates RV enlargement with RV wall motion abnormalities and RV apical aneurysm formation. MRI may show fatty replacement of the ventricle, thinning of the RV free wall with increased fibrosis, and associated wall motion abnormalities. Because of the presence of extensive amounts of fat normally covering the epicardium in the region of the RV, caution must be used to avoid overinterpreting the MRI in trying to determine the appropriate diagnosis. Patients tend to have multiple VT morphologies. The VT will typically have an LBBB type QRS pattern in V_1 and tend to have poor R-wave progression in V_1 through V_6, consistent with an RV free-wall origin. Areas of low electrogram voltage that are identified during RV catheter endocardial sinus rhythm voltage mapping may be helpful in confirming the diagnosis. Importantly, endocardial biopsy may

not identify the presence of fatty replacement or fibrosis unless directed to the basal RV free wall. The familial forms of this syndrome have been linked to a number of desmosomal protein mutations. A distinct genetic form of this syndrome, Naxos disease, consists of arrhythmogenic RV dysplasia coupled with palmar-plantar keratosis and woolly hair and is associated with a high risk of SCD in adolescents and young adults.

TREATMENT	Arrhythmogenic Right Ventricular Cardiomyopathy/Dysplasia

The threshold for ICD implantation in patients with an established diagnosis of ARVCM/D is low. An ICD typically is implanted in patients deemed to have a persistent VT risk, those who have had spontaneous or inducible rapid VTs, and those who show concomitant LV cardiomyopathy. Treatment options for recurrent VT in patients with ARVCM/D include the use of the antiarrhythmic agent sotalol. Beta blockers serve as useful adjunctive therapy when coupled with other antiarrhythmic agents. Catheter ablative therapy directed at mappable sustained ventricular arrhythmias is also highly successful in controlling recurrent VT. In selected patients with multiple VT morphologies and unstable VT, linear ablation lesions directed at endocardial scars and, if required, targeting late potentials in epicardial scars, defined by catheter-based bipolar voltage mapping, provide significant amelioration of the recurrent VT episodes.

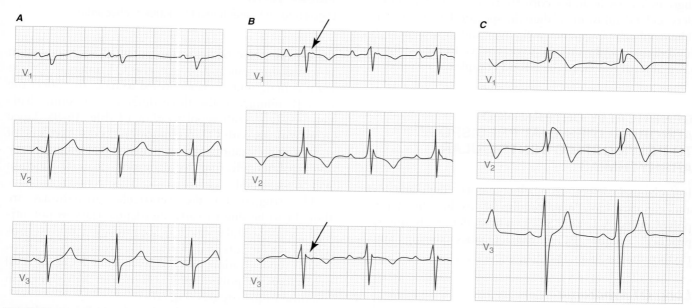

FIGURE 16-14

Leads V_1 to V_3 in sinus rhythm from a normal subject (**A**), from a patient with arrhythmogenic right ventricular cardiomyopathy showing epsilon waves (*arrow*) and T-wave inversion (**B**), and from a patient with Brugada syndrome with ST-segment elevation in V_1 and V_2 (**C**).

VT after operative tetralogy of Fallot repair

VT may also occur after surgical repair of tetralogy of Fallot. Patients typically develop VT many years after the surgery. VT tends to occur in patients with evidence of RV systolic dysfunction. The VT mechanism and location are typically a macroreentrant circuit around the right ventriculotomy scar to the valve annuli. Catheter ablation creating linear lesions that extend from either the pulmonic or the tricuspid annulus to the ventriculotomy scar is typically effective in preventing arrhythmia recurrences. An ICD is usually implanted in patients who manifest rapid VT, have persistent inducible VT after ablation, or have concomitant LV dysfunction.

Fascicular tachycardia caused by digoxin toxicity

Digoxin toxicity can produce increased ventricular ectopy and, when coupled with bradyarrhythmias caused by digoxin toxicity, may predispose to sustained polymorphic ventricular arrhythmias and VF. The signature VT associated with digoxin toxicity is bidirectional VT **(Fig. 16-15)**. This unique VT is due to triggered activity associated with calcium overload resulting from the inhibition of Na$^+$, K$^+$-ATPase by digoxin. Bidirectional VT originates from the left anterior and posterior fascicles, creating a relatively narrow QRS right bundle branch (RBB) configuration with a beat-to-beat alternating right and left frontal plane QRS axis. This VT seldom is observed in the absence of digoxin toxicity. Treatment for bidirectional VT or other hemodynamically significant arrhythmias due to digoxin excess includes correction of electrolyte disorders and IV infusion of digoxin-specific Fab fragments. The antibody fragments will, over the course of 1 h, bind digoxin and eliminate toxic effects. In the setting of normal renal function, the bound complex is secreted.

GENETICALLY DETERMINED ABNORMALITIES THAT PREDISPOSE TO POLYMORPHIC VENTRICULAR ARRHYTHMIAS

Ion channel defects that affect cardiac depolarization and repolarization may predispose to life-threatening polymorphic VT and SCD. These defects frequently produce unique ECG characteristics during sinus rhythm that facilitate the diagnosis.

Long QT syndrome

The congenital form of LQTS consists of defects in cardiac ion channels that are responsible for cardiac repolarization. Defects that enhance sodium or calcium inward currents or inhibit outward potassium currents during

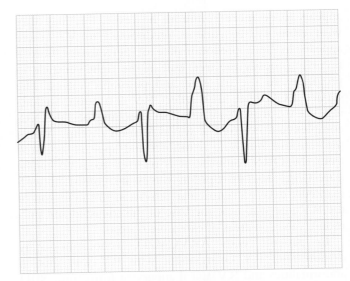

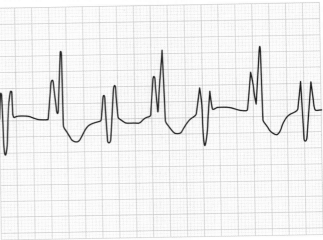

FIGURE 16-15

Digoxin toxic bidirectional fascicular tachycardia.

the plateau phase of the action potential lengthen action potential duration and, hence, the QT interval. Of the eight genetic mutations identified to date, five affect the α or β subunits of the three different potassium channels involved with repolarization **(Table 16-8)**. Since many patients with QT prolongation do not have one of the defined mutations, it is anticipated that other genetic abnormalities affecting repolarization channel function will be identified.

The triggers for the ventricular arrhythmias are thought to be due to early afterdepolarizations potentiated by intracellular calcium accumulation from a prolonged action potential plateau. Heterogeneity of myocardial repolarization indexed by a longer QT interval predisposes to polymorphic ventricular arrhythmias in response to the triggers (Fig. 16-9).

In most patients with LQTS, the QT interval corrected for heart rate using Bazett's formula is >460 ms in men and >480 ms in women with LQTS. Marked lengthening of the QT interval to >500 ms is clearly

TABLE 16-8

INHERITED ARRHYTHMIA DISORDERS: "CHANNELOPATHIES" WITH HIGH RISK OF VENTRICULAR ARRHYTHMIAS

DISORDER	GENE	PROTEIN/CHANNEL AFFECTED
LQT1	*KCNQ1*	I_{Ks} channel α subunit
LQT2	*KCNH2 (HERG)*	I_{Kr} channel α subunit
LQT3	*SCN5A*	I_{na} channel α subunit
LQT4	*ANK2*	Ankyrin-B
LQT5	*KCNE1*	I_{Ks} channel β subunit
LQT6	*KCNE2*	I_{Kr} channel β subunit
LQT7	*KCNJ2*	I_{K1} channel α subunit
LQT8	*CACNA1C*	I_{Ca} channel α subunit
Jervell LN1	*KCNQ1*	I_{Ks} channel β subunit
Jervell LN2	*KCNE1*	I_{Kr} channel β subunit
Brugada syndrome	*SCN5A*	I_{Na} channel
Catecholaminergic VT	*Ry R2*	Ryanodine receptor, calsequestrin receptor
SQTS1	*KCNH2 (HERG)*	I_{Kr} channel α subunit
SQTS2	*KCNQ1(KvLQT1)*	I_{Ks} channel α subunit
SQTS3	*KCNJ2*	I_{K1} channel

Abbreviations: LQT, long QT (interval); SQT, short QT (interval).

associated with a greater arrhythmia risk in patients with LQTS. Many affected individuals may have QT intervals that intermittently measure within a normal range or fail to shorten appropriately with exercise. Some individuals manifest the syndrome only when exposed to a drug, such as sotalol, that alters channel function.

The genotype associated with LQTS appears to influence prognosis, and identification of the genotype appears to help optimize clinical management. The first three genotypic designations of the mutations identified, LQT1, LQT2, and LQT3, appear to account for >99% of patients with clinically relevant LQTSs. Surface ECG characteristics may be helpful in distinguishing the three most common genotypes, with genetic testing being definitive.

LQT1 represents the most common genotypic abnormality. Patients with LQT1 fail to shorten or actually prolong their QT interval with exercise. The T wave in patients with LQT1 tends to be broad and constitutes the majority of the prolonged QT interval. The most common trigger for potentiating cardiac arrhythmias in patients with LQT1 is exercise, followed by emotional stress.

More than 80% of male patients have their first cardiac event by age 20, so competitive exercise should be restricted and swimming avoided for these patients. Patients tend to respond to beta blocker therapy. Patients with two LQT1 alleles have Jervell and Lange-Nielsen syndrome, with more dramatic QT prolongation and deafness and a worse arrhythmia prognosis.

LQT2 is the second most common genotypic abnormality. The T wave tends to be notched and bifid. In LQT2 patients, the most common precipitant is emotional stress, followed by sleep or auditory stimulation. Despite the occurrence during sleep, patients typically respond to beta blocker therapy.

LQT3 is due to a mutation in the gene that encodes the cardiac sodium channel on chromosome 3. Prolongation of the action potential duration occurs because of failure to inactivate this channel. LQT3 patients have either late-onset peaked biphasic T waves or asymmetric peaked T waves. The arrhythmia events tend to be more life threatening, and thus the prognosis for LQT3 is the poorest of all the LQTs. Male patients appear to have the worst prognosis among patients with LQT3. Most events in LQT3 patients occur during sleep, suggesting that they are at higher risk during periods of slow heart rates. Beta blockers are not recommended, and exercise is not restricted in LQT3.

TREATMENT   Long QT Syndrome

The institution of ICD therapy should be strongly considered in any patient with LQTS who has demonstrated any life-threatening arrhythmia. Patients with syncope with a confirmed diagnosis based on unequivocal ECG criteria or positive genetic testing should also be given the same strong consideration. Primary prevention with prophylactic ICD implantation should be considered in male patients with LQT3 and in all patients with marked QT prolongation (>500 ms), particularly when coupled with an immediate family history of SCD. Future epidemiologic investigation may provide firmer guidelines to sort patients further on the basis of risks such as age, gender, arrhythmia history, and genetic characteristics. In all patients with documented or suspected LQTS, drugs that prolong the QT interval must be avoided. For an updated list of drugs, see www.qtdrugs.org.

Acquired LQTS

Patients with a genetic predisposition related to what appear to be sporadic mutations and/or single nucleotide polymorphisms can develop marked QT prolongation in response to drugs that alter repolarization currents. The QT prolongation and associated polymorphic ventricular tachycardia (TDP) are seen more frequently in women and may be a manifestation of subclinical LQTS. Drug-induced long QT and TDP frequently are potentiated by the development of hypokalemia and bradycardia. The offending drugs typically block the potassium I_{Kr} channel (Table 16-5). Since most drug effects are dose dependent, important drug-drug interactions that alter metabolism and/or alterations in elimination kinetics because of hepatic or renal dysfunction frequently contribute to the arrhythmias.

TREATMENT   Acquired Long QT Syndrome

Acute therapy for acquired LQTS is directed at eliminating the offending drug therapy, reversing metabolic abnormalities by the infusion of magnesium and/or potassium, and preventing pause-dependent arrhythmias by temporary pacing or the cautious infusion of isoproterenol. Class IB antiarrhythmic agents (e.g., lidocaine) that do not cause QT prolongation may also be used, though they are frequently ineffective. Supportive therapy to allay anxiety and prevent pain with required DC shock therapy for sustained arrhythmias and efforts to facilitate drug elimination are important.

Short QT syndrome

A gain in function of repolarization currents can result in a shortening of atrial and ventricular refractoriness and marked QT shortening on the surface ECG (Table 16-8). The T wave tends to be tall and peaked. A QT interval <320 ms is required to establish the diagnosis of this uncommon syndrome. Mutations in the *HERG*, *KvLQT1*, and *KCNJ2* genes have been identified. Patients with the syndrome are predisposed to both AF and VF. ICD implantation is recommended.

Double counting of QRS and T waves may lead to inappropriate ICD shocks. Drug therapy with quinidine has been used to lengthen the QT interval and reduce the amplitude of the T wave. This therapy is being evaluated to determine long-term efficacy in preventing arrhythmias in this syndrome.

Brugada syndrome

The major clinical features of Brugada syndrome include manifest, transient, or concealed ST segment elevation in V_1 to V_3 that typically can be provoked with the sodium channel-blocking drugs ajmaline, flecainide, and procainamide and a risk of polymorphic ventricular arrhythmias. It appears that a diminished inward sodium current in the region of the RV outflow tract epicardium is responsible for Brugada syndrome (Table 16-8). A loss of the action potential dome in the RV epicardium due to unopposed I_{To} potassium outward current results in dramatic shortening of the action potential. The large potential difference between the normal endocardium and rapidly depolarized RV outflow epicardium gives rise to ST-segment elevation in V_1–V_3 in sinus rhythm and predisposes to local ventricular reentry (Fig. 16-14). The majority of genetic abnormalities responsible for the syndrome have not been described; however, in ~20% of patients, mutations of *SCN5A* genes have been identified. Although identified in both genders and all races with an autosomal dominant inheritance pattern, the arrhythmia syndrome is most common in young male patients (~75%) and is thought to be responsible for the sudden and unexpected nocturnal death syndrome (SUDS) described in Southeast Asian men. The ventricular arrhythmia characteristically occurs with rest or during sleep. Fever and other sodium channel-blocking drugs have also precipitated ventricular arrhythmias.

The presence of spontaneous coved–type ST elevation in the right precordial leads and a history of syncope or aborted sudden cardiac death are predictors of an adverse outcome. Because of the overlap in *SCN5A* mutations, the association of Brugada syndrome with phenotypic LQT3 and conduction disturbances has been noted.

TREATMENT   Brugada Syndrome

A drug challenge with procainamide may be important to establish the diagnosis and the probable cause of unexplained syncope when the surface ECG is equivocal (saddleback ST elevation pattern). Ajmaline and intravenous flecainide, which are not available in the United States, may have higher sensitivities for identifying the syndrome. Successful acute management of recurrent

VT has been reported with isoproterenol or quinidine administration, although experience has been limited. Patients who do not benefit from beta blockers and chronic suppression with quinidine, which may lengthen epicardial action potential duration by blocking I_{TO} current, may be considered for ICD implantation. ICD treatment to manage recurrences and prevent sudden death is recommended for all patients who have had documented arrhythmia episodes and patients with syncope and positive spontaneous or provoked coved-type ECG ST-segment changes in V_1–V_3. Family members should undergo ECG screening for the presence of the abnormality. The role of programmed cardiac stimulation and the use of ICD therapy in asymptomatic patients with the Brugada-type ECG pattern remain somewhat controversial, as is provocative drug infusion and programmed stimulation in patients with borderline abnormalities and no arrhythmia symptoms. Longer-term follow-up in a larger group of these relatively low-risk patients may be required before definitive recommendations can be provided. Counseling on controversies that exist, the potential risk of fever, and inadvertent administration of tricyclic antidepressants should be considered. Genetic testing may be helpful in confirming the presence of the genetic abnormality in family members of patients who manifest the arrhythmia syndrome.

Catecholaminergic polymorphic VT

A mutation of the myocardial ryanodine release channel, which effectively creates a "leak" in calcium from the sarcoplasmic reticulum, has been identified in patients with catecholaminergic VT (Table 16-8). The accumulation of intracellular calcium potentiates delayed afterdepolarizations and triggered activity. Patients can manifest bidirectional VT, nonsustained polymorphic VT, or recurrent VF. Both an autosomal dominant familial form and sporadic forms of the disease have been described. More recently, an autosomal recessive variant associated with a mutation in the sarcoplasmic reticulum calcium-buffering protein calsequestrin has also been identified. The arrhythmias are precipitated by exercise and emotional stress (Fig. 16–16). Exercise restriction is warranted. Treatment with beta blockers and ICD implantation has been recommended. Prevention of inappropriate or easily triggered ICD

shocks by proper ICD programming is essential to prevent VT storm from endogenous catecholamine release.

SPECIAL CONSIDERATION: APPROACH TO TACHYARRHYTHMIAS IN ATHLETES

The first manifestation of a tachyarrhythmia, whether benign or malignant, may occur during athletic activity. Fortunately, successful cardiopulmonary resuscitation of life-threatening ventricular arrhythmias has increased with the use of automatic external defibrillators at major sporting events and schools. Rarely, VF may be precipitated by blunt precordial blows without structural injury to the heart or chest wall (commotio cordis).

The approach to the athlete should begin with an assessment of the severity and significance of symptoms. Syncope with exertion should be assumed to be caused by a potentially lethal arrhythmia. A thorough cardiac evaluation and restricted participation in competitive sports are in order until a less life-threatening diagnosis can be established. ECG recording at the time of the symptomatic events usually can establish the diagnosis, although it may be difficult to obtain.

In patients with syncope and no ECG-documented arrhythmia, a systematic attempt to define a cardiac structural or primarily electrical abnormality with a routine ECG and a transthoracic echocardiogram is in order. Common structural abnormalities associated with fatal or life-threatening ventricular arrhythmias include hypertrophic cardiomyopathy, arrhythmogenic cardiomyopathy, and acute myocarditis. Coronary anomalies should be suspected if the arrhythmia symptoms are preceded in onset by chest pain. The 12-lead ECG should be screened for the presence of preexcitation, QT prolongation, a Brugada-type ECG pattern or epsilon waves, and T-wave inversions consistent with a nonischemic RV or LV cardiomyopathy or myocarditis. Additional ECG monitoring may be required. A stress test may be appropriate to provoke arrhythmias, especially if there are recurrent symptoms. It is critical to achieve the level of exercise that precipitated the arrhythmia, which for some athletes may be a challenge for the exercise lab.

Management of an athlete with cardiac arrhythmias may be a challenge, with a tendency to discourage participation in competitive sports and institute treatment whenever there is a perception of increased risk. Guidelines for restricting athletic activity have

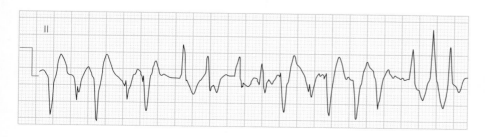

FIGURE 16-16
Catecholaminergic polymorphic ventricular tachycardia noted during an exercise stress test.

TABLE 16-9

RECOMMENDATIONS FOR COMPETITIVE ATHLETES WITH SELECTED CARDIOVASCULAR ABNORMALITIES

CLINICAL ENTITY	CLINICAL CRITERIA	SPORTS PERMITTED
Gene carriers for arrhythmia syndromes without phenotype VT		All sports
Long QT syndrome	>0.47 s in men, >0.48 s in women	Low-intensity competitive sports
Brugada syndrome		Low-intensity competitive sports
Catecholaminergic polymorphic VT		No competitive sports
Asymptomatic Wolff-Parkinson-White syndrome	Electrophysiological study not mandatory	All sports except restriction in dangerous environments
Premature ventricular complexes		All competitive sports when no increase in PVCs or symptoms occur with exercise
Nonsustained ventricular tachycardia	No structural heart disease	All competitive sports
Nonsustained ventricular tachycardia	Structural heart disease	Only low-intensity competitive sports

Source: Adapted from ACC Bethesda Conference #36 from Pelliccia et al: J Am Coll Cardiol 52:1990–1996, 2008.

been promulgated on the basis of expert consensus and evidence-based data and can facilitate management once a diagnosis has been established (Table 16-9). Treatment should be based on standards established for each arrhythmia syndrome. Curative catheter ablative therapy should be applied if indicated. ICD therapy, if required, is incompatible with contact sports because of the potential for blunt trauma and consequent damage to the device. Although ICDs are effective, their psychosocial impact, the potential for inappropriate shocks for sinus tachycardia, and lead-related complications must be recognized.

CHAPTER 17

HEART FAILURE AND COR PULMONALE

Douglas L. Mann   ■   Murali Chakinala

HEART FAILURE

DEFINITION

Heart failure (HF) is a clinical syndrome that occurs in patients who, because of an inherited or acquired abnormality of cardiac structure and/or function, develop a constellation of clinical symptoms (dyspnea and fatigue) and signs (edema and rales) that lead to frequent hospitalizations, a poor quality of life, and a shortened life expectancy.

EPIDEMIOLOGY

HF is a burgeoning problem worldwide, with more than 20 million people affected. The overall prevalence of HF in the adult population in developed countries is 2%. HF prevalence follows an exponential pattern, rising with age, and affects 6–10% of people over age 65. Although the relative incidence of HF is lower in women than in men, women constitute at least one-half the cases of HF because of their longer life expectancy. In North America and Europe, the lifetime risk of developing HF is approximately one in five for a 40-year-old. The overall prevalence of HF is thought to be increasing, in part because current therapies for cardiac disorders, such as myocardial infarction (MI), valvular heart disease, and arrhythmias, are allowing patients to survive longer. Very little is known about the prevalence or risk of developing HF in emerging nations because of the lack of population-based studies in those countries. Although HF once was thought to arise primarily in the setting of a depressed left ventricular (LV) ejection fraction (EF), epidemiologic studies have shown that approximately one-half of patients who develop HF have a normal or preserved EF (EF ≥40–50%). Accordingly, HF patients are now broadly categorized into one of two groups:

(1) HF with a depressed EF (commonly referred to as *systolic failure*) or (2) HF with a preserved EF (commonly referred to as *diastolic failure*).

ETIOLOGY

As shown in Table 17-1, any condition that leads to an alteration in LV structure or function can predispose a patient to developing HF. Although the etiology of HF in patients with a preserved EF differs from that of patients with depressed EF, there is considerable overlap between the etiologies of these two conditions. In industrialized countries, coronary artery disease (CAD) has become the predominant cause in men and women and is responsible for 60–75% of cases of HF. Hypertension contributes to the development of HF in 75% of patients, including most patients with CAD. Both CAD and hypertension interact to augment the risk of HF, as does diabetes mellitus.

In 20–30% of the cases of HF with a depressed EF, the exact etiologic basis is not known. These patients are referred to as having nonischemic, dilated, or idiopathic cardiomyopathy if the cause is unknown (Chap. 21). Prior viral infection or toxin exposure (e.g., alcoholic or chemotherapeutic) also may lead to a dilated cardiomyopathy. Moreover, it is becoming increasingly clear that a large number of cases of dilated cardiomyopathy are secondary to specific genetic defects, most notably those in the cytoskeleton. Most forms of familial dilated cardiomyopathy are inherited in an autosomal dominant fashion. Mutations of genes that encode cytoskeletal proteins (desmin, cardiac myosin, vinculin) and nuclear membrane proteins (laminin) have been identified thus far. Dilated cardiomyopathy also is associated with Duchenne's, Becker's, and limb-girdle muscular dystrophies. Conditions that lead to a high cardiac output (e.g., arteriovenous fistula, anemia) are seldom responsible for the development of HF in a normal heart;

TABLE 17-1

ETIOLOGIES OF HEART FAILURE

Depressed Ejection Fraction (<40%)

Coronary artery disease	Nonischemic dilated cardiomyopathy
Myocardial infarction[a]	Familial/genetic disorders
Myocardial ischemia[a]	Infiltrative disorders[a]
Chronic pressure overload	Toxic/drug-induced damage
Hypertension[a]	Metabolic disorder[a]
Obstructive valvular disease[a]	Viral
Chronic volume overload	Chagas' disease
Regurgitant valvular disease	Disorders of rate and rhythm
Intracardiac (left-to-right) shunting	Chronic bradyarrhythmias
Extracardiac shunting	Chronic tachyarrhythmias

Preserved Ejection Fraction (>40–50%)

Pathologic hypertrophy	Restrictive cardiomyopathy
Primary (hypertrophic cardiomyopathies)	Infiltrative disorders (amyloidosis, sarcoidosis)
Secondary (hypertension)	Storage diseases (hemochromatosis)
Aging	Fibrosis
	Endomyocardial disorders

Pulmonary Heart Disease

Cor pulmonale
Pulmonary vascular disorders

High-Output States

Metabolic disorders	Excessive blood-flow requirements
Thyrotoxicosis	Systemic arteriovenous shunting
Nutritional disorders (beriberi)	Chronic anemia

[a]Indicates conditions that can also lead to heart failure with a preserved ejection fraction.

however, in the presence of underlying structural heart disease, these conditions can lead to overt HF.

GLOBAL CONSIDERATIONS

Rheumatic heart disease remains a major cause of HF in Africa and Asia, especially in the young. Hypertension is an important cause of HF in the African and African-American populations. Chagas' disease is still a major cause of HF in South America. Not surprisingly, anemia is a frequent concomitant factor in HF in many developing nations. As developing nations undergo socioeconomic development, the epidemiology of HF is becoming similar to that of Western Europe and North America, with CAD

emerging as the single most common cause of HF. Although the contribution of diabetes mellitus to HF is not well understood, diabetes accelerates atherosclerosis and often is associated with hypertension.

PROGNOSIS

Despite many recent advances in the evaluation and management of HF, the development of symptomatic HF still carries a poor prognosis. Community-based studies indicate that 30–40% of patients die within 1 year of diagnosis and 60–70% die within 5 years, mainly from worsening HF or as a sudden event (probably because of a ventricular arrhythmia). Although it is difficult to predict prognosis in an individual, patients with symptoms at rest (New York Heart Association [NYHA] class IV) have a 30–70% annual mortality rate, whereas patients with symptoms with moderate activity (NYHA class II) have an annual mortality rate of 5–10%. Thus, functional status is an important predictor of patient outcome (Table 17-2).

TABLE 17-2

NEW YORK HEART ASSOCIATION CLASSIFICATION

FUNCTIONAL CAPACITY	OBJECTIVE ASSESSMENT
Class I	Patients with cardiac disease but without resulting limitation of physical activity. Ordinary physical activity does not cause undue fatigue, palpitations, dyspnea, or anginal pain.
Class II	Patients with cardiac disease resulting in slight limitation of physical activity. They are comfortable at rest. Ordinary physical activity results in fatigue, palpitation, dyspnea, or anginal pain.
Class III	Patients with cardiac disease resulting in marked limitation of physical activity. They are comfortable at rest. Less than ordinary activity causes fatigue, palpitation, dyspnea, or anginal pain.
Class IV	Patients with cardiac disease resulting in inability to carry on any physical activity without discomfort. Symptoms of heart failure or the anginal syndrome may be present even at rest. If any physical activity is undertaken, discomfort is increased.

Source: Adapted from New York Heart Association, Inc., *Diseases of the Heart and Blood Vessels: Nomenclature and Criteria for Diagnosis,* 6th ed. Boston, Little Brown, 1964, p. 114.

PATHOGENESIS

Figure 17-1 provides a general conceptual framework for considering the development and progression of HF with a depressed EF. As shown, HF may be viewed as a progressive disorder that is initiated after an *index event* either damages the heart muscle, with a resultant loss of functioning cardiac myocytes, or, alternatively, disrupts the ability of the myocardium to generate force, thereby preventing the heart from contracting normally. This index event may have an abrupt onset, as in the case of a myocardial infarction (MI); it may have a gradual or insidious onset, as in the case of hemodynamic pressure or volume overloading; or it may be hereditary, as in the case of many of the genetic cardiomyopathies. Regardless of the nature of the inciting event, the feature that is common to each of these index events is that they all in some manner produce a decline in the pumping capacity of the heart. In most instances, patients remain asymptomatic or minimally symptomatic after the initial decline in pumping capacity of the heart or develop symptoms only after the dysfunction has been present for some time.

Although the precise reasons why patients with LV dysfunction may remain asymptomatic is not certain,

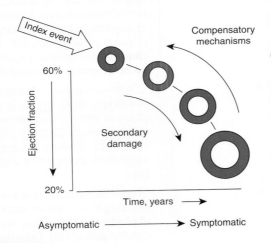

FIGURE 17-1
Pathogenesis of heart failure with a depressed ejection fraction. Heart failure begins after an index event produces an initial decline in the heart's pumping capacity. After this initial decline in pumping capacity, a variety of compensatory mechanisms are activated, including the adrenergic nervous system, the renin-angiotensin-aldosterone system, and the cytokine system. In the short term, these systems are able to restore cardiovascular function to a normal homeostatic range with the result that the patient remains asymptomatic. However, with time the sustained activation of these systems can lead to secondary end-organ damage within the ventricle, with worsening left ventricular remodeling and subsequent cardiac decompensation. (*From D Mann: Circulation 100:999, 1999.*)

one potential explanation is that a number of compensatory mechanisms become activated in the presence of cardiac injury and/or LV dysfunction allowing patients to sustain and modulate LV function for a period of months to years. The list of compensatory mechanisms that have been described thus far include (1) activation of the renin-angiotensin-aldosterone (RAA) and adrenergic nervous systems, which are responsible for maintaining cardiac output through increased retention of salt and water (**Fig. 17-2**), and (2) increased myocardial contractility. In addition, there is activation of a family of countervailing vasodilatory molecules, including the atrial and brain natriuretic peptides (ANP and BNP), prostaglandins (PGE_2 and PGI_2), and nitric oxide (NO), that offsets the excessive peripheral vascular vasoconstriction. Genetic background, sex, age, or environment may influence these compensatory mechanisms, which are able to modulate LV function within a physiologic/homeostatic range so that the functional capacity of the patient is preserved or is depressed only minimally. Thus, patients may remain asymptomatic or minimally symptomatic for a period of years; however, at some point patients become overtly symptomatic, with a resultant striking increase in morbidity and mortality rates. Although the exact mechanisms that are responsible for this transition are not known, as will be discussed later in this chapter, the transition to symptomatic HF is accompanied by increasing activation of neurohormonal, adrenergic, and cytokine systems that lead to a series of adaptive changes within the myocardium collectively referred to as *LV remodeling.*

In contrast to our understanding of the pathogenesis of HF with a depressed EF, our understanding of the mechanisms that contribute to the development of HF with a preserved EF is still evolving. That is, although diastolic dysfunction (see later in this chapter) was thought to be the only mechanism responsible for the development of HF with a preserved EF, community-based studies suggest that additional extracardiac mechanisms may be important, such as increased vascular stiffness and impaired renal function.

BASIC MECHANISMS OF HEART FAILURE
Systolic dysfunction

LV remodeling develops in response to a series of complex events that occur at the cellular and molecular levels (**Table 17-3**). These changes include (1) myocyte hypertrophy, (2) alterations in the contractile properties of the myocyte, (3) progressive loss of myocytes through necrosis, apoptosis, and autophagic cell death, (4) β-adrenergic desensitization, (5) abnormal myocardial energetics and metabolism, and (6) reorganization of the extracellular matrix with dissolution of the

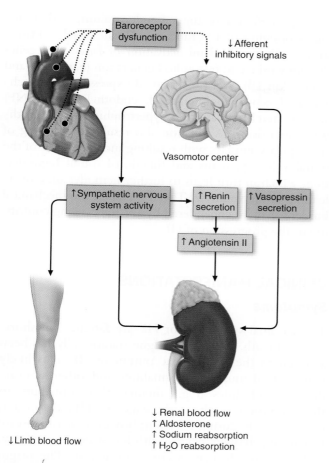

Vasomotor center

↓ Renal blood flow
↑ Aldosterone
↑ Sodium reabsorption
↑ H₂O reabsorption

↓Limb blood flow

FIGURE 17-2

Activation of neurohormonal systems in heart failure.
The decreased cardiac output in HF patients results in an "unloading" of high-pressure baroceptors (circles) in the left ventricle, carotid sinus, and aortic arch. This unloading of the peripheral baroreceptors leads to a loss of inhibitory parasympathetic tone to the central nervous system (CNS), with a resultant generalized increase in efferent sympathetic tone, and nonosmotic release of arginine vasopressin (AVP) from the pituitary. AVP (or antidiuretic hormone [ADH]) is a powerful vasoconstrictor that increases the permeability of the renal collecting ducts, leading to the reabsorption of free water. These afferent signals to the CNS also activate efferent sympathetic nervous system pathways that innervate the heart, kidney, peripheral vasculature, and skeletal muscles.

Sympathetic stimulation of the kidney leads to the release of renin, with a resultant increase in the circulating levels of angiotensin II and aldosterone. The activation of the renin-angiotensin-aldosterone system promotes salt and water retention and leads to vasoconstriction of the peripheral vasculature, myocyte hypertrophy, myocyte cell death, and myocardial fibrosis. Although these neurohormonal mechanisms facilitate short-term adaptation by maintaining blood pressure, and hence perfusion to vital organs, the same neurohormonal mechanisms are believed to contribute to end-organ changes in the heart and the circulation and to the excessive salt and water retention in advanced HF. (*Modified from A Nohria et al: Neurohormonal, renal and vascular adjustments, in Atlas of Heart Failure: Cardiac Function and Dysfunction, 4th ed, WS Colucci [ed]. Philadelphia, Current Medicine Group 2002, p. 104.*)

TABLE 17-3
OVERVIEW OF LEFT VENTRICULAR REMODELING

Alterations in Myocyte Biology

Excitation-contraction coupling
Myosin heavy chain (fetal) gene expression
β-adrenergic desensitization
Hypertrophy
Myocytolysis
Cytoskeletal proteins

Myocardial Changes

Myocyte loss
  Necrosis
  Apoptosis
  Autophagy

Alterations in Extracellular Matrix

Matrix degradation
Myocardial fibrosis

Alterations in Left Ventricular Chamber Geometry

Left ventricular (LV) dilation
Increased LV sphericity
LV wall thinning
Mitral valve incompetence

Source: Adapted from D Mann: Pathophysiology of heart failure, in *Braunwald's Heart Disease*, 8th ed, PL Libby et al (eds). Philadelphia, Elsevier, 2008, p. 550.

organized structural collagen weave surrounding myocytes and subsequent replacement by an interstitial collagen matrix that does not provide structural support to the myocytes. The biologic stimuli for these profound changes include mechanical stretch of the myocyte, circulating neurohormones (e.g., norepinephrine, angiotensin II), inflammatory cytokines (e.g., tumor necrosis factor [TNF]), other peptides and growth factors (e.g., endothelin), and reactive oxygen species (e.g., superoxide). The sustained overexpression of these biologically active molecules is believed to contribute to the progression of HF by virtue of the deleterious effects they exert on the heart and circulation. Indeed, this insight forms the clinical rationale for using pharmacologic agents that antagonize these systems (e.g., angiotensin-converting enzyme [ACE] inhibitors and beta blockers) in treating patients with HF.

In order to understand how the changes that occur in the failing cardiac myocyte contribute to depressed LV systolic function in HF, it is instructive first to review the biology of the cardiac muscle cell (Chap. 1). Sustained neurohormonal activation and mechanical overload result in transcriptional and posttranscriptional changes in the genes and proteins that regulate excitation-contraction coupling and cross-bridge interaction (see Figs. 1-6 and 1-7). The changes that regulate excitation-contraction include decreased function of sarcoplasmic reticulum Ca^{2+} adenosine triphosphatase (SERCA2A), resulting in decreased calcium uptake into the sarcoplasmic reticulum (SR), and hyperphosphorylation of the ryanodine receptor, leading to calcium leakage from the SR. The changes that occur in the cross-bridges include decreased expression of α-myosin heavy chain and increased expression of β-myosin heavy chain, myocytolysis, and disruption of the cytoskeletal links between the sarcomeres and the extracellular matrix. Collectively, these changes impair the ability of the myocyte to contract and therefore contribute to the depressed LV systolic function observed in patients with HF.

Diastolic dysfunction

Myocardial relaxation is an adenosine triphosphate (ATP)-dependent process that is regulated by uptake of cytoplasmic calcium into the SR by SERCA2A and extrusion of calcium by sarcolemmal pumps (see Fig. 1-7). Accordingly, reductions in ATP concentration, as occurs in ischemia, may interfere with these processes and lead to slowed myocardial relaxation. Alternatively, if LV filling is delayed because LV compliance is reduced (e.g., from hypertrophy or fibrosis), LV filling pressures will similarly remain elevated at end diastole (see Fig. 1-11). An increase in heart rate disproportionately shortens the time for diastolic filling, which may lead to elevated LV filling pressures, particularly in noncompliant ventricles. Elevated LV end-diastolic filling pressures result in increases in pulmonary capillary pressures, which can contribute to the dyspnea experienced by patients with diastolic dysfunction. In addition to impaired myocardial relaxation, increased myocardial stiffness secondary to cardiac hypertrophy and increased myocardial collagen content may contribute to diastolic failure. Importantly, diastolic dysfunction can occur alone or in combination with systolic dysfunction in patients with HF.

Left ventricular remodeling

Ventricular remodeling refers to the changes in LV mass, volume, and shape and the composition of the heart that occur after cardiac injury and/or abnormal hemodynamic loading conditions. LV remodeling may contribute independently to the progression of HF by virtue of the mechanical burdens that are engendered by the changes in the geometry of the remodeled LV. In addition to the increase in LV end-diastolic volume, LV wall thinning occurs as the left ventricle begins to dilate. The increase in wall thinning, along with the increase in afterload created by LV dilation, leads to a functional *afterload mismatch* that may contribute further to a decrease in stroke volume. Moreover, the high end-diastolic wall stress might be expected to lead to

(1) hypoperfusion of the subendocardium, with resultant worsening of LV function, (2) increased oxidative stress, with the resultant activation of families of genes that are sensitive to free radical generation (e.g., TNF and interleukin 1β), and (3) sustained expression of stretch-activated genes (angiotensin II, endothelin, and TNF) and/or stretch activation of hypertrophic signaling pathways. Increasing LV dilation also results in tethering of the papillary muscles with resulting incompetence of the mitral valve apparatus and functional mitral regurgitation, which in turn leads to further hemodynamic overloading of the ventricle. Taken together, the mechanical burdens that are engendered by LV remodeling contribute to the progression of HF.

CLINICAL MANIFESTATIONS

Symptoms

The cardinal symptoms of HF are fatigue and shortness of breath. Although fatigue traditionally has been ascribed to the low cardiac output in HF, it is likely that skeletal-muscle abnormalities and other noncardiac comorbidities (e.g., anemia) also contribute to this symptom. In the early stages of HF, dyspnea is observed only during exertion; however, as the disease progresses, dyspnea occurs with less strenuous activity, and it ultimately may occur even at rest. The origin of dyspnea in HF is probably multifactorial (Chap. 5). The most important mechanism is pulmonary congestion with accumulation of interstitial or intraalveolar fluid, which activates juxtacapillary J receptors, which in turn stimulate the rapid, shallow breathing characteristic of cardiac dyspnea. Other factors that contribute to dyspnea on exertion include reductions in pulmonary compliance, increased airway resistance, respiratory muscle and/or diaphragm fatigue, and anemia. Dyspnea may become less frequent with the onset of right ventricular (RV) failure and tricuspid regurgitation.

▬ Orthopnea

Orthopnea, which is defined as dyspnea occurring in the recumbent position, is usually a later manifestation of HF than is exertional dyspnea. It results from redistribution of fluid from the splanchnic circulation and lower extremities into the central circulation during recumbency, with a resultant increase in pulmonary capillary pressure. Nocturnal cough is a common manifestation of this process and a frequently overlooked symptom of HF. Orthopnea generally is relieved by sitting upright or sleeping with additional pillows. Although orthopnea is a relatively specific symptom of HF, it may occur in patients with abdominal obesity or ascites and patients with pulmonary disease whose lung mechanics favor an upright posture.

Paroxysmal nocturnal dyspnea (PND)

This term refers to acute episodes of severe shortness of breath and coughing that generally occur at night and awaken the patient from sleep, usually 1–3 h after the patient retires. PND may be manifest by coughing or wheezing, possibly because of increased pressure in the bronchial arteries leading to airway compression, along with interstitial pulmonary edema that leads to increased airway resistance. Whereas orthopnea may be relieved by sitting upright at the side of the bed with the legs in a dependent position, patients with PND often have persistent coughing and wheezing even after they have assumed the upright position. *Cardiac asthma* is closely related to PND, is characterized by wheezing secondary to bronchospasm, and must be differentiated from primary asthma and pulmonary causes of wheezing.

Cheyne-Stokes respiration

Also referred to as periodic respiration or cyclic respiration, Cheyne-Stokes respiration is present in 40% of patients with advanced HF and usually is associated with low cardiac output. Cheyne-Stokes respiration is caused by a diminished sensitivity of the respiratory center to arterial P_{CO_2}. There is an apneic phase, during which arterial P_{O_2} falls and arterial P_{CO_2} rises. These changes in the arterial blood gas content stimulate the depressed respiratory center, resulting in hyperventilation and hypocapnia, followed by recurrence of apnea. Cheyne-Stokes respirations may be perceived by the patient or the patient's family as severe dyspnea or as a transient cessation of breathing.

Acute pulmonary edema

See Chap. 28.

Other symptoms

Patients with HF also may present with gastrointestinal symptoms. Anorexia, nausea, and early satiety associated with abdominal pain and fullness are common complaints and may be related to edema of the bowel wall and/or a congested liver. Congestion of the liver and stretching of its capsule may lead to right-upper-quadrant pain. Cerebral symptoms such as confusion, disorientation, and sleep and mood disturbances may be observed in patients with severe HF, particularly elderly patients with cerebral arteriosclerosis and reduced cerebral perfusion. Nocturia is common in HF and may contribute to insomnia.

PHYSICAL EXAMINATION

A careful physical examination is always warranted in the evaluation of patients with HF. The purpose of the examination is to help determine the cause of HF as well as to assess the severity of the syndrome. Obtaining additional information about the hemodynamic profile and the response to therapy and determining the prognosis are important additional goals of the physical examination.

General appearance and vital signs

In mild or moderately severe HF, the patient appears to be in no distress at rest except for feeling uncomfortable when lying flat for more than a few minutes. In more severe HF, the patient must sit upright, may have labored breathing, and may not be able to finish a sentence because of shortness of breath. Systolic blood pressure may be normal or high in early HF, but it generally is reduced in advanced HF because of severe LV dysfunction. The pulse pressure may be diminished, reflecting a reduction in stroke volume. Sinus tachycardia is a nonspecific sign caused by increased adrenergic activity. Peripheral vasoconstriction leading to cool peripheral extremities and cyanosis of the lips and nail beds is also caused by excessive adrenergic activity.

Jugular veins

(See also Chap. 9) Examination of the jugular veins provides an estimation of right atrial pressure. The jugular venous pressure is best appreciated with the patient lying recumbent, with the head tilted at 45°. The jugular venous pressure should be quantified in centimeters of water (normal ≤8 cm) by estimating the height of the venous column of blood above the sternal angle in centimeters and then adding 5 cm. In the early stages of HF, the venous pressure may be normal at rest but may become abnormally elevated with sustained (~1 min) pressure on the abdomen (positive abdominojugular reflux). Giant *v* waves indicate the presence of tricuspid regurgitation.

Pulmonary examination

Pulmonary crackles (rales or crepitations) result from the transudation of fluid from the intravascular space into the alveoli. In patients with pulmonary edema, rales may be heard widely over both lung fields and may be accompanied by expiratory wheezing (cardiac asthma). When present in patients without concomitant lung disease, rales are specific for HF. Importantly, rales are frequently absent in patients with chronic HF, even when LV filling pressures are elevated, because of increased lymphatic drainage of alveolar fluid. Pleural effusions result from the elevation of pleural capillary pressure and the resulting transudation of fluid into the pleural cavities. Since the pleural veins drain into both the systemic and the pulmonary veins, pleural effusions occur most commonly with biventricular failure. Although pleural effusions are often bilateral in HF, when they are unilateral, they occur more frequently in the right pleural space.

Cardiac examination

Examination of the heart, although essential, frequently does not provide useful information about the severity of HF. If cardiomegaly is present, the point of maximal impulse (PMI) usually is displaced below the fifth intercostal space and/or lateral to the midclavicular line, and the impulse is palpable over two interspaces. Severe LV hypertrophy leads to a sustained PMI. In some patients, a third heart sound (S_3) is audible and palpable at the apex. Patients with enlarged or hypertrophied right ventricles may have a sustained and prolonged left parasternal impulse extending throughout systole. An S_3 (or *protodiastolic gallop*) is most commonly present in patients with volume overload who have tachycardia and tachypnea, and it often signifies severe hemodynamic compromise. A fourth heart sound (S_4) is not a specific indicator of HF but is usually present in patients with diastolic dysfunction. The murmurs of mitral and tricuspid regurgitation are frequently present in patients with advanced HF.

Abdomen and extremities

Hepatomegaly is an important sign in patients with HF. When it is present, the enlarged liver is frequently tender and may pulsate during systole if tricuspid regurgitation is present. Ascites, a late sign, occurs as a consequence of increased pressure in the hepatic veins and the veins draining the peritoneum. Jaundice, also a late finding in HF, results from impairment of hepatic function secondary to hepatic congestion and hepatocellular hypoxemia and is associated with elevations of both direct and indirect bilirubin.

Peripheral edema is a cardinal manifestation of HF, but it is nonspecific and usually is absent in patients who have been treated adequately with diuretics. Peripheral edema is usually symmetric and dependent in HF and occurs predominantly in the ankles and the pretibial region in ambulatory patients. In bedridden patients, edema may be found in the sacral area (*presacral edema*) and the scrotum. Long-standing edema may be associated with indurated and pigmented skin.

Cardiac cachexia

With severe chronic HF, there may be marked weight loss and cachexia. Although the mechanism of cachexia is not entirely understood, it is probably multifactorial and includes elevation of the resting metabolic rate; anorexia, nausea, and vomiting due to congestive hepatomegaly and abdominal fullness; elevation of circulating concentrations of cytokines such as TNF; and impairment of intestinal absorption due to congestion of the intestinal veins. When present, cachexia augurs a poor overall prognosis.

DIAGNOSIS

The diagnosis of HF is relatively straightforward when the patient presents with classic signs and symptoms of HF; however, the signs and symptoms of HF are neither specific nor sensitive. Accordingly, the key to making the diagnosis is to have a high index of suspicion, particularly for high-risk patients. When these patients present with signs or symptoms of HF, additional laboratory testing should be performed.

Routine laboratory testing

Patients with new-onset HF and those with chronic HF and acute decompensation should have a complete blood count, a panel of electrolytes, blood urea nitrogen, serum creatinine, hepatic enzymes, and a urinalysis. Selected patients should have assessment for diabetes mellitus (fasting serum glucose or oral glucose tolerance test), dyslipidemia (fasting lipid panel), and thyroid abnormalities (thyroid-stimulating hormone level).

Electrocardiogram (ECG)

A routine 12-lead ECG is recommended. The major importance of the ECG is to assess cardiac rhythm and determine the presence of LV hypertrophy or a prior MI (presence or absence of Q waves) as well as to determine QRS width to ascertain whether the patient may benefit from resynchronization therapy (see later). A normal ECG virtually excludes LV systolic dysfunction.

Chest x-ray

A chest x-ray provides useful information about cardiac size and shape, as well as the state of the pulmonary vasculature, and may identify noncardiac causes of the patient's symptoms. Although patients with acute HF have evidence of pulmonary hypertension, interstitial edema, and/or pulmonary edema, the majority of patients with chronic HF do not. The absence of these findings in patients with chronic HF reflects the increased capacity of the lymphatics to remove interstitial and/or pulmonary fluid.

Assessment of LV function

Noninvasive cardiac imaging (Chap. 12) is essential for the diagnosis, evaluation, and management of

HF. The most useful test is the two-dimensional (2-D) echocardiogram/Doppler, which can provide a semi-quantitative assessment of LV size and function as well as the presence or absence of valvular and/or regional wall motion abnormalities (indicative of a prior MI). The presence of left atrial dilation and LV hypertrophy, together with abnormalities of LV diastolic filling provided by pulse-wave and tissue Doppler, is useful for the assessment of HF with a preserved EF. The 2-D echocardiogram/Doppler is also invaluable in assessing RV size and pulmonary pressures, which are critical in the evaluation and management of cor pulmonale (see later). Magnetic resonance imaging (MRI) also provides a comprehensive analysis of cardiac anatomy and function and is now the gold standard for assessing LV mass and volumes. MRI also is emerging as a useful and accurate imaging modality for evaluating patients with HF, both in terms of assessing LV structure and for determining the cause of HF (e.g., amyloidosis, ischemic cardiomyopathy, hemochromatosis).

The most useful index of LV function is the EF (stroke volume divided by end-diastolic volume). Because the EF is easy to measure by noninvasive testing and easy to conceptualize, it has gained wide acceptance among clinicians. Unfortunately, the EF has a number of limitations as a true measure of contractility, since it is influenced by alterations in afterload and/or preload. Nonetheless, with the exceptions indicated above, when the EF is normal ($\geq 50\%$), systolic function is usually adequate, and when the EF is significantly depressed (<30–40%), contractility is usually depressed.

Biomarkers

Circulating levels of natriuretic peptides are useful adjunctive tools in the diagnosis of patients with HF. Both B-type natriuretic peptide (BNP) and N-terminal pro-BNP, which are released from the failing heart, are relatively sensitive markers for the presence of HF with depressed EF; they also are elevated in HF patients with a preserved EF, albeit to a lesser degree. However, it is important to recognize that natriuretic peptide levels increase with age and renal impairment, are more elevated in women, and can be elevated in right HF from any cause. Levels can be falsely low in obese patients and may normalize in some patients after appropriate treatment. At present, serial measurements of BNP are not recommended as a guide to HF therapy. Other biomarkers, such as troponin T and I, C-reactive protein, TNF receptors, and uric acid, may be elevated in HF and provide important prognostic information. Serial measurements of one or more biomarkers ultimately may help guide therapy in HF, but they are not currently recommended for this purpose.

Exercise testing

Treadmill or bicycle exercise testing is not routinely advocated for patients with HF, but either is useful for assessing the need for cardiac transplantation in patients with advanced HF (Chap. 18). A peak oxygen uptake (V_{O_2}) <14 mL/kg per min is associated with a relatively poor prognosis. Patients with a V_{O_2} <14 mL/kg per min have been shown, in general, to have better survival when transplanted than when treated medically.

DIFFERENTIAL DIAGNOSIS

HF resembles but should be distinguished from (1) conditions in which there is circulatory congestion secondary to abnormal salt and water retention but in which there is no disturbance of cardiac structure or function (e.g., renal failure) and (2) noncardiac causes of pulmonary edema (e.g., acute respiratory distress syndrome). In most patients who present with classic signs and symptoms of HF, the diagnosis is relatively straightforward. However, even experienced clinicians have difficulty differentiating the dyspnea that arises from cardiac and pulmonary causes (Chap. 5). In this regard, noninvasive cardiac imaging, biomarkers, pulmonary function testing, and chest x-ray may be useful. A very low BNP or N-terminal pro-BNP may be helpful in excluding a cardiac cause of dyspnea in this setting. Ankle edema may arise secondary to varicose veins, obesity, renal disease, or gravitational effects. When HF develops in patients with a preserved EF, it may be difficult to determine the relative contribution of HF to the dyspnea that occurs in chronic lung disease and/or obesity.

TREATMENT   Heart Failure

HF should be viewed as a continuum that is composed of four interrelated stages. *Stage A* includes patients who are at high risk for developing HF but do not have structural heart disease or symptoms of HF (e.g., patients with diabetes mellitus or hypertension). *Stage B* includes patients who have structural heart disease but do not have symptoms of HF (e.g., patients with a previous MI and asymptomatic LV dysfunction). *Stage C* includes patients who have structural heart disease and have developed symptoms of HF (e.g., patients with a previous MI with dyspnea and fatigue). *Stage D* includes patients with refractory HF requiring special interventions (e.g., patients with refractory HF who are awaiting cardiac transplantation). In this continuum, every effort should be made to prevent HF not only by treating the preventable causes of HF (e.g., hypertension) but also by treating the patient in stages B and C with drugs that prevent disease progression (e.g., ACE inhibitors and beta blockers) and by symptomatic management of patients in stage D.

DEFINING AN APPROPRIATE THERAPEUTIC STRATEGY FOR CHRONIC HF Once patients have developed structural heart disease, their therapy depends on their NYHA functional classification (Table 17-2). Although this classification system is notoriously subjective and has large interobserver variability, it has withstood the test of time and continues to be widely applied to patients with HF. For patients who have developed LV systolic dysfunction but remain asymptomatic (class I), the goal should be to slow disease progression by blocking neurohormonal systems that lead to cardiac remodeling (see later). For patients who have developed symptoms (class II–IV), the primary goal should be to alleviate fluid retention, lessen disability, and reduce the risk of further disease progression and death. These goals generally require a strategy that combines diuretics (to control salt and water retention) with neurohormonal interventions (to minimize cardiac remodeling).

MANAGEMENT OF HF WITH DEPRESSED EJECTION FRACTION (<40%)

General Measures Clinicians should aim to screen for and treat comorbidities such as hypertension, CAD, diabetes mellitus, anemia, and sleep-disordered breathing, as these conditions tend to exacerbate HF. HF patients should be advised to stop smoking and to limit alcohol consumption to two standard drinks per day in men or one per day in women. Patients suspected of having an alcohol-induced cardiomyopathy should be urged to abstain from alcohol consumption indefinitely. Extremes of temperature and heavy physical exertion should be avoided. Certain drugs are known to make HF worse and should be avoided (Table 17-4). For example, nonsteroidal anti-inflammatory drugs, including cyclooxygenase 2 inhibitors, are not recommended in patients with chronic HF because the risk of renal failure and fluid retention is markedly increased in the presence of reduced renal function or ACE inhibitor therapy. Patients should receive immunization with influenza and pneumococcal vaccines to prevent respiratory infections. It is equally important to educate the patient and family about HF, the importance of proper diet, and the importance of compliance with the medical regimen. Supervision of outpatient care by a specially trained nurse or physician assistant and/or in specialized HF clinics has been found to be helpful, particularly in patients with advanced disease.

Activity Although heavy physical labor is not recommended in HF, routine modest exercise has been shown to be beneficial in patients with NYHA class I–III HF. For euvolemic patients, regular isotonic exercise such as walking or riding a stationary-bicycle ergometer, as tolerated, should be encouraged. Exercise training results in reduced HF symptoms, increased exercise capacity, and improved quality of life.

TABLE 17-4

FACTORS THAT MAY PRECIPITATE ACUTE DECOMPENSATION IN PATIENTS WITH CHRONIC HEART FAILURE

Dietary indiscretion
Myocardial ischemia/infarction
Arrhythmias (tachycardia or bradycardia)
Discontinuation of HF therapy
Infection
Anemia
Initiation of medications that worsen HF
    Calcium antagonists (verapamil, diltiazem)
    Beta blockers
    Nonsteroidal anti-inflammatory drugs
    Antiarrhythmic agents (all class I agents, sotalol [class III])
    Anti-TNF antibodies
Alcohol consumption
Pregnancy
Worsening hypertension
Acute valvular insufficiency

Abbreviations: HF, heart failure; TNF, tumor necrosis factor.

Diet Dietary restriction of sodium (2–3 g daily) is recommended in all patients with HF and preserved or depressed EF. Further restriction (<2 g daily) may be considered in moderate to severe HF. Fluid restriction is generally unnecessary unless the patient develops hyponatremia (<130 meq/L), which may develop because of activation of the renin-angiotensin system, excessive secretion of antidiuretic hormone, or loss of salt in excess of water from diuretic use. Fluid restriction (<2 L/day) should be considered in hyponatremic patients or those whose fluid retention is difficult to control despite high doses of diuretics and sodium restriction. Vasopressin antagonists also may be useful in severe hyponatremia. Caloric supplementation is recommended for patients with advanced HF and unintentional weight loss or muscle wasting (cardiac cachexia); however, anabolic steroids are not recommended for these patients because of the potential problems with volume retention. The use of dietary supplements ("nutriceuticals") should be avoided in the management of symptomatic HF because of the lack of proven benefit and the potential for significant (adverse) interactions with proven HF therapies.

Diuretics Many of the clinical manifestations of moderate to severe HF result from excessive salt and water retention that leads to volume expansion and congestive symptoms. Diuretics (Table 17-5) are the only pharmacologic agents that can adequately control fluid retention in advanced HF, and they should be used to restore and maintain normal volume status in patients with congestive symptoms (dyspnea, orthopnea,

TABLE 17-5

DRUGS FOR THE TREATMENT OF CHRONIC HEART FAILURE (EF <40%)

	INITIATING DOSE	MAXIMAL DOSE
Diuretics		
Furosemide	20–40 mg qd or bid	400 mg/d[a]
Torsemide	10–20 mg qd bid	200 mg/d[a]
Bumetanide	0.5–1 mg qd or bid	10 mg/d[a]
Hydrochlorthiazide	25 mg qd	100 mg/d[a]
Metolazone	2.5–5 mg qd or bid	20 mg/d[a]
Angiotensin-Converting Enzyme Inhibitors		
Captopril	6.25 mg tid	50 mg tid
Enalapril	2.5 mg bid	10 mg bid
Lisinopril	2.5–5 mg qd	20–35 mg qd
Ramipril	1.25–2.5 mg bid	2.5–5 mg bid
Trandolapril	0.5 mg qd	4 mg qd
Angiotensin Receptor Blockers		
Valsartan	40 mg bid	160 mg bid
Candesartan	4 mg qd	32 mg qd
Irbesartan	75 mg qd	300 mg qd[b]
Losartan	12.5 mg qd	50 mg qd
β Receptor Blockers		
Carvedilol	3.125 mg bid	25–50 mg bid
Bisoprolol	1.25 mg qd	10 mg qd
Metoprolol succinate CR	12.5–25 mg qd	Target dose 200 mg qd
Additional Therapies		
Spironolactone	12.5–25 mg qd	25–50 mg qd
Eplerenone	25 mg qd	50 mg qd
Combination of hydralazine/ isosorbide dinitrate	10–25 mg/ 10 mg tid	75 mg/ 40 mg tid
Fixed dose of hydralazine/ isosorbide dinitrate	37.5 mg/20 mg (one tablet) tid	75 mg/40 mg (two tablets) tid
Digoxin	0.125 mg qd	≤0.375 mg/d[b]

[a]Dose must be titrated to reduce the patient's congestive symptoms.
[b]Target dose not established.

edema) or signs of elevated filling pressures (rales, jugular venous distention, peripheral edema). Furosemide, torsemide, and bumetanide act at the loop of Henle (*loop diuretics*) by reversibly inhibiting the reabsorption of Na^+, K^+, and Cl^- in the thick ascending limb of Henle's loop; thiazides and metolazone reduce the reabsorption of Na^+ and Cl^- in the first half of the distal convoluted tubule; and potassium-sparing diuretics such as spironolactone act at the level of the collecting duct.

Although all diuretics increase sodium excretion and urinary volume, they differ in their potency and pharmacologic properties. Whereas loop diuretics increase the fractional excretion of sodium by 20–25%, thiazide diuretics increase it by only 5–10% and tend to lose their effectiveness in patients with moderate or severe renal insufficiency (creatinine >2.5 mg/dL). Hence, loop diuretics generally are required to restore normal volume status in patients with HF. Diuretics should be initiated in low doses (Table 17-5) and then carefully titrated upward to relieve signs and symptoms of fluid overload in an attempt to obtain the patient's "dry weight." This typically requires multiple dose adjustments over many days and occasionally weeks in patients with severe fluid overload. Intravenous administration of diuretics may be necessary to relieve congestion acutely and can be done safely in the outpatient setting. Once the congestion has been relieved, treatment with diuretics should be continued to prevent the recurrence of salt and water retention.

Refractoriness to diuretic therapy may represent patient nonadherence, a direct effect of chronic diuretic use on the kidney, or progression of underlying HF. The addition of thiazides or metolazone, once or twice daily, to loop diuretics may be considered in patients with persistent fluid retention despite high-dose loop diuretic therapy. Metolazone is generally more potent and much longer-acting than the thiazides in this setting as well as in patients with chronic renal insufficiency. However, chronic daily use, especially of metolazone, should be avoided if possible because of the potential for electrolyte shifts and volume depletion. Ultrafiltration and dialysis may be used in cases of refractory fluid retention that are unresponsive to high doses of diuretics and have been shown to be helpful in the short term.

Adverse Effects Diuretics have the potential to produce electrolyte and volume depletion as well as worsening azotemia. In addition, they may lead to worsening neurohormonal activation and disease progression. One of the most important adverse consequences of diuresis is alterations in potassium homeostasis (hypokalemia or hyperkalemia), which increase the risk of life-threatening arrhythmias. In general, both loop- and thiazide-type diuretics lead to hypokalemia, whereas spironolactone, eplerenone, and triamterene lead to hyperkalemia.

PREVENTING DISEASE PROGRESSION (Table 17-5) Drugs that interfere with excessive activation of the RAA system and the adrenergic nervous system can relieve the symptoms of HF with a depressed EF by stabilizing and/or reversing cardiac remodeling. In this regard, ACE inhibitors and beta blockers have emerged as the cornerstones of modern therapy for HF with a depressed EF.

ACE Inhibitors There is overwhelming evidence that ACE inhibitors should be used in symptomatic and asymptomatic patients **(Figs. 17-3** and **17-4)** with a depressed EF (<40%). ACE inhibitors interfere with the renin-angiotensin system by inhibiting the enzyme that is responsible for the conversion of angiotensin I to angiotensin II. However, because ACE inhibitors also inhibit kininase II, they may lead to the upregulation of bradykinin, which may further enhance the beneficial effects of angiotensin suppression. ACE inhibitors stabilize LV remodeling, improve symptoms, reduce hospitalization, and prolong life. Because fluid retention can attenuate the effects of ACE inhibitors, it is preferable to optimize the dose of diuretic before starting the ACE inhibitor. However, it may be necessary to reduce the dose of diuretic during the initiation of ACE inhibition to

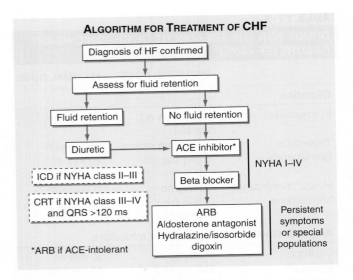

ALGORITHM FOR TREATMENT OF CHF

FIGURE 17-4

Treatment algorithm for chronic heart failure patients with a depressed ejection fraction. After the clinical diagnosis of HF is made, it is important to treat the patient's fluid retention before starting an ACE inhibitor (or an ARB if the patient is ACE-intolerant). Beta blockers should be started after the fluid retention has been treated and/or the ACE inhibitor has been uptitrated. If the patient remains symptomatic, an ARB, an aldosterone antagonist, or digoxin can be added as "triple therapy." The fixed-dose combination of hydralazine/isosorbide dinitrate should be added to an ACE inhibitor and a beta blocker in African-American patients with NYHA class II–IV HF. Device therapy should be considered in addition to pharmacologic therapy in appropriate patients. HF, heart failure; ACE, angiotensin-converting enzyme; ARB, angiotensin receptor blocker; NYHA, New York Heart Association; CRT, cardiac resynchronization therapy; ICD, implantable cardiac defibrillator.

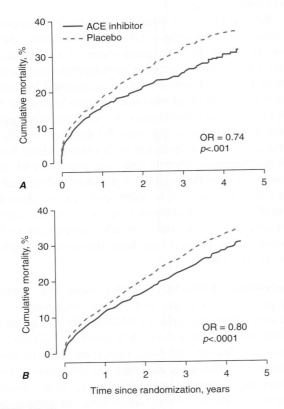

FIGURE 17-3

Meta-analysis of angiotensin-converting enzyme (ACE) inhibitors in heart failure patients with a depressed ejection fraction. *A.* The Kaplan-Meier curves for mortality for 5966 HF patients with a depressed EF treated with an ACE inhibitor after acute myocardial infarction (three trials). ***B.*** The Kaplan-Meier curves for mortality for 12,763 HF patients with a depressed EF treated with an ACE inhibitor in five clinical trials, including postinfarction trials. The benefits of ACE inhibitors were observed early and persisted long term. (*Modified from MD Flather et al: Lancet 355:1575, 2000.*)

prevent symptomatic hypotension. ACE inhibitors should be initiated in low doses, followed by gradual increments if the lower doses have been well tolerated. The doses of ACE inhibitors should be increased until they are similar to those which have been shown to be effective in clinical trials (Table 17-5). Higher doses are more effective than lower doses in preventing hospitalization.

Adverse Effects The majority of adverse effects are related to suppression of the renin-angiotensin system. The decreases in blood pressure and mild azotemia that may occur during the initiation of therapy generally are well tolerated and do not require a decrease in the dose of the ACE inhibitor. However, if hypotension is accompanied by dizziness or if the renal dysfunction becomes severe, it may be necessary to reduce the dose of the inhibitor. Potassium retention may also become problematic if the patient is receiving potassium supplements or a potassium-sparing diuretic. Potassium retention that is not responsive to these measures may require a reduction in the dose of an ACE inhibitor.

The side effects of ACE inhibitors related to kinin potentiation include a nonproductive cough (10–15% of patients) and angioedema (1% of patients). In patients who cannot tolerate ACE inhibitors because of cough or angioedema, angiotensin receptor blockers (ARBs) are the recommended first line of therapy (see later). Patients intolerant of ACE inhibitors because of hyperkalemia or renal insufficiency are likely to experience the same side effects with ARBs. In these cases, the combination of hydralazine and an oral nitrate should be considered (Table 17-5).

Angiotensin Receptor Blockers These drugs are well tolerated in patients who are intolerant of ACE inhibitors because of cough, skin rash, and angioedema. ARBs should be used in symptomatic and asymptomatic patients with an EF <40% who are ACE-intolerant for reasons other than hyperkalemia or renal insufficiency (Table 17-5). Although ACE inhibitors and ARBs inhibit the renin-angiotensin system, they do so by different mechanisms. Whereas ACE inhibitors block the enzyme responsible for converting angiotensin I to angiotensin II, ARBs block the effects of angiotensin II on the angiotensin type 1 receptor. Some clinical trials have demonstrated a therapeutic benefit from the addition of an ARB to an ACE inhibitor in patients with chronic HF. When given in concert with beta blockers, ARBs reverse the process of LV remodeling, improve patient symptoms, prevent hospitalization, and prolong life.

Adverse Effects Both ACE inhibitors and ARBs have similar effects on blood pressure, renal function, and potassium. Therefore, the problems of symptomatic hypotension, azotemia, and hyperkalemia are similar for both of these agents.

β-Adrenergic Receptor Blockers Beta-blocker therapy represents a major advance in the treatment of patients with a depressed EF (Fig. 17-5). These drugs interfere with the harmful effects of sustained activation of the adrenergic nervous system by competitively antagonizing one or more adrenergic receptors (α_1, β_1, and β_2). Although there are a number of potential benefits to blocking all three receptors, most of the deleterious effects of adrenergic activation are mediated by the β_1 receptor. When given in concert with ACE inhibitors, beta blockers reverse the process of LV remodeling, improve patient symptoms, prevent hospitalization, and prolong life. Therefore, beta blockers are indicated for patients with symptomatic or asymptomatic HF and a depressed EF <40%.

Analogous to the use of ACE inhibitors, beta blockers should be initiated in low doses (Table 17-5), followed by gradual increments in the dose if lower doses have been well tolerated. The dose of beta blocker should be increased until the doses used are similar to those which have been reported to be effective in clinical trials (Table 17-5). However, unlike ACE inhibitors, which may be titrated upward relatively rapidly, the

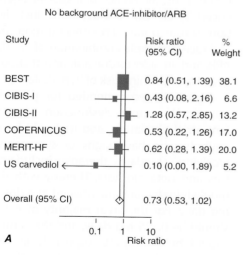 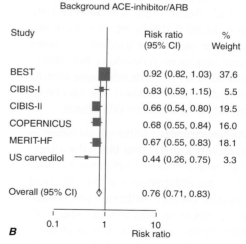

FIGURE 17-5

Meta-analysis of beta blockers on mortality rates in HF patients with a depressed EF. Effect of beta blockers vs. placebo in patients who were not (**A**) or who were (**B**) receiving an angiotensin-converting enzyme (ACE) inhibitor or an angiotensin receptor blocker (ARB) at baseline in six clinical trials. There was a similar impact of beta-blocker therapy on the endpoints of all-cause mortality as well as death and heart failure hospitalization in both the presence and the absence of ACE inhibitor or ARB at baseline. BEST, Beta-Blocker Evaluation of Survival Trial (bucindolol); CIBIS, Cardiac Insufficiency Bisoprolol Study (bisoprolol); COPERNICUS, Carvedilol prOsPEctive RaNdomIzed Cumulative Survival (carvedilol); MERIT-HF, Metoprolol CR/XL RaNdomized Intervention Trial in Heart Failure (metoprolol CR/XL). (*Modified from H Krum et al: Eur Heart J 26:2154, 2005.*)

CHAPTER 17 Heart Failure and Cor Pulmonale

titration of beta blockers should proceed no more rapidly than at 2-week intervals, because the initiation and/or increased dosing of these agents may lead to worsening fluid retention consequent to the withdrawal of adrenergic support to the heart and the circulation. Thus, it is important to optimize the dose of diuretics before starting therapy with beta blockers. If worsening fluid retention does occur, it is likely to do so within 3–5 days of the initiation of therapy, and it will be manifest as an increase in body weight and/or symptoms of worsening HF. The increased fluid retention usually can be managed by increasing the dose of diuretics. In some patients the dose of the beta blocker may have to be reduced.

Contrary to early reports, the aggregate results of clinical trials suggest that beta-blocker therapy is well tolerated by the great majority (≥85%) of HF patients, including patients with comorbid conditions such as diabetes mellitus, chronic obstructive lung disease, and peripheral vascular disease. Nonetheless, there is a subset of patients (10–15%) who remain intolerant to beta blockers because of worsening fluid retention or symptomatic hypotension or bradycardia.

Adverse Effects The adverse effects of beta-blocker use generally are related to the predictable complications that arise from interfering with the adrenergic nervous system. These reactions generally occur within several days of the initiation of therapy and generally are responsive to adjustments of concomitant medications, as described earlier in this chapter. Therapy with beta blockers can lead to bradycardia and/or exacerbate heart block. Accordingly, the dose of beta blocker should be reduced if the heart rate decreases to <50 beats/min and/or second- or third-degree heart block or symptomatic hypotension develops. Beta blockers are not recommended for patients who have asthma with active bronchospasm. Beta blockers that also block the α_1 receptor can lead to vasodilatory side effects.

Aldosterone Antagonists Although classified as potassium-sparing diuretics, drugs that block the effects of aldosterone (spironolactone or eplerenone) have beneficial effects that are independent of the effects of these agents on sodium balance. Although ACE inhibition may transiently decrease aldosterone secretion, with chronic therapy there is a rapid return of aldosterone to levels similar to those before ACE inhibition. Accordingly, the administration of an aldosterone antagonist is recommended for patients with NYHA class IV or class III (previously class IV) HF who have a depressed EF (<35%) and are receiving standard therapy, including diuretics, ACE inhibitors, and beta blockers. The dose of aldosterone antagonist should be increased until the doses used are similar to those which have been shown to be effective in clinical trials (Table 17-5).

Adverse Effects The major problem with the use of aldosterone antagonists is the development of life-threatening hyperkalemia, which is more prone to occur in patients who are receiving potassium supplements or who have underlying renal insufficiency. Aldosterone antagonists are not recommended when the serum creatinine is >2.5 mg/dL (or creatinine clearance is <30 mL/min) or when the serum potassium is >5 mmol/L. Painful gynecomastia may develop in 10–15% of patients who use spironolactone, in which case eplerenone may be substituted.

SPECIAL POPULATIONS The combination of hydralazine and isosorbide dinitrate (Table 17-5) is recommended as part of standard therapy in addition to beta blockers and ACE inhibitors for African Americans with NYHA class II–IV HF. Although the exact mechanism for the effects of this combination is not known, it is believed to be secondary to the beneficial effects of NO on the peripheral circulation.

MANAGEMENT OF PATIENTS WHO REMAIN SYMPTOMATIC Additional pharmacologic therapy should be considered in patients who have persistent symptoms or progressive worsening despite optimized therapy with an ACE inhibitor and a beta blocker. Agents that may be considered as part of additional therapy include an ARB, spironolactone, the combination of hydralazine and isosorbide dinitrate, and digitalis. The optimal choice of additional drug therapy to improve the outcome further has not been firmly established. Thus, the choice of a specific agent will be influenced by clinical considerations, including renal function, serum potassium concentration, blood pressure, and race. The triple combination of an ACE inhibitor, an ARB, and an aldosterone antagonist should not be used because of the high risk of hyperkalemia.

Digoxin is recommended for patients with symptomatic LV systolic dysfunction who have concomitant atrial fibrillation, and it should be considered for patients who have signs or symptoms of HF while receiving standard therapy, including ACE inhibitors and beta blockers. Therapy with digoxin is commonly initiated and maintained at a dose of 0.125–0.25 mg daily. For the great majority of patients, the dose should be 0.125 mg daily, and the serum digoxin level should be <1 ng/mL, especially in elderly patients, patients with impaired renal function, and patients with a low lean body mass. Higher doses (and serum concentrations) appear to be less beneficial. There is no indication for using loading doses of digoxin to initiate therapy in patients with HF.

ANTICOAGULATION AND ANTIPLATELET THERAPY Patients with HF have an increased risk for arterial or venous thromboembolic events. In clinical

HF trials, the rate of stroke ranges from 1.3% to 2.4% per year. Depressed LV function is believed to promote relative stasis of blood in dilated cardiac chambers with increased risk of thrombus formation. Treatment with warfarin (goal international normalized ratio [INR] 2–3) is recommended for patients with HF and chronic or paroxysmal atrial fibrillation or with a history of systemic or pulmonary emboli, including stroke or transient ischemic attack. Patients with symptomatic or asymptomatic ischemic cardiomyopathy and documented recent large anterior MI or recent MI with documented LV thrombus should be treated with warfarin (goal INR 2–3) for the initial 3 months after the MI unless there are contraindications to its use.

Aspirin is recommended in HF patients with ischemic heart disease for the prevention of MI and death. However, lower doses of aspirin (75 or 81 mg) may be preferable because of the concern of worsening of HF at higher doses.

MANAGEMENT OF CARDIAC ARRHYTHMIAS

(See also Chap. 16) Atrial fibrillation occurs in 15–30% of patients with HF and is a common cause of cardiac decompensation. Most antiarrhythmic agents, with the exception of amiodarone and dofetilide, have negative inotropic effects and are proarrhythmic. Amiodarone is a class III antiarrhythmic that has few or no negative inotropic and/or proarrhythmic effects and is effective against most supraventricular arrhythmias. Amiodarone is the preferred drug for restoring and maintaining sinus rhythm, and it may improve the success of electrical cardioversion in patients with HF. Amiodarone increases the level of phenytoin and digoxin and prolongs the INR in patients taking warfarin. Therefore, it is often necessary to reduce the dose of these drugs by as much as 50% when initiating therapy with amiodarone. The risk of adverse events such as hyperthyroidism, hypothyroidism, pulmonary fibrosis, and hepatitis is relatively low, particularly when lower doses of amiodarone are used (100–200 mg/d).

Implantable cardiac defibrillators (ICDs; see later) are highly effective in treating recurrences of sustained ventricular tachycardia and/or ventricular fibrillation in HF patients with recurrent arrhythmias and/or cardiac syncope, and they may be used as stand-alone therapy or in combination with amiodarone and/or a beta blocker (Chap. 16). There is no role for treating ventricular arrhythmias with an antiarrhythmic agent without an ICD.

DEVICE THERAPY

Cardiac Resynchronization Approximately one-third of patients with a depressed EF and symptomatic HF (NYHA class III–IV) manifest a QRS duration >120 ms. This ECG finding of abnormal inter- or intraventricular conduction has been used to identify patients with dyssynchronous ventricular contraction. The mechanical consequences of ventricular dyssynchrony include suboptimal ventricular filling, a reduction in LV contractility, prolonged duration (and therefore greater severity) of mitral regurgitation, and paradoxical septal wall motion. *Biventricular pacing*, also termed *cardiac resynchronization therapy* (CRT), stimulates both ventricles nearly simultaneously, thereby improving the coordination of ventricular contraction and reducing the severity of mitral regurgitation. When CRT is added to optimal medical therapy in patients in sinus rhythm, there is a significant decrease in patient mortality rates and hospitalization and a reversal of LV remodeling, as well as improved quality of life and exercise capacity. Accordingly, CRT is recommended for patients in sinus rhythm with an EF <35% and a QRS >120 ms and those who remain symptomatic (NYHA III–IV) despite optimal medical therapy. The benefits of CRT in patients with atrial fibrillation have not been clearly established.

Implantable Cardiac Defibrillators (See also Chap. 16) The prophylactic implantation of ICDs in patients with mild to moderate HF (NYHA class II–III) has been shown to reduce the incidence of sudden cardiac death in patients with ischemic or nonischemic cardiomyopathy. Accordingly, implantation of an ICD should be considered for patients in NYHA class II–III HF with a depressed EF of <35% who are already on optimal background therapy, including an ACE inhibitor (or ARB), a beta blocker, and an aldosterone antagonist. An ICD may also be combined with a biventricular pacemaker in patients with NYHA class III–IV HF.

MANAGEMENT OF HF WITH A PRESERVED EJECTION FRACTION (>40–50%)

Despite the wealth of information with respect to the evaluation and management of HF with a depressed EF, there are no proven and/or approved pharmacologic or device therapies for the management of patients with HF and a preserved EF. Therefore, it is recommended that initial treatment efforts should be focused, wherever possible, on the underlying disease process (e.g., myocardial ischemia, hypertension) associated with HF with preserved EF. Precipitating factors such as tachycardia and atrial fibrillation should be treated as quickly as possible through rate control and restoration of sinus rhythm when appropriate. Dyspnea may be treated by reducing total blood volume (dietary sodium restriction and diuretics), decreasing central blood volume (nitrates), or blunting neurohormonal activation with ACE inhibitors, ARBs, and/or beta blockers. Treatment with diuretics and nitrates should be initiated at low doses to avoid hypotension and fatigue.

ACUTE DECOMPENSATED HF

Defining an Appropriate Therapeutic Strategy The therapeutic goals for the management of acute decompensated HF (ADHF) therapy are to (1) stabilize the hemodynamic derangements that provoked the symptoms responsible for the hospitalization, (2) identify and treat the reversible factors that precipitated decompensation, and (3) reestablish an effective outpatient medical regimen that will prevent disease progression and relapse. In most instances this will require hospitalization, often in an intensive care unit (ICU) setting. Every effort should be made to identify the precipitating causes, such as infection, arrhythmias, dietary indiscretion, pulmonary embolism, infective endocarditis, occult myocardial ischemia/infarction, and environmental and/or emotional stress (Table 17-4), since removal of these precipitating events is critical to the success of treatment.

The two primary hemodynamic determinants of ADHF are elevated LV filling pressures and a depressed cardiac output. Frequently, the depressed cardiac output is accompanied by an increase in systemic vascular resistance (SVR) as a result of excessive neurohormonal activation. Because these hemodynamic derangements may occur singly or together, patients with acute HF generally present with one of four basic hemodynamic profiles (Fig. 17-6): normal LV filling pressure with normal perfusion (Profile A), elevated LV filling pressure with normal perfusion (Profile B), elevated LV filling

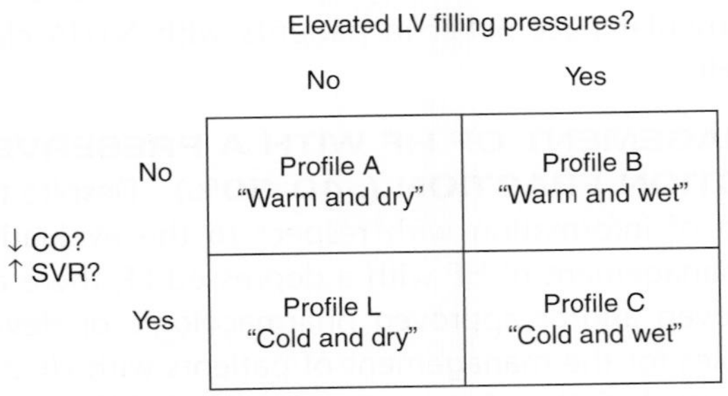

FIGURE 17-6

Hemodynamic profiles in patients with acute heart failure. Most patients can be categorized into one of the four hemodynamic profiles by performing a brief bedside examination that includes examination of the neck veins, lungs, and peripheral extremities. More definitive hemodynamic information may be obtained by performing invasive hemodynamic monitoring, particularly if the patient is gravely ill or if the clinical presentation is unclear. This hemodynamic classification provides a useful guide for selecting the initial optimal therapies for the management of acute HF. LV, left ventricular; CO, cardiac output; SVR, systemic vascular resistance. (*Modified from KL Grady et al: Circulation 102:2443, 2000.*)

pressures with decreased perfusion (Profile C), and normal or low LV filling pressure with decreased tissue perfusion (Profile L).

Accordingly, the therapeutic approach to treating patients with acute HF should be tailored to reflect the patient's hemodynamic presentation. The goal should be, whenever possible, to restore the patient to a normal hemodynamic profile (Profile A). In many instances, the patient's hemodynamic presentation can be approximated from the clinical examination. For example, patients with elevated LV filling pressures may have signs of fluid retention (rales, elevated neck veins, peripheral edema) and are referred to as being "wet," whereas patients with a depressed cardiac output and an elevated SVR generally have poor tissue perfusion manifested by cool distal extremities and are referred to as being "cold." Nonetheless, it should be emphasized that patients with chronic heart failure may not have rales or evidence of peripheral edema at the time of the initial presentation with acute decompensation, and this may lead to the underrecognition of elevated filling pressures. In these patients, it may be appropriate to perform invasive hemodynamic monitoring.

Patients who are not congested and have normal tissue perfusion are referred to as being "dry" and "warm," respectively. When acute HF patients present to the hospital with Profile A, their symptoms are often due to conditions other than HF (e.g., pulmonary or hepatic disease or transient myocardial ischemia). More commonly, however, acute HF patients present with congestive symptoms ("warm and wet" [Profile B]), in which case treatment of the elevated filling pressures with diuretics and vasodilators is warranted to reduce LV filling pressures. Profile B includes most patients with acute pulmonary edema. The treatment of this life-threatening condition is described in Chap. 28.

Patients also may present with congestion and a significantly elevated SVR and reduction of cardiac output ("cold and wet" [Profile C]). In these patients, cardiac output can be increased and LV filling pressures reduced by using intravenous vasodilators. Intravenous inotropic agents with vasodilating action (dobutamine, low-dose dopamine, milrinone [Table 17-6]) augment cardiac output by stimulating myocardial contractility as well as by functionally unloading the heart.

Patients who present with Profile L ("cold and dry") should be carefully evaluated by right-heart catheterization for the presence of an occult elevation of LV filling pressures. If LV filling pressures are low (pulmonary capillary wedge pressure [PCWP] <12 mmHg), a cautious trial of fluid repletion may be considered. The goals of further therapy depend on the clinical situation. Therapy to reach the aforementioned goals may not be possible in some patients, particularly if they have disproportionate RV dysfunction or if they develop cardiorenal

TABLE 17-6

DRUGS FOR THE TREATMENT FOR ACUTE HEART FAILURE		
	INITIATING DOSE	**MAXIMAL DOSE**
Vasodilators		
Nitroglycerin	20 μg/min	40–400 μg/min
Nitroprusside	10 μg/min	30–350 μg/min
Nesiritide	Bolus 2 μg/kg	0.01–0.03 μg/kg per min[a]
Inotropes		
Dobutamine	1–2 μg/kg per min	2–10 μg/kg per min[b]
Milrinone	Bolus 50 μg/kg	0.1–0.75 μg/kg per min[b]
Dopamine	1–2 μg/kg per min	2–4 μg/kg per min[b]
Levosimendan	Bolus 12 μg/kg	0.1–0.2 μg/kg per min[c]
Vasoconstrictors		
Dopamine for hypotension	5 μg/kg per min	5–15 μg/kg per min
Epinephrine	0.5 μg/kg per min	50 μg/kg per min
Phenylephrine	0.3 μg/kg per min	3 μg/kg per min
Vasopressin	0.05 units/min	0.1–0.4 units/min

[a]Usually <4 μg/kg/min.
[b]Inotropes will also have vasodilatory properties.
[c]Approved outside the United States for management of acute heart failure.

syndrome, in which renal function deteriorates during aggressive diuresis. Worsening renal dysfunction occurs in approximately 25% of patients hospitalized with HF and is associated with prolonged hospital stays and higher mortality rates after discharge.

Pharmacologic Management of Acute HF
(Table 17-6)

Vasodilators After diuretics, intravenous vasodilators are the most useful medications for the management of acute HF. By stimulating guanylyl cyclase within smooth-muscle cells, nitroglycerin, nitroprusside, and nesiritide exert dilating effects on arterial resistance and venous capacitance vessels, which results in a lowering of LV filling pressure, a reduction in mitral regurgitation, and improved forward cardiac output without increasing heart rate or causing arrhythmias. Hypotension is the most common side effect of all vasodilating agents.

Intravenous *nitroglycerin* generally is begun at 20 μg/min and is increased in 20-μg increments until patient symptoms are improved or PCWP is decreased to 16 mmHg without reducing systolic blood pressure below 80 mmHg. The most common side effect of IV or oral nitrates is headache, which, if mild, can be treated with analgesics and often resolves during continued therapy. *Nitroprusside* generally is initiated at 10 μg/min and increased by 10–20 μg every 10–20 min as tolerated, with the same hemodynamic goals as described above. The rapidity of onset and offset, with a half-life of approximately 2 min, facilitates early establishment of an individual patient's optimal level of vasodilation in the ICU. The major limitation of nitroprusside is side effects from cyanide toxicity, which manifests predominantly as gastrointestinal and central nervous system manifestations and is most likely to occur in patients receiving >250 μg/min for over 48 h.

Nesiritide, the newest vasodilator, is a recombinant form of brain-type natriuretic peptide, which is an endogenous peptide secreted primarily from the LV in response to an increase in wall stress. Nesiritide is given as a bolus (2 μg/kg) followed by a fixed-dose infusion (0.01–0.03 μg/kg per min). Nesiritide effectively lowers LV filling pressures and improves symptoms during the treatment of acute HF. Headache is less common with nesiritide than with nitroglycerin. Although termed a *natriuretic peptide*, nesiritide has not been associated with major diuresis when used alone in clinical trials. It does, however, appear to potentiate the effect of concomitant diuretics such that the total required diuretic dose may be slightly lower. There have, however, been recent concerns about the adverse effects of neseritide on renal function in acute decompensated HF which may be related to the initial bolus.

Inotropic Agents Positive inotropic agents produce direct hemodynamic benefits by stimulating cardiac contractility as well as by producing peripheral vasodilation. Collectively, these hemodynamic effects result in an improvement in cardiac output and a fall in LV filling pressures.

Dobutamine, which is the most commonly used inotropic agent for the treatment of acute HF, exerts its effects by stimulating β_1 and β_2 receptors, with little effect on α_1 receptors. Dobutamine is given as a continuous infusion at an initial infusion rate of 1–2 μg/kg per min. Higher doses (>5 μg/kg per min) are frequently necessary for severe hypoperfusion; however, there is little added benefit to increasing the dose above 10 μg/kg per min. Patients maintained on chronic infusions for >72 h generally develop tachyphylaxis and require increasing doses.

Milrinone is a phosphodiesterase III inhibitor that leads to increased cyclic AMP by inhibiting its breakdown. Milrinone may act synergistically with β-adrenergic agonists to achieve a greater increase in cardiac output than is achieved with either agent alone, and it may also be more effective than dobutamine in increasing cardiac output in the presence of beta blockers. Milrinone may be administered as a bolus dose of 50 μg/kg per min, followed by a continuous infusion rate of 0.1–0.75 μg/kg per min. If the patient has a low blood pressure, many clinicians will omit the bolus dose. Because milrinone is a more effective vasodilator than dobutamine, it produces a greater reduction in LV filling pressures, albeit with a greater risk of hypotension.

Although short-term use of inotropes provides hemodynamic benefits, these agents are more prone to cause tachyarrhythmias and ischemic events than vasodilators are. Therefore, inotropes are most appropriately used in clinical settings in which vasodilators and diuretics are not helpful, such as in patients with poor systemic perfusion and/or cardiogenic shock, patients requiring short-term hemodynamic support after an MI or surgery, and patients awaiting cardiac transplantation, or palliative care as in patients with advanced HF. If patients require sustained use of intravenous inotropes, strong consideration should be given to the use of an ICD to safeguard against the proarrhythmic effects of these agents.

Vasoconstrictors Vasoconstrictors are used to support systemic blood pressure in patients with HF. Of the three agents that are commonly used (Table 17-6), dopamine is generally the first choice for therapy in situations in which modest inotropy and pressor support are required. Dopamine is an endogenous catecholamine that stimulates β_1 and α_1 receptors and dopaminergic receptors (DA_1 and DA_2) in the heart and circulation. The effects of dopamine are dose-dependent. Low doses of dopamine (<2 μg/kg per min) stimulate the DA_1 and DA_2 receptors and cause vasodilation of the splanchnic and renal vasculature. Moderate doses (2–4 μg/kg per min) stimulate the β_1 receptors and cause an increase in cardiac output with little or no change in heart rate or SVR. At higher doses (≥5 μg/kg per min) the effects of dopamine on the α_1 receptors overwhelm the dopaminergic receptors, and vasoconstriction ensues, leading to an increase in SVR, LV filling pressures, and heart rate. Significant additional inotropic and blood pressure support can be provided by epinephrine, phenylephrine, and vasopressin (Table 17-6); however, prolonged use of these agents can lead to renal and hepatic failure and can cause gangrene of the limbs. Therefore, these agents should not be administered except in true emergency situations.

Vasopressin Antagonists Vasopressin levels are often elevated in patients with HF and LV dysfunction and may contribute to the hyponatremia that develops in HF patients. Vasopressin antagonists reduce body weight and edema and normalize serum sodium in patients with hyponatremia but have not been associated with improved patient outcomes in clinical trials.

Tolvaptan (oral) and conivaptan (IV) are currently approved for the treatment of hyponatremia but are not approved for the treatment of HF.

Mechanical and Surgical Interventions If pharmacologic interventions fail to stabilize a patient with refractory HF, mechanical and surgical interventions may provide effective circulatory support. These interventions include intraaortic balloon counter pulsation, percutaneous and surgically implanted LV assist devices, and cardiac transplantation (Chap. 18).

Planning for Hospital Discharge Patient education should take place during the entire hospitalization, with a specific focus on salt and fluid status and obtaining daily weights, in addition to medication schedules. Although the majority of patients hospitalized with HF can be stabilized and returned to a good level of function on an oral regimen designed to maintain stability, 30–50% of patients discharged with a diagnosis of HF are rehospitalized within 3–6 months. Although there are multiple reasons for rehospitalization, failure to meet criteria for discharge is perhaps the most common. Criteria for discharge should include at least 24 h of stable fluid status, blood pressure, and renal function on the oral regimen planned for home. Before discharge, patients should be free of dyspnea or symptomatic hypotension while at rest, washing, and walking on the ward.

COR PULMONALE

DEFINITION

Cor pulmonale, often referred to as *pulmonary heart disease*, is defined as dilation and hypertrophy of the right ventricle in response to diseases of the pulmonary vasculature and/or lung parenchyma. Historically, this definition has excluded congenital heart disease and those diseases in which the right heart fails secondary to dysfunction of the left side of the heart.

ETIOLOGY AND EPIDEMIOLOGY

Cor pulmonale develops in response to acute or chronic changes in the pulmonary vasculature and/or the lung parenchyma that are sufficient to cause pulmonary hypertension. The true prevalence of cor pulmonale is difficult to ascertain for two reasons. First, not all patients with chronic lung disease will develop cor pulmonale, and second, our ability to diagnose pulmonary hypertension and cor pulmonale by routine physical examination and laboratory testing is relatively insensitive. However, advances in 2-D echo/Doppler imaging and biomarkers (BNP) make it easier to screen for and detect cor pulmonale.

TABLE 17-7

ETIOLOGY OF CHRONIC COR PULMONALE

Diseases Leading to Hypoxemic Vasoconstriction

Chronic bronchitis
Chronic obstructive pulmonary disease
Cystic fibrosis
Chronic hypoventilation
    Obesity
    Neuromuscular disease
    Chest wall dysfunction
Living at high altitudes

Diseases That Cause Occlusion of the Pulmonary Vascular Bed

Thromboembolic disease, acute or chronic
Pulmonary arterial hypertension
Pulmonary venoocclusive disease

Diseases That Lead to Parenchymal Disease

Chronic bronchitis
Chronic obstructive pulmonary disease
Bronchiectasis
Cystic fibrosis
Pneumoconiosis
Sarcoidosis
Interstitial lung disease

Once patients with chronic pulmonary or pulmonary vascular disease develop cor pulmonale, the prognosis worsens. Although chronic obstructive pulmonary disease (COPD) and chronic bronchitis are responsible for approximately 50% of the cases of cor pulmonale in North America, any disease that affects the pulmonary vasculature (Chap. 40) or parenchyma can lead to cor pulmonale. Table 17-7 provides a list of common diseases that may lead to cor pulmonale. In contrast to COPD, the elevation in pulmonary artery pressure appears to be substantially higher in the interstitial lung diseases, in which there is an inverse correlation between pulmonary artery pressure and the diffusion capacity for carbon monoxide, as well as patient survival. When cor pulmonale occurs in conjunction with obstructive sleep apnea, typically COPD or a hypoventilation syndrome (e.g., obesity hypoventilation syndrome [OHS]) is present concurrently.

PATHOPHYSIOLOGY AND BASIC MECHANISMS

Although many conditions can lead to cor pulmonale, the common pathophysiologic mechanism in each case is pulmonary hypertension that is sufficient to lead to RV dilation, with or without the development of concomitant RV hypertrophy. The systemic consequences of cor pulmonale relate to alterations in cardiac output as well as salt and water homeostasis. Anatomically, the RV is a thin-walled, compliant chamber that is better suited to handle volume overload than pressure overload. Thus, the sustained pressure overload imposed by pulmonary hypertension and increased pulmonary vascular resistance eventually causes the RV to fail.

The response of the RV to pulmonary hypertension depends on the acuteness and severity of the pressure overload. Acute cor pulmonale occurs after a sudden and severe stimulus (e.g., massive pulmonary embolus), with RV dilatation and failure but no RV hypertrophy. Chronic cor pulmonale, however, is associated with a more slowly evolving and progressive pulmonary hypertension that leads to initial modest RV hypertrophy and subsequent RV dilation.

Decompensation of chronic cor pulmonale can be aggravated by intermittent events that induce pulmonary vasoconstriction and RV afterload, such as hypoxemia and especially hypercarbia-induced respiratory acidosis (e.g., OHS), as well as sustained events, including COPD exacerbations, acute pulmonary emboli, and positive-pressure (mechanical) ventilation. RV failure also can be precipitated by alterations in RV volume that occur in various settings, including increased salt and fluid retention, atrial arrhythmias, polycythemia, sepsis, and a large left-to-right (extracardiac) shunt. The most common mechanisms that lead to pulmonary hypertension, are vasoconstriction, activation of the clotting cascade, and obliteration of pulmonary arterial vessels, are discussed in Chap. 40.

CLINICAL MANIFESTATIONS

Symptoms

The symptoms of chronic cor pulmonale generally are related to the underlying pulmonary disorder. Dyspnea, the most common symptom, is usually the result of the increased work of breathing secondary to changes in elastic recoil of the lung (fibrosing lung diseases), altered respiratory mechanics (e.g., overinflation with COPD), or inefficient ventilation (e.g., primary pulmonary vascular disease). Orthopnea and paroxysmal nocturnal dyspnea are rarely symptoms of isolated right HF and usually point toward concurrent left heart dysfunction. Rarely, these symptoms reflect increased work of breathing in the supine position resulting from compromised diaphragmatic excursion. Tussive or effort-related syncope may occur because of the inability of the RV to deliver blood adequately to the left side of the heart. Abdominal pain and ascites that occur with cor pulmonale are similar to the right-heart failure that ensues in chronic HF. Lower-extremity edema may occur secondary to neurohormonal activation, elevated RV filling pressures, or increased levels of carbon dioxide and hypoxemia, which can lead to peripheral vasodilation and edema formation.

Signs

Many of the signs encountered in cor pulmonale are also present in HF patients with a depressed EF, including tachypnea, elevated jugular venous pressures, hepatomegaly, and lower-extremity edema. Patients may have prominent *v* waves in the jugular venous pulse as a result of tricuspid regurgitation. Other cardiovascular signs include an RV heave palpable along the left sternal border or in the epigastrium. The increase in intensity of the holosystolic murmur of tricuspid regurgitation with inspiration ("Carvallo's sign") may be lost eventually as RV failure worsens. Cyanosis is a late finding in cor pulmonale and is secondary to a low cardiac output with systemic vasoconstriction and ventilation–perfusion mismatches in the lung.

DIAGNOSIS

The most common cause of right-heart failure is not pulmonary parenchymal or vascular disease but left heart failure. Therefore, it is important to evaluate the patient for LV systolic and diastolic dysfunction. The ECG in severe pulmonary hypertension shows P pulmonale, right axis deviation, and RV hypertrophy. Radiographic examination of the chest may show enlargement of the main pulmonary artery, the hilar vessels, and the descending right pulmonary artery. Spirometry and lung volumes can identify obstructive and/or restrictive defects indicative of parenchymal lung diseases; arterial blood gases can demonstrate hypoxemia and/or hypercapnia. Spiral computed tomography (CT) scans of the chest are useful in diagnosing acute thromboembolic disease; however, ventilation–perfusion lung scanning remains best suited for diagnosing *chronic thromboembolic disease.* A high-resolution CT scan of the chest can identify interstitial lung disease.

Two-dimensional echocardiography is useful for measuring RV thickness and chamber dimensions as well as the anatomy of the pulmonary and tricuspid valves. Location of the RV behind the sternum and its crescent shape challenge assessment of RV function by echocardiography, especially when parenchymal lung disease is present. Calculated measures of RV function (e.g., tricuspid annular plane systolic excursion [TAPSE] or the Tei Index) supplement more subjective assessments of RV function. The interventricular septum may move paradoxically during systole in the presence of pulmonary hypertension. As noted, Doppler echocardiography can be used to assess pulmonary artery pressures. MRI is also useful for assessing RV structure and function, particularly in patients who are difficult to image with 2-D echocardiography because of severe lung disease. Right-heart catheterization is useful for confirming the diagnosis of pulmonary hypertension and for excluding elevated left-heart pressures (measured as the PCWP) as a cause for right-heart failure. BNP and N-terminal BNP levels are elevated in patients with cor pulmonale secondary to RV stretch and may be dramatically elevated in acute pulmonary embolism.

| TREATMENT | Cor Pulmonale |

The primary treatment goal of cor pulmonale is to target the underlying pulmonary disease, since this will decrease pulmonary vascular resistance and lessen RV afterload. Most pulmonary diseases that lead to chronic cor pulmonale are advanced and therefore are less amenable to treatment. General principles of treatment include decreasing work of breathing by using noninvasive mechanical ventilation and bronchodilation, as well as treating any underlying infection. Adequate oxygenation (oxygen saturation ≥90–92%) and correcting respiratory acidosis are vital for decreasing pulmonary vascular resistance and reducing demands on the RV. Patients should be transfused if they are anemic, and phlebotomy may be considered in extreme cases of polycythemia.

Diuretics are effective in RV failure, and indications are similar to those for chronic HF. One caveat of chronic diuretic use is to avoid inducing contraction alkalosis and worsening hypercapnia. Digoxin is of uncertain benefit in the treatment of cor pulmonale and may lead to arrhythmias in the setting of tissue hypoxemia and acidosis. Therefore, if digoxin is administered, it should be given at low doses and monitored carefully.

Pulmonary vasodilators can effectively improve symptoms through modest reduction of pulmonary pressures and RV afterload when isolated pulmonary arterial hypertension is present. Vasodilators are unproven in cases of pulmonary hypertension and cor pulmonale due to parenchymal lung diseases or hypoventilation syndromes. The treatment of pulmonary hypertension is discussed in Chap. 40.

CHAPTER 18

CARDIAC TRANSPLANTATION AND PROLONGED ASSISTED CIRCULATION

Sharon A. Hunt ■ Hari R. Mallidi

Advanced or end-stage heart failure is an increasingly frequent sequela, as progressively more effective palliation for the earlier stages of heart disease and prevention of sudden death associated with heart disease become more widely recognized and employed (Chap. 17). When patients with end-stage or refractory heart failure are identified, the physician is faced with the decision of advising compassionate end-of-life care or choosing to recommend extraordinary life-extending measures. For the occasional patient who is relatively young and without serious comorbidities, the latter may represent a reasonable option. Current therapeutic options are limited to cardiac transplantation (with the option of mechanical cardiac assistance as a "bridge" to transplantation) or (at least in theory) the option of permanent mechanical assistance of the circulation. In the future, it is possible that genetic modulation of ventricular function or cell-based cardiac repair will be options for such patients. Currently, both approaches are considered to be experimental.

CARDIAC TRANSPLANTATION

Surgical techniques for orthotopic transplantation of the heart were devised in the 1960s and taken into the clinical arena in 1967. The procedure did not gain widespread clinical acceptance until the introduction of "modern" and more effective immunosuppression in the early 1980s. By the 1990s, the demand for transplantable hearts met, and then exceeded, the available donor supply and leveled off at about 4000 heart transplants annually worldwide, according to data from the Registry of the International Society for Heart and Lung Transplantation (ISHLT). Subsequently, heart transplant activity in the United States has remained stable at ~2200/year, but worldwide activity reported to this registry has decreased somewhat. This apparent decline in numbers may be a result of the fact that reporting is legally mandated in the United States, but not elsewhere, and several countries have started their own databases.

SURGICAL TECHNIQUE

Donor and recipient hearts are excised in virtually identical operations with incisions made across the atria and atrial septum at the midatrial level (leaving the posterior walls of the atria in place) and across the great vessels just above the semilunar valves. The donor heart is generally "harvested" in an anatomically identical manner by a separate surgical team and transported from the donor hospital in a bag of iced saline solution and then is reanastomosed into the waiting recipient in the orthotopic or normal anatomic position. The only change in surgical technique since this method was first described has been a movement in recent years to move the right atrial anastamosis back to the level of the superior and inferior vena cavae to better preserve right atrial geometry and prevent atrial arrhythmias. Both methods of implantation leave the recipient with a surgically denervated heart that does not respond to any direct sympathetic or parasympathetic stimuli but does respond to circulating catecholamines. The physiologic responses of the denervated heart to the demands of exercise are atypical but quite adequate to carry on normal physical activity.

DONOR ALLOCATION SYSTEM

In the United States, the allocation of donor organs is accomplished under the supervision of the United Network for Organ Sharing (UNOS), a private organization under contract to the federal government. The United States is divided geographically into eleven regions for donor heart allocation. Allocation of donor hearts within a region is decided according to a system of priority that takes into account (1) the severity of illness, (2) geographic distance from the donor, and (3) patient time on the waiting list. A physiologic limit of ~3 h of "ischemic" (out-of-body) time for hearts precludes a national sharing of hearts. This allocation system design is reissued annually and is responsive to input from a variety of constituencies, including both donor families and transplant professionals.

At the current time, highest priority according to severity of illness is assigned to patients requiring hospitalization at the transplant center for IV inotropic support with a pulmonary artery catheter in place for hemodynamic monitoring or to patients requiring mechanical circulatory support (i.e., intraaortic balloon pump [IABP], right or left ventricular assist device [RVAD, LVAD], extracorporeal membrane oxygenation [ECMO], or mechanical ventilation). Second highest priority is given to patients requiring ongoing inotropic support, but without a pulmonary artery catheter in place. All other patients have priority according to their time accrued on the waiting list, and matching is achieved only according to ABO blood group compatibility and gross body size compatibility, although some patients who are "presensitized" and have pre-existing anti-HLA antibodies (commonly multiparous women or patients previously multiply transfused) undergo prospective cross-matching with the donor. While HLA matching of donor and recipient would be ideal, the relatively small numbers of patients, as well as the time constraints involved, make such matching impractical.

INDICATIONS/CONTRAINDICATIONS

Heart failure is an increasingly common cause of death, particularly in the elderly. Most patients who reach what has recently been categorized as stage D, or refractory end-stage heart failure, are appropriately treated with compassionate end-of-life care. A subset of such patients who are younger and without significant comorbidities can be considered as candidates for heart transplantation. Exact criteria vary in different centers but generally take into consideration the patient's physiologic age and the existence of comorbidities such as peripheral or cerebrovascular disease, obesity, diabetes, cancer, or chronic infection.

RESULTS

A registry organized by the ISHLT has tracked worldwide and U.S. survival rates after heart transplantation since 1982. The most recent update reveals 83% and 76% survival 1 and 3 years posttransplant, or a posttransplant "half-life" of 10 years (Fig. 18-1). The quality of life in these patients is generally excellent, with well over 90% of patients in the registry returning to normal and unrestricted function following transplantation.

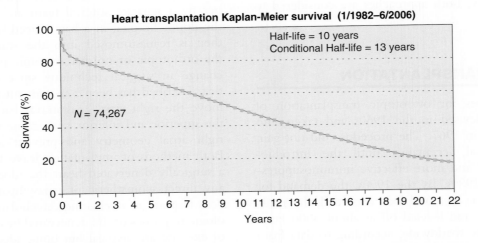

Heart transplantation Kaplan-Meier survival (1/1982–6/2006)

Half-life = 10 years
Conditional Half-life = 13 years

N = 74,267

Survival (%) — Years

FIGURE 18-1

Survival was calculated using the Kaplan-Meier method, which incorporates information from all transplants for whom any follow-up has been provided. Because many patients are still alive and some patients have been lost to follow-up, the survival rates are estimates rather than exact rates because the time of death is not known for all patients. Therefore, 95% confidence limits are provided. (*From J Heart Lung Transplant* 2008; 27:937–983.)

IMMUNOSUPPRESSION

Medical regimens employed to provide suppression of the normal immune response to a solid organ allograft vary from center to center and are in a constant state of evolution, as more effective agents with improved side-effect profiles and less toxicity are introduced. All currently used regimens are nonspecific, providing general hyporeactivity to foreign antigens rather than donor-specific hyporeactivity, and also providing the attendant, and unwanted, susceptibility to infections and malignancy. Most cardiac transplant programs currently use a three-drug regimen including a calcineurin inhibitor (cyclosporine or tacrolimus), an inhibitor of T cell proliferation or differentiation (azathioprine, mycophenolate mofetil, or sirolimus), and at least a short initial course of glucocorticoids. Many programs also include an initial "induction" course of polyclonal or monoclonal anti-T cell antibodies in the perioperative period to decrease the frequency or severity of early posttransplant rejection. Most recently introduced have been monoclonal antibodies (daclizumab and basiliximab) that block the interleukin 2 receptor and may provide prevention of allograft rejection without additional global immunosuppression.

Diagnosis of cardiac allograft rejection is usually made with the use of endomyocardial biopsy, either done on a surveillance basis or in response to clinical deterioration. Biopsy surveillance is performed on a regular basis in most programs for the first year postoperatively and for the first 5 years in many programs. Therapy consists of augmentation of immunosuppression, the intensity and duration of which is dictated by the severity of the rejection.

LATE POSTTRANSPLANT MANAGEMENT ISSUES

Increasing numbers of heart transplant patients are surviving for years following transplantation and constitute a population of patients with a number of long-term management issues.

Allograft coronary artery disease

Despite usually having young donor hearts, cardiac allograft recipients are prone to develop coronary artery disease (CAD). This CAD is generally a diffuse, concentric, and longitudinal process that is quite different from "ordinary" atherosclerotic CAD, which is more focal and often eccentric. The underlying etiology is most likely primarily immunologic injury of the vascular endothelium, but a variety of risk factors influence its existence and progression and include nonimmunologic factors such as dyslipidemia, diabetes mellitus, and cytomegalovirus (CMV) infection. It is hoped that newer and improved immunosuppressive modalities will

reduce the incidence and impact of these devastating complications, which currently account for the majority of late posttransplant deaths. Thus far, the immunosuppressive agents mycophenolate mofetil and the mammalian target of rapamycin (mTOR) inhibitors sirolimus and everolimus have been shown to be associated with short-term lesser incidence and extent of coronary intimal thickening; in anecdotal reports, institution of sirolimus was associated with some reversal of the disease. The use of statins has also been shown to be associated with a reduced incidence of this vasculopathy, and these drugs are now almost universally used in transplant recipients unless contraindicated. Palliation of the disease with percutaneous interventions is probably safe and effective in the short term, although the disease often advances relentlessly. Because of the denervated status of the organ, patients rarely experience angina pectoris, even with advanced stages of the disease.

Retransplantation is the only definitive form of therapy for advanced allograft CAD, but the scarcity of donor hearts makes the decision to pursue retransplantation a difficult one in an individual patient, as well as a difficult ethical issue.

Malignancy

The occurrence of an increased incidence of malignancy is a well-recognized sequela of any program of chronic immunosuppression, and organ transplantation is no exception. Lymphoproliferative disorders are among the most frequent posttransplant complications and, in most cases, seem to be driven by the Epstein-Barr virus. Effective therapy includes reduction of immunosuppression (a clear "double-edged sword" in the setting of a life-sustaining organ), antiviral agents, and traditional chemo- and radiotherapy. Most recently, specific antilymphocyte (CD20) therapy has shown great promise. Cutaneous malignancies (both basal cell and squamous cell carcinomas) also occur with increased frequency in transplant recipients and can pursue very aggressive courses. The role of decreasing immunosuppression for treatment of these cancers is far less clear.

Infections

The use of currently available nonspecific immunosuppressive modalities to prevent allograft rejection naturally results in an increased susceptibility to infectious complications in transplant recipients. Although their incidence has decreased since the introduction of cyclosporine, infections with unusual and opportunistic organisms remain the major cause of death during the first postoperative year and remain a threat to the chronically immunosuppressed patient throughout life. Effective therapy depends on careful surveillance for early signs and symptoms of opportunistic infection and an extremely aggressive approach to obtaining a specific diagnosis as well as expertise in recognizing the more common clinical presentations of CMV, *Aspergillus*, and other opportunistic infectious agents.

PROLONGED ASSISTED CIRCULATION

The modern era of mechanical circulatory support can be traced back to 1953, when cardiopulmonary bypass was first used in a clinical setting and ushered in the possibility of brief periods of circulatory support to permit open-heart surgery. Subsequently, a variety of extracorporeal pumps to provide circulatory support for brief periods of time have been developed. The use of a mechanical device to support the circulation for more than a few hours initially developed slowly, with the implant of a total artificial heart in 1969 in Texas by Cooley. This patient survived for 60 h until a donor organ became available, at which point he was transplanted. Unfortunately, the patient died of pulmonary complications after transplantation. The entire field of mechanical replacement of the heart took a decade-long hiatus until the 1980s, when total artificial hearts were reintroduced with much publicity; however, they failed to produce the hoped-for treatment of end-stage heart disease. Starting in the 1970s, parallel to the development of the total artificial heart, there was intense research in the development of ventricular assist devices, which provide mechanical assistance to (rather than replacement of) the failing ventricle (currently, newer versions of the total artificial heart are in preliminary clinical trials).

Although conceived of initially as alternatives to biologic replacement of the heart, LVADs were introduced as, and are still employed primarily as, temporary "bridges" to heart transplantation in candidates who begin to fail medical therapy before a donor heart becomes available. Several devices are approved by the U.S. Food and Drug Administration (FDA) and are currently in widespread use. Those that are implantable within the body are compatible with hospital discharge and offer the patient a chance for life at home while waiting for a donor heart. However successful such "bridging" is for the individual patient, it does nothing to alleviate the scarcity of donor hearts; the ultimate goal in the field remains that of providing a reasonable alternative to biologic replacement of the heart—one that is widely and easily available and cost-effective.

CURRENT INDICATIONS AND APPLICATIONS OF VENTRICULAR ASSIST DEVICES

Currently, there are two major indications for long-term ventricular assistance. First, patients with chronic end-stage heart failure are eligible for mechanical support if they are at risk of imminent death from cardiogenic shock. Second, if patients have a left ventricular ejection fraction <25%, peak VO$_2$ <14 mL/kg/min, or are dependent on inotropic therapy or support with intraaortic balloon counterpulsation, they may be eligible for mechanical support. If they are eligible for heart transplantation, the mechanical circulatory assistance is termed "bridge to transplantation." By contrast, if the patient has a contraindication to heart transplantation, the device therapy is deemed to be "destination" left ventricular assistance therapy.

AVAILABLE DEVICES

In the United States, there are currently four FDA-approved devices that are used as bridges to transplantation in adults. Of these four devices, one is also approved for use as destination therapy or long-term mechanical support of the heart. There are a number of other devices that are approved only for short-term support for post-cardiac surgery shock or for patients with cardiogenic shock secondary to acute myocardial infarction or fulminant myocarditis; these will not be considered here. None of the long-term devices as yet are totally implantable and, because of this need for transcutaneous connections, all share a common problem with infectious complications. Likewise, all share some tendency to thromboembolic complications as well as the expected possibility of mechanical device failure common to any machine.

The CardioWest total artificial heart (TAH) (Syncardia, Tucson, AZ) is a pneumatic, biventricular, orthotopically implanted total artificial heart with an externalized driveline connecting it to its console. It consists of two spherical polyurethane chambers with polyurethane diaphragms. Inflow and outflow conduits are constructed of Dacron and contain Medtronic-Hall (Medtronic, Inc., Minneapolis, MN) valves. It is currently the only FDA-approved device for use as a bridge to transplantation in patients who have severe biventricular failure.

The Thoratec LVAD (Thoratec Corp., Pleasanton, CA) is an extracorporeal pump that takes blood from a large cannula placed in the left ventricular apex and propels it forward through an outflow cannula inserted into the ascending aorta. The pump itself sits in the paracorporeal position on the abdomen and is attached to a device console cart with wheels, allowing for limited ambulation. The extracorporeal nature of this pump allows it to be used in small adults for whom intracorporeal pumps would be too large.

The Novacor LVAD (WorldHeart, Inc., Oakland, CA) also takes blood from the left ventricular apex through a cannula and propels it into the ascending aorta through a second cannula. With this device, the pump itself is placed in a surgically created pocket in the peritoneal fascia in the abdomen. A driveline that connects to the power source is tunneled subcutaneously and usually exits in the right upper quadrant of the abdomen.

The HeartMate XVE LVAD (Thoratec Corp., Pleasanton, CA) is an intracorporeal left ventricular assist device that has an externalized driveline. The pump sits in the anterior abdominal wall with cannulae that traverse across the diaphragm. There is a drainage cannula in the left ventricular apex, and the blood is expelled from the pump into the ascending aorta via a synthetic vascular graft. This device may be used as a bridge to transplantation and patients may be discharged from the hospital with this device to await transplantation. The HeartMate XVE LVAD is now one of two FDA-approved devices for destination therapy.

The HeartMate II LVAS (Thoratec Corp., Pleasanton, CA) similarly uses a drainage cannula in the left ventricular apex to drain blood into a small chamber, where the blood is driven by an electrically powered motor that spins a rotor, accelerating blood outflow into the ascending aorta (Fig. 18-2). This device is currently the only FDA-approved axial-flow pump that can be used both as a bridge to transplantation and as destination therapy. There are several other axial-flow pumps currently being investigated. These devices have fewer moving parts than previous devices and provide nonpulsatile blood flow. All current axial-flow pumps continue to require transcutaneous connections to power the electric motor. Newer, third-generation devices, which also provide nonpulsatile flow, work through a different mechanism than the axial-flow pumps and are currently being investigated. These devices are even smaller than the currently available axial-flow pumps, and their mechanism of action involves less trauma to blood cells, which may result in better durability and decreased long-term complications.

RESULTS

The use of these devices in the United States is limited mainly to patients with post-cardiac surgery shock and to those who are bridged to transplantation. The results of bridging to transplantation with the available devices are quite good, with nearly 75% of younger patients receiving a transplant by 1 year and having excellent posttransplant survival rates.

Publication of the REMATCH (Randomized Evaluation of Mechanical Assistance in the Treatment of Heart Failure) trial in 2001 documented a somewhat improved survival rate in nontransplant candidates with end-stage heart disease randomized to a HeartMate XVE LVAD (albeit with a high rate of complications, especially neurologic ones) as opposed to continued medical therapy; this led to renewed interest in also using the devices as nonbiologic permanent replacement of heart function, as well as to FDA approval of one device for this indication. This outcome, in turn, led the ISHLT to initiate a Mechanical Circulatory Support database in 2002, which collects voluntary data from 60 international centers and contained data from 655 patients in its most recent publication. Only 12% of these patients had the device placed with the intention of permanent, or "destination," use, with survival rates of only 65% at 6 months and 34% at 1 year.

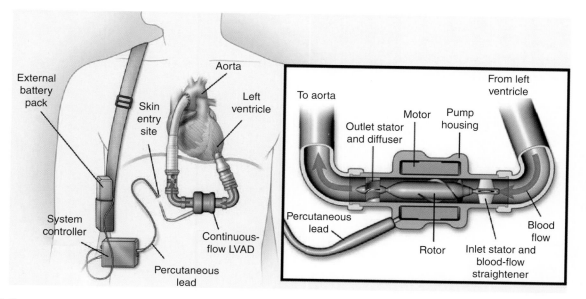

FIGURE 18-2

Diagram of HeartMate II left ventricular assist device. (*Reprinted with permission from Thoratec Corp., Pleasanton, CA.*)

Several studies have evaluated the benefit of LVAD therapy as a bridge to transplantation, with the most recent data taken from a series of 133 patients who underwent implantation of a HeartMate II device. In this group of patients, 80% achieved the principal outcome (defined as survival to transplantation, recovery of heart function, or ongoing device support) at 180 days. With increased experience and improved outcomes using LVADs as a bridge to transplantation, the ability to maintain end-organ function and limit the progression of pulmonary hypertension, or even decrease pulmonary vascular resistance, makes mechanical unloading an attractive option when compared with continued inotropic support. The early bridge-to-transplantation experience demonstrated reduced posttransplantation survival when compared with medical management; however, more recent experience has shown equivalent outcomes following transplantation. This result is likely secondary to a trend toward earlier device implantation, prior to the onset of irreversible end-organ damage.

CHAPTER 19

CONGENITAL HEART DISEASE IN THE ADULT

John S. Child ■ Jamil Aboulhosn

A little over a hundred years ago, Sir William Osler, in his classic textbook *The Principles and Practice of Medicine* (New York, Appleton & Co, 1892, pp 659–663), devoted only five pages to "Congenital Affections of the Heart," with the first sentence declaring, that "[t]hese [disorders] have only limited clinical interest, as in a large proportion of cases the anomaly is not compatible with life, and in others nothing can be done to remedy the defect or even to relieve symptoms." Fortunately, in the intervening century, considerable progress has been made in understanding the basis for these disorders and their effective treatment.

The most common birth defects are cardiovascular in origin. These malformations are due to complex multifactorial genetic and environmental causes, but recognized chromosomal aberrations and mutations of single genes account for <10% of all cardiac malformations. Congenital heart disease (CHD) complicates ~1% of all live births in the general population—about 40,000 births/year—but occurs more frequently in the offspring (about 4–5%) of women with CHD. Owing to the remarkable surgical advances over the last 60 years, >90% of afflicted neonates and children now reach adulthood; women with CHD may now frequently successfully bear children after competent repairs. As such, the population with CHD is steadily increasing. Women with aortic disease (e.g., aortic coarctation or Marfan's syndrome) risk aortic dissection. Patients with cyanotic heart disease, pulmonary hypertension, or Marfan's syndrome with a dilated aortic root generally should not become pregnant; those with correctable lesions should be counseled about the risks of pregnancy with an uncorrected malformation versus repair and later pregnancy.

More than 1 million adults with operated or unoperated CHD live in the United States today and, thus, outnumber the 800,000 children with CHD. Because true surgical cures are rare, and all repairs—be they palliative or corrective—may leave residua, sequelae, or complications, most require some degree of lifetime expert surveillance. The anatomic and physiologic changes in the heart and circulation due to any specific CHD lesion are not static but, rather, progress from prenatal life to adulthood. Malformations that are benign or escape detection in childhood may become clinically significant in the adult. For example, a functionally normal congenitally bicuspid aortic valve may thicken and calcify with time, resulting in significant aortic stenosis; a well-tolerated left-to-right shunt of an atrial septal defect (ASD) may result in cardiac decompensation or pulmonary hypertension only after the fourth to fifth decade.

CARDIAC DEVELOPMENT (ALSO SEE CHAPTER 1)

CHD is generally the result of aberrant embryonic development of a normal structure or failure of such a structure to progress beyond an early stage of embryonic or fetal development. This brief section serves to introduce the reader to normal development so that defects may be better understood; by necessity, it is not exhaustive. Cardiogenesis is a finely tuned process with transcriptional control of a complex group of regulatory proteins that activate or inhibit their gene targets in a location- and time-dependent manner. At about 3 weeks of embryonic development, two cardiac cords form and become canalized; at that point, the primordial cardiac tube develops from two sources (cardiac crescent or the first heart field, pharyngeal mesoderm or the second heart field); by 21 days, these fuse into a single cardiac tube beginning at the cranial end. The cardiac tube then elongates and develops discrete constrictions with the following segments from caudal to cranial location: *sinus venosus* receives the umbilical, vitelline, and common cardinal veins: *atrium, ventricle, bulbus cordis, truncus arteriosus, aortic sac,* and the *aortic arches.* The cardiac tube is fixed at the sinus venosus and arterial ends.

Subsequently, in the next few weeks, differential growth of cells causes the tube to elongate and loop as an "S" with the bulboventricular portion moving rightward and the atrium and sinus venosus moving posterior to the ventricle. The primitive atrium and ventricle communicate via the atrioventricular canal from which the endocardial cushion develops into two parts (ventrally and dorsally). The cushions fuse and divide the atrioventricular canal into two atrioventricular inlets and also migrate to help form the ventricular septum. The primitive atrium is divided first by a *septum primum* membrane, which grows down from the superior wall to the cushions; as this fusion occurs, the midportion resorbs in the center forming the *ostium secundum.* Rightward of the *septum primum,* a second *septum secundum* membrane grows down from the ventral-cranial wall toward—but not reaching—the cushions, and covering most, but not all, of the *ostium secundum,* resulting in a flap of the *foramen ovale.* The primitive ventricle is partitioned by a finely tuned set of events. The interventricular septum grows up toward the cushions, and the cushions form an upper inlet septum; between the two portions is a hole called the interventricular foramen. The left and right ventricles begin to develop side by side, and the atria and their respective inlet valves align over their ventricles. Finally, these two parts of the septum fuse with the bulboventricular ridges, which, once having septated the truncus arteriosus, extend into the ventricle. The bulbocordis divides into a subaortic portion as the muscular conus resorbs, while the subpulmonary section has elongation of its muscular conus. Spiral division of the common truncus arteriosus rotates and aligns the pulmonary artery and aortic portions over their respective outflow tracts, the aortic valve moving posterior over the left ventricle (LV) outflow tract and the pulmonary valve moving anterior over the right ventricle (RV) outflow tract, with a wraparound relationship of the two great arteries.

Early on, the venous systems are bilateral and symmetric and enter 2 horns of the sinus venosus. Ultimately, except for the coronary sinus, most of the left-sided portions and the left sinus–venosus horn regress and the systemic venous system empties into the right horn via the inferior and superior vena cavae. The pulmonary venous system, initially connecting to the systemic venous system, develops as buds from the developing lungs fuse together in the *pulmonary venous* confluence at which point the connection to the systemic system regresses. Simultaneously, a projection from the back wall of the left atrium (the *common pulmonary vein*) grows posteriorly to merge with the confluence, which then becomes a part of the posterior left atrial wall.

The truncus arteriosus and aortic sac initially develop six paired symmetric arches, which curve posteriorly and become the paired dorsal aortae. The detailed description of the selective regression of some of the arches is not presented in this chapter. In brief summary, this process results in the development of arch 3 as the internal carotid arteries, left arch 4 as the aortic arch and right subclavian artery, and part of arch 6 as the patent ductus arteriosus. The two dorsal thoracic aortae fuse in the abdomen with persistence of the left dorsal aorta.

SPECIFIC CARDIAC DEFECTS

Tables 19-1, 19-2, and 19-3 list CHD malformations as simple, intermediate, or complex. Simple defects generally are single lesions with a shunt or a valvular malformation. Intermediate defects may have two or more simple defects. Complex defects generally have components of an intermediate defect plus more complex cardiac and vascular anatomy, often with cyanosis, and frequently with transposition complexes. The goal of these tables is to suggest when cardiology consultation or advanced CHD specialty care is needed. Patients with complex CHD (which includes most "named" surgeries that usually involve complex CHD) should virtually always be managed in conjunction with an experienced specialty adult CHD center. Patients with intermediate lesions should have an initial consultation and subsequent occasional intermittent follow-up with a cardiologist. Patients with simple lesions often may be managed

TABLE 19-1

SIMPLE ADULT CONGENITAL HEART DISEASE
Native disease
Uncomplicated congenital aortic valve disease
Mild congenital mitral valve disease (e.g., except parachute valve, cleft leaflet)
Uncomplicated small atrial septal defect
Uncomplicated small ventricular septal defect
Mild pulmonic stenosis
Repaired conditions
Previously ligated or occluded ductus arteriosus
Repaired secundum or sinus venosus atrial septal defect without residua
Repaired ventricular septal defect without residua

TABLE 19-2

INTERMEDIATE COMPLEXITY CONGENITAL HEART DISEASE

Ostium primum or sinus venosus atrial septal defect
Anomalous pulmonary venous drainage, partial or total
Atrioventricular canal defects (partial or complete)
Ventricular septal defect, complicated (e.g., absent or abnormal valves or with associated obstructive lesions, aortic regurgitation)
Coarctation of the aorta
Pulmonic valve stenosis (moderate to severe)
Infundibular right ventricular outflow obstruction of significance
Pulmonary valve regurgitation (moderate to severe)
Patent ductus arteriosus (nonclosed)—moderate to large
Sinus of Valsalva fistula/aneurysm
Subvalvular or supravalvular aortic stenosis

by a well-informed internist or general cardiologist, although consultation with a specifically trained adult congenital cardiologist is occasionally advisable.

ATRIAL SEPTAL DEFECT

ASD is a common cardiac anomaly that may be first encountered in the adult and occurs more frequently in females. *Sinus venosus* ASD occurs high in the atrial septum near the entry of the superior vena cava into the right atrium and is associated frequently with anomalous pulmonary venous connection from the right lung to the superior vena cava or right atrium. *Ostium primum* ASDs lie adjacent to the atrioventricular valves, either of which may be deformed and regurgitant. Ostium primum ASDs are common in Down syndrome; the more complex atrioventricular septal defects with a common atrioventricular valve and a posterior defect of the basal portion of the interventricular septum are more typical of this chromosomal defect. The most common *ostium secundum* ASD involves the fossa ovalis and is midseptal in location; this should not be confused with a *patent foramen ovale*.

TABLE 19-3

COMPLEX ADULT CONGENITAL HEART DISEASE

Cyanotic congenital heart diseases (all forms)
Eisenmenger's syndrome
Ebstein's anomaly
Tetralogy of Fallot or pulmonary atresia (all forms)
Transposition of the great arteries
Single ventricle; tricuspid or mitral atresia
Double-outlet ventricle
Truncus arteriosus
Fontan or Rastelli procedures

Anatomic obliteration of the foramen ovale ordinarily follows its functional closure soon after birth, but residual "probe patency" is a common normal variant; ASD denotes a true deficiency of the atrial septum and implies functional and anatomic patency. The magnitude of the left-to-right shunt depends on the ASD size, ventricular diastolic properties, and the relative impedance in the pulmonary and systemic circulations. The left-to-right shunt causes diastolic overloading of the right ventricle and increased pulmonary blood flow. Patients with ASD are usually asymptomatic in early life, although there may be some physical underdevelopment and an increased tendency for respiratory infections; cardiorespiratory symptoms occur in many older patients. Beyond the fourth decade, a significant number of patients develop atrial arrhythmias, pulmonary arterial hypertension, bidirectional and then right-to-left shunting of blood, and right heart failure. Patients exposed to the chronic environmental hypoxemia of high altitude tend to develop pulmonary hypertension at younger ages. In older patients, left-to-right shunting across the ASD increases as progressive systemic hypertension and/or coronary artery disease (CAD) result in reduced compliance of the left ventricle.

Physical examination

Examination usually reveals a prominent RV impulse and palpable pulmonary artery pulsation. The first heart sound is normal or split, with accentuation of the tricuspid valve closure sound. Increased flow across the pulmonic valve is responsible for a mid-systolic pulmonary outflow murmur. The second heart sound is widely split and is relatively fixed in relation to respiration. A mid-diastolic rumbling murmur, loudest at the fourth intercostal space and along the left sternal border, reflects increased flow across the tricuspid valve. In ostium primum ASD, an apical holosystolic murmur indicates associated mitral or tricuspid regurgitation or a ventricular septal defect (VSD).

These findings are altered when increased pulmonary vascular resistance causes diminution of the left-to-right shunt. Both the pulmonary outflow and tricuspid inflow murmurs decrease in intensity, the pulmonic component of the second heart sound and a systolic ejection sound are accentuated, the two components of the second heart sound may fuse, and a diastolic murmur of pulmonic regurgitation appears. Cyanosis and clubbing accompany the development of a right-to-left shunt (see "Ventricular Septal Defect" later). In adults with an ASD and atrial fibrillation, the physical findings may be confused with mitral stenosis with pulmonary hypertension because the tricuspid diastolic flow murmur and widely split second heart sound may be mistakenly thought to represent the diastolic murmur of mitral stenosis and the mitral "opening snap," respectively.

Electrocardiogram

In ostium secundum ASD, electrocardiogram (ECG) usually shows right-axis deviation and an rSr′ pattern in the right precordial leads representing enlargement of the RV outflow tract. An ectopic atrial pacemaker or first-degree heart block may occur with the sinus venous ASD. In ostium primum ASD, the RV conduction defect is accompanied by left superior axis deviation and counterclockwise rotation of the frontal plane QRS loop. Varying degrees of RV and right atrial (RA) enlargement or hypertrophy may occur with each type of defect, depending on the height of the pulmonary artery pressure. *Chest x-ray* shows an enlarged right atrium and right ventricle, and pulmonary artery and its branches; increased pulmonary vascular markings of left-to-right shunt vascularity will diminish if pulmonary vascular disease develops.

Echocardiogram

Echocardiography reveals pulmonary arterial and RV and RA dilatation with abnormal (paradoxical) ventricular septal motion in the presence of a significant right heart volume overload. The ASD may be visualized directly by two-dimensional imaging, color-flow imaging, or echo-contrast. In most institutions, two-dimensional echocardiography and Doppler examination have supplanted cardiac catheterization. Transesophageal echocardiography is indicated if the transthoracic echocardiogram is ambiguous, which is often the case with sinus venosus defects, or during catheter device closure (**Fig. 19-1**). Cardiac catheterization is performed if inconsistencies exist in the clinical data, if significant pulmonary hypertension or associated malformations are suspected, or if CAD is a possibility.

TREATMENT   Atrial Septal Defect

Operative repair, usually with a patch of pericardium or of prosthetic material or percutaneous transcatheter device closure, if the ASD is of an appropriate size and shape, should be advised for all patients with uncomplicated secundum ASD with significant left-to-right shunting, i.e., pulmonary-to-systemic flow ratios ≥2:1. Excellent results may be anticipated, at low risk, even in patients >40 years, in the absence of severe pulmonary hypertension. In ostium primum ASD, cleft mitral valves may require repair in addition to patch closure of the ASD. Closure should not be carried out in patients with small defects and trivial left-to-right shunts or in those with severe pulmonary vascular disease without a significant left-to-right shunt.

Patients with sinus venosus or ostium secundum ASDs rarely die before the fifth decade. During the fifth and sixth decades, the incidence of progressive symptoms, often leading to severe disability, increases substantially. Medical management should include prompt

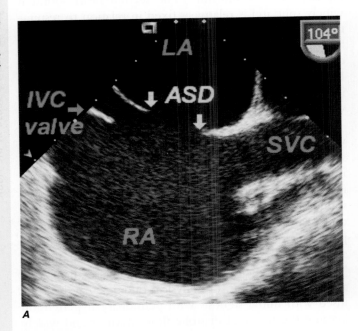

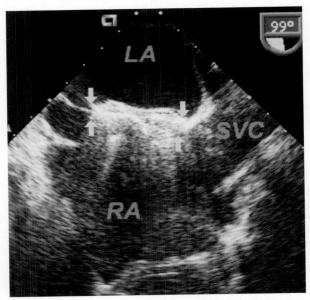

FIGURE 19-1
Secundum atrial septal defect. Transesophageal echocardiogram of secundum ASD and device closure. **A.** The atrial septal defect (ASD) between the left atrium (LA) and right atrium (RA) is shown. **B.** A percutaneous catheter–delivered device has occluded the defect. IVC, inferior vena cava; SVC, superior vena cava.

treatment of respiratory tract infections; antiarrhythmic medications for atrial fibrillation or supraventricular tachycardia; and the usual measures for hypertension, coronary disease, or heart failure (Chap. 17), if these complications occur. The risk of infective endocarditis is quite low unless the defect is complicated by valvular regurgitation or has recently been repaired with a patch or device (Chap. 25).

Ventricular septal defect

A VSD is one of the most common of all cardiac birth defects, either as isolated defects or as a component of a combination of anomalies. The VSD is usually single and situated in the membranous or midmuscular portion of the septum. The functional disturbance depends on its size and on the status of the pulmonary vascular bed. Only small- or moderate-size VSDs are seen initially in adulthood, as most patients with an isolated large VSD come to medical or surgical attention early in life.

A wide spectrum exists in the natural history of VSD, ranging from spontaneous closure to congestive cardiac failure and death in infancy. Included within this spectrum are the possible development of pulmonary vascular obstruction, RV outflow tract obstruction, aortic regurgitation, or infective endocarditis. Spontaneous closure is more common in patients born with a small VSD, which occurs in early childhood in most. The pulmonary vascular bed is often a principal determinant of the clinical manifestations and course of a given VSD and feasibility of surgical repair. Increased pulmonary arterial pressure results from increased pulmonary blood flow and/or resistance, the latter usually the result of obstructive, obliterative structural changes within the pulmonary vascular bed. It is important to quantitate and compare pulmonary-to-systemic flows and resistances in patients with severe pulmonary hypertension. The term *Eisenmenger's syndrome* is applied to patients with a large communication between the two circulations at the aortopulmonary, ventricular, or atrial levels and bidirectional or predominantly right-to-left shunts because of high resistance and obstructive pulmonary hypertension.

Patients with large VSDs and pulmonary hypertension are at greatest risk for developing pulmonary vascular obstruction. Large VSDs should be corrected surgically early in life when pulmonary vascular disease is still reversible or not yet developed. In patients with Eisenmenger syndrome, symptoms in adult life consist of exertional dyspnea, chest pain, syncope, and hemoptysis. The right-to-left shunt leads to cyanosis, clubbing, and erythrocytosis (see later). The degree to which pulmonary vascular resistance is elevated before operation is a critical factor determining prognosis. If

the pulmonary vascular resistance is one-third or less of the systemic value, progression of pulmonary vascular disease after operation is unusual; however, if a moderate to severe increase in pulmonary vascular resistance exists preoperatively, either no change or a progression of pulmonary vascular disease is common postoperatively. Pregnancy is contraindicated in Eisenmenger syndrome. The mother's health is most at risk if she has a cardiovascular lesion associated with pulmonary vascular disease and pulmonary hypertension (e.g., Eisenmenger physiology or mitral stenosis) or LV outflow tract obstruction (e.g., aortic stenosis), but she is also at risk of death with any malformation that may cause heart failure or a hemodynamically important arrhythmia. The fetus is most at risk with maternal cyanosis, heart failure, or pulmonary hypertension.

RV outflow tract obstruction develops in ~5–10% of patients who present in infancy with a moderate to large left-to-right shunt. With time, as subvalvular RV outflow tract obstruction progresses, the findings in these patients whose VSD remains sizable begin to resemble more closely those of the cyanotic tetralogy of Fallot. In ~5% of patients, aortic valve regurgitation results from insufficient cusp tissue or prolapse of the cusp through the interventricular defect; the aortic regurgitation then complicates and dominates the clinical course. Two-dimensional *echocardiography* with spectral and color Doppler examination defines the number and location of defects in the ventricular septum and associated anomalies and the hemodynamic physiology of the defect(s). Hemodynamic and angiographic study may be occasionally required to assess the status of the pulmonary vascular bed and clarify details of the altered anatomy.

TREATMENT   **Ventricular Septal Defect**

Surgery is not recommended for patients with normal pulmonary arterial pressures with small shunts (pulmonary-to-systemic flow ratios of <1.5 to 2:1). Operative correction or transcatheter closure is indicated when there is a moderate to large left-to-right shunt with a pulmonary-to-systemic flow ratio >1.5:1 or 2:1, in the absence of prohibitively high levels of pulmonary vascular resistance.

In the Eisenmenger VSD patient, pulmonary arterial vasodilators and both single-lung transplantation with intracardiac defect repair and total heart-lung transplantation show promise for improvement in symptoms (Chap. 18). Chronic hypoxemia in cyanotic CHD results in secondary *erythrocytosis* due to increased erythropoietin production (Chap. 6). The term *polycythemia* is a misnomer; white cell counts are normal and platelet counts

---

are normal to decreased. Compensated erythrocytosis with iron-replete equilibrium hematocrits rarely result in symptoms of hyperviscosity at hematocrits <65% and occasionally not even with hematocrits ≥70%. For this reason, therapeutic phlebotomy is rarely required in compensated erythrocytosis. In contrast, patients with decompensated erythrocytosis fail to establish equilibrium with unstable, rising hematocrits and recurrent hyperviscosity symptoms. Therapeutic phlebotomy, a two-edged sword, allows temporary relief of symptoms but limits oxygen delivery, begets instability of the hematocrit, and compounds the problem by iron depletion. Iron-deficiency symptoms are usually indistinguishable from those of hyperviscosity; progressive symptoms after recurrent phlebotomy are usually due to iron depletion with hypochromic microcytosis. Iron depletion results in a larger number of smaller (microcytic) hypochromic red cells that are less capable of carrying oxygen and less deformable in the microcirculation; with more of them relative to plasma volume, viscosity is greater than for an equivalent hematocrit with fewer, larger, iron-replete, deformable cells. As such, iron-depleted erythrocytosis results in increasing symptoms due to decreased oxygen delivery to the tissues.

Hemostasis is abnormal in cyanotic CHD, due, in part, to the increased blood volume and engorged capillaries, abnormalities in platelet function, and sensitivity to aspirin or nonsteroidal anti–inflammatory agents, as well as abnormalities of the extrinsic and intrinsic coagulation system. Oral contraceptives are often contraindicated for cyanotic women because of the enhanced risk of vascular thrombosis. Adults with cyanotic CHD do not appear to be at increased risk for stroke unless there are excessive injudicious phlebotomies, inappropriate use of aspirin or anticoagulants, or the presence of atrial arrhythmias or infective endocarditis. Symptoms of hyperviscosity can be produced in any cyanotic patient with erythrocytosis if dehydration reduces plasma volume. Phlebotomy for symptoms of hyperviscosity not due to dehydration or iron deficiency is a simple outpatient removal of 500 mL of blood over 45 min with isovolumetric replacement with isotonic saline. Acute phlebotomy without volume replacement is contraindicated. Iron repletion in decompensated iron-depleted erythrocytosis reduces iron-deficiency symptoms, but must be done gradually to avoid an excessive rise in hematocrit and resulting hyperviscosity.

Patent ductus arteriosus

The ductus arteriosus is a vessel leading from the bifurcation of the pulmonary artery to the aorta just distal to the left subclavian artery. Normally, the vascular channel is open in the fetus but closes immediately after birth. The flow across the ductus is determined by the pressure and resistance relationships between the systemic and pulmonary circulations and by the cross-sectional area and length of the ductus. In most adults with this anomaly, pulmonary pressures are normal and a gradient and shunt from aorta to pulmonary artery persist throughout the cardiac cycle, resulting in a characteristic thrill and a continuous "machinery" murmur with late systolic accentuation at the upper left sternal edge. In adults who were born with a large left-to-right shunt through the ductus arteriosus, pulmonary vascular obstruction (Eisenmenger syndrome) with pulmonary hypertension, right-to-left shunting, and cyanosis have usually developed. Severe pulmonary vascular disease results in reversal of flow through the ductus; unoxygenated blood is shunted to the descending aorta; and the toes—but not the fingers—become cyanotic and clubbed, a finding termed *differential cyanosis*. The leading causes of death in adults with patent ductus are cardiac failure and infective endocarditis; occasionally severe pulmonary vascular obstruction may cause aneurysmal dilatation, calcification, and rupture of the ductus.

TREATMENT   Patent Ductus Arteriosus

In the absence of severe pulmonary vascular disease and predominant left-to-right shunting of blood, the patent ductus should be surgically ligated or divided. Transcatheter closure using coils, buttons, plugs, and umbrellas has become commonplace for appropriately shaped defects. Thoracoscopic surgical approaches are considered experimental. Operation should be deferred for several months in patients treated successfully for infective endocarditis because the ductus may remain somewhat edematous and friable.

Aortic root–to–right-heart shunts

The three most common causes of aortic root–to–right-heart shunts are congenital aneurysm of an aortic sinus of Valsalva with fistula, coronary arteriovenous fistula, and anomalous origin of the left coronary artery from the pulmonary trunk. *Aneurysm of an aortic sinus of Valsalva* consists of a separation or lack of fusion between the media of the aorta and the annulus of the aortic valve. Rupture usually occurs in the third or fourth decade of life; most often, the aorticocardiac fistula is between the right coronary cusp and the right ventricle; but occasionally, when the noncoronary cusp is involved, the fistula drains into the right atrium. Abrupt rupture causes chest pain, bounding pulses, a continuous murmur accentuated in diastole, and volume overload of the heart. Diagnosis is confirmed by two-dimensional and Doppler echocardiographic studies; cardiac catheterization quantitates the left-to-right shunt, and thoracic aortography visualizes the fistula. Medical management is directed at cardiac failure, arrhythmias, or endocarditis. At operation, the aneurysm is closed and amputated, and the aortic wall is reunited with the heart, either by direct suture or with a patch or prosthesis.

Coronary arteriovenous fistula, an unusual anomaly, consists of a communication between a coronary artery and another cardiac chamber, usually the coronary sinus, right atrium, or right ventricle. The shunt is usually of small magnitude and myocardial blood flow is not usually compromised; if the shunt is large, there may be a coronary "steal" syndrome with myocardial ischemia and possible angina or ventricular arrhythmias. Potential complications include infective endocarditis; thrombus formation with occlusion or distal embolization with myocardial infarction; rupture of an aneurysmal fistula; and, rarely, pulmonary hypertension and congestive failure. A loud, superficial, continuous murmur at the lower or midsternal border usually prompts a further evaluation of asymptomatic patients. Doppler echocardiography demonstrates the site of drainage; if the site of origin is proximal, it may be detectable by two-dimensional echocardiography. Angiography (classic catheterization, CT, or magnetic resonance angiography) permits identification of the size and anatomic features of the fistulous tract, which may be closed by suture or transcatheter obliteration.

The third anomaly causing a shunt from the aortic root to the right heart is *anomalous origin of the left coronary artery from the pulmonary artery*. Myocardial infarction and fibrosis commonly lead to death within the first year, although up to 20% of patients survive to adolescence and beyond without surgical correction. The diagnosis is supported by the ECG findings of an anterolateral myocardial infarction and left ventricular hypertrophy (LVH). Operative management of adults consists of coronary artery bypass with an internal mammary artery graft or saphenous vein–coronary artery graft.

Congenital aortic stenosis

Malformations that cause obstruction to LV outflow include congenital valvular aortic stenosis, discrete subaortic stenosis, or supravalvular aortic stenosis. Bicuspid aortic valves are more common in males than in females. The congenital bicuspid aortic valve, which may initially be functionally normal, is one of the most common congenital malformations of the heart and may go undetected in early life. Because bicuspid valves may develop stenosis or regurgitation with time or be the site of infective endocarditis, the lesion may be difficult to distinguish in older adults from acquired rheumatic or degenerative calcific aortic valve disease. The dynamics of blood flow associated with a congenitally deformed, rigid aortic valve commonly lead to thickening of the cusps and, in later life, to calcification. Hemodynamically significant

obstruction causes concentric hypertrophy of the LV wall. The ascending aorta is often dilated, misnamed "poststenotic" dilatation; this is due to histologic abnormalities of the aortic media similar to those in Marfan's syndrome and may result in aortic dissection. Diagnosis is made by echocardiography, which reveals the morphology of the aortic valve and aortic root and quantitates severity of stenosis or regurgitation. The clinical manifestations and hemodynamic abnormalities are discussed in Chap. 20.

TREATMENT Valvular Aortic Stenosis

Medical management includes prophylaxis against infective endocarditis and, in patients with diminished cardiac reserve, the administration of digoxin and diuretics and sodium restriction while awaiting operation. A dilated aortic root may require beta blockers. Aortic valve replacement is indicated in adults with critical obstruction, i.e., with an aortic valve area <0.45 cm²/m², with symptoms secondary to LV dysfunction or myocardial ischemia, or with hemodynamic evidence of LV dysfunction. In asymptomatic children or adolescents or young adults with critical aortic stenosis without valvular calcification or these features, aortic balloon valvuloplasty is often useful (Chap. 36). If surgery is contraindicated in older patients because of a complicating medical problem such as malignancy or renal or hepatic failure, balloon valvuloplasty may provide short-term improvement. This procedure may serve as a bridge to aortic valve replacement in patients with severe heart failure.

Subaortic stenosis

The *discrete* form of subaortic stenosis consists of a membranous diaphragm or fibromuscular ring encircling the LV outflow tract just beneath the base of the aortic valve. The jet impact from the subaortic stenotic jet on the underside of the aortic valve often begets progressive aortic valve fibrosis and valvular regurgitation. Echocardiography demonstrates the anatomy of the subaortic obstruction; Doppler studies show turbulence proximal to the aortic valve and can quantitate the pressure gradient and severity of aortic regurgitation. Treatment consists of complete excision of the membrane or fibromuscular ring.

Supravalvular aortic stenosis

This is a localized or diffuse narrowing of the ascending aorta originating just above the level of the coronary arteries at the superior margin of the sinuses of Valsalva. In contrast to other forms of aortic stenosis, the coronary arteries are subjected to elevated systolic pressures from the left ventricle, are often dilated and tortuous, and are susceptible to premature atherosclerosis. In most patients, a genetic defect for the anomaly is located in the same chromosomal region as elastin on chromosome 7. Supravalvular aortic stenosis is the most commonly associated cardiac defect in Williams-Beuren syndrome, typically comprising the following: "elfin" facies, low nasal bridge, cheerful demeanor, mental retardation with retained language skills and love of music, supravalvular aortic stenosis, and transient hypercalcemia.

Coarctation of the aorta

Narrowing or constriction of the lumen of the aorta may occur anywhere along its length but is most common distal to the origin of the left subclavian artery near the insertion of the ligamentum arteriosum. Coarctation occurs in ~7% of patients with congenital heart disease, is more common in males than females, and is particularly frequent in patients with gonadal dysgenesis (e.g., Turner syndrome). Clinical manifestations depend on the site and extent of obstruction and the presence of associated cardiac anomalies; most commonly a bicuspid aortic valve. Circle of Willis aneurysms may occur in up to 10%, and pose a high risk of sudden rupture and death.

Most children and young adults with isolated, discrete coarctation are asymptomatic. Headache, epistaxis, cold extremities, and claudication with exercise may occur, and attention is usually directed to the cardiovascular system when a heart murmur or hypertension in the upper extremities and absence, marked diminution, or delayed pulsations in the femoral arteries are detected on physical examination. Enlarged and pulsatile collateral vessels may be palpated in the intercostal spaces anteriorly, in the axillae, or posteriorly in the interscapular area. The upper extremities and thorax may be more developed than the lower extremities. A mid-systolic murmur over the left interscapular space may become continuous if the lumen is narrowed sufficiently to result in a high-velocity jet across the lesion throughout the cardiac cycle. Additional systolic and continuous murmurs over the lateral thoracic wall may reflect increased flow through dilated and tortuous collateral vessels. The ECG usually reveals LV hypertrophy. Chest x-ray may show a dilated left subclavian artery high on the left mediastinal border and a dilated ascending aorta. Indentation of the aorta at the site of coarctation and pre- and poststenotic dilatation (the "3" sign) along the left paramediastinal shadow are essentially pathognomonic. Notching of the third to ninth ribs, an important radiographic sign, is due to inferior rib erosion by dilated collateral vessels (Figs. 19-2 and 19-3). Two-dimensional echocardiography from suprasternal windows identifies the site of coarctation; Doppler quantitates the pressure gradient. Transesophageal echocardiography and MRI or three-dimensional CT allow visualization of the length and severity of the

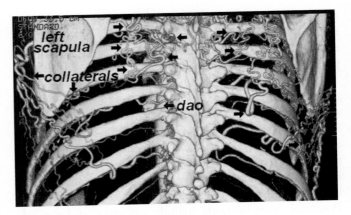

FIGURE 19-2

Aortic coarctation. The extensive collaterals (*left*) underneath the ribs and in the periscapular region are shown on a posterior view of a three-dimensional CT angiogram, which are responsible for rib notching on chest x-ray. dao, descending aorta.

obstruction and associated collateral arteries (Figs. 19-2 and 19-3). In adults, cardiac catheterization is indicated primarily to evaluate the coronary arteries or to perform catheter-based intervention (angioplasty and stent of the coarctation).

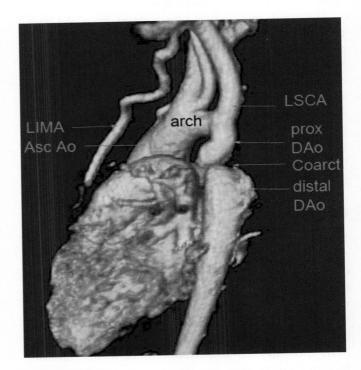

FIGURE 19-3

Aortic coarctation. The coarctation (Coarct) of the aorta is shown in the typical "adult" location in the descending aorta (DAo) just distal to the dilated left subclavian artery (LSCA) in this three-dimensional reconstruction of an MR angiogram. There is a post-coarct aneurysm that is in part due to intrinsic aortic medial tissue weakness. The left internal mammary artery (LIMA) is dilated. Asc Ao, ascending aorta; prox, proximal.

The chief hazards of proximal aortic severe hypertension include cerebral aneurysms and hemorrhage, aortic dissection and rupture, premature coronary arteriosclerosis, and LV failure; infective endarteritis may occur on the coarctation site or endocarditis may settle on an associated bicuspid aortic valve, which is estimated to be present in up to 75% of patients.

TREATMENT Coarctation of the Aorta

Treatment is surgical or involves percutaneous catheter balloon dilatation with stent placement; the details of selection of therapy are beyond this review. Late postoperative systemic hypertension in the absence of residual coarctation is related partly to the duration of preoperative hypertension. Follow-up of rest and exercise blood pressures is important; many have systolic hypertension only during exercise, in part due to a diffuse vasculopathy. All operated or stented coarctation patients deserve a high-quality MRI or CT procedure in follow-up.

Pulmonary stenosis with intact ventricular septum

Obstruction to RV outflow may be localized to the supravalvular, valvular, or subvalvular levels or occur at a combination of these sites. Multiple sites of narrowing of the peripheral pulmonary arteries are a feature of *rubella embryopathy* and may occur with both the familial and sporadic forms of supravalvular aortic stenosis. Valvular pulmonic stenosis (PS) is the most common form of isolated RV obstruction.

The severity of the obstructing lesion, rather than the site of narrowing, is the most important determinant of the clinical course. In the presence of a normal cardiac output, a peak systolic pressure gradient <30 mmHg indicates mild PS and >50 mmHg indicates severe PS; processes between these limits are considered to indicate moderate stenosis. Patients with mild PS are generally asymptomatic and demonstrate little or no progression in the severity of obstruction with age. In patients with more significant stenosis, the severity may increase with time. Symptoms vary with the degree of obstruction. Fatigue, dyspnea, RV failure, and syncope may limit the activity of older patients, in whom moderate or severe obstruction may prevent an augmentation of cardiac output with exercise. In patients with severe obstruction, the systolic pressure in the RV may exceed that in the LV, because the ventricular septum is intact. RV ejection is prolonged with moderate or severe stenosis, and the sound of pulmonary valve closure is delayed and soft. RV hypertrophy reduces the compliance of that chamber, and a forceful RA contraction is necessary to augment RV filling. A fourth heart

sound; prominent *a* waves in the jugular venous pulse; and, occasionally, presystolic pulsations of the liver reflect vigorous atrial contraction. The clinical diagnosis is supported by a left parasternal lift and harsh systolic crescendo–decrescendo murmur and thrill at the upper left sternal border, typically preceded by a systolic ejection sound if the obstruction is due to a mobile non-dysplastic pulmonary valve. The holosystolic murmur of tricuspid regurgitation may accompany severe PS, especially in the presence of congestive heart failure. Cyanosis usually reflects right-to-left shunting through a patent foramen ovale or ASD. In patients with supravalvular or peripheral pulmonary arterial stenosis, the murmur is systolic or continuous and is best heard over the area of narrowing, with radiation to the peripheral lung fields.

In mild cases, the ECG is normal, whereas moderate and severe stenoses are associated with RV hypertrophy. The chest x-ray with mild or moderate PS shows a heart of normal size with normal lung vascularity. In pulmonary valvular stenosis, dilatation of the main and left pulmonary arteries occurs in part due to the direction of the PS jet and in part due to intrinsic tissue weakness. With severe obstruction, RV hypertrophy is generally evident. The pulmonary vascularity may be reduced with severe stenosis, RV failure, and/or a right-to-left shunt at the atrial level. Two-dimensional echocardiography visualizes pulmonary-valve morphology; the outflow tract pressure gradient is quantitated by Doppler echocardiography.

TREATMENT Pulmonary Stenosis

The cardiac catheter technique of balloon valvuloplasty (Chap. 13) is usually effective. Direct surgical relief of moderate and severe obstruction may be accomplished at a low risk. Multiple stenoses of the peripheral pulmonary arteries are usually inoperable, but narrowing of a proximal branch or at the bifurcation of the main pulmonary trunk may be surgically corrected or undergo balloon dilatation and stenting.

Tetralogy of Fallot

The four components of the tetralogy of Fallot are malaligned VSD, obstruction to RV outflow, aortic override of the VSD, and RV hypertrophy due to the RV's response to aortic pressure via the large VSD **(Fig. 19-4)**.

The severity of RV outflow obstruction determines the clinical presentation. The severity of hypoplasia of the RV outflow tract varies from mild to complete (pulmonary atresia). Pulmonary valve stenosis and supravalvular and peripheral pulmonary arterial obstruction may

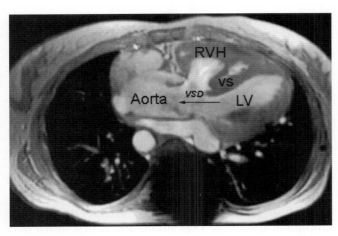

FIGURE 19-4
Tetralogy of Fallot. Magnetic resonance angiogram. A mid-systolic frame showing the malaligned ventricular septal defect (VSD) with the aorta overriding the ventricular septal defect. LV, left ventricle; RVH, RV hypertrophy; VS, ventricular septum.

coexist; rarely, there is unilateral absence of a pulmonary artery (usually the left). A right-sided aortic arch and descending thoracic aorta occur in ~25%.

The relationship between the resistance of blood flow from the ventricles into the aorta and into the pulmonary artery plays a major role in determining the hemodynamic and clinical picture. When the RV outflow obstruction is severe, pulmonary blood flow is reduced markedly, and a large volume of desaturated systemic venous blood shunts right–to–left across the VSD. Severe cyanosis and erythrocytosis occur, and symptoms of systemic hypoxemia are prominent. In many infants and children, the obstruction is mild but progressive.

The ECG shows RV hypertrophy. Chest x–ray shows a normal-sized, boot-shaped heart (*coeur en sabot*) with a prominent right ventricle and a concavity in the region of the pulmonary conus. Pulmonary vascular markings are typically diminished, and the aortic arch and knob may be on the right side. Two-dimensional echocardiography demonstrates the malaligned VSD with the overriding aorta and the site and severity of PS, which may be subpulmonic (fixed or dynamic), at the pulmonary valve or in the main or branch pulmonary arteries. Classic contrast angiography may provide details regarding the RV outflow tract, pulmonary valve and annulus, and caliber of the main branches of the pulmonary artery as well of possible associated aortopulmonary collaterals. Coronary arteriography identifies the anatomy and course of the coronary arteries. In experienced centers, these issues are often well demonstrated in adults by MRI (Fig. 19-4) or CT angiography with three-dimensional reconstruction.

TREATMENT   Tetralogy of Fallot

For a variety of reasons, only a few adults with tetralogy of Fallot have not had some form of previous surgical intervention. Reoperation in adults is most commonly for severe pulmonary regurgitation. Long-term concerns about ventricular function persist. Ventricular and atrial arrhythmias may require medical treatment or electrophysiologic study and ablation. Interventional catheterization may be needed in selected patients (i.e., angioplasty and stenting of branch pulmonary stenosis). The aortic root has a medial tissue defect; it is commonly enlarged and associated with aortic regurgitation. Endocarditis remains a risk despite surgical repair.

Complete transposition of the great arteries

This condition is commonly called *dextro-* or *D-transposition of the great arteries*. The aorta arises rightward anteriorly from the right ventricle, and the pulmonary artery emerges leftward and posteriorly from the LV, which results in two separate parallel circulations; some communication between them must exist after birth to sustain life. Most patients have an interatrial communication, two-thirds have a patent ductus arteriosus, and about one-third have an associated VSD. Transposition is more common in males and accounts for ~10% of cyanotic heart disease. The course is determined by the degree of tissue hypoxemia, the ability of each ventricle to sustain an increased workload in the presence of reduced coronary arterial oxygenation, the nature of the associated cardiovascular anomalies, and the status of the pulmonary vascular bed. By the third decade of life, ~30% of patients will have developed decreased RV function and progressive tricuspid regurgitation, which may lead to congestive heart failure. Pulmonary vascular obstruction develops by 1 to 2 years of age in patients with an associated large VSD or large patent ductus arteriosus in the absence of obstruction to LV outflow.

TREATMENT   Transposition of the Great Arteries

The balloon or blade catheter or surgical creation or enlargement of an interatrial communication in the neonate is the simplest procedure for providing increased intracardiac mixing of systemic and pulmonary venous blood. Systemic pulmonary–artery anastomosis may be indicated in the patient with severe obstruction to LV outflow and diminished pulmonary blood flow. Intracardiac repair may be accomplished by rearranging the venous returns (intraatrial switch, i.e., Mustard or Senning operation) so that the systemic venous blood is directed to the mitral valve and, thence, to the left ventricle and pulmonary artery, while the pulmonary venous blood is diverted through the tricuspid valve and right ventricle to the aorta. The late survival after these repairs is good, but arrhythmias (e.g., atrial flutter) or conduction defects (e.g., sick sinus syndrome) occur in ~50% of such patients by 30 years after the intraatrial switch surgery. Progressive dysfunction of the systemic subaortic right ventricle, tricuspid regurgitation, ventricular arrhythmias, or cardiac arrest and late sudden death are worrisome features. Preferably, this malformation is corrected in infancy by transposing both coronary arteries to the posterior artery and transecting, contraposing, and anastomosing the aorta and pulmonary arteries (arterial-switch operation). For those patients with a VSD in whom it is necessary to bypass a severely obstructed LV outflow tract, corrective operation employs an intracardiac ventricular baffle and extracardiac prosthetic conduit to replace the pulmonary artery (Rastelli procedure).

Single ventricle

This is a family of complex lesions with both atrioventricular valves or a common atrioventricular valve opening to a single ventricular chamber. Associated anomalies include abnormal great artery positional relationships, pulmonic valvular or subvalvular stenosis, and subaortic stenosis. Survival to adulthood depends on a relatively normal pulmonary blood flow, yet normal pulmonary resistance and good ventricular function. Modifications of the Fontan approach are generally applied to carefully selected patients with creation of a pathway(s) from the systemic veins to the pulmonary arteries.

Tricuspid atresia

This malformation is characterized by atresia of the tricuspid valve; an interatrial communication; and, frequently, hypoplasia of the right ventricle and pulmonary artery. The clinical picture is usually dominated by severe cyanosis due to obligatory admixture of systemic and pulmonary venous blood in the left ventricle. The ECG characteristically shows RA enlargement, left-axis deviation, and LV hypertrophy.

Atrial septostomy and palliative operations to increase pulmonary blood flow, often by anastomosis of a systemic artery or vein to a pulmonary artery, may allow survival to the second or third decade. A Fontan atriopulmonary or total cavopulmonary connection may then allow functional correction in those patients with normal or low pulmonary arterial resistance pressure and good LV function.

Ebstein's anomaly

Characterized by a downward displacement of the tricuspid valve into the right ventricle, due to anomalous attachment of the tricuspid leaflets, the Ebstein tricuspid valve tissue is dysplastic and results in tricuspid regurgitation. The abnormally situated tricuspid orifice produces an "atrialized" portion of the RV lying between the atrioventricular ring and the origin of the valve, which is continuous with the RA chamber. Often, the RV is hypoplastic. Although the clinical manifestations are variable, some patients come to initial attention because of either (1) progressive cyanosis from right-to-left atrial shunting, (2) symptoms due to tricuspid regurgitation and RV dysfunction, or (3) paroxysmal atrial tachyarrhythmias with or without atrioventricular bypass tracts (Wolff-Parkinson-White [WPW] syndrome). Diagnostic findings by two-dimensional echocardiography include the abnormal positional relation between the tricuspid and mitral valves with abnormally increased apical displacement of the septal tricuspid leaflet. Tricuspid regurgitation is quantitated by Doppler examination. Surgical approaches include prosthetic replacement of the tricuspid valve when the leaflets are tethered or repair of the native valve.

Congenitally corrected transposition

The two fundamental anatomic abnormalities in this malformation are transposition of the ascending aorta and pulmonary trunk and inversion of the ventricles. This arrangement results in desaturated systemic venous blood passing from the right atrium through the mitral valve to the LV and into the pulmonary trunk, whereas oxygenated pulmonary venous blood flows from the left atrium through the tricuspid valve to the RV and into the aorta. Thus, the circulation is corrected functionally. The clinical presentation, course, and prognosis of patients with congenitally corrected transposition vary depending on the nature and severity of any complicating intracardiac anomalies and of development of dysfunction of the systemic subaortic RV. Progressive RV dysfunction and tricuspid regurgitation may also develop in one-third of patients by age 30; Ebstein-type anomalies of the left-side tricuspid atrioventricular valve are common. VSD or PS due to obstruction to outflow from the right-sided subpulmonary (anatomic left) ventricle may coexist. Complete heart block occurs at a rate of 2–10% per decade. The diagnosis of the malformation and associated lesions can be established by comprehensive two-dimensional echocardiography and Doppler examination.

Malpositions of the heart

Positional anomalies refer to conditions in which the cardiac apex is in the right side of the chest (dextrocardia), or at the midline (mesocardia), or in which there is a normal location of the heart in the left side of the chest but abnormal position of the viscera (isolated levocardia).

Knowledge of the position of the abdominal organs and of the branching pattern of the main stem bronchi is important in categorizing these malpositions. When dextrocardia occurs without situs inversus, when the visceral situs is indeterminate, or if isolated levocardia is present, associated, often complex, multiple cardiac anomalies are usually present. In contrast, mirror-image dextrocardia is usually observed with complete situs inversus, which occurs most frequently in individuals whose hearts are otherwise normal.

SURGICALLY MODIFIED CONGENITAL HEART DISEASE

Owing to the enormous strides in cardiovascular surgical techniques that have occurred in the past 60 years, a large number of long-term survivors of corrective operations in infancy and childhood have reached adulthood. These patients are often challenging because of the diversity of anatomic, hemodynamic, and electrophysiologic residua and sequelae of cardiac operations.

The proper care of the survivor of operation for CHD requires that the clinician understand the details of the malformation before operation; pay meticulous attention to the details of the operative procedure; and recognize the postoperative residua (conditions left totally or partially uncorrected), the sequelae (conditions caused by surgery), and the complications that may have resulted from the operation. Except for ligation of an uncomplicated patent ductus arteriosus, almost every other surgical repair leaves behind or causes some abnormality of the heart and circulation that may range from trivial to serious. Intraoperative transesophageal echocardiography assists in detecting unsuspected lesions, in monitoring the repair, and in verifying a satisfactory result or directing further repair. Thus, even with results that are considered clinically to be good to excellent, continued long-term postoperative follow-up is advisable.

Cardiac operations importantly involving the atria, such as closure of ASD, repair of total or partial anomalous pulmonary venous return, or venous switch corrections of complete transposition of the great arteries (the Mustard or Senning operations), may be followed years later by sinus node or atrioventricular node dysfunction or by atrial arrhythmias (especially atrial flutter). Intraventricular surgery may also result in electrophysiologic consequences, including complete heart block necessitating pacemaker insertion to avoid sudden death. Valvular problems may arise late after initial cardiac operation. An example is the progressive stenosis of an initially nonobstructive bicuspid aortic valve in the patient who underwent aortic coarctation repair. Such aortic valves may also be the site of infective endocarditis. After repair of the ostium primum ASD, the cleft mitral valve may become progressively regurgitant. Tricuspid regurgitation may also

be progressive in the postoperative patient with tetralogy of Fallot if RV outflow tract obstruction was not relieved adequately at initial surgery. In many patients with surgically modified CHD, inadequate relief of an obstructive lesion, or a residual regurgitant lesion, or a residual shunt will cause or hasten the onset of clinical signs and symptoms of myocardial dysfunction. Despite a good hemodynamic repair, many patients with a subaortic RV develop RV decompensation and signs of left heart failure. In many patients, particularly those who were cyanotic for many years before operation, a preexisting compromise in ventricular performance is due to the original underlying malformation.

A final category of postoperative problems involves the use of prosthetic valves, patches, or conduits in the operative repair. The special risks include infective endocarditis, thrombus formation, and premature degeneration and calcification of the prosthetic materials. There are many patients in whom extracardiac conduits are required to correct the circulation functionally and often to carry blood to the lungs from the right atrium or right ventricle. These conduits may develop intraluminal obstruction, and, if they include a prosthetic valve, it may show progressive calcification and thickening. Many such patients face reintervention (interventional cardiac catheterization or surgical reoperation) one or more times in their lives. Such care should be directed to centers specializing in adults with complex congenital cardiovascular malformations. The effect of pregnancy in postoperative patients depends on the outcome of the repair, including the presence and severity of residua, sequelae, or complications. Contraception is an important topic with such patients. Tubal ligation should be considered in those in whom pregnancy is strictly contraindicated.

Endocarditis prophylaxis

Two major predisposing causes of infective endocarditis are a susceptible cardiovascular substrate and a source of bacteremia. The clinical and bacteriologic profile of infective endocarditis in patients with CHD has changed with the advent of intracardiac surgery and of prosthetic devices. Prophylaxis includes both antimicrobial and hygienic measures. Meticulous dental and skin care are required. Routine antimicrobial prophylaxis is recommended for bacteremic dental procedures or instrumentation through an infected site in most patients with operated CHD, particularly if foreign material, such as a prosthetic valve, conduit, surgically constructed shunt, etc., is in place. In the case of patches, in the absence of a high-pressure patch leak, prophylaxis is usually recommended for 6 months until there is endothelialization. Individuals with unrepaired cyanotic heart disease are also generally recommended to receive prophylaxis (Chap. 25).

CHAPTER 20

VALVULAR HEART DISEASE

Patrick O'Gara ■ Joseph Loscalzo

The role of the physical examination in the evaluation of patients with valvular heart disease is also considered in Chaps. 9 and 10; of electrocardiography (ECG) in Chap. 11; of echocardiography and other noninvasive imaging techniques in Chap. 12; and of cardiac catheterization and angiography in Chap. 13.

MITRAL STENOSIS

ETIOLOGY AND PATHOLOGY

Rheumatic fever is the leading cause of mitral stenosis (MS) (Table 20-1). Other less common etiologies of obstruction to left atrial outflow include congenital mitral valve stenosis, cor triatriatum, mitral annular calcification with extension onto the leaflets, systemic lupus erythematosus, rheumatoid arthritis, left atrial myxoma, and infective endocarditis with large vegetations. Pure or predominant MS occurs in approximately 40% of all patients with rheumatic heart disease and a history of rheumatic fever. In other patients with rheumatic heart disease, lesser degrees of MS may accompany mitral regurgitation (MR) and aortic valve disease. With reductions in the incidence of acute rheumatic fever, particularly in temperate climates and developed countries, the incidence of MS has declined considerably over the past few decades. However, it remains a major problem in developing nations, especially in tropical and semitropical climates.

In rheumatic MS, the valve leaflets are diffusely thickened by fibrous tissue and/or calcific deposits. The mitral commissures fuse, the chordae tendineae fuse and shorten, the valvular cusps become rigid, and these changes, in turn, lead to narrowing at the apex of the funnel-shaped ("fish-mouth") valve. Although the initial insult to the mitral valve is rheumatic, the later changes may be a nonspecific process resulting from trauma to the valve caused by altered flow patterns due to the initial deformity. Calcification of the stenotic mitral valve immobilizes the leaflets and narrows the orifice further. Thrombus formation and arterial embolization may arise from the calcific valve itself, but in patients with atrial fibrillation (AF), thrombi arise more frequently from the dilated left atrium (LA), particularly from within the left atrial appendage.

PATHOPHYSIOLOGY

In normal adults, the area of the mitral valve orifice is 4–6 cm². In the presence of significant obstruction, i.e., when the orifice area is reduced to <~2 cm², blood can flow from the LA to the left ventricle (LV) only if propelled by an abnormally elevated left atrioventricular pressure gradient, the hemodynamic hallmark of MS. When the mitral valve opening is reduced to <1 cm², often referred to as "severe" MS, an LA pressure of ~25 mmHg is required to maintain a normal cardiac output (CO). The elevated pulmonary venous and pulmonary arterial (PA) wedge pressures reduce pulmonary compliance, contributing to exertional dyspnea. The first bouts of dyspnea are usually precipitated by clinical events that increase the rate of blood flow across the mitral orifice, resulting in further elevation of the LA pressure (see later in this chapter).

To assess the severity of obstruction hemodynamically, both the transvalvular pressure gradient and the flow rate must be measured (Chap. 13). The latter depends not only on the CO but on the heart rate, as well. An increase in heart rate shortens diastole proportionately more than systole and diminishes the time available for flow across the mitral valve. Therefore, at any given level of CO, tachycardia, including that associated with rapid AF, augments the transvalvular pressure gradient and elevates further the LA pressure. Similar considerations apply to the pathophysiology of tricuspid stenosis.

TABLE 20-1

MAJOR CAUSES OF VALVULAR HEART DISEASES

VALVE LESION	ETIOLOGIES	VALVE LESION	ETIOLOGIES
Mitral stenosis	Rheumatic fever	Tricuspid stenosis	Rheumatic
	Congenital		Congenital
	Severe mitral annular calcification	Tricuspid regurgitation	Primary
	SLE, RA		Rheumatic
Mitral regurgitation	Acute		Endocarditis
	Endocarditis		Myxomatous (TVP)
	Papillary muscle rupture (post-MI)		Carcinoid
	Trauma		Radiation
	Chordal rupture/leaflet flail (MVP, IE)		Congenital (Ebstein's)
	Chronic		Trauma
	Myxomatous (MVP)		Papillary muscle injury (post-MI)
	Rheumatic fever		Secondary
	Endocarditis (healed)		RV and tricuspid annular dilatation
	Mitral annular calcification		Multiple causes of RV enlargement
	Congenital (cleft, AV canal)		(e.g., long-standing pulmonary HTN)
	HOCM with SAM		Chronic RV apical pacing
	Ischemic (LV remodeling)	Pulmonic stenosis	Congenital
	Dilated cardiomyopathy		Carcinoid
	Radiation	Pulmonic regurgitation	Valve disease
Aortic stenosis	Congenital (bicuspid, unicuspid)		Congenital
	Degenerative calcific		Postvalvotomy
	Rheumatic fever		Endocarditis
	Radiation		Annular enlargement
Aortic regurgitation	Valvular		Pulmonary hypertension
	Congenital (bicuspid)		Idiopathic dilation
	Endocarditis		Marfan's syndrome
	Rheumatic fever		
	Myxomatous (prolapse)		
	Traumatic		
	Syphilis		
	Ankylosing spondylitis		
	Root disease		
	Aortic dissection		
	Cystic medial degeneration		
	Marfan's syndrome		
	Bicuspid aortic valve		
	Nonsyndromic familial aneurysm		
	Aortitis		
	Hypertension		

Abbreviations: AV, atrioventricular; HOCM, hypertrophic obstructive cardiomyopathy; HTN, hypertension; IE, infective endocarditis; LV, ventricular; MI, myocardial infarction; MVP, mitral valve prolapse; RA, rheumatoid arthritis; RV, right ventricular; SAM, systolic anterior motion of the anterior mitral valve leaflet; SLE, systemic lupus erythematosus; TVP, tricuspid valve prolapse.

The LV diastolic pressure and ejection fraction (EF) are normal in isolated MS. In MS and sinus rhythm, the elevated LA and PA wedge pressures exhibit a prominent atrial contraction pattern (*a* wave) and a gradual pressure decline after the *v* wave and mitral valve opening (*y* descent). In severe MS and whenever pulmonary vascular resistance is significantly increased, the pulmonary arterial pressure (PAP) is elevated at rest and rises further during exercise, often causing secondary elevations of right ventricular (RV) end-diastolic pressure and volume.

Cardiac output

In patients with moderate MS (mitral valve orifice 1–1.5 cm²), the CO is normal or almost so at rest, but rises subnormally during exertion. In patients with severe MS (valve area <1 cm²), particularly those in whom pulmonary vascular resistance is markedly elevated, the CO is subnormal at rest and may fail to rise or may even decline during activity.

Pulmonary hypertension

The clinical and hemodynamic features of MS are influenced importantly by the level of the PAP. Pulmonary hypertension results from: (1) passive backward transmission of the elevated LA pressure; (2) pulmonary arteriolar constriction (the so-called "second stenosis"), which presumably is triggered by LA and pulmonary venous hypertension (reactive pulmonary hypertension);

(3) interstitial edema in the walls of the small pulmonary vessels; and (4) at end stage, organic obliterative changes in the pulmonary vascular bed. Severe pulmonary hypertension results in RV enlargement, secondary tricuspid regurgitation (TR), and pulmonic regurgitation (PR), as well as right-sided heart failure.

SYMPTOMS

In temperate climates, the latent period between the initial attack of rheumatic carditis (in the increasingly rare circumstances in which a history of one can be elicited) and the development of symptoms due to MS is generally about two decades; most patients begin to experience disability in the fourth decade of life. Studies carried out before the development of mitral valvotomy revealed that once a patient with MS became seriously symptomatic, the disease progressed continuously to death within 2–5 years.

In patients whose mitral orifices are large enough to accommodate a normal blood flow with only mild elevations of LA pressure, marked elevations of this pressure leading to dyspnea and cough may be precipitated by sudden changes in the heart rate, volume status, or CO, as, for example, with severe exertion, excitement, fever, severe anemia, paroxysmal AF and other tachycardias, sexual intercourse, pregnancy, and thyrotoxicosis. As MS progresses, lesser degrees of stress precipitate dyspnea, the patient becomes limited in daily activities, and orthopnea and paroxysmal nocturnal dyspnea develop. The development of permanent AF often marks a turning point in the patient's course and is generally associated with acceleration of the rate at which symptoms progress.

Hemoptysis results from rupture of pulmonary-bronchial venous connections secondary to pulmonary venous hypertension. It occurs most frequently in patients who have elevated LA pressures without markedly elevated pulmonary vascular resistances and is rarely fatal. *Recurrent pulmonary emboli*, sometimes with infarction, are an important cause of morbidity and mortality rates late in the course of MS. *Pulmonary infections*, i.e., bronchitis, bronchopneumonia, and lobar pneumonia, commonly complicate untreated MS, especially during the winter months.

Pulmonary changes

In addition to the aforementioned changes in the pulmonary vascular bed, fibrous thickening of the walls of the alveoli and pulmonary capillaries occurs commonly in MS. The vital capacity, total lung capacity, maximal breathing capacity, and oxygen uptake per unit of ventilation are reduced. Pulmonary compliance falls further as pulmonary capillary pressure rises during exercise.

Thrombi and emboli

Thrombi may form in the left atria, particularly within the enlarged atrial appendages of patients with MS. Systemic embolization, the incidence of which is 10–20%, occurs more frequently in patients with AF, in patients >65 years of age, and in those with a reduced CO. However, systemic embolization may be the presenting feature in otherwise asymptomatic patients with only mild MS.

PHYSICAL FINDINGS

(See also Chaps. 9 and 10)

Inspection and palpation

In patients with severe MS, there may be a malar flush with pinched and blue facies. In patients with sinus rhythm and severe pulmonary hypertension or associated tricuspid stenosis (TS), the jugular venous pulse reveals prominent *a* waves due to vigorous right atrial systole. The systemic arterial pressure is usually normal or slightly low. An RV tap along the left sternal border signifies an enlarged RV. A diastolic thrill may rarely be present at the cardiac apex, with the patient in the left lateral recumbent position.

Auscultation

The first heart sound (S_1) is usually accentuated and slightly delayed. The pulmonic component of the second heart sound (P_2) also is often accentuated, and the two components of the second heart sound (S_2) are closely split. The opening snap (OS) of the mitral valve is most readily audible in expiration at, or just medial to, the cardiac apex. This sound generally follows the sound of aortic valve closure (A_2) by 0.05–0.12 s. The time interval between A_2 and OS varies inversely with the severity of the MS. The OS is followed by a low-pitched, rumbling, diastolic murmur, heard best at the apex with the patient in the left lateral recumbent position (see Fig. 9-5); it is accentuated by mild exercise (e.g., a few rapid sit-ups) carried out just before auscultation. In general, the duration of this murmur correlates with the severity of the stenosis in patients with preserved CO. In patients with sinus rhythm, the murmur often reappears or becomes louder during atrial systole (presystolic accentuation). Soft, grade I or II/VI systolic murmurs are commonly heard at the apex or along the left sternal border in patients with pure MS and do not necessarily signify the presence of MR. Hepatomegaly, ankle edema, ascites, and pleural effusion, particularly in the right pleural cavity, may occur in patients with MS and RV failure.

Associated lesions

With severe pulmonary hypertension, a pansystolic murmur produced by functional TR may be audible along the left sternal border. This murmur is usually louder during inspiration and diminishes during forced expiration (Carvallo's sign). When the CO is markedly reduced in MS, the typical auscultatory findings, including the diastolic rumbling murmur, may not be detectable (silent MS), but they may reappear as compensation is restored. The *Graham Steell murmur* of PR, a high-pitched, diastolic, decrescendo blowing murmur along the left sternal border, results from dilation of the pulmonary valve ring and occurs in patients with mitral valve disease and severe pulmonary hypertension. This murmur may be indistinguishable from the more common murmur produced by aortic regurgitation (AR), although it may increase in intensity with inspiration and is accompanied by a loud and often palpable P_2.

LABORATORY EXAMINATION

ECG

In MS and sinus rhythm, the P wave usually suggests LA enlargement (see Fig. 11-8). It may become tall and peaked in lead II and upright in lead V_1 when severe pulmonary hypertension or TS complicates MS and right atrial (RA) enlargement occurs. The QRS complex is usually normal. However, with severe pulmonary hypertension, right-axis deviation and RV hypertrophy are often present.

Echocardiogram

(See also Chap. 12) Transthoracic echocardiography (TTE) with color flow and spectral Doppler imaging provides critical information, including measurements of mitral inflow velocity during early (E wave) and late (A wave in patients in sinus rhythm) diastolic filling, estimates of the transvalvular peak and mean gradients and of the mitral orifice area, the presence and severity of any associated MR, the extent of leaflet calcification and restriction, the degree of distortion of the subvalvular apparatus, and the anatomic suitability for percutaneous mitral balloon valvotomy (percutaneous mitral balloon valvuloplasty [PMBV]; see later). In addition, TTE provides an assessment of LV and RV function, chamber sizes, an estimation of the pulmonary artery pressure (PAP) based on the tricuspid regurgitant jet velocity, and an indication of the presence and severity of any associated valvular lesions. Transesophageal echocardiography (TEE) provides superior images and should be employed when TTE is inadequate for guiding management decisions. TEE is especially indicated to exclude the presence of left atrial thrombus prior to PMBV.

Chest x-ray

The earliest changes are straightening of the upper left border of the cardiac silhouette, prominence of the main pulmonary arteries, dilation of the upper lobe pulmonary veins, and posterior displacement of the esophagus by an enlarged LA. Kerley B lines are fine, dense, opaque, horizontal lines that are most prominent in the lower and midlung fields and that result from distention of interlobular septae and lymphatics with edema when the resting mean LA pressure exceeds approximately 20 mmHg.

DIFFERENTIAL DIAGNOSIS

Like MS, significant MR may also be associated with a prominent diastolic murmur at the apex due to increased antegrade transmitral flow, but in patients with isolated MR, this diastolic murmur commences slightly later than in patients with MS, and there is often clear-cut evidence of LV enlargement. An opening snap and increased P_2 are absent, and S_1 is soft or absent. An apical pansystolic murmur of at least grade III/VI intensity as well as an S_3 suggest significant MR. Similarly, the apical mid-diastolic murmur associated with severe AR (*Austin Flint murmur*) may be mistaken for MS but can be differentiated from it because it is not intensified in presystole and becomes softer with administration of amyl nitrite. TS, which occurs rarely in the absence of MS, may mask many of the clinical features of MS or be clinically silent; when present, the diastolic murmur of TS increases with inspiration.

Atrial septal defect (Chap. 19) may be mistaken for MS; in both conditions there is often clinical, ECG, and chest x-ray evidence of RV enlargement and accentuation of pulmonary vascularity. However, the absence of LA enlargement and of Kerley B lines and the demonstration of fixed splitting of S_2 with a grade 2 or 3 midsystolic murmur at the mid to upper left sternal border all favor atrial septal defect over MS. Atrial septal defects with large left-to-right shunts may result in functional TS because of the enhanced diastolic flow.

Left atrial myxoma (Chap. 23) may obstruct LA emptying, causing dyspnea, a diastolic murmur, and hemodynamic changes resembling those of MS. However, patients with an LA myxoma often have features suggestive of a systemic disease, such as weight loss, fever, anemia, systemic emboli, and elevated serum IgG and interleukin 6 (IL-6) concentrations. The auscultatory findings may change markedly with body position. The diagnosis can be established by the demonstration of a characteristic echo-producing mass in the LA with TTE.

CARDIAC CATHETERIZATION

Left and right heart catheterization is useful when there is a discrepancy between the clinical and TTE findings that cannot be resolved with either TEE or cardiac magnetic resonance (CMR) imaging. The growing experience with CMR for the assessment of patients with valvular heart disease may decrease the need for invasive catheterization. Catheterization is helpful in assessing associated lesions, such as aortic stenosis (AS) and AR. Catheterization and coronary angiography are not usually necessary to aid in decision making about surgery in patients younger than 65 years of age, with typical findings of severe mitral obstruction on physical examination and TTE. In men older than 40 years of age, women older than 45 years of age, and younger patients with coronary risk factors, especially those with positive noninvasive stress tests for myocardial ischemia, coronary angiography is advisable preoperatively to identify patients with critical coronary obstructions that should be bypassed at the time of operation. Computed tomographic coronary angiography (CTCA) (Chap. 12) is now often used to screen preoperatively for the presence of coronary artery disease (CAD) in patients with valvular heart disease and low pretest likelihood of CAD. Catheterization and left ventriculography are indicated in most patients who have undergone PMBV or previous mitral valve surgery, and who have redeveloped limiting symptoms, especially if questions regarding the severity of the valve lesion(s) remain after echocardiography.

TREATMENT   Mitral Stenosis

(See **Fig. 20-1**) Penicillin prophylaxis of group A β-hemolytic streptococcal infections (Chap. 26) for secondary prevention of rheumatic fever is important for at-risk patients with rheumatic MS (**Table 20-2**). Recommendations for infective endocarditis prophylaxis have recently changed. In symptomatic patients, some improvement usually occurs with restriction of sodium intake and small doses of oral diuretics. Beta blockers, nondihydropyridine calcium channel blockers (e.g., verapamil or diltiazem), and digitalis glycosides are useful in slowing the ventricular rate of patients with AF. Warfarin to an international normalized ratio (INR) of 2–3 should be administered indefinitely to patients with MS, who have AF or a history of thromboembolism. The routine use of warfarin in patients in sinus rhythm with LA enlargement (maximal dimension >5.5 cm) with or without spontaneous echo contrast is more controversial.

If AF is of relatively recent onset in a patient whose MS is not severe enough to warrant PMBV or surgical commissurotomy, reversion to sinus rhythm

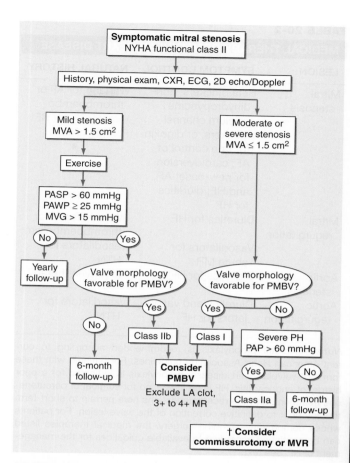

FIGURE 20-1

Management strategy for patients with mitral stenosis (MS) and mild symptoms. †There is controversy as to whether patients with severe MS (MVA <1 cm²) and severe pulmonary hypertension (PH) (PASP >60 mmHg) should undergo percutaneous mitral balloon valvotomy (PMBV) or mitral valve replacement (MVR) to prevent right ventricular failure. CXR, chest x-ray; ECG, electrocardiogram; echo, echocardiography; LA, left atrial; MR, mitral regurgitation; MVA, mitral valve area; MVG, mean mitral valve pressure gradient; NYHA, New York Heart Association; PASP, pulmonary artery systolic pressure; PAWP, pulmonary artery wedge pressure; 2-D, two-dimensional. (*From RO Bonow et al: J Am Coll Cardiol 48:e1, 2006; with permission.*)

pharmacologically or by means of electrical countershock is indicated. Usually, cardioversion should be undertaken after the patient has had at least 3 consecutive weeks of anticoagulant treatment to a therapeutic INR. If cardioversion is indicated more urgently, then intravenous heparin should be provided and TEE performed to exclude the presence of left atrial thrombus before the procedure. Conversion to sinus rhythm is rarely successful or sustained in patients with severe MS, particularly those in whom the LA is especially enlarged or in whom AF has been present for more than 1 year.

TABLE 20-2

MEDICAL THERAPY OF VALVULAR HEART DISEASE

LESION	SYMPTOM CONTROL	NATURAL HISTORY
Mitral stenosis	Beta blockers, non-dihydropyridine calcium channel blockers, or digoxin for rate control of AF; cardioversion for new-onset AF and HF; diuretics for HF	Warfarin for AF or thromboembolism; PCN for RF prophylaxis
Mitral regurgitation	Diuretics for HF	Warfarin for AF or thromboembolism
	Vasodilators for acute MR	Vasodilators for HTN
Aortic stenosis	Diuretics for HF	No proven therapy
Aortic regurgitation	Diuretics and vasodilators for HF	Vasodilators for HTN

Note: Antibiotic prophylaxis is recommended according to current American Heart Association guidelines. For patients with these forms of valvular heart disease, prophylaxis is indicated for a prior history of endocarditis. HF is an indication for surgical or percutaneous treatment, and the recommendations here pertain to short-term therapy prior to definitive correction of the valve lesion. For patients whose comorbidities prohibit surgery, the medical therapies listed can be continued according to available guidelines for the management of HF. See text.

Abbreviations: AF, atrial fibrillation; HF, heart failure; HTN, systemic hypertension; PCN, penicillin; RF, rheumatic fever.

Source: Adapted from NA Boon, P Bloomfield: Heart 87:395, 2002; with permission.

MITRAL VALVOTOMY Unless there is a contraindication, mitral valvotomy is indicated in symptomatic [New York Heart Association (NYHA) Functional Class II–IV] patients with isolated MS, whose effective orifice (valve area) is <~1 cm²/m² body surface area, or <1.5 cm² in normal-sized adults. Mitral valvotomy can be carried out by two techniques: PMBV and surgical valvotomy. In PMBV (**Figs. 20-2** and **20-3**), a catheter is directed into the LA after transseptal puncture, and a single balloon is directed across the valve and inflated in the valvular orifice. Ideal patients have relatively pliable leaflets with little or no commissural calcium. In addition, the subvalvular structures should not be significantly scarred or thickened, and there should be no left atrial thrombus. The short- and long-term results of this procedure in appropriate patients are similar to those of surgical valvotomy, but with less morbidity and a lower periprocedural mortality rate. Event-free survival in younger (<45 years) patients with pliable valves is

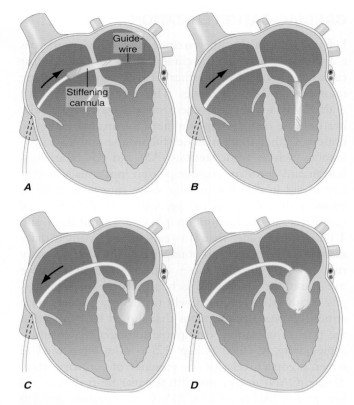

FIGURE 20-2

Inoue balloon technique for percutaneous mitral balloon valvotomy. A. After transseptal puncture, the deflated balloon catheter is advanced across the interatrial septum, then across the mitral valve and into the left ventricle. **B–D.** The balloon is inflated stepwise within the mitral orifice.

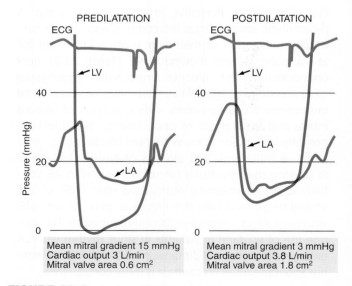

FIGURE 20-3

Simultaneous left atrial (LA) and left ventricular (LV) pressure before and after percutaneous mitral balloon valvuloplasty (PMBV) in a patient with severe mitral stenosis. (*Courtesy of Raymond G. McKay, MD; with permission.*)

excellent, with rates as high as 80–90% over 3–7 years. Therefore, PMBV has become the procedure of choice for such patients when it can be performed by a skilled operator in a high-volume center.

Transthoracic echocardiography is helpful in identifying patients for the percutaneous procedure, and TEE is performed routinely to exclude left atrial thrombus at the time of the scheduled procedure. An "echo score" has been developed to help guide decision making. The score accounts for the degree of leaflet thickening, calcification, and mobility, and for the extent of subvalvular thickening. A lower score predicts a higher likelihood of successful PMBV.

In patients in whom PMBV is not possible or unsuccessful, or in many patients with restenosis, an "open" valvotomy using cardiopulmonary bypass is necessary. In addition to opening the valve commissures, it is important to loosen any subvalvular fusion of papillary muscles and chordae tendineae and to remove large deposits of calcium, thereby improving valvular function, as well as to remove atrial thrombi. The perioperative mortality rate is ~2%.

Successful valvotomy is defined by a 50% reduction in the mean mitral valve gradient and a doubling of the mitral valve area. Successful valvotomy, whether balloon or surgical, usually results in striking symptomatic and hemodynamic improvement and prolongs survival. However, there is no evidence that the procedure improves the prognosis of patients with slight or no functional impairment. Therefore, unless recurrent systemic embolization or severe pulmonary hypertension has occurred (PA systolic pressures >50 mmHg at rest or >60 mmHg with exercise), valvotomy is *not* recommended for patients who are entirely asymptomatic and/or who have mild stenosis (mitral valve area >1.5 cm^2). When there is little symptomatic improvement after valvotomy, it is likely that the procedure was ineffective, that it induced MR, or that associated valvular or myocardial disease was present. About half of all patients undergoing surgical mitral valvotomy require reoperation by 10 years. In the pregnant patient with MS, valvotomy should be carried out if pulmonary congestion occurs despite intensive medical treatment. PMBV is the preferred strategy in this setting and is performed with TEE and no or minimal x-ray exposure.

Mitral valve replacement (MVR) is necessary in patients with MS and significant associated MR, those in whom the valve has been severely distorted by previous transcatheter or operative manipulation, or those in whom the surgeon does not find it possible to improve valve function significantly with valvotomy. MVR is now routinely performed with preservation of the chordal attachments to optimize LV functional recovery. Perioperative mortality rates with MVR vary with age, LV function, the presence of CAD, and

TABLE 20-3

MORTALITY RATES AFTER VALVE SURGERY[a]

OPERATION	NUMBER	UNADJUSTED OPERATIVE MORTALITY (%)
AVR (isolated)	20,168	3.2
MVR (isolated)	4,616	5.0
AVR + CAB	16,678	5.0
MVR + CAB	2,479	8.8
AVR + MVR	1,239	9.0
MVP	5,617	1.8
MVP + CAB	4,932	4.8
TV surgery	6,235	9.2
PV surgery	480	6.0

[a]Data are for calendar year 2008, in which 912 sites reported a total of 276,308 procedures. Data are available from the Society of Thoracic Surgeons at *http://www.sts.org/documents/pdf/ndb/2ndHarvestExecutiveSummary_2009.pdf*.

Abbreviations: AVR, aortic valve replacement; CAB, coronary artery bypass; MVR, mitral valve replacement; MVP, mitral valve repair; TV surgery, tricuspid valve repair and replacement; PV surgery, pulmonic valve repair and replacement.

associated comorbidities. They average 5% overall but are lower in young patients and may be twice as high in patients >65 years of age with comorbidity rates (Table 20-3). Since there are also long-term complications of valve replacement, patients in whom preoperative evaluation suggests the possibility that MVR may be required should be operated on only if they have severe MS—i.e., an orifice area ≤1 cm^2—and are in NYHA class III, i.e., symptomatic with ordinary activity despite optimal medical therapy. The overall 10-year survival of surgical survivors is ~70%. Long-term prognosis is worse in patients >65 years of age and those with marked disability and marked depression of the CO preoperatively. Pulmonary hypertension and RV dysfunction are additional risk factors for poor outcome.

MITRAL REGURGITATION

ETIOLOGY

MR may result from an abnormality or disease process that affects any one or more of the five functional components of the mitral valve apparatus (leaflets, annulus, chordae tendineae, papillary muscles, and subjacent myocardium) (Table 20-1). Acute MR can occur in the setting of acute myocardial infarction (MI) with papillary muscle rupture (Chap. 35), following blunt chest wall trauma, or during the course of infective endocarditis. With acute

MI, the posteromedial papillary muscle is involved much more frequently than the anterolateral papillary muscle because of its singular blood supply. Transient, acute MR can occur during periods of active ischemia and bouts of angina pectoris. Rupture of chordae tendineae can result in "acute-on-chronic MR" in patients with myxomatous degeneration of the valve apparatus.

Chronic MR can result from rheumatic disease, mitral valve prolapse (MVP), extensive mitral annular calcification, congenital valve defects, hypertrophic obstructive cardiomyopathy (HOCM), and dilated cardiomyopathy (Chap. 21). The rheumatic process produces rigidity, deformity, and retraction of the valve cusps and commissural fusion, as well as shortening, contraction, and fusion of the chordae tendineae. The MR associated with both MVP and HOCM is usually dynamic in nature. MR in HOCM occurs as a consequence of anterior papillary muscle displacement and systolic anterior motion of the anterior mitral valve leaflet into the narrowed LV outflow tract. Annular calcification is especially prevalent among patients with advanced renal disease and is commonly observed in women >65 years of age with hypertension and diabetes. MR may occur as a congenital anomaly (Chap. 19), most commonly as a defect of the endocardial cushions (atrioventricular cushion defects). A cleft anterior mitral valve leaflet accompanies primum atrial septal defect. Chronic MR is frequently secondary to ischemia and may occur as a consequence of ventricular remodeling, papillary muscle displacement, and leaflet tethering, or with fibrosis of a papillary muscle, in patients with healed myocardial infarction(s) and ischemic cardiomyopathy. Similar mechanisms of annular dilation and ventricular remodeling contribute to the MR that occurs among patients with nonischemic forms of dilated cardiomyopathy once the left ventricular end-diastolic dimension reaches 6 cm.

Irrespective of cause, chronic severe MR is often progressive, since enlargement of the LA places tension on the posterior mitral leaflet, pulling it away from the mitral orifice and thereby aggravating the valvular dysfunction. Similarly, LV dilation increases the regurgitation, which, in turn, enlarges the LA and LV further, causing chordal rupture and resulting in a vicious circle; hence the aphorism, "mitral regurgitation begets mitral regurgitation."

PATHOPHYSIOLOGY

The resistance to LV emptying (LV afterload) is reduced in patients with MR. As a consequence, the LV is decompressed into the LA during ejection, and with the reduction in LV size during systole, there is a rapid decline in LV tension. The initial compensation to MR is more complete LV emptying. However, LV volume increases progressively with time as the severity of the regurgitation increases and as LV contractile function deteriorates. This increase in LV volume is often accompanied by a reduced forward CO, although LV compliance is often increased and, thus, LV diastolic pressure does not increase until late in the course. The regurgitant volume varies directly with the LV systolic pressure and the size of the regurgitant orifice; as mentioned earlier, the latter, in turn, is influenced by the extent of LV and mitral annular dilation. Since ejection fraction (EF) rises in severe MR in the presence of normal LV function, even a modest reduction in this parameter (<60%) reflects significant dysfunction.

During early diastole, as the distended LA empties, there is a particularly rapid y descent in the absence of accompanying MS. A brief, early diastolic LA-LV pressure gradient (often generating a rapid filling sound [S_3] and mid-diastolic murmur masquerading as MS) may occur in patients with pure MR as a result of the very rapid flow of blood across a normal-sized mitral orifice.

Semiquantitative estimates of left ventricular ejection fraction (LVEF), CO, PA systolic pressure, regurgitant volume, regurgitant fraction (RF), and the effective regurgitant orifice area can be obtained during a careful Doppler echocardiographic examination. These measurements can also be obtained with CMR. Left and right heart catheterization with contrast ventriculography is used less frequently. Severe, nonischemic MR is defined by a regurgitant volume ≥60 mL/beat, regurgitant fraction (RF) ≥50%, and effective regurgitant orifice area ≥0.40 cm². Severe ischemic MR is usually associated with an effective regurgitant orifice area of >0.3 cm².

LA compliance

In acute severe MR, the regurgitant volume is delivered into a normal-sized LA having normal or reduced compliance. As a result, LA pressures rise markedly for any increase in LA volume. The v wave in the LA pressure pulse is usually prominent, LA and pulmonary venous pressures are markedly elevated, and pulmonary edema is common. Because of the rapid rise in LA pressures during ventricular systole, the murmur of acute MR is early in timing and decrescendo in configuration ending well before S_2, as a reflection of the progressive diminution in the LV-LA pressure gradient. LV systolic function in acute MR may be normal, hyperdynamic, or reduced, depending on the clinical context.

Patients with chronic severe MR, on the other hand, develop marked LA enlargement and *increased* LA compliance with little if any increase in LA and pulmonary venous pressures for any increase in LA volume. The LA v wave is relatively less prominent. The murmur of chronic MR is classically holosystolic in timing and plateau in configuration, as a reflection of the near-constant LV-LA pressure gradient. These patients usually complain of severe fatigue and exhaustion secondary to a low forward CO, while symptoms resulting from pulmonary congestion are less prominent initially; AF is almost invariably present once the LA dilates significantly.

SYMPTOMS

Patients with chronic mild-to-moderate isolated MR are usually asymptomatic. This form of LV volume overload is well tolerated. Fatigue, exertional dyspnea, and orthopnea are the most prominent complaints in patients with chronic severe MR. Palpitations are common and may signify the onset of AF. Right-sided heart failure, with painful hepatic congestion, ankle edema, distended neck veins, ascites, and secondary TR, occurs in patients with MR who have associated pulmonary vascular disease and marked pulmonary hypertension. Conversely, acute pulmonary edema is common in patients with acute severe MR.

PHYSICAL FINDINGS

In patients with chronic severe MR, the arterial pressure is usually normal, although the carotid arterial pulse may show a sharp upstroke owing to the reduced forward cardiac output. A systolic thrill is often palpable at the cardiac apex, the LV is hyperdynamic with a brisk systolic impulse and a palpable rapid-filling wave (S_3), and the apex beat is often displaced laterally.

In patients with acute severe MR, the arterial pressure may be reduced with a narrow pulse pressure, the jugular venous pressure and wave forms may be normal or increased and exaggerated, the apical impulse is not displaced, and signs of pulmonary congestion are prominent.

Auscultation

S_1 is generally absent, soft, or buried in the holosystolic murmur of chronic MR. In patients with severe MR, the aortic valve may close prematurely, resulting in wide but physiologic splitting of S_2. A low-pitched S_3 occurring 0.12–0.17 s after the aortic valve closure sound, i.e., at the completion of the rapid-filling phase of the LV, is believed to be caused by the sudden tensing of the papillary muscles, chordae tendineae, and valve leaflets. It may be followed by a short, rumbling, mid-diastolic murmur, even in the absence of structural MS. A fourth heart sound is often audible in patients with *acute* severe MR who are in sinus rhythm. A presystolic murmur is not ordinarily heard with isolated MR.

A systolic murmur of at least grade III/VI intensity is the most characteristic auscultatory finding in chronic severe MR. It is usually holosystolic (see Fig. 9-5A), but as previously noted it is decrescendo and ceases in mid- to late systole in patients with acute severe MR. The systolic murmur of chronic MR is usually most prominent at the apex and radiates to the axilla. However, in patients with ruptured chordae tendineae or primary involvement of the posterior mitral leaflet with prolapse or flail, the regurgitant jet is eccentric, directed anteriorly, and strikes the LA wall adjacent to the aortic root. In this situation, the systolic murmur is transmitted to the base of the heart and, therefore, may be confused with the murmur of AS. In patients with ruptured chordae tendineae, the systolic murmur may have a cooing or "seagull" quality, while a flail leaflet may produce a murmur with a musical quality. The systolic murmur of chronic MR not due to MVP is intensified by isometric exercise (hand grip) but is reduced during the strain phase of the Valsalva maneuver because of the associated decrease in LV preload.

LABORATORY EXAMINATION

ECG

In patients with sinus rhythm, there is evidence of LA enlargement, but RA enlargement also may be present when pulmonary hypertension is severe. Chronic severe MR is generally associated with AF. In many patients, there is no clear-cut ECG evidence of enlargement of either ventricle. In others, the signs of eccentric LV hypertrophy are present.

Echocardiogram

TTE is indicated to assess the mechanism of the MR and its hemodynamic severity. LV function can be assessed from LV end-diastolic and end-systolic volumes and EF. Observations can be made regarding leaflet structure and function, chordal integrity, LA and LV size, annular calcification, and regional and global LV systolic function. Doppler imaging should demonstrate the width or area of the color flow MR jet within the LA, the intensity of the continuous wave Doppler signal, the pulmonary venous flow contour, the early peak mitral inflow velocity, and the quantitative measures of regurgitant volume, RF, and effective regurgitant orifice area. In addition, the PA pressures can be estimated from the TR jet velocity. TTE is also indicated to follow the course of patients with chronic MR and to provide rapid assessment for any clinical change. The echocardiogram in patients with MVP is described in the next section. TEE provides greater detail than TTE (see Fig. 12-5).

Chest x-ray

The LA and LV are the dominant chambers in chronic MR. Late in the course of the disease, the LA may be massively enlarged and forms the right border of the cardiac silhouette. Pulmonary venous congestion, interstitial edema, and Kerley B lines are sometimes noted. Marked calcification of the mitral leaflets occurs commonly in patients with long–standing, combined rheumatic MR and MS. Calcification of the mitral annulus may be visualized, particularly on the lateral view of the chest. Patients with acute severe MR may have asymmetric pulmonary edema if the regurgitant jet is directed predominantly to the orifice of an upper lobe pulmonary vein.

TREATMENT 〉 **Mitral Regurgitation**

MEDICAL TREATMENT (See **Fig. 20-4** and Table 20-2) The management of chronic severe MR depends to some degree on its cause. Warfarin should be provided once AF intervenes with a target INR of 2–3. Cardioversion should be considered depending on the clinical context and left atrial size. In contrast to the acute setting, there are no large, long-term prospective studies to substantiate the use of vasodilators for the

treatment of chronic, isolated severe MR with preserved LV systolic function *in the absence of systemic hypertension*. The severity of MR in the setting of an ischemic or nonischemic dilated cardiomyopathy may diminish with aggressive, evidence-based treatment of heart failure, including the use of diuretics, beta blockers, angiotensin-converting enzyme (ACE) inhibitors, digitalis, and biventricular pacing (cardiac resynchronization therapy [CRT]). Asymptomatic patients with severe MR in sinus rhythm with normal LV size and systolic function should avoid isometric forms of exercise.

Patients with acute severe MR require urgent stabilization and preparation for surgery. Diuretics, intravenous vasodilators (particularly sodium nitroprusside), and even intraaortic balloon counterpulsation may be needed for patients with post-MI papillary muscle rupture or other forms of acute severe MR.

SURGICAL TREATMENT In the selection of patients with chronic, nonischemic, severe MR for surgical treatment, the often slowly progressive nature of the condition must be balanced against the immediate and long-term risks associated with operation. These risks are significantly lower for primary valve repair than for valve replacement (Table 20-3). Repair usually consists of valve reconstruction using a variety of valvuloplasty techniques and insertion of an annuloplasty ring. Repair

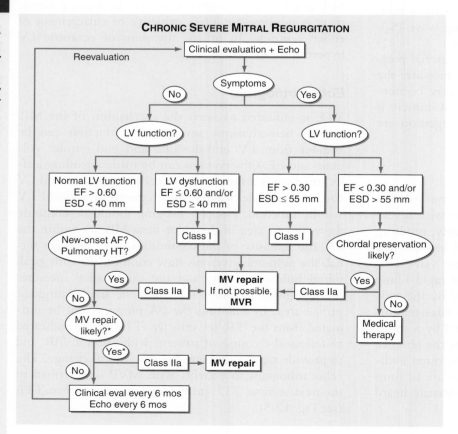

FIGURE 20-4

Management strategy for patients with chronic severe nonischemic mitral regurgitation. *Mitral valve (MV) repair may be performed in asymptomatic patients with normal left ventricular (LV) function if performed by an experienced surgical team and if the likelihood of successful MV repair is >90%. AF, atrial fibrillation; Echo, echocardiography; EF, ejection fraction; ESD, end-systolic dimension; eval, evaluation; HT, hypertension; MVR, mitral valve replacement. (*From RO Bonow et al: J Am Coll Cardiol 48:e1, 2006; with permission.*)

spares the patient the long-term adverse consequences of valve replacement, i.e., thromboembolic and hemorrhagic complications in the case of mechanical prostheses and late valve failure necessitating repeat valve replacement in the case of bioprostheses. In addition, by preserving the integrity of the papillary muscles, subvalvular apparatus, and chordae tendineae, mitral repair and valvuloplasty maintain LV function to a relatively greater degree.

Surgery for chronic, nonischemic, severe MR is indicated once symptoms occur, especially if valve repair is feasible (Fig. 20-4). Other indications for early consideration of mitral valve repair include recent-onset AF and pulmonary hypertension, defined as a PA pressure ≥50 mmHg at rest or ≥60 mmHg with exercise. Surgical treatment of chronic, nonischemic severe MR is indicated for asymptomatic patients when LV dysfunction is progressive, with LVEF falling below 60% and/or end-systolic dimension increasing beyond 40 mm. These aggressive recommendations for surgery are predicated on the outstanding results achieved with mitral valve repair, particularly when applied to patients with myxomatous disease, such as that associated with prolapse or flail leaflet. Indeed, primary valvuloplasty repair of patients younger than 75 years with normal LV systolic function and no CAD can now be performed by experienced surgeons with <1% perioperative mortality risk. Repair is feasible in up to 95% of patients with myxomatous disease. Long-term durability is excellent; the incidence of reoperative surgery for failed primary repair is ~1% per year for 10 years after surgery. For patients with AF, left or bi-atrial Maze surgery or radio-frequency isolation of the pulmonary veins is often performed to reduce the risk of recurrent, postoperative AF.

The surgical management of patients with ischemic MR is more complicated and almost always involves simultaneous coronary artery revascularization. Although current surgical practice includes annuloplasty repair with an undersized ring for patients with moderate or greater degrees of MR at the time of coronary artery bypass surgery, the efficacy of this approach has not been established in prospective, randomized trials. There is also uncertainty as to whether or not valve repair or replacement is the preferred strategy, given the higher incidence of residual or recurrent MR after repair in this context compared with outcomes in patients with organic (myxomatous) disease. In patients with significantly impaired LV function (EF <30%), the risk of surgery increases, the recovery of LV performance is incomplete, and the long-term survival is reduced. However, conservative management has little to offer these patients, so operative treatment may be indicated, and the clinical and hemodynamic improvement that follows surgical treatment of patients with advanced disease is occasionally dramatic, especially when severe

CAD is present and bypass grafting can be performed. The routine performance of valve repair in patients with significant MR in the setting of severe, dilated cardiomyopathy has not been shown to improve long-term survival. Patients with acute severe MR can often be stabilized temporarily with appropriate medical therapy, but surgical correction will be necessary, emergently in the case of papillary muscle rupture and within days to weeks in most other settings.

When surgical treatment is contemplated, left and right heart catheterization and left ventriculography *may* be helpful in confirming the presence of severe MR in patients in whom there is a discrepancy between the clinical and TTE findings that cannot be resolved with TEE or CMR. Coronary angiography identifies patients who require concomitant coronary revascularization.

PERCUTANEOUS MITRAL VALVE REPAIR

A transcatheter approach to the treatment of either organic or functional MR may be feasible in selected patients with appropriate anatomy, although the proper role of current techniques remains under active investigation. One approach involves the deployment of a clip delivered via transeptal puncture that grasps the leading edges of the mitral leaflets in their midportion (anterior scallop 2–posterior scallop 2 or A2-P2, **Fig. 20-5**). The length and width of the gap between these leading edges have dictated patient eligibility in the trials reported to date. Preliminary results with this technically demanding technique have been favorable. A second approach involves the deployment of a device within the coronary sinus that can be adjusted to reduce its circumference, thus secondarily decreasing the circumference

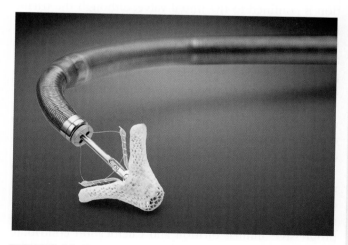

FIGURE 20-5

Clip used to grasp the free edges of the anterior and posterior leaflets in their midsections during percutaneous repair of selected patients with mitral regurgitation. (*Courtesy of Abbott Vascular. © 2010 Abbott Laboratories. All rights reserved.*)

of the mitral annulus and the effective orifice area of the valve, much like a surgically implanted ring. Variations in the anatomic relationship of the coronary sinus to the mitral annulus and circumflex coronary artery have limited the applicability of this technique. Attempts to reduce the septal-lateral dimension of a dilated annulus using adjustable cords placed across the LV in a subvalvular location have also been investigated.

MITRAL VALVE PROLAPSE

MVP, also variously termed the *systolic click-murmur syndrome, Barlow's syndrome, floppy-valve syndrome,* and *billowing mitral leaflet syndrome,* is a relatively common but highly variable clinical syndrome resulting from diverse pathologic mechanisms of the mitral valve apparatus. Among these are excessive or redundant mitral leaflet tissue, which is commonly associated with myxomatous degeneration and greatly increased concentrations of certain glycosaminoglycans.

In most patients with MVP, the cause is unknown, but in some it appears to be a genetically determined collagen disorder. A reduction in the production of type III collagen has been incriminated, and electron microscopy has revealed fragmentation of collagen fibrils.

MVP is a frequent finding in patients with heritable disorders of connective tissue, including Marfan's syndrome, osteogenesis imperfecta, and Ehlers-Danlos syndrome. MVP may be associated with thoracic skeletal deformities similar to but not as severe as those in Marfan's syndrome, such as a high-arched palate and alterations of the chest and thoracic spine, including the so-called straight back syndrome.

In most patients with MVP, myxomatous degeneration is confined to the mitral valve, although the tricuspid and aortic valves may also be affected. The posterior mitral leaflet is usually more affected than the anterior, and the mitral valve annulus is often dilated. In many patients, elongated, redundant, or ruptured chordae tendineae cause or contribute to the regurgitation.

MVP also may occur rarely as a sequel to acute rheumatic fever, in ischemic heart disease, and in various cardiomyopathies, as well as in 20% of patients with ostium secundum atrial septal defect.

MVP may lead to excessive stress on the papillary muscles, which, in turn, leads to dysfunction and ischemia of the papillary muscles and the subjacent ventricular myocardium. Rupture of chordae tendineae and progressive annular dilation and calcification contribute to valvular regurgitation, which then places more stress on the diseased mitral valve apparatus, thereby creating a vicious circle. The ECG changes (see later in this chapter) and ventricular arrhythmias appear to result from regional ventricular dysfunction related to the increased stress placed on the papillary muscles.

CLINICAL FEATURES

MVP is more common in women and occurs most frequently between the ages of 15 and 30 years; the clinical course is most often benign. MVP may also be observed in older (>50 years) patients, often men, in whom MR is often more severe and requires surgical treatment. There is an increased familial incidence for some patients, suggesting an autosomal dominant form of inheritance with incomplete penetrance. MVP varies in its clinical expression, ranging from only a systolic click and murmur with mild prolapse of the posterior leaflet to severe MR due to chordal rupture and leaflet flail. The degree of myxomatous change of the leaflets can also vary widely. In many patients, the condition progresses over years or decades; in others it worsens rapidly as a result of chordal rupture or endocarditis.

Most patients are asymptomatic and remain so for their entire lives. However, in North America, MVP is now the most common cause of isolated severe MR requiring surgical treatment. Arrhythmias, most commonly ventricular premature contractions and paroxysmal supraventricular and ventricular tachycardia, as well as AF, have been reported and may cause palpitations, light-headedness, and syncope. Sudden death is a very rare complication and occurs most often in patients with severe MR and depressed LV systolic function. There may be an excess risk of sudden death among patients with a flail leaflet. Many patients have chest pain that is difficult to evaluate; it is often substernal, prolonged, and not related to exertion, but may rarely resemble angina pectoris. Transient cerebral ischemic attacks secondary to emboli from the mitral valve due to endothelial disruption have been reported. Infective endocarditis may occur in patients with MR and/or leaflet thickening.

Auscultation

The most important finding is the mid- or late (nonejection) systolic click, which occurs 0.14 s or more after S_1 and is thought to be generated by the sudden tensing of slack, elongated chordae tendineae or by the prolapsing mitral leaflet when it reaches its maximum excursion. Systolic clicks may be multiple and may be followed by a high-pitched, late systolic crescendo-decrescendo murmur, which occasionally is "whooping" or "honking" and is heard best at the apex. The click and murmur occur earlier with standing, during the strain phase of the Valsalva maneuver, and with any intervention that decreases LV volume, exaggerating the propensity of mitral leaflet prolapse. Conversely, squatting and isometric exercises, which increase LV volume, diminish MVP; the click-murmur complex is delayed, moves away from S_1, and may even disappear. Some patients have a mid-systolic click without a murmur;

others have a murmur without a click. Still others have both sounds at different times.

LABORATORY EXAMINATION

The ECG most commonly is normal but may show biphasic or inverted T waves in leads II, III, and aVF, and occasionally supraventricular or ventricular premature beats. TTE is particularly effective in identifying the abnormal position and prolapse of the mitral valve leaflets. A useful echocardiographic definition of MVP is systolic displacement (in the parasternal long axis view) of the mitral valve leaflets by at least 2 mm into the LA superior to the plane of the mitral annulus. Color flow and continuous wave Doppler imaging is helpful to evaluate the associated MR and provide semiquantitative estimates of severity. The jet lesion of MR due to MVP is most often eccentric, and assessment of RF and effective regurgitant orifice area can be difficult. TEE is indicated when more accurate information is required and is performed routinely for intraoperative guidance for valve repair. Invasive left ventriculography is rarely necessary but can also show prolapse of the posterior and sometimes of both mitral valve leaflets.

TREATMENT   Mitral Valve Prolapse

Infective endocarditis prophylaxis is indicated only for patients with a prior history of endocarditis. Beta blockers sometimes relieve chest pain and control palpitations. If the patient is symptomatic from severe MR, mitral valve repair (or rarely, replacement) is indicated (Fig. 20-4). Antiplatelet agents, such as aspirin, should be given to patients with transient ischemic attacks, and if these are not effective, anticoagulants, such as warfarin, should be considered. Warfarin is also indicated once AF intervenes.

AORTIC STENOSIS

AS occurs in about one-fourth of all patients with chronic valvular heart disease; approximately 80% of adult patients with symptomatic valvular AS are male.

ETIOLOGY AND PATHOGENESIS

(Table 20-1) AS in adults is due to degenerative calcification of the aortic cusps and occurs most commonly on a substrate of congenital disease (bicuspid aortic valve [BAV]), chronic (tri-)leaflet deterioration, or previous rheumatic inflammation. A recent pathologic study of specimens removed at the time of aortic valve replacement for AS showed that 53% were bicuspid and 4% unicuspid. Contrary to previous teachings, the process of aortic valve deterioration and calcification is not a passive one, but rather one that shares many features with vascular atherosclerosis, including endothelial dysfunction, lipid accumulation, inflammatory cell activation, cytokine release, and upregulation of several signaling pathways (Fig. 20-6). Eventually, valvular myofibroblasts differentiate phenotypically into osteoblasts and actively produce bone matrix proteins that allow for the deposition of calcium hydroxyapatite crystals. Genetic polymorphisms involving the vitamin D receptor, the estrogen receptor in postmenopausal women, interleukin 10, and apolipoprotein E4 have been linked to the development of calcific AS, and a strong familial clustering of cases has been reported from western France. Several traditional atherosclerotic risk factors have also been associated with the development and progression of calcific AS, including low-density lipoprotein (LDL)-cholesterol, lipoprotein a (Lp[a]), diabetes mellitus, smoking, chronic kidney disease, and the metabolic syndrome. The presence of aortic valve sclerosis (focal thickening and calcification of the leaflets not severe enough to cause obstruction) is associated with an excess risk of cardiovascular death and MI among persons older than age 65. Approximately 30% of persons older than 65 years exhibit aortic valve sclerosis, whereas 2% exhibit frank stenosis.

Rheumatic disease of the aortic leaflets produces commissural fusion, sometimes resulting in a bicuspid-appearing valve. This condition, in turn, makes the leaflets more susceptible to trauma and ultimately leads to fibrosis, calcification, and further narrowing. By the time the obstruction to LV outflow causes serious clinical disability, the valve is usually a rigid calcified mass, and careful examination may make it difficult or even impossible to determine the etiology of the underlying process. Rheumatic AS is almost always associated with involvement of the mitral valve and with AR. Mediastinal radiation can also result in late scarring, fibrosis, and calcification of the leaflets with AS.

BICUSPID AORTIC VALVE DISEASE

A bicuspid aortic valve (BAV) is the most common congenital heart valve defect and occurs in 0.5–1.4% of the population with a 2–4:1 male to female predominance. The inheritance pattern appears to be autosomal dominant with incomplete penetrance, although some have questioned an X-linked component as suggested by the prevalence of BAV disease among patients with Turner's syndrome. The prevalence of BAV disease among first-degree relatives of an affected individual is approximately 10%. A single gene defect to explain the majority of cases has not been identified, although a mutation in the *NOTCH1* gene has been described in some families.

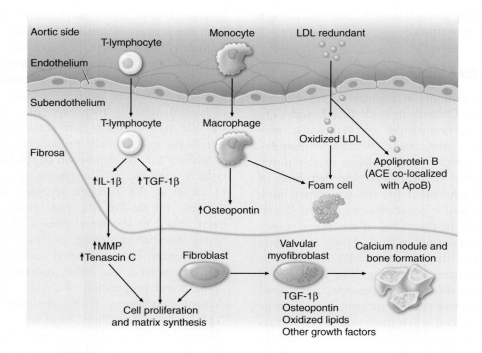

FIGURE 20-6

Pathogenesis of calcific aortic stenosis. Inflammatory cells infiltrate across the endothelial barrier and release cytokines that act on fibroblasts to promote cellular proliferation and matrix remodeling. LDL is oxidatively modified and taken up by macrophage scavengers to become foam cells. Angiotensin-converting enzyme colocalizes with Apo-B. A subset of myofibroblasts differentiate into an osteoblast phenotype capable of promoting bone formation. ACE, angiotensin-converting enzyme; ApoB, apolipoprotein B; LDL, low-density lipoprotein; IL, interleukin; MMP, matrix metalloproteinase; TGF, transforming growth factor. (*From RV Freeman, CM Otto: Circulation 111:3316, 2005; with permission.*)

Abnormalities in endothelial nitric oxide synthase and NKX2.5 have been implicated, as well. Aortic coarctation or medial degeneration with ascending aortic aneurysm formation occurs commonly among patients with BAV disease. Patients with BAV disease have larger aortas than patients with comparable tricuspid aortic valve disease. The aortopathy develops independent of the hemodynamic severity of the valve lesion and is a risk factor for dissection. A BAV can be a component of more complex congenital heart disease with or without other left heart obstructing lesions.

OTHER FORMS OF OBSTRUCTION TO LEFT VENTRICULAR OUTFLOW

In addition to valvular AS, three other lesions may be responsible for obstruction to LV outflow: *hypertrophic obstructive cardiomyopathy* (Chap. 21), *discrete fibromuscular/membranous subaortic stenosis*, and *supravalvular AS* (Chap. 19). The causes of left ventricular outflow obstruction can be differentiated on the basis of the cardiac examination and Doppler echocardiographic findings.

PATHOPHYSIOLOGY

The obstruction to LV outflow produces a systolic pressure gradient between the LV and aorta. When severe obstruction is suddenly produced experimentally, the LV responds by dilation and reduction of stroke volume. However, in some patients, the obstruction may be present at birth and/or increase gradually over the course of many years, and LV contractile performance is maintained by the presence of concentric LV hypertrophy. Initially, this serves as an adaptive mechanism because it reduces toward normal the systolic stress developed by the myocardium, as predicted by the Laplace relation ($S = Pr/h$, where S = systolic wall stress, P = pressure, r = radius, and h = wall thickness). A large transaortic valve pressure gradient may exist for many years without a reduction in CO or LV dilation; ultimately, however, excessive hypertrophy becomes maladaptive, LV systolic function declines, abnormalities of diastolic function progress, and irreversible myocardial fibrosis develops.

A mean systolic pressure gradient >40 mmHg with a normal CO or an effective aortic orifice area <~1 cm^2

(or ~<0.6 cm^2/m^2 body surface area in a normal-sized adult)—i.e., less than approximately one-third of the normal orifice area—is generally considered to represent severe obstruction to LV outflow. The elevated LV end-diastolic pressure observed in many patients with severe AS and preserved EF signifies the presence of diminished compliance of the hypertrophied LV. Although the CO at rest is within normal limits in most patients with severe AS, it usually fails to rise normally during exercise. Loss of an appropriately timed, vigorous atrial contraction, as occurs in AF or atrioventricular dissociation, may cause rapid progression of symptoms. Late in the course, contractile function deteriorates because of afterload excess, the CO and LV–aortic pressure gradient decline, and the mean LA, PA, and RV pressures rise. LV performance can be further compromised by superimposed CAD.

The hypertrophied LV causes an increase in myocardial oxygen requirements. In addition, even in the absence of obstructive CAD, coronary blood flow is impaired to the extent that ischemia can be precipitated under conditions of excess demand. Capillary density is reduced relative to wall thickness, compressive forces are increased, and the elevated LV end-diastolic pressure reduces the coronary driving pressure. The subendocardium is especially vulnerable to ischemia by this mechanism.

SYMPTOMS

AS is rarely of clinical importance until the valve orifice has narrowed to approximately 1 cm^2. Even severe AS may exist for many years without producing any symptoms because of the ability of the hypertrophied LV to generate the elevated intraventricular pressures required to maintain a normal stroke volume. Once symptoms occur, valve replacement is indicated.

Most patients with pure or predominant AS have gradually increasing obstruction over years, but do not become symptomatic until the sixth to eighth decades. Adult patients with BAV disease, however, develop significant valve dysfunction and symptoms one to two decades sooner. Exertional dyspnea, angina pectoris, and syncope are the three cardinal symptoms. Often, there is a history of insidious progression of fatigue and dyspnea associated with gradual curtailment of activities. *Dyspnea* results primarily from elevation of the pulmonary capillary pressure caused by elevations of LV diastolic pressures secondary to reduced left ventricular compliance and impaired relaxation. *Angina pectoris* usually develops somewhat later and reflects an imbalance between the augmented myocardial oxygen requirements and reduced oxygen availability. CAD may or may not be present, although its coexistence is common among AS patients older than age 65. *Exertional syncope* may result from a decline in arterial pressure caused by vasodilation

in the exercising muscles and inadequate vasoconstriction in nonexercising muscles in the face of a fixed CO, or from a sudden fall in CO produced by an arrhythmia.

Because the CO at rest is usually well maintained until late in the course, marked fatigability, weakness, peripheral cyanosis, cachexia, and other clinical manifestations of a low CO are usually not prominent until this stage is reached. Orthopnea, paroxysmal nocturnal dyspnea, and pulmonary edema, i.e., symptoms of LV failure, also occur only in the advanced stages of the disease. Severe pulmonary hypertension leading to RV failure and systemic venous hypertension, hepatomegaly, AF, and TR are usually late findings in patients with isolated severe AS.

When AS and MS coexist, the reduction in CO induced by MS lowers the pressure gradient across the aortic valve and, thereby, masks many of the clinical findings produced by AS.

PHYSICAL FINDINGS

The rhythm is generally regular until late in the course; at other times, AF should suggest the possibility of associated mitral valve disease. The systemic arterial pressure is usually within normal limits. In the late stages, however, when stroke volume declines, the systolic pressure may fall and the pulse pressure narrow. The peripheral arterial pulse rises slowly to a delayed peak (*pulsus parvus et tardus*). A thrill or anacrotic "shudder" may be palpable over the carotid arteries, more commonly the left. In the elderly, the stiffening of the arterial wall may mask this important physical sign. In many patients, the *a* wave in the jugular venous pulse is accentuated. This results from the diminished distensibility of the RV cavity caused by the bulging, hypertrophied interventricular septum.

The LV impulse is usually displaced laterally. A double apical impulse (with a palpable S$_4$) may be recognized, particularly with the patient in the left lateral recumbent position. A systolic thrill may be present at the base of the heart to the right of the sternum when leaning forward or in the suprasternal notch.

Auscultation

An early systolic ejection sound is frequently audible in children, adolescents, and young adults with congenital BAV disease. This sound usually disappears when the valve becomes calcified and rigid. As AS increases in severity, LV systole may become prolonged so that the aortic valve closure sound no longer precedes the pulmonic valve closure sound, and the two components may become synchronous, or aortic valve closure may even follow pulmonic valve closure, causing paradoxical splitting of S$_2$ (Chap. 9). The sound of aortic valve closure can be heard most frequently in patients with

AS who have pliable valves, and calcification diminishes the intensity of this sound. Frequently, an S_4 is audible at the apex and reflects the presence of LV hypertrophy and an elevated LV end-diastolic pressure; an S_3 generally occurs late in the course, when the LV dilates and its systolic function becomes severely compromised.

The murmur of AS is characteristically an ejection (mid)-systolic murmur that commences shortly after the S_1, increases in intensity to reach a peak toward the middle of ejection, and ends just before aortic valve closure. It is characteristically low pitched, rough and rasping in character, and loudest at the base of the heart, most commonly in the second right intercostal space. It is transmitted upward along the carotid arteries. Occasionally it is transmitted downward and to the apex, where it may be confused with the systolic murmur of MR (Gallavardin effect). In almost all patients with severe obstruction and preserved CO, the murmur is at least grade III/VI. In patients with mild degrees of obstruction or in those with severe stenosis with heart failure and low CO in whom the stroke volume and, therefore, the transvalvular flow rate are reduced, the murmur may be relatively soft and brief.

LABORATORY EXAMINATION

ECG

In most patients with severe AS there is LV hypertrophy. In advanced cases, ST-segment depression and T-wave inversion (LV "strain") in standard leads I and aVL and in the left precordial leads are evident. However, there is no close correlation between the ECG and the hemodynamic severity of obstruction, and the absence of ECG signs of LV hypertrophy does not exclude severe obstruction. Many patients with AS have systemic hypertension, which can also contribute to the development of hypertrophy.

Echocardiogram

The key findings on TTE are thickening, calcification, and reduced systolic opening of the valve leaflets and LV hypertrophy. Eccentric closure of the aortic valve cusps is characteristic of congenitally bicuspid valves. TEE imaging usually displays the obstructed orifice extremely well, but it is not routinely required for accurate characterization. The valve gradient and aortic valve area can be estimated by Doppler measurement of the transaortic velocity. Severe AS is defined by a valve area <1 cm², whereas moderate AS is defined by a valve area of 1–1.5 cm² and mild AS by a valve area of 1.5–2 cm². Aortic valve sclerosis, conversely, is accompanied by a jet velocity of less than 2.5 meters/s (peak gradient <25 mmHg). LV dilation and reduced systolic shortening reflect impairment of LV function. There is

increasing experience with the use of longitudinal strain and strain rate to characterize earlier changes in LV systolic function, well before a decline in EF can be appreciated. Doppler indices of impaired diastolic function are frequently seen.

Echocardiography is useful for identifying coexisting valvular abnormalities; for differentiating valvular AS from other forms of LV outflow obstruction; and for measurement of the aortic root and proximal ascending aortic dimension. These aortic measurements are particularly important for patients with BAV disease. Dobutamine stress echocardiography is useful for the evaluation of patients with AS and severe LV systolic dysfunction (EF <0.35), in whom the severity of the AS can often be difficult to judge.

Chest x-ray

The chest x-ray may show no or little overall cardiac enlargement for many years. Hypertrophy without dilation may produce some rounding of the cardiac apex in the frontal projection and slight backward displacement in the lateral view. A dilated proximal ascending aorta may be seen along the upper right heart border in the frontal view. Aortic valve calcification may be discernible in the lateral view, but is usually readily apparent on fluoroscopic examination or by echocardiography; the absence of valvular calcification in an adult suggests that severe valvular AS is *not* present. In later stages of the disease, as the LV dilates there is increasing roentgenographic evidence of LV enlargement, pulmonary congestion, and enlargement of the LA, PA, and right heart chambers.

Catheterization

Right and left heart catheterization for invasive assessment of AS is now performed infrequently but can be useful when there is a discrepancy between the clinical and Doppler echocardiographic findings. Appropriate concerns have been raised that attempts to cross the aortic valve for measurement of left ventricular pressures are associated with a risk of cerebral embolization. Catheterization is also useful in three distinct categories of patients: (1) *patients with multivalvular disease,* in whom the role played by each valvular deformity should be defined to aid in the planning of operative treatment; (2) *young, asymptomatic patients with noncalcific congenital AS,* to define the severity of obstruction to LV outflow, since operation or percutaneous aortic balloon valvoplasty (PABV) may be indicated in these patients if severe AS is present, even in the absence of symptoms; balloon valvotomy may follow left heart catheterization in the same sitting; and (3) *patients in whom it is suspected that the obstruction to LV outflow may not be at the level of the aortic valve* but rather at the sub- or supravalvular level.

Coronary angiography is indicated to detect or exclude CAD in appropriate patients with severe AS who are being considered for surgery. The incidence of significant CAD for which bypass grafting is indicated at the time of aortic valve replacement (AVR) exceeds 50% among adult patients.

NATURAL HISTORY

Death in patients with severe AS occurs most commonly in the seventh and eighth decades. Based on data obtained at postmortem examination in patients before surgical treatment became widely available, the average time to death after the onset of various symptoms was as follows: angina pectoris, 3 years; syncope, 3 years; dyspnea, 2 years; congestive heart failure, 1.5–2 years. Moreover, in >80% of patients who died with AS, symptoms had existed for <4 years. Among adults dying with valvular AS, sudden death, which presumably resulted from an arrhythmia, occurred in 10–20%; however, most sudden deaths occurred in patients who had previously been symptomatic. Sudden death as the first manifestation of severe AS is very uncommon (<1% per year) in asymptomatic adult patients. Calcific AS is a progressive disease, with an annual reduction in valve area averaging 0.1 cm² and annual increases in the peak jet velocity and mean valve gradient averaging 0.3 meters/s and 7 mmHg, respectively (Table 20-2, **Fig. 20-7**).

TREATMENT   Aortic Stenosis

MEDICAL TREATMENT   In patients with severe AS (valve area <1 cm²), strenuous physical activity and competitive sports should be avoided, even in the asymptomatic stage. Care must be taken to avoid dehydration and hypovolemia to protect against a significant reduction in CO. Medications used for the treatment of hypertension or CAD, including beta blockers and ACE inhibitors, are generally safe for asymptomatic patients with preserved left ventricular systolic function. Nitroglycerin is helpful in relieving angina pectoris in patients with CAD. Retrospective studies have shown that patients with degenerative calcific AS who receive HMG-CoA reductase inhibitors ("statins") exhibit slower progression of leaflet calcification and aortic valve area reduction than those who do not. However, randomized prospective studies with either high-dose atorvastatin or combination simvastatin/ezetimibe have failed to show a measurable effect on valve-related outcomes. The use of statin medications should continue to be driven by considerations regarding primary and secondary prevention of CAD. ACE inhibitors have not been studied prospectively for AS-related outcomes. The need for endocarditis prophylaxis is restricted to AS patients with a prior history of endocarditis.

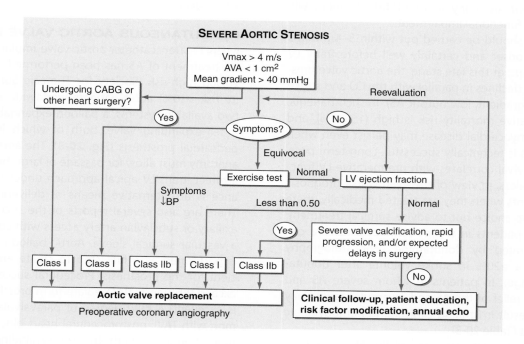

FIGURE 20-7

Management strategy for patients with severe aortic stenosis. Preoperative coronary angiography should be performed routinely as determined by age, symptoms, and coronary risk factors. Cardiac catheterization and angiography may also be helpful when there is a discrepancy between clinical findings and echocardiography. AVA, aortic valve area; BP, blood pressure; CABG, coronary artery bypass graft surgery; echo, echocardiography; LV, left ventricle; Vmax, maximal velocity across aortic valve by Doppler echocardiography. (*From RO Bonow et al: Circulation 114:450, 2006. Modified from CM Otto: J Am Coll Cardiol 47:2141, 2006.*)

SURGICAL TREATMENT Asymptomatic patients with calcific AS and severe obstruction should be followed carefully for the development of symptoms and by serial echocardiograms for evidence of deteriorating LV function. Operation is indicated in patients with severe AS (valve area <1 cm^2 or 0.6 cm^2/m^2 body surface area) who are symptomatic, those who exhibit LV dysfunction (EF <50%), as well as those with BAV disease and an aneurysmal or expanding aortic root (maximal dimension >4.5 cm or annual increase in size >0.5 cm/year), even if they are asymptomatic. Patients with asymptomatic moderate or severe AS who are referred for CABG surgery should also have AVR. In patients without heart failure, the operative risk of AVR is approximately 3% (Table 20-3) but increases as a function of age and the need for concomitant coronary revascularization with bypass grafting. The indications for AVR in the asymptomatic patient have been the subject of intense debate over the past 5 years, as surgical outcomes in selected patients have continued to improve. Relative indications for which surgery can be considered include an abnormal response to treadmill exercise; rapid progression of AS, especially when urgent access to medical care might be compromised; very severe AS defined by a valve area <0.6 cm^2; and severe LV hypertrophy suggested by a wall thickness of >15 mm. Exercise testing can be safely performed in the asymptomatic patient, as many as one-third of whom will show signs of functional impairment.

Operation should be carried out within 3–4 months of symptom onset and certainly well before frank LV failure develops; at this late stage, the aortic valve pressure gradient declines in parallel with the CO and stroke volume (low gradient, low output AS). In such patients, the perioperative mortality risk is high (15–20%), and evidence of myocardial disease may persist even when the operation is technically successful. Long-term postoperative survival correlates with preoperative LV function. Nonetheless, in view of the even worse prognosis of such patients when they are treated medically, there is usually little choice but to advise surgical treatment, especially in patients in whom contractile reserve can be demonstrated by dobutamine echocardiography (defined by a ≥20% in stroke volume after dobutamine challenge). In patients in whom severe AS and CAD coexist, relief of the AS and revascularization may sometimes result in striking clinical and hemodynamic improvement (Table 20-3).

Because many patients with calcific AS are elderly, particular attention must be directed to the adequacy of hepatic, renal, and pulmonary function before AVR is recommended. Age alone is not a contraindication to AVR for AS. The mortality rate depends to a substantial extent on the patient's preoperative clinical and hemodynamic

state. The 10-year survival rate of patients with AVR is approximately 60%. Approximately 30% of bioprosthetic valves evidence primary valve failure in 10 years, requiring re-replacement, and an approximately equal percentage of patients with mechanical prostheses develop significant hemorrhagic complications as a consequence of treatment with anticoagulants. Homograft AVR is usually reserved for patients with aortic valve endocarditis.

The Ross procedure involves replacement of the diseased aortic valve with the autologous pulmonic valve and implantation of a homograft in the native pulmonic position. Its use has declined considerably in the United States because of the technical complexity of the procedure and the incidence of late postoperative aortic root dilation and autograft failure with AR. There is also a low incidence of homograft stenosis.

PERCUTANEOUS BALLOON AORTIC VALVULOPLASTY This procedure is preferable to operation in many children and young adults with congenital, noncalcific AS (Chap. 19). It is not commonly used in adults with severe calcific AS because of a very high restenosis rate (80% within 1 year) and the risk of procedural complications, but on occasion it has been used successfully as a "bridge to operation" in patients with severe LV dysfunction and shock who are too ill to tolerate surgery.

PERCUTANEOUS AORTIC VALVE REPLACEMENT Transcatheter aortic valve implantation (TAVI) for treatment of AS has been performed in more than 20,000 high-risk (Society for Thoracic Surgery mortality risk >10%) adult patients worldwide using one of two available systems, a balloon-expandable valve and a self-expanding valve, both of which incorporate a pericardial prosthesis (Fig. 20-8). The aorto-iliofemoral anatomy must allow for passage of large-bore catheters; a direct, trans-LV apical approach under surgical guidance is an alternative means of delivering the valve. There are also several reports of the successful use of axillary or subclavian artery access with construction of a vascular surgical sleeve. Aortic balloon valvuloplasty is performed as a first step to create an orifice sufficient for the prosthesis. Procedural success rates now exceed 90%, and intermediate-term prosthetic function is excellent. A mild degree of paravalvular AR is common with TAVI; postprocedural heart block is observed more frequently with the self-expanding valve. Preliminary results with TAVI have been very favorable (Fig. 20-9), and it is anticipated that this technology, now clinically available in Canada and Europe, will gain regulatory approval in the United States for the treatment of patients with severe AS considered too high

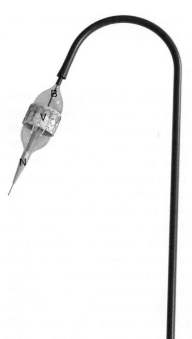

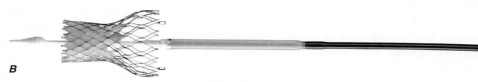

FIGURE 20-8

(*A*) Balloon-expandable and (*B*) and self-expanding valves for percutaneous aortic valve replacement. B, inflated balloon; N, nose cone; V, valve. (*Part A, courtesy of Edwards Lifesciences, Irvine, CA; with permission. RetroFlex 3 is a trademark of Edwards Lifesciences Corporation. Part B, © Medtronic, Inc. 2010. Medtronic CoreValve Transcatheter Aortic Valve. CoreValve is a registered trademark of Medtronic, Inc.*)

A

risk for surgical AVR. For elderly patients with symptomatic, severe AS who are deemed too high risk for surgery, TAVI has been shown in a randomized prospective trial to prolong life and improve functionality. The use of these devices for the treatment of prosthetic valve failure not due to paravalvular regurgitation ("valve-in-valve"), as an alternative to reoperative valve replacement, is also under active study.

AORTIC REGURGITATION

ETIOLOGY

(Table 20-1) AR may be caused by primary valve disease or by primary aortic root disease.

Primary valve disease

Rheumatic disease results in thickening, deformity, and shortening of the individual aortic valve cusps, changes

CHAPTER 20 Valvular Heart Disease

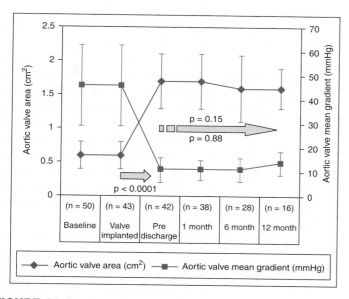

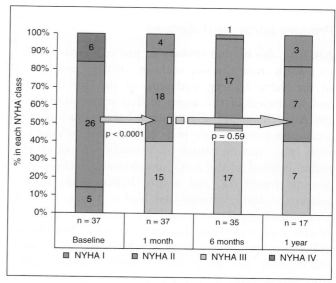

FIGURE 20-9

Twelve-month outcomes following percutaneous aortic valve replacement. (*Adapted from JG Webb et al: Circulation 116:755, 2007; with permission.*)

237

that prevent their proper opening during systole and closure during diastole. A rheumatic origin is much less common in patients with isolated AR who do not have associated rheumatic mitral valve disease. Patients with congenital BAV disease may develop predominant AR, and approximately 20% of patients will require aortic valve surgery between 10 and 40 years of age. Congenital fenestrations of the aortic valve occasionally produce mild AR. Membranous subaortic stenosis often leads to thickening and scarring of the aortic valve leaflets with secondary AR. Prolapse of an aortic cusp, resulting in progressive chronic AR, occurs in approximately 15% of patients with ventricular septal defect (Chap. 19) but may also occur as an isolated phenomenon or as a consequence of myxomatous degeneration sometimes associated with mitral and/or tricuspid valve involvement.

AR may result from infective endocarditis, which can develop on a valve previously affected by rheumatic disease, a congenitally deformed valve, or on a normal aortic valve, and may lead to perforation or erosion of one or more leaflets. The aortic valve leaflets may become scarred and retracted during the course of syphilis or ankylosing spondylitis and contribute further to the AR that derives primarily from the associated root disease. Although traumatic rupture or avulsion of the aortic valve is an uncommon cause of acute AR, it does represent the most frequent serious lesion in patients surviving nonpenetrating cardiac injuries. The coexistence of hemodynamically significant AS with AR usually excludes all the rarer forms of AR because it occurs almost exclusively in patients with rheumatic or congenital AR. In patients with AR due to primary valvular disease, dilation of the aortic annulus may occur secondarily and lead to worsening regurgitation.

Primary aortic root disease

AR may also be due entirely to marked aortic dilation, i.e., aortic root disease, without primary involvement of the valve leaflets; widening of the aortic annulus and separation of the aortic leaflets are responsible for the AR (Chap. 38). Cystic medial degeneration of the ascending aorta, which may or may not be associated with other manifestations of Marfan's syndrome; idiopathic dilation of the aorta; annuloaortic ectasia; osteogenesis imperfecta; and severe hypertension may all widen the aortic annulus and lead to progressive AR. Occasionally, AR is caused by retrograde dissection of the aorta involving the aortic annulus. Syphilis and ankylosing spondylitis, both of which may affect aortic valves, may also be associated with cellular infiltration and scarring of the media of the thoracic aorta, leading to aortic dilation, aneurysm formation, and severe regurgitation. In syphilis of the aorta, now a very rare condition, the involvement of the intima may narrow the coronary ostia, which in turn may be responsible for myocardial ischemia.

PATHOPHYSIOLOGY

The total stroke volume ejected by the LV (i.e., the sum of the effective forward stroke volume and the volume of blood that regurgitates back into the LV) is increased in patients with AR. In patients with severe AR, the volume of regurgitant flow may equal the effective forward stroke volume. In contrast to MR, in which a portion of the LV stroke volume is delivered into the low-pressure LA, in AR the entire LV stroke volume is ejected into a high-pressure zone, the aorta. An increase in the LV end-diastolic volume (increased preload) constitutes the major hemodynamic compensation for AR. The dilation and eccentric hypertrophy of the LV allow this chamber to eject a larger stroke volume without requiring any increase in the relative shortening of each myofibril. Therefore, severe AR may occur with a normal effective forward stroke volume and a normal left ventricular EF (total [forward plus regurgitant] stroke volume/end-diastolic volume), together with an elevated LV end-diastolic pressure and volume. However, through the operation of Laplace's law, LV dilation increases the LV systolic tension required to develop any given level of systolic pressure. Chronic AR is, thus, a state in which LV preload and afterload are both increased. Ultimately, these adaptive measures fail. As LV function deteriorates, the end-diastolic volume rises further and the forward stroke volume and EF decline. Deterioration of LV function often precedes the development of symptoms. Considerable thickening of the LV wall also occurs with chronic AR, and at autopsy the hearts of these patients may be among the largest encountered, sometimes weighing >1000 g.

The reverse pressure gradient from aorta to LV, which drives the AR flow, falls progressively during diastole, accounting for the decrescendo nature of the diastolic murmur. Equilibration between aortic and LV pressures may occur toward the end of diastole in patients with chronic severe AR, particularly when the heart rate is slow. In patients with acute severe AR, the LV is unprepared for the regurgitant volume load. LV compliance is normal or reduced, and LV diastolic pressures rise rapidly, occasionally to levels >40 mmHg. The LV pressure may exceed the LA pressure toward the end of diastole, and this reversed pressure gradient closes the mitral valve prematurely.

In patients with chronic severe AR, the effective forward CO usually is normal or only slightly reduced at rest, but often it fails to rise normally during exertion. An early sign of LV dysfunction is a reduction in the EF. In advanced stages there may be considerable elevation of the LA, PA wedge, PA, and RV pressures and lowering of the forward CO at rest.

Myocardial ischemia may occur in patients with AR because myocardial oxygen requirements are elevated by LV dilation, hypertrophy, and elevated LV systolic tension, and coronary blood flow may be compromised. A large fraction of coronary blood flow occurs during diastole, when arterial pressure is low, thereby reducing coronary perfusion or driving pressure. This combination of increased oxygen demand and reduced supply may cause myocardial ischemia, particularly of the subendocardium, even in the absence of concomitant CAD.

HISTORY

Approximately three-fourths of patients with pure or predominant valvular AR are men; women predominate among patients with primary valvular AR who have associated rheumatic mitral valve disease. A history compatible with infective endocarditis may sometimes be elicited from patients with rheumatic or congenital involvement of the aortic valve, and the infection often precipitates or seriously aggravates preexisting symptoms.

In patients with *acute severe AR,* as may occur in infective endocarditis, aortic dissection, or trauma, the LV cannot dilate sufficiently to maintain stroke volume, and LV diastolic pressure rises rapidly with associated marked elevations of LA and PA wedge pressures. Pulmonary edema and/or cardiogenic shock may develop rapidly.

Chronic severe AR may have a long latent period, and patients may remain relatively asymptomatic for as long as 10–15 years. However, uncomfortable awareness of the heartbeat, especially on lying down, may be an early complaint. Sinus tachycardia, during exertion or with emotion, or premature ventricular contractions may produce particularly uncomfortable palpitations as well as head pounding. These complaints may persist for many years before the development of exertional dyspnea, usually the first symptom of diminished cardiac reserve. The dyspnea is followed by orthopnea, paroxysmal nocturnal dyspnea, and excessive diaphoresis. Anginal chest pain even in the absence of CAD may occur in patients with severe AR, even in younger patients. Anginal pain may develop at rest as well as during exertion. Nocturnal angina may be a particularly troublesome symptom, and it may be accompanied by marked diaphoresis. The anginal episodes can be prolonged and often do not respond satisfactorily to sublingual nitroglycerin. Systemic fluid accumulation, including congestive hepatomegaly and ankle edema, may develop late in the course of the disease.

PHYSICAL FINDINGS

In chronic severe AR, the jarring of the entire body and the bobbing motion of the head with each systole can be appreciated, and the abrupt distention and collapse of the larger arteries are easily visible. The examination should be directed toward the detection of conditions predisposing to AR, such as bicuspid valve, endocarditis, Marfan's syndrome, and ankylosing spondylitis.

Arterial pulse

A rapidly rising "water-hammer" pulse, which collapses suddenly as arterial pressure falls rapidly during late systole and diastole (Corrigan's pulse), and capillary pulsations, an alternate flushing and paling of the skin at the root of the nail while pressure is applied to the tip of the nail (Quincke's pulse), are characteristic of chronic severe AR. A booming "pistol-shot" sound can be heard over the femoral arteries (Traube's sign), and a to-and-fro murmur (Duroziez's sign) is audible if the femoral artery is lightly compressed with a stethoscope.

The arterial pulse pressure is widened as a result of both systolic hypertension and a lowering of the diastolic pressure. The measurement of arterial diastolic pressure with a sphygmomanometer may be complicated by the fact that systolic sounds are frequently heard with the cuff completely deflated. However, the level of cuff pressure at the time of muffling of the Korotkoff sounds (phase IV) generally corresponds fairly closely to the true intraarterial diastolic pressure. As the disease progresses and the LV end-diastolic pressure rises, the arterial diastolic pressure may actually rise as well, because the aortic diastolic pressure cannot fall below the LV end-diastolic pressure. For the same reason, acute severe AR may also be accompanied by only a slight widening of the pulse pressure. Such patients are invariably tachycardic as the heart rate increases in an attempt to preserve the CO.

Palpation

In patients with chronic severe AR, the LV impulse is heaving and displaced laterally and inferiorly. The systolic expansion and diastolic retraction of the apex are prominent. A diastolic thrill may be palpable along the left sternal border in thin-chested individuals, and a prominent systolic thrill may be palpable in the suprasternal notch and transmitted upward along the carotid arteries. This systolic thrill and the accompanying murmur do not necessarily signify the coexistence of AS. In many patients with pure AR or with combined AS and AR, the carotid arterial pulse is bisferiens, i.e., with two systolic waves separated by a trough (see Fig. 9-2D).

Auscultation

In patients with severe AR, the aortic valve closure sound (A_2) is usually absent. A systolic ejection sound is audible in patients with BAV disease, and occasionally an S$_4$ also may be heard. The murmur of chronic AR is typically a high-pitched, blowing, decrescendo diastolic murmur, heard best in the third intercostal space along the left sternal border (see Fig. 9-5B). In patients with mild AR, this murmur is brief, but as the severity increases, it generally becomes louder and longer, indeed holodiastolic. When the murmur is soft, it can be heard best with the diaphragm of the stethoscope and with the patient sitting up, leaning forward, and with the breath held in forced expiration. In patients in whom the AR is caused by primary valvular disease, the diastolic murmur is usually louder along the left than the right sternal border. However, when the murmur is heard best along the right sternal border, it suggests that the AR is caused by aneurysmal dilation of the aortic root. "Cooing" or musical diastolic murmurs suggest eversion of an aortic cusp vibrating in the regurgitant stream.

A mid-systolic ejection murmur is frequently audible in isolated AR. It is generally heard best at the base of the heart and is transmitted along the carotid arteries. This murmur may be quite loud without signifying aortic obstruction. A third murmur sometimes heard in patients with severe AR is the *Austin Flint murmur,* a soft, low-pitched, rumbling mid-to-late diastolic murmur. It is probably produced by the diastolic displacement of the anterior leaflet of the mitral valve by the AR stream and is not associated with hemodynamically significant mitral obstruction. The auscultatory features of AR are intensified by strenuous and sustained hand grip, which augments systemic vascular resistance.

In acute severe AR, the elevation of LV end-diastolic pressure may lead to early closure of the mitral valve, a soft S$_1$, a pulse pressure that is not particularly wide, and a soft, short, early diastolic murmur of AR.

LABORATORY EXAMINATION

ECG

In patients with chronic severe AR, the ECG signs of LV hypertrophy become manifest (Chap. 11). In addition, these patients frequently exhibit ST-segment depression and T-wave inversion in leads I, aVL, V$_5$, and V$_6$ ("LV strain"). Left-axis deviation and/or QRS prolongation denote diffuse myocardial disease, generally associated with patchy fibrosis, and usually signify a poor prognosis.

Echocardiogram

LV size is increased in chronic AR and systolic function is normal or even supernormal until myocardial contractility declines, as signaled by a decrease in ejection or increase in the end-systolic dimension. A rapid, high-frequency diastolic fluttering of the anterior mitral leaflet produced by the impact of the regurgitant jet is a characteristic finding. The echocardiogram is also useful in determining the cause of AR, by detecting dilation of the aortic annulus and root, aortic dissection (see Fig. 12-5), or primary leaflet pathology. With severe AR, the central jet width assessed by color flow Doppler imaging exceeds 65% of the left ventricular outflow tract, the regurgitant volume is ≥60 mL/beat, the regurgitant fraction is ≥50%, and there is diastolic flow reversal in the proximal descending thoracic aorta. The continuous wave Doppler profile shows a rapid deceleration time in patients with acute severe AR, due to the rapid increase in LV diastolic pressure. Surveillance transthoracic echocardiography forms the cornerstone of longitudinal follow-up and allows for the early detection of changes in LV size and/or function. For patients in whom echocardiography is limited by poor acoustical windows or inadequate semiquantitative assessment, gated cardiac MR imaging can be performed. This modality also allows for accurate assessment of aortic size and contour.

Chest x-ray

In chronic severe AR, the apex is displaced downward and to the left in the frontal projection. In the left anterior oblique and lateral projections, the LV is displaced posteriorly and encroaches on the spine. When AR is caused by primary disease of the aortic root, aneurysmal dilation of the aorta may be noted, and the aorta may fill the retrosternal space in the lateral view. Echocardiography, cardiac MR, and CT angiography are more sensitive than the chest x-ray for the detection of aortic root enlargement.

Cardiac catheterization and angiography

When needed, right and left heart catheterization with contrast aortography can provide confirmation of the magnitude of regurgitation and the status of LV function. Coronary angiography is performed routinely in appropriate patients prior to surgery.

TREATMENT   Aortic Regurgitation

ACUTE AORTIC REGURGITATION   (See Fig. 20-10) Patients with acute severe AR may respond to intravenous diuretics and vasodilators (such as sodium nitroprusside), but stabilization is usually short-lived and operation is indicated urgently. Intraaortic balloon counterpulsation is contraindicated. Beta blockers are also best avoided so as not to reduce the CO further or slow the heart rate. Surgery is the treatment of choice and is usually necessary within 24 h of diagnosis.

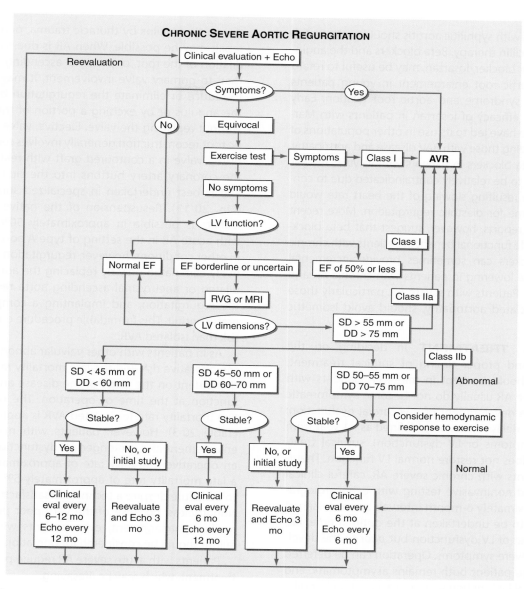

CHRONIC SEVERE AORTIC REGURGITATION

FIGURE 20-10

Management strategy for patients with chronic severe aortic regurgitation. Preoperative coronary angiography should be performed routinely, as determined by age, symptoms, and coronary risk factors. Cardiac catheterization and angiography may also be helpful when there is a discrepancy between clinical and echocardiographic findings. "Stable" refers to stable echocardiographic measurements. In some centers, serial follow-up may be performed with radionuclide ventriculography (RVG) or magnetic resonance imaging (MRI) rather than echocardiography (echo) to assess left ventricular (LV) volume and systolic function. AVR, aortic valve replacement; DD, end-diastolic dimension; EF, ejection fraction; eval, evaluation; SD, end-systolic dimension. (*Modified from RO Bonow et al: Circulation 114:450, 2006.*)

CHRONIC AORTIC REGURGITATION Early symptoms of dyspnea and effort intolerance respond to treatment with diuretics; vasodilators (ACE inhibitors, dihydropyridine calcium channel blockers, or hydralazine) may be useful as well. Surgery can then be performed in a more controlled setting. The use of vasodilators to extend the compensated phase of chronic severe AR before the onset of symptoms or the development of LV dysfunction is more controversial. Expert consensus is strong regarding the need to control systolic blood pressure (goal <140 mmHg) in patients with chronic AR, and vasodilators are an excellent first choice as antihypertensive agents. It is often difficult to achieve adequate control because of the increased stroke volume that accompanies severe AR. Cardiac arrhythmias and systemic infections are poorly tolerated in patients with severe AR and must be treated promptly and vigorously. Although nitroglycerin and long-acting nitrates are not as helpful in relieving anginal pain as they are in patients with ischemic heart disease, they are worth a trial. Patients with syphilitic aortitis should receive a full course of penicillin therapy. Beta blockers and the angiotensin receptor blocker, losartan, may be useful to retard the rate of aortic root enlargement in young patients with Marfan's syndrome and aortic root dilation. Early reports of the efficacy of losartan in patients with Marfan's syndrome have led to its use in other populations of patients, including those with BAV disease and aortopathy. The use of beta blockers in patients with valvular AR was previously felt to be relatively contraindicated due to concerns that the resulting slowing of the heart rate would allow more time for diastolic regurgitation. More recent observational reports, however, suggest that beta blockers may provide functional benefit in patients with chronic AR. Beta blockers can sometimes provide incremental blood pressure lowering in patients with chronic AR and hypertension. Patients with severe AR, particularly those with an associated aortopathy, should avoid isometric exercises.

SURGICAL TREATMENT In deciding on the advisability and proper timing of surgical treatment, two points should be kept in mind: (1) patients with chronic severe AR usually do not become symptomatic until *after* the development of myocardial dysfunction; and (2) when delayed too long (defined as >1 year from onset of symptoms or LV dysfunction), surgical treatment often does not restore normal LV function. Therefore, in patients with chronic severe AR, careful clinical follow-up and noninvasive testing with echocardiography at approximately 6-month intervals are necessary if operation is to be undertaken at the optimal time, i.e., *after* the onset of LV dysfunction but *prior* to the development of severe symptoms. Operation can be deferred as long as the patient both remains asymptomatic and retains normal LV function without severe chamber dilation (end-diastolic dimension >75 mm).

AVR is indicated for the treatment of severe AR in symptomatic patients irrespective of LV function. In general, the operation should be carried out in asymptomatic patients with severe AR and progressive LV dysfunction defined by an LVEF <50%, an LV end-systolic dimension >55 mm or end-systolic volume >55 mL/m², or an LV diastolic dimension >75 mm. Smaller dimensions may be appropriate thresholds in individuals of smaller stature. Patients with severe AR without indications for operation should be followed by clinical and echocardiographic examination every 3–12 months.

Surgical options for management of aortic valve and root disease have expanded considerably over the past decade. AVR with a suitable mechanical or tissue prosthesis is generally necessary in patients with rheumatic AR and in many patients with other forms of regurgitation. Rarely, when a leaflet has been perforated during infective endocarditis or torn from its attachments to the aortic annulus by thoracic trauma, primary surgical repair may be possible. When AR is due to aneurysmal dilation of the root, or proximal ascending aorta, rather than to primary valve involvement, it may be possible to reduce or eliminate the regurgitation by narrowing the annulus or by excising a portion of the aortic root without replacing the valve. Elective, valve-sparing aortic root reconstruction generally involves reimplantation of the valve in a contoured graft with reattachment of the coronary artery buttons into the side of the graft and is best undertaken in specialized surgical centers (Fig. 20-11). Resuspension of the native aortic valve leaflets is possible in approximately 50% of patients with acute AR in the setting of type A aortic dissection. In other conditions, however, regurgitation can be effectively eliminated only by replacing the aortic valve, the dilated or aneurysmal ascending aorta responsible for the regurgitation, and implanting a composite valve-graft conduit. This formidable procedure entails a higher risk than isolated AVR.

As in patients with other valvular abnormalities, both the operative risk and the late mortality rate are largely dependent on the stage of the disease and myocardial function at the time of operation. The overall operative mortality rate for isolated AVR is approximately 3% (Table 20-3). However, patients with marked cardiac enlargement and prolonged LV dysfunction experience an operative mortality rate of approximately 10% and a late mortality rate of approximately 5% per year due to LV failure despite a technically satisfactory operation. Nonetheless, because of the very poor prognosis with medical management, even patients with LV systolic failure should be considered for operation.

Patients with acute severe AR require prompt surgical treatment, which may be lifesaving.

TRICUSPID STENOSIS

TS, which is much less prevalent than MS in North America and Western Europe, is generally rheumatic in origin and more common in women than men. It does not occur as an isolated lesion and is usually associated with MS. Hemodynamically significant TS occurs in 5–10% of patients with severe MS; rheumatic TS is commonly associated with some degree of TR. Nonrheumatic causes of TS are rare.

PATHOPHYSIOLOGY

A diastolic pressure gradient between the RA and RV defines TS. It is augmented when the transvalvular blood flow increases during inspiration and declines during expiration. A mean diastolic pressure gradient of 4 mmHg is usually sufficient to elevate the mean RA

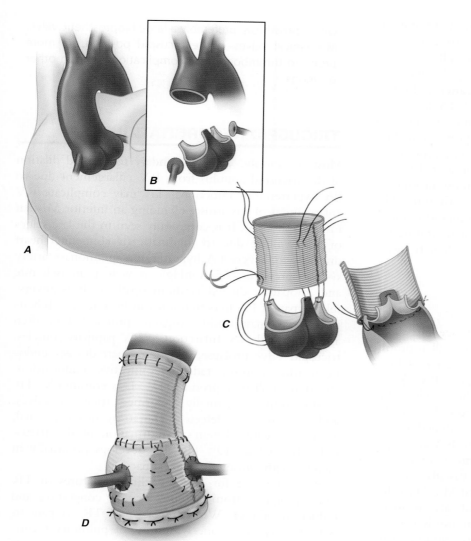

FIGURE 20-11
Valve-sparing aortic root reconstruction (David procedure). (*From P Steltzer et al [eds]: Valvular Heart Disease: A Companion to Braunwald's Heart Disease, 3rd ed, Fig 12-27, p. 200.*)

pressure to levels that result in systemic venous congestion. Unless sodium intake has been restricted and diuretics administered, this venous congestion is associated with hepatomegaly, ascites, and edema, sometimes severe. In patients with sinus rhythm, the RA *a* wave may be extremely tall and may even approach the level of the RV systolic pressure. The *y* descent is prolonged. The CO at rest is usually depressed, and it fails to rise during exercise. The low CO is responsible for the normal or only slightly elevated LA, PA, and RV systolic pressures despite the presence of MS. Thus, the presence of TS can mask the hemodynamic and clinical features of any associated MS.

SYMPTOMS

Because the development of MS generally precedes that of TS, many patients initially have symptoms of pulmonary congestion and fatigue. Characteristically, patients with severe TS complain of relatively little dyspnea for

the degree of hepatomegaly, ascites, and edema that they have. However, fatigue secondary to a low CO and discomfort due to refractory edema, ascites, and marked hepatomegaly are common in patients with TS and/or TR. In some patients, TS may be suspected for the first time when symptoms of right-sided failure persist after an adequate mitral valvotomy.

PHYSICAL FINDINGS

Because TS usually occurs in the presence of other obvious valvular disease, the diagnosis may be missed unless it is considered. Severe TS is associated with marked hepatic congestion, often resulting in cirrhosis, jaundice, serious malnutrition, anasarca, and ascites. Congestive hepatomegaly and, in cases of severe tricuspid valve disease, splenomegaly are present. The jugular veins are distended, and in patients with sinus rhythm there may be giant *a* waves. The *v* waves are less conspicuous, and because tricuspid obstruction impedes RA emptying during diastole, there is a slow γ descent. In patients with sinus rhythm there may be prominent presystolic pulsations of the enlarged liver as well.

On auscultation, an OS of the tricuspid valve may rarely be heard approximately 0.06 s after pulmonic valve closure. The diastolic murmur of TS has many of the qualities of the diastolic murmur of MS, and because TS almost always occurs in the presence of MS, it may be missed. However, the tricuspid murmur is generally heard best along the left lower sternal border and over the xiphoid process, and is most prominent during presystole in patients with sinus rhythm. The murmur of TS is augmented during inspiration, and it is reduced during expiration and particularly during the strain phase of the Valsalva maneuver, when tricuspid transvalvular flow is reduced.

LABORATORY EXAMINATION

The ECG features of RA enlargement (see Fig. 11-8) include tall, peaked P waves in lead II, as well as prominent, upright P waves in lead V_1. The *absence* of ECG evidence of right ventricular hypertrophy (RVH) in a patient with right-sided heart failure who is believed to have MS should suggest associated tricuspid valve disease. The chest x-ray in patients with combined TS and MS shows particular prominence of the RA and superior vena cava without much enlargement of the PA and with less evidence of pulmonary vascular congestion than occurs in patients with isolated MS. On echocardiographic examination, the tricuspid valve is usually thickened and domes in diastole; the transvalvular gradient can be estimated routinely by continuous wave Doppler echocardiography. TTE provides additional information regarding mitral valve structure and function, LV and RV size and function, and PA pressure.

TREATMENT	Tricuspid Stenosis

Patients with TS generally exhibit marked systemic venous congestion; intensive salt restriction, bed rest, and diuretic therapy are required during the preoperative period. Such a preparatory period may diminish hepatic congestion and thereby improve hepatic function sufficiently so that the risks of operation, particularly bleeding, are diminished. Surgical relief of the TS should be carried out, preferably at the time of surgical mitral valvotomy or MVR, in patients with moderate or severe TS who have mean diastolic pressure gradients exceeding ~4 mmHg and tricuspid orifice areas <1.5–2 cm². TS is almost always accompanied by significant TR. Operative repair may permit substantial improvement of tricuspid valve function. If repair cannot be accomplished, the tricuspid valve may have to be replaced

with a prosthesis, preferably a large bioprosthetic valve. Mechanical valves in the tricuspid position are more prone to thromboembolic complications than in other positions.

TRICUSPID REGURGITATION

Most commonly, TR is secondary to marked dilation of the tricuspid annulus from RV enlargement due to PA hypertension. Functional TR may complicate RV enlargement of any cause, including an inferior MI that involves the RV. It is commonly seen in the late stages of heart failure due to rheumatic or congenital heart disease with severe PA hypertension (pulmonary artery systolic pressure >55 mmHg), as well as in ischemic and idiopathic dilated cardiomyopathies. It is reversible in part if PA hypertension can be relieved. Rheumatic fever may produce organic (primary) TR, often associated with TS. Infarction of RV papillary muscles, tricuspid valve prolapse, carcinoid heart disease, endomyocardial fibrosis, radiation, infective endocarditis, and trauma all may produce TR. Less commonly, TR results from congenitally deformed tricuspid valves, and it occurs with defects of the atrioventricular canal, as well as with Ebstein's malformation of the tricuspid valve (Chap. 19). TR also develops eventually in patients with chronic RV apical pacing.

As is the case for TS, the clinical features of TR result primarily from systemic venous congestion and reduction of CO. With the onset of TR in patients with PA hypertension, symptoms of pulmonary congestion diminish, but the clinical manifestations of right-sided heart failure become intensified. The neck veins are distended with prominent *v* waves and rapid γ descents, marked hepatomegaly, ascites, pleural effusions, edema, systolic pulsations of the liver, and a positive hepatojugular reflex. A prominent RV pulsation along the left parasternal region and a blowing holosystolic murmur along the lower left sternal margin, which may be intensified during inspiration and reduced during expiration or the strain of the Valsalva maneuver, are characteristic findings; AF is usually present.

The ECG may show changes characteristic of the lesion responsible for the enlargement of the RV that leads to TR, e.g., an inferior Q-wave MI or RVH. Echocardiography may be helpful by demonstrating RV dilation and prolapsing, flail, scarred, or displaced tricuspid leaflets; the diagnosis and assessment of TR can be made by color flow Doppler imaging (see Fig. 12-8). Severe TR is accompanied by hepatic vein systolic flow reversal. Continuous wave Doppler of the TR velocity profile is useful in estimating PA systolic pressure. Roentgenographic examination usually reveals enlargement of both the RA and RV.

In patients with severe TR, the CO is usually markedly reduced, and the RA pressure pulse may exhibit no x descent during early systole but a prominent c-v wave with a rapid γ descent. The mean RA and the RV end-diastolic pressures are often elevated.

| **TREATMENT** | **Tricuspid Regurgitation** |

Isolated TR, in the absence of PA hypertension, such as that occurring as a consequence of infective endocarditis or trauma, is usually well tolerated and does not require operation. Indeed, even total excision of an infected tricuspid valve may be well tolerated for several years if the PA pressure and resistance are normal. Treatment of the underlying cause of left heart failure usually reduces the severity of functional TR, by reducing the size of the tricuspid annulus. In patients with mitral valve disease and TR secondary to PA hypertension and RV enlargement, effective surgical correction of the mitral valve abnormality results in lowering of the PA pressures and a gradual reduction or disappearance of the TR without direct treatment of the tricuspid valve. However, recovery may be more rapid in patients with severe functional TR if, at the time of mitral valve surgery and especially when there is enlargement of the tricuspid valve annulus, tricuspid valve annuloplasty (generally with the insertion of a ring) or in the rare instance of severe organic tricuspid valve disease, tricuspid valve replacement, is performed (Table 20-3). Tricuspid valve annuloplasty or replacement may rarely be required for severe, primary TR.

PULMONIC VALVE DISEASE

The pulmonic valve is affected by rheumatic fever far less frequently than are the other valves, and it is uncommonly a nidus for infective endocarditis. The most common *acquired* abnormality affecting the pulmonic valve is regurgitation secondary to dilation of the pulmonic valve ring as a consequence of severe PA hypertension. This dilation produces the *Graham Steell murmur,* a high-pitched, decrescendo, diastolic blowing murmur along the left sternal border, which is difficult to differentiate from the far more common murmur produced by AR. Pulmonic regurgitation is usually of little hemodynamic significance; indeed, surgical removal or destruction of the pulmonic valve by infective endocarditis does not produce heart failure unless significant PA hypertension is also present.

Carcinoid syndrome may cause pulmonic stenosis and/or regurgitation. Pulmonic regurgitation occurs universally among patients who have undergone childhood repair of tetralogy of Fallot with reconstruction of the RV outflow tract. Congenital pulmonic stenosis is discussed in Chap. 19.

Percutaneous pulmonic valve replacement has been successfully performed in many patients with severe PR after childhood repair of tetralogy of Fallot or pulmonic valve stenosis or atresia. This procedure was introduced clinically prior to percutaneous aortic valve replacement.

MULTIPLE AND MIXED VALVULAR HEART DISEASE

Many acquired and congenital cardiac lesions may result in stenosis and/or regurgitation of one or more heart valves. For example, rheumatic fever may present with mitral (MS, MR, MS and MR), aortic (AS, AR, AS and AR), and/or tricuspid (TS, TR, TS and TR) valve involvement. The common association of secondary TR with significant mitral valve disease has been discussed previously. Aortic valve infective endocarditis may secondarily involve the mitral apparatus. Mediastinal radiation may result in aortic, mitral, and even tricuspid valve disease, most often with mixed stenosis and regurgitation. Ergotamines, and the previously used combination of fenfluramine and phentermine, may result in mixed valve lesions, as are also seen in patients with carcinoid heart disease. Patients with Marfan's syndrome may have both AR from root dilation and MR due to MVP.

The clinical assessment of patients with multiple or mixed valve disease can be challenging. With combined mitral and aortic valve disease, the hemodynamic derangements associated with the mitral lesion(s) may mask the full expression of the aortic valve disease. For example, severe mitral stenosis may decrease LV preload to the extent that the severity of AS or AR can be underappreciated. Alternatively, the development of AF during the course of MS can lead to sudden worsening in a patient whose aortic valve disease was not previously felt to be significant. In patients with mixed MS/MR or AS/AR, the regurgitant lesion usually predominates, and can be followed primarily as the trigger for surgical or transcatheter intervention as appropriate. Nevertheless, there are frequent exceptions to the rules, and careful assessment is indicated. The LV in a patient with hypertrophy in the setting of both AS and AR may not be able to dilate in response to the volume load imposed by the regurgitant lesion and, thus, show signs or lead to the development of symptoms of compromise at a relatively earlier point in the natural history. Serial echocardiography can aid in decision making.

Similar considerations pertain to the evaluation of patients with heart valve disease and other cardiac and systemic disorders that can contribute to impaired exercise tolerance, such as hypertension, coronary artery disease, obesity, sleep apnea, and skeletal muscle deconditioning.

VALVE REPLACEMENT AND REPAIR

The results of valve replacement surgery are dependent on (1) the patient's myocardial function and general medical condition at the time of operation; (2) the technical abilities of the operative team and the quality of the postoperative care; and (3) the durability, hemodynamic characteristics, and thrombogenicity of the prosthesis. Increased perioperative mortality rate is associated with advanced age and comorbidity rate (e.g., pulmonary or renal disease, the need for nonvalvular cardiovascular surgery, diabetes mellitus) as well as with greater levels of preoperative functional disability and PA hypertension. Late complications of valve replacement include thromboemboli, bleeding due to anticoagulants, mechanical valve thrombosis, pannus ingrowth, paravalvular leak, hemolysis, structural deterioration, infective endocarditis, and prosthesis–patient mismatch (functional prosthetic valve stenosis that occurs when the prosthesis is too small relative to the patient's anatomy).

The choice between a tissue and mechanical prosthesis is essentially a trade-off between the risk of structural valve deterioration and the possible need for reoperation with a tissue valve versus the obligate need for lifelong anticoagulation and its attendant risks with a mechanical valve. The incidence of structural valve deterioration varies inversely with patient age and may be accelerated further by pregnancy or end-stage renal disease. Failure of a tissue prosthesis results in the need for reoperation in up to 30% of patients by 10 years and in 50% by 15 years. Rates of structural valve deterioration are higher for mitral than for aortic bioprostheses. This phenomenon may be due in part to the greater closing pressure to which a mitral prosthesis is exposed.

Traditionally, a mechanical prosthesis was considered preferable for a patient younger than age 65 who could take anticoagulants reliably. Bioprostheses were recommended for older patients (>65 years) who did not otherwise have an indication for anticoagulation (e.g., AF). Recent surveys of cardiac surgery in the United States, as reflected in the Society of Thoracic Surgeons database, show a clear and progressive trend favoring the implantation of bioprosthetic valves in younger (<65 years) patients. Reasons for this development include improved durability of newer generation bioprostheses, decreased risk of death or major complication at time of reoperation, the hazards of long-term anticoagulation, and patient preference to avoid anticoagulation for lifestyle reasons. Patient preference must be factored into any decision regarding the type of valve replacement. A mechanical prosthesis is reasonable for aortic or mitral valve replacement in patients younger than 65 years without a contraindication to anticoagulation. A bioprosthesis is equally reasonable for aortic or mitral valve replacement in patients younger than 65 years who elect this strategy for lifestyle reasons with full knowledge of the likely need for reoperation over time.

Bioprostheses remain the preferred valve choice for patients older than 65 years, in both the aortic and mitral position. Bioprosthetic valves are also indicated for women who expect to become pregnant, as well as for others who refuse to take anticoagulation or for whom anticoagulation may be contraindicated. Types of bioprostheses include xenografts (e.g., porcine aortic valves; cryopreserved, mounted bovine pericardial valves), homograft (allograft) aortic valves obtained from cadavers, and pulmonary autografts transplanted into the aortic position (Ross procedure). Homograft replacement may be preferred for the management of complicated aortic valve infective endocarditis.

In patients without contraindications to anticoagulants, particularly those younger than 65 years, a mechanical prosthesis is reasonable. Many surgeons now select the St. Jude prosthesis, a double-disk tilting prosthesis, for replacement of both aortic and mitral valves because of favorable hemodynamic characteristics and possible association with lower thrombogenicity. A tissue valve is preferred for tricuspid replacement.

The decision to proceed with valve replacement should be finalized only after an experienced surgeon has agreed that valve repair is either not appropriate or not feasible. As noted previously, valve repair techniques have improved considerably over the past 10–15 years, for both mitral and aortic lesions. Primary repair is often associated with a lower risk of postoperative LV functional impairment, particularly for patients with MR, and avoids the long-term risks of a prosthesis.

Antibiotic prophylaxis prior to dental procedures that involve manipulation of gingival tissue or the periapical region of teeth or perforation of the oral mucosa is indicated for patients after valve replacement or ring annuloplasty. Prosthetic valve and ventricular function should be assessed with transthoracic echocardiography 3 months after surgery and a baseline complete blood count, reticulocyte count, and serum lactate dehydrogenase (LDH) test obtained to serve as a baseline set of values should the question of hemolysis arise in the future. The intensity of anticoagulation should follow recommended guidelines.

GLOBAL BURDEN OF VALVULAR HEART DISEASE

 Primary valvular heart disease ranks well below coronary heart disease, stroke, hypertension, obesity, and diabetes as major threats to the public health. Nevertheless, it is the source of significant morbidity and mortality rates. Rheumatic fever is the dominant cause of valvular heart disease in developing countries. Its prevalence has been estimated to range from as low as 1 per 100,000 school-age children in Costa Rica to as high as 150 per 100,000 in China. Rheumatic heart disease accounts for 12–65% of hospital admissions related to cardiovascular disease and 2–10% of hospital discharges in some developing countries. Prevalence and mortality rates vary among communities even within the same country as a function of crowding and the availability of medical resources and population-wide programs for detection and treatment of group A streptococcal pharyngitis. In economically deprived areas, tropical and subtropical climates (particularly on the Indian subcontinent), Central America, and the Middle East, rheumatic valvular disease progresses more rapidly than in more developed nations and frequently causes serious symptoms in patients younger than 20 years of age. This accelerated natural history may be due to repeated infections with more virulent strains of rheumatogenic streptococci. Approximately 16 million people live with rheumatic heart disease worldwide. As of 2000, worldwide death rates for rheumatic heart disease approximated 5.5 per 100,000 population ($n = 332,000$), with the highest rates reported from Southeast Asia (7.6 per 100,000).

Although there have been recent reports of isolated outbreaks of streptococcal infection in North America, valve disease in developed countries is now dominated by degenerative or inflammatory processes that lead to valve thickening, calcification, and dysfunction. The prevalence of valvular heart disease increases with age. Important left-sided valve disease may affect as many as 12–13% of adults older than the age of 75. In the United States, there were 1.5 million hospital discharges with any diagnosis of valvular heart disease in 2005, and 94,000 of these were related to surgical procedures for heart valve disease (mostly involving the aortic and mitral valves).

The incidence of infective endocarditis (Chap. 25) has increased with the aging of the population, the more widespread prevalence of vascular grafts and intracardiac devices, the emergence of more virulent multidrug-resistant microorganisms, and the growing epidemic of diabetes. Infective endocarditis has become a more frequent cause of acute valvular regurgitation. Bicuspid aortic valve disease affects as many as 0.5–1.4% of the population, and an increasing number of childhood survivors of congenital heart disease present later in life with valvular dysfunction. The global burden of valvular heart disease is expected to progress.

As is true for other health conditions, disparities in access to and quality of care for patients with valvular heart disease have been well documented. Management decisions and outcome differences based on age, gender, and race require educational efforts across all levels of providers.

CHAPTER 21
CARDIOMYOPATHY AND MYOCARDITIS

Lynne Warner Stevenson ■ Joseph Loscalzo

DEFINITION AND CLASSIFICATION

Cardiomyopathy is a disease of the heart muscle. It is estimated that cardiomyopathy accounts for 5–10% of the 5–6 million patients already diagnosed with heart failure in the United States. This term is intended to exclude cardiac dysfunction that results from other structural heart disease, such as coronary artery disease, primary valve disease, or severe hypertension; however, in general usage the phrase *ischemic cardiomyopathy* is sometimes applied to describe diffuse dysfunction occurring in the presence of multivessel coronary artery disease, and *nonischemic cardiomyopathy* to describe cardiomyopathy from other causes. As of 2006, cardiomyopathies are defined as "a heterogeneous group of diseases of the myocardium associated with mechanical and/or electrical dysfunction that usually (but not invariably) exhibit inappropriate ventricular hypertrophy or dilatation and are due to a variety of causes that frequently are genetic."[1]

The traditional classification of cardiomyopathies into a triad of dilated, restrictive, and hypertrophic was based initially on autopsy specimens and later on echocardiographic findings. Dilated and hypertrophic cardiomyopathies can be distinguished on the basis of left ventricular wall thickness and cavity dimension; however, restrictive cardiomyopathy can have variably increased wall thickness and chamber dimensions that range from reduced to slightly increased, with prominent atrial enlargement. Restrictive cardiomyopathy is now defined more on the basis of abnormal diastolic function, which is also present but initially less prominent in dilated and hypertrophic cardiomyopathy. Restrictive cardiomyopathy can overlap in presentation, gross morphology, and etiology with both hypertrophic and dilated cardiomyopathies **(Table 21-1)**.

Expanding information renders this classification triad based on phenotype increasingly inadequate to define disease or therapy. Identification of more genetic determinants of cardiomyopathy has suggested a four-way classification scheme of etiology as primary (affecting primarily the heart) and secondary to other systemic disease. The primary causes are then divided into genetic, mixed genetic and acquired, and acquired; however, in current practice the genetic information is often unavailable at the time of initial presentation, particularly in the absence of extracardiac manifestations. Many mutated genes can be associated with the same general phenotype, and one defective gene may manifest as multiple phenotypes. In addition, the bases of evidence for most therapies are still driven by clinical phenotypes. Although the proposed genetic classification does not yet guide many current clinical strategies, it will become increasingly relevant as classification of disease moves beyond individual organ pathology to more integrated systems approaches.

GENERAL PRESENTATION

For all cardiomyopathies, the early symptoms often relate to exertional intolerance with breathlessness or fatigue, usually from inadequate cardiac reserve during exercise. These symptoms may initially go unnoticed or be attributed to other causes, commonly pulmonary. As fluid retention leads to elevation of resting filling pressures, shortness of breath may occur during routine daily activity, such as dressing, and may manifest as dyspnea or cough in the supine position. Although often considered the hallmark of congestion, peripheral edema may not appear despite severe fluid retention, particularly in younger patients. The nonspecific term *congestive heart failure* describes only the resulting syndrome of fluid retention, which is common to the three types of cardiomyopathy and also to other cardiac diseases associated with elevated filling pressures. Despite the different

[1]From BJ Maron et al: Circulation 113:1807, 2006.

TABLE 21-1

PRESENTATION WITH SYMPTOMATIC CARDIOMYOPATHY

	DILATED	RESTRICTIVE	HYPERTROPHIC
Ejection fraction (normal >55%)	Usually <30% when symptoms severe	25–50%	>60%
Left ventricular diastolic dimension (normal <55 mm)	≥60 mm	<60 mm (may be decreased)	Often decreased
Left ventricular wall thickness	Decreased	Normal or increased	Markedly increased
Atrial size	Increased	Increased; may be massive	Increased; related to abnormal
Valvular regurgitation	Related to annular dilation; mitral appears earlier, during decompensation; tricuspid regurgitation in late stages	Related to endocardial involvement; frequent mitral and tricuspid regurgitation, rarely severe	Related to valve-septum interaction; mitral regurgitation
Common first symptoms	Exertional intolerance	Exertional intolerance, fluid retention early	Exertional intolerance; may have chest pain
Congestive symptoms[a]	Left before right, except right prominent in young adults	Right often dominates	Left-sided congestion may develop late
Arrhythmia	Ventricular tachyarrhythmia; conduction block in Chagas' disease, and some families; atrial fibrillation.	Ventricular uncommon except in sarcoidosis conduction block in sarcoidosis and amyloidosis; atrial fibrillation.	Ventricular tachyarrhythmias; atrial fibrillation

[a]Left-sided symptoms of pulmonary congestion; dyspnea on exertion, orthopnea, paroxysmal nocturnal dyspnea. Right-sided symptoms of systemic versus congestion: discomfort on bending, hepatic and abdominal distention, peripheral edema.

structural basis, all three types of cardiomyopathy can be associated with atrioventricular valve regurgitation, typical and atypical chest pain, atrial and ventricular tachyarrhythmias, and embolic events (Table 21-1). Initial evaluation begins with a detailed clinical history and examination, looking for clues to cardiac, extracardiac, and familial disease (Table 21-2). The initial evaluation, prognosis, and therapy are generally defined by the severity of cardiac and clinical dysfunction, with some distinctive features according to etiology.

GENETIC ETIOLOGIES OF CARDIOMYOPATHY

The estimated prevalence of a genetic etiology for cardiomyopathy continues to increase with increasing awareness of the importance of the family history and the availability of genetic testing. Well recognized in hypertrophic cardiomyopathy, heritability is present in at least 30% of dilated cardiomyopathies without other clear etiology. Careful family history should elicit not only known cardiomyopathy and heart failure, but also family members who have had sudden death, often incorrectly attributed to "a massive heart attack," who have had atrial fibrillation or pacemaker implantation by middle age, or who have muscular dystrophy. The family history should be reviewed at subsequent intervals

particularly regarding siblings and cousins, who may tend to manifest disease at similar ages.

Most familial cardiomyopathies are inherited in an autosomal dominant pattern, with occasional autosomal recessive and X-linked inheritance (Table 21-3). The penetrance and phenotype of a given mutation varies with other genetic, epigenetic, and environmental determinants. Some mutations are associated with primary conduction system disease as well as dilated cardiomyopathy (CDDC). With rare exceptions, such as the replacements for defective metabolic enzymes, current therapy is based on the phenotype rather than the genetic defect. However, knowledge of the genetic defect may influence prognosis and in some cases provide indication for implantable defibrillators.

Defects in sarcomeric proteins of myosin, actin, and troponin are the best characterized. While the majority of these are associated with hypertrophic cardiomyopathy, an increasing number of sarcomeric mutations have now been implicated in dilated cardiomyopathy, and some have also been associated with left ventricular noncompaction. Thus far, few mutations have been identified in excitation-contraction coupling proteins, perhaps because they are too crucial for survival to allow variation.

Many of the proteins encoded by abnormal structural genes span more than one functional area of the myocyte (Fig. 21-1). Proteins contributing to the Z-disk

TABLE 21-2

INITIAL EVALUATION OF CARDIOMYOPATHY

Clinical Evaluation

Thorough history and physical examination to identify cardiac and noncardiac disorders[a]

Detailed family history of heart failure, cardiomyopathy, skeletal myopathy, conduction disorders and tachyarrhythmias, sudden death

History of alcohol, illicit drugs, chemotherapy or radiation therapy[a]

Assessment of ability to perform routine and desired activities[a]

Assessment of volume status, orthostatic blood pressure, body mass index[a]

Laboratory Evaluation

Electrocardiogram[a]

Chest radiograph[a]

Two-dimensional and Doppler echocardiogram[a]

Chemistry:
    Serum sodium,[a] potassium,[a] calcium,[a] magnesium[a]
    Fasting glucose (glycohemoglobin in DM)
    Creatinine,[a] blood urea nitrogen[a]
    Albumin,[a] total protein,[a] liver function tests[a]
    Lipid profile
    Thyroid-stimulating hormone[a]
    Serum iron, transferrin saturation
    Urinalysis
    Creatine kinase

Hematology:
    Hemoglobin/hematocrit[a]
    White blood cell count with differential,[a] including eosinophils
    Erythrocyte sedimentation rate

Initial Evaluation Only in Patients Selected for Possible Specific Diagnosis

Titers for infection in presence of clinical suspicion:
    Acute viral (coxsackievirus, echovirus, influenza virus)
    Human immunodeficiency virus,
    Chagas' disease, Lyme disease, toxoplasmosis

Catheterization with coronary angiography in patients with angina who are candidates for intervention[a]

Serologies for active rheumatologic disease

Endomyocardial biopsy including sample for electron microscopy when suspecting specific diagnosis with therapeutic implications

Screening for sleep-disordered breathing

[a]Level I Recommendations from ACC/AHA Practice Guidelines for Chronic Heart Failure in the adult.
Source: From SA Hunt et al: Circulation 112:e154, 2005.

organize and stabilize the sarcomeres. Multiple other proteins are involved in connecting and maintaining the cytoskeleton of the myocyte. For example, desmin forms intermediate filaments that connect the nuclear and plasma membranes, Z-lines, and the intercalated disks between muscle cells. Desmin mutations impair the transmission of force and signaling for both cardiac and skeletal muscle, and are, thus, associated with a peripheral myopathy as well as a dilated

cardiomyopathy. Most of the identified genetic defects in the Z-disk and cytoskeleton are associated with dilated cardiomyopathy.

Proteins in the sarcolemmal membrane are associated with dilated cardiomyopathy. The best known is the X-linked dystrophin, abnormalities of which cause Duchenne's and Becker's muscle dystrophy. (Interestingly, abnormal dystrophin can be acquired when the coxsackievirus cleaves dystrophin during viral myocarditis.) This protein provides a network that supports the sarcolemma and also connects to the sarcomere. The progressive functional defect in both cardiac and skeletal muscle reflects vulnerability to mechanical stress. Dystrophin is associated at the membrane with a complex of other proteins, such as metavinculin, abnormalities of which cause dilated cardiomyopathy with autosomal dominant inheritance. Defects in the sarcolemmal channel proteins (*channelopathies*) are generally associated with primary arrhythmias, but mutations in SCN5A, distinct from those which cause the Brugada or long-QT syndromes, have been implicated in dilated cardiomyopathy.

Nuclear membrane protein defects in the myocyte can also cause skeletal myopathy in either autosomal dominant (lamin proteins) or X-linked (emerin) patterns. These are associated with a high prevalence of atrial arrhythmias and conduction system disease which, in some family members, occur without detectable cardiomyopathy.

Intercalated disks between cardiac myocytes allow mechanical and electrical coupling between cells and also connect to desmin filaments within the cell. Mutations in proteins of the desmosomal complex compromise attachment of the myocytes, which can become disconnected and die, to be replaced by fat and fibrous tissue. These areas are highly arrhythmogenic and may go on to aneurysm formation. Although it is more noticeable in the thinner right ventricle, this condition often affects both ventricles. As desmosomes are also important for elasticity of hair and skin, some defective desmosomal proteins are associated with striking "woolly hair" and thickened skin on the palms and soles.

Owing to the conservation of signaling pathways in multiple systems, we may expect to discover more extracardiac manifestations of genetic abnormalities initially considered to manifest exclusively in the heart. In contrast, the monogenic disorders of metabolism that affect the heart are already clearly recognized to affect multiple organ systems (Table 21-4). The most important currently are those defective enzymes for which specific enzyme replacement therapy can now ameliorate the course of disease, as with alpha-galactosidase-A (Fabry's disease). Abnormalities of mitochondrial DNA (maternally transmitted) impair energy production with multiple clinical manifestations, including impaired cognitive function and skeletal myopathy. The phenotypic

TABLE 21-3

INHERITED GENETIC DEFECTS ASSOCIATED WITH CARDIOMYOPATHY

	GENE PRODUCT	INHERITANCE	CARDIAC PHENOTYPE	ISOLATED CARDIAC PHENOTYPE	EXTRACARDIAC MANIFESTATIONS
Sarcomere	MYH7 (β myosin heavy chain)	AD	HCM, DCM, LVNC	yes	Skeletal myopathy
	MYBPC3 (myosin-binding protein C)	AD	HCM, (DCM)	yes	
	TNNT2 (cardiac troponin T)	AD	HCM, DCM, LVNC	yes	
	TNNI3 (cardiac troponin I)	AD, AR	HCM, DCM, RCM	yes	
	TTN (Titin)	AD	HCM, DCM	yes	
	TPM1 (α-tropomyosin)	AD	HCM, DCM	yes	
	TNNC1 (slow troponin C)	AD	DCM	yes	
	ACTC (α-actin)	AD	HCM, DCM, (LVNC)	yes	
	MYL2 (myosin regulatory light chain)	AD	HCM	yes	Skeletal myopathy
	MYL3 (myosin essential light chain)	AD	HCM	yes	
	MYH6 (α-myosin heavy chain)	AD	HCM, (DCM)	yes	
Z-disk and Cytoskeleton	DES (Desmin)	AD	DCM	yes	Skeletal myopathy
	LDB3 (Cypher-ZASP)	AD	DCM, LVNC	yes	Skeletal myopathy
	MYOZ2 (Myozenin)	AD	HCM	yes	
	TCAP (Telethonin)	AD	DCM, HCM	yes	
	ANKRD1 (CARP)	AD	HCM, (DCM)	yes	
	CSRP3 (MLP)	AD	DCM, (HCM)	yes	
	OBSCN (Obscurin)	AD	HCM	yes	
	ACTN2 (α-actinin-2)	AD	DCM	yes	
	CRYAB (αB-crystallin)	AD	DCM	yes	
Nuclear Membrane	LMNA (Lamin A/C)	AD	CDDC	yes	Skeletal myopathy
	EMD (Emerin)	X-linked	CDDC	no	Skeletal myopathy, contractures
	TMPO (Thymopoietin)	AD	DCM	yes	
Excitation-Contraction Coupling	PLN (Phospholamban)	AD	DCM	yes	
	SCN5A (NAV 1.5)	AD	CDDC	yes	
	RYR2 (cardiac ryanodine receptor)	AD	ARVC	yes	

(continued)

TABLE 21-3

INHERITED GENETIC DEFECTS ASSOCIATED WITH CARDIOMYOPATHY (*CONTINUED*)

	GENE PRODUCT	INHERITANCE	CARDIAC PHENOTYPE	ISOLATED CARDIAC PHENOTYPE	EXTRACARDIAC MANIFESTATIONS
Cellular Metabolism	PRKAG2 (γ-subunit of AMP Kinase)	AD	HCM+	yes	
	LAMP2 (lysosomal associated membrane protein)	X-linked	HCM+	no[a]	Danon's disease: skeletal myopathy, cognitive impairment
	TAZ (Tafazzin)	X-linked	DCM, LVNC	no	Barth's syndrome: skeletal myopathy, cognitive impairment, neutropenia
	FXN (Frataxin)	AR	HCM	no	Friedreich's ataxia: ataxia, diabetes mellitus type 2
	ABCC9 (sulfonylurea receptor 2)	AD	DCM	yes	
	TMEM43 (transmembrane protein 43)	AD	ARVC	yes	
	GLA (α-galactosidase-A) (other systemic metabolic defects, see Table 21-4)	X-linked	HCM	yes	Fabry's disease: renal failure, angiokeratomas and painful neuropathy
Mitochondria	Mitochondrial DNA	Maternal transmission	DCM, HCMc	no	MELAS, MERRF, Kearns-Sayre syndrome, ocular myopathy
Sarcolemmal Membrane	DMD (Dystrophin)	X-linked	DCM	no[a]	Duchenne's and Becker's muscular dystrophy
	DMPK (dystrophica myotonica protein kinase)	AD	DCM	no	Myotonic dystrophy type 1
	SGCD (δ-sarcoglycan)	AD	DCM	yes	
	VCL (Metavinculin)	AD	DCM	yes	
Desmosome	DSP (Desmoplakin)	AD, AR	ARVC	yes	Carvajal syndrome (AR)
	DSG2 (Desmoglein 2)	AD	ARVC	yes	
	DSC2 (Desmocollin 2)	AD	ARVC	yes	
	PKP2 (Plakophilin 2)	AD	ARVC	yes	
	JUP (Plakoglobin)	AD, AR	ARVC	yes	Naxos syndrome (AR)
Other	EYA4 (Eyes absent 4)	AD	DCM	no	Sensorineural deafness
	RBM20 (RNA-binding motif 20)	AD	DCM	yes	
	PSEN1 (Presenilin-1,2)	AD	DCM	yes	Dementia

[a]Indicates that isolated cardiac phenotype can occur in women with the X-linked defects.

Abbreviations: AD, autosomal dominant; AR, autosomal recessive; ARVC, arrhythmogenic right ventricular cardiomyopathy; CDDC, conduction disease with dilated cardiomyopathy; DCM, dilated cardiomyopathy; HCM+, HCM with preexcitation; HCMc, HCM with conduction disease; LVNC, left ventricular noncompaction; MELAS, (mitochondrial) myopathy, encephalopathy, lactic acidosis, and stroke-like episodes syndrome; MERRF, myoclonic epilepsy with ragged red fibers; RCM, restrictive cardiomyopathy.

Source: From Neal Lakdawala, MD, Cardiovascular Genetics, Brigham and Women's Hospital.

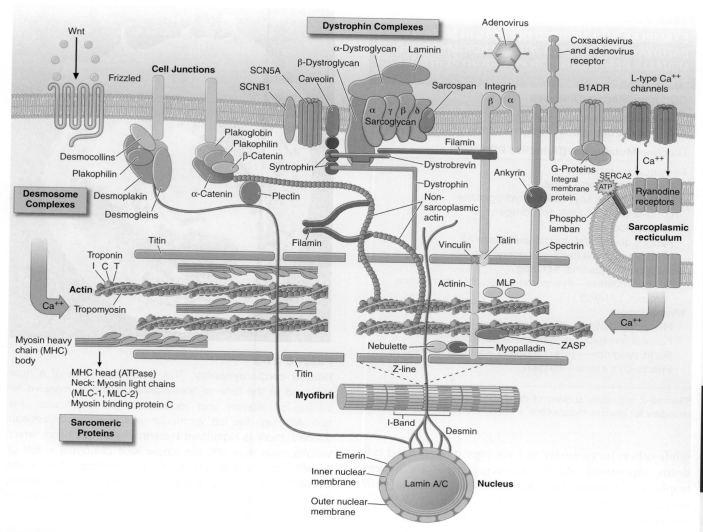

FIGURE 21-1

Drawing of myocyte indicating multiple sites of abnormal gene products associated with cardiomyopathy. Major functional groups include the sarcomeric proteins (actin, myosin, tropomyosin, and the associated regulatory proteins), the dystrophin complex stabilizing and connecting the cell membrane to intracellular structures, the desmosome complexes associated with cell-cell connections and stability, and multiple cytoskeletal proteins that integrate and stabilize the myocyte. ATP, adenosine triphosphate. (*Figure adapted from Jeffrey A. Towbin, MD, University of Cincinnati, with permission.*)

expression is highly variable depending on the distribution of the maternal mitochondria during embryonic development. Heritable systemic diseases, such as familial amyloidosis and hemochromatosis, can affect the heart without abnormal expression of specific cardiac genes.

For any patient with suspected or proven genetic disease, family members should be considered and evaluated in a longitudinal fashion. Screening includes an echocardiogram and electrocardiogram (ECG). The indications and implications for confirmatory specific genetic testing vary depending upon the specific mutation. The profound questions raised by families about diseases shared and passed down merit serious and sensitive discussion, ideally provided by a trained genetic counselor.

DILATED CARDIOMYOPATHY

An enlarged left ventricle with decreased systolic function as measured by left ventricular ejection fraction characterizes dilated cardiomyopathy (**Figs. 21-2, 21-3, and 21-4**). *Systolic failure* is more marked than the frequently accompanying diastolic dysfunction, although the latter may be functionally severe in the setting of marked volume overload. The syndrome of dilated cardiomyopathy has multiple etiologies (**Table 21-5**). Up to one-third of cases may be familial, as discussed later. Acquired cardiomyopathy is often attributed to a brief primary injury such as infection or toxin exposure. Some myocytes may die during the initial injury,

TABLE 21-4

EXAMPLES OF INHERITED DEFECTS IN METABOLIC PATHWAYS ASSOCIATED WITH CARDIOMYOPATHY, USUALLY RESTRICTIVE OR PSEUDOHYPERTROPHIC PHENOTYPE

Glycogen Storage Diseases

II—Pompe's (alpha 1,4 glucosidase)
III –Forbes: debranching enzyme (amylo 1,6 glucosidase)

Glucose Metabolism (Defective PRKAG2[a])

Fatty acid metabolism
  Carnitine transport defect
  Medium-chain Acyl-CoA dehydrogenase
  Long-chain Acyl-CoA dehydrogenase
Sphingolipidoses
  Fabry's disease (alpha galactosidase A)
  Gaucher disease (beta-glucocerebroside)
Disorders of lysosomal function
  Danon's disease—(lysosome-associated membrane protein, LAMP2)
Miscellaneous
  Hemochromatosis—Fe metabolism
  Familial amyloidosis—abnormal transthyretin
  Barth syndrome—tafazzin defect affecting cardiolipin
  Friedreich's ataxia—frataxin

[a]Gamma-2 regulatory subunit of the AMP-activated protein kinase important for glucose metabolism.

while others survive only to have later programmed cell death, (apoptosis). As the surviving myocytes hypertrophy to accommodate the increased burden of wall stress, local and circulating factors stimulate deleterious responses that contribute to progression of disease, even in the absence of further primary injury. Dynamic remodeling of the interstitial scaffolding affects diastolic function and the amount of ventricular dilation. Mitral regurgitation commonly develops as the valvular apparatus is distorted by ventricular dilation and sometimes by focal injury to underlying myocardium and is usually substantial by the time heart failure is severe. Many cases that present "acutely" have progressed silently through these stages over months to years.

Regardless of the nature and degree of direct cell injury, the resulting functional impairment often includes some contribution from secondary responses that may be reversible. The potential reversibility of cardiomyopathy in the absence of ongoing injury remains a subject of active controversy. Almost half of all patients with truly recent onset cardiomyopathy demonstrate substantial spontaneous recovery. Some patients have dramatic improvement to near-normal ejection fractions during pharmacologic therapy, particularly notable with the β-adrenergic antagonists coupled with renin-angiotensin system inhibition. Interest in the potential for recovery of cardiomyopathy in the absence of coronary artery disease has been further stimulated by occasional "recovery" of left ventricular function in young patients

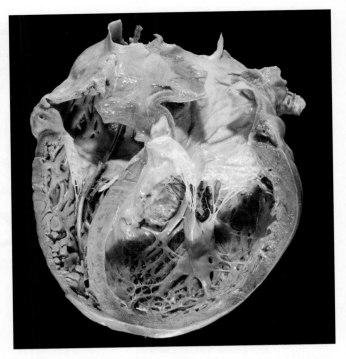

FIGURE 21-2

Dilated cardiomyopathy. This gross specimen of a heart removed at the time of transplantation shows massive left ventricular dilation and moderate right ventricular dilation. Although the left ventricular wall in particular appears thinned, there is significant hypertrophy of this heart, which weighs more than 800 gm (upper limit of normal = 360 g). A defibrillator lead is seen traversing the tricuspid valve into the right ventricular apex. (*Image courtesy of Robert Padera, MD, PhD, Department of Pathology, Brigham and Women's Hospital, Boston.*)

after a year or more of mechanical circulatory support. The diagnosis and therapy for dilated cardiomyopathy is generally dictated by the stage of heart failure (Chap. 17), with specific aspects discussed with the relevant etiology later in this chapter.

INFECTIVE MYOCARDITIS

Myocarditis is an inflammatory process, most commonly attributed to infectious organisms that can invade the myocardium directly, produce cardiotoxins, and trigger chronic inflammatory responses. Infective myocarditis has been reported with almost all types of infectious agents, but is most commonly associated with viral infections, the protozoan *Trypanosoma cruzi* in South America, and endomyocardial fibrosis in equatorial Africa.

Viral myocarditis in murine models begins with acute infection. After viruses enter the circulation through the respiratory or gastrointestinal tract, they can infect other organs possessing specific receptors, such as the coxsackie-adenovirus receptor on the heart. Viral invasion and replication can lead directly to myocardial injury and lysis. Viral proteases have multiple actions, of which

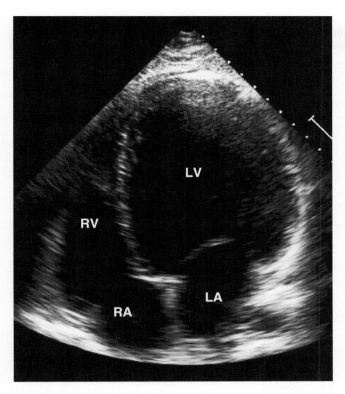

FIGURE 21-3
Dilated cardiomyopathy. This echocardiogram of a young man with dilated cardiomyopathy shows massive global dilation and thinning of the walls of the left ventricle (LV). The left atrium (LA) is also enlarged compared to normal. Note that the echocardiographic and pathologic images are vertically opposite, such that the LV is by convention on the top right in the echocardiographic image and bottom right in the pathologic images. (*Image courtesy of Justina Wu, MD, Brigham and Women's Hospital, Boston.*)

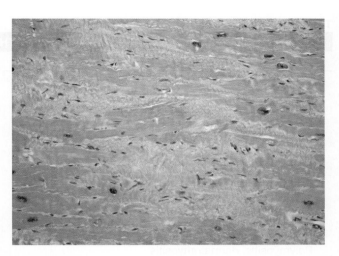

FIGURE 21-4
Dilated cardiomyopathy. Microscopic specimen of a dilated cardiomyopathy showing the nonspecific changes of interstitial fibrosis and myocyte hypertrophy characterized by increased myocyte size and enlarged, irregular nuclei. Hematoxylin and eosin stained section, 100× original magnification. (*Image courtesy of Robert Padera, MD, PhD, Department of Pathology, Brigham and Women's Hospital, Boston.*)

one is to degrade the protein, dystrophin, in the myocyte membrane complex that is genetically abnormal in some muscular dystrophies. Viral antigens activate immune responses that help to contain the initial infection but may persist into later phases. Components include nonspecific cytokines, specific antibodies, and cytotoxic T-lymphocytes, which in some cases recognize myocyte proteins. There is varying evidence for a latent phase of ongoing infection with persistence of the viral genome and some viral proteins. The relative contributions of viral persistence and deleterious host immune responses to progressive dysfunction have not been clearly delineated in human disease (Fig. 21-5). The late stages are dominated by nonspecific secondary changes in gene expression, and by local and systemic neurohormonal responses, as seen for other etiologies of heart failure.

Although viral myocarditis is generally considered to be an acquired cardiomyopathy, families have been reported whose clinical disease appeared after a syndrome consistent with viral myocarditis. One possible explanation for this apparent mixed etiology is that some genetic variants of myocardial cell surface receptors bind more avidly to certain viruses, particularly coxsackievirus and adenovirus.

The typical clinical picture of myocarditis is a young adult with progressive dyspnea and weakness over a few days to weeks after a recent viral syndrome with fevers and often myalgias indicative of skeletal muscle inflammation. Some patients present with atypical or anginal-type chest pain, or with pleuritic, positional chest pain due to pericarditis with some degree of underlying myocarditis. Patients in whom ventricular tachyarrhythmias dominate the presentation may have viral myocarditis but should be evaluated for sarcoidosis or giant cell myocarditis. Patients presenting with pulmonary or systemic embolic events from intracardiac thrombi generally already have chronic, severe cardiac dysfunction.

A small number of patients present with *acute fulminant myocarditis*, with rapid progression from a severe febrile respiratory syndrome to cardiogenic shock from which multiple organ system failure, including coagulopathy, may develop. Such patients have often been discharged from the emergency department with antibiotic therapy only to return in extremis. Prompt triage is vital to provide aggressive support with high-level intravenous inotropic therapy and on occasion, mechanical circulatory support; importantly, more than half of patients with this acute presentation can survive with marked improvement within the first few weeks, often returning to near-normal systolic function.

Many patients presenting with heart failure after a viral illness actually have a long-standing cardiomyopathy that was acutely exacerbated but not caused by the new viral illness. Heart failure from any cause

TABLE 21-5

MAJOR CAUSES OF DILATED CARDIOMYOPATHY (WITH COMMON EXAMPLES)

Inflammatory Myocarditis	Metabolic[a]
Infective 　Viral (coxsackie, adenovirus, HIV, hepatitis C) 　Parasitic (*T. cruzi*—Chagas' disease, toxoplasmosis) 　Bacterial (diphtheria) 　Spirochetal (*Borellia burgdorferi*—Lyme disease) 　Rickettsial—(Q fever) 　Fungal (with systemic infection) Noninfective 　Granulomatous inflammatory disease 　　Sarcoidosis 　　Giant cell myocarditis 　Hypersensitivity myocarditis 　Polymyositis, dermatomyositis 　Collagen vascular disease 　Peripartum cardiomyopathy 　Transplant rejection	Nutritional deficiencies: thiamine, selenium, carnitine Electrolyte deficiencies: calcium, phosphate, magnesium Endocrinopathy: 　Thyroid disease 　Pheochromocytoma 　Diabetes Obesity Hemochromatosis
	Inherited Metabolic Pathway Defects (See Table 21-4)
	Familial[a] (See Table 21-3)
Toxic	Skeletal and cardiac myopathy Dystrophin-related dystrophy (Duchenne's, Becker's) Mitochondrial myopathies (e.g., Kearns-Sayre syndrome) Arrhythmogenic ventricular dysplasia Hemochromatosis Associated with other systemic diseases Susceptibility to immune-mediated myocarditis
Alcohol Catecholamines: amphetamines, cocaine Chemotherapeutic agents: (anthracyclines, trastuzumab) 　Interferon 　Other therapeutic agents (hydroxychloroquine, 　　chloroquine) Drugs of misuse (emetine, anabolic steroids) Heavy metals: lead, mercury Occupational exposure: hydrocarbons, arsenicals	**Overlap with Restrictive Cardiomyopathy**
	"Minimally dilated cardiomyopathy" Hemochromatosis Amyloidosis Hypertrophic cardiomyopathy ("burned-out")
	"Idiopathic"[a]
	Miscellaneous (Shared Elements of above Etiologies)
	Arrhythmogenic right ventricular dysplasia (may also affect 　left ventricle)[a] Left ventricular noncompaction[a] Peripartum cardiomyopathy

[a]Some specific cases can be linked now to specific genetic mutation in a familial cardiomyopathy; others with similar phenotypes that appear to be acquired or idiopathic may represent genetic factors not yet identified.

often worsens transiently during infection, presumably due to the myocardial depressant effects of circulating cytokines. Marked left ventricular dilation and the presence of severely elevated left-ventricular filling pressures without frank pulmonary edema suggest chronic, slowly progressive disease, which is often further supported by a history of gradual changes in exercise tolerance before the viral syndrome.

For the usual subacute presentation, the diagnosis of cardiomyopathy is confirmed by echocardiography, and further evaluation is directed to ascertain whether myocarditis is present. Troponin is often mildly elevated, and creatine kinase may be released from the cardiac injury or skeletal muscle involvement. In some cases, cardiac catheterization is performed to rule out acute ischemia. Magnetic resonance imaging is increasingly used for the diagnosis of myocarditis, which is supported by evidence of increased tissue edema and gadolinium enhancement, particularly in the mid-wall distinct from the usual coronary artery territories.

Endomyocardial biopsy criteria for myocarditis require lymphocytic infiltration with evidence of myocyte necrosis (Fig. 21-6), but are met in only about 10–20% of classic presentations. Most biopsies in fulminant myocarditis show only marked tissue edema without a cellular infiltrate, and it is likely that many less acute cases may similarly be characterized by tissue edema and cytokine depression of myocardial function, possibly including some antibody-mediated endothelial injury, without marked cellular infiltrates. Acute and convalescent viral titers are usually sent but are more likely to be important from the public health standpoint than for the individual.

Viral myocarditis treatment is initially directed toward stabilizing the hemodynamic status and then toward adjusting neurohormonal antagonists for the treatment of heart failure as tolerated. Presentation with fulminant disease requires rapid evaluation and therapy as discussed earlier. For patients with subacute presentation, randomized trials have shown no benefit

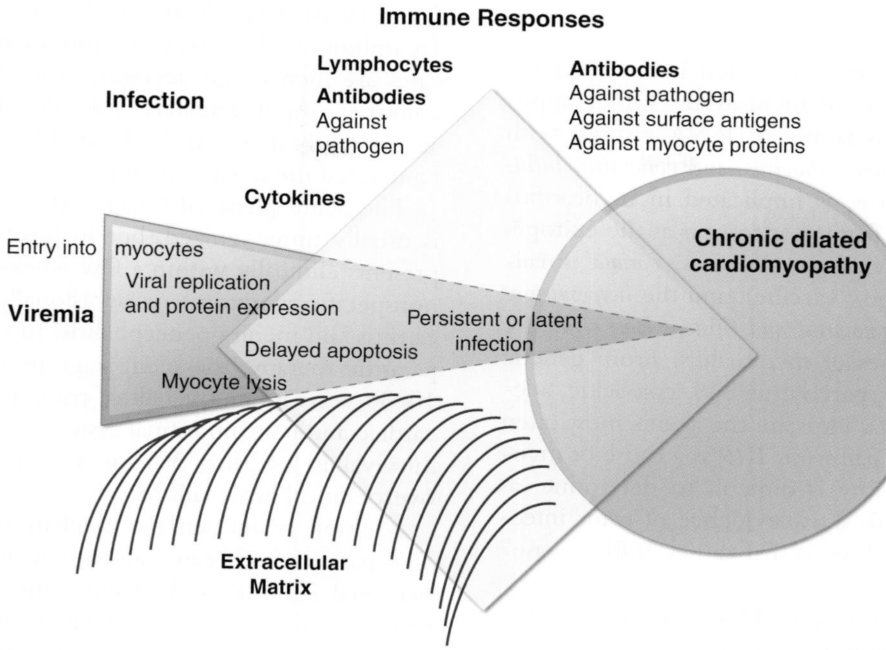

Immune Responses

Infection

Lymphocytes
Antibodies
Against pathogen

Antibodies
Against pathogen
Against surface antigens
Against myocyte proteins

Cytokines

Entry into myocytes

Viral replication and protein expression

Chronic dilated cardiomyopathy

Viremia

Persistent or latent infection

Delayed apoptosis

Myocyte lysis

Extracellular Matrix

FIGURE 21-5

Schematic diagram demonstrating the possible progression from infection through direct, secondary, and autoimmune responses to dilated cardiomyopathy. Most of the supporting evidence for this sequence is derived from animal models. It is not known to what degree persistent infection and/or ongoing immune responses contribute to ongoing myocardial injury in the chronic phase.

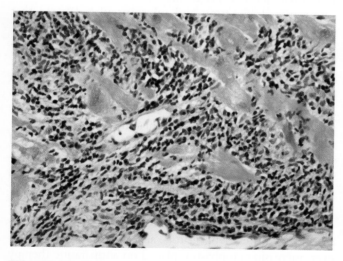

FIGURE 21-6

Acute myocarditis. Microscopic image of an endomyocardial biopsy showing massive infiltration with mononuclear cells and occasional eosinophils associated with clear myocyte damage. The myocyte nuclei are enlarged and reactive. Such extensive involvement of the myocardium would lead to extensive replacement fibrosis even if the inflammatory response could be suppressed. Hematoxylin and eosin stained section, 200× original magnification. (*Image courtesy of Robert Padera, MD, PhD, Department of Pathology, Brigham and Women's Hospital, Boston.*)

of immunosuppression with glucocorticoid combinations or intravenous immunoglobulin, even when the biopsy is positive for lymphocytic infiltrates; yet, immunosuppression is often used even in the absence of evidence of benefit, in part due to perceived analogy to acute cardiac transplant rejection. Animal models have shown that viral replication and myocardial injury can be worsened by immunosuppression during the early phase of infection; however, patients with persistent inflammatory myocarditis and a progressive downhill course over weeks may be treated empirically with glucocorticoids in an attempt to avoid the need for cardiac transplantation.

The true prognosis of viral myocarditis is not known, as most unrecognized cases probably resolve spontaneously, while others progress to cardiomyopathy without other obvious cause. However, among patients who have truly recent onset cardiomyopathy of less than 3–6 months' duration without other apparent etiology, almost half will have major improvement in left ventricular ejection fraction during the subsequent 6–12 months. Those patients in whom left ventricular ejection fraction and dimensions return to normal are usually considered to have residual subclinical cardiomyopathy. Neurohormonal antagonist therapy is usually continued indefinitely as tolerated, with dose adjustments to avoid side effects.

Specific viruses

In humans, viruses are often suspected but rarely confirmed as the direct cause of myocarditis. Often implicated is the picornavirus family of RNA viruses, with the enteroviruses *Coxsackie, echovirus,* and *poliovirus. Influenza,* another RNA virus, is implicated in myocarditis with varying frequency from year to year as the epitopes change. Of the DNA viruses, *adenovirus, variola* (smallpox) and *vaccinia* (smallpox vaccine), and the *herpesviruses* (*Varicella zoster, Cytomegalovirus, and Epstein-Barr virus*) are well recognized as causes of myocarditis. From genetic analyses of biopsy tissue, parvovirus B19, coxsackie, adenovirus, and Epstein-Barr virus are the agents most often implicated. The role of *parvovirus B19* as a cause of myocarditis or cardiomyopathy is difficult to determine, as almost half of individuals show evidence of prior infection with this small DNA virus that causes "fifth disease" in children.

Human immunodeficiency virus (HIV) has been associated with echocardiographic abnormalities in 10–40% patients with clinical disease. Cardiomyopathy in HIV may result from cardiac involvement with other associated viruses, such as cytomegalovirus and hepatitis C. Antiviral drugs to treat chronic HIV can cause cardiomyopathy, both directly as cardiotoxins and through drug hypersensitivity. The clinical picture may be complicated by pericardial effusions and pulmonary hypertension. There is a high frequency of lymphocytic myocarditis found at autopsy, and viral particles have been demonstrated in the myocardium in some cases, consistent with direct causation.

Hepatitis C has been repeatedly implicated in cardiomyopathy, particularly in Germany and Asia. Cardiac function may improve after interferon therapy. As this cytokine itself often depresses cardiac function transiently, careful coordination of administration and ongoing clinical evaluation are critical. Involvement of the heart with hepatitis B is uncommon but can be seen when associated with systemic vasculitis (polyarteritis nodosa).

Other viral infections in which cardiac involvement is specifically implicated, beyond the depression of cardiac function during any systemic cytokine activation, include *mumps, respiratory syncytial virus,* the *arboviruses (dengue fever and yellow fever),* and *arenaviruses (Lassa fever).*

Parasitic myocarditis

Chagas' disease is the third most common parasitic infection in the world and the most common cause of cardiomyopathy. The protozoan *Trypanosoma cruzi* (*T. cruzi*) is usually transmitted by the bite of the reduviid bug, endemic in the rural areas of South and Central America. Transmission can also occur through blood transfusion, organ donation, from mother to fetus, and occasionally orally. While programs to eradicate the insect vector have decreased the prevalence from about 16 million to less than 10 million in South America, cases are increasingly recognized in Western developed countries. Approximately 100,000 affected individuals are currently living in the United States, most of whom contracted the disease in endemic areas.

The acute phase of Chagas' disease with parasitemia is usually unrecognized, but in fewer than 5% of cases presents clinically within a few weeks of infection, with nonspecific symptoms or occasionally with acute myocarditis and meningoencephalitis. In the absence of antiparasitic therapy, the silent stage progresses slowly over 10–30 years in almost half of patients to manifest in the cardiac and gastrointestinal systems in the chronic stages. Survival is less than 30% at 5 years after the onset of overt clinical heart failure.

Multiple pathogenetic mechanisms are implicated. The parasite itself can cause myocyte lysis and primary neuronal damage, and specific immune responses may recognize the parasites or related antigens and lead to chronic immune activation in the absence of detectable parasites. Molecular techniques have revealed persistent parasite DNA fragments in infected individuals. Further evidence for persistent infection is the eruption of parasitic skin lesions during immunosuppression after cardiac transplantation. As in postviral myocarditis, the relative roles of persistent infection and of secondary autoimmune injury have not been resolved (Fig. 21-5). An additional factor in progression of Chagas' disease is the autonomic dysfunction and microvascular damage that may contribute to cardiac and gastrointestinal disease.

Features typical of Chagas' disease are conduction system abnormalities, particularly sinus node and atrioventricular (AV) node dysfunction and right bundle branch block. Atrial fibrillation and ventricular tachyarrhythmias also occur. Small ventricular aneurysms are common, particularly at the apex. The dilated ventricles are particularly thrombogenic, giving rise to pulmonary and systemic emboli. The serologic enzyme-linked immunosorbent assay (ELISA) for the IgM has largely replaced the previous complement fixation test for diagnosis.

Treatment of the advanced stages focused on the clinical manifestations of the disease, with heart failure regimens, pacemaker-defibrillators, and anticoagulation; however, increasing emphasis is placed on antiparasitic therapy even in chronic disease. The most common effective antiparasitic therapies are benznidazole and nifurtimox, both associated with multiple severe reactions, including dermatitis, gastrointestinal distress, and neuropathy. Patients without major extracardiac disease have occasionally undergone transplantation, after which they require lifelong therapy to suppress reactivation of infection.

African trypanosomiasis infection results from the tsetse fly bite and can occur in travelers exposed during trips to Africa. The West African form is caused by *Trypanosoma brucei gambiense* and progresses silently over years.

The East African form caused by *T. brucei rhodesiense* can progress rapidly through perivascular infiltration to myocarditis and heart failure, with frequent arrhythmias. The diagnosis is made by identification of trypanosomes in blood, lymph nodes, or other affected sites. Development of optimal drug regimens remains limited, and depends on the type and the stage (hemolymphatic or neurologic).

Toxoplasmosis is contracted through undercooked infected beef or pork, transmission from feline feces, organ transplantation, transfusion, or maternal-fetal transmission. Immunocompromised hosts are at greatest risk for reactivation of latent infection from cysts. The cysts have been found in up to 40% of autopsies of patients dying from HIV infection. Toxoplasmosis may present with encephalitis or chorioretinitis, and in the heart can cause myocarditis, pericardial effusion, constrictive pericarditis, and heart failure. The diagnosis may be suspected in an immunocompromised patient with myocarditis and serologic evidence of toxoplasmosis. Fortuitous sampling may reveal the cysts in the myocardium. Combination therapy can include pyrimethamine and sulfadiazine or clindamycin.

Trichinellosis is caused by *Trichinella spiralis* larva ingested with undercooked meat. Larva migrating into skeletal muscles cause myalgias, weakness, and fever. Periorbital and facial edema, and conjunctival and retinal hemorrhage may also be seen. Although the larva may occasionally invade the myocardium, clinical heart failure is rare, and when observed, attributed to the eosinophilic inflammatory response. The diagnosis is made from the specific serum antibody and is further supported by the presence of eosinophilia. Treatment includes antihelminthic drugs and glucocorticoids if inflammation is severe.

Cardiac involvement with *Echinococcus* is rare, but cysts can form and rupture in the myocardium and pericardium.

Bacterial infections

Most bacterial infections can involve the heart occasionally through direct invasion and abscess formation, but do so rarely. More commonly, contractility is depressed globally in severe infection and sepsis through systemic inflammatory responses. *Diphtheria* specifically affects the heart in almost one-half of cases and is the most common cause of death in patients with this infection. Once a disease of children, the prevalence of vaccines has shifted the incidence of this disease to countries where immunization is not routine and to older populations who have lost their immunity. The bacillus releases a toxin that impairs protein synthesis and may particularly affect the conduction system. The specific antitoxin should be administered as soon as possible, with higher priority than antibiotic therapy. Other systemic bacterial infections that can involve the heart include *brucellosis, chlamydophila, legionella, meningococcus, mycoplasma, psittacosis,*

and *salmonellosis,* for which treatment is directed at the systemic infection.

Clostridial infections cause myocardial damage from the released toxin. Gas bubbles can be detected in the myocardium, and occasionally abscesses can form in the myocardium and pericardium. *Streptococcal infection* with β-hemolytic streptococci is most commonly associated with acute rheumatic fever, and is characterized by inflammation and fibrosis of cardiac valves and systemic connective tissue, but can also lead to a myocarditis with focal or diffuse infiltrates of mononuclear cells.

Tuberculosis can involve the myocardium directly as well as through tuberculous pericarditis, but rarely does so when the disease is treated with antibiotics. *Whipple's disease* is caused by *Tropheryma whippleii*. The usual manifestations are in the gastrointestinal tract, but pericarditis, coronary arteritis, valvular lesions, and occasionally clinical heart failure may also occur. Multidrug antituberculous regimens are effective, but the disease tends to relapse even with appropriate treatment.

Other infections

Spirochetal myocarditis has been diagnosed from myocardial biopsies containing *Borrelia burgdorferi* that causes *Lyme disease*. Lyme carditis most often presents with arthritis and conduction system disease that resolves within 1–2 weeks of antibiotic treatment, only rarely causing clinical heart failure.

Fungal myocarditis can occur due to hematogenous or direct spread of infection from other sites, as has been described for aspergillosis, actinomycosis, blastomycosis, candidiasis, coccidioidomycosis, cryptococcosis, histoplasmosis, and mucormycosis. However, cardiac infection is rarely the dominant clinical feature of these infections.

The **rickettsial infections**, *Q fever, Rocky Mountain spotted fever,* and *scrub typhus,* are frequently accompanied by ECG changes, but most clinical manifestations relate to systemic vascular involvement.

NONINFECTIVE MYOCARDITIS

Myocardial inflammation can occur without apparent preceding infection. The paradigm of noninfectious inflammation without infection is cardiac transplant rejection, from which we have learned that myocardial depression can develop and reverse quickly, that noncellular mediators such as antibodies and cytokines play a major role in addition to lymphocytes, and that myocardial antigens are exposed by prior physical injury and viral infection.

The most commonly diagnosed noninfectious inflammation is granulomatous myocarditis, including both sarcoidosis and giant cell myocarditis. Sarcoidosis is a multisystem disease most commonly affecting the lungs, presenting in young adults with higher prevalence in African-American males. Patients with pulmonary sarcoid are at high risk for cardiac involvement, but cardiac sarcoidosis may also occur without clinical lung disease in middle-aged whites of both genders. Regional clustering of the disease supports the suspicion that the granulomatous reaction is triggered by an infectious or environmental allergen not yet identified.

The sites and density of cardiac granulomata, the time course, and the degree of extracardiac involvement are remarkably variable. Patients may present with rapid onset heart failure and ventricular tachyarrhythmias, conduction block, chest pain syndromes, or minor cardiac findings in the setting of ocular involvement, an infiltrative skin rash, or a nonspecific febrile illness. They may also present less acutely after months to years of fluctuating cardiac symptoms. When ventricular tachycardia or conduction block dominate the initial presentation of heart failure without coronary artery disease, suspicion should be high for these granulomatous myocardites.

Depending on the time course, the ventricles may appear restrictive or dilated, at times with right ventricular predominance. Small ventricular aneurysms are common. Computed tomography of the chest often reveals pulmonary lymphadenopathy even in the absence of clinical lung disease. Metabolic imaging (positron emission tomography [PET]) of the whole chest can highlight active sarcoid lesions that are avid for glucose. Magnetic resonance imaging (MRI) of the heart can identify areas likely to be inflammatory. To rule out chronic granulomatous infections, the diagnosis usually requires pathologic confirmation. Biopsy of enlarged mediastinal nodes may provide the highest yield. The scattered granulomata of sarcoidosis can be missed on cardiac biopsy (Fig. 21-7).

Immunosuppressive treatment for sarcoidosis is initiated with high-dose glucocorticoids, which are often more effective for arrhythmias than for the heart failure. Pacemakers and implantable defibrillators are generally indicated to prevent life-threatening heart block or ventricular tachycardia, respectively. Because the inflammation often resolves into extensive fibrosis that impairs cardiac function and provides pathways for reentrant arrhythmias, the prognosis is best when the granulomata are not extensive.

Giant cell myocarditis is less common than sarcoidosis, but accounts for 10–20% of biopsy-positive cases of myocarditis. Giant cell myocarditis typically presents with rapidly progressive heart failure and tachyarrhythmias. Diffuse granulomatous lesions are surrounded by extensive inflammatory infiltrate unlikely to be missed on endomyocardial biopsy. Associated conditions are thymomas, thyroiditis, pernicious anemia, other autoimmune diseases, and occasionally recent infections.

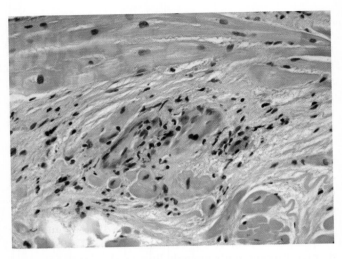

FIGURE 21-7

Sarcoidosis. Microscopic image of an endomyocardial biopsy showing a noncaseating granuloma and associated interstitial fibrosis typical of sarcoidosis. No microorganisms were present on special stains, and no foreign material was identified. Hematoxylin and eosin stained section, 200× original magnification. (*Image courtesy of Robert Padera, MD, PhD, Department of Pathology, Brigham and Women's Hospital, Boston.*)

Glucocorticoid therapy is less effective than for sarcoidosis, and is sometimes combined with other immunosuppressive agents. The course is generally of rapid deterioration requiring urgent transplantation. Although the severity of presentation and myocardial histology are more fulminant than sarcoidosis, the occasional finding of giant cell myocarditis after sarcoidosis suggests that they may in some cases represent different stages of a similar disease.

Hypersensitivity myocarditis is usually an unexpected diagnosis, made when the biopsy reveals infiltration with lymphocytes and mononuclear cells with a high proportion of eosinophils. (Sometimes called eosinophilic myocarditis, this should not be confused with hypereosinophilic syndrome in which very high circulating, often clonal populations of eosinophils cause endomyocardial fibrosis.) Most commonly the reaction is attributed to antibiotics, particularly those taken chronically, but thiazides, anticonvulsants, indomethacin, and methyldopa have also been implicated. High-dose glucocorticoids can be curative.

Myocarditis can be associated with systemic inflammatory diseases such as polymyositis and *dermatomyositis*. While sometimes considered as an explanation for cardiac findings in patients with other inflammatory disease, such as systemic lupus erythematosus, the more common causes are pericarditis, vasculitis, pulmonary hypertension, or accelerated coronary artery disease.

Peripartum cardiomyopathy develops during the last trimester or within the first 6 months after pregnancy, with a frequency between 1:3000 and 1:15,000 deliveries. The mechanisms remain controversial, but inflammation has been implicated. Risk factors are increased maternal age, increased parity, twin pregnancy, malnutrition, use of tocolytic therapy for premature labor, and preeclampsia or toxemia of pregnancy. As the increased circulatory demand of pregnancy can aggravate other cardiac disease that was clinically unrecognized, it is crucial to the diagnosis that there be no evidence for preexisting cardiac disorder.

Heart failure early after delivery was previously common in Nigeria, when the custom for new mothers included salt ingestion while reclining on a warm bed, which likely impaired mobilization of the excess circulating volume after delivery. In the Western world, lymphocytic myocarditis has often been found on myocardial biopsy. This inflammation has been hypothesized to reflect increased susceptibility to viral myocarditis or an autoimmune myocarditis due to cross-reactivity of anti-uterine antibodies against cardiac muscle. Another mechanism involving a prolactin cleavage fragment has been proposed based on an animal model.

TOXIC CARDIOMYOPATHY

Cardiotoxicity has been reported with multiple environmental and pharmacologic agents. Often these associations are seen only with very high levels of exposure or acute overdoses, respectively, in which acute electrocardiographic and hemodynamic abnormalities may reflect both direct drug effect and systemic toxicity.

Alcohol is the most common toxin implicated in chronic dilated cardiomyopathy. Excess consumption may contribute to more than 10% of cases of heart failure, including exacerbation of cases with other primary etiologies such as valvular disease or previous infarction. Toxicity is attributed both to alcohol and to its primary metabolite acetaldehyde. Polymorphisms of the genes encoding alcohol dehydrogenase and the angiotensin-converting enzyme increase the likelihood of alcoholic cardiomyopathy. Superimposed vitamin deficiencies and toxic alcohol additives are rarely implicated. The alcohol consumption necessary to produce cardiomyopathy in an otherwise normal heart has been estimated to be six drinks (about 4 ounces of pure ethanol) daily for 5–10 years, but frequent binge drinking may also be sufficient. Many patients with alcoholic cardiomyopathy are fully functional without apparent stigmata of alcoholism.

Diastolic dysfunction, mild ventricular dilation, and subclinical depression of contractility can be seen before the development of clinical heart failure. Atrial fibrillation occurs commonly. The cardiac impairment in severe alcoholic cardiomyopathy is the sum of both permanent damage and a substantial component that is reversible after cessation of alcohol consumption. Medical therapy includes neurohormonal antagonists and diuretics as needed for fluid management. Withdrawal

should be supervised to avoid exacerbations of heart failure or arrhythmias, and ongoing support arranged. Even with severe disease, marked improvement can occur within 3–6 months of abstinence. Implantable defibrillators are generally deferred until an adequate period of abstinence, after which they may not be necessary if the ejection fraction has improved. With continued consumption, the prognosis is grim.

Cocaine, amphetamines, and related catecholaminergic stimulants can produce chronic cardiomyopathy as well as acute ischemia and tachyarrhythmias. Pathology reveals tiny microinfarcts consistent with small vessel ischemia. Similar findings can be seen with pheochromocytoma.

Chemotherapy agents are the most common drugs implicated in cardiomyopathy. Judicious use of these drugs requires balancing the risks of the malignancy and the risks of cardiotoxicity, as many cancers have a chronic course with prognosis no worse than heart failure.

Anthracyclines cause characteristic histologic changes of vacuolar degeneration and myofibrillar loss. Generation of reactive oxygen species involving heme compounds is currently the favored explanation for myocyte injury and fibrosis. Disruption of the large titin protein may contribute to loss of sarcomere organization. There are three different presentations of anthracycline-induced cardiomyopathy. Acute heart failure developing during administration of a single dose can be severe, but may clinically resolve in a few weeks. Early onset doxorubicin cardiotoxicity develops in about 3% of patients during or shortly after a chronic course, relating closely to total dose. It may be rapidly progressive, but may also improve to restore reasonable ventricular function. The chronic presentation differs according to whether therapy was given before or after puberty. Patients who received doxorubicin while still growing may have inadequate development of the heart to support cardiac function into the early twenties. Late after adult exposure, patients may develop the gradual onset of symptoms or an acute onset precipitated by a reversible insult, such as influenza or atrial fibrillation. Doxorubicin cardiotoxicity leads to a relatively nondilated ventricle, perhaps due to the accompanying fibrosis. Thus, the stroke volume may be severely reduced with an ejection fraction of 30–40%, which would be well tolerated in a patient with a more dilated ventricle typical of other cardiomyopathies. Therapy is that for heart failure, with careful suppression of "inappropriate" sinus tachycardia, and attention to postural hypotension that can occur in these patients. Once thought to have an inexorable downward course, some patients with doxorubicin cardiotoxicity improve under careful management to near-normal clinical function for many years.

Trastuzumab is a monoclonal antibody that interferes with cell surface receptors crucial for some tumor growth and for cardiac adaptation. The incidence of cardiotoxicity is lower than for anthracyclines but enhanced by coadministration with them. Although considered to be more often reversible, trastuzumab cardiotoxicity does not always resolve, and some patients progress to clinical heart failure and death. As with anthracycline cardiotoxicity, therapy is as usual for heart failure, but it is not clear whether or not the spontaneous rate of improvement is enhanced by neurohormonal antagonists.

Cardiotoxicity with *cyclophosphamide* and *ifosfamide* generally occurs acutely and with very high doses. 5-Fluorouracil, cisplatin, and some other alkylating agents can cause recurrent coronary spasm that occasionally leads to depressed contractility. Many small molecule *tyrosine kinase inhibitors* are under development for different malignancies. Although these agents are "targeted" at specific tumor receptors or pathways, the biologic conservation of signaling pathways can cause inhibitors to have "off-target" effects that include the heart and vasculature. Acute administration of *interferon-α* can cause hypotension and arrhythmias. Clinical heart failure occurring during repeated chronic administration usually resolves after discontinuation.

Other therapeutic drugs that can cause cardiotoxicity during chronic use include hydroxychloroquine, chloroquine, emetine, and antiretroviral therapies.

Toxic exposures are most commonly implicated in arrhythmias or respiratory injury acutely during accidents. Chronic exposures that can cause cardiotoxicity include hydrocarbons, fluorocarbons, arsenicals, lead, and mercury.

METABOLIC CAUSES OF DILATED CARDIOMYOPATHY

Endocrine disorders affect multiple organ systems, including the heart. *Hyperthyroidism and hypothyroidism* do not often cause clinical heart failure in an otherwise normal heart, but commonly exacerbate heart failure. The most common, current reason for thyroid abnormalities in the heart failure population is the use of amiodarone, a drug with substantial iodine content. Clinical signs of thyroid disease may be masked, so tests of thyroid function are part of the routine evaluation of cardiomyopathy. Hypothyroidism should be treated with very slow escalation of doses to avoid exacerbating tachyarrhythmias and heart failure. Hyperthyroidism should always be considered with new onset atrial fibrillation or ventricular tachycardia, or atrial fibrillation in which the rapid ventricular response is difficult to control. Hyperthyroidism and heart failure are a dangerous combination that merits very close supervision, often hospitalization, during titration of antithyroid medications, which may lead to precipitous worsening of heart failure. *Pheochromocytoma* is rare, but should be considered when a patient has heart failure and very labile blood pressure and heart rate, sometimes with episodic palpitations. Most patients with pheochromocytoma have postural hypotension. In addition to α-adrenergic receptor antagonists, definitive therapy requires surgical extirpation. Very high renin states, such as those caused by renal artery stenosis, can lead to modest depression in ejection fraction with little or no ventricular dilation and markedly labile symptoms with flash pulmonary edema, related to sudden shifts in vascular tone and intravascular volume.

Controversies remain regarding whether *diabetes* and *obesity* are sufficient to cause cardiomyopathy. Most heart failure in diabetes results from epicardial coronary disease, with further increase in coronary artery risk due to accompanying hypertension and renal dysfunction. Cardiomyopathy may result in part from insulin resistance and increased advanced-glycosylation end products, which impair both systolic and diastolic function. However, much of the dysfunction can be attributed to scattered focal ischemia resulting from distal coronary artery tapering and limited microvascular perfusion even without proximal focal stenoses. Diabetes is a typical factor, along with hypertension, advanced age, and female gender, in heart failure with "preserved" ejection fraction.

The existence of a cardiomyopathy due to *obesity* is generally accepted. In addition to cardiac involvement from associated diabetes, hypertension, and vascular inflammation of the metabolic syndrome, obesity alone is associated with impaired excretion of excess volume load, which, over time, can lead to increased wall stress and secondary adaptive neurohumoral responses. The rapid clearance of natriuretic peptides by adipose tissue may contribute to fluid retention. In the absence of another obvious cause of cardiomyopathy in an obese patient with systolic dysfunction without marked ventricular dilation, effective weight reduction is often associated with major improvement in ejection fraction and clinical function.

Nutritional deficiencies can occasionally cause dilated cardiomyopathy but are not commonly implicated in developed Western countries. *Beri-beri heart disease* due to thiamine deficiency can result from poor nutrition in undernourished populations, and in patients deriving most of their calories from alcohol, and has been reported in teenagers subsisting only on highly processed foods. This disease is initially a vasodilated state with very high output heart failure that can later progress to a low output state; thiamine repletion can lead to prompt recovery of cardiovascular function. Abnormalities in *carnitine* metabolism can cause dilated or restrictive cardiomyopathies, usually in children. Deficiency of trace elements such as *selenium* can cause cardiomyopathy (Keshan's disease).

Calcium is essential for excitation-contraction coupling, serving as an inotrope when administered. Chronic deficiencies of calcium, such as can occur with hypoparathyroidism (particularly postsurgical) or intestinal dysfunction (from diarrheal syndromes and following extensive resection), can cause severe chronic heart failure that responds over days or weeks to vigorous calcium repletion. *Phosphate* is a component of high-energy compounds needed for efficient energy transfer and multiple signaling pathways. Hypophosphatemia can develop during starvation and early refeeding following a prolonged fast, and occasionally during hyperalimentation. *Magnesium* is a cofactor for thiamine-dependent reactions and for the sodium–potassium adenosine triphosphatase (ATPase), but hypomagnesemia rarely becomes sufficiently profound to cause clinical cardiomyopathy.

Hemochromatosis is variably classified as a metabolic or storage disease. It is included among the causes of restrictive cardiomyopathy, but the clinical presentation is often that of a dilated cardiomyopathy. The autosomal recessive form is related to the HFE gene. With up to 10% of the population heterozygous for one mutation, the clinical prevalence might be as high as 1 in 500. The lower rates observed highlight the limited penetrance of the disease, suggesting the role of additional genetic and environmental factors for clinical expression. The clinical syndrome includes cirrhosis, diabetes, and hypogonadism. Hemochromatosis can also be acquired from iron overload due to hemolytic anemia and transfusions. Excess iron is deposited in the perinuclear compartment of cardiomyocytes, with resulting disruption of intracellular architecture and mitochondrial function. Diagnosis is easily made from measurement of serum iron and transferrin saturation, with a threshold of >60% for men, and >45–50% for women. Magnetic resonance imaging can help to quantitate iron stores in the liver and heart, and endomyocardial biopsy tissue can be stained for iron (**Fig. 21-8**). If diagnosed early, hemochromatosis can often be managed by repeated phlebotomy to remove iron. For more severe iron overload, iron chelation therapy with desferrioxamine (deferoxamine) or deferasirox can help to improve cardiac function if myocyte loss and replacement fibrosis are not too severe. Inborn disorders of metabolism occasionally present with dilated cardiomyopathy, although are most often associated with restrictive cardiomyopathy (Table 21-4).

FAMILIAL DILATED CARDIOMYOPATHY

The recognized frequency of familial involvement in dilated cardiomyopathy has now increased to an estimated 30% (Table 21-3). The most recognizable familial syndromes are the *muscular dystrophies*. Both Duchenne's and the milder Becker's dystrophy result from abnormalities in the X-linked dystrophin gene of the sarcolemmal membrane. Skeletal myopathy is present in multiple other genetic cardiomyopathies (Table 21-3), some

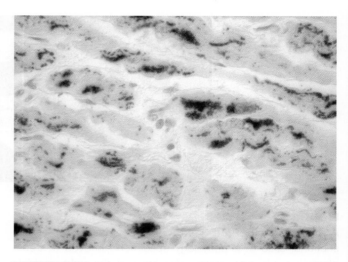

FIGURE 21-8

Hemochromatosis. Microscopic image of an endomyocardial biopsy showing extensive iron deposition within the cardiac myocytes with the Prussian blue stain (400× original magnification). (*Image courtesy of Robert Padera, MD, PhD, Department of Pathology, Brigham and Women's Hospital, Boston.*)

of which are associated with creatine kinase elevations. Mitochondrial myopathies are associated with varying degrees of skeletal involvement, biopsies of which show the characteristic "ragged red fiber" appearance. Some patients with mitochondrial myopathy have characteristic drooping eyelids. The energy deficits associated with mitochondrial abnormalities lead to multiple systemic syndromes. Other familial metabolic defects more often present as restrictive disease, but can sometimes be identified on electron microscopy of endomyocardial biopsies.

Families with a history of atrial arrhythmias, conduction system disease, and cardiomyopathy may have abnormalities of the nuclear membrane lamin proteins. While all dilated cardiomyopathies carry a risk of sudden death, a family history of cardiomyopathy with sudden death raises suspicion for a particularly arrhythmogenic mutation; affected family members may be considered for implantable defibrillators even before meeting the reduced ejection fraction threshold for primary prevention of sudden death.

A prominent family history of sudden death or ventricular tachycardia before clinical cardiomyopathy suggests genetic defects in the desmosomal proteins causing *arrhythmogenic ventricular dysplasia* (**Fig. 21-9**). Originally described as affecting the right ventricle (arrhythmogenic right ventricular dysplasia [ARVD]), this disorder can affect either or both ventricles. Patients often present first with ventricular tachycardia. Genetic defects in proteins of the desmosomal complex disrupt myocyte junctions and adhesions, leading to replacement of myocardium by deposits of fat. Thin ventricular walls may be recognized on echocardiography but are better visualized on MRI. The same protein also affects hair

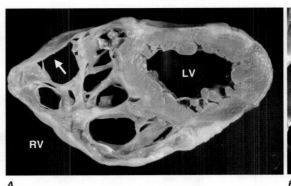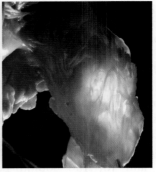

A   **B**

FIGURE 21-9
Arrhythmogenic right ventricular dysplasia. (A) Cross-sectional slice of a pathology specimen removed at transplantation, showing severe dysplasia of the right ventricle (RV) with extensive fatty replacement of right ventricular myocardium. The remarkably thin right ventricular free wall is revealed by transillumination (**B**). (*Images courtesy of Gayle Winters, MD, and Richard Mitchell, MD, PhD, Division of Pathology, Brigham and Women's Hospital, Boston.*)

and skin, leading in some cases to a distinct syndrome of "woolly hair," and thickened palms and soles. Implantable defibrillators are usually indicated to prevent sudden death. There is variable progression to right, left, or biventricular failure.

Left ventricular noncompaction is a condition of unknown prevalence that is increasingly revealed by better imaging techniques, first by two-dimensional echocardiography and more recently by magnetic resonance imaging. The diagnostic criteria includes the presence of multiple trabeculations in the left ventricle distal to the papillary muscles, creating a "spongy" appearance of the apex; it has been associated with multiple genetic variants in the sarcomeric and other proteins such as tafazzin. The condition may be diagnosed incidentally or in patients carrying previous diagnoses of dilated, restrictive, or hypertrophic cardiomyopathy. The three cardinal clinical features are ventricular arrhythmias, embolic events, and heart failure. Treatment generally includes anticoagulation and consideration for an implantable defibrillator.

Some families inherit a susceptibility to viral-induced myocarditis. This propensity may relate to abnormalities in cell surface receptors, such as the coxsackie-adenovirus receptor, that bind viral proteins. Some may have partial homology with viral proteins such that an autoimmune response is triggered against the myocardium.

The therapy of familial dilated cardiomyopathy is dictated primarily by the stage of clinical disease and the risk for sudden death. In some cases, the familial etiology facilitates prognostic decisions, particularly regarding the likelihood of recovery after a new diagnosis, which is unlikely for familial disease and frequent if the disease is acquired. The rate of progression of disease is to some extent heritable, although marked variation can be seen; however, there have been cases of remarkable clinical remission after acute presentation, likely after a reversible insult, such as infective myocarditis.

Genetic testing is less robust for dilated cardiomyopathy, for which our current understanding is similar to that for hypertrophic cardiomyopathy a decade ago. Newer molecular techniques, animal models, and data banks of cardiomyopathy patients are all contributing to the rapid expansion of the data presented in Table 21-3. However, serendipitous identification of inherited cardiomyopathy, its systemic signature, and clinical course remain crucial to continue to advance the field, one family and one gene at a time.

TAKO-TSUBO CARDIOMYOPATHY

The apical ballooning syndrome, or stress-induced cardiomyopathy, occurs typically in older women after sudden intense emotional or physical stress. The ventricle shows global ventricular dilation with basal contraction, forming the shape of the narrow-necked jar (*tako-tsubo*) used in Japan to trap octopi. Originally described there, it is increasingly recognized in other countries and may go unrecognized during intensive care unit (ICU) admission for noncardiac conditions. Presentations include pulmonary edema, hypotension, and chest pain with ECG changes mimicking an acute infarction. The left ventricular dysfunction extends beyond a specific coronary artery distribution and generally resolves within days to weeks, but may recur in up to 10% of patients. Animal models and ventricular biopsies suggest that this acute cardiomyopathy may result from intense sympathetic activation with heterogeneity of myocardial autonomic innervation, diffuse microvascular spasm, and/or direct catecholamine toxicity. Coronary angiography may be required to rule out acute coronary occlusion. No therapies have been proven beneficial, but reasonable strategies include nitrates for pulmonary edema, intraaortic balloon pump if needed for low output, combined alpha and beta blockers rather than selective beta blockade if hemodynamically stable, and magnesium for arrhythmias related to QT prolongation. Anticoagulation is generally withheld due to the occasional occurrence of ventricular rupture.

IDIOPATHIC DILATED CARDIOMYOPATHY

Idiopathic dilated cardiomyopathy is a diagnosis of exclusion, when all other known factors have been excluded. Approximately two-thirds of dilated cardiomyopathies are still labeled as idiopathic; however, a substantial proportion of these may reflect unrecognized genetic disease. Continued reconsideration of etiology often reveals specific causes later in a patient's course.

OVERLAP BETWEEN CARDIOMYOPATHIES

The limitations of our phenotypic classification are revealed through the multiple overlaps between the etiologies and presentations of the three types. Cardiomyopathy with reduced systolic function but without severe dilation can represent early dilated cardiomyopathy, "minimally dilated cardiomyopathy," or restrictive diseases without marked increases in ventricular wall thickness. For example, sarcoidosis and hemochromatosis can present as dilated or restrictive disease. Early stages of amyloidosis sometimes appear as dilated cardiomyopathy, but can also be mistaken for hypertrophic cardiomyopathy. Progression of hypertrophic cardiomyopathy into a "burned-out" phase occurs occasionally, with decreased contractility and modest ventricular dilation. Overlaps are particularly common with the inherited metabolic disorders, which can present as any of the three major phenotypes (Fig. 21-4).

RESTRICTIVE CARDIOMYOPATHY

The least common of the triad of cardiomyopathies is restrictive cardiomyopathy, which is dominated by abnormal diastolic function, often with mildly decreased contractility and ejection fraction (usually >30–50%). Both atria are enlarged, sometimes massively. Modest left ventricular dilation can be present, usually with an end-diastolic dimension <6 cm. End-diastolic pressures are elevated in both ventricles, with preservation of cardiac output until late in the disease. Subtle exercise intolerance is usually the first symptom but is often not recognized until after clinical presentation with congestive symptoms. The restrictive diseases often present with relatively more right-sided symptoms, such as edema, abdominal discomfort, and ascites, although filling pressures are elevated in both ventricles. The cardiac impulse is less displaced than in dilated cardiomyopathy

TABLE 21-6

CAUSES OF RESTRICTIVE CARDIOMYOPATHIES

Infiltrative (Between Myocytes)

Amyloidosis
  Primary (light-chain amyloid)
  Familial (abnormal transthyretin)[a]
  Senile (normal transthyretin or atrial peptides)
Inherited metabolic defects[a] (see Table 21-4)

Storage (Within Myocytes)

Hemochromatosis (iron)[a]
Inherited metabolic defects[a] (see Table 21-4)
  Fabry's disease
  Glycogen storage disease (II, III)

Fibrotic

Radiation
Scleroderma

Endomyocardial

Possibly related fibrotic diseases
  Tropical endomyocardial fibrosis
  Hypereosinophilic syndrome (Löffler's endocarditis)
Carcinoid syndrome
Radiation
Drugs: e.g., serotonin, ergotamine

Overlap with Other Cardiomyopathies

Hypertrophic cardiomyopathy/"pseudohypertrophic"[a]
"Minimally dilated" cardiomyopathy
  Early-stage dilated cardiomyopathy
  Partial recovery from dilated cardiomyopathy
Sarcoidosis

Idiopathic[a]

[a]Can be familial.

and less dynamic than in hypertrophic cardiomyopathy. A fourth heart sound is more common than a third heart sound in sinus rhythm, but atrial fibrillation is common. Jugular venous pressures often show rapid Y descents, and may increase during inspiration (positive Kussmaul's sign). Most restrictive cardiomyopathies are due to infiltration of abnormal substances between myocytes, storage of abnormal metabolic products within myocytes, or fibrotic injury (Table 21-6).

INFILTRATIVE DISEASE

Amyloidosis is the major cause of restrictive cardiomyopathy (Figs. 21-10, 21-11, and 21-12), most often due to "primary amyloidosis" caused by abnormal production of immunoglobulin light chains. Familial amyloidosis results from an autosomal dominant mutation in transthyretin, a carrier protein for thyroxine and retinol, that is more common in African Americans than whites. Amyloidosis secondary to other chronic diseases rarely involves the heart. Senile amyloidosis with deposition of normal transthyretin or atrial natriuretic peptide usually has an

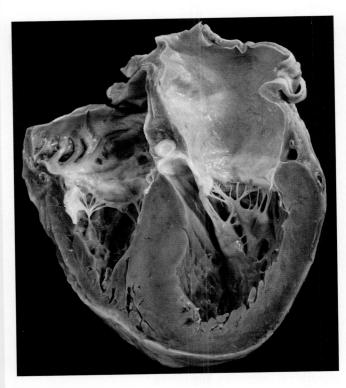

FIGURE 21-10

Restrictive cardiomyopathy—amyloidosis. Gross specimen of a heart with amyloidosis. The heart is firm and rubbery with a waxy cut surface. The atria are markedly dilated and the left atrial endocardium, normally smooth, has yellow-brown amyloid deposits that give texture to the surface. (*Image courtesy of Robert Padera, MD, PhD, Department of Pathology, Brigham and Women's Hospital, Boston.*)

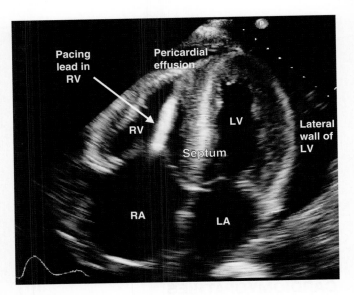

FIGURE 21-11

Restrictive cardiomyopathy—amyloidosis. Echocardiogram showing thickened walls of both ventricles without major chamber dilation. The atria are markedly dilated, consistent with chronically elevated ventricular filling pressures. In this example, there is a characteristic hyper-refractile "glittering" of the myocardium typical of amyloid infiltration, which is often absent (especially with more recent echocardiographic systems of better resolution). The mitral and tricuspid valves are thickened. A pacing lead is visible in the right ventricle and a pericardial effusion is evident. Note that the echocardiographic and pathologic images are vertically opposite, such that the LV is by convention on the top right in the echocardiographic image and bottom right in the pathologic images. (*Image courtesy of Justina Wu, MD, Brigham and Women's Hospital, Boston.*)

indolent course and is very common beyond the seventh decade.

Amyloid fibrils infiltrate the myocardium, especially around the conduction system and coronary vessels. Typical clinical features are conduction block, autonomic neuropathy, renal involvement, and occasionally thickened skin lesions. Cardiac amyloid is suspected from thickened ventricular walls in conjunction with an electrocardiogram that shows low voltage. A characteristic refractile brightness in the septum on echocardiography is suggestive, but neither sensitive nor specific. Both atria are dilated, often dramatically so. The diagnosis of primary or familial can be made from biopsies of an abdominal fat pad or the rectum, but cardiac amyloidosis is most reliably identified from the myocardium (Fig. 21-12). Therapy is largely symptomatic, using diuretics as needed to treat fluid retention, which often requires high doses. Digoxin bound to the amyloid fibrils can reach toxic levels, and should therefore be used only in very low doses, if at all. There is no evidence regarding use of neurohormonal antagonists in amyloid heart disease, where the possible theoretical benefit has to be balanced against their potential

side effects in light of frequent autonomic neuropathy and dependence on heart rate reserve. The risk of intracardiac thrombi may warrant chronic anticoagulation. Once heart failure develops, the median survival is 6–12 months in primary amyloidosis. Multiple myeloma is treated with chemotherapy (prednisone, melphalan, bortezomib), the extent of which is usually limited by the potential of worsening cardiac dysfunction. Colchicine can be of some benefit in inflammation-associated (AA) amyloid. Transthyretin-associated cardiac amyloid requires heart and liver transplantation, while senile cardiac amyloid is treated with conventional heart failure regimens. Immunoglobulin–associated amyloid has occasionally been treated with sequential heart transplantation and delayed bone marrow transplant, with frequent recurrence of amyloid in the transplanted heart.

DISORDERS OF METABOLIC PATHWAYS

Multiple genetic disorders of metabolic pathways can cause myocardial disease, due to infiltration of abnormal products or cells containing them between the

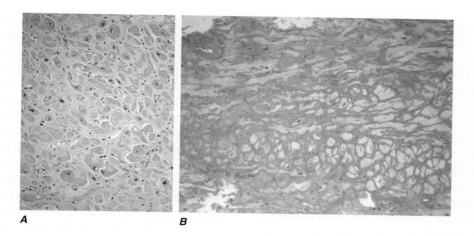

A   *B*

FIGURE 21-12

Amyloidosis—microscopic images of amyloid involving the myocardium. The left panel (hematoxylin-eosin stain) shows glassy, grey-pink amorphous material infiltrating between cardiomyocytes, which stain a darker pink. The right panel shows a sulfated blue stain that highlights the amyloid green and stains the cardiac myocytes yellow. (The Congo red stain can also be used to highlight amyloid; under polarized light, amyloid will have an apple-green birefringence when stained with Congo red.) Images at 100× original magnification. (*Image courtesy of Robert Padera, MD, PhD, Department of Pathology, Brigham and Women's Hospital, Boston.*)

myocytes, and storage disease, due to their accumulation within cells (Tables 21-4 and 21-6). The restrictive phenotype is most common but mildly dilated cardiomyopathy may occur. Hypertrophic cardiomyopathy may be mimicked by the myocardium thickened with these abnormal products causing "pseudohypertrophy." Most of these diseases are diagnosed during childhood.

Fabry's disease results from a deficiency of the lysosomal enzyme alpha-galactosidase A caused by one of more than 160 mutations. This disorder of glycosphingolipid metabolism is an X-linked recessive disorder that may also cause clinical disease in female carriers. Glycolipid accumulation may be limited to the cardiac tissues or may also involve the skin and kidney. Electron microscopy of endomyocardial biopsy tissue shows diagnostic vesicles containing concentric lamellar figures **(Fig. 21-13).** Diagnosis is crucial because enzyme replacement can reduce abnormal deposits and improve cardiac and clinical function. Enzyme replacement can also improve the course of Gaucher's disease, in which cerebroside-rich cells accumulate in multiple organs due to a deficiency of beta-glucosidase. Cerebroside-rich cells infiltrate the heart, which can also lead to a hemorrhagic pericardial effusion and valvular disease.

Glycogen storage diseases lead to accumulation of lysosomal storage products and intracellular glycogen accumulation, particularly with *glycogen storage disease type III,* due to a defective debranching enzyme. There are more than 10 types of *mucopolysaccharidoses,* in which autosomal dominant or X-linked deficiencies of lysosomal enzymes lead to the accumulation of glycosaminoglycans in the skeleton, nervous system, and heart. With characteristic facies, short stature, and frequent cognitive impairment, most individuals are diagnosed early in childhood and die before adulthood.

Carnitine is an essential cofactor in long-chain fatty acid metabolism. Multiple defects have been described that lead to carnitine deficiency, causing intracellular lipid inclusions and restrictive or dilated cardiomyopathy, often presenting in children. Fatty acid oxidation requires many metabolic steps with specific enzymes that can be deficient, with complex interactions with carnitine. Depending on the defect, cardiac and skeletal

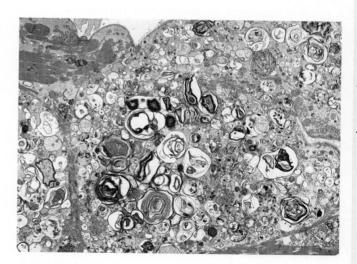

FIGURE 21-13

Fabry's disease. Transmission electron micrograph of a right ventricular endomyocardial biopsy specimen at high magnification showing the characteristic concentric lamellar inclusions of glycosphingolipids accumulating as a result of deficiency of the lysosomal enzyme alpha-galactosidase A. Image taken at 15,000× original magnification. (*Image courtesy of Robert Padera, MD, PhD, Department of Pathology, Brigham and Women's Hospital, Boston.*)

myopathy can be ameliorated with replacement of fatty acid intermediates and carnitine.

Two monogenic metabolic cardiomyopathies have recently been described as causes of increased ventricular wall thickness without an increase of muscle subunits or an increase in contractility. Mutations in the gamma-2 regulatory subunit of the adenosine monophosphate (AMP)-activated protein kinase important for glucose metabolism (PRKAG2) have been associated with a high prevalence of conduction abnormalities, such as AV block and ventricular preexcitation (Wolff-Parkinson-White syndrome). Several defects have been reported in an X-linked lysosome-associated membrane protein (LAMP2). This defect can be maternally transmitted or sporadic and has occasionally been isolated to the heart, although it often leads to a syndrome of skeletal myopathy, mental retardation, and hepatic dysfunction referred to as *Danon's disease*. Left ventricular hypertrophy appears early, often in childhood, and can progress rapidly to end-stage heart failure with low ejection fraction. Electron microscopy of these metabolic disorders shows that the myocytes are enlarged by multiple intracellular vacuoles of metabolic by-products.

FIBROTIC RESTRICTIVE CARDIOMYOPATHY

Progressive fibrosis can cause restrictive myocardial disease without dilation. Thoracic radiation, common for breast and lung cancer or mediastinal lymphoma, can produce early or late restrictive cardiomyopathy. Patients with *radiation cardiomyopathy* may present with a possible diagnosis of constrictive pericarditis, as the two conditions often coexist. Careful hemodynamic evaluation and, often, endomyocardial biopsy should be performed if considering pericardial stripping surgery, which is unlikely to be successful in the presence of underlying restrictive cardiomyopathy.

Scleroderma causes small vessel spasm and ischemia that can lead to a small, stiff heart with reduced ejection fraction without dilation. Doxorubicin causes direct myocyte injury usually leading to dilated cardiomyopathy, but the limited degree of dilation may result from increased fibrosis, which restricts remodeling.

ENDOMYOCARDIAL DISEASE

The physiologic picture of elevated filling pressures with atrial enlargement and preserved ventricular contractility with normal or reduced ventricular volumes can also result from extensive fibrosis of the endocardium, without transmural myocardial disease. For patients who have not lived in the equatorial regions, this picture is rare, and when seen is usually associated with a history of chronic hypereosinophilic syndrome (*Löffler's endocarditis*), which is more common in men than women. In this disease, persistent

hypereosinophilia of >1500 eos/mm^3 for at least 6 months can cause an acute phase of eosinophilic injury in the endocardium, with systemic illness and injury to other organs. There is usually no obvious cause, but the hypereosinophilia can occasionally be explained by allergic, parasitic, or malignant disease. It is postulated to be followed by a period in which cardiac inflammation is replaced by evidence of fibrosis with superimposed thrombosis. In severe disease, the dense fibrotic layer can obliterate the ventricular apices and extend to thicken and tether the atrioventricular valve leaflets. The clinical disease may present with heart failure, embolic events, and atrial arrhythmias. While plausible, the sequence of transition has not been clearly demonstrated.

In tropical countries, up to one-quarter of heart failure may be due to *endomyocardial fibrosis,* affecting either or both ventricles. This condition shares with the previous condition the partial obliteration of the ventricular apex with fibrosis extending into the valvular inflow tract and leaflets; however, it is not clear that the etiologies are the same for all cases. Pericardial effusions frequently accompany endomyocardial fibrosis but are not common in Löffler's endocarditis. For endomyocardial fibrosis, there is no gender difference, but a higher prevalence in African-American populations. While tropical endomyocardial fibrosis could represent the end stage of previous hypereosinophilic disease triggered by endemic parasites, neither prior parasitic infection nor hypereosinophilia is usually documented. Geographic nutritional deficiencies have also been proposed as an etiology.

Medical treatment focuses on glucocorticoids and chemotherapy to suppress hypereosinophilia when present. Fluid retention may become increasingly resistant to diuretic therapy. Anticoagulation is recommended. Atrial fibrillation is associated with worse symptoms and prognosis, but may be difficult to suppress. Surgical resection of the apices and replacement of the fibrotic valves can improve symptoms, but surgical morbidity and mortality and later recurrence rates are high.

The serotonin secreted by *carcinoid* tumors can produce fibrous plaques in the endocardium and right-sided cardiac valves, occasionally affecting left-sided valves, as well. Valvular lesions may be stenotic or regurgitant. Systemic symptoms include flushing and diarrhea. Liver disease from hepatic metastases may play a role by limiting hepatic function and thereby allowing more serotonin to reach the venous circulation.

HYPERTROPHIC CARDIOMYOPATHY

Hypertrophic cardiomyopathy is characterized by marked left ventricular hypertrophy in the absence of other causes, such as hypertension or valve disease (**Figs. 21-14** and **21-15**). The systolic function as measured by

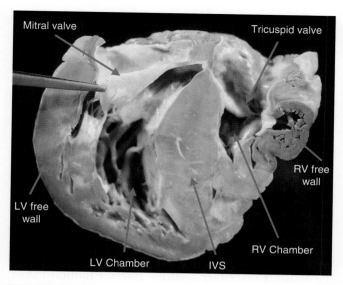

FIGURE 21-14

Hypertrophic cardiomyopathy. Gross specimen of a heart with hypertrophic cardiomyopathy removed at the time of transplantation, showing asymmetric septal hypertrophy (septum much thicker than left ventricular free wall) with the septum bulging into the left ventricular outflow tract causing obstruction. The forceps are retracting the anterior leaflet of the mitral valve, demonstrating the characteristic plaque of systolic anterior motion, manifest as endocardial fibrosis on the interventricular septum in a mirror-image pattern to the valve leaflet. There is patchy replacement fibrosis, and small thick walled arterioles can be appreciated grossly, especially in the interventricular septum. IVS, interventricular septum; LV, left ventricle; RV, right ventricle. (*Image courtesy of Robert Padera, MD, PhD, Department of Pathology, Brigham and Women's Hospital, Boston.*)

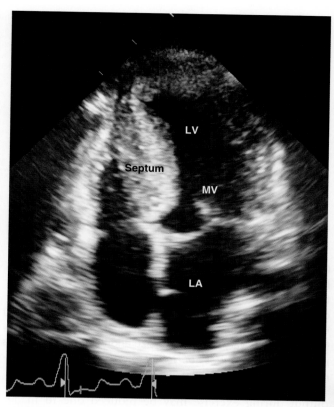

FIGURE 21-15

Hypertrophic cardiomyopathy. This echocardiogram of hypertrophic cardiomyopathy shows asymmetric hypertrophy of the septum compared to the lateral wall of the left ventricle (LV). The mitral valve is moving anteriorly toward the hypertrophied septum in systole. The left atrium (LA) is enlarged. Note that the echocardiographic and pathologic images are vertically opposite, such that the LV is by convention on the top right in the echocardiographic image and bottom right in the pathologic images. (*Image courtesy of Justina Wu, MD, Brigham and Women's Hospital, Boston.*)

ejection fraction is often supranormal, at times with virtual obliteration of the left ventricular cavity during systole. The hypertrophy may be asymmetric, involving the septum more than the free wall of the ventricle. Approximately one-third of symptomatic patients demonstrate a resting intraventricular gradient that impedes outflow during systole and is exacerbated by increased contractility. This was previously termed *hypertrophic obstructive cardiomyopathy* (HOCM), as distinguished from *nonobstructive hypertrophic cardiomyopathy*. Other terms that have been used include *asymmetric septal hypertrophy* (ASH) and *idiopathic hypertrophic subaortic stenosis* (IHSS). However, the accepted terminology is now hypertrophic cardiomyopathy with or without an obstructive gradient. Classically, the microscopic picture shows marked disarray of individual fibers in a characteristic whorled pattern and disarray, also at the level of the larger bundles, interspersed with fibrosis (Fig. 21-16).

The prevalence of hypertrophic cardiomyopathy is 1:500 adults. Approximately one-half of these cases occur in a recognizable autosomal dominant pattern, and spontaneous mutations also arise. This is the best characterized genetic cardiomyopathy, for which more than 400 individual mutations have been identified in 11 sarcomeric genes. More than 80% of the mutations are in the beta-myosin heavy chain, the cardiac myosin-binding protein C, or cardiac troponin T. Some families may demonstrate a higher incidence of early progression to end-stage heart failure or death, suggesting that their mutations are more "malignant." However, the heterogeneity of phenotypic expression within and between families confirms the influence of modifying factors from other genes and the environment.

Hypertrophic cardiomyopathy is characterized hemodynamically by diastolic dysfunction, originally attributed to the hypertrophy, fibrosis, and intraventricular gradient when present. However, studies of asymptomatic family members indicate that diastolic dysfunction is a more fundamental abnormality that can precede evidence of hypertrophy. Resting ejection fraction and cardiac output are usually normal, but peak cardiac

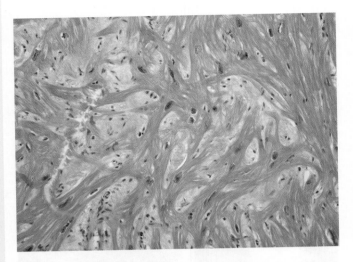

FIGURE 21-16
Hypertrophic cardiomyopathy. Microscopic image of hypertrophic cardiomyopathy showing the characteristic disordered myocyte architecture with swirling and branching rather than the usual parallel arrangement of myocyte fibers. Myocyte nuclei vary markedly in size and interstitial fibrosis is present. (*Image courtesy of Robert Padera, MD, PhD, Department of Pathology, Brigham and Women's Hospital, Boston.*)

output during exercise may be reduced due to inadequate ventricular filling at high heart rates.

DIAGNOSIS

Hypertrophic cardiomyopathy usually presents between the ages of 20 and 40 years. Dyspnea on exertion is the most common presenting symptom, reflecting elevated intracardiac filling pressures. Chest pain with either an atypical or typical exertional pattern occurs in more than half of symptomatic patients and is attributed to myocardial ischemia from high demand and abnormal intramural coronary arteries in the hypertrophied myocardium. Palpitations may result from atrial fibrillation or ventricular arrhythmias. Much less common are episodes of presyncope or syncope, often related to heavy exertion. Of grave concern is the possibility that the first manifestation of disease may be sudden death from ventricular tachycardia or fibrillation. Hypertrophic cardiomyopathy is the most common lesion found at autopsy of young athletes dying suddenly.

The physical examination typically reveals a harsh murmur heard best at the left lower sternal border, arising from both the outflow tract turbulence during ventricular ejection and the commonly associated mitral regurgitation. The gradient and the murmur may be enhanced by maneuvers that decrease ventricular volume, such as the Valsalva maneuver, or standing after squatting. They may be decreased by increasing ventricular volume or vascular resistance, such as with squatting

or hand grip. A fourth heart sound is commonly heard due to decreased ventricular compliance. In patients with a significant outflow tract gradient, palpation of the carotid pulse may reveal a bifid systolic impulse, from early and delayed ejection. Patients with chronic, severe elevations in filling pressures may show signs of systemic fluid retention.

The electrocardiogram usually shows left ventricular hypertrophy, often with prominent septal Q waves that can be misdiagnosed as indicative of infarction. The diagnosis of hypertrophic cardiomyopathy is confirmed by echocardiography demonstrating left ventricular hypertrophy, which may or may not be more marked in the septum (Fig. 21-15). Intraventricular gradients to outflow can be identified by Doppler echocardiography at rest or during provocative maneuvers, such as the Valsalva maneuver. Systolic anterior motion (SAM) of the mitral valve is a classic finding on the echocardiogram. Mitral regurgitation may become severe. Cardiac catheterization can be performed to quantify the gradient, which characteristically increases after a premature ventricular contraction.

Apical hypertrophic cardiomyopathy is a variant that is uncommon in the United States; however, this variant accounts for about one-fourth of patients with hypertrophic cardiomyopathy in Japan. The electrocardiogram shows deep T-wave inversions in the precordial leads, and the echocardiogram shows a characteristic spade-like appearance with apical obliteration. It has been associated with a specific genetic defect in cardiac actin (Glu 101 Lys), but may occur with other sarcomere mutations.

The differential diagnosis of hypertrophic cardiomyopathy is limited in most patients once other cardiovascular causes for secondary hypertrophy are excluded. However, other diseases that result in thickened myocardium can appear indistinguishable on echocardiography, and are considered "pseudohypertrophic," particularly the inherited metabolic diseases (Table 21-4). The differential diagnosis between hypertrophic and restrictive cardiomyopathy may be particularly difficult when considering a diagnosis of "burned-out" hypertrophic cardiomyopathy in which systolic function has decreased. Overlap with infiltrative and restrictive myocardial diseases should be considered in the evaluation of increased left ventricular wall thickness on echocardiography, particularly when clinical features are atypical for classic hypertrophic cardiomyopathy. The metabolic defects in PRKAG2, alpha-galactosidase (Fabry's disease), and LAMP2 mutations (Tables 21-3 and 21-4) should routinely be considered during evaluation of apparent hypertrophic cardiomyopathy. With late onset without a family history of hypertrophic cardiomyopathy, amyloidosis should be carefully considered.

TREATMENT Hypertrophic Cardiomyopathy

Therapy of hypertrophic cardiomyopathy is directed to symptom management and the prevention of sudden death (Fig. 21-17); it is not known whether treatment will decrease disease progression in asymptomatic family members. Exertional dyspnea and chest pain are treated by medication to reduce heart rate and ventricular contractility with hopes of improving diastolic filling patterns. Beta-adrenergic blocking drugs and verapamil are most commonly used as initial therapy. These agents both act to decrease heart rate and increase the length of time for diastolic filling, as well as to decrease the inotropic state. If there is fluid retention, diuretic therapy will usually be necessary, but requires careful titration to avoid hypovolemia, particularly in the presence of a resting or inducible obstruction to ventricular outflow. When symptoms persist and an outflow gradient is present, addition of disopyramide is sometimes effective. Amiodarone can also improve symptoms, but is usually initiated for control of arrhythmias rather than symptoms. Anticoagulation is recommended to prevent embolic events for patients who have had atrial fibrillation.

Symptoms that limit routine daily life despite adjustment of medical therapies develop in fewer than 5–10% of patients, generally those with substantial obstruction to ventricular outflow. Further therapies are directed to reduce this obstruction by changing ventricular

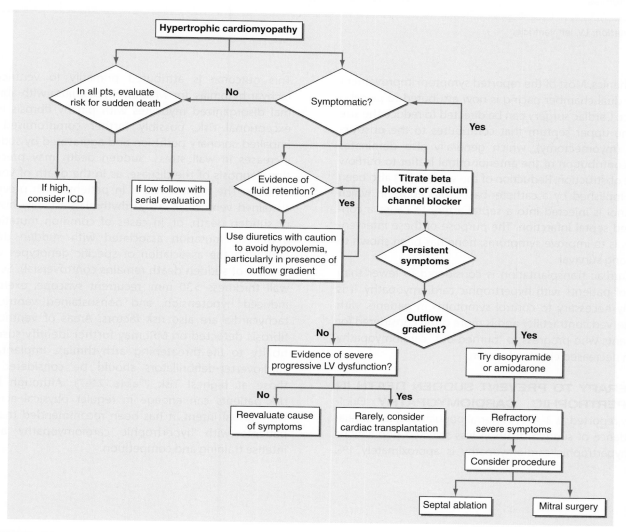

FIGURE 21-17

Treatment algorithm for hypertrophic cardiomyopathy depending on the presence and severity of symptoms, and the presence of an intraventricular gradient with obstruction to outflow. Note that all patients with hypertrophic cardiomyopathy should be evaluated for risk of sudden death, whether or not they require treatment for symptoms. ICD, implantable cardioverter-defibrillator; LV, left ventricular.

TABLE 21-7

RISK FACTORS FOR SUDDEN DEATH IN HYPERTROPHIC CARDIOMYOPATHY

MAJOR RISK FACTOR		SCREENING TECHNIQUE
History of cardiac arrest or spontaneous sustained ventricular tachycardia		History
Syncope	Usually with or after exertion	History
Family history of sudden cardiac death	Or possibly with a documented gene mutation associated with high risk	Family history
Spontaneous nonsustained ventricular tachycardia	>3 beats at rate >120	Exercise or 24–48 h ambulatory recording
LV thickness >30 mm	Present in about 10% of patients, but many sudden deaths occur with wall thickness <30 mm	Echocardiography
Abnormal blood pressure response to exercise	Systolic blood pressure fall or failure to increase at peak exercise	Maximal upright exercise testing

Abbreviation: LV, left ventricle.

mechanics. Most of the reported symptom improvement with dual chamber pacing is now attributed to placebo effect. Cardiac surgery can be directed to reduce the size of the upper septum that contributes to the obstruction (myomectomy), which generally also dominates the contribution of the anterior mitral leaflet to outflow tract obstruction. Reduction of the septum has also been accomplished by a catheter-based procedure in which ethanol is injected into a septal artery to cause a controlled septal infarction. The purpose of these interventions is to improve symptoms; none has been shown to prolong survival.

Cardiac transplantation is considered in fewer than 5% of patients with hypertrophic cardiomyopathy. It is rarely necessary to control symptoms in patients with preserved contractility and is more often considered for patients who progress to "burned-out" cardiomyopathy with decreased ejection fraction.

THERAPY TO PREVENT SUDDEN DEATH IN HYPERTROPHIC CARDIOMYOPATHY Originally reported as 3–4% in referral populations, the annual incidence of sudden death in less selected populations of hypertrophic cardiomyopathy is approximately 1%.

This outcome is attributed primarily to ventricular tachyarrhythmias, for which a myocardium with abnormal disorganized myocytes with patchy fibrosis is at exceptional risk, possibly further compromised by impaired coronary perfusion and aggravated by sudden increases in wall stress. Sudden death may precede the diagnosis of the disease, as in the death of young athletes. The highest risk is in patients with previous sustained ventricular tachyarrhythmias, a family history of sudden death, or, in cases of common mutations, a genetic mutation associated with sudden death (although the association of specific genotypes with the risk of sudden death remains controversial). Septal wall thickness >30 mm, recurrent syncope, exercise-induced hypotension, and nonsustained ventricular tachycardia are also risk factors. Areas of ventricular fibrosis detected on MRI may further identify susceptibility to life-threatening arrhythmias. Implantable cardioverter-defibrillators should be considered for those at highest risk (Table 21-7). Although low-risk patients can engage in regular physical activity with casual intent, it has been recommended that all patients with hypertrophic cardiomyopathy avoid intense training and competition.

CHAPTER 22

PERICARDIAL DISEASE

Eugene Braunwald

NORMAL FUNCTIONS OF THE PERICARDIUM

The normal pericardium is a double-layered sac; the visceral pericardium is a serous membrane that is separated by a small quantity (15–50 mL) of fluid, an ultrafiltrate of plasma, from the fibrous parietal pericardium. The normal pericardium, by exerting a restraining force, prevents sudden dilation of the cardiac chambers, especially the right atrium and ventricle, during exercise and with hypervolemia. It also restricts the anatomic position of the heart, minimizes friction between the heart and surrounding structures, prevents displacement of the heart and kinking of the great vessels, and probably retards the spread of infections from the lungs and pleural cavities to the heart. Nevertheless, total absence of the pericardium, either congenital or after surgery, does not produce obvious clinical disease. In partial left pericardial defects, the main pulmonary artery and left atrium may bulge through the defect; very rarely, herniation and subsequent strangulation of the left atrium may cause sudden death.

ACUTE PERICARDITIS

Acute pericarditis, by far the most common pathologic process involving the pericardium, may be classified both clinically and etiologically (Table 22-1). There are four principal diagnostic features:

1. *Chest pain* is an important but not invariable symptom in various forms of acute pericarditis (Chap. 4); it is usually present in the acute infectious types and in many of the forms presumed to be related to hypersensitivity or autoimmunity. Pain is often absent in slowly developing tuberculous, post-irradiation, neoplastic, and uremic pericarditis. The pain of acute pericarditis is often severe, retrosternal and left precordial, and referred to the neck, arms, or left shoulder. Often the pain is pleuritic, consequent to accompanying pleural inflammation (i.e., sharp and aggravated by inspiration and coughing), but sometimes it is a steady, constricting pain that radiates into either arm or both arms and resembles that of myocardial ischemia; therefore, confusion with acute myocardial infarction (AMI) is common. Characteristically, however, pericardial pain may be relieved by sitting up and leaning forward and is intensified by lying supine. The differentiation of AMI from acute pericarditis becomes perplexing when, with acute pericarditis, serum biomarkers of myocardial damage such as creatine kinase and troponin rise, presumably because of concomitant involvement of the epicardium in the inflammatory process (an epi-myocarditis) with resulting myocyte necrosis. However, these elevations, if they occur, are quite modest given the extensive electrocardiographic ST-segment elevation in pericarditis. This dissociation is useful in differentiating between these conditions.

2. A *pericardial friction rub* is audible in about 85% of these patients, may have up to three components per cardiac cycle, is high pitched, and is described as rasping, scratching, or grating (Chap. 9); it can be elicited sometimes when the diaphragm of the stethoscope is applied firmly to the chest wall at the left lower sternal border. It is heard most frequently at end expiration with the patient upright and leaning forward. The rub is often inconstant, and the

TABLE 22-1

CLASSIFICATION OF PERICARDITIS

Clinical Classification

I. Acute pericarditis (<6 weeks)
   A. Fibrinous
   B. Effusive (serous or sanguineous)
II. Subacute pericarditis (6 weeks to 6 months)
   A. Effusive-constrictive
   B. Constrictive
III. Chronic pericarditis (>6 months)
   A. Constrictive
   B. Effusive
   C. Adhesive (nonconstrictive)

Etiologic Classification

I. Infectious pericarditis
   A. Viral (coxsackievirus A and B, echovirus, mumps, adenovirus, hepatitis, HIV)
   B. Pyogenic (pneumococcus, streptococcus, staphylococcus, *Neisseria, Legionella*)
   C. Tuberculous
   D. Fungal (histoplasmosis, coccidioidomycosis, *Candida*, blastomycosis)
   E. Other infections (syphilitic, protozoal, parasitic)
II. Noninfectious pericarditis
   A. Acute myocardial infarction
   B. Uremia
   C. Neoplasia
     1. Primary tumors (benign or malignant, mesothelioma)
     2. Tumors metastatic to pericardium (lung and breast cancer, lymphoma, leukemia)
   D. Myxedema
   E. Cholesterol
   F. Chylopericardium
   G. Trauma
     1. Penetrating chest wall
     2. Nonpenetrating
   H. Aortic dissection (with leakage into pericardial sac)
   I. Postirradiation
   J. Familial Mediterranean fever
   K. Familial pericarditis
     1. Mulibrey nanism[a]
   L. Acute idiopathic
   M. Whipple's disease
   N. Sarcoidosis
III. Pericarditis presumably related to hypersensitivity or autoimmunity
   A. Rheumatic fever
   B. Collagen vascular disease (systemic lupus erythematosus, rheumatoid arthritis, ankylosing spondylitis, scleroderma, acute rheumatic fever, granulomatosis with polyangiitis (Wegener's))
   C. Drug-induced (e.g., procainamide, hydralazine, phenytoin, isoniazide, minoxidil, anticoagulants, methysergide)
   D. Post-cardiac injury
     1. Postmyocardial infarction (Dressler's syndrome)
     2. Postpericardiotomy
     3. Posttraumatic

[a]An autosomal recessive syndrome characterized by growth failure, muscle hypotonia, hepatomegaly, ocular changes, enlarged cerebral ventricles, mental retardation, ventricular hypertrophy, and chronic constrictive pericarditis.

loud to-and-fro leathery sound may disappear within a few hours, possibly to reappear on the next day. A pericardial rub is heard throughout the respiratory cycle, whereas a pleural rub disappears when respiration is suspended.

3. The *electrocardiogram* (ECG) in acute pericarditis without massive effusion usually displays changes secondary to acute subepicardial inflammation (**Fig. 22-1**). It typically evolves through four stages. In stage 1, there is widespread elevation of the ST segments, often with upward concavity, involving two or three standard limb leads and V_2 to V_6, with reciprocal depressions only in aVR and sometimes V_1, as well as depression of the PR segment below the TP segment reflecting atrial involvement. Usually, there are no significant changes in QRS complexes. In stage 2, after several days, the ST segments return to normal, and only then, or even later, do the T waves become inverted (stage 3). Ultimately, weeks or months after the onset of acute pericarditis, the ECG returns to normal in stage 4. In contrast, in AMI, ST elevations are convex, and reciprocal depression is usually more prominent; QRS changes occur, particularly the development of Q waves, as well as notching and loss of R-wave amplitude, and T-wave inversions are usually seen within hours *before* the ST segments have become isoelectric. Sequential ECGs are useful in distinguishing acute pericarditis from AMI. In the latter, elevated ST segments return to normal within hours (Chaps. 34 and 35).

Early repolarization is a normal variant and may also be associated with widespread ST-segment elevation, most prominent in left precordial leads. However, in this condition the T waves are usually tall and the ST/T ratio is <0.25; importantly, this ratio is higher in acute pericarditis.

4. *Pericardial effusion* is usually associated with pain and/or the ECG changes mentioned earlier, as well as with an enlargement of the cardiac silhouette. Pericardial effusion is especially important clinically when it develops within a relatively short time as it may lead to cardiac tamponade (see later). Differentiation from cardiac enlargement may be difficult on physical examination, but heart sounds may be fainter with pericardial effusion. The friction rub may disappear, and the apex impulse may vanish, but sometimes it remains palpable, albeit medial to the left border of cardiac dullness. The base of the left lung may be compressed by pericardial fluid, producing *Ewart's sign*, a patch of dullness and increased fremitus (and egophony) beneath the angle of the left scapula. The chest roentgenogram may show a "water bottle" configuration of the cardiac silhouette (**Fig. 22-2**) but may be normal.

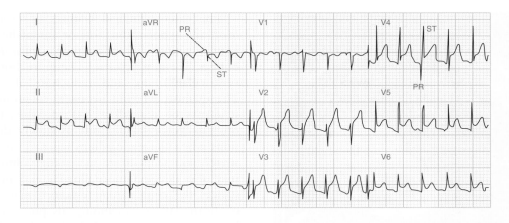

FIGURE 22-1

Acute pericarditis often produces diffuse ST-segment elevations (in this case in leads I, II, aVF, and V_2 to V_6) due to a ventricular current of injury. Note also the characteristic PR-segment deviation (opposite in polarity to the ST segment) due to a concomitant atrial injury current.

Diagnosis

Echocardiography (Chap. 12) is the most widely used imaging technique since it is sensitive, specific, simple, and noninvasive; may be performed at the bedside; and can identify accompanying cardiac tamponade (see later) **(Fig. 22-3)**. The presence of pericardial fluid is recorded by two-dimensional transthoracic echocardiography as a relatively echo-free space between the posterior pericardium and left ventricular epicardium in patients with small effusions and as a space between the anterior right ventricle and the parietal pericardium just beneath the anterior chest wall in those with larger effusions. In the latter, the heart may swing freely within the

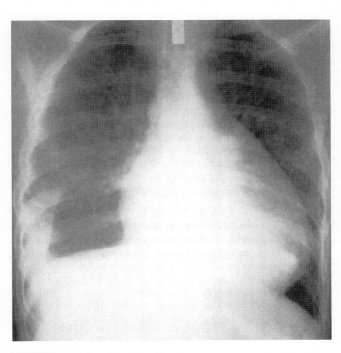

FIGURE 22-2

Chest radiogram from a patient with a pericardial effusion showing typical "water bottle" heart. There is also a right pleural effusion. (*From SS Kabbani, M LeWinter, in MH Crawford et al [eds]: Cardiology. London, Mosby, 2001.*)

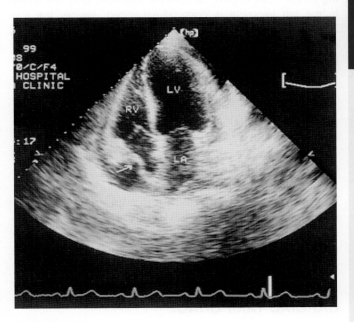

FIGURE 22-3

Apical four-chamber echocardiogram recorded in a patient with a moderate pericardial effusion and evidence of hemodynamic compromise. The frame is recorded in early ventricular systole, immediately after atrial contraction. Note that the right atrial wall is indented inward and its curvature is frankly reversed (*arrow*), implying elevated intrapericardial pressure above right atrial pressure. LA, left atrium; LV, left ventricle; RV, right ventricle. (*From WF Armstrong: Echocardiography, in DP Zipes et al [eds]: Braunwald's Heart Disease, 7th ed. Philadelphia, Elsevier, 2005.*)

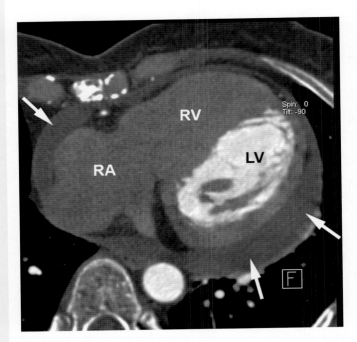

FIGURE 22-4

Chronic pericardial effusion in a 54-year-old female patient with Hodgkin's disease seen in contrast-enhanced 64-slice CT. The arrows point at the pericardial effusion (LV, left ventricle; RV, right ventricle; RA, right atrium). Due to the timing of the scan relative to contrast injection, only the blood in the left ventricle is contrast-enhanced, hence, the low attenuation in the right-sided chambers. (*From Achenbach S, Daniel WG: Computed Tomography of the Heart, in P Libby et al [eds]: Braunwald's Heart Disease, 8th ed. Philadelphia, Elsevier, 2008.*)

pericardial sac. When severe, the extent of this motion alternates and may be associated with electrical alternans. Echocardiography allows localization and estimation of the quantity of pericardial fluid.

The diagnosis of pericardial fluid or thickening may be confirmed by computed tomography (CT) or magnetic resonance imaging (MRI) **(Fig. 22-4)**. These techniques may be superior to echocardiography in detecting loculated pericardial effusions, pericardial thickening, and the presence of pericardial masses.

CARDIAC TAMPONADE

The accumulation of fluid in the pericardial space in a quantity sufficient to cause serious obstruction to the inflow of blood to the ventricles results in cardiac tamponade. This complication may be fatal if it is not recognized and treated promptly. The three most common causes of tamponade are neoplastic disease, idiopathic pericarditis, and renal failure. Tamponade may also result from bleeding into the pericardial space after cardiac operations, trauma, and treatment of patients with acute pericarditis with anticoagulants.

The three principal features of tamponade (*Beck's triad*) are hypotension, soft or absent heart sounds, and jugular venous distention with a prominent *x* descent but an absent *y* descent. There are both limitation of ventricular filling and reduction of cardiac output. The quantity of fluid necessary to produce this critical state may be as small as 200 mL when the fluid develops rapidly or >2000 mL in slowly developing effusions when the pericardium has had the opportunity to stretch and adapt to an increasing volume. Tamponade may also develop more slowly, and in these circumstances the clinical manifestations may resemble those of heart failure, including dyspnea, orthopnea, and hepatic engorgement. A high index of suspicion for cardiac tamponade is required since in many instances no obvious cause for pericardial disease is apparent, and it should be considered in any patient with otherwise unexplained enlargement of the cardiac silhouette, hypotension, and elevation of jugular venous pressure. There may be reduction in amplitude of the QRS complexes, and *electrical alternans* of the P, QRS, or T waves should raise the suspicion of cardiac tamponade.

Table 22-2 lists the features that distinguish acute cardiac tamponade from constrictive pericarditis.

Paradoxical pulse

This important clue to the presence of cardiac tamponade consists of a greater than normal (10 mmHg) inspiratory decline in systolic arterial pressure. When severe, it may be detected by palpating weakness or disappearance of the arterial pulse during inspiration, but usually sphygmomanometric measurement of systolic pressure during slow respiration is required.

Since both ventricles share a tight incompressible covering, i.e., the pericardial sac, the inspiratory enlargement of the right ventricle in cardiac tamponade compresses and reduces left ventricular volume; leftward bulging of the interventricular septum further reduces the left ventricular cavity as the right ventricle enlarges during inspiration. Thus, in cardiac tamponade the normal inspiratory augmentation of right ventricular volume causes an exaggerated reciprocal reduction in left ventricular volume. Also, respiratory distress increases the fluctuations in intrathoracic pressure, which exaggerates the mechanism just described. Right ventricular infarction (Chap. 35) may resemble cardiac tamponade with hypotension, elevated jugular venous pressure, an absent *y* descent in the jugular venous pulse, and, occasionally, pulsus paradoxus. The differences between these two conditions are shown in Table 22-2.

Paradoxical pulse occurs not only in cardiac tamponade but also in approximately one-third of patients with constrictive pericarditis (see later). This physical finding is not pathognomonic of pericardial disease because it may be observed in some cases of hypovolemic shock,

TABLE 22-2

FEATURES THAT DISTINGUISH CARDIAC TAMPONADE FROM CONSTRICTIVE PERICARDITIS AND SIMILAR CLINICAL DISORDERS

CHARACTERISTIC	TAMPONADE	CONSTRICTIVE PERICARDITIS	RESTRICTIVE CARDIOMYOPATHY	RVMI
Clinical				
Pulsus paradoxus	Common	Usually absent	Rare	Rare
Jugular veins				
Prominent y descent	Absent	Usually present	Rare	Rare
Prominent x descent	Present	Usually present	Present	Rare
Kussmaul's sign	Absent	Present	Present	Present
Third heart sound	Absent	Absent	Rare	May be present
Pericardial knock	Absent	Often present	Absent	Absent
Electrocardiogram				
Low ECG voltage	May be present	May be present	May be present	Absent
Electrical alternans	May be present	Absent	Absent	Absent
Echocardiography				
Thickened pericardium	Absent	Present	Absent	Absent
Pericardial calcification	Absent	Often present	Absent	Absent
Pericardial effusion	Present	Absent	Absent	Absent
RV size	Usually small	Usually normal	Usually normal	Enlarged
Myocardial thickness	Normal	Normal	Usually increased	Normal
Right atrial collapse and RVDC	Present	Absent	Absent	Absent
Increased early filling, ↑ mitral flow velocity	Absent	Present	Present	May be present
Exaggerated respiratory variation in flow velocity	Present	Present	Absent	Absent
CT/MRI				
Thickened/calcific pericardium	Absent	Present	Absent	Absent
Cardiac catheterization				
Equalization of diastolic pressures	Usually present	Usually present	Usually absent	Absent or present
Cardiac biopsy helpful?	No	No	Sometimes	No

Abbreviations: ECG, electrocardiograph; RV, right ventricle; RVDC, right ventricular diastolic collapse; RVMI, right ventricular myocardial infarction.

Source: From GM Brockington et al: Cardiol Clin 8:645, 1990; with permission.

acute and chronic obstructive airway disease, and pulmonary embolus.

Low-pressure tamponade refers to mild tamponade in which the intrapericardial pressure is increased from its slightly subatmospheric levels to +5 to +10 mmHg; in some instances, hypovolemia coexists. As a consequence, the central venous pressure is normal or only slightly elevated, whereas arterial pressure is unaffected and there is no paradoxical pulse. These patients are asymptomatic or complain of mild weakness and

dyspnea. The diagnosis is aided by echocardiography, and both hemodynamic and clinical manifestations improve after pericardiocentesis.

Diagnosis

Since immediate treatment of cardiac tamponade may be lifesaving, prompt measures to establish the diagnosis by echocardiography should be undertaken (Fig. 22-3). When pericardial effusion causes tamponade, Doppler ultrasound shows that tricuspid and pulmonic valve flow velocities increase markedly during inspiration, whereas pulmonic vein, mitral, and aortic flow velocities diminish. Often the right ventricular cavity is reduced in diameter, and there is late diastolic inward motion (collapse) of the right ventricular free wall and the right atrium. Transesophageal echocardiography may be necessary to diagnose a loculated or hemorrhagic effusion responsible for cardiac tamponade.

TREATMENT Cardiac Tamponade

Patients with acute pericarditis should be observed frequently for the development of an effusion; if a large effusion is present, the patient should be hospitalized and pericardiocentesis carried out or the patient should be watched closely for signs of tamponade. Arterial and venous pressures and heart rate should be monitored or followed carefully, and serial echocardiograms obtained.

PERICARDIOCENTESIS If manifestations of tamponade appear, echocardiographically or fluoroscopically guided pericardiocentesis using an apical, parasternal, or, most commonly, subxiphoid approach must be carried out at once as reduction of the elevated intrapericardial pressure may be lifesaving. Intravenous saline may be administered as the patient is being readied for the procedure, but the pericardiocentesis must not be delayed. If possible, intrapericardial pressure should be measured before fluid is withdrawn, and the pericardial cavity should be drained as completely as possible. A small, multiholed catheter advanced over the needle inserted into the pericardial cavity may be left in place to allow draining of the pericardial space if fluid reaccumulates. Surgical drainage through a limited (subxiphoid) thoracotomy may be required in recurrent tamponade, when it is necessary to remove loculated effusions, and/or when it is necessary to obtain tissue for diagnosis.

Pericardial fluid obtained from an effusion often has the physical characteristics of an exudate. Bloody fluid is most commonly due to neoplasm in the United States and tuberculosis in developing nations but may also be found in the effusion of acute rheumatic fever, postcardiac injury, and postmyocardial infarction, as well as in the pericarditis associated with renal failure or dialysis. Transudative pericardial effusions may occur in heart failure.

The pericardial fluid should be analyzed for red and white blood cells, and cytologic studies for cancer, microscopic studies, and cultures should be obtained. The presence of DNA of Mycobacterium tuberculosis determined by polymerase chain reaction or an elevated adenosine deaminase activity (>30 U/L) strongly supports the diagnosis of tuberculous pericarditis.

VIRAL OR IDIOPATHIC FORM OF ACUTE PERICARDITIS

In many instances, acute pericarditis occurs in association with illnesses of known or presumed viral origin and probably is caused by the same agent. Commonly, there is an antecedent infection of the respiratory tract, and viral isolation and serologic studies are negative. In some cases, coxsackievirus A or B or the virus of influenza, echovirus, mumps, herpes simplex, chickenpox, adenovirus, cytomegalovirus, Epstein-Barr, or HIV has been isolated from pericardial fluid and/or appropriate elevations in viral antibody titers have been noted. Pericardial effusion is a common cardiac manifestation of HIV; it is usually secondary to infection (often mycobacterial) or neoplasm, most frequently lymphoma. Most frequently, a viral causation cannot be established; the term *idiopathic acute pericarditis* is then appropriate. Viral or idiopathic acute pericarditis occurs at all ages but is more common in young adults and is often associated with pleural effusions and pneumonitis. The almost simultaneous development of fever and precordial pain, often 10 to 12 days after a presumed viral illness, constitutes an important feature in the differentiation of acute pericarditis from AMI, in which chest pain precedes fever. The constitutional symptoms are usually mild to moderate, and a pericardial friction rub is often audible. The disease ordinarily runs its course in a few days to 4 weeks. The ST-segment alterations in the ECG usually disappear after 1 or more weeks, but the abnormal T waves may persist for several years and be a source of confusion in persons without a clear history of pericarditis.

Pleuritis and pneumonitis frequently accompany pericarditis. Accumulation of some pericardial fluid is common, and both tamponade and constrictive pericarditis are possible complications. Recurrent (relapsing) pericarditis occurs in about one-fourth of patients with acute idiopathic pericarditis. In a smaller number, there are multiple recurrences.

TREATMENT Idiopathic Acute Pericarditis

In acute idiopathic pericarditis there is no specific therapy, but bed rest and anti-inflammatory treatment with aspirin (2–4 g/d) may be given. If this is ineffective, one of the nonsteroidal anti-inflammatory drugs (NSAIDs), such as ibuprofen (400–600 mg tid), indomethacin (25–50 mg tid), or colchicine (0.6 mg bid), is often effective. Glucocorticoids (e.g., prednisone, 40–80 mg daily) usually suppress the clinical manifestations of the acute illness and may be useful in patients in whom purulent bacterial pericarditis has been excluded and in patients with pericarditis secondary to connective tissue disorders and renal failure (see later). Anticoagulants should be avoided since their use could cause bleeding into the pericardial cavity and tamponade.

After the patient has been asymptomatic and afebrile for about a week, the dose of the NSAID may be tapered gradually. Colchicine may prevent recurrences, but when recurrences are multiple, frequent, and disabling; continued beyond 2 years; and are not controlled by glucocorticoids, pericardiectomy may be necessary to terminate the illness.

Postcardiac injury syndrome

Acute pericarditis may appear in a variety of circumstances that have one common feature: previous injury to the myocardium with blood in the pericardial cavity. The syndrome may develop after a cardiac operation (postpericardiotomy syndrome), after blunt or penetrating cardiac trauma (Chap. 23), or after perforation of the heart with a catheter. Rarely, it follows AMI.

The clinical picture mimics acute viral or idiopathic pericarditis. The principal symptom is the pain of acute pericarditis, which usually develops 1 to 4 weeks after the cardiac injury (1 to 3 days after AMI) but sometimes appears only after an interval of months. Recurrences are common and may occur up to 2 years or more after the injury. Pericarditis, fever with temperature up to 39°C (102.2°F), pleuritis, and pneumonitis are the outstanding features, and the bout of illness usually subsides in 1 or 2 weeks. The pericarditis may be of the fibrinous variety, or it may be a pericardial effusion, which is often serosanguineous but rarely causes tamponade. Leukocytosis, an increased sedimentation rate, and ECG changes typical of acute pericarditis may also occur.

This syndrome is probably the result of a hypersensitivity reaction to antigen that originates from injured myocardial tissue and/or pericardium. Circulating myocardial antisarcolemmal and antifibrillar autoantibodies occur frequently, but their precise role in the development of this syndrome has not been defined. Viral infection may also play an etiologic role, since antiviral antibodies are often elevated in patients who develop this syndrome after cardiac surgery.

Often no treatment is necessary aside from aspirin and analgesics. When the illness is followed by a series of disabling recurrences, therapy with an NSAID, colchicine, or a glucocorticoid is usually effective.

DIFFERENTIAL DIAGNOSIS

Since there is no specific test for *acute idiopathic pericarditis*, the diagnosis is one of exclusion. Consequently, all other disorders that may be associated with acute fibrinous pericarditis must be considered. A common diagnostic error is mistaking acute viral or idiopathic

pericarditis for AMI and vice versa. When acute fibrinous pericarditis is associated with AMI (Chap. 35), it is characterized by fever, pain, and a friction rub in the first 4 days after the development of the infarct. ECG abnormalities (such as the appearance of Q waves, brief ST-segment elevations with reciprocal changes, and earlier T-wave changes in AMI) and the extent of the elevations of myocardial enzymes are helpful in differentiating pericarditis from AMI.

Pericarditis secondary to postcardiac injury is differentiated from acute idiopathic pericarditis chiefly by timing. If it occurs within a few days or weeks of an AMI, a chest blow, a cardiac perforation, or a cardiac operation, it may be justified to conclude that the two are probably related.

It is important to distinguish *pericarditis due to collagen vascular disease* from acute idiopathic pericarditis. Most important in the differential diagnosis is the pericarditis due to systemic lupus erythematosus (SLE) or drug-induced (procainamide or hydralazine) lupus. When pericarditis occurs in the absence of any obvious underlying disorder, the diagnosis of SLE may be suggested by a rise in the titer of antinuclear antibodies. Acute pericarditis is an occasional complication of *rheumatoid arthritis*, *scleroderma*, and *polyarteritis nodosa*, and other evidence of these diseases is usually obvious. Asymptomatic pericardial effusion is also common in these disorders. The pericarditis of *acute rheumatic fever* is generally associated with evidence of severe pancarditis and with cardiac murmurs (Chap. 26).

Pyogenic (purulent) pericarditis is usually secondary to cardiothoracic operations, by extension of infection from the lungs or pleural cavities, from rupture of the esophagus into the pericardial sac, or from rupture of a ring abscess in a patient with infective endocarditis, or it can occur if septicemia complicates aseptic pericarditis. It is usually accompanied by fever, chills, septicemia, and evidence of infection elsewhere and generally has a poor prognosis. The diagnosis is made by examination of the pericardial fluid. Acute pericarditis may also complicate the viral, pyogenic, mycobacterial, and fungal infections that occur with HIV infection.

Pericarditis of renal failure occurs in up to one-third of patients with chronic uremia (*uremic pericarditis*), is also seen in patients undergoing chronic dialysis with normal levels of blood urea and creatinine, and is termed *dialysis-associated pericarditis*. These two forms of pericarditis may be fibrinous and are generally associated with an effusion that may be sanguineous. A pericardial friction rub is common, but pain is usually absent or mild. Treatment with an NSAID and intensification of dialysis are usually adequate. Occasionally, tamponade occurs and pericardiocentesis is required. When the pericarditis of renal failure is recurrent or persistent, a pericardial window should be created or pericardiectomy may be necessary.

Pericarditis due to *neoplastic diseases* results from extension or invasion of metastatic tumors (most commonly carcinoma of the lung and breast, malignant melanoma, lymphoma, and leukemia) to the pericardium; pain, atrial arrhythmias, and tamponade are complications that occur occasionally. Diagnosis is made by pericardial fluid cytology or pericardial biopsy. *Mediastinal irradiation* for neoplasm may cause acute pericarditis and/or chronic constrictive pericarditis. Unusual causes of acute pericarditis include syphilis, fungal infection (histoplasmosis, blastomycosis, aspergillosis, and candidiasis), and parasitic infestation (amebiasis, toxoplasmosis, echinococcosis, trichinosis).

CHRONIC PERICARDIAL EFFUSIONS

Chronic pericardial effusions are sometimes encountered in patients without an antecedent history of acute pericarditis. They may cause few symptoms per se, and their presence may be detected by finding an enlarged cardiac silhouette on chest roentgenogram. Tuberculosis is a common cause.

Other causes

Myxedema may be responsible for chronic pericardial effusion that is sometimes massive but rarely, if ever, causes cardiac tamponade. The cardiac silhouette is markedly enlarged, and an echocardiogram distinguishes cardiomegaly from pericardial effusion. The diagnosis of myxedema can be confirmed by tests for thyroid function. Myxedematous pericardial effusion responds to thyroid hormone replacement.

Neoplasms, systemic lupus erythematosus (SLE), rheumatoid arthritis, mycotic infections, radiation therapy to the chest, pyogenic infections, and chylopericardium may also cause chronic pericardial effusion and should be considered and specifically sought in such patients.

Aspiration and analysis of the pericardial fluid are often helpful in diagnosis. Pericardial fluid should be analyzed as described earlier. Grossly sanguineous pericardial fluid results most commonly from a neoplasm, tuberculosis, renal failure, or slow leakage from an aortic aneurysm. Pericardiocentesis may resolve large effusions, but pericardiectomy may be required with recurrence. Intrapericardial instillation of sclerosing agents or antineoplastic agents may be used to prevent reaccumulation of fluid.

CHRONIC CONSTRICTIVE PERICARDITIS

This disorder results when the healing of an acute fibrinous or serofibrinous pericarditis or the resorption of a chronic pericardial effusion is followed by obliteration of the pericardial cavity with the formation of granulation tissue. The latter gradually contracts and forms a firm scar, which may be calcified, encasing the heart and interfering with filling of the ventricles. In developing nations where the condition is prevalent, a high percentage of cases are of tuberculous origin, but this is now an uncommon cause in North America. Chronic constrictive pericarditis may follow acute or relapsing viral or idiopathic pericarditis, trauma with organized blood clot, cardiac surgery of any type, mediastinal irradiation, purulent infection, histoplasmosis, neoplastic disease (especially breast cancer, lung cancer, and lymphoma), rheumatoid arthritis, SLE, and chronic renal failure with uremia treated by chronic dialysis. In many patients the cause of the pericardial disease is undetermined, and in them an asymptomatic or forgotten bout of viral pericarditis, acute or idiopathic, may have been the inciting event.

The basic physiologic abnormality in patients with chronic constrictive pericarditis is the inability of the ventricles to fill because of the limitations imposed by the rigid, thickened pericardium. In constrictive pericarditis, ventricular filling is unimpeded during early diastole but is reduced abruptly when the elastic limit of the pericardium is reached, whereas in cardiac tamponade, ventricular filling is impeded throughout diastole. In both conditions, ventricular end-diastolic and stroke volumes are reduced and the end-diastolic pressures in both ventricles and the mean pressures in the atria, pulmonary veins, and systemic veins are all elevated to similar levels (i.e., within 5 mmHg of one another). Despite these hemodynamic changes, myocardial function may be normal or only slightly impaired in chronic constrictive pericarditis. However, the fibrotic process may extend into the myocardium and cause myocardial scarring and atrophy, and venous congestion may then be due to the combined effects of the pericardial and myocardial lesions.

In constrictive pericarditis, the right and left atrial pressure pulses display an M-shaped contour, with prominent x and y descents. The y descent, which is absent or diminished in cardiac tamponade, is the most prominent deflection in constrictive pericarditis; it reflects rapid early filling of the ventricles. The y descent is interrupted by a rapid rise in atrial pressure during early diastole, when ventricular filling is impeded by the constricting pericardium. These characteristic changes are transmitted to the jugular veins, where they may be recognized by inspection. In constrictive pericarditis, the ventricular pressure pulses in both ventricles exhibit characteristic "square root" signs during diastole. These hemodynamic changes, although characteristic, are not pathognomonic of constrictive pericarditis and may also be observed in cardiomyopathies characterized by restriction of ventricular filling (Chap. 21) (Table 22-2).

CLINICAL AND LABORATORY FINDINGS

Weakness, fatigue, weight gain, increased abdominal girth, abdominal discomfort, a protuberant abdomen, and edema are common. The patient often appears chronically ill, and in advanced cases there are anasarca, skeletal muscle wasting, and cachexia. Exertional dyspnea is common, and orthopnea may occur, although it is usually not severe. Acute left ventricular failure (acute pulmonary edema) is very uncommon. The cervical veins are distended and may remain so even after intensive diuretic treatment, and venous pressure may fail to decline during inspiration (*Kussmaul's sign*). The latter is common in chronic pericarditis but may also occur in tricuspid stenosis, right ventricular infarction, and restrictive cardiomyopathy.

The pulse pressure is normal or reduced. In about one-third of cases, a paradoxical pulse can be detected. Congestive hepatomegaly is pronounced and may impair hepatic function and cause jaundice; ascites is common and is usually more prominent than dependent edema. The apical pulse is reduced and may retract in systole (*Broadbent's sign*). The heart sounds may be distant; an early third heart sound (i.e., a pericardial knock, occurring at the cardiac apex 0.09–0.12 s after aortic valve closure) is often conspicuous; it occurs with the abrupt cessation of ventricular filling. A systolic murmur of tricuspid regurgitation may be present.

The *ECG* frequently displays low voltage of the QRS complexes and diffuse flattening or inversion of the T waves. Atrial fibrillation is present in about one-third of patients. The *chest roentgenogram* shows a normal or slightly enlarged heart; pericardial calcification is most common in tuberculous pericarditis. Pericardial calcification may, however, occur in the absence of constriction.

Inasmuch as the usual physical signs of cardiac disease (murmurs, cardiac enlargement) may be inconspicuous or absent in chronic constrictive pericarditis, hepatic enlargement and dysfunction associated with jaundice and intractable ascites may lead to a mistaken diagnosis of hepatic cirrhosis. This error can be avoided if the neck veins are inspected carefully in patients with ascites and hepatomegaly. Given a clinical picture resembling hepatic cirrhosis, but with the added feature of distended neck veins, a careful search for thickening of the pericardium by imaging (see Fig. 12-6) should be carried out and may disclose this curable or remediable form of heart disease.

The transthoracic *echocardiogram* typically shows pericardial thickening, dilation of the inferior vena cava and hepatic veins, and a sharp halt in ventricular filling in early diastole, with normal ventricular systolic function and flattening of the left ventricular posterior wall. Atrial enlargement may be seen, especially in patients with long-standing constrictive physiology. There is a distinctive pattern of transvalvular flow velocity on Doppler flow-velocity echocardiography. During inspiration there is an exaggerated reduction in blood flow velocity in the pulmonary veins and across the mitral valve and a leftward shift of the ventricular septum; the opposite occurs during expiration. Diastolic flow velocity in the vena cavae into the right atrium and across the tricuspid valve increases in an exaggerated manner during inspiration and declines during expiration (**Fig. 22-5**). However, echocardiography cannot definitively exclude the diagnosis of constrictive pericarditis. MRI and CT scanning (**Fig. 22-6**) are more accurate than echocardiography in establishing or excluding the presence of a thickened pericardium. Pericardial thickening and even pericardial calcification, however, are not synonymous with constrictive pericarditis since they may occur without seriously impairing ventricular filling.

DIFFERENTIAL DIAGNOSIS

Like chronic constrictive pericarditis, cor pulmonale (Chap. 17) may be associated with severe systemic venous hypertension but little pulmonary congestion; the heart is usually not enlarged, and a paradoxical pulse may be present. However, in cor pulmonale, advanced parenchymal pulmonary disease is usually obvious and venous pressure *falls* during inspiration (i.e., Kussmaul's sign is negative). *Tricuspid stenosis* (Chap. 20) may also simulate chronic constrictive pericarditis; congestive hepatomegaly, splenomegaly, ascites, and venous distention may be equally prominent. However, in tricuspid stenosis, a characteristic murmur as well as the murmur of accompanying mitral stenosis is usually present.

Because constrictive pericarditis can be corrected surgically, it is important to distinguish chronic

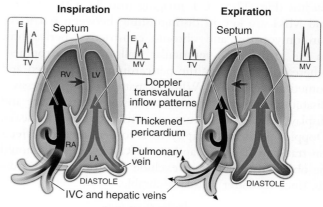

FIGURE 22-5

Constrictive pericarditis. Doppler schema of respirophasic changes in mitral and tricuspid inflow. Reciprocal patterns of ventricular filling are assessed on pulsed Doppler examination of mitral valve (MV) and tricuspid valve (TV) inflow. (*Courtesy of Bernard E. Bulwer, MD; with permission.*)

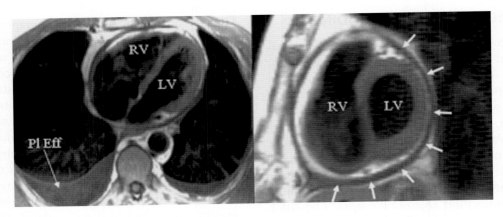

FIGURE 22-6

Cardiovascular magnetic resonance in a patient with constrictive pericarditis. On the right is a basal short-axis view of the ventricles showing a thickened pericardium encasing the heart (*arrows*). On the left is a transaxial view, again showing the thickened pericardium, particularly over the right heart, but also a pleural effusion (Pl Eff). LV, left ventricle; RV, right ventricle. (*From D Pennell: Cardiovascular Magnetic Resonance, in P Libby et al [eds]: Braunwald's Heart Disease, 8th ed. Philadelphia, Elsevier, 2005.*)

constrictive pericarditis from restrictive cardiomyopathy (Chap. 21), which has a similar physiologic abnormality (i.e., restriction of ventricular filling). In many patients with restrictive cardiomyopathy the ventricular wall is thickened as shown on echocardiographic examination (Table 22-2). The features favoring the diagnosis of restrictive cardiomyopathy over chronic constrictive pericarditis include a well-defined apex beat, cardiac enlargement, and pronounced orthopnea with attacks of acute left ventricular failure, left ventricular hypertrophy, gallop sounds (in place of a pericardial knock), bundle branch block, and, in some cases, abnormal Q waves on the ECG. The typical echocardiographic features of constrictive pericarditis (see earlier) are useful in the differential diagnosis in chronic constrictive pericarditis (Fig. 22-5). CT imaging (usually with contrast) and MRI are key in distinguishing between restrictive cardiomyopathy and chronic constrictive pericarditis. In the former, the ventricular walls are hypertrophied, whereas in the latter, the pericardium is thickened and sometimes calcified. When a patient has progressive, disabling, and unresponsive congestive heart failure and displays any of the features of constrictive heart disease, Doppler echocardiography to record respiratory effects on transvalvular flow and an MRI or CT scan should be obtained to detect or exclude constrictive pericarditis, since the latter is usually curable.

TREATMENT   Constrictive Pericarditis

Pericardial resection is the only definitive treatment of constrictive pericarditis and should be as complete as possible. Dietary sodium restriction and diuretics are useful during preoperative preparation. Coronary arteriography should be carried out preoperatively in patients older than 50 years of age to exclude unsuspected coronary artery disease. The benefits derived from cardiac decortication are usually progressive over a period of months. The risk of this operation depends on the extent of penetration of the myocardium by the fibrotic and calcific process, the severity of myocardial atrophy, the extent of secondary impairment of hepatic and/or renal function, and the patient's general condition. Operative mortality is in the range of 5% to 10%; the patients with the most severe disease are at highest risk. Therefore, surgical treatment should, if possible, be carried out relatively early in the course.

Subacute effusive-constrictive pericarditis

This form of pericardial disease is characterized by the combination of a tense effusion in the pericardial space and constriction of the heart by thickened pericardium. It shares a number of features both with chronic pericardial effusion producing cardiac compression and with pericardial constriction. It may be caused by tuberculosis (see later), multiple attacks of acute idiopathic pericarditis, radiation, traumatic pericarditis, renal failure, scleroderma, and neoplasms. The heart is generally enlarged, and a paradoxical pulse and a prominent *x* descent (without a prominent *y* descent) are present in the atrial and jugular venous pressure pulses. After pericardiocentesis, the physiologic findings may change from those of cardiac tamponade to those of pericardial constriction. Furthermore, the intrapericardial pressure and the central venous pressure may decline, but not to normal. The diagnosis can be established by pericardiocentesis followed by pericardial biopsy.

Wide excision of both the visceral and parietal pericardium is usually effective therapy.

Tuberculous pericardial disease

This chronic infection is a common cause of chronic pericardial effusion, although less so in the United States than in Africa, Asia, the Middle East, and other parts of the developing world where active tuberculosis is endemic. The clinical picture is that of a chronic, systemic illness in a patient with pericardial effusion. It is important to consider this diagnosis in a patient with known tuberculosis, with HIV, and with fever, chest pain, weight loss, and enlargement of the cardiac silhouette of undetermined origin. If the etiology of chronic pericardial effusion remains obscure despite detailed analysis of the pericardial fluid (see earlier), a pericardial biopsy, preferably by a limited thoracotomy, should be performed. If definitive evidence is still lacking but the specimen shows granulomas with caseation, antituberculous chemotherapy is indicated.

If the biopsy specimen shows a thickened pericardium, pericardiectomy should be carried out to prevent the development of constriction. Tubercular cardiac constriction should be treated surgically while the patient is receiving antituberculous chemotherapy.

OTHER DISORDERS OF THE PERICARDIUM

Pericardial cysts appear as rounded or lobulated deformities of the cardiac silhouette, most commonly at the right cardiophrenic angle. They do not cause symptoms, and their major clinical significance lies in the possibility of confusion with a tumor, ventricular aneurysm, or massive cardiomegaly. *Tumors* involving the pericardium are most commonly secondary to malignant neoplasms originating in or invading the mediastinum, including carcinoma of the bronchus and breast, lymphoma, and melanoma. The most common *primary* malignant tumor is the mesothelioma. The usual clinical picture of malignant pericardial tumor is an insidiously developing, often bloody pericardial effusion. Surgical exploration is required to establish a definitive diagnosis and to carry out definitive or, more commonly, palliative treatment.

CHAPTER 23

TUMORS AND TRAUMA OF THE HEART

Eric H. Awtry ■ Wilson S. Colucci

TUMORS OF THE HEART

PRIMARY TUMORS

Primary tumors of the heart are rare. Approximately three-quarters are histologically benign, and the majority of these tumors are myxomas. Malignant tumors, almost all of which are sarcomas, account for 25% of primary cardiac tumors (Table 23-1). All cardiac tumors, regardless of pathologic type, have the potential to cause life-threatening complications. Many tumors are now surgically curable; thus, early diagnosis is imperative.

Clinical presentation

Cardiac tumors may present with a wide array of cardiac and noncardiac manifestations. These manifestations depend in large part on the location and size of the tumor and are often nonspecific features of more common forms of heart disease, such as chest pain, syncope, heart failure, murmurs, arrhythmias, conduction disturbances, and pericardial effusion with or without tamponade. Additionally, embolic phenomena and constitutional symptoms may occur.

Myxoma

Myxomas are the most common type of primary cardiac tumor in all age groups, accounting for one-third to one-half of all cases at postmortem and about three-quarters of the tumors treated surgically. They occur at all ages, most commonly in the third through sixth decades, with a female predilection. Approximately 90% of myxomas are sporadic; the remainder are familial with autosomal dominant transmission. The familial variety often occurs as part of a syndrome complex

TABLE 23-1

RELATIVE INCIDENCE OF PRIMARY TUMORS OF THE HEART

TYPE	NUMBER	PERCENT
Benign	199	58.0
Myxoma	114	33.2
Rhabdomyoma	20	5.8
Fibroma	20	5.8
Hemangioma	17	5.0
Atrioventricular nodal	10	2.9
Granular cell	4	1.2
Lipoma	2	0.6
Paraganglioma	2	0.6
Myocytic hamartoma	2	0.6
Histiocytoid cardiomyopathy	2	0.6
Inflammatory psuedotumor	2	0.6
Other benign tumors	4	1.2
Malignant	144	42.0
Sarcoma	137	39.9
Lymphoma	7	2.1

Source: Modified from A Burke, R Virmani: *Atlas of Tumor Pathology: Tumors of the Heart and Great Vessels.* Washington, DC, Armed Forces Institute of Pathology 1996, p. 231; with permission.

(Carney complex) that includes (1) myxomas (cardiac, skin, and/or breast), (2) lentigines and/or pigmented nevi, and (3) endocrine overactivity (primary nodular adrenal cortical disease with or without Cushing's syndrome, testicular tumors, and/or pituitary adenomas with gigantism or acromegaly). Certain constellations of findings have been referred to as the *NAME* syndrome (nevi, atrial myxoma, myxoid neurofibroma, and ephelides) or the *LAMB* syndrome (lentigines, atrial myxoma, and blue nevi), although these syndromes probably represent subsets of the Carney complex. The genetic basis of this complex has not been elucidated completely; however, patients frequently have inactivating mutations in the tumor-suppressor gene *PRKAR1A*, which encodes the protein kinase A type I-α regulatory subunit.

Pathologically, myxomas are gelatinous structures that consist of myxoma cells embedded in a stroma rich in glycosaminoglycans. Most are solitary, are located in the atria (particularly the left atrium, where they usually arise from the interatrial septum in the vicinity of the fossa ovalis), and are often pedunculated on a fibrovascular stalk. In contrast to sporadic tumors, familial or syndromic tumors tend to occur in younger individuals, are often multiple, may be ventricular in location, and are more likely to recur after initial resection.

Myxomas commonly present with obstructive signs and symptoms. The most common clinical presentation mimics that of mitral valve disease: either stenosis owing to tumor prolapse into the mitral orifice or regurgitation resulting from tumor-induced valvular trauma. Ventricular myxomas may cause outflow obstruction similar to that caused by subaortic or subpulmonic stenosis. The symptoms and signs of myxoma may be sudden in onset or positional in nature, owing to the effects of gravity on tumor position. A characteristic low-pitched sound, a "tumor plop," may be appreciated on auscultation during early or mid-diastole and is thought to result from the impact of the tumor against the mitral valve or ventricular wall. Myxomas also may present with peripheral or pulmonary emboli or with constitutional signs and symptoms, including fever, weight loss, cachexia, malaise, arthralgias, rash, digital clubbing, Raynaud's phenomenon, hypergammaglobulinemia, anemia, polycythemia, leukocytosis, elevated erythrocyte sedimentation rate, thrombocytopenia, and thrombocytosis. These factors account for the frequent misdiagnosis of patients with myxomas as having endocarditis, collagen vascular disease, or a paraneoplastic syndrome.

Two-dimensional transthoracic or omniplane transesophageal echocardiography is useful in the diagnosis of cardiac myxoma and allows assessment of tumor size and determination of the site of tumor attachment, both of which are important considerations in the planning of surgical excision (Fig. 23-1). CT and MRI may provide important information regarding size, shape, composition, and surface characteristics of the tumor (Fig. 23-2).

Although cardiac catheterization and angiography were previously performed routinely before tumor resection, they no longer are considered mandatory when adequate noninvasive information is available and other cardiac disorders (e.g., coronary artery disease) are not considered likely. Additionally, catheterization of the chamber from which the tumor arises carries the risk of tumor embolization. Because myxomas may be familial, echocardiographic screening of first-degree relatives is appropriate, particularly if the patient is young and has multiple tumors or evidence of myxoma syndrome.

TREATMENT | **Myxoma**

Surgical excision utilizing cardiopulmonary bypass is indicated regardless of tumor size and is generally curative. Myxomas recur in 12–22% of familial cases but in only 1–2% of sporadic cases. Tumor recurrence most likely is due to multifocal lesions in the former and inadequate resection in the latter.

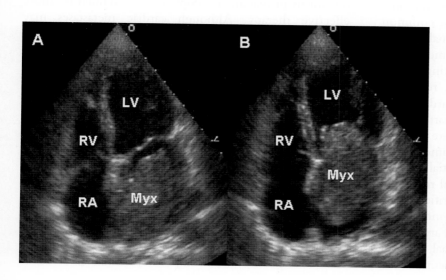

FIGURE 23-1

Transthoracic echocardiogram demonstrating a large atrial myxoma. The myxoma (Myx) fills the entire left atrium in systole (*panel A*) and prolapses across the mitral valve and into the left ventricle (LV) during diastole (*panel B*). RA, right atrium; RV, right ventricle. (*Courtesy of Dr. Michael Tsang; with permission.*)

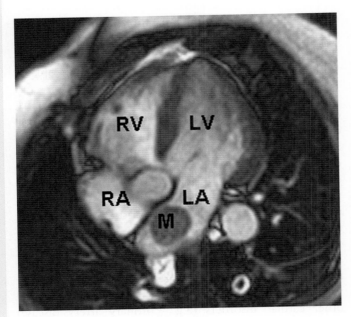

FIGURE 23-2

Cardiac MRI demonstrating a rounded mass (M) within the left atrium (LA). Pathologic evaluation at the time of surgery revealed it to be an atrial myxoma. LV, left ventricle; RA, right atrium; RV, right ventricle.

Other benign tumors

Cardiac *lipomas*, although relatively common, are usually incidental findings at postmortem examination; however, they may grow as large as 15 cm and may present with symptoms owing to mechanical interference with cardiac function, arrhythmias, or conduction disturbances or as an abnormality of the cardiac silhouette on chest x-ray. *Papillary fibroelastomas* are the most common tumors of the cardiac valves. Although usually clinically silent, they can cause valve dysfunction and may embolize distally, resulting in transient ischemic attacks, stroke, or myocardial infarction. Therefore, these tumors should be resected even when asymptomatic. *Rhabdomyomas* and *fibromas* are the most common cardiac tumors in infants and children and usually occur in the ventricles, where they may produce mechanical obstruction to blood flow, thereby mimicking valvular stenosis, congestive heart failure (CHF), restrictive or hypertrophic cardiomyopathy, or pericardial constriction. Rhabdomyomas are probably hamartomatous growths, are multiple in 90% of cases, and are strongly associated with tuberous sclerosis. These tumors have a tendency to regress completely or partially; only tumors that cause obstruction require surgical resection. Fibromas are usually single, are often calcified, tend to grow and cause obstructive symptoms, and should be resected. *Hemangiomas* and *mesotheliomas* are generally small tumors, most often intramyocardial in location, and may cause atrioventricular (AV) conduction

disturbances and even sudden death as a result of their propensity to develop in the region of the AV node. Other benign tumors arising from the heart include *teratoma*, *chemodectoma*, *neurilemoma*, *granular cell myoblastoma*, and *bronchogenic cysts*.

Sarcoma

Almost all primary cardiac malignancies are sarcomas, which may be of several histologic types. In general, these tumors are characterized by rapid progression that culminates in the patient's death within weeks to months from the time of presentation as a result of hemodynamic compromise, local invasion, or distant metastases. Sarcomas commonly involve the right side of the heart, are characterized by rapid growth, frequently invade the pericardial space, and may obstruct the cardiac chambers or venae cavae. Sarcomas also may occur on the left side of the heart and may be mistaken for myxomas.

TREATMENT Sarcoma

At the time of presentation these tumors have often spread too extensively to allow for surgical excision. Although there are scattered reports of palliation with surgery, radiotherapy, and/or chemotherapy, the response of cardiac sarcomas to these therapies is generally poor. The one exception appears to be cardiac lymphosarcomas, which may respond to a combination of chemo- and radiotherapy.

TUMORS METASTATIC TO THE HEART

Tumors metastatic to the heart are much more common than primary tumors, and their incidence is likely to increase as the life expectancy of patients with various forms of malignant neoplasms is extended by more effective therapy. Although cardiac metastases may occur with any tumor type, the relative incidence is especially high in malignant melanoma and, to a somewhat lesser extent, leukemia and lymphoma. In absolute terms, the most common primary originating sites of cardiac metastases are carcinoma of the breast and lung, reflecting the high incidence of those cancers. Cardiac metastases almost always occur in the setting of widespread primary disease, and most often there is either primary or metastatic disease elsewhere in the thoracic cavity. Nevertheless, cardiac metastasis occasionally may be the initial presentation of an extrathoracic tumor.

Cardiac metastases may occur via hematogenous or lymphangitic spread or by direct tumor invasion. They generally manifest as small, firm nodules; diffuse infiltration also may occur, especially with sarcomas or hematologic neoplasms. The pericardium is most often involved, followed by myocardial involvement of any chamber and, rarely, by involvement of the endocardium or cardiac valves.

Cardiac metastases are clinically apparent only ~10% of the time, are usually not the cause of the patient's presentation, and rarely are the cause of death. The vast majority occur in the setting of a previously recognized malignant neoplasm. When symptomatic, cardiac metastases may result in a variety of clinical features, including dyspnea, acute pericarditis, cardiac tamponade, ectopic tachyarrhythmias, heart block, and CHF. As with primary cardiac tumors, the clinical presentation reflects more the location and size of the tumor than its histologic type. Many of these signs and symptoms may also result from myocarditis, pericarditis, or cardiomyopathy induced by radiotherapy or chemotherapy.

Electrocardiographic (ECG) findings are nonspecific. On chest x-ray, the cardiac silhouette is most often normal but may be enlarged or exhibit a bizarre contour. Echocardiography is useful for identifying pericardial effusions and visualizing larger metastases, although CT and radionuclide imaging with gallium or thallium may define the tumor burden more clearly. Cardiac MRI offers superb image quality and plays a central role in the diagnostic evaluation of cardiac metastases and cardiac tumors in general. Pericardiocentesis may allow for a specific cytologic diagnosis in patients with malignant pericardial effusions. Angiography is rarely necessary but may delineate discrete lesions.

TREATMENT ▷ Tumors Metastatic to the Heart

Most patients with cardiac metastases have advanced malignant disease; thus, therapy is generally palliative and consists of treatment of the primary tumor. Symptomatic malignant pericardial effusions should be drained by pericardiocentesis. Concomitant instillation of a sclerosing agent (e.g., tetracycline) may delay or prevent reaccumulation of the effusion, and creation of a pericardial window allows drainage of the effusion to the pleural space.

TRAUMATIC CARDIAC INJURY

Traumatic cardiac injury may be caused by either penetrating or nonpenetrating trauma. *Penetrating injuries* most often result from gunshot or knife wounds, and the site of entry is usually obvious. *Nonpenetrating injuries* most often occur during motor vehicle accidents, either from a rapid deceleration injury or from impact of the chest against the steering wheel, and may be associated with significant cardiac injury even in the absence of external signs of thoracic trauma.

Myocardial contusions are the most common form of nonpenetrating cardiac injury and may initially be overlooked in trauma patients as the clinical focus is directed toward other, more obvious injuries. Myocardial necrosis may occur as a direct result of the blunt injury or as a result of traumatic coronary laceration or thrombosis. The contused myocardium is pathologically similar to infarcted myocardium and may be associated with atrial or ventricular arrhythmias; conduction disturbances, including bundle branch block; or ECG abnormalities resembling those of infarction or pericarditis. Thus, it is important to consider contusion as a cause of otherwise unexplained ECG changes in a trauma patient. Serum creatine kinase, myocardial bound (CK-MB) isoenzyme levels are increased in ~20% of patients who experience blunt chest trauma but may be falsely elevated in the presence of massive skeletal muscle injury. Cardiac troponin levels are more specific for identifying cardiac injury in this setting. Echocardiography is useful in detecting structural and functional sequelae of contusion, including wall motion abnormalities, pericardial effusion, valvular dysfunction, and ventricular rupture.

Rupture of the cardiac valves or their supporting structures, most commonly of the tricuspid or mitral valve, leads to acute valvular incompetence. This complication is usually heralded by the development of a loud murmur, may be associated with rapidly progressive heart failure, and can be diagnosed by either transthoracic or transesophageal echocardiography.

The most serious consequence of nonpenetrating cardiac injury is myocardial rupture, which may result in hemopericardium and tamponade (free wall rupture) or intracardiac shunting (ventricular septal rupture). Although it generally is fatal, up to 40% of patients with cardiac rupture have been reported to survive long enough to reach a specialized trauma center. Hemopericardium also may result from traumatic rupture of a pericardial vessel or a coronary artery. Additionally, a pericardial effusion may develop weeks or even months after blunt chest trauma as a manifestation of the postcardiac injury syndrome, which resembles the post-pericardiotomy syndrome (Chap. 22).

Blunt, nonpenetrating, often innocent-appearing injuries to the chest may trigger ventricular fibrillation even in absence of overt signs of injury. This syndrome, referred to as *commotio cordis*, occurs most often in adolescents during sporting events (e.g., baseball, hockey, football, and lacrosse) and probably results from an impact to the chest wall overlying the heart during the susceptible phase of repolarization just before the peak of the T wave. Survival depends on prompt defibrillation.

Rupture of the aorta, usually just above the aortic valve or at the site of the ligamentum arteriosum, is a common consequence of nonpenetrating chest trauma and is the most common vascular deceleration injury.

The clinical presentation is similar to that of aortic dissection (Chap. 38); the arterial pressure and pulse amplitude may be increased in the upper extremities and decreased in the lower extremities, and chest x-ray may reveal mediastinal widening. Occasionally, aortic rupture is contained by the aortic adventitia, resulting in a false, or *pseudo-*, aneurysm that may be discovered months or years after the initial injury.

Sudden emotional or physical trauma may precipitate a transient catecholamine-mediated cardiomyopathy referred to as *Tako-Tsubo syndrome* or the *apical ballooning syndrome* (Chap. 21).

Penetrating injuries of the heart produced by knife or bullet wounds usually result in rapid clinical deterioration and frequently in death as a result of hemopericardium/pericardial tamponade or massive hemorrhage. Nonetheless, up to half of such patients may survive long enough to reach a specialized trauma center if immediate resuscitation is performed. Prognosis in these patients relates to the mechanism of injury, their clinical condition at presentation, and the specific cardiac chamber(s) involved. Iatrogenic cardiac or coronary arterial perforation may complicate placement of central venous or intracardiac catheters, pacemaker leads, or intracoronary stents and is associated with a better prognosis than are other forms of penetrating cardiac trauma.

Traumatic rupture of a great vessel from penetrating injury is usually associated with hemothorax and, less often, hemopericardium. Local hematoma formation may compress major vessels and produce ischemic symptoms, and AV fistulas may develop, occasionally resulting in high-output CHF.

Occasionally, patients who survive penetrating cardiac injuries may subsequently present with a new cardiac murmur or CHF as a result of mitral regurgitation or an intracardiac shunt (i.e., ventricular or atrial septal defect, aortopulmonary fistula, or coronary AV fistula) that was undetected at the time of the initial injury or developed subsequently. Therefore, trauma patients should be examined carefully several weeks after the injury. If a mechanical complication is suspected, it can be confirmed by echocardiography or cardiac catheterization.

TREATMENT   Traumatic Cardiac Injury

The treatment of an uncomplicated myocardial contusion is similar to the medical therapy for a myocardial infarction, except that anticoagulation is contraindicated, and should include monitoring for the development of arrhythmias and mechanical complications such as cardiac rupture (Chap. 35). Acute myocardial failure resulting from traumatic valve rupture usually requires urgent operative correction. Immediate thoracotomy should be carried out for most cases of penetrating injury or if there is evidence of cardiac tamponade and/or shock regardless of the type of trauma. Pericardiocentesis may be lifesaving in patients with tamponade but is usually only a temporizing measure while awaiting definitive surgical therapy. Pericardial hemorrhage often leads to constriction (Chap. 22), which must be treated by surgical decortication.

CHAPTER 24
CARDIAC MANIFESTATIONS OF SYSTEMIC DISEASE

Eric H. Awtry ■ **Wilson S. Colucci**

The common systemic disorders that have associated cardiac manifestations are summarized in Table 24-1.

DIABETES MELLITUS

Diabetes mellitus, both insulin- and non–insulin-dependent, is an independent risk factor for coronary artery disease (CAD; Chap. 30) and accounts for 14–50% of new cases of cardiovascular disease. Furthermore, CAD is the most common cause of death in adults with diabetes mellitus. In the diabetic population the incidence of CAD relates to the duration of diabetes and the level of glycemic control, and its pathogenesis involves endothelial dysfunction, increased lipoprotein peroxidation, increased inflammation, a prothrombotic state, and associated metabolic abnormalities.

Diabetic patients are more likely to have a myocardial infarction, have a greater burden of CAD, have larger infarct size, and have more postinfarct complications, including heart failure, shock, and death, than are nondiabetics. Importantly, diabetic patients are more likely to have atypical ischemic symptoms; nausea, dyspnea, pulmonary edema, arrhythmias, heart block, or syncope may be their anginal equivalent. Additionally, "silent ischemia," resulting from autonomic nervous system dysfunction, is more common in diabetic patients, accounting for up to 90% of their ischemic episodes. Thus, one must have a low threshold for suspecting CAD in diabetic patients. The treatment of diabetic patients with CAD must include aggressive risk factor management. Pharmacologic therapy and revascularization are similar in diabetic patients and nondiabetics except that diabetic patients have higher morbidity and mortality rates associated with revascularization, have an increased risk of restenosis after percutaneous coronary intervention (PCI),

and probably have improved survival when treated with surgical bypass compared with PCI for multivessel CAD.

Patients with diabetes mellitus also may have abnormal left ventricular systolic and diastolic function, reflecting concomitant epicardial CAD and/or hypertension, coronary microvascular disease, endothelial dysfunction, ventricular hypertrophy, and autonomic dysfunction. A restrictive cardiomyopathy may be present with abnormal myocardial relaxation and elevated ventricular filling pressures. Histologically, interstitial fibrosis is seen, and intramural arteries may demonstrate intimal thickening, hyaline deposition, and inflammatory changes. Diabetic patients have an increased risk of developing clinical heart failure, which probably contributes to their excessive cardiovascular morbidity and mortality rates. There is some evidence that insulin therapy may ameliorate diabetes-related myocardial dysfunction.

MALNUTRITION AND VITAMIN DEFICIENCY

Malnutrition

In patients whose intake of protein, calories, or both is severely deficient, the heart may become thin, pale, and hypokinetic with myofibrillar atrophy and interstitial edema. The systolic pressure and cardiac output fall, and the pulse pressure narrows. Generalized edema is common and relates to a variety of factors, including reduced serum oncotic pressure and myocardial dysfunction. Such profound states of protein and calorie malnutrition, termed *kwashiorkor* and *marasmus,* respectively, are most common in underdeveloped countries. However, significant nutritional heart disease also may occur in developed nations, particularly in patients with chronic diseases such as AIDS, patients with

TABLE 24-1

COMMON SYSTEMIC DISORDERS AND THEIR ASSOCIATED CARDIAC MANIFESTATIONS

SYSTEMIC DISORDER	COMMON CARDIAC MANIFESTATIONS
Diabetes mellitus	CAD, atypical angina, CMP, systolic or diastolic CHF
Protein-calorie malnutrition	Dilated CMP, CHF
Thiamine deficiency	High-output failure, dilated CMP
Hyperhomocysteinemia	Premature atherosclerosis
Obesity	CMP, systolic or diastolic CHF
Hyperthyroidism	Palpitations, SVT, atrial fibrillation, hypertension
Hypothyroidism	Hypotension, bradycardia, dilated CMP, CHF, pericardial effusion
Malignant carcinoid	Tricuspid and pulmonary valve disease, right heart failure
Pheochromocytoma	Hypertension, palpitations, CHF
Acromegaly	Systolic or diastolic heart failure
Rheumatoid arthritis	Pericarditis, pericardial effusions, coronary arteritis, myocarditis, valvulitis
Seronegative arthropathies	Aortitis, aortic and mitral insufficiency, conduction abnormalities
Systemic lupus erythematosus	Pericarditis, Libman-Sacks endocarditis, myocarditis, arterial and venous thrombosis
HIV	Myocarditis, dilated CMP, pericardial effusion
Amyloidosis	CHF, restrictive CMP, valvular regurgitation, pericardial effusion
Sarcoidosis	CHF, dilated or restrictive CMP, ventricular arrhythmias, heart block
Hemochromatosis	CHF, arrhythmias, heart block
Marfan syndrome	Aortic aneurysm and dissection, aortic insufficiency, mitral valve prolapse
Ehlers-Danlos syndrome	Aortic and coronary aneurysms, mitral and tricuspid valve prolapse

Abbreviations: CAD, coronary artery disease; CHF, congestive heart failure; CMP, cardiomyopathy; SVT, supraventricular tachycardia.

anorexia nervosa, and patients with severe cardiac failure in whom gastrointestinal hypoperfusion and venous congestion may lead to anorexia and malabsorption. Open-heart surgery poses increased risk in malnourished patients, and those patients may benefit from preoperative hyperalimentation.

Thiamine deficiency (beriberi)

Generalized malnutrition often is accompanied by thiamine deficiency; however, this hypovitaminosis also may occur in the presence of an adequate protein and caloric intake, particularly in the Far East, where polished rice deficient in thiamine may be a major dietary component. In Western nations where the use of thiamine-enriched flour is widespread, clinical thiamine deficiency is limited primarily to alcoholics, food faddists, and patients receiving chemotherapy. Nonetheless, when thiamine stores are measured using the thiamine-pyrophosphate effect (TPPE), thiamine deficiency has been found in 20–90% of patients with chronic heart failure. This deficiency appears to result from both reduced dietary intake and a diuretic-induced increase in the urinary excretion of thiamine. The acute administration of thiamine to these patients increases the left ventricular ejection fraction and the excretion of salt and water.

Clinically, patients with thiamine deficiency usually have evidence of generalized malnutrition, peripheral neuropathy, glossitis, and anemia. The classic associated cardiovascular syndrome is characterized by high-output heart failure, tachycardia, and often elevated biventricular filling pressures. The major cause of the high-output state is vasomotor depression leading to reduced systemic vascular resistance, the precise mechanism of which is not understood. The cardiac examination reveals a wide pulse pressure, tachycardia, a third heart sound, and, frequently, an apical systolic murmur. The electrocardiogram (ECG) may reveal decreased voltage, a prolonged QT interval, and T-wave abnormalities. The chest x-ray generally reveals cardiomegaly and signs of congestive heart failure (CHF). The response to thiamine is often dramatic, with an increase in systemic vascular resistance, a decrease in cardiac output, clearing of pulmonary congestion, and a reduction in heart size often occurring in 12–48 h. Although the response to inotropes and diuretics may be poor before thiamine therapy, these agents may be important *after* thiamine is given, since the left ventricle may not be able to handle the increased work load presented by the return of vascular tone.

Vitamins B_6, B_{12}, and folate deficiency

Vitamins B_6, B_{12}, and folate are cofactors in the metabolism of homocysteine. Their deficiency probably contributes to the majority of cases of hyperhomocysteinemia, a disorder associated with increased atherosclerotic risk. Supplementation of these vitamins has reduced the incidence of hyperhomocysteinemia in the United States; however, the clinical cardiovascular benefit of normalizing elevated homocysteine levels has not been proved.

OBESITY

Severe obesity, especially abdominal obesity, is associated with an increase in cardiovascular morbidity and mortality rates. Although obesity itself is not considered a disease, it is associated with an increased prevalence of hypertension, glucose intolerance, and atherosclerotic CAD. In addition, obese patients have a distinct cardiovascular abnormality characterized by increased total and central blood volumes, increased cardiac output, and elevated left ventricular filling pressure. The elevated cardiac output appears to be required to support the metabolic demands of the excess adipose tissue. Left ventricular filling pressure is often at the upper limits of normal at rest and rises excessively with exercise. In part as a result of chronic volume overload, eccentric cardiac hypertrophy with cardiac dilation and ventricular dysfunction may develop. In addition, altered levels of adipokines secreted by adipose tissue may contribute to adverse myocardial remodeling via direct effects on cardiac myocytes and other cells. Pathologically, there is left and, in some cases, right ventricular hypertrophy and generalized cardiac dilation. Pulmonary congestion, peripheral edema, and exercise intolerance may all ensue; however, the recognition of these findings may be difficult in massively obese patients.

Weight reduction is the most effective therapy and results in reduction in blood volume and the return of cardiac output toward normal. However, rapid weight reduction may be dangerous, as cardiac arrhythmias and sudden death owing to electrolyte imbalance have been described. Treatment with angiotensin-converting enzyme inhibitors, sodium restriction, and diuretics may be useful to control heart failure symptoms. This form of heart disease should be distinguished from Pickwickian syndrome, which may share several of the cardiovascular features of heart disease secondary to severe obesity but, in addition, frequently has components of central apnea, hypoxemia, pulmonary hypertension, and cor pulmonale.

THYROID DISEASE

Thyroid hormone exerts a major influence on the cardiovascular system by a number of direct and indirect mechanisms, and, not surprisingly, cardiovascular effects are prominent in both hypo- and hyperthyroidism. Thyroid hormone causes increases in total-body metabolism and oxygen consumption that indirectly increase the cardiac workload. In addition, thyroid hormone exerts direct inotropic, chronotropic, and dromotropic effects that are similar to those seen with adrenergic stimulation (e.g., tachycardia, increased cardiac output); they are mediated at least partly by both transcriptional and nontranscriptional effects of thyroid hormone on myosin, calcium-activated ATPase, Na$^+$-K$^+$-ATPase, and myocardial β-adrenergic receptors.

Hyperthyroidism

Common cardiovascular manifestations of hyperthyroidism include palpitations, systolic hypertension, and fatigue. Sinus tachycardia is present in ~40% of hyperthyroid patients, and atrial fibrillation in ~15%. Physical examination may reveal a hyperdynamic precordium, a widened pulse pressure, increases in the intensity of the first heart sound and the pulmonic component of the second heart sound, and a third heart sound. An increased incidence of mitral valve prolapse has been described in hyperthyroid patients, in which case a mid-systolic murmur may be heard at the left sternal border with or without a mid-systolic click. A systolic pleuro-pericardial friction rub (*Means-Lerman scratch*) may be heard at the left second intercostal space during expiration and is thought to result from the hyperdynamic cardiac motion.

Elderly patients with hyperthyroidism may present with only cardiovascular manifestations of thyrotoxicosis such as sinus tachycardia, atrial fibrillation, and hypertension, all of which may be resistant to therapy until the hyperthyroidism is controlled. Angina pectoris and CHF are unusual with hyperthyroidism unless there is coexistent heart disease; in such cases, symptoms often resolve with treatment of the hyperthyroidism.

Hypothyroidism

Cardiac manifestations of hypothyroidism include a reduction in cardiac output, stroke volume, heart rate, blood pressure, and pulse pressure. Pericardial effusions are present in about one-third of patients, rarely progress to tamponade, and probably result from increased capillary permeability. Other clinical signs include cardiomegaly, bradycardia, weak arterial pulses, distant heart sounds, and pleural effusions. Although the signs and symptoms of myxedema may mimic those of CHF, in the absence of other cardiac disease, myocardial failure is uncommon. The ECG generally reveals sinus bradycardia and low voltage and may show prolongation of the QT interval, decreased P-wave voltage, prolonged AV conduction time, intraventricular conduction disturbances, and nonspecific ST-T-wave abnormalities. Chest x-ray may show cardiomegaly, often with a "water bottle" configuration; pleural effusions; and, in some cases, evidence of CHF. Pathologically, the heart is pale and dilated and often demonstrates myofibrillar swelling, loss of striations, and interstitial fibrosis.

Patients with hypothyroidism frequently have elevations of cholesterol and triglycerides, resulting in premature atherosclerotic CAD. Before treatment with thyroid hormone, patients with hypothyroidism frequently do not have angina pectoris, presumably because of the low metabolic demands caused by their condition. However, angina and myocardial infarction may be precipitated during initiation of thyroid hormone replacement, especially in elderly patients with underlying heart disease. Therefore, replacement should be done with care, starting with low doses that are increased gradually.

MALIGNANT CARCINOID

Carcinoid tumors most often originate in the small bowel and elaborate a variety of vasoactive amines (e.g., serotonin), kinins, indoles, and prostaglandins that are believed to be responsible for the diarrhea, flushing, and labile blood pressure that characterize the carcinoid syndrome. Some 50% of patients with carcinoid syndrome have cardiac involvement, usually manifesting as abnormalities of the right-sided cardiac structures. These patients invariably have hepatic metastases that allow vasoactive substances to circumvent hepatic metabolism. Left-sided cardiac involvement is rare and indicates either pulmonary carcinoid or an intracardiac shunt. Pathologically, carcinoid lesions are fibrous plaques that consist of smooth-muscle cells embedded in a stroma of glycosaminoglycans and collagen. They occur on the cardiac valves, where they cause valvular dysfunction, as well as on the endothelium of the cardiac chambers and great vessels.

Carcinoid heart disease most often presents as tricuspid regurgitation, pulmonic stenosis, or both. In some cases a high cardiac output state may occur, presumably as a result of a decrease in systemic vascular resistance resulting from vasoactive substances released by the tumor. Treatment with somatostatin analogues (e.g., octreotide) or interferon α improves symptoms and survival in patients with carcinoid heart disease but does not appear to improve valvular abnormalities. In some severely symptomatic patients, valve replacement is indicated. Coronary artery spasm, presumably due to a circulating vasoactive substance, may occur in patients with carcinoid syndrome.

PHEOCHROMOCYTOMA

In addition to causing labile or sustained hypertension, the high circulating levels of catecholamines resulting from a pheochromocytoma may cause direct myocardial injury. Focal myocardial necrosis and inflammatory cell infiltration are present in ~50% of patients who die with pheochromocytoma and may contribute to clinically significant left ventricular failure and pulmonary edema. In addition, associated hypertension results in left ventricular hypertrophy. Left ventricular dysfunction and CHF may resolve after removal of the tumor.

ACROMEGALY

Exposure of the heart to excessive growth hormone may cause CHF as a result of high cardiac output, diastolic dysfunction owing to ventricular hypertrophy (with increased left ventricular chamber size or wall thickness), or global systolic dysfunction. Hypertension occurs in up to one-third of patients with acromegaly and is characterized by suppression of the renin-angiotensin-aldosterone axis and increases in total-body sodium and plasma volume. Some form of cardiac disease occurs in about one-third of patients with acromegaly and is associated with a doubling of the risk of cardiac death.

RHEUMATOID ARTHRITIS AND THE COLLAGEN VASCULAR DISEASES

Rheumatoid arthritis

Rheumatoid arthritis may be associated with inflammatory changes in any or all cardiac structures, although pericarditis is the most common clinical entity. Pericardial effusions are found on echocardiography in 10–50% of patients with rheumatoid arthritis, particularly those with subcutaneous nodules. Nonetheless, only a small fraction of these patients have symptomatic pericarditis, and when present, it usually follows a benign course, only occasionally progressing to cardiac tamponade or constrictive pericarditis. The pericardial fluid is generally exudative, with decreased concentrations of complement and glucose and elevated cholesterol. Coronary arteritis with intimal inflammation and edema is present in ~20% of cases but only rarely results in angina pectoris or myocardial infarction. Inflammation and granuloma formation may affect the cardiac valves, most often the mitral and aortic valves, and may cause clinically significant regurgitation owing to valve deformity. Myocarditis is uncommon and rarely results in cardiac dysfunction.

Treatment is directed at the underlying rheumatoid arthritis and may include glucocorticoids. Urgent pericardiocentesis should be performed in patients with tamponade, but pericardiectomy usually is required in cases of pericardial constriction.

Seronegative arthropathies

The seronegative arthropathies, including ankylosing spondylitis, reactive arthritis, psoriatic arthritis, and the arthritides associated with ulcerative colitis and regional enteritis, are all strongly associated with the HLA-B27 histocompatibility antigen and may be accompanied by a pancarditis and proximal aortitis. The aortic inflammation usually is limited to the aortic root but may extend to involve the aortic valve, mitral valve, and ventricular myocardium, resulting in aortic and mitral regurgitation, conduction abnormalities, and ventricular dysfunction. One-tenth of these patients have significant aortic insufficiency, and one-third have conduction disturbances; both are more common in patients with peripheral joint involvement and long-standing disease. Treatment with aortic valve replacement and permanent pacemaker implantation may be required. Occasionally, aortic regurgitation precedes the onset of arthritis, and therefore, the diagnosis of a seronegative arthritis should be considered in young males with isolated aortic regurgitation.

Systemic lupus erythematosus (SLE)

A significant percentage of patients with SLE have cardiac involvement. Pericarditis is common, occurring in about two-thirds of patients, and generally follows a benign course, although rarely tamponade or constriction may result. The characteristic endocardial lesions of SLE are verrucous valvular abnormalities known as *Libman-Sacks endocarditis*. They most often are located on the left-sided cardiac valves, particularly on the ventricular surface of the posterior mitral leaflet, and are made up almost entirely of fibrin. These lesions may embolize or become infected but rarely cause hemodynamically important valvular regurgitation. Myocarditis generally parallels the activity of the disease and, although common histologically, seldom results in clinical heart failure unless associated with hypertension. Although arteritis of epicardial coronary arteries may occur, it rarely results in myocardial ischemia. There is, however, an increased incidence of coronary atherosclerosis that probably is related more to associated risk factors and glucocorticoid use than to SLE itself. Patients with the antiphospholipid antibody syndrome may have a higher incidence of cardiovascular abnormalities, including valvular regurgitation, venous and arterial thrombosis, premature stroke, myocardial infarction, pulmonary hypertension, and cardiomyopathy.

CHAPTER 25

INFECTIVE ENDOCARDITIS

Adolf W. Karchmer

The prototypic lesion of infective endocarditis, the *vegetation* (Fig. 25-1), is a mass of platelets, fibrin, microcolonies of microorganisms, and scant inflammatory cells. Infection most commonly involves heart valves (either native or prosthetic) but may also occur on the low-pressure side of a ventricular septal defect, on the mural endocardium where it is damaged by aberrant jets of blood or foreign bodies, or on intracardiac devices themselves. The analogous process involving arteriovenous shunts, arterioarterial shunts (patent ductus arteriosus), or a coarctation of the aorta is called *infective endarteritis*.

Endocarditis may be classified according to the temporal evolution of disease, the site of infection, the cause of infection, or a predisposing risk factor such as injection drug use. While each classification criterion provides therapeutic and prognostic insight, none is sufficient alone. *Acute endocarditis* is a hectically febrile illness that rapidly damages cardiac structures, hematogenously seeds extracardiac sites, and, if untreated, progresses to death within weeks. *Subacute endocarditis* follows an indolent course; causes structural cardiac damage only slowly, if at all; rarely metastasizes; and is gradually progressive unless complicated by a major embolic event or ruptured mycotic aneurysm.

In developed countries, the incidence of endocarditis ranges from 2.6 to 7 cases per 100,000 population per year and has remained relatively stable during recent decades. While congenital heart diseases remain a constant predisposition, predisposing conditions in developed countries have shifted from chronic rheumatic heart disease (which remains a common predisposition in developing countries) to illicit IV drug use, degenerative valve disease, and intracardiac devices. The incidence of endocarditis is notably increased among the elderly. In developed countries, 30–35% of cases of native valve endocarditis (NVE) are associated with health care, and 16–30% of all cases of endocarditis involve prosthetic valves. The risk of prosthesis infection is greatest during the first 6–12 months after valve replacement; gradually declines to a low, stable rate thereafter; and is similar for mechanical and bioprosthetic devices.

ETIOLOGY

Although many species of bacteria and fungi cause sporadic episodes of endocarditis, a few bacterial species cause the majority of cases (Table 25-1). Because of their different portals of entry, the pathogens involved vary somewhat with the clinical types of endocarditis. The oral cavity, skin, and upper respiratory tract are the respective primary portals for the viridans streptococci, staphylococci, and HACEK organisms (*Haemophilus*, *Actinobacillus*, *Cardiobacterium*, *Eikenella*, and *Kingella*; *Haemophilus aphrophilus* and *Actinobacillus actinomycetemcomitans* have been reclassified into the genus *Aggregatibacter*). *Streptococcus gallolyticus* (formerly *S. bovis*) originates from the gastrointestinal tract, where it is associated with polyps and colonic tumors, and

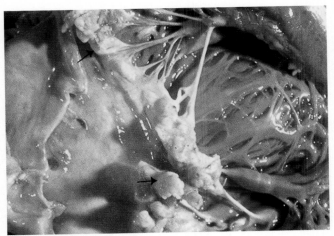

FIGURE 25-1
Vegetations (*arrows*) due to viridans streptococcal endocarditis involving the mitral valve.

TABLE 25-1

ORGANISMS CAUSING MAJOR CLINICAL FORMS OF ENDOCARDITIS

| | PERCENTAGE OF CASES | | | | | | | |
| | NATIVE VALVE ENDOCARDITIS | | PROSTHETIC VALVE ENDOCARDITIS AT INDICATED TIME OF ONSET (MONTHS) AFTER VALVE SURGERY | | | ENDOCARDITIS IN INJECTION DRUG USERS | | |
ORGANISM	COMMUNITY-ACQUIRED ($n = 1718$)	HEALTH CARE-ASSOCIATED ($n = 788$)	<2 ($n = 144$)	2–12 ($n = 31$)	>12 ($n = 194$)	RIGHT-SIDED ($n = 346$)	LEFT-SIDED ($n = 204$)	TOTAL ($n = 675$)[a]
Streptococci[b]	40	9	1	9	31	5	15	12
Pneumococci	2	—	—	—	—	—	—	—
Enterococci	9	13	8	12	11	2	24	9
Staphylococcus aureus	28	53[c]	22	12	18	77	23	57
Coagulase-negative staphylococci	5	12	33	32	11			
Fastidious gram-negative coccobacilli (HACEK group)[d]	3	—	—		6	—	—	—
Gram-negative bacilli	1	2	13	3	6	5	13	7
Candida spp.	<1	2	8	12	1	—	12	4
Polymicrobial/ miscellaneous	3	4	3	6	5	8	10	7
Diphtheroids	—	<1	6	—	3	—	—	0.1
Culture-negative	9	5	5	6	8	3	3	3

[a]The total number of cases is larger than the sum of right- and left-sided cases because the location of infection was not specified in some cases.
[b]Includes viridans streptococci; *Streptococcus gallolyticus*; other nongroup A, groupable streptococci; and *Abiotrophia* spp. (nutritionally variant, pyridoxal-requiring streptococci).
[c]Methicillin resistance is common among these *S. aureus* strains.
[d]Includes *Haemophilus* spp., *Aggregatibacter actinomycetemcomitans*, *Cardiobacterium hominis*, *Eikenella* spp., and *Kingella* spp.
Note: Data are compiled from multiple studies.

enterococci enter the bloodstream from the genito-urinary tract. Health care–associated NVE, commonly caused by *Staphylococcus aureus*, coagulase-negative staphylococci (CoNS), and enterococci, has a noso-comial onset (55%) or a community onset (45%) in patients who have had extensive contact with the health care system over the preceding 90 days. Endocarditis complicates 6–25% of episodes of catheter-associated *S. aureus* bacteremia; the higher rates are detected by careful transesophageal echocardiography (TEE) screening (see "Echocardiography," later).

Prosthetic valve endocarditis (PVE) arising within 2 months of valve surgery is generally nosocomial, the result of intraoperative contamination of the prosthesis or a bacteremic postoperative complication. This noso-comial origin is reflected in the primary microbial causes: *S. aureus*, CoNS, facultative gram-negative bacilli, diph-theroids, and fungi. The portals of entry and organisms causing cases beginning >12 months after surgery are similar to those in community-acquired NVE. PVE due to CoNS that presents 2–12 months after surgery often

represents delayed-onset nosocomial infection. Regard-less of the time of onset after surgery, at least 68–85% of CoNS strains that cause PVE are resistant to methicillin.

Transvenous pacemaker– or implanted defibrillator–associated endocarditis is usually nosocomial. The major-ity of episodes occur within weeks of implantation or generator change and are caused by *S. aureus* or CoNS, both of which are commonly resistant to methicillin.

Endocarditis occurring among injection drug users, especially that involving the tricuspid valve, is commonly caused by *S. aureus*, many strains of which are resistant to methicillin. Left-sided valve infections in addicts have a more varied etiology. In addition to the usual causes of endocarditis, these cases are caused by *Pseudomonas aeru-ginosa* and *Candida* species and sporadically by unusual organisms such as *Bacillus*, *Lactobacillus*, and *Corynebacte-rium* species. Polymicrobial endocarditis occurs among injection drug users. HIV infection in drug users does not significantly influence the causes of endocarditis.

From 5% to 15% of patients with endocarditis have negative blood cultures; in one-third to one-half of these cases, cultures are negative because of prior antibiotic exposure. The remainder of these patients are infected by fastidious organisms, such as nutritionally variant organisms (now designated *Granulicatella* and *Abiotrophia* species), HACEK organisms, *Coxiella burnetii*, and *Bartonella* species. Some fastidious organisms occur in characteristic geographic settings (e.g., *C. burnetii* and *Bartonella* species in Europe, *Brucella* species in the Middle East). *Tropheryma whipplei* causes an indolent, culture-negative, afebrile form of endocarditis.

PATHOGENESIS

The endothelium, unless damaged, is resistant to infection by most bacteria and to thrombus formation. Endothelial injury (e.g., at the site of impact of high-velocity blood jets or on the low-pressure side of a cardiac structural lesion) allows either direct infection by virulent organisms or the development of an uninfected platelet-fibrin thrombus—a condition called *nonbacterial thrombotic endocarditis* (NBTE). The thrombus subsequently serves as a site of bacterial attachment during transient bacteremia. The cardiac conditions most commonly resulting in NBTE are mitral regurgitation, aortic stenosis, aortic regurgitation, ventricular septal defects, and complex congenital heart disease. NBTE also arises as a result of a hypercoagulable state; this phenomenon gives rise to the clinical entity of *marantic endocarditis* (uninfected vegetations seen in patients with malignancy and chronic diseases) and to bland vegetations complicating systemic lupus erythematosus and the antiphospholipid antibody syndrome.

Organisms that cause endocarditis generally enter the bloodstream from mucosal surfaces, the skin, or sites of focal infection. Except for more virulent bacteria (e.g., *S. aureus*) that can adhere directly to intact endothelium or exposed subendothelial tissue, microorganisms in the blood adhere at sites of NBTE. If resistant to the bactericidal activity of serum and the microbicidal peptides released locally by platelets, the organisms proliferate and induce platelet deposition and a procoagulant state at the site by eliciting tissue factor from the endothelium or, in the case of *S. aureus*, from monocytes as well. Fibrin deposition combines with platelet aggregation and microorganism proliferation to generate an infected vegetation. The organisms that commonly cause endocarditis have surface adhesin molecules, collectively called microbial surface components recognizing adhesin matrix molecules (MSCRAMMs), that mediate adherence to NBTE sites or injured endothelium. Fibronectin-binding proteins present on many gram-positive bacteria, clumping factor (a fibrinogen- and fibrin-binding surface protein) on *S. aureus*, and glucans or FimA (a member of the family of oral mucosal adhesins) on streptococci facilitate adherence. Fibronectin-binding proteins are required for *S. aureus*

invasion of intact endothelium; thus these surface proteins may facilitate infection of previously normal valves. In the absence of host defenses, organisms enmeshed in the growing platelet-fibrin vegetation proliferate to form dense microcolonies. Organisms deep in vegetations are metabolically inactive (nongrowing) and relatively resistant to killing by antimicrobial agents. Proliferating surface organisms are shed into the bloodstream continuously.

The pathophysiologic consequences and clinical manifestations of endocarditis—other than constitutional symptoms, which probably result from cytokine production—arise from damage to intracardiac structures; embolization of vegetation fragments, leading to infection or infarction of remote tissues; hematogenous infection of sites during bacteremia; and tissue injury due to the deposition of circulating immune complexes or immune responses to deposited bacterial antigens.

CLINICAL MANIFESTATIONS

The clinical syndrome of infective endocarditis is highly variable and spans a continuum between acute and subacute presentations. NVE (whether acquired in the community or in association with health care), PVE, and endocarditis due to injection drug use share clinical and laboratory manifestations (Table 25-2). The causative microorganism is primarily responsible for the temporal course of endocarditis. β-Hemolytic streptococci, *S. aureus*, and pneumococci typically result in an acute course, although *S. aureus* occasionally causes subacute disease. Endocarditis caused by *Staphylococcus lugdunensis* (a coagulase-negative species) or by enterococci may present acutely. Subacute endocarditis is typically caused by viridans streptococci, enterococci, CoNS, and the HACEK group. Endocarditis caused by *Bartonella* species, *T. whipplei*, or *C. burnetii* is exceptionally indolent.

The clinical features of endocarditis are nonspecific. However, these symptoms in a febrile patient with valvular abnormalities or a behavior pattern that predisposes to endocarditis (e.g., injection drug use) suggest the diagnosis, as do bacteremia with organisms that frequently cause endocarditis, otherwise-unexplained arterial emboli, and progressive cardiac valvular incompetence. In patients with subacute presentations, fever is typically low grade and rarely exceeds 39.4°C (103°F); in contrast, temperatures of 39.4°–40°C (103°–104°F) are often noted in acute endocarditis. Fever may be blunted or absent in patients who are elderly or severely debilitated or who have marked cardiac or renal failure.

Cardiac manifestations

Although heart murmurs are usually indicative of the predisposing cardiac pathology rather than of endocarditis, valvular damage and ruptured chordae may result in new regurgitant murmurs. In acute endocarditis

TABLE 25-2

CLINICAL AND LABORATORY FEATURES OF INFECTIVE ENDOCARDITIS

FEATURE	FREQUENCY, %
Fever	80–90
Chills and sweats	40–75
Anorexia, weight loss, malaise	25–50
Myalgias, arthralgias	15–30
Back pain	7–15
Heart murmur	80–85
New/worsened regurgitant murmur	20–50
Arterial emboli	20–50
Splenomegaly	15–50
Clubbing	10–20
Neurologic manifestations	20–40
Peripheral manifestations (Osler's nodes, subungual hemorrhages, Janeway lesions, Roth's spots)	2–15
Petechiae	10–40
Laboratory manifestations	
Anemia	70–90
Leukocytosis	20–30
Microscopic hematuria	30–50
Elevated erythrocyte sedimentation rate	60–90
Elevated C-reactive protein level	>90
Rheumatoid factor	50
Circulating immune complexes	65–100
Decreased serum complement	5–40

involving a normal valve, murmurs may be absent initially but ultimately are detected in 85% of cases. Congestive heart failure (CHF) develops in 30–40% of patients; it is usually a consequence of valvular dysfunction but occasionally is due to endocarditis-associated myocarditis or an intracardiac fistula. Heart failure due to aortic valve dysfunction progresses more rapidly than does that due to mitral valve dysfunction. Extension of infection beyond valve leaflets into adjacent annular or myocardial tissue results in perivalvular abscesses, which in turn may cause intracardiac fistulae with new murmurs. Abscesses may burrow from the aortic valve annulus through the epicardium, causing pericarditis, or into the upper ventricular septum, where they may interrupt the conduction system, leading to varying degrees of heart block. Perivalvular abscesses arising from the mitral valve rarely interrupt conduction pathways near the atrioventricular node or in the proximal bundle of His. Emboli to a coronary artery occur in 2% of patients and may result in myocardial infarction.

Noncardiac manifestations

The classic nonsuppurative peripheral manifestations of subacute endocarditis are related to the duration of infection and, with early diagnosis and treatment, have become infrequent. In contrast, septic embolization mimicking some of these lesions (subungual hemorrhage, Osler's nodes) is common in patients with acute *S. aureus* endocarditis (**Fig. 25-2**). Musculoskeletal pain usually remits promptly with treatment but must be distinguished from focal metastatic infections (e.g., spondylodiscitis), which may complicate 10–15% of cases. Hematogenously seeded focal infection is most often clinically evident in the skin, spleen, kidneys, skeletal system, and meninges. Arterial emboli are clinically apparent in up to 50% of patients. Endocarditis caused by *S. aureus*, vegetations >10 mm in diameter (as measured by echocardiography), and infection involving the mitral valve are independently associated with an increased risk of embolization. Emboli occurring late, during, or after effective therapy do not in themselves constitute evidence of failed antimicrobial treatment. Cerebrovascular emboli presenting as strokes or occasionally as encephalopathy complicate 15–35% of cases of endocarditis. One-half of these events precede the diagnosis of endocarditis. The frequency of stroke is 8 per 1000 patient-days during the week prior to diagnosis; the figure falls to 4.8 and 1.7 per 1000 patient-days during the first and second weeks of effective antimicrobial therapy, respectively. This decline exceeds that which can be attributed to change in vegetation size. Only 3% of strokes occur after 1 week of effective therapy. Other neurologic complications include aseptic or purulent meningitis, intracranial hemorrhage due to hemorrhagic infarcts or ruptured mycotic aneurysms, and seizures. (*Mycotic aneurysms* are focal dilations of arteries occurring at points in the artery wall that have been

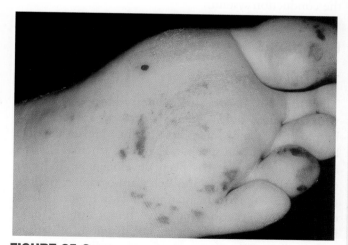

FIGURE 25-2
Septic emboli with hemorrhage and infarction due to acute *Staphylococcus aureus* endocarditis. (*Used with permission of L. Baden.*)

CHAPTER 25 Infective Endocarditis

weakened by infection in the vasa vasorum or where septic emboli have lodged.) Microabscesses in brain and meninges occur commonly in *S. aureus* endocarditis; surgically drainable intracerebral abscesses are infrequent.

Immune complex deposition on the glomerular basement membrane causes diffuse hypocomplementemic glomerulonephritis and renal dysfunction, which typically improve with effective antimicrobial therapy. Embolic renal infarcts cause flank pain and hematuria but rarely cause renal dysfunction.

Manifestations of specific predisposing conditions

Almost 50% of endocarditis cases associated with injection drug use are limited to the tricuspid valve and present with fever but with faint or no murmur. In 75% of cases, septic emboli cause cough, pleuritic chest pain, nodular pulmonary infiltrates, or occasionally pyopneumothorax. Infection of the aortic or mitral valves on the left side of the heart presents with the typical clinical features of endocarditis.

Health care–associated endocarditis has typical manifestations if it is not associated with a retained intracardiac device or masked by the symptoms of concurrent comorbid illness. Transvenous pacemaker– or implanted defibrillator–associated endocarditis may be associated with obvious or cryptic generator pocket infection and results in fever, minimal murmur, and pulmonary symptoms due to septic emboli.

Late-onset PVE presents with typical clinical features. In cases arising within 60 days of valve surgery (early onset), typical symptoms may be obscured by comorbidity associated with recent surgery. In both early-onset and more delayed presentations, paravalvular infection is common and often results in partial valve dehiscence, regurgitant murmurs, CHF, or disruption of the conduction system.

DIAGNOSIS

The Duke criteria

The diagnosis of infective endocarditis is established with certainty only when vegetations are examined histologically and microbiologically. Nevertheless, a highly sensitive and specific diagnostic schema—known as the *Duke criteria*—has been developed on the basis of clinical, laboratory, and echocardiographic findings (Table 25-3). Documentation of two major criteria, of one major criterion and three minor criteria, or of five minor criteria allows a clinical diagnosis of definite endocarditis. The diagnosis of endocarditis is rejected if an alternative diagnosis is established, if symptoms resolve and do not recur with ≤4 days of antibiotic therapy, or if surgery or autopsy after ≤4 days of

antimicrobial therapy yields no histologic evidence of endocarditis. Illnesses not classified as definite endocarditis or rejected as such are considered cases of possible infective endocarditis when either one major criterion

TABLE 25-3

THE DUKE CRITERIA FOR THE CLINICAL DIAGNOSIS OF INFECTIVE ENDOCARDITIS[a]

Major Criteria

1. Positive blood culture
   Typical microorganism for infective endocarditis from two separate blood cultures
      Viridans streptococci, *Streptococcus gallolyticus*, HACEK group, *Staphylococcus aureus*, or
      Community-acquired enterococci in the absence of a primary focus, *or*
   Persistently positive blood culture, defined as recovery of a microorganism consistent with infective endocarditis from:
      Blood cultures drawn >12 h apart; *or*
      All of 3 or a majority of ≥4 separate blood cultures, with first and last drawn at least 1 h apart
   Single positive blood culture for *Coxiella burnetii* or phase I IgG antibody titer of >1:800
2. Evidence of endocardial involvement
   Positive echocardiogram[b]
      Oscillating intracardiac mass on valve or supporting structures or in the path of regurgitant jets or in implanted material, in the absence of an alternative anatomic explanation, *or*
      Abscess, *or*
      New partial dehiscence of prosthetic valve, *or*
   New valvular regurgitation (increase or change in preexisting murmur not sufficient)

Minor Criteria

1. Predisposition: predisposing heart condition or injection drug use
2. Fever ≥38.0°C (≥100.4°F)
3. Vascular phenomena: major arterial emboli, septic pulmonary infarcts, mycotic aneurysm, intracranial hemorrhage, conjunctival hemorrhages, Janeway lesions
4. Immunologic phenomena: glomerulonephritis, Osler's nodes, Roth's spots, rheumatoid factor
5. Microbiologic evidence: positive blood culture but not meeting major criterion as noted previously[c] or serologic evidence of active infection with organism consistent with infective endocarditis

[a]Definite endocarditis is defined by documentation of two major criteria, of one major criterion and three minor criteria, or of five minor criteria. See text for further details.
[b]Transesophageal echocardiography is recommended for assessing possible prosthetic valve endocarditis or complicated endocarditis.
[c]Excluding single positive cultures for coagulase-negative staphylococci and diphtheroids, which are common culture contaminants, and organisms that do not cause endocarditis frequently, such as gram-negative bacilli.
Note: HACEK, *Haemophilus* spp., *Aggregatibacter actinomycetemcomitans*, *Cardiobacterium hominis*, *Eikenella corrodens*, *Kingella* spp.
Source: Adapted from JS Li et al: Clin Infect Dis 30:633, 2000, with permission from the University of Chicago Press.

and one minor criterion or three minor criteria are fulfilled. Requiring the identification of clinical features of endocarditis for classification as possible infective endocarditis increases the specificity of the schema without significantly reducing its sensitivity.

The roles of bacteremia and echocardiographic findings in the diagnosis of endocarditis are emphasized in the Duke criteria. The requirement for multiple positive blood cultures over time is consistent with the continuous low-density bacteremia characteristic of endocarditis. Among patients with untreated endocarditis who ultimately have a positive blood culture, 95% of all blood cultures are positive. The diagnostic criteria attach significance to the species of organism isolated from blood cultures. To fulfill a major criterion, the isolation of an organism that causes both endocarditis and bacteremia in the absence of endocarditis (e.g., *S. aureus*, enterococci) must take place repeatedly (i.e., persistent bacteremia) and in the absence of a primary focus of infection. Organisms that rarely cause endocarditis but commonly contaminate blood cultures (e.g., diphtheroids, CoNS) must be isolated repeatedly if their isolation is to serve as a major criterion.

Blood cultures

Isolation of the causative microorganism from blood cultures is critical for diagnosis, determination of antimicrobial susceptibility, and planning of treatment. In the absence of prior antibiotic therapy, three 2-bottle blood culture sets, separated from one another by at least 1 h, should be obtained from different venipuncture sites over 24 h. If the cultures remain negative after 48–72 h, two or three additional blood culture sets should be obtained, and the laboratory should be consulted for advice regarding optimal culture techniques. Pending culture results, empirical antimicrobial therapy should be withheld initially from hemodynamically stable patients with suspected subacute endocarditis, especially those who have received antibiotics within the preceding 2 weeks; thus, if necessary, additional blood culture sets can be obtained without the confounding effect of empirical treatment. Patients with acute endocarditis or with deteriorating hemodynamics who may require urgent surgery should be treated empirically immediately after three sets of blood cultures are obtained over several hours.

Non-blood-culture tests

Serologic tests can be used to implicate causally some organisms that are difficult to recover by blood culture: *Brucella*, *Bartonella*, *Legionella*, *Chlamydophila psittaci*, and *C. burnetii*. Pathogens can also be identified in vegetations by culture, microscopic examination with special stains (i.e., the periodic acid–Schiff stain for *T. whipplei*),

or direct fluorescence antibody techniques and by the use of polymerase chain reaction (PCR) to recover unique microbial DNA or 16S rRNA that, when sequenced, allows identification of organisms.

Echocardiography

Echocardiography allows anatomic confirmation of infective endocarditis, sizing of vegetations, detection of intracardiac complications, and assessment of cardiac function (Fig. 25-3). Transthoracic echocardiography (TTE) is noninvasive and exceptionally specific; however, it cannot image vegetations <2 mm in diameter, and in 20% of patients it is technically inadequate because of emphysema or body habitus. TTE detects vegetations in only 65% of patients with definite clinical endocarditis. Moreover, TTE is not adequate for evaluating prosthetic valves or detecting intracardiac complications. TEE is safe and detects vegetations in >90% of patients with definite endocarditis; nevertheless, initial studies may be false-negative in 6–18% of endocarditis patients. When endocarditis is likely, a negative TEE result does not exclude the diagnosis but rather warrants repetition of the study in 7–10 days. TEE is the optimal method for the diagnosis of PVE or the detection of myocardial abscess, valve perforation, or intracardiac fistulae.

Experts favor echocardiographic evaluation of all patients with a clinical diagnosis of endocarditis; however, the test should not be used to screen patients with a low probability of endocarditis (e.g., patients with unexplained fever). An American Heart Association approach to the use of echocardiography for evaluation of patients with suspected endocarditis is illustrated in Fig. 25-4.

Other studies

Many laboratory studies that are not diagnostic—i.e., complete blood count, creatinine determination, liver function tests, chest radiography, and electrocardiography—are nevertheless important in the management of patients with endocarditis. The erythrocyte sedimentation rate, C-reactive protein level, and circulating immune complex titer are commonly increased in endocarditis (Table 25-2). Cardiac catheterization is useful primarily to assess coronary artery patency in older individuals who are to undergo surgery for endocarditis.

TREATMENT Infective Endocarditis

ANTIMICROBIAL THERAPY It is difficult to eradicate bacteria from the vegetation because local host defenses are deficient and because the largely non-growing, metabolically inactive bacteria are less easily

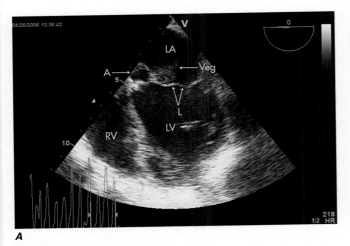

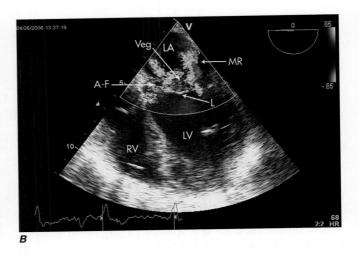

FIGURE 25-3

Imaging of a mitral valve infected with *Staphylococcus aureus* by low-esophageal four-chamber-view transesophageal echocardiography (TEE). **A.** Two-dimensional echocardiogram showing a large vegetation with an adjacent echolucent abscess cavity. **B.** Color-flow Doppler image showing severe mitral regurgitation through both the abscess-fistula and the central valve orifice. A, abscess; A-F, abscess-fistula; L, valve leaflets; LA, left atrium; LV, left ventricle; MR, mitral central valve regurgitation; RV, right ventricle; veg, vegetation. (*With permission of Andrew Burger, MD*)

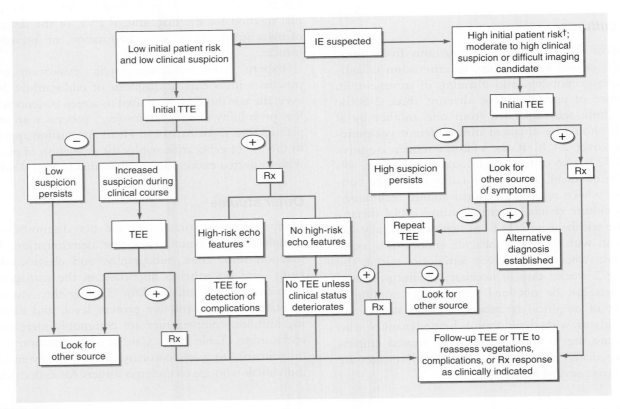

FIGURE 25-4

The diagnostic use of transesophageal and transtracheal echocardiography (TEE and TTE, respectively). †High initial patient risk for endocarditis as listed in Table 25-8 or evidence of intracardiac complications (new regurgitant murmur, new electrocardiographic conduction changes, or congestive heart failure). *High-risk echocardiographic features include large vegetations, valve insufficiency, paravalvular infection, or ventricular dysfunction. Rx indicates initiation of antibiotic therapy. (*Reproduced with permission from Diagnosis and Management of Infective Endocarditis and Its Complications. Circulation 98:2936, 1998. © 1998 American Heart Association.*)

killed by antibiotics. To cure endocarditis, all bacteria in the vegetation must be killed; therefore, therapy must be bactericidal and prolonged. Antibiotics are generally given parenterally to achieve serum concentrations that, through passive diffusion, lead to effective concentrations in the depths of the vegetation. To select effective therapy requires knowledge of the susceptibility of the causative microorganisms. The decision to initiate treatment empirically must balance the need to establish a microbiologic diagnosis against the potential progression of disease or the need for urgent surgery (see "Blood Cultures," earlier). Simultaneous infection at other sites (such as meningitis), allergies, end-organ dysfunction, interactions with concomitant medications, and risks of adverse events must be considered in the selection of therapy.

Although given for several weeks longer, the regimens recommended for the treatment of endocarditis involving prosthetic valves (except for staphylococcal infections) are similar to those used to treat NVE (Table 25-4). Recommended doses and durations of therapy should be adhered to unless alterations are required by end-organ dysfunction or adverse events.

Organism-Specific Therapies

Streptococci Optimal therapy for streptococcal endocarditis is based on the minimal inhibitory concentration (MIC) of penicillin for the causative isolate (Table 25-4). The 2-week penicillin/gentamicin or ceftriaxone/gentamicin regimens should not be used to treat complicated NVE or PVE. The regimen recommended for relatively penicillin-resistant streptococci is advocated for treatment of group B, C, or G streptococcal endocarditis. Nutritionally variant organisms (*Granulicatella* or *Abiotrophia* species) and *Gemella morbillorum* are treated with the regimen for moderately penicillin-resistant streptococci, as is PVE caused by these organisms or by streptococci with a penicillin MIC of >0.1 µg/mL (Table 25-4).

Enterococci Enterococci are resistant to oxacillin, nafcillin, and the cephalosporins and are only inhibited—not killed—by penicillin, ampicillin, teicoplanin (not available in the United States), and vancomycin. To kill enterococci requires the synergistic interaction of a cell wall–active antibiotic (penicillin, ampicillin, vancomycin, or teicoplanin) that is effective at achievable serum concentrations and an aminoglycoside (gentamicin or streptomycin) to which the isolate does not exhibit high-level resistance. An isolate's resistance to cell wall–active agents or its ability to replicate in the presence of gentamicin at ≥500 µg/mL or streptomycin at 1000–2000 µg/mL—a phenomenon called *high-level aminoglycoside resistance*—indicates that the ineffective

antimicrobial agent cannot participate in the interaction to produce killing. High-level resistance to gentamicin predicts that tobramycin, netilmicin, amikacin, and kanamycin also will be ineffective. In fact, even when enterococci are not highly resistant to gentamicin, it is difficult to predict the ability of these other aminoglycosides to participate in synergistic killing; consequently, they should not in general be used to treat enterococcal endocarditis. High concentrations of ampicillin plus ceftriaxone or cefotaxime, by expanded binding of penicillin-binding proteins, kill *E. faecalis* in vitro and in animal models of endocarditis.

Enterococci causing endocarditis must be tested for high-level resistance to streptomycin and gentamicin, β-lactamase production, and susceptibility to penicillin and ampicillin (MIC, <8 µg/mL) and to vancomycin (MIC, ≤4 µg/mL). If the isolate produces β-lactamase, ampicillin/sulbactam or vancomycin can be used as the cell wall–active component; if the penicillin/ampicillin MIC is ≥8 µg/mL, vancomycin can be considered; and if the vancomycin MIC is ≥8 µg/mL, penicillin or ampicillin can be considered. In the absence of high-level resistance, gentamicin or streptomycin should be used as the aminoglycoside (Table 25-4). If there is high-level resistance to both these drugs, no aminoglycoside should be given; instead, an 8- to 12-week course of a single cell wall–active agent—or, for *E. faecalis*, high doses of ampicillin combined with ceftriaxone or cefotaxime—is suggested. If this alternative therapy fails or the isolate is resistant to all of the commonly used agents, surgical treatment is advised. The role of newer agents potentially active against multidrug-resistant enterococci (quinupristin/dalfopristin [*E. faecium* only], linezolid, and daptomycin) in the treatment of endocarditis has not been established. Although the dose of gentamicin used to achieve bactericidal synergy in treating enterococcal endocarditis is smaller than that used in standard therapy, nephrotoxicity is not uncommon during treatment for 4–6 weeks. Regimens in which the aminoglycoside component is discontinued at 2–3 weeks because of toxicity have been curative. Thus, discontinuation of the aminoglycoside is recommended when nephrotoxicity develops in patients who have responded satisfactorily to therapy. Alternatively, the ampicillin-ceftriaxone regimen can be used to treat *E. faecalis* endocarditis if nephrotoxicity develops or is exceptionally threatening.

Staphylococci The regimens used to treat staphylococcal endocarditis (Table 25-4) are based not on coagulase production but rather on the presence or absence of a prosthetic valve or foreign device, the native valve(s) involved, and the susceptibility of the isolate to penicillin, methicillin, and vancomycin. All staphylococci are considered penicillin resistant until shown

TABLE 25-4

ANTIBIOTIC TREATMENT FOR INFECTIVE ENDOCARDITIS CAUSED BY COMMON ORGANISMS[a]

ORGANISM	DRUG (DOSE, DURATION)	COMMENTS
Streptococci		
Penicillin-susceptible[b] streptococci, S. gallolyticus	• Penicillin G (2–3 mU IV q4h for 4 weeks) • Ceftriaxone (2 g/d IV as a single dose for 4 weeks) • Vancomycin[c] (15 mg/kg IV q12h for 4 weeks) • Penicillin G (2–3 mU IV q4h) or ceftriaxone (2 g IV qd) for 2 weeks *plus* Gentamicin[d] (3 mg/kg qd IV or IM, as a single dose[e] or divided into equal doses q8h for 2 weeks)	— Can use ceftriaxone in patients with non-immediate penicillin allergy Use vancomycin in patients with severe or immediate β-lactam allergy Avoid 2-week regimen when risk of amino-glycoside toxicity is increased and in prosthetic valve or complicated endocarditis
Relatively penicillin-resistant[f] streptococci	• Penicillin G (4 mU IV q4h) or ceftriaxone (2 g IV qd) for 4 weeks *plus* Gentamicin[d] (3 mg/kg qd IV or IM, as a single dose[e] or divided into equal doses q8h for 2 weeks) • Vancomycin[c] as noted above for 4 weeks	Penicillin alone at this dose for 6 weeks or with gentamicin during initial 2 weeks preferred for prosthetic valve endocarditis caused by streptococci with penicillin MICs of ≤0.1 μg/mL —
Moderately penicillin-resistant[g] streptococci, nutritionally variant organisms, or *Gemella morbillorum*	• Penicillin G (4–5 mU IV q4h) or ceftriaxone (2 g IV qd) for 6 weeks *plus* Gentamicin[d] (3 mg/kg qd IV or IM as a single dose[e] or divided into equal doses q8h for 6 weeks) • Vancomycin[c] as noted above for 4 weeks	Preferred for prosthetic valve endocarditis caused by streptococci with penicillin MICs of >0.1 μg/mL
Enterococci[h]		
	• Penicillin G (4–5 mU IV q4h) *plus* Gentamicin[d] (1 mg/kg IV q8h), both for 4–6 weeks • Ampicillin (2 g IV q4h) *plus* Gentamicin[d] (1 mg/kg IV q8h), both for 4–6 weeks • Vancomycin[c] (15 mg/kg IV q12h) *plus* Gentamicin[d] (1 mg/kg IV q8h), both for 4–6 weeks	Can use streptomycin (7.5 mg/kg q12h) in lieu of gentamicin if there is not high-level resistance to streptomycin — Use vancomycin plus gentamicin for penicillin-allergic patients, or desensitize to penicillin
Staphylococci		
Methicillin-susceptible, infecting native valves (no foreign devices)	• Nafcillin or oxacillin (2 g IV q4h for 4–6 weeks) • Cefazolin (2 g IV q8h for 4–6 weeks) • Vancomycin[c] (15 mg/kg IV q12h for 4–6 weeks)	Can use penicillin (4 mU q4h) if isolate is penicillin susceptible (does not produce β-lactamase) Can use cefazolin regimen for patients with nonimmediate penicillin allergy Use vancomycin for patients with immediate (urticarial) or severe penicillin allergy
Methicillin-resistant, infecting native valves (no foreign devices)	• Vancomycin[c] (15 mg/kg IV q8–12h for 4–6 weeks)	No role for routine use of rifampin
Methicillin-susceptible, infecting prosthetic valves	• Nafcillin or oxacillin (2 g IV q4h for 6–8 weeks) *plus* Gentamicin[d] (1 mg/kg IM or IV q8h for 2 weeks) *plus* Rifampin[i] (300 mg PO q8h for 6–8 weeks)	Use gentamicin during initial 2 weeks; determine susceptibility to gentamicin before initiating rifampin (see text); if patient is highly allergic to penicillin, use regimen for methicillin-resistant staphylococci; if β-lactam allergy is of the minor, nonimmediate type, can substitute cefazolin for oxacillin/nafcillin
Methicillin-resistant, infecting prosthetic valves	• Vancomycin[c] (15 mg/kg IV q12h for 6–8 weeks) *plus* Gentamicin[d] (1 mg/kg IM or IV q8h for 2 weeks) *plus* Rifampin[i] (300 mg PO q8h for 6–8 weeks)	Use gentamicin during initial 2 weeks; determine gentamicin susceptibility before initiating rifampin (see text)

(continued)

TABLE 25-4

ANTIBIOTIC TREATMENT FOR INFECTIVE ENDOCARDITIS CAUSED BY COMMON ORGANISMS*a* (*CONTINUED*)

ORGANISM	DRUG (DOSE, DURATION)	COMMENTS
HACEK Organisms		
	• Ceftriaxone (2 g/d IV as a single dose for 4 weeks)	Can use another third-generation cephalosporin at comparable dosage
	• Ampicillin/sulbactam (3 g IV q6h for 4 weeks)	—

*a*Doses are for adults with normal renal function. Doses of gentamicin, streptomycin, and vancomycin must be adjusted for reduced renal function. Ideal body weight is used to calculate doses of gentamicin and streptomycin per kilogram (men = 50 kg + 2.3 kg per inch over 5 feet; women = 45.5 kg + 2.3 kg per inch over 5 feet).

*b*MIC, ≤0.1 μg/mL.

*c*Vancomycin dose is based on actual body weight. Adjust for trough level of 10–15 μg/mL for streptococcal and enterococcal infections and 15–20 μg/mL for staphylococcal infections.

*d*Aminoglycosides should not be administered as single daily doses for enterococcal endocarditis and should be introduced as part of the initial treatment. Target peak and trough serum concentrations of divided-dose gentamicin 1 h after a 20- to 30-min infusion or IM injection are ~3.5 μg/mL and ≤1 μg/mL, respectively; target peak and trough serum concentrations of streptomycin (timing as with gentamicin) are 20–35 μg/mL and <10 μg/mL, respectively.

*e*Netilmicin (4 mg/kg qd, as a single dose) can be used in lieu of gentamicin.

*f*MIC, >0.1 μg/mL and <0.5 μg/mL.

*g*MIC, ≥0.5 μg/mL and <8 μg/mL.

*h*Antimicrobial susceptibility must be evaluated; see text.

*i*Rifampin increases warfarin and dicumarol requirements for anticoagulation.

not to produce penicillinase. Similarly, methicillin resistance has become so prevalent among staphylococci that therapy should be initiated with a regimen for methicillin-resistant organisms and subsequently revised if the strain proves to be susceptible to methicillin. The addition of 3–5 days of gentamicin (if the isolate is susceptible) to a β-lactam antibiotic to enhance therapy for native mitral or aortic valve endocarditis has been optional. While the addition of gentamicin minimally hastens eradication of bacteremia, it does not improve survival rates, and even abbreviated gentamicin therapy may be associated with nephrotoxicity and thus is not recommended. Gentamicin generally is not added to the vancomycin regimen in this setting.

For treatment of endocarditis caused by methicillin-resistant *S. aureus* (MRSA), vancomycin dosing to achieve trough concentrations of 15–20 μg/mL is recommended, with the recognition that this regimen may be associated with nephrotoxicity. Although resistance to vancomycin among staphylococci is rare, reduced vancomycin susceptibility among MRSA strains is increasingly encountered. Isolates with a vancomycin MIC of 4–16 μg/mL have intermediate susceptibility and are referred to as vancomycin-intermediate *S. aureus* (VISA). Isolates with an MIC of 2 μg/mL may harbor subpopulations with higher MICs. These isolates, called hetero-resistant VISA (hVISA), are not detectable by routine susceptibility testing. Because of the pharmacokinetics/pharmacodynamics of vancomycin, killing of MRSA with a vancomycin MIC of 2 μg/mL is unpredictable even with aggressive vancomycin dosing. Although not approved by the U.S. Food and Drug Administration (FDA), daptomycin (6 mg/kg [or, as some experts prefer, 8–10 mg/kg] IV once daily) has been recommended as an alternative to vancomycin, particularly for endocarditis caused by VISA, hVISA, and isolates with a vancomycin MIC of 2 μg/mL. These isolates should be tested to document daptomycin susceptibility. Treatment of endocarditis in which bacteremia persists despite this therapy is beyond the scope of this chapter and requires consultation with an infectious disease specialist. The efficacy of linezolid for left-sided MRSA endocarditis has not been established.

Methicillin-susceptible *S. aureus* endocarditis that is uncomplicated and limited to the tricuspid or pulmonic valve—a condition occurring almost exclusively in injection drug users—can often be treated with a 2-week course that combines oxacillin or nafcillin (but not vancomycin) with gentamicin. Patients with prolonged fever (≥5 days) during therapy or multiple septic pulmonary emboli should receive standard therapy. Right-sided endocarditis caused by MRSA is treated for 4 weeks with a standard vancomycin regimen or with daptomycin (6 mg/kg as a single daily dose).

Staphylococcal PVE is treated for 6–8 weeks with a multidrug regimen. Rifampin is an essential component because it kills staphylococci that are adherent to foreign material in a biofilm. Two other agents (selected on the basis of susceptibility testing) are combined with rifampin to prevent in vivo emergence of resistance.

Because many staphylococci (particularly MRSA and *S. epidermidis*) are resistant to gentamicin, susceptibility to gentamicin or an alternative agent should be established before rifampin treatment is begun. If the isolate is resistant to gentamicin, then another aminoglycoside, a fluoroquinolone (chosen on the basis of susceptibility), or another active agent should be substituted for gentamicin.

Other Organisms In the absence of meningitis, endocarditis caused by *S. pneumoniae* with a penicillin MIC of ≤1 μg/mL can be treated with IV penicillin (4 million units every 4 h), ceftriaxone (2 g/d as a single dose), or cefotaxime (at a comparable dosage). Infection caused by pneumococcal strains with a penicillin MIC of ≥2 μg/mL should be treated with vancomycin. Until the strain's susceptibility to penicillin is established, therapy should consist of vancomycin plus ceftriaxone, especially if concurrent meningitis is suspected. *P. aeruginosa* endocarditis is treated with an antipseudomonal penicillin (ticarcillin or piperacillin) and high doses of tobramycin (8 mg/kg per day in three divided doses). Endocarditis caused by Enterobacteriaceae is treated with a potent β-lactam antibiotic plus an aminoglycoside. Corynebacterial endocarditis is treated with penicillin plus an aminoglycoside (if the organism is susceptible to the aminoglycoside) or with vancomycin, which is highly bactericidal for most strains. Therapy for *Candida* endocarditis consists of amphotericin B plus flucytosine and early surgery; long-term (if not indefinite) suppression with an oral azole is advised. Caspofungin treatment of *Candida* endocarditis has been effective in sporadic cases; nevertheless, the role of echinocandins in this setting has not been established.

Empirical Therapy In the design and execution of therapy without culture data (i.e., before culture results are known or when cultures are negative), clinical clues (e.g., site of infection, patient's predispositions), as well as epidemiologic clues to etiology must be considered. Thus, empirical therapy for acute endocarditis in an injection drug user should cover MRSA and gram-negative bacilli. Treatment with vancomycin plus gentamicin, initiated immediately after blood is obtained for cultures, covers these as well as many other potential causes. Similarly, treatment of health care–associated endocarditis must cover MRSA. In the treatment of culture-negative episodes, marantic endocarditis must be excluded and fastidious organisms sought by serologic testing. In the absence of prior antibiotic therapy, it is unlikely that *S. aureus*, CoNS, or enterococcal infection will present with negative blood cultures; thus, in this situation, recommended empirical therapy targets not these organisms but rather nutritionally variant organisms, the HACEK group, and *Bartonella* species. Pending the availability of diagnostic data, blood culture–negative subacute

NVE is treated either with ampicillin-sulbactam (12 g every 24 h) or with ceftriaxone plus gentamicin; doxycycline (100 mg twice daily) is added for *Bartonella* coverage. Vancomycin, gentamicin, cefepime, and rifampin should be used if prosthetic valves in place for ≤1 year are involved. Empirical therapy for infected prosthetic valves in place for >1 year is similar to that for culture-negative PVE. If negative cultures have been confounded by prior antibiotic administration, broader empirical therapy may be indicated, with particular attention to pathogens likely to be inhibited by the specific prior therapy.

Outpatient Antimicrobial Therapy Fully compliant patients who have sterile blood cultures, no fever, and no clinical or echocardiographic findings that suggest an impending complication may complete therapy as outpatients. Careful follow-up and a stable home setting are necessary, as are predictable IV access and use of antimicrobial agents that are stable in solution.

Monitoring Antimicrobial Therapy The serum bactericidal titer—the highest dilution of the patient's serum during therapy that kills 99.9% of the standard inoculum of the infecting organism—is no longer recommended for assessment of standard regimens. However, in the treatment of endocarditis caused by unusual organisms, this measurement may provide a patient-specific assessment of in vivo antibiotic effect. Serum concentrations of aminoglycosides and vancomycin should be monitored.

Antibiotic toxicities, including allergic reactions, occur in 25–40% of patients and commonly arise during the third week of therapy. Blood tests to detect renal, hepatic, and hematologic toxicity should be performed periodically.

Blood cultures should be repeated daily until sterile, rechecked if there is recrudescent fever, and performed again 4–6 weeks after therapy to document cure. Blood cultures become sterile within 2 days after the start of appropriate therapy when infection is caused by viridans streptococci, enterococci, or HACEK organisms. In *S. aureus* endocarditis, β-lactam therapy results in sterile cultures in 3–5 days, whereas with MRSA endocarditis positive cultures may persist for 7–9 days with vancomycin treatment. MRSA bacteremia persisting despite an adequate dosage of vancomycin may indicate infection due to a strain with reduced vancomycin susceptibility and therefore may point to a need for alternative therapy. When fever persists for 7 days despite appropriate antibiotic therapy, patients should be evaluated for paravalvular abscess, extracardiac abscesses (spleen, kidney), or complications (embolic events). Recrudescent fever raises the question of these complications but also of drug reactions or complications of hospitalization. Vegetations become smaller with effective therapy; however, 3 months after cure, 50% are unchanged and 25% are slightly larger.

SURGICAL TREATMENT Intracardiac and central nervous system complications of endocarditis are important causes of morbidity and death. In some cases, effective treatment for these complications requires surgery. The indications for cardiac surgical treatment of endocarditis (Table 25-5) have been derived from observational studies and expert opinion. The strength of individual indications vary; thus, the risks and benefits as well as the timing of surgery must be individualized (Table 25-6). From 25% to 40% of patients with left-sided endocarditis undergo cardiac surgery during active infection, with slightly higher surgery rates with PVE than with NVE. Clinical events resulting from intracardiac complications, which are most reliably detected by TEE, justify most surgery. In the absence of randomized trials to evaluate a survival benefit for surgical intervention, the effect of surgery has been assessed in studies comparing populations of medically and surgically treated patients matched for the necessity of surgery (indication), with adjustments for predictors of death (comorbidity) and time of the surgical intervention. Although study results vary, surgery for currently advised indications appears to convey a significant survival benefit (27–55%) that becomes apparent only with follow-up for ≥6 months after the intervention. During the initial weeks after surgery, mortality risk is actually increased (disease-plus

TABLE 25-5

INDICATIONS FOR CARDIAC SURGICAL INTERVENTION IN PATIENTS WITH ENDOCARDITIS

Surgery required for optimal outcome

Moderate to severe congestive heart failure due to valve dysfunction

Partially dehisced unstable prosthetic valve

Persistent bacteremia despite optimal antimicrobial therapy

Lack of effective microbicidal therapy (e.g., fungal or *Brucella* endocarditis)

S. aureus prosthetic valve endocarditis with an intracardiac complication

Relapse of prosthetic valve endocarditis after optimal antimicrobial therapy

Surgery to be strongly considered for improved outcome[a]

Perivalvular extension of infection

Poorly responsive *S. aureus* endocarditis involving the aortic or mitral valve

Large (>10-mm diameter) hypermobile vegetations with increased risk of embolism

Persistent unexplained fever (≥10 days) in culture-negative native valve endocarditis

Poorly responsive or relapsed endocarditis due to highly antibiotic-resistant enterococci or gram-negative bacilli

[a]Surgery must be carefully considered; findings are often combined with other indications to prompt surgery.

TABLE 25-6

TIMING OF CARDIAC SURGICAL INTERVENTION IN PATIENTS WITH ENDOCARDITIS

	INDICATION FOR SURGICAL INTERVENTION	
	---	---
TIMING	**STRONG SUPPORTING EVIDENCE**	**CONFLICTING EVIDENCE, BUT MAJORITY OF OPINIONS FAVOR SURGERY**
Emergent (same day)	Acute aortic regurgitation plus preclosure of mitral valve Sinus of Valsalva abscess ruptured into right heart Rupture into pericardial sac	
Urgent (within 1–2 days)	Valve obstruction by vegetation Unstable (dehisced) prosthesis Acute aortic or mitral regurgitation with heart failure (New York Heart Association class III or IV) Septal perforation Perivalvular extension of infection with/without new electrocardiographic conduction system changes Lack of effective antibiotic therapy	Major embolus plus persisting large vegetation (>10 mm in diameter)
Elective (earlier usually preferred)	Progressive paravalvular prosthetic regurgitation Valve dysfunction plus persisting infection after ≥7–10 days of antimicrobial therapy Fungal (mold) endocarditis	Staphylococcal PVE Early PVE (≤2 months after valve surgery) Fungal endocarditis (*Candida* spp.) Antibiotic-resistant organisms

Note: PVE, prosthetic valve endocarditis.

Source: Adapted from L Olaison, G Pettersson: Infect Dis Clin North Am 16:453, 2002.

surgery-related mortality). With less demanding surgical indications, this combined mortality risk may erode potential long-term benefits. Benefit is greatest for NVE complicated by heart failure or myocardial abscess and is less clear for PVE; this difference may reflect sample size in the relevant studies.

Congestive Heart Failure Moderate to severe refractory CHF caused by new or worsening valve dysfunction is the major indication for cardiac surgical treatment of endocarditis. At 6 months of follow-up, patients with left-sided endocarditis and moderate to severe heart failure due to valve dysfunction who are treated only medically have a 50% mortality rate; the figure is 15% among matched patients who undergo surgery. The survival benefit with surgery is seen in both NVE and PVE. Surgery can relieve functional stenosis due to large vegetations or restore competence to damaged regurgitant valves by repair or replacement.

Perivalvular Infection This complication, which is most common with aortic valve infection, occurs in 10–15% of native valve and 45–60% of prosthetic valve infections. It is suggested by persistent unexplained fever during appropriate therapy, new electrocardiographic conduction disturbances, and pericarditis. TEE with color Doppler is the test of choice to detect perivalvular abscesses (sensitivity, ≥85%). For optimal outcome, surgery is required, especially when fever persists, fistulae develop, prostheses are dehisced and unstable, and invasive infection relapses after appropriate treatment. Cardiac rhythm must be monitored since high-grade heart block may require insertion of a pacemaker.

Uncontrolled Infection Continued positive blood cultures or otherwise-unexplained persistent fevers (in patients with either blood culture–positive or –negative endocarditis) despite optimal antibiotic therapy may reflect uncontrolled infection and may warrant surgery. Surgical treatment is also advised for endocarditis caused by organisms for which experience indicates that effective antimicrobial therapy is lacking (e.g., yeasts, fungi, *P. aeruginosa*, other highly resistant gram-negative bacilli, *Brucella* species, and probably *C. burnetii*).

S. aureus Endocarditis The mortality rate for *S. aureus* PVE exceeds 50% with medical treatment but is reduced to 25% with surgical treatment. In patients with intracardiac complications associated with *S. aureus* PVE, surgical treatment reduces the mortality rate twentyfold. Surgical treatment should be considered for patients with *S. aureus* native aortic or mitral valve infection who have TTE-demonstrable vegetations and remain septic during the initial week of therapy. Isolated tricuspid valve endocarditis, even with persistent fever, rarely requires surgery.

Prevention of Systemic Emboli Death and persisting morbidity due to emboli are largely limited to patients suffering occlusion of cerebral or coronary arteries. Echocardiographic determination of vegetation size and anatomy, although predictive of patients at high risk of systemic emboli, does not identify those patients in whom the benefits of surgery to prevent emboli clearly exceed the risks of the surgical procedure. Net benefits from surgery to prevent emboli are most likely when other surgical benefits can be achieved simultaneously—e.g., repair of a moderately dysfunctional valve or debridement of a paravalvular abscess. Only 3.5% of patients undergo surgery solely to prevent systemic emboli. Valve repair avoiding insertion of a prosthesis makes the benefit-to-risk ratio of surgery to address vegetations more favorable.

Timing of Cardiac Surgery In general, when indications for surgical treatment of infective endocarditis are identified, surgery should not be delayed simply to permit additional antibiotic therapy, since this course of action increases the risk of death (Table 25-6). After 14 days of recommended antibiotic therapy, excised valves are culture-negative in 99% and 50% of patients with streptococcal and *S. aureus* endocarditis, respectively. Recrudescent endocarditis on a new implanted prosthetic valve follows surgery for active NVE and PVE in 2% and 6–15% of patients, respectively. These frequencies do not justify the risk of adverse outcome with delayed surgery, particularly in patients with severe heart failure, valve dysfunction, and staphylococcal infections. Delay is justified only when infection is controlled and CHF is resolved with medical therapy.

Among patients who have experienced a neurologic complication of endocarditis, further neurologic deterioration can occur as a consequence of cardiac surgery. The risk of neurologic deterioration is related to the type of neurologic complication and the interval between the complication and surgery. Whenever feasible, cardiac surgery should be delayed for 2–3 weeks after a nonhemorrhagic embolic infarction and for 4 weeks after a cerebral hemorrhage. A ruptured mycotic aneurysm should be treated before cardiac surgery.

Antibiotic Therapy after Cardiac Surgery Bacteria visible in Gram-stained preparations of excised valves do not necessarily indicate a failure of antibiotic therapy. Organisms have been detected on Gram's stain—or their DNA has been detected by PCR—in excised valves from 45% of patients who have successfully completed the recommended therapy for endocarditis. In only 7% of these patients are the organisms, most of which are unusual and antibiotic resistant, cultured from the valve. Despite the detection of organisms or their DNA, relapse of endocarditis after surgery is uncommon. Thus, when valve cultures are negative in uncomplicated NVE caused by susceptible organisms, the duration of preoperative plus postoperative treatment should equal the total duration of recommended therapy, with ~2 weeks of treatment administered after surgery. For endocarditis complicated by paravalvular abscess, partially treated PVE, or cases with culture-positive valves, a full course of therapy should be given postoperatively.

Extracardiac Complications Splenic abscess develops in 3–5% of patients with endocarditis. Effective therapy requires either image-guided percutaneous drainage or splenectomy. Mycotic aneurysms occur in 2–15% of endocarditis patients; one-half of these cases involve the cerebral arteries and present as headaches, focal neurologic symptoms, or hemorrhage. Cerebral aneurysms should be monitored by angiography. Some will resolve with effective antimicrobial therapy, but those that persist, enlarge, or leak should be treated surgically if possible. Extracerebral aneurysms present as local pain, a mass, local ischemia, or bleeding; these aneurysms are treated by resection.

OUTCOME

Older age, severe comorbid conditions and diabetes, delayed diagnosis, involvement of prosthetic valves or the aortic valve, an invasive (*S. aureus*) or antibiotic-resistant (*P. aeruginosa*, yeast) pathogen, intracardiac and major neurologic complications, and an association with health care adversely affect outcome. Death and poor outcome often are related not to failure of antibiotic therapy but rather to the interactions of comorbidities and endocarditis-related end-organ complications. Overall survival rates for patients with NVE caused by viridans streptococci, HACEK organisms, or enterococci (susceptible to synergistic therapy) are 85–90%. For *S. aureus* NVE in patients who do not inject drugs, survival rates are 55–70%, whereas 85–90% of injection drug users survive this infection. PVE beginning within 2 months of valve replacement results in mortality rates of 40–50%, whereas rates are only 10–20% in later-onset cases.

PREVENTION

In the past, in an effort to prevent endocarditis (long a goal in clinical practice), expert committees have supported systemic antibiotic administration prior to many bacteremia-inducing procedures. In the absence of human trials, a reappraisal of the indirect evidence for antibiotic prophylaxis for endocarditis by the American Heart Association has culminated in guidelines that reverse prior recommendations and restrict prophylactic antibiotic use. At best, the benefit of antibiotic prophylaxis is minimal. Most endocarditis cases do not follow a procedure. In case-control studies, dental treatments—widely considered as predisposing to endocarditis—occur no more frequently before endocarditis than in matched controls. Furthermore, the frequency and magnitude of bacteremia associated with dental procedures and routine daily activities (e.g., tooth brushing and flossing) are similar. Because dental procedures are infrequent, exposure of cardiac structures to bacteremic oral-cavity organisms is notably greater from routine daily activities than from dental care. The relation of gastrointestinal and genitourinary procedures to subsequent endocarditis is more tenuous than that of dental procedures. In addition, cost-effectiveness and cost-benefit estimates suggest that antibiotic prophylaxis represents a poor use of resources.

Studies in animal models suggest that antibiotic prophylaxis may be effective. Thus it is possible that rare cases of endocarditis are prevented. Weighing the potential benefits, potential adverse events, and costs associated with antibiotic prophylaxis, the American Heart Association and the European Society of Cardiology now recommend prophylactic antibiotics (**Table 25-7**) only for those patients at highest risk for severe morbidity or death from endocarditis (**Table 25-8**). Maintaining good dental hygiene is essential. Prophylaxis is recommended only when there is manipulation of gingival tissue or the periapical region of the teeth or perforation of the oral mucosa (including surgery on the respiratory tract). Prophylaxis is not advised for patients undergoing

TABLE 25-7

ANTIBIOTIC REGIMENS FOR PROPHYLAXIS OF ENDOCARDITIS IN ADULTS WITH HIGH-RISK CARDIAC LESIONS[a,b]

A. Standard oral regimen
   1. Amoxicillin: 2 g PO 1 h before procedure
B. Inability to take oral medication
   1. Ampicillin: 2 g IV or IM within 1 h before procedure
C. Penicillin allergy
   1. Clarithromycin or azithromycin: 500 mg PO 1 h before procedure
   2. Cephalexin[c]: 2 g PO 1 h before procedure
   3. Clindamycin: 600 mg PO 1 h before procedure
D. Penicillin allergy, inability to take oral medication
   1. Cefazolin[c] or ceftriaxone[c]: 1 g IV or IM 30 min before procedure
   2. Clindamycin: 600 mg IV or IM 1 h before procedure

[a]Dosing for children: for amoxicillin, ampicillin, cephalexin, or cefadroxil, use 50 mg/kg PO; cefazolin, 25 mg/kg IV; clindamycin, 20 mg/kg PO, 25 mg/kg IV; clarithromycin, 15 mg/kg PO; and vancomycin, 20 mg/kg IV.
[b]For high-risk lesions, see Table 25-8. Prophylaxis is not advised for other lesions.
[c]Do not use cephalosporins in patients with immediate hypersensitivity (urticaria, angioedema, anaphylaxis) to penicillin.
Source: W Wilson et al: Circulation 116:1736, 2007.

TABLE 25-8

HIGH-RISK CARDIAC LESIONS FOR WHICH ENDOCARDITIS PROPHYLAXIS IS ADVISED BEFORE DENTAL PROCEDURES

Prosthetic heart valves

Prior endocarditis

Unrepaired cyanotic congenital heart disease, including palliative shunts or conduits

Completely repaired congenital heart defects during the 6 months after repair

Incompletely repaired congenital heart disease with residual defects adjacent to prosthetic material

Valvulopathy developing after cardiac transplantation

Source: W Wilson et al: Circulation 116:1736, 2007.

gastrointestinal or genitourinary tract procedures. High-risk patients should be treated before or when they undergo procedures on an infected genitourinary tract or on infected skin and soft tissue. The British Society for Antimicrobial Chemotherapy continues to recommend prophylaxis for at-risk patients undergoing selected gastrointestinal and genitourinary procedures. In contrast, the National Institute for Health and Clinical Excellence in the United Kingdom found no convincing evidence that antibiotic prophylaxis was cost-effective and advised discontinuation of the practice (see *www.nice.org.uk/guidance/CG64*).

CHAPTER 26

ACUTE RHEUMATIC FEVER

Jonathan R. Carapetis

Acute rheumatic fever (ARF) is a multisystem disease resulting from an autoimmune reaction to infection with group A streptococcus. Although many parts of the body may be affected, almost all of the manifestations resolve completely. The exception is cardiac valvular damage (rheumatic heart disease [RHD]), which may persist after the other features have disappeared.

GLOBAL CONSIDERATIONS

ARF and RHD are diseases of poverty. They were common in all countries until the early twentieth century, when their incidence began to decline in industrialized nations. This decline was largely attributable to improved living conditions—particularly less crowded housing and better hygiene—which resulted in reduced transmission of group A streptococci. The introduction of antibiotics and improved systems of medical care had a supplemental effect. Recurrent outbreaks of ARF began in the 1980s in the Rocky Mountain states of the United States, where elevated rates persist.

The virtual disappearance of ARF and reduction in the incidence of RHD in industrialized countries during the twentieth century unfortunately was not replicated in developing countries, where these diseases continue unabated. RHD is the most common cause of heart disease in children in developing countries and is a major cause of mortality and morbidity in adults as well. It has been estimated that between 15 and 19 million people worldwide are affected by RHD, with approximately one-quarter of a million deaths occurring each year. Some 95% of ARF cases and RHD deaths now occur in developing countries.

Although ARF and RHD are relatively common in all developing countries, they occur at particularly elevated rates in certain regions. These "hot spots" are sub-Saharan Africa, Pacific nations, Australasia, and the Indian subcontinent (Fig. 26-1). Unfortunately, most developing countries do not currently have coordinated, register-based RHD control programs, which are proven to be cost-effective in reducing the burden of RHD. Enhancing awareness of RHD and mobilizing resources for its control in developing countries is an issue requiring international attention.

EPIDEMIOLOGY

ARF is mainly a disease of children aged 5–14 years. Initial episodes become less common in older adolescents and young adults and are rare in persons aged >30 years. By contrast, recurrent episodes of ARF remain relatively common in adolescents and young adults. This pattern contrasts with the prevalence of RHD, which peaks between 25 and 40 years. There is no clear gender association for ARF, but RHD more commonly affects females, sometimes up to twice as frequently as males.

PATHOGENESIS

ORGANISM FACTORS

Based on currently available evidence, ARF is exclusively caused by infection of the upper respiratory tract with group A streptococci. Although classically, certain M-serotypes (particularly types 1, 3, 5, 6, 14, 18, 19, 24, 27, and 29) were associated with ARF, in high-incidence regions, it is now thought that any strain of group A streptococcus has the potential to cause ARF. Potential role of skin infection and of groups C and G streptococci are currently being investigated.

HOST FACTORS

Approximately 3–6% of any population may be susceptible to ARF, and this proportion does not vary dramatically between populations. Findings of familial

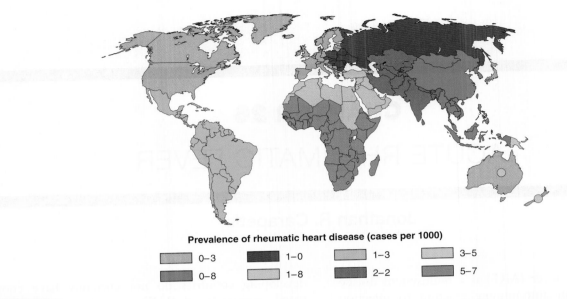

Prevalence of rheumatic heart disease (cases per 1000)

0–3	1–0	1–3	3–5
0–8	1–8	2–2	5–7

FIGURE 26-1

Prevalence of rheumatic heart disease in children aged 5–14 years. Circles within Australia and New Zealand represent indigenous populations, and also Pacific Islanders in New Zealand. (*From JR Carapetis et al: Lancet Infect Dis. Copyright 2005; with permission from Elsevier.*)

clustering of cases and concordance in monozygotic twins—particularly for chorea—confirm that susceptibility to ARF is an inherited characteristic. Particular human leukocyte antigen (HLA) class II alleles appear to be strongly associated with susceptibility. Associations have also been described with high levels of circulating mannose-binding lectin and polymorphisms of transforming growth factor β_1 gene and immunoglobulin genes. High-level expression of a particular alloantigen present on B cells, D8-17, has been found in patients with a history of ARF in many populations, with intermediate-level expression in first-degree family members, suggesting that this may be a marker of inherited susceptibility.

THE IMMUNE RESPONSE

When a susceptible host encounters a group A streptococcus, an autoimmune reaction results, which leads to damage to human tissues as a result of cross-reactivity between epitopes on the organism and the host (Fig. 26-2). Cross-reactive epitopes are present in the streptococcal M protein and the *N*-acetylglucosamine of group A streptococcal carbohydrate and are immunologically similar to molecules in human myosin, tropomyosin, keratin, actin, laminin, vimentin, and *N*-acetylglucosamine. It is currently thought that the initial damage is due to cross-reactive antibodies attaching at the cardiac valve endothelium, allowing the entry of primed CD4+ T cells, leading to subsequent T cell–mediated inflammation.

CLINICAL FEATURES

There is a latent period of ~3 weeks (1–5 weeks) between the precipitating group A streptococcal infection and the appearance of the clinical features of ARF. The exceptions are chorea and indolent carditis, which may follow prolonged latent periods lasting up to 6 months. Although many patients report a prior sore throat, the preceding group A streptococcal infection is commonly subclinical; in these cases it can only be confirmed using streptococcal antibody testing. The most common clinical presentation of ARF is polyarthritis and fever. Polyarthritis is present in 60–75% of cases and carditis in 50–60%. The prevalence of chorea in ARF varies substantially between populations, ranging from <2% to 30%. Erythema marginatum and subcutaneous nodules are now rare, being found in <5% of cases.

HEART INVOLVEMENT

Up to 60% of patients with ARF progress to RHD. The endocardium, pericardium, or myocardium may be affected. Valvular damage is the hallmark of rheumatic carditis. The mitral valve is almost always affected, sometimes together with the aortic valve; isolated aortic valve involvement is rare. Early valvular damage leads to regurgitation. Over ensuing years, usually as a result of recurrent episodes, leaflet thickening, scarring, calcification, and valvular stenosis may develop (Fig. 26-3). Videos 26-1 and 26-2 can be accessed at the following link: http://www.mhprofessional.com/mediacenter/.

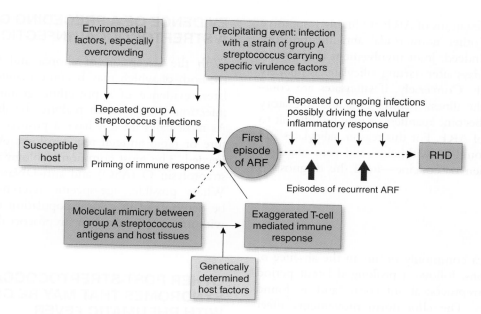

FIGURE 26-2

Pathogenetic pathway for acute rheumatic fever and rheumatic heart disease. (*From JR Carapetis et al: Lancet 366:155, 2005. Copyright 2005; with permission from Elsevier.*)

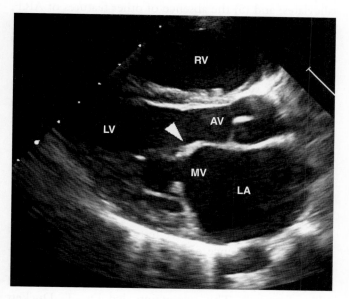

FIGURE 26-3

Transthoracic echocardiographic image from a 5-year-old boy with chronic rheumatic heart disease. This diastolic image demonstrates leaflet thickening, restriction of the anterior mitral valve leaflet tip, and doming of the body of the leaflet toward the interventricular septum. This appearance (marked by the arrowhead) is commonly described as a "hockey stick" or an "elbow" deformity. AV, aortic valve; LA, left atrium; LV, left ventricle; MV, mitral valve; RV, right ventricle. (*Courtesy of Dr. Bo Remenyi, Department of Paediatric and Congential Cardiac Services, Starship Children's Hospital, Auckland, New Zealand.*)

Therefore the characteristic manifestation of carditis in previously unaffected individuals is mitral regurgitation, sometimes accompanied by aortic regurgitation. Myocardial inflammation may affect electrical conduction pathways, leading to P-R interval prolongation (first-degree AV block or rarely higher-level block) and softening of the first heart sound.

JOINT INVOLVEMENT

To qualify as a major manifestation, joint involvement in ARF must be arthritic, i.e., objective evidence of inflammation, with hot, swollen, red and/or tender joints, and involvement of more than one joint (i.e., polyarthritis). The typical arthritis is migratory, moving from one joint to another over a period of hours. ARF almost always affects the large joints—most commonly the knees, ankles, hips, and elbows—and is asymmetric. The pain is severe and usually disabling until anti-inflammatory medication is commenced.

Less severe joint involvement is also relatively common but qualifies only as a minor manifestation. Arthralgia without objective joint inflammation usually affects large joints in the same migratory pattern as polyarthritis. In some populations, aseptic monoarthritis may be a presenting feature of ARF. This may occur because of early commencement of anti-inflammatory medication before the typical migratory pattern is established.

The joint manifestations of ARF are highly responsive to salicylates and other nonsteroidal anti-inflammatory drugs (NSAIDs). Indeed, joint involvement that persists more than 1 or 2 days after starting salicylates is unlikely to be due to ARF. Conversely, if salicylates are commenced early in the illness, before fever and migratory polyarthritis have become manifest, it may be difficult to make a diagnosis of ARF. For this reason, salicylates and other NSAIDs should be withheld—and pain managed with acetaminophen or codeine—until the diagnosis is confirmed.

CHOREA

Sydenham's chorea commonly occurs in the absence of other manifestations, follows a prolonged latent period after group A streptococcal infection, and is found mainly in females. The choreiform movements affect particularly the head (causing characteristic darting movements of the tongue) and the upper limbs. They may be generalized or restricted to one side of the body (hemi-chorea). The chorea varies in severity. In mild cases it may be evident only on careful examination, while in the most severe cases the affected individuals are unable to perform activities of daily living and are at risk of injuring themselves. Chorea eventually resolves completely, usually within 6 weeks.

SKIN MANIFESTATIONS

The classic rash of ARF is *erythema marginatum*, which begins as pink macules that clear centrally, leaving a serpiginous, spreading edge. The rash is evanescent, appearing and disappearing before the examiner's eyes. It occurs usually on the trunk, sometimes on the limbs, but almost never on the face.

Subcutaneous nodules occur as painless, small (0.5–2 cm), mobile lumps beneath the skin overlying bony prominences, particularly of the hands, feet, elbows, occiput, and occasionally the vertebrae. They are a delayed manifestation, appearing 2–3 weeks after the onset of disease, last for just a few days up to 3 weeks, and are commonly associated with carditis.

OTHER FEATURES

Fever occurs in most cases of ARF, although rarely in cases of pure chorea. Although high-grade fever (≥39°C) is the rule, lower-grade temperature elevations are not uncommon. Elevated acute-phase reactants are also present in most cases. C-reactive protein (CRP) and erythrocyte sedimentation rate (ESR) are often dramatically elevated. Occasionally, the peripheral leukocyte count is mildly elevated.

EVIDENCE OF A PRECEDING GROUP A STREPTOCOCCAL INFECTION

With the exception of chorea and low-grade carditis, both of which may become manifest many months later, evidence of a preceding group A streptococcal infection is essential in making the diagnosis of ARF. As most cases do not have a positive throat swab culture or rapid antigen test, serologic evidence is usually needed. The most common serologic tests are the anti-streptolysin O (ASO) and anti-DNase B (ADB) titers. Where possible, age-specific reference ranges should be determined in a local population of healthy people without a recent group A streptococcal infection.

OTHER POST-STREPTOCOCCAL SYNDROMES THAT MAY BE CONFUSED WITH RHEUMATIC FEVER

Post-streptococcal reactive arthritis (PSRA) is differentiated from ARF on the basis of: (1) small-joint involvement that is often symmetric; (2) a short latent period following streptococcal infection (usually <1 week); (3) occasional causation by nongroup A β-hemolytic streptococcal infection; (4) slower responsiveness to salicylates; and (5) the absence of other features of ARF, particularly carditis.

Pediatric autoimmune neuropsychiatric disorders associated with streptococcal infection (PANDAS) is a term that links a range of tic disorders and obsessive-compulsive symptoms with group A streptococcal infections. People with PANDAS are said not to be at risk of carditis, unlike patients with Sydenham's chorea. The diagnoses of PANDAS and PSRA should rarely be made in populations with a high incidence of ARF.

CONFIRMING THE DIAGNOSIS

Because there is no definitive test, the diagnosis of ARF relies on the presence of a combination of typical clinical features together with evidence of the precipitating group A streptococcal infection, and the exclusion of other diagnoses. This uncertainty led Dr. T. Duckett Jones in 1944 to develop a set of criteria (subsequently known as the *Jones criteria*) to aid in the diagnosis. An expert panel convened by the World Health Organization (WHO) clarified the use of the Jones criteria in ARF recurrences (Table 26-1). Because each revision of the Jones criteria since 1944 has reduced sensitivity and increased specificity, in response to the decline in incidence of ARF in high-income countries, there is now concern that they may be too insensitive for countries where ARF incidence remains high. As a result, some countries (e.g., Australia and New Zealand) have

TABLE 26-1

2002–2003 WORLD HEALTH ORGANIZATION CRITERIA FOR THE DIAGNOSIS OF RHEUMATIC FEVER AND RHEUMATIC HEART DISEASE (BASED ON THE 1992 REVISED JONES CRITERIA)

DIAGNOSTIC CATEGORIES	CRITERIA
Primary episode of rheumatic fever[a]	Two major or one major and two minor manifestations plus evidence of preceding group A streptococcal infection
Recurrent attack of rheumatic fever in a patient without established rheumatic heart disease	Two major or one major and two minor manifestations plus evidence of preceding group A streptococcal infection
Recurrent attack of rheumatic fever in a patient with established rheumatic heart disease[b]	Two minor manifestations plus evidence of preceding group A streptococcal infection[c]
Rheumatic chorea Insidious onset rheumatic carditis[b]	Other major manifestations or evidence of group A streptococcal infection not required
Chronic valve lesions of rheumatic heart disease (patients presenting for the first time with pure mitral stenosis or mixed mitral valve disease and/or aortic valve disease)[d]	Do not require any other criteria to be diagnosed as having rheumatic heart disease
Major manifestations	Carditis Polyarthritis Chorea Erythema marginatum Subcutaneous nodules
Minor manifestations	Clinical: fever, polyarthralgia Laboratory: elevated erythrocyte sedimentation rate or leukocyte count[e] Electrocardiogram: prolonged P-R interval
Supporting evidence of a preceding streptococcal infection within the last 45 days	Elevated or rising anti-streptolysin O or other streptococcal antibody, or A positive throat culture, or Rapid antigen test for group A streptococcus, or Recent scarlet fever[e]

[a]Patients may present with polyarthritis (or with only polyarthralgia or monoarthritis) and with several (three or more) other minor manifestations, together with evidence of recent group A streptococcal infection. Some of these cases may later turn out to be rheumatic fever. It is prudent to consider them as cases of "probable rheumatic fever" (once other diagnoses are excluded) and advise regular secondary prophylaxis. Such patients require close follow-up and regular examination of the heart. This cautious approach is particularly suitable for patients in vulnerable age groups in high incidence settings.
[b]Infective endocarditis should be excluded.
[c]Some patients with recurrent attacks may not fulfill these criteria.
[d]Congenital heart disease should be excluded.
[e]1992 Revised Jones criteria do not include elevated leukocyte count as a laboratory minor manifestation (but do include elevated C-reactive protein), and do not include recent scarlet fever as supporting evidence of a recent streptococcal infection.
Source: Reprinted with permission from WHO Expert Consultation on Rheumatic Fever and Rheumatic Heart Disease (2001: Geneva, Switzerland): *Rheumatic Fever and Rheumatic Heart Disease: Report of a WHO Expert Consultation* (WHO Tech Rep Ser, 923). Geneva, World Health Organization, 2004.

developed their own, more sensitive, diagnostic criteria for ARF in their populations (links available at the *RHDnet* website *www.worldheart.org/rhd*).

TREATMENT ▶ **Acute Rheumatic Fever**

Patients with possible ARF should be followed closely to ensure that the diagnosis is confirmed, treatment of heart failure and other symptoms is undertaken, and preventive measures including commencement of secondary prophylaxis, inclusion on an ARF registry, and health education are commenced. Echocardiography should be performed on all possible cases to aid in making the diagnosis and to determine the severity at baseline of any carditis. Other tests that should be performed are listed in **Table 26-2**.

There is no treatment for ARF that has been proven to alter the likelihood of developing, or the severity of, RHD. With the exception of treatment of heart failure, which may be lifesaving in cases of severe carditis, the treatment of ARF is symptomatic.

ANTIBIOTICS All patients with ARF should receive antibiotics sufficient to treat the precipitating group A streptococcal infection. Penicillin is the drug of choice

TABLE 26-2

RECOMMENDED TESTS IN CASES OF POSSIBLE ACUTE RHEUMATIC FEVER

Recommended for all cases

  White blood cell count

  Erythrocyte sedimentation rate

  C-reactive protein

  Blood cultures if febrile

  Electrocardiogram (repeat in 2 weeks and 2 months if prolonged P-R interval or other rhythm abnormality)

  Chest x-ray if clinical or echocardiographic evidence of carditis

  Echocardiogram (consider repeating after 1 month if negative)

  Throat swab (preferably before giving antibiotics)—culture for group A streptococcus

  Anti-streptococcal serology: both anti-streptolysin O and anti-DNase B titres, if available (repeat 10–14 days later if 1st test not confirmatory)

Tests for alternative diagnoses, depending on clinical features

  Repeated blood cultures if possible endocarditis

  Joint aspirate (microscopy and culture) for possible septic arthritis

  Copper, ceruloplasmin, anti-nuclear antibody, drug screen for choreiform movements

  Serology and auto-immune markers for arboviral, auto-immune or reactive arthritis

Source: Reprinted with permission from National Heart Foundation of Australia: *Diagnosis and Management of Acute Rheumatic Fever and Rheumatic Heart Disease in Australia: Complete Evidence-Based Review and Guideline.* Melbourne, National Heart Foundation of Australia, 2009.

and can be given orally (as phenoxymethyl penicillin, 500 mg [250 mg for children ≤27 kg] PO twice daily, or amoxicillin 50 mg/kg [max 1 g] daily, for 10 days] or as a single dose of 1.2 million units (600,000 units for children ≤27 kg) IM benzathine penicillin G.

SALICYLATES AND NSAIDS These may be used for the treatment of arthritis, arthralgia, and fever, once the diagnosis is confirmed. They are of no proven value in the treatment of carditis or chorea. Aspirin is the drug of choice. An initial dose of 80–100 mg/kg per day in children (4–8 g/d in adults) in 4–5 divided doses is often needed for the first few days up to 2 weeks. A lower dose should be used if symptoms of salicylate toxicity emerge, such as nausea, vomiting, or tinnitus. When the acute symptoms are substantially resolved, the dose can be reduced to 60–70 mg/kg per day for a further 2–4 weeks. Fever, joint manifestations, and elevated acute-phase reactants sometimes recur up to 3 weeks after the medication is discontinued. This does not indicate a recurrence and can be managed by recommencing salicylates for a brief period. Although less well studied, naproxen at a dose of 10–20 mg/kg per day has been reported to lead to good symptomatic response.

CONGESTIVE HEART FAILURE Glucocorticoids The use of glucocorticoids in ARF remains controversial. Two meta-analyses have failed to demonstrate a benefit of glucocorticoids compared to placebo or salicylates in improving the short- or longer-term outcome of carditis. However, the studies included in these meta-analyses all took place >40 years ago and did not use medications in common usage today. Many clinicians treat cases of severe carditis (causing heart failure) with glucocorticoids in the belief that they may reduce the acute inflammation and result in more rapid resolution of failure. However, the potential benefits of this treatment should be balanced against the possible adverse effects, including gastrointestinal bleeding and fluid retention. If used, prednisone or prednisolone are recommended at doses of 1–2 mg/kg per day (maximum, 80 mg). Glucocorticoids are often only required for a few days or up to a maximum of 3 weeks.

MANAGEMENT OF HEART FAILURE See Chap. 17.

BED REST Traditional recommendations for long-term bed rest, once the cornerstone of management, are no longer widely practiced. Instead, bed rest should be prescribed as needed while arthritis and arthralgia are present, and for patients with heart failure. Once symptoms are well controlled, gradual mobilization can commence as tolerated.

CHOREA Medications to control the abnormal movements do not alter the duration or outcome of chorea. Milder cases can usually be managed by providing a calm environment. In patients with severe chorea, carbamazepine or sodium valproate are preferred to haloperidol. A response may not be seen for 1–2 weeks, and a successful response may only be to reduce rather than resolve the abnormal movements. Medication should be continued for 1–2 weeks after symptoms subside.

INTRAVENOUS IMMUNOGLOBULIN (IVIg) Small studies have suggested that IVIg may lead to more rapid resolution of chorea but has shown no benefit on the short- or long-term outcome of carditis in ARF without chorea. In the absence of better data, IVIg is *not* recommended except in cases of severe chorea refractory to other treatments.

PROGNOSIS

Untreated, ARF lasts on average 12 weeks. With treatment, patients are usually discharged from hospital within 1–2 weeks. Inflammatory markers should be monitored every 1–2 weeks until they have normalized (usually within 4–6 weeks), and an echocardiogram should be performed after 1 month to determine if there has been progression of carditis. Cases with more severe carditis need close clinical and echocardiographic monitoring in the longer term.

Once the acute episode has resolved, the priority in management is to ensure long-term clinical follow-up and adherence to a regimen of secondary prophylaxis. Patients should be entered onto the local ARF registry (if present) and contact made with primary care practitioners to ensure a plan for follow-up and administration of secondary prophylaxis before the patient is discharged. Patients and their families should also be educated about their disease, emphasizing the importance of adherence to secondary prophylaxis. If carditis is present, they should also be informed of the need for antibiotic prophylaxis against endocarditis for dental and surgical procedures.

PREVENTION

PRIMARY PREVENTION

Ideally, primary prevention would entail elimination of the major risk factors for streptococcal infection, particularly overcrowded housing. This is difficult to achieve in most places where ARF is common.

Therefore, the mainstay of primary prevention for ARF remains primary prophylaxis (i.e., the timely and complete treatment of group A streptococcal sore throat with antibiotics). If commenced within 9 days of sore throat onset, a course of penicillin (as outlined earlier for treatment of ARF) will prevent almost all cases of ARF that would otherwise have developed. This important strategy relies on individuals presenting for medical care when they have a sore throat, the availability of trained health and microbiology staff along with the materials and infrastructure to take throat swabs, and a reliable supply of penicillin. Unfortunately, many of these elements are not available in developing countries.

SECONDARY PREVENTION

The mainstay of controlling ARF and RHD is secondary prevention. Because patients with ARF are at dramatically higher risk than the general population of developing a further episode of ARF after a group A streptococcal infection, they should receive long-term penicillin prophylaxis to prevent recurrences. The best

TABLE 26-3

AMERICAN HEART ASSOCIATION RECOMMENDATIONS FOR DURATION OF SECONDARY PROPHYLAXIS[a]

CATEGORY OF PATIENT	DURATION OF PROPHYLAXIS
Rheumatic fever without carditis	For 5 years after the last attack or 21 years of age (whichever is longer)
Rheumatic fever with carditis but no residual valvular disease	For 10 years after the last attack, or 21 years of age (whichever is longer)
Rheumatic fever with persistent valvular disease, evident clinically or on echocardiography	For 10 years after the last attack, or 40 years of age (whichever is longer). Sometimes lifelong prophylaxis.

[a]These are only recommendations and must be modified by individual circumstances as warranted. Note that other organizations have slightly different recommendations (see www.worldheart.org/rhd for links).

Source: Adapted from AHA Scientific Statement Prevention of Rheumatic Fever and Diagnosis and Treatment of Acute Streptococcal Pharyngitis. Circulation 119:1541, 2009.

antibiotic for secondary prophylaxis is benzathine penicillin G (1.2 million units, or 600,000 units if ≤27 kg) delivered every 4 weeks. It can be given every 3 weeks, or even every 2 weeks, to persons considered to be at particularly high risk, although in settings where good compliance with 4-weekly dosing can be achieved, more frequent dosing is rarely needed. Oral penicillin V (250 mg) can be given twice daily instead but is somewhat less effective than benzathine penicillin G. Penicillin-allergic patients can receive erythromycin (250 mg) twice daily.

The duration of secondary prophylaxis is determined by many factors, in particular the duration since the last episode of ARF (recurrences become less likely with increasing time), age (recurrences are less likely with increasing age), and the severity of RHD (if severe, it may be prudent to avoid even a very small risk of recurrence because of the potentially serious consequences) (Table 26-3). Secondary prophylaxis is best delivered as part of a coordinated RHD control program, based around a registry of patients. Registries improve the ability to follow patients and identify those who default from prophylaxis and institute strategies to improve adherence.

CHAPTER 26 Acute Rheumatic Fever

CHAPTER 27

CHAGAS' DISEASE

Louis V. Kirchhoff ■ Anis Rassi, Jr.

Although the genus *Trypanosoma* contains many species of protozoans, only *T. cruzi*, *T. brucei gambiense*, and *T. brucei rhodesiense* cause disease in humans. *T. cruzi* is the etiologic agent of Chagas' disease in the Americas; *T. b. gambiense* and *T. b. rhodesiense* cause African trypanosomiasis.

CHAGAS' DISEASE

DEFINITION

Chagas' disease, or American trypanosomiasis, is a zoonosis caused by the protozoan parasite *T. cruzi*. Acute Chagas' disease is usually a mild febrile illness that results from initial infection with the organism. After spontaneous resolution of the acute illness, most infected persons remain for life in the indeterminate phase of chronic Chagas' disease, which is characterized by subpatent parasitemia, easily detectable antibodies to *T. cruzi*, and an absence of associated signs and symptoms. In 10–30% of chronically infected patients, cardiac and/or gastrointestinal lesions develop that can result in serious morbidity and even death.

LIFE CYCLE AND TRANSMISSION

T. cruzi is transmitted among its mammalian hosts by hematophagous triatomine insects, often called reduviid bugs. The insects become infected by sucking blood from animals or humans who have circulating parasites. Ingested organisms multiply in the gut of the triatomines, and infective forms are discharged with the feces at the time of subsequent blood meals. Transmission to a second vertebrate host occurs when breaks in the skin, mucous membranes, or conjunctivae become contaminated with bug feces that contain infective parasites. *T. cruzi* can also be transmitted by the transfusion of blood donated by infected persons, by organ transplantation, from mother to unborn child, by ingestion of contaminated food or drink, and in laboratory accidents.

PATHOLOGY

Initial infection at the site of parasite entry is characterized by local histologic changes that include the presence of parasites within leukocytes and cells of subcutaneous tissues and the development of interstitial edema, lymphocytic infiltration, and reactive hyperplasia of adjacent lymph nodes. After dissemination of the organisms through the lymphatics and the bloodstream, primarily muscles (including the myocardium) **(Fig. 27-1)** and ganglion cells may become heavily parasitized. The characteristic pseudocysts present in sections of infected tissues are intracellular aggregates of multiplying parasites.

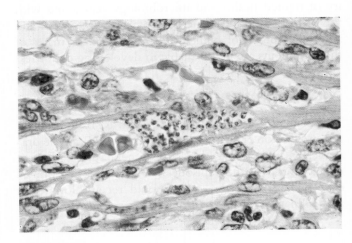

FIGURE 27-1

***Trypanosoma cruzi* in the heart muscle of a child who died of acute Chagas' myocarditis.** An infected myocyte containing several dozen *T. cruzi* amastigotes is in the center of the field (hematoxylin and eosin, 900×).

In individuals with chronic *T. cruzi* infections who develop related clinical manifestations, the heart is the organ most commonly affected. Changes include thinning of the ventricular walls, biventricular enlargement, apical aneurysms, and mural thrombi. Widespread lymphocytic infiltration, diffuse interstitial fibrosis, and atrophy of myocardial cells are often apparent, but parasites are difficult to find in myocardial tissue by conventional histologic methods. Conduction-system abnormalities often affect the right branch and the left anterior branch of the bundle of His. In chronic Chagas' disease of the gastrointestinal tract (megadisease), the esophagus and colon may exhibit varying degrees of dilatation. On microscopic examination, focal inflammatory lesions with lymphocytic infiltration are seen, and the number of neurons in the myenteric plexus may be markedly reduced. Accumulating evidence implicates the persistence of parasites and the accompanying chronic inflammation—rather than autoimmune mechanisms—as the basis for the pathology in patients with chronic *T. cruzi* infection.

EPIDEMIOLOGY

T. cruzi is found only in the Americas. Wild and domestic mammals harboring *T. cruzi* and infected triatomines are found in spotty distributions from the southern United States to southern Argentina. Humans become involved in the cycle of transmission when infected vectors take up residence in the primitive wood, adobe, and stone houses common in much of Latin America. Thus, human *T. cruzi* infection is a health problem primarily among the poor in rural areas of Mexico and Central and South America. Most new *T. cruzi* infections in rural settings occur in children, but the incidence is unknown because most cases go undiagnosed. Historically, transfusion-associated transmission of *T. cruzi* was a serious public health problem in many endemic countries. However, with some notable exceptions, transmission by this route has been essentially eliminated as effective programs for the screening of donated blood have been implemented. Several dozen patients with HIV and chronic *T. cruzi* infections who underwent acute recrudescence of the latter have been described. These patients generally presented with *T. cruzi* brain abscesses, a manifestation of the illness that does not occur in immunocompetent persons. Currently, it is estimated that 8 million people are chronically infected with *T. cruzi* and that 14,000 deaths due to the illness occur each year. The resulting morbidity and mortality make Chagas' disease the most important parasitic disease burden in Latin America.

In recent years, the rate of *T. cruzi* transmission has decreased markedly in several endemic countries as a result of successful programs involving vector control, blood-bank screening, and education of at-risk populations. A major program, which began in 1991 in the "southern cone" nations of South America (Uruguay, Paraguay, Bolivia, Brazil, Chile, and Argentina), has provided the framework for much of this progress. Uruguay and Chile were certified free of transmission by the main domiciliary vector species (*Triatoma infestans*) in the late 1990s, and Brazil was declared transmission-free in 2006. Transmission has been reduced markedly in Argentina as well. Similar control programs have been initiated in the countries of northern South America and in the Central American nations.

Acute Chagas' disease is rare in the United States. Five cases of autochthonous transmission and five instances of transmission by blood transfusion have been reported. Moreover, *T. cruzi* was transmitted to five recipients of organs from three *T. cruzi*–infected donors. Two of these recipients became infected through cardiac transplants. Acute Chagas' disease has not been reported in tourists returning to the United States from Latin America, although three such instances have been reported in Europe. In contrast, the prevalence of chronic *T. cruzi* infections in the United States has increased considerably in recent years. An estimated 23 million immigrants from Chagas'-endemic countries currently live in the United States, ~17 million of whom are Mexicans. The total number of *T. cruzi*–infected persons living in the United States is estimated to be 300,000. Screening of the U.S. blood supply for *T. cruzi* infection began in January 2007. The overall prevalence of *T. cruzi* infection among donors is about 1 in 29,000, and to date more than 1200 infected donors have been identified and deferred permanently (see "Diagnosis," later in this chapter).

CLINICAL COURSE

The first signs of acute Chagas' disease develop at least 1 week after invasion by the parasites. When the organisms enter through a break in the skin, an indurated area of erythema and swelling (the chagoma), accompanied by local lymphadenopathy, may appear. *Romaña's sign*—the classic finding in acute Chagas' disease, which consists of unilateral painless edema of the palpebrae and periocular tissues—can result when the conjunctiva is the portal of entry. These initial local signs may be followed by malaise, fever, anorexia, and edema of the face and lower extremities. Generalized lymphadenopathy and hepatosplenomegaly may develop. Severe myocarditis develops rarely; most deaths in acute Chagas' disease are due to heart failure. Neurologic signs are not common, but meningoencephalitis occurs occasionally, especially in children <2 years old. Usually within 4–8 weeks, acute signs and symptoms resolve spontaneously in virtually all patients, who then enter the asymptomatic or indeterminate phase of chronic *T. cruzi* infection.

Symptomatic chronic Chagas' disease becomes apparent years or even decades after the initial infection. The heart is commonly involved, and symptoms are caused by rhythm disturbances, segmental or dilated cardiomyopathy, and thromboembolism. Right bundle-branch block is a common electrocardiographic abnormality, but other types of intraventricular and atrioventricular blocks, premature ventricular contractions, and tachy- and bradyarrhythmias occur frequently. Cardiomyopathy often results in biventricular heart failure with a predominance of right-sided failure at advanced stages. Embolization of mural thrombi to the brain or other areas may take place. Sudden death is the main cause of death in Chagas' heart disease. Patients with megaesophagus suffer from dysphagia, odynophagia, chest pain, and regurgitation. Aspiration can occur (especially during sleep) in patients with severe esophageal dysfunction, and repeated episodes of aspiration pneumonitis are common. Weight loss, cachexia, and pulmonary infection can result in death. Patients with megacolon are plagued by abdominal pain and chronic constipation, which predisposes to fecaloma formation. Advanced megacolon can cause obstruction, volvulus, septicemia, and death.

DIAGNOSIS

The diagnosis of acute Chagas' disease requires the detection of parasites. Microscopic examination of fresh anticoagulated blood or the buffy coat is the simplest way to see the motile organisms. Parasites also can be seen in Giemsa-stained thin and thick blood smears. Microhematocrit tubes containing acridine orange as a stain can be used for the same purpose. When used by experienced personnel, all of these methods yield positive results in a high proportion of cases of acute Chagas' disease. Serologic testing plays no role in diagnosing acute Chagas' disease.

Chronic Chagas' disease is diagnosed by the detection of specific IgG antibodies that bind to *T. cruzi* antigens. Demonstration of the parasite is not of primary importance. In Latin America, ~30 assays are commercially available, including several based on recombinant antigens. Although these tests usually show good sensitivity and reasonable specificity, false-positive reactions may occur—typically with samples from patients who have other infectious and parasitic diseases or autoimmune disorders. In addition, confirmatory testing has presented a persistent challenge. For these reasons, the World Health Organization recommends that specimens be tested in at least two assays and that well-characterized positive and negative comparison samples be included in each run. The radioimmune precipitation assay (Chagas RIPA) is a highly sensitive and specific confirmatory method for detecting antibodies

to *T. cruzi* (approved under the Clinical Laboratory Improvement Amendment and available in the authors' laboratory). In December 2006, the U.S. Food and Drug Administration (FDA) approved a test to screen blood and organ donors for *T. cruzi* infection (Ortho *T. cruzi* ELISA Test System, Ortho-Clinical Diagnostics, Raritan, NJ). Since January 2007, the vast majority of U.S. blood donors have been screened with the Ortho test, and positive units have undergone confirmatory testing in the Chagas RIPA. A second test for donor screening was approved by the FDA in April 2010 (Abbott PRISM® Chagas Assay, Abbott Laboratories, Abbott Park, IL). The use of PCR assays to detect *T. cruzi* DNA in chronically infected persons has been studied extensively. The sensitivity of this approach has not been shown to be reliably greater than that of serology, and no PCR assays are commercially available.

TREATMENT	Chagas' Disease

Therapy for Chagas' disease is still unsatisfactory. For many years now, only two drugs—nifurtimox and benznidazole—have been available for this purpose. Unfortunately, both drugs lack efficacy and may cause bothersome side effects.

In acute Chagas' disease, nifurtimox markedly reduces the duration of symptoms and parasitemia and decreases the mortality rate. Nevertheless, limited studies have shown that only ~70% of acute infections are cured parasitologically by a full course of treatment. Common adverse effects of nifurtimox include anorexia, nausea, vomiting, weight loss, and abdominal pain. Neurologic reactions to the drug may include restlessness, disorientation, insomnia, twitching, paresthesia, polyneuritis, and seizures. These symptoms usually disappear when the dosage is reduced or treatment is discontinued. The recommended daily dosage is 8–10 mg/kg for adults, 12.5–15 mg/kg for adolescents, and 15–20 mg/kg for children 1–10 years of age. The drug should be given orally in four divided doses each day, and therapy should be continued for 90–120 days. Nifurtimox is available from the Drug Service of the Centers for Disease Control and Prevention (CDC) in Atlanta (telephone number, 404-639-3670).

The efficacy of benznidazole is similar or even superior to that of nifurtimox. A cure rate of 90% among congenitally infected infants treated before their first birthday has been reported. Adverse effects include rash, peripheral neuropathy, and rarely granulocytopenia. The recommended oral dosage is 5 mg/kg per day for 60 days for adults and 5–10 mg/kg per day for 60 days for children, with administration of two or three divided doses. Benznidazole is generally considered the drug of choice in Latin America.

The question of whether adults in the indeterminate or chronic symptomatic phase of Chagas' disease should be treated with nifurtimox or benznidazole has been debated for years. The fact that parasitologic cure rates in chronically infected persons are notably inferior to those in patients with acute or recent chronic infection is central to this controversy. No convincing evidence from randomized controlled trials indicates that nifurtimox or benznidazole treatment of adults in the indeterminate or chronic symptomatic phase reduces either the appearance and progression of symptoms or mortality rates. On the basis of results of some observational studies, a panel of experts convened by the CDC in 2006 recommended that adults <50 years old with presumably long-standing indeterminate *T. cruzi* infections—or even with mild to moderate disease—be offered treatment. A large randomized clinical trial (the BENEFIT multicenter trial) designed to assess the parasitologic and clinical efficacy of benznidazole in adults (18–75 years old) with chronic Chagas' heart disease (without advanced lesions) is being performed in Brazil, Argentina, Colombia, and Bolivia, but results are not yet available. In contrast, randomized studies have shown that treatment of children is useful, and the current consensus of Latin American authorities is that all *T. cruzi*–infected persons up to 18 years old and all adults known to have become infected recently should be given benznidazole or nifurtimox.

The usefulness of antifungal azoles for the treatment of Chagas' disease has been studied in laboratory animals and to a lesser extent in humans. To date, none of these drugs has exhibited a level of anti–*T. cruzi* activity that would justify its use in humans. Several newer drugs in this class have shown promise in animal studies and are likely to undergo human trials in the near future.

Patients who develop cardiac and/or gastrointestinal disease in association with *T. cruzi* infection should be referred to appropriate subspecialists for further evaluation and treatment. Cardiac transplantation is an option for patients with end-stage chagasic cardiomyopathy; more than 150 such transplantations have been done in Brazil and the United States. The survival rate among Chagas' disease cardiac transplant recipients seems to be higher than that among persons receiving cardiac transplants for other reasons. This better outcome may be due to the fact that lesions are limited to the heart in most patients with symptomatic chronic Chagas' disease.

PREVENTION

Since drug therapy has limitations and vaccines are not available, the control of *T. cruzi* transmission in endemic countries depends on the reduction of domiciliary vector populations by spraying of insecticides, improvements in housing, and education of at-risk persons. As noted earlier, these measures, coupled with serologic screening of blood donors, have markedly reduced transmission of the parasite in many endemic countries. Tourists would be wise to avoid sleeping in dilapidated houses in rural areas of endemic countries. Mosquito nets and insect repellent can provide additional protection.

In view of the possibly serious consequences of chronic *T. cruzi* infection, it would be prudent for all immigrants from endemic regions who are living in the United States to be tested for evidence of infection. Identification of persons harboring the parasite would permit periodic electrocardiographic monitoring, which can be important because pacemakers benefit some patients who develop ominous rhythm disturbances. The possibility of congenital transmission is yet another justification for screening. *T. cruzi* is classified as a Risk Group 2 agent in the United States and a Risk Group 3 agent in some European countries. Laboratory staff should work with the parasite or infected vectors at containment levels consistent with the risk group designation in their areas.

CHAPTER 28

CARDIOGENIC SHOCK
AND PULMONARY EDEMA

Judith S. Hochman ■ David H. Ingbar

Cardiogenic shock and pulmonary edema are life-threatening conditions that should be treated as medical emergencies. The most common etiology for both is severe left ventricular (LV) dysfunction that leads to pulmonary congestion and/or systemic hypoperfusion (Fig. 28-1). The pathophysiology of pulmonary edema is discussed in Chap. 5.

CARDIOGENIC SHOCK

Cardiogenic shock (CS) is characterized by systemic hypoperfusion due to severe depression of the cardiac index (<2.2 [L/min]/m²) and sustained systolic arterial hypotension (<90 mmHg) despite an elevated filling pressure (pulmonary capillary wedge pressure [PCWP] >18 mmHg). It is associated with in-hospital mortality rates >50%. The major causes of CS are listed in Table 28-1. Circulatory failure based on cardiac dysfunction may be caused by primary myocardial failure, most commonly secondary to acute myocardial infarction (MI) (Chap. 35), and less frequently by cardiomyopathy or myocarditis (Chap. 21), cardiac tamponade (Chap. 22), or critical valvular heart disease (Chap. 20).

Incidence

CS is the leading cause of death of patients hospitalized with MI. Early reperfusion therapy for acute MI decreases the incidence of CS. The rate of CS complicating acute MI was 20% in the 1960s, stayed at ~8% for >20 years, but decreased to 5–7% in the first decade of this millennium. Shock typically is associated with ST elevation MI (STEMI) and is less common with non-ST elevation MI (Chap. 35).

LV failure accounts for ~80% of cases of CS complicating acute MI. Acute severe mitral regurgitation

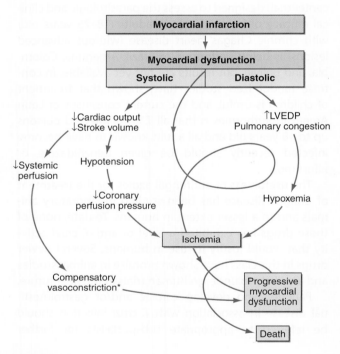

FIGURE 28-1

Pathophysiology of cardiogenic shock. Systolic and diastolic myocardial dysfunction results in a reduction in cardiac output and often pulmonary congestion. Systemic and coronary hypoperfusion occur, resulting in progressive ischemia. Although a number of compensatory mechanisms are activated in an attempt to support the circulation, these compensatory mechanisms may become maladaptive and produce a worsening of hemodynamics. *Release of inflammatory cytokines after myocardial infarction may lead to inducible nitric oxide expression, excess nitric oxide, and inappropriate vasodilation. This causes further reduction in systemic and coronary perfusion. A vicious spiral of progressive myocardial dysfunction occurs that ultimately results in death if it is not interrupted. LVEDP, left ventricular end-diastolic pressure. (*From SM Hollenberg et al: Ann Intern Med 131:47, 1999.*)

TABLE 28-1

ETIOLOGIES OF CARDIOGENIC SHOCK (CS)[a] AND CARDIOGENIC PULMONARY EDEMA

Etiologies of Cardiogenic Shock or Pulmonary Edema

Acute myocardial infarction/ischemia
  LV failure
  VSR
  Papillary muscle/chordal rupture—severe MR
  Ventricular free wall rupture with subacute tamponade
  Other conditions complicating large MIs
    Hemorrhage
    Infection
    Excess negative inotropic or vasodilator medications
    Prior valvular heart disease
    Hyperglycemia/ketoacidosis

Post-cardiac arrest

Post-cardiotomy

Refractory sustained tachyarrhythmias

Acute fulminant myocarditis

End-stage cardiomyopathy

Left ventricular apical ballooning

Takotsubo's cardiomyopathy

Hypertrophic cardiomyopathy with severe outflow obstruction

Aortic dissection with aortic insufficiency or tamponade

Pulmonary embolus

Severe valvular heart disease
  Critical aortic or mitral stenosis
  Acute severe aortic or MR

Toxic-metabolic
  Beta-blocker or calcium channel antagonist overdose

Other Etiologies of Cardiogenic Shock[b]

RV failure due to:
  Acute myocardial infarction
  Acute coronary pulmonale
Refractory sustained bradyarrhythmias
Pericardial tamponade
Toxic/metabolic
  Severe acidosis, severe hypoxemia

[a]The etiologies of CS are listed. Most of these can cause pulmonary edema instead of shock or pulmonary edema with CS.
[b]These cause CS but not pulmonary edema.
Abbreviations: LV, left ventricular; VSR, ventricular septal rupture; MR, mitral regurgitation; MI, myocardial infarction; RV, right ventricular.

(MR), ventricular septal rupture (VSR), predominant right ventricular (RV) failure, and free wall rupture or tamponade account for the remainder.

Pathophysiology

CS is characterized by a vicious circle in which depression of myocardial contractility, usually due to ischemia, results in reduced cardiac output and arterial pressure

(BP), which result in hypoperfusion of the myocardium and further ischemia and depression of cardiac output (Fig. 28-1). Systolic myocardial dysfunction reduces stroke volume and, together with diastolic dysfunction, leads to elevated LV end-diastolic pressure and PCWP as well as to pulmonary congestion. Reduced coronary perfusion leads to worsening ischemia and progressive myocardial dysfunction and a rapid downward spiral, which, if uninterrupted, is often fatal. A systemic inflammatory response syndrome may accompany large infarctions and shock. Inflammatory cytokines, inducible nitric oxide synthase, and excess nitric oxide and peroxynitrite may contribute to the genesis of CS as they do to that of other forms of shock. Lactic acidosis from poor tissue perfusion and hypoxemia from pulmonary edema may result from pump failure and then contribute to the vicious circle by worsening myocardial ischemia and hypotension. Severe acidosis (pH <7.25) reduces the efficacy of endogenous and exogenously administered catecholamines. Refractory sustained ventricular or atrial tachyarrhythmias can cause or exacerbate CS.

Patient profile

In patients with acute MI, older age, female sex, prior MI, diabetes, and anterior MI location are all associated with an increased risk of CS. Shock associated with a first inferior MI should prompt a search for a mechanical cause. Reinfarction soon after MI increases the risk of CS. Two-thirds of patients with CS have flow-limiting stenoses in all three major coronary arteries, and 20% have stenosis of the left main coronary artery. CS may rarely occur in the absence of significant stenosis, as seen in LV apical ballooning/Takotsubo's cardiomyopathy.

Timing

Shock is present on admission in only one-quarter of patients who develop CS complicating MI; one-quarter develop it rapidly thereafter, within 6 h of MI onset. Another quarter develop shock later on the first day. Subsequent onset of CS may be due to reinfarction, marked infarct expansion, or a mechanical complication.

Diagnosis

Due to the unstable condition of these patients, supportive therapy must be initiated simultaneously with diagnostic evaluation (Fig. 28-2). A focused history and physical examination should be performed, blood specimens sent to the laboratory, and an electrocardiogram (ECG) and chest x-ray obtained.

Echocardiography is an invaluable diagnostic tool in patients suspected of CS.

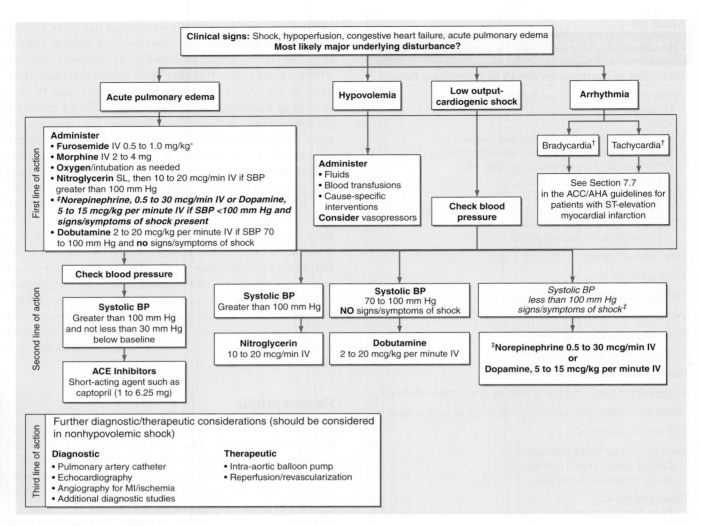

FIGURE 28-2

The emergency management of patients with cardio-genic shock, acute pulmonary edema, or both is outlined. *Furosemide: <0.5 mg/kg for new-onset acute pulmonary edema without hypervolemia; 1 mg/kg for acute on chronic volume overload, renal insufficiency. †For management of bradycardia and tachycardia, see Chaps. 15 and 16. ‡Indicates modification from published guidelines. ACE, angiotensin-converting enzyme; BP, blood pressure; MI, myocardial infarction. (*Modified from Guidelines 2000 for Cardiopulmonary Resuscitation and Emergency Cardiovascular Care. Part 7: The era of reperfusion: Section 1: Acute coronary syndromes [acute myocardial infarction]. The American Heart Association in collaboration with the International Liaison Committee on Resuscitation. Circulation 102:1172, 2000.*)

Clinical findings

Most patients have continuing chest pain and dyspnea and appear pale, apprehensive, and diaphoretic. Mentation may be altered, with somnolence, confusion, and agitation. The pulse is typically weak and rapid, often in the range of 90–110 beats/min, or severe bradycardia due to high-grade heart block may be present. Systolic blood pressure is reduced (<90 mmHg) with a narrow pulse pressure (<30 mmHg), but occasionally BP may be maintained by very high systemic vascular resistance. Tachypnea, Cheyne-Stokes respirations, and jugular venous distention may be present. The precordium is typically quiet, with a weak apical pulse. S_1 is usually soft, and an S_3 gallop may be audible.

Acute, severe MR and VSR usually are associated with characteristic systolic murmurs (Chap. 35). Rales are audible in most patients with LV failure causing CS. Oliguria (urine output <30 mL/h) is common.

Laboratory findings

The white blood cell count is typically elevated with a left shift. In the absence of prior renal insufficiency, renal function is initially normal, but blood urea nitrogen and creatinine rise progressively. Hepatic transaminases may be markedly elevated due to liver hypoperfusion. Poor tissue perfusion may result in an anion-gap acidosis and elevation of the lactic acid level. Before support with supplemental O_2, arterial blood gases usually demonstrate hypoxemia and metabolic acidosis, which may be compensated by respiratory alkalosis. Cardiac markers, creatine phosphokinase and its MB fraction, and troponins I and T are markedly elevated.

Electrocardiogram

In CS due to acute MI with LV failure, Q waves and/or >2-mm ST elevation in multiple leads or left bundle branch block are usually present. More than one-half of all infarcts associated with shock are anterior. Global ischemia due to severe left main stenosis usually is accompanied by severe (e.g., >3 mm) ST depressions in multiple leads.

Chest roentgenogram

The chest x-ray typically shows pulmonary vascular congestion and often pulmonary edema, but these findings may be absent in up to a third of patients. The heart size is usually normal when CS results from a first MI but is enlarged when it occurs in a patient with a previous MI.

Echocardiogram

A two-dimensional echocardiogram with color-flow Doppler (Chap. 12) should be obtained promptly in patients with suspected CS to help define its etiology. Doppler mapping demonstrates a left-to-right shunt in patients with VSR and the severity of MR when the latter

is present. Proximal aortic dissection with aortic regurgitation or tamponade may be visualized, or evidence for pulmonary embolism may be obtained.

Pulmonary artery catheterization

There is controversy regarding the use of pulmonary artery (Swan-Ganz) catheters in patients with established or suspected CS (Chap. 13). Their use is generally recommended for measurement of filling pressures and cardiac output to confirm the diagnosis and optimize the use of IV fluids, inotropic agents, and vasopressors in persistent shock (Table 28-2). Blood samples for O$_2$ saturation measurement should be obtained from the right atrium, right ventricle, and pulmonary artery to rule out a left-to-right shunt. Mixed venous O$_2$ saturations are low and arteriovenous (AV) O$_2$ differences are elevated, reflecting low cardiac index and high fractional O$_2$ extraction. However, when a systemic inflammatory response syndrome accompanies CS, AV O$_2$ differences may not be elevated. The PCWP is elevated. However, use of sympathomimetic amines may return these measurements and the systemic BP to normal. Systemic vascular resistance may be low, normal, or elevated in CS. Equalization of right- and left-sided filling pressures (right atrial and PCWP) suggests cardiac tamponade as the cause of CS (Chap. 22).

TABLE 28-2

HEMODYNAMIC PATTERNS[a]

	RA, mmHg	RVS, mmHg	RVD, mmHg	PAS, mmHg	PAD, mmHg	PCW, mmHg	CI, (L/min)/m²	SVR, (dyn · s)/cm⁵
Normal values	<6	<25	0–12	<25	0–12	<6–12	≥2.5	(800–1600)
MI without pulmonary edema[b]	—	—	—	—	—	~13 (5–18)	~2.7 (2.2–4.3)	—
Pulmonary edema	↔↑	↔↑	↔↑	↑	↑	↑	↔↓	↑
Cardiogenic shock								
LV failure	↔↑	↔↑	↔↑	↔↑	↑	↑	↓	↔↑
RV failure[c]	↑	↓↔↑[d]	↑	↓↔↑[d]	↔↓↑[d]	↓↔↑[d]	↓	↑
Cardiac tamponade	↑	↔↑	↑	↔↑	↔↑	↔↑	↓	↑
Acute mitral regurgitation	↔↑	↑	↔↑	↑	↑	↑	↔↓	↔↑
Ventricular septal rupture	↑	↔↑	↑	↔↑	↔↑	↔↑	↑PBF ↓SBF	↔↑
Hypovolemic shock	↓	↔↓	↔↓	↓	↓	↓	↓	↑
Septic shock	↓	↔↓	↔↓	↓	↓	↓	↑	↓

[a]There is significant patient-to-patient variation. Pressure may be normalized if cardiac output is low.
[b]Forrester et al classified nonreperfused MI patients into four hemodynamic subsets. (From Forrester JS et al: N Engl J Med 295:1356, 1976.) PCWP and CI in clinically stable subset 1 patients are shown. Values in parentheses represent range.
[c]"Isolated" or predominant RV failure.
[d]PCW and PA pressures may rise in RV failure after volume loading due to RV dilation, right-to-left shift of the interventricular septum, resulting in impaired LV filling. When biventricular failure is present, the patterns are similar to those shown for LV failure.
Abbreviations: CI, cardiac index; MI, myocardial infarction; P/SBF, pulmonary/systemic blood flow; PAS/D, pulmonary artery systolic/diastolic; PCW, pulmonary capillary wedge; RA, right atrium; RVS/D, right ventricular systolic/diastolic; SVR, systemic vascular resistance.
Source: Table prepared with the assistance of Krishnan Ramanathan, MD.

CHAPTER 28 Cardiogenic Shock and Pulmonary Edema

■■■ **Left heart catheterization and coronary angiography**

Measurement of LV pressure and definition of the coronary anatomy provide useful information and are indicated in most patients with CS complicating MI. Cardiac catheterization should be performed when there is a plan and capability for immediate coronary intervention (see later) or when a definitive diagnosis has not been made by other tests.

TREATMENT ▶ **Acute Myocardial Infarction**

GENERAL MEASURES (Fig. 28-2) In addition to the usual treatment of acute MI (Chap. 35), initial therapy is aimed at maintaining adequate systemic and coronary perfusion by raising systemic BP with vasopressors and adjusting volume status to a level that ensures optimum LV filling pressure. There is interpatient variability, but the values that generally are associated with adequate perfusion are systolic BP ~90 mmHg or mean BP >60 mmHg and PCWP >20 mmHg. Hypoxemia and acidosis must be corrected; most patients require ventilatory support with either endotracheal intubation or noninvasive ventilation to correct these abnormalities and reduce the work of breathing (see "Pulmonary Edema," later). Negative inotropic agents should be discontinued, and the doses of renally cleared medications adjusted. Hyperglycemia should be controlled with insulin. Bradyarrhythmias may require transvenous pacing. Recurrent ventricular tachycardia or rapid atrial fibrillation may require immediate treatment (Chap. 16).

VASOPRESSORS Various IV drugs may be used to augment BP and cardiac output in patients with CS. All have important disadvantages, and none has been shown to change the outcome in patients with established shock. *Norepinephrine* is a potent vasoconstrictor and inotropic stimulant that is useful for patients with CS. As first line of therapy norepinephrine was associated with fewer adverse events, including arrhythmias, compared to a dopamine randomized trial of patients with several eteologies of circulatory shock. Although it did not significantly improve survival compared to dopamine, its relative safety suggests that norepinephrine is reasonable as initial vasopressor therapy. Norepinephrine should be started at a dose of 2 to 4 μg/min and titrated upward as necessary. If systemic perfusion or systolic pressure cannot be maintained at >90 mmHg with a dose of 15 μg/min, it is unlikely that a further increase will be beneficial.

Dopamine has varying hemodynamic effects based on the dose; at low doses (≤2 μg/kg per min), it dilates the renal vascular bed, although its outcome benefits at this low dose have not been demonstrated conclusively; at moderate doses (2–10 μg/kg per min), it has positive chronotropic and inotropic effects as a consequence of β-adrenergic receptor stimulation. At higher doses, a vasoconstrictor effect results from α-receptor stimulation. It is started at an infusion rate of 2–5 μg/kg per min, and the dose is increased every 2–5 min to a maximum of 20–50 μg/kg per min. *Dobutamine* is a synthetic sympathomimetic amine with positive inotropic action and minimal positive chronotropic activity at low doses (2.5 μg/kg per min) but moderate chronotropic activity at higher doses. Although the usual dose is up to 10 μg/kg per min, its vasodilating activity precludes its use when a vasoconstrictor effect is required.

AORTIC COUNTERPULSATION In CS, mechanical assistance with an intraaortic balloon pumping (IABP) system capable of augmenting both arterial diastolic pressure and cardiac output is helpful in rapidly stabilizing patients. A sausage-shaped balloon is introduced percutaneously into the aorta via the femoral artery; the balloon is automatically inflated during early diastole, augmenting coronary blood flow. The balloon collapses in early systole, reducing the afterload against which the LV ejects. IABP improves hemodynamic status temporarily in most patients. In contrast to vasopressors and inotropic agents, myocardial O_2 consumption is reduced, ameliorating ischemia. IABP is useful as a stabilizing measure in patients with CS before and during cardiac catheterization and percutaneous coronary intervention (PCI) or before urgent surgery. IABP is contraindicated if aortic regurgitation is present or aortic dissection is suspected. Ventricular assist devices may be considered for eligible young patients with refractory shock as a bridge to cardiac transplantation (Chap. 18).

REPERFUSION-REVASCULARIZATION The rapid establishment of blood flow in the infarct-related artery is essential in the management of CS and forms the centerpiece of management. The randomized SHOCK Trial demonstrated that 132 lives were saved per 1000 patients treated with early revascularization with PCI or coronary artery bypass graft (CABG) compared with initial medical therapy including IABP with fibrinolytics followed by delayed revascularization. The benefit is seen across the risk strata and is sustained up to 11 years after an MI. Early revascularization with PCI or CABG is a class I recommendation for patients age <75 years with ST elevation or left bundle branch block MI who develop CS within 36 h of MI and who can be revascularized within 18 h of the development of CS. When mechanical revascularization is not possible, IABP and fibrinolytic therapy are recommended. Older patients who are suitable candidates for aggressive care also should be offered early revascularization.

Prognosis

Within this high-risk condition, there is a wide range of expected death rates based on age, severity of hemodynamic abnormalities, severity of the clinical manifestations of hypoperfusion, and the performance of early revascularization.

SHOCK SECONDARY TO RIGHT VENTRICULAR INFARCTION

Although transient hypotension is common in patients with RV infarction and inferior MI (Chap. 35), persistent CS due to RV failure accounts for only 3% of CS complicating MI. The salient features of RV shock are absence of pulmonary congestion, high right atrial pressure (which may be seen only after volume loading), RV dilation and dysfunction, only mildly or moderately depressed LV function, and predominance of single-vessel proximal right coronary artery occlusion. Management includes IV fluid administration to optimize right atrial pressure (10–15 mmHg); avoidance of excess fluids, which cause a shift of the interventricular septum into the LV; sympathomimetic amines; IABP; and the early reestablishment of infarct-artery flow.

MITRAL REGURGITATION

(See also Chap. 35) Acute severe MR due to papillary muscle dysfunction and/or rupture may complicate MI and result in CS and/or pulmonary edema. This complication most often occurs on the first day, with a second peak several days later. The diagnosis is confirmed by echo-Doppler. Rapid stabilization with IABP is recommended, with administration of dobutamine as needed to raise cardiac output. Reducing the load against which the LV pumps (afterload) reduces the volume of regurgitant flow of blood into the left atrium. Mitral valve surgery is the definitive therapy and should be performed early in the course in suitable candidates.

VENTRICULAR SEPTAL RUPTURE

(See also Chap. 35) Echo-Doppler demonstrates shunting of blood from the left to the right ventricle and may visualize the opening in the interventricular septum. Timing and management are similar to those for MR with IABP support and surgical correction for suitable candidates.

FREE WALL RUPTURE

Myocardial rupture is a dramatic complication of STEMI that is most likely to occur during the first week after the onset of symptoms; its frequency increases with the age of the patient. The clinical presentation typically is a sudden loss of pulse, blood pressure, and consciousness but sinus rhythm on ECG (pulseless electrical activity) due to cardiac tamponade (Chap. 22). Free wall rupture may also result in CS due to subacute tamponade when the pericardium temporarily seals the rupture sites. Definitive surgical repair is required.

ACUTE FULMINANT MYOCARDITIS

(See also Chap. 21) Myocarditis can mimic acute MI with ST deviation or bundle branch block on the ECG and marked elevation of cardiac markers. Acute myocarditis causes CS in a small proportion of cases. These patients are typically younger than those with CS due to acute MI and often do not have typical ischemic chest pain. Echocardiography usually shows global LV dysfunction. Initial management is the same as for CS complicating acute MI (Fig. 28-2) but does not involve coronary revascularization.

PULMONARY EDEMA

The etiologies and pathophysiology of pulmonary edema are discussed in Chap. 5.

Diagnosis

Acute pulmonary edema usually presents with the rapid onset of dyspnea at rest, tachypnea, tachycardia, and severe hypoxemia. Rales and wheezing due to airway compression from peribronchial cuffing may be audible. Hypertension is usually present due to release of endogenous catecholamines.

It is often difficult to distinguish between cardiogenic and noncardiogenic causes of acute pulmonary edema. *Echocardiography* may identify systolic and diastolic ventricular dysfunction and valvular lesions. Pulmonary edema associated with electrocardiographic ST elevation and evolving Q waves is usually diagnostic of acute MI and should prompt immediate institution of MI protocols and coronary artery reperfusion therapy (Chap. 35). Brain natriuretic peptide levels, when substantially elevated, support heart failure as the etiology of acute dyspnea with pulmonary edema (Chap. 17).

The use of a *Swan-Ganz catheter* permits measurement of PCWP and helps differentiate high-pressure (cardiogenic) from normal-pressure (noncardiogenic) causes of pulmonary edema. Pulmonary artery catheterization is indicated when the etiology of the pulmonary edema is uncertain, when it is refractory to therapy, or when it is accompanied by hypotension. Data derived from use of a catheter often alter the treatment plan, but the impact on mortality rates has not been demonstrated.

TREATMENT   Pulmonary Edema

The treatment of pulmonary edema depends on the specific etiology. In light of the acute, life-threatening nature of the condition, a number of measures must be applied immediately to support the circulation, gas exchange, and lung mechanics. In addition, conditions that frequently complicate pulmonary edema, such as infection, acidemia, anemia, and renal failure, must be corrected.

SUPPORT OF OXYGENATION AND VENTI-LATION   Patients with acute cardiogenic pulmonary edema generally have an identifiable cause of acute LV failure—such as arrhythmia, ischemia/infarction, or myocardial decompensation (Chap. 17)—that can be rapidly treated, with improvement in gas exchange. In contrast, noncardiogenic edema usually resolves much less quickly, and most patients require mechanical ventilation.

Oxygen Therapy   Support of oxygenation is essential to ensure adequate O_2 delivery to peripheral tissues, including the heart.

Positive-Pressure Ventilation   Pulmonary edema increases the work of breathing and the O_2 requirements of this work, imposing a significant physiologic stress on the heart. When oxygenation or ventilation is not adequate in spite of supplemental O_2, positive-pressure ventilation by face or nasal mask or by endotracheal intubation should be initiated. Noninvasive ventilation can rest the respiratory muscles, improve oxygenation and cardiac function, and reduce the need for intubation. In refractory cases, mechanical ventilation can relieve the work of breathing more completely than can noninvasive ventilation. Mechanical ventilation with positive end-expiratory pressure can have multiple beneficial effects on pulmonary edema: (1) decreases both preload and afterload, thereby improving cardiac function, (2) redistributes lung water from the intraalveolar to the extraalveolar space, where the fluid interferes less with gas exchange, and (3) increases lung volume to avoid atelectasis.

REDUCTION OF PRELOAD   In most forms of pulmonary edema, the quantity of extravascular lung water is determined by both the PCWP and the intravascular volume status.

Diuretics   The "loop diuretics" furosemide, bumetanide, and torsemide are effective in most forms of pulmonary edema, even in the presence of hypoalbuminemia, hyponatremia, or hypochloremia. Furosemide is also a venodilator that reduces preload rapidly, before any diuresis, and is the diuretic of choice. The initial dose of furosemide should be ≤0.5 mg/kg, but a higher dose (1 mg/kg) is required in patients with renal insufficiency, chronic diuretic use, or hypervolemia or after failure of a lower dose.

Nitrates   Nitroglycerin and isosorbide dinitrate act predominantly as venodilators but have coronary vasodilating properties as well. They are rapid in onset and effective when administered by a variety of routes. Sublingual nitroglycerin (0.4 mg × 3 every 5 min) is first-line therapy for acute cardiogenic pulmonary edema. If pulmonary edema persists in the absence of hypotension, sublingual may be followed by IV nitroglycerin, commencing at 5–10 µg/min. IV nitroprusside (0.1–5 µg/kg per min) is a potent venous and arterial vasodilator. It is useful for patients with pulmonary edema and hypertension but is not recommended in states of reduced coronary artery perfusion. It requires close monitoring and titration using an arterial catheter for continuous BP measurement.

Morphine   Given in 2- to 4-mg IV boluses, morphine is a transient venodilator that reduces preload while relieving dyspnea and anxiety. These effects can diminish stress, catecholamine levels, tachycardia, and ventricular afterload in patients with pulmonary edema and systemic hypertension.

Angiotensin-Converting Enzyme (ACE) Inhibitors   ACE inhibitors reduce both afterload and preload and are recommended for hypertensive patients. A low dose of a short-acting agent may be initiated and followed by increasing oral doses. In acute MI with heart failure, ACE inhibitors reduce short- and long-term mortality rates.

Other Preload-Reducing Agents   IV recombinant brain natriuretic peptide (nesiritide) is a potent vasodilator with diuretic properties and is effective in the treatment of cardiogenic pulmonary edema. It should be reserved for refractory patients and is not recommended in the setting of ischemia or MI.

Physical Methods   Reduction of venous return reduces preload. Patients without hypotension should be maintained in the sitting position with the legs dangling along the side of the bed.

Inotropic and Inodilator Drugs   The sympathomimetic amines dopamine and dobutamine (see earlier) are potent inotropic agents. The bipyridine phosphodiesterase-3 inhibitors (inodilators), such as milrinone (50 µg/kg followed by 0.25–0.75 µg/kg per min), stimulate myocardial contractility while promoting peripheral and pulmonary vasodilation. Such agents are indicated in patients with cardiogenic pulmonary edema and severe LV dysfunction.

Digitalis Glycosides   Once a mainstay of treatment because of their positive inotropic action (Chap. 17), digitalis glycosides are rarely used at present. However, they may be useful for control of ventricular rate in patients with rapid atrial fibrillation or flutter and LV dysfunction, since they do not have the negative inotropic effects of other drugs that inhibit atrioventricular nodal conduction.

Intraaortic Counterpulsation IABP may help relieve cardiogenic pulmonary edema. It is indicated as a stabilizing measure when acute severe mitral regurgitation or ventricular septal rupture causes refractory pulmonary edema, especially in preparation for surgical repair. IABP or LV-assist devices (Chap. 18) are useful as bridging therapy to cardiac transplantation in patients with refractory pulmonary edema secondary to myocarditis or cardiomyopathy.

Treatment of Tachyarrhythmias and Atrial-Ventricular Resynchronization (See also Chap. 16) Sinus tachycardia or atrial fibrillation can result from elevated left atrial pressure and sympathetic stimulation. Tachycardia itself can limit LV filling time and raise left atrial pressure further. Although relief of pulmonary congestion will slow the sinus rate or ventricular response in atrial fibrillation, a primary tachyarrhythmia may require cardioversion. In patients with reduced LV function and without atrial contraction or with lack of synchronized atrioventricular contraction, placement of an atrioventricular sequential pacemaker should be considered (Chap. 15).

Stimulation of Alveolar Fluid Clearance Recent mechanistic studies on alveolar epithelial ion transport have defined a variety of ways to upregulate the clearance of solute and water from the alveolar space. In patients with acute lung injury (noncardiogenic pulmonary edema), IV β-adrenergic agonist treatment decreases extravascular lung water, but the outcome benefit is uncertain.

SPECIAL CONSIDERATIONS
The Risk of Iatrogenic Cardiogenic Shock In the treatment of pulmonary edema vasodilators lower BP, and, particularly when used in combination, their use may lead to hypotension, coronary artery hypoperfusion, and shock (Fig. 28-1). In general, patients with a *hypertensive* response to pulmonary edema tolerate and benefit from these medications. In normotensive patients, low doses of single agents should be instituted sequentially, as needed.

Acute Coronary Syndromes (See also Chap. 35) Acute STEMI complicated by pulmonary edema is associated with in-hospital mortality rates of 20–40%. After immediate stabilization, coronary artery blood flow must be reestablished rapidly. When available, primary PCI is preferable; alternatively, a fibrinolytic agent should be administered. Early coronary angiography and revascularization by PCI or CABG also are indicated for patients with non-ST elevation acute coronary syndrome. IABP use may be required to stabilize patients for coronary angiography if hypotension develops or for refractory pulmonary edema in patients with LV failure who are candidates for revascularization.

Unusual Types of Edema Specific etiologies of pulmonary edema may require particular therapy. Reexpansion pulmonary edema can develop after removal of air or fluid that has been in the pleural space for some time. These patients may develop hypotension or oliguria resulting from rapid fluid shifts into the lung. Diuretics and preload reduction are contraindicated, and intravascular volume repletion often is needed while supporting oxygenation and gas exchange.

High-altitude pulmonary edema often can be prevented by use of dexamethasone, calcium channel-blocking drugs, or long-acting inhaled β$_2$-adrenergic agonists. Treatment includes descent from altitude, bed rest, oxygen, and, if feasible, inhaled nitric oxide; nifedipine may also be effective.

For pulmonary edema resulting from upper airway obstruction, recognition of the obstructing cause is key, since treatment then is to relieve or bypass the obstruction.

CHAPTER 29

CARDIOVASCULAR COLLAPSE, CARDIAC ARREST, AND SUDDEN CARDIAC DEATH

Robert J. Myerburg ■ Agustin Castellanos

OVERVIEW AND DEFINITIONS

Sudden cardiac death (SCD) is defined *as natural death due to cardiac causes* in a person who may or may not have previously recognized heart disease but in whom the time and mode of death are *unexpected*. In the context of time, "sudden" is defined for most clinical and epidemiologic purposes as *1 h or less* between a change in clinical status heralding the onset of the terminal clinical event and the cardiac arrest itself. An exception is unwitnessed deaths, in which pathologists may expand the definition of time to 24 h after the victim was last seen to be alive and stable.

The overwhelming majority of natural deaths are caused by cardiac disorders. However, it is common for underlying heart diseases—often far advanced—to go unrecognized before the fatal event. As a result, up to two-thirds of all SCDs occur as the first clinical expression of previously undiagnosed disease or in patients with known heart disease, the extent of which suggests low risk. The magnitude of sudden *cardiac* death as a public health problem is highlighted by the estimate that ~50% of all cardiac deaths are sudden and unexpected, accounting for a total SCD burden estimated to range from <200,000 to >450,000 deaths each year in the United States. SCD is a direct consequence of cardiac arrest, which may be reversible if addressed promptly. Since resuscitation techniques and emergency rescue systems are available to respond to victims of out-of-hospital cardiac arrest, which was uniformly fatal in the past, understanding the SCD problem has practical clinical importance.

Because of community-based interventions, victims may remain biologically alive for days or even weeks after a cardiac arrest that has resulted in irreversible central nervous system damage. Confusion in terms can be avoided by adhering strictly to definitions of cardiovascular collapse, cardiac arrest, and death (Table 29-1). Although cardiac arrest is often potentially reversible by appropriate and timely interventions, death is biologically, legally, and literally an absolute and irreversible event. Death may be delayed in a survivor of cardiac arrest, but "survival after sudden death" is an irrational term. When biologic death of a cardiac arrest victim is delayed because of interventions, the relevant pathophysiologic event remains the sudden and unexpected cardiac arrest that leads ultimately to death, even though delayed by interventions. The language used should reflect the fact that the index event was a cardiac arrest and that death was due to its delayed consequences. Accordingly, for statistical purposes, deaths that occur during hospitalization or within 30 days after resuscitated cardiac arrest are counted as sudden deaths.

CLINICAL DEFINITION OF FORMS OF CARDIOVASCULAR COLLAPSE

Cardiovascular collapse is a general term connoting loss of sufficient cerebral blood flow to maintain consciousness due to acute dysfunction of the heart and/or peripheral vasculature. It may be caused by vasodepressor syncope (vasovagal syncope, postural hypotension with syncope, neurocardiogenic syncope, a transient severe bradycardia, or cardiac arrest. The latter is distinguished from the transient forms of cardiovascular collapse in that it usually requires an intervention to restore spontaneous blood flow. In contrast, vasodepressor syncope and other primary bradyarrhythmic syncopal events are transient and non-life-threatening, with spontaneous return of consciousness.

The most common electrical mechanism for cardiac arrest is ventricular fibrillation (VF), which is responsible for 50–80% of cardiac arrests. Severe persistent brady-arrhythmias, asystole, and pulseless electrical activity

TABLE 29-1

DISTINCTION BETWEEN CARDIOVASCULAR COLLAPSE, CARDIAC ARREST, AND DEATH

TERM	DEFINITION	QUALIFIERS	MECHANISMS
Cardiovascular collapse	Sudden loss of effective blood flow due to cardiac and/or peripheral vascular factors that may reverse spontaneously (e.g., neurocardiogenic syncope, vasovagal syncope) or require interventions (e.g., cardiac arrest)	Nonspecific term: includes cardiac arrest and its consequences and transient events that characteristically revert spontaneously	Same as "cardiac arrest," plus vasodepressor syncope or other causes of transient loss of blood flow
Cardiac arrest	Abrupt cessation of cardiac mechanical function, which may be reversible by a prompt intervention but will lead to death in its absence	Rare spontaneous reversions; likelihood of successful intervention relates to mechanism of arrest, clinical setting, and prompt return of circulation	Ventricular fibrillation, ventricular tachycardia, asystole, bradycardia, pulseless electrical activity, mechanical factors
Sudden cardiac death	Sudden, irreversible cessation of all biological functions	None	

Source: Modified from RJ Myerburg, A Castellanos: Cardiac arrest and sudden cardiac death, in *Braunwald's Heart Disease*, 8th ed, P Libby et al (eds). Philadelphia, Saunders, 2008, with permission of publisher.

(PEA: organized electrical activity, unusually slow, without mechanical response, formerly called electromechanical dissociation [EMD]) cause another 20–30%. Pulseless sustained ventricular tachycardia (a rapid arrhythmia distinct from PEA) is a less common mechanism. Acute low cardiac output states, having a precipitous onset, also may present clinically as a cardiac arrest. These hemodynamic causes include massive acute pulmonary emboli, internal blood loss from a ruptured aortic aneurysm, intense anaphylaxis, and cardiac rupture with tamponade after myocardial infarction (MI). Sudden deaths due to these causes are not included in the SCD category.

ETIOLOGY, INITIATING EVENTS, AND CLINICAL EPIDEMIOLOGY

Clinical, epidemiologic, and pathologic studies have provided information on the underlying *structural abnormalities* in victims of SCD and identified subgroups at high risk for SCD. In addition, studies of clinical physiology have begun to identify *transient functional factors* that may convert a long-standing underlying structural abnormality from a stable to an unstable state, leading to the onset of cardiac arrest (**Table 29-2**).

Cardiac disorders constitute the most common causes of sudden *natural* death. After an initial peak incidence of sudden death between birth and 6 months of age (the sudden infant death syndrome [SIDS]), the incidence of sudden death declines sharply and remains low through childhood and adolescence. Among adolescents

and young adults, the incidence of SCD is approximately 1 per 100,000 population per year. The incidence begins to increase in adults over age 30 years, reaching a second peak in the age range 45–75 years, when it approximates 1–2 per 1000 per year among the unselected adult population. Increasing age within this range is associated with increasing risk for sudden *cardiac* death (**Fig. 29-1A**). From 1 to 13 years of age, only one of five sudden *natural* deaths is due to cardiac causes. Between 14 and 21 years of age, the proportion increases to 30%, and it rises to 88% in the middle-aged and elderly.

Young and middle-aged men and women have different susceptibilities to SCD, but the sex differences decrease with advancing age. The difference in risk for SCD parallels the differences in age-related risks for other manifestations of coronary heart disease (CHD) between men and women. As the gender gap for manifestations of CHD closes in the sixth to eighth decades of life, the excess risk of SCD in males progressively narrows. Despite the lower incidence among younger women, coronary risk factors such as cigarette smoking, diabetes, hyperlipidemia, and hypertension are highly influential, and SCD remains an important clinical and epidemiologic problem. The incidence of SCD among the African-American population appears to be higher than it is among the white population; the reasons remain uncertain.

Genetic factors contribute to the risk of acquiring CHD and its expression as acute coronary syndromes, including SCD. In addition, however, there are data

TABLE 29-2

CARDIAC ARREST AND SUDDEN CARDIAC DEATH

Structural Associations and Causes

I. Coronary heart disease
   A. Coronary artery abnormalities
      1. Chronic atherosclerotic lesions
      2. Acute (active) lesions (plaque fissuring, platelet aggregation, acute thrombosis)
      3. Anomalous coronary artery anatomy
   B. Myocardial Infarction
      1. Healed
      2. Acute

II. Myocardial hypertrophy
   A. Secondary
   B. Hypertrophic cardiomyopathy
      1. Obstructive
      2. Nonobstructive

III. Dilated cardiomyopathy—primary muscle disease

IV. Inflammatory and infiltrative disorders
   A. Myocarditis
   B. Noninfectious inflammatory diseases
   C. Infiltrative diseases

V. Valvular heart disease

VI. Electrophysiologic abnormalities, structural
   A. Anomalous pathways in Wolff-Parkinson-White syndrome
   B. Conducting system disease

VII. Inherited disorders associated with electrophysiological abnormalities (congenital long QT syndromes, right ventricular dysplasia, Brugada syndrome, catecholaminergic polymorphic ventricular tachycardia, etc.)

Functional Contributing Factors

I. Alterations of coronary blood flow
   A. Transient ischemia
   B. Reperfusion after ischemia

II. Low cardiac output states
   A. Heart failure
      1. Chronic
      2. Acute decompensation
   B. Shock

III. Systemic metabolic abnormalities
   A. Electrolyte imbalance (e.g., hypokalemia)
   B. Hypoxemia, acidosis

IV. Neurologic disturbances
   A. Autonomic fluctuations: central, neural, humoral
   B. Receptor function

V. Toxic responses
   A. Proarrhythmic drug effects
   B. Cardiac toxins (e.g., cocaine, digitalis intoxication)
   C. Drug interactions

suggesting a familial predisposition to SCD as a specific form of expression of CHD. A parental history of SCD as an initial coronary event increases the probability of a similar expression in the offspring. In a number of less common syndromes, such as hypertrophic cardiomyopathy, congenital long QT interval syndromes, right ventricular dysplasia, and the syndrome of right bundle branch block and nonischemic ST-segment elevations (Brugada syndrome), there is a specific inherited risk of ventricular arrhythmias and SCD (Chap. 16).

The structural causes of and functional factors contributing to the SCD syndrome are listed in Table 29-2. Worldwide, and especially in Western cultures, coronary atherosclerotic heart disease is the most common structural abnormality associated with SCD in middle-aged and older adults. Up to 80% of all SCDs in the United States are due to the consequences of coronary atherosclerosis. The nonischemic cardiomyopathies (dilated and hypertrophic, collectively; Chap. 14) account for another 10–15% of SCDs, and all the remaining diverse etiologies cause only 5–10% of all SCDs. The inherited arrhythmia syndromes (see earlier and Table 29-2) are proportionally more common causes in adolescents and young adults. For some of these syndromes, such as hypertrophic cardiomyopathy (Chap. 21), the risk of SCD increases significantly after the onset of puberty.

Transient ischemia in a previously scarred or hypertrophied heart, hemodynamic and fluid and electrolyte disturbances, fluctuations in autonomic nervous system activity, and transient electrophysiologic changes caused by drugs or other chemicals (e.g., proarrhythmia) have all been implicated as mechanisms responsible for the transition from electrophysiologic stability to instability. In addition, reperfusion of ischemic myocardium may cause transient electrophysiologic instability and arrhythmias.

PATHOLOGY

Data from postmortem examinations of SCD victims parallel the clinical observations on the prevalence of CHD as the major structural etiologic factor. More than 80% of SCD victims have pathologic findings of CHD. The pathologic description often includes a combination of long-standing, extensive atherosclerosis of the epicardial coronary arteries and unstable coronary artery lesions, which include various permutations of eroded, fissured, or ruptured plaques; platelet aggregates; hemorrhage; and/or thrombosis. As many as 70–75% of males who die suddenly have preexisting healed MIs, whereas only 20–30% have recent acute MIs, despite the prevalence of unstable plaques and thrombi. The latter suggests transient ischemia as the mechanism of onset. Regional or global left ventricular (LV) hypertrophy often coexists with prior MIs.

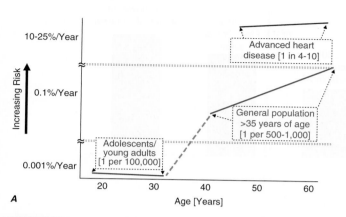

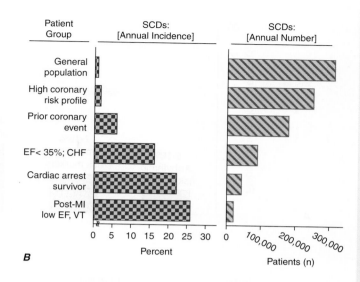

FIGURE 29-1

Panel A demonstrates age-related risk for SCD. For the general population age 35 years and older, SCD risk is 0.1–0.2% per year (1 per 500–1000 population). Among the general population of adolescents and adults younger than age 30 years, the overall risk of SCD is 1 per 100,000 population, or 0.001% per year. The risk of SCD increases dramatically beyond age 35 years. The greatest rate of increase is between 40 and 65 years (vertical axis is discontinuous). Among patients older than 30 years of age, with advanced structural heart disease and markers of high risk for cardiac arrest, the event rate may exceed 25% per year, and age-related risk attenuates. (*Modified from Myerburg and Castellanos 2008, with permission of publisher.*) **Panel B** demonstrates the incidence of SCD in population subgroups and the relation of total number of events per year to incidence figures. Approximations of subgroup incidence figures and the related population pool from which they are derived are presented. Approximately 50% of all cardiac deaths are sudden and unexpected. The incidence triangle on the left ("Percent/Year") indicates the approximate percentage of sudden and nonsudden deaths in each of the population subgroups indicated, ranging from the lowest percentage in unselected adult populations (0.1–2% per year) to the highest percentage in patients with VT or VF during convalescence after an MI (approximately 50% per year). The triangle on the right indicates the total number of events per year in each of these groups to reflect incidence in context with the size of the population subgroups. The highest risk categories identify the smallest number of total annual events, and the lowest incidence category accounts for the largest number of events per year. EF, ejection fraction; VT, ventricular tachycardia; VF, ventricular fibrillation; MI, myocardial infarction. (*After RJ Myerburg et al: Circulation 85:2, 1992.*)

PREDICTION AND PREVENTION OF CARDIAC ARREST AND SUDDEN CARDIAC DEATH

SCD accounts for approximately one-half the total number of cardiovascular deaths. As shown in Fig. 29-1B, the very high-risk subgroups provide more focused populations ("percent per year") for predicting cardiac arrest or SCD, but the representation of such subgroups within the overall population burden of SCD, indicated by the absolute number of events ("events per year"), is relatively small. The requirements for achieving a major population impact are effective prevention of underlying diseases and/or new epidemiologic probes that will allow better resolution of specific high-risk subgroups within the large general populations.

Strategies for predicting and preventing SCD are classified as primary and secondary. *Primary prevention*, as defined in various implantable defibrillator trials, refers to the attempt to identify individual patients at specific risk for SCD and institute preventive strategies. *Secondary prevention* refers to measures taken to prevent recurrent cardiac arrest or death in individuals who have survived a previous cardiac arrest. A third category consists of interventions intended to abort sudden cardiac arrests, thus avoiding their progression to death. This focuses primarily on out-of-hospital response strategies.

The primary prevention strategies currently used depend on the magnitude of risk among the various population subgroups. Because the annual incidence of SCD among the unselected adult population is limited to 1–2 per 1000 population per year (Fig. 29-1) and >30% of all SCDs due to coronary artery disease occur as the first clinical manifestation of the disease (Fig. 29-2A), the only currently practical strategies are profiling for risk of developing CHD and risk factor control (Fig. 29-2B). The most powerful long-term risk factors include age, cigarette smoking, elevated serum cholesterol, diabetes mellitus, elevated blood pressure, LV hypertrophy, and nonspecific electrocardiographic abnormalities. Markers of inflammation (e.g., levels of

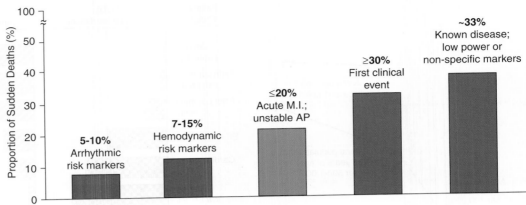

Target	Examples	Goal	Sensitivity
• ASHD risk factors	• Framingham risk index	• Predict evolution of disease	• Very low
• Anatomic screening	• CT imaging	• Identify CAD	• Moderate for anatomy
• Clinical markers	• EF; angiography	• Define extent of disease	• High for extent of disease; variable for specificity of risk
	• AM; EPS	• Identify arrhythmia markers	• Low-to-intermediate for screening
	• History of heart failure	• Define high risk subgroups	• High for specific groups
• Transient risk predictors	• EP and hemodynamic variations	• Clinical markers of instability	• Primary predictive value unknown
	• Autonomic fluctuations	• Quantify autonomic triggers	• Uncertain; some measures useful (?)
	• Predictors of ischemia	• Predict unstable plaques	• Unknown; potentially high
• Individual risk predictors	• Familial/genetic profiles	• Predict specific SCD risk before disease expression	• High potential for future profiling

FIGURE 29-2

Population subsets, risk predictors, and distribution of sudden cardiac deaths (SCDs) according to clinical circumstances. A. The population subset with high-risk arrhythmia markers in conjunction with low ejection fraction is a group at high risk of SCD but accounts for <10% of the total SCD burden attributable to coronary artery disease. In contrast, nearly two-thirds of all SCD victims present with SCD as the first and only manifestation of underlying disease or have known disease but are considered relatively low risk because of the absence of high-risk markers. **B.** Risk profile for prediction and prevention of SCD is difficult. The highest absolute numbers of

events occur among the general population who may have risk factors for coronary heart disease or expressions of disease that do not predict high risk. This results in a low sensitivity for predicting and preventing SCD. New approaches that include epidemiologic modeling of transient risk factors and methods of predicting individual patient risk offer hope for greater sensitivity in the future. AP, angina pectoris; ASHD, arteriosclerotic heart disease; CAD, coronary artery disease; EPS, electrophysiologic study; HRV, heart rate variability. (*Modified from Myerburg RJ: J Cardiovasc Electrophysiol 2001; 12:369–381, reproduced with permission of the publisher.*)

C-reactive protein) that may predict plaque destabilization have been added to risk classifications. The presence of multiple risk factors progressively increases incidence, but not sufficiently or specifically enough to warrant therapies targeted to potentially fatal arrhythmias (Fig. 29-1A). However, recent studies offer the hope that genetic markers for specific risk may become available. These studies suggest that a family history of SCD associated with acute coronary syndromes predicts a higher likelihood of cardiac arrest as the initial manifestation of coronary artery disease in first-degree family members.

After coronary artery disease has been identified in a patient, additional strategies for risk profiling become available (Fig. 29-2B), but the majority of SCDs occur among the large unselected groups rather than in the

specific high-risk subgroups that become evident among populations with established disease (compare events per year with percent per year in Fig. 29-1B). After a major cardiovascular event, such as acute coronary syndromes, recent onset of heart failure, and survival after out-of-hospital cardiac arrest, the highest risk of death occurs during the initial 6–18 months after the event and then plateaus toward the baseline risk associated with the extent of underlying disease. However, many of the early deaths are nonsudden, diluting the potential benefit of strategies targeted specifically to SCD. Thus, although post-MI beta-blocker therapy has an identifiable benefit for both early SCD and nonsudden mortality risk, a total mortality benefit for ICD therapy early after MI has not been observed.

Among patients in the acute, convalescent, and chronic phases of myocardial infarction (Chap. 35), subgroups at high absolute risk of SCD can be identified. During the acute phase, the potential risk of cardiac arrest from onset through the first 48 h may be as high as 15%, emphasizing the importance for patients to respond promptly to the onset of symptoms. Those who survive acute-phase VF, however, are not at continuing risk for recurrent cardiac arrest indexed to that event. During the convalescent phase after MI (3 days to ~6 weeks), an episode of sustained ventricular tachycardia (VT) or VF, which is usually associated with a large infarct, predicts a natural history mortality risk of >25% at 12 months. At least one-half of the deaths are sudden. Aggressive intervention techniques may reduce this incidence.

After passage into the chronic phase of MI, the longer-term risk for total mortality and SCD mortality is predicted by a number of factors (Fig. 29-2B). The most important for both SCD and nonsudden death is the extent of myocardial damage sustained as a result of the acute MI. This is measured by the magnitude of reduction of the ejection fraction (EF) and/ or the occurrence of heart failure. Various studies have demonstrated that ventricular arrhythmias identified by ambulatory monitoring contribute significantly to this risk, especially in patients with an EF <40%. In addition, inducibility of VT or VF during electrophysiologic testing of patients who have ambient ventricular arrhythmias (premature ventricular contractions [PVCs] and nonsustained VT) and an EF <35 or 40% is a strong predictor of SCD risk. Patients in this subgroup are now considered candidates for implantable cardioverter defibrillators (ICDs) (see later). Risk falls off sharply with EFs >40% after MI and the absence of ambient arrhythmias and conversely is high with EFs <30% even without the ambient arrhythmia markers.

The cardiomyopathies (dilated and hypertrophic, Chap. 21) are the second most common category of diseases associated with risk of SCD, after CHD (Table 29-2). Some risk factors have been identified, largely related to extent of disease, documented ventricular arrhythmias, and symptoms of arrhythmias (e.g., syncope). The less common causes of SCD include valvular heart disease (primarily aortic) and inflammatory and infiltrative disorders of the myocardium. The latter include viral myocarditis, sarcoidosis, and amyloidosis.

Among adolescents and young adults, rare inherited disorders such as hypertrophic cardiomyopathy, the long QT interval syndromes, right ventricular dysplasia, and Brugada syndrome have received attention as important causes of SCD because of advances in genetics and the ability to identify some of those at risk before a fatal event. The subgroup of young competitive athletes has received special attention. The incidence of SCD among athletes appears to be higher than it is for the general adolescent and young adult population, perhaps up to 1 in 75,000. Hypertrophic cardiomyopathy (Chap. 21) is the most common cause in the United States, compared with Italy, where more comprehensive screening programs remove potential victims from the population of athletes.

Secondary prevention strategies should be applied to surviving victims of a cardiac arrest that was not associated with an acute MI or a transient risk of SCD (e.g., drug exposures, correctable electrolyte imbalances). Multivessel coronary artery disease and dilated cardiomyopathy, especially with markedly reduced left ventricular EF predict a 1- to 2-year risk of recurrence of an SCD or cardiac arrest of up to 30% in the absence of specific interventions (see later). The presence of life-threatening arrhythmias with long QT syndromes or right ventricular dysplasia are also associated with increased risks.

CLINICAL CHARACTERISTICS OF CARDIAC ARREST

PRODROME, ONSET, ARREST, DEATH

SCD may be presaged by days to months of increasing angina, dyspnea, palpitations, easy fatigability, and other nonspecific complaints. However, these *prodromal symptoms* are generally predictive of any major cardiac event; they are not specific for predicting SCD.

The *onset of the clinical transition*, leading to cardiac arrest, is defined as an acute change in cardiovascular status preceding cardiac arrest by up to 1 h. When the onset is instantaneous or abrupt, the probability that the arrest is cardiac in origin is >95%. Continuous electrocardiographic (ECG) recordings fortuitously obtained at the onset of a cardiac arrest commonly demonstrate changes in cardiac electrical activity during the minutes or hours before the event. There is a tendency for the heart rate to increase and for advanced grades of PVCs to evolve. Most cardiac arrests that are caused by VF begin with a run of nonsustained or sustained VT, which then degenerates into VF.

The probability of achieving successful resuscitation from cardiac arrest is related to the interval from onset of loss of circulation to institution of resuscitative efforts, the setting in which the event occurs, the mechanism (VF, VT, PEA, asystole), and the clinical status of the patient before the cardiac arrest. Return of circulation and survival rates as a result of defibrillation decrease almost linearly from the first minute to 10 min. After 5 min, survival rates are no better than 25–30% in out-of-hospital settings. Those settings in which it is possible to institute prompt cardiopulmonary resuscitation (CPR) followed by prompt defibrillation provide a better chance of a successful outcome. However, the outcome in intensive care units and other in-hospital environments is heavily influenced by the patient's preceding clinical status. The immediate outcome is good for cardiac arrest occurring in the intensive care unit in the presence of an acute cardiac event or transient metabolic disturbance, but survival among patients with far-advanced chronic cardiac disease or advanced noncardiac diseases (e.g., renal failure, pneumonia, sepsis, diabetes, cancer) is low and not much better in the in-hospital than in the out-of-hospital setting. Survival from unexpected cardiac arrest in unmonitored areas in a hospital is not much better than that it is for witnessed out-of-hospital arrests. Since implementation of community response systems, survival from out-of-hospital cardiac arrest has improved although it still remains low, under most circumstances. Survival probabilities in public sites exceed those in the home environment.

The success rate for initial resuscitation and survival to hospital discharge after an out-of-hospital cardiac arrest depends heavily on the mechanism of the event. When the mechanism is pulseless VT, the outcome is best; VF is the next most successful; and asystole and PEA generate dismal outcome statistics. Advanced age also adversely influences the chances of successful resuscitation.

Progression to biologic death is a function of the mechanism of cardiac arrest and the length of the delay before interventions. VF or asystole without CPR within the first 4–6 min has a poor outcome even if defibrillation is successful because of superimposed brain damage; there are few survivors among patients who had no life support activities for the first 8 min after onset. Outcome statistics are improved by lay bystander intervention (basic life support—see later) before definitive interventions (advanced life support) especially when followed by early successful defibrillation. In regard to the latter, evaluations of deployment of automatic external defibrillators (AEDs) in communities (e.g., police vehicles, large buildings, airports, and stadiums) are beginning to generate encouraging data. Increased deployment is to be encouraged.

Death during the hospitalization after a successfully resuscitated cardiac arrest relates closely to the severity of central nervous system injury. Anoxic encephalopathy and infections subsequent to prolonged respirator dependence account for 60% of the deaths. Another 30% occur as a consequence of low cardiac output states that fail to respond to interventions. Recurrent arrhythmias are the least common cause of death, accounting for only 10% of in-hospital deaths.

In the setting of acute MI (Chap. 35), it is important to distinguish between primary and secondary cardiac arrests. *Primary cardiac arrests* are those which occur in the absence of hemodynamic instability, and *secondary cardiac arrests* are those which occur in patients in whom abnormal hemodynamics dominate the clinical picture before

cardiac arrest. The success rate for immediate resuscitation in primary cardiac arrest during acute MI in a monitored setting should exceed 90%. In contrast, as many as 70% of patients with secondary cardiac arrest succumb immediately or during the same hospitalization.

<hr>

TREATMENT   **Cardiac Arrest**

An individual who collapses suddenly is managed in five stages: (1) initial evaluation and basic life support if arrest is confirmed, (2) public access defibrillation (when available), (3) advanced life support, (4) postresuscitation care, and (5) long-term management. The initial response, including confirmation of loss of circulation, followed by basic life support and public access defibrillation, can be carried out by physicians, nurses, paramedical personnel, and trained laypersons. There is a requirement for increasingly specialized skills as the patient moves through the stages of advanced life support, postresuscitation care, and long-term management.

INITIAL EVALUATION AND BASIC LIFE SUPPORT Confirmation that a sudden collapse is indeed due to a cardiac arrest includes prompt observations of the state of consciousness, respiratory movements, skin color, and the presence or absence of pulses in the carotid or femoral arteries. For lay responders, the pulse check is no longer recommended. As soon as a cardiac arrest is suspected, confirmed, or even considered to be impending, calling an emergency rescue system (e.g., 911) is the immediate priority. With the development of AEDs that are easily used by nonconventional emergency responders, an additional layer for response has evolved (see later).

Agonal respiratory movements may persist for a short time after the onset of cardiac arrest, but it is important to observe for severe stridor with a persistent pulse as a clue to aspiration of a foreign body or food. If this is suspected, a Heimlich maneuver (see later) may dislodge the obstructing body. A precordial blow, or "thump," delivered firmly with a clenched fist to the junction of the middle and lower thirds of the sternum may occasionally revert VT or VF, but there is concern about converting VT to VF. Therefore, it is recommended to use precordial thumps as a life support technique only when monitoring and defibrillation are available. This conservative application of the technique remains controversial.

The third action during the initial response is to clear the airway. The head is tilted back and the chin lifted so that the oropharynx can be explored to clear the airway. Dentures or foreign bodies are removed, and the Heimlich maneuver is performed if there is reason to suspect that a foreign body is lodged in the oropharynx. If respiratory arrest precipitating cardiac arrest is suspected, a second precordial thump is delivered after the airway is cleared.

Basic life support, more popularly known as CPR, is intended to maintain organ perfusion until definitive interventions can be instituted. The elements of CPR are the maintenance of ventilation of the lungs and compression of the chest. Mouth-to-mouth respiration may be used if no specific rescue equipment is immediately available (e.g., plastic oropharyngeal airways, esophageal obturators, masked Ambu bag). Conventional ventilation techniques during single-responder CPR require that the lungs be inflated twice in succession after every 30 chest compressions. Recent data suggest that interrupting chest compressions to perform mouth-to-mouth respiration may be less effective than a continuous chest compression strategy.

Chest compression is based on the assumption that cardiac compression allows the heart to maintain a pump function by sequential filling and emptying of its chambers, with competent valves maintaining forward direction of flow. The palm of one hand is placed over the lower sternum, with the heel of the other resting on the dorsum of the lower hand. The sternum is depressed, with the arms remaining straight, at a rate of approximately 100 per min. Sufficient force is applied to depress the sternum 4–5 cm, and relaxation is abrupt.

AUTOMATED EXTERNAL DEFIBRILLATION (AED)

AEDs that are easily used by nonconventional responders, such as nonparamedic firefighters, police officers, ambulance drivers, trained security guards, and minimally trained or untrained laypersons, have been developed. This advance has inserted another level of response into the cardiac arrest paradigm. A number of studies have demonstrated that AED use by nonconventional responders in strategic response systems and public access lay responders can improve cardiac arrest survival rates. This strategy is based on shortening the time to the first defibrillation attempt while awaiting the arrival of advanced life support.

ADVANCED CARDIAC LIFE SUPPORT (ACLS)

ACLS is intended to achieve adequate ventilation, control cardiac arrhythmias, stabilize blood pressure and cardiac output, and restore organ perfusion. The activities carried out to achieve these goals include (1) defibrillation/cardioversion and/or pacing, (2) intubation with an endotracheal tube, and (3) insertion of an intravenous line. The speed with which defibrillation/cardioversion is achieved is an important element in successful resuscitation, both for restoration of spontaneous circulation and for protection of the central nervous system. Immediate defibrillation should precede intubation and insertion of an intravenous line; CPR should be carried out while the defibrillator

is being charged. As soon as a diagnosis of VF or VT is established, a shock of at least 300 J should be delivered when one is using a monophasic waveform device or 120–150 J with a biphasic waveform. Additional shocks are escalated to a maximum of 360 J monophasic (200 J biphasic) if the initial shock does not successfully revert VT or VF. However, it is now recommended that five cycles of CPR be carried out before repeated shocks, if the first shock fails to restore an organized rhythm, or 60–90 s of CPR before the first shock if 5 min has elapsed between the onset of cardiac arrest and ability to deliver a shock (see 2005 update of guidelines for cardiopulmonary resuscitation and emergency cardiac care at *http://circ.ahajournals.org/content/vol112/24_suppl.toc*).

Epinephrine, 1 mg intravenously, is given after failed defibrillation, and attempts to defibrillate are repeated. The dose of epinephrine may be repeated after intervals of 3–5 min (Fig. 29-3A). Vasopressin (a single 40-unit dose given IV) has been suggested as an alternative to epinephrine.

If the patient is less than fully conscious upon reversion or if two or three attempts fail, prompt intubation, ventilation, and arterial blood gas analysis should be carried out. Ventilation with O_2 (room air if O_2 is not immediately available) may promptly reverse hypoxemia and acidosis. A patient who is persistently acidotic after successful defibrillation and intubation should be given 1 meq/kg $NaHCO_3$ initially and an additional 50% of the dose repeated every 10–15 min. However, it should not be used routinely.

After initial unsuccessful defibrillation attempts or with persistent/recurrent electrical instability, antiarrhythmic therapy should be instituted. Intravenous amiodarone has emerged as the initial treatment of choice (150 mg over 10 min, followed by 1 mg/min for up to 6 h and 0.5 mg/min thereafter) (Fig. 29-3A). For cardiac arrest due to VF in the early phase of an acute coronary syndrome, a bolus of 1 mg/kg of lidocaine may be given intravenously as an alternative, and the dose may be repeated in 2 min. It also may be tried in patients in whom amiodarone is unsuccessful. Intravenous procainamide (loading infusion of 100 mg/5 min to a total dose of 500–800 mg, followed by continuous infusion at 2–5 mg/min) is now rarely used in this setting but may be tried for persisting, hemodynamically stable arrhythmias. Intravenous calcium gluconate is no longer considered safe or necessary for routine administration. It is used only in patients in whom acute hyperkalemia is known to be the triggering event for resistant VF, in the presence of known hypocalcemia, or in patients who have received toxic doses of calcium channel antagonists.

Cardiac arrest due to bradyarrhythmias or asystole (B/A cardiac arrest) is managed differently (Fig. 29-3B). The patient is promptly intubated, CPR is continued, and an attempt is made to control hypoxemia and acidosis.

CHAPTER 29 Cardiovascular Collapse, Cardiac Arrest, and Sudden Cardiac Death

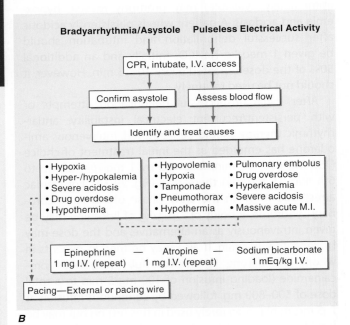

VENTRICULAR FIBRILLATION OR PULSELESS VENTRICULAR TACHYCARDIA

Immediate defibrillation within 5 minutes of onset; 60-90 seconds of CPR before defibrillation for delay ≥5 minutes

If return of circulation fails

5 cycles of CPR followed by repeat shock; repeat sequence twice if needed

If return of circulation fails

Continue CPR, Intubate, I.V. Access

Epinephrine, 1 mg I.V. -or- Vasopressin, 40 units I.V; follow with repeat defibrillation at maximum energy within 30-60 seconds as required; repeat epinephrine

If return of circulation fails

Epinephrine, ↑ dose | Antiarrhythmics | NaHCO₃, 1 mEq/kg (↑ K⁺)

Amiodarone: 150 mg over 10 min, 1 mg/min
Lidocaine: 1.5 mg/kg; repeat in 3-5 min

Magnesium sulfate: 1-2 gm I.V. (polymorphic VT)
Procainamide: 30 mg/min, to 17 mg/kg (limited use-see text)

If return of circulation fails

Defibrillate, CPR: Drug –Shock –Drug –Shock

A

Bradyarrhythmia/Asystole   Pulseless Electrical Activity

CPR, intubate, I.V. access

Confirm asystole | Assess blood flow

Identify and treat causes

- Hypoxia
- Hyper-/hypokalemia
- Severe acidosis
- Drug overdose
- Hypothermia

- Hypovolemia
- Hypoxia
- Tamponade
- Pneumothorax
- Hypothermia

- Pulmonary embolus
- Drug overdose
- Hyperkalemia
- Severe acidosis
- Massive acute M.I.

Epinephrine — Atropine — Sodium bicarbonate
1 mg I.V. (repeat) 1 mg I.V. (repeat) 1 mEq/kg I.V.

Pacing—External or pacing wire

B

FIGURE 29-3

A. **The algorithm of ventricular fibrillation** or pulseless ventricular tachycardia begins with defibrillation attempts. If that fails, it is followed by epinephrine and then antiarrhythmic drugs. See text for details. ***B.*** **The algorithms for bradyarrhythmia/asystole** (*left*) or pulseless electrical activity (*right*) are dominated first by continued life support and a search for reversible causes. Subsequent therapy is nonspecific and is accompanied by a low success rate. See text for details. CPR, cardiopulmonary resuscitation; MI, myocardial infarction.

Epinephrine and/or atropine are given intravenously or by an intracardiac route. External pacing devices are used to attempt to establish a regular rhythm. The success rate may be good when B/A arrest is due to acute inferior wall myocardial infarction or to correctable airway obstruction or drug-induced respiratory depression or with prompt resuscitation efforts. For acute airway obstruction, prompt removal of foreign bodies by the Heimlich maneuver or, in hospitalized patients, by intubation and suctioning of obstructing secretions in the airway is often successful. The prognosis is generally very poor in other causes of this form of cardiac arrest, such as end-stage cardiac or noncardiac diseases. Treatment of PEA is similar to that for bradyarrhythmias, but its outcome is also dismal.

POSTRESUSCITATION CARE This phase of management is determined by the clinical setting of the cardiac arrest. *Primary VF* in acute MI (not accompanied by low-output states) (Chap. 35) is generally very responsive to life support techniques and easily controlled after the initial event. In the in-hospital setting, respirator support is usually not necessary or is needed for only a short time, and hemodynamics stabilize promptly after defibrillation or cardioversion. In *secondary VF* in acute MI (those events in which hemodynamic abnormalities predispose to the potentially fatal arrhythmia), resuscitative efforts are less often successful, and in patients who are successfully resuscitated, the recurrence rate is high. The clinical picture and outcome are dominated by hemodynamic instability and the ability to control hemodynamic dysfunction. Bradyarrhythmias, asystole, and PEA are commonly secondary events in hemodynamically unstable patients. The in-hospital phase of care of an out-of-hospital cardiac arrest survivor is dictated by specific clinical circumstances. The most difficult is the presence of anoxic encephalopathy, which is a strong predictor of in-hospital death. A recent addition to the management of this condition is induced hypothermia to reduce metabolic demands and cerebral edema.

The outcome after in-hospital cardiac arrest associated with noncardiac diseases is poor, and in the few successfully resuscitated patients, the postresuscitation course is dominated by the nature of the underlying disease. Patients with end-stage cancer, renal failure, acute central nervous system disease, and uncontrolled infections, as a group, have a survival rate of <10% after in-hospital cardiac arrest. Some major exceptions are patients with transient airway obstruction, electrolyte disturbances, proarrhythmic effects of drugs, and severe metabolic abnormalities, most of whom may have a good chance of survival if they can be resuscitated promptly and stabilized while the transient abnormalities are being corrected.

LONG-TERM MANAGEMENT AFTER SURVIVAL OF OUT-OF-HOSPITAL CARDIAC ARREST Patients who survive cardiac arrest without irreversible damage to the central nervous system and who achieve hemodynamic stability should have diagnostic testing to define appropriate therapeutic interventions for their long-term management. This aggressive approach is driven by the fact that survival after out-of-hospital cardiac arrest is followed by a 10–25% mortality rate during the first 2 years after the event, and there are data suggesting that significant survival benefits can be achieved by prescription of an implantable cardioverter-defibrillator (ICD).

Among patients in whom an acute ST elevation MI, or transient and reversible myocardial ischemia, is identified as the specific mechanism triggering an out-of-hospital cardiac arrest, the management is dictated in part by the transient nature of life-threatening arrhythmia risk during the acute coronary syndrome (ACS) and in part by the extent of permanent myocardial damage that results. Cardiac arrest during the acute ischemic phase is not an ICD indication, but survivors of cardiac arrest not associated with an ACS do benefit. In addition, patients who survive MI with an ejection fraction less than 30–35% appear to benefit from ICDs.

For patients with cardiac arrest determined to be due to a treatable transient ischemic mechanism, particularly with higher EFs, catheter interventional, surgical, and/or pharmacologic anti-ischemic therapy is generally accepted for long-term management.

Survivors of cardiac arrest due to other categories of disease, such as the hypertrophic or dilated cardiomyopathies and the various rare inherited disorders (e.g., right ventricular dysplasia, long QT syndrome, Brugada syndrome, catecholaminergic polymorphic VT, and so-called idiopathic VF), are all considered ICD candidates.

PREVENTION OF SCD IN HIGH-RISK INDIVIDUALS WITHOUT PRIOR CARDIAC ARREST

Post-MI patients with EFs <35% and other markers of risk such as ambient ventricular arrhythmias, inducible ventricular tachyarrhythmias in the electrophysiology laboratory, and a history of heart failure are considered candidates for ICDs 30 days or more after the MI. Total mortality benefits in the range of a 20–35% reduction over 2–5 years have been observed in a series of clinical trials. One study suggested that an EF <30% was a sufficient marker of risk to indicate ICD benefit, and another demonstrated benefit for patients with Functional Class 2 or 3 heart failure and ejection fractions ≤35%, regardless of etiology (ischemic or nonischemic) or the presence of ambient or induced arrhythmias (see Chaps. 16 and 17). There appears to be a gradient of increasing ICD benefit with EFs ranging lower than the threshold indications. However, patients with very low EFs (e.g., <20%) may receive less benefit.

Decision making for primary prevention in disorders other than coronary artery disease and dilated cardiomyopathy is generally driven by observational data and judgment based on clinical observations. Controlled clinical trials providing evidence-based indicators for ICDs are lacking for these smaller population subgroups. In general, for the rare disorders listed earlier, indicators of arrhythmic risk such as syncope, documented ventricular tachyarrhythmias, aborted cardiac arrest or a family history of premature SCD in some conditions, and a number of other clinical or ECG markers may be used as indicators for ICDs.

CHAPTER 29

Cardiovascular Collapse, Cardiac Arrest, and Sudden Cardiac Death

SECTION V

DISORDERS OF THE VASCULATURE

CHAPTER 30

THE PATHOGENESIS, PREVENTION, AND TREATMENT OF ATHEROSCLEROSIS

Peter Libby

PATHOGENESIS

Atherosclerosis remains the major cause of death and premature disability in developed societies. Moreover, current predictions estimate that by the year 2020 cardiovascular diseases, notably atherosclerosis, will become the leading global cause of total disease burden. Although many generalized or systemic risk factors predispose to its development, atherosclerosis affects various regions of the circulation preferentially and has distinct clinical manifestations that depend on the particular circulatory bed affected. Atherosclerosis of the coronary arteries commonly causes myocardial infarction (MI) (Chap. 35) and angina pectoris (Chap. 33). Atherosclerosis of the arteries supplying the central nervous system frequently provokes strokes and transient cerebral ischemia. In the peripheral circulation, atherosclerosis causes intermittent claudication and gangrene and can jeopardize limb viability. Involvement of the splanchnic circulation can cause mesenteric ischemia. Atherosclerosis can affect the kidneys either directly (e.g., renal artery stenosis) or as a common site of atheroembolic disease (Chap. 38).

Even within a particular arterial bed, stenoses due to atherosclerosis tend to occur focally, typically in certain predisposed regions. In the coronary circulation, for example, the proximal left anterior descending coronary artery exhibits a particular predilection for developing atherosclerotic disease. Similarly, atherosclerosis preferentially affects the proximal portions of the renal arteries and, in the extracranial circulation to the brain, the carotid bifurcation. Indeed, atherosclerotic lesions often form at branching points of arteries which are regions of disturbed blood flow. Not all manifestations of atherosclerosis result from stenotic, occlusive disease. Ectasia and the development of aneurysmal disease, for example, frequently occur in the aorta (Chap. 38). In addition to focal, flow-limiting stenoses, nonocclusive intimal atherosclerosis also occurs diffusely in affected arteries, as shown by intravascular ultrasound and postmortem studies.

Atherogenesis in humans typically occurs over a period of many years, usually many decades. Growth of atherosclerotic plaques probably does not occur in a smooth, linear fashion but discontinuously, with periods of relative quiescence punctuated by periods of rapid evolution. After a generally prolonged "silent" period, atherosclerosis may become clinically manifest. The clinical expressions of atherosclerosis may be *chronic*, as in the development of stable, effort-induced angina pectoris or predictable and reproducible intermittent claudication. Alternatively, a dramatic *acute* clinical event such as MI, stroke, or sudden cardiac death may first herald the presence of atherosclerosis. Other individuals may never experience clinical manifestations of arterial disease despite the presence of widespread atherosclerosis demonstrated postmortem.

INITIATION OF ATHEROSCLEROSIS

An integrated view of experimental results in animals and studies of human atherosclerosis suggests that the "fatty streak" represents the initial lesion of atherosclerosis. These early lesions most often seem to arise from focal increases in the content of lipoproteins within regions of the intima. This accumulation of lipoprotein particles may not result simply from increased permeability, or "leakiness," of the overlying endothelium (Fig. 30-1). Rather, the lipoproteins may collect in the intima of arteries because they bind to constituents of the extracellular matrix, increasing the residence time of the lipid-rich particles within the arterial wall.

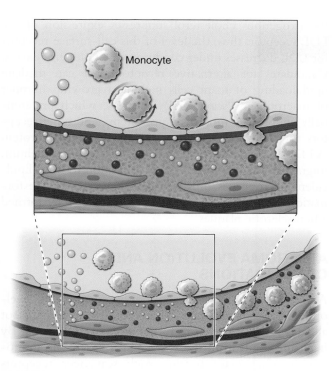

FIGURE 30-1

Cross-sectional view of an artery depicting steps in development of an atheroma, from left to right. The *upper panel* shows a detail of the boxed area below. The endothelial monolayer overlying the intima contacts blood. Hypercholesterolemia promotes accumulation of LDL particles (*light spheres*) in the intima. The lipoprotein particles often associate with constituents of the extracellular matrix, notably proteoglycans. Sequestration within the intima separates lipoproteins from some plasma antioxidants and favors oxidative modification. Such modified lipoprotein particles (*darker spheres*) may trigger a local inflammatory response that signals subsequent steps in lesion formation. The augmented expression of various adhesion molecules for leukocytes recruits monocytes to the site of a nascent arterial lesion.

Once adherent, some white blood cells migrate into the intima. The directed migration of leukocytes probably depends on chemoattractant factors, including modified lipoprotein particles themselves and chemoattractant cytokines (depicted by the smaller spheres), such as the chemokine macrophage chemoattractant protein-1 produced by vascular wall cells in response to modified lipoproteins. Leukocytes in the evolving fatty streak can divide and exhibit augmented expression of receptors for modified lipoproteins (scavenger receptors). These mononuclear phagocytes ingest lipids and become foam cells, represented by a cytoplasm filled with lipid droplets. As the fatty streak evolves into a more complicated atherosclerotic lesion, smooth-muscle cells migrate from the media (*bottom of lower panel hairline*) through the internal elastic membrane (*solid wavy line*) and accumulate within the expanding intima, where they lay down extracellular matrix that forms the bulk of the advanced lesion (*bottom panel, right side*).

Lipoproteins that accumulate in the extracellular space of the intima of arteries often associate with glycosaminoglycans of the arterial extracellular matrix, an interaction that may slow the egress of these lipid-rich particles from the intima. Lipoprotein particles in the extracellular space of the intima, particularly those retained by binding to matrix macromolecules, may undergo oxidative modifications. Considerable evidence supports a pathogenic role for products of oxidized lipoproteins in atherogenesis. Lipoproteins sequestered from plasma antioxidants in the extracellular space of the intima become particularly susceptible to oxidative modification, giving rise to hydroperoxides, lysophospholipids, oxysterols, and aldehydic breakdown products of fatty acids and phospholipids. Modifications of the apoprotein moieties may include breaks in the peptide backbone as well as derivatization of certain amino acid residues. Local production of hypochlorous acid by myeloperoxidase associated with inflammatory cells within the plaque yields chlorinated species such as chlorotyrosyl moieties. High-density lipoprotein (HDL) particles modified by HOCl-mediated chlorination function poorly as cholesterol acceptors, a finding that links oxidative stress with impaired reverse cholesterol transport, which is one likely mechanism of the antiatherogenic action of HDL (see later). Considerable evidence supports the presence of such oxidation products in atherosclerotic lesions. A particular member of the phospholipase family, lipoprotein-associated phospholipase A_2 (LpPL A_2), can generate proinflammatory lipids, including lysophosphatidyl choline-bearing oxidized lipid moieties from oxidized phospholipids found in oxidized low-density lipoproteins (LDLs). An inhibitor of this enzyme is in clinical development.

Leukocyte recruitment

Accumulation of leukocytes characterizes the formation of early atherosclerotic lesions (Fig. 30-1). Thus, from its very inception, atherogenesis involves elements of inflammation, a process that now provides a unifying theme in the pathogenesis of this disease. The inflammatory cell types typically found in the evolving atheroma include monocyte-derived macrophages and lymphocytes. A number of adhesion molecules or receptors for leukocytes expressed on the surface of the arterial endothelial cell probably participate in the recruitment of leukocytes to the nascent atheroma. Constituents of oxidatively modified low-density lipoprotein can augment the expression of leukocyte adhesion molecules. This example illustrates how the accumulation of lipoproteins in the arterial intima may link mechanistically with leukocyte recruitment, a key event in lesion formation.

Laminar shear forces such as those encountered in most regions of normal arteries also can suppress the expression of leukocyte adhesion molecules. Sites of predilection for atherosclerotic lesions (e.g., branch points) often have disturbed flow. Ordered, pulsatile laminar shear of normal blood flow augments the production of nitric oxide by endothelial cells. This molecule, in addition to its vasodilator properties, can act at the low levels constitutively produced by arterial endothelium as a local anti-inflammatory autacoid, e.g., limiting local adhesion molecule expression. Exposure of endothelial cells to laminar shear stress increases the transcription of Krüppel-like factor 2 (KLF2) and reduces the expression of a thioredoxin-interacting protein (Txnip) that inhibits the activity of the endogenous antioxidant thioredoxin. KLF2 augments the activity of endothelial nitric oxide synthase, and reduced Txnip levels boost the function of thioredoxin. Laminar shear stress also stimulates endothelial cells to produce superoxide dismutase, an antioxidant enzyme. These examples indicate how hemodynamic forces may influence the cellular events that underlie atherosclerotic lesion initiation and potentially explain the favored localization of atherosclerotic lesions at sites that experience disturbance to laminar shear stress.

Once captured on the surface of the arterial endothelial cell by adhesion receptors, the monocytes and lymphocytes penetrate the endothelial layer and take up residence in the intima. In addition to products of modified lipoproteins, cytokines (protein mediators of inflammation) can regulate the expression of adhesion molecules involved in leukocyte recruitment. For example, interleukin 1 (IL-1) or tumor necrosis factor α (TNF-α) induce or augment the expression of leukocyte adhesion molecules on endothelial cells. Because products of lipoprotein oxidation can induce cytokine release from vascular wall cells, this pathway may provide an additional link between arterial accumulation of lipoproteins and leukocyte recruitment. Chemoattractant cytokines such as monocyte chemoattractant protein 1 appear to direct the migration of leukocytes into the arterial wall.

Foam-cell formation

Once resident within the intima, the mononuclear phagocytes mature into macrophages and become lipid-laden foam cells, a conversion that requires the uptake of lipoprotein particles by receptor-mediated endocytosis. One might suppose that the well-recognized "classic" receptor for LDL mediates this lipid uptake; however, humans or animals lacking effective LDL receptors due to genetic alterations (e.g., familial hypercholesterolemia) have abundant arterial lesions and extraarterial xanthomata rich in macrophage-derived foam cells. In addition,

the exogenous cholesterol suppresses expression of the LDL receptor; thus, the level of this cell-surface receptor for LDL decreases under conditions of cholesterol excess. Candidates for alternative receptors that can mediate lipid loading of foam cells include a growing number of macrophage "scavenger" receptors, which preferentially endocytose modified lipoproteins, and other receptors for oxidized LDL or very low-density lipoprotein (VLDL). Monocyte attachment to the endothelium, migration into the intima, and maturation to form lipid-laden macrophages thus represent key steps in the formation of the fatty streak, the precursor of fully formed atherosclerotic plaques.

ATHEROMA EVOLUTION AND COMPLICATIONS

Although the fatty streak commonly precedes the development of a more advanced atherosclerotic plaque, not all fatty streaks progress to form complex atheromata. By ingesting lipids from the extracellular space, the mononuclear phagocytes bearing such scavenger receptors may remove lipoproteins from the developing lesion. Some lipid-laden macrophages may leave the artery wall, exporting lipid in the process. Lipid accumulation, and hence the propensity to form an atheroma, ensues if the amount of lipid entering the artery wall exceeds that removed by mononuclear phagocytes or other pathways.

Export by phagocytes may constitute one response to local lipid overload in the evolving lesion. Another mechanism, reverse cholesterol transport mediated by high-density lipoproteins, probably provides an independent pathway for lipid removal from atheroma. This transfer of cholesterol from the cell to the HDL particle involves specialized cell-surface molecules such as the ATP binding cassette (ABC) transporters. *ABCA1*, the gene mutated in Tangier disease, a condition characterized by very low HDL levels, transfers cholesterol from cells to nascent HDL particles and ABCG1 to mature HDL particles. "Reverse cholesterol transport" mediated by these ABC transporters allows HDL loaded with cholesterol to deliver it to hepatocytes by binding to scavenger receptor B 1 or other receptors. The liver cell can metabolize the sterol to bile acids that can be excreted. This export pathway from macrophage foam cells to peripheral cells such as hepatocytes explains part of the antiatherogenic action of HDLs. (Anti-inflammatory and antioxidant properties also may contribute to the atheroprotective effects of HDLs.) Thus, macrophages may play a vital role in the dynamic economy of lipid accumulation in the arterial wall during atherogenesis.

Some lipid-laden foam cells within the expanding intimal lesion perish. Some foam cells may die as a result of programmed cell death, or *apoptosis*. This death of mononuclear phagocytes results in the formation of the lipid-rich center, often called the *necrotic core*, in established atherosclerotic plaques. Macrophages loaded with modified lipoproteins may elaborate cytokines and growth factors that can further signal some of the cellular events in lesion complication. Whereas accumulation of lipid-laden macrophages characterizes the fatty streak, buildup of fibrous tissue formed by extracellular matrix typifies the more advanced atherosclerotic lesion. The smooth-muscle cell synthesizes the bulk of the extracellular matrix of the complex atherosclerotic lesion. A number of growth factors or cytokines elaborated by mononuclear phagocytes can stimulate smooth-muscle cell proliferation and production of extracellular matrix. Cytokines found in the plaque, including IL-1 and TNF-α, can induce local production of growth factors, including forms of platelet-derived growth factor (PDGF), fibroblast growth factors, and others, which may contribute to plaque evolution and complication. Other cytokines, notably interferon γ (IFN-γ) derived from activated T cells within lesions, can limit the synthesis of interstitial forms of collagen by smooth-muscle cells. These examples illustrate how atherogenesis involves a complex mix of mediators that in the balance determines the characteristics of particular lesions.

The arrival of smooth-muscle cells and their elaboration of extracellular matrix probably provide a critical transition, yielding a fibrofatty lesion in place of a simple accumulation of macrophage-derived foam cells. For example, PDGF elaborated by activated platelets, macrophages, and endothelial cells can stimulate the migration of smooth-muscle cells normally resident in the tunica media into the intima. Such growth factors and cytokines produced locally can stimulate the proliferation of resident smooth-muscle cells in the intima as well as those that have migrated from the media. Transforming growth factor β (TGF-β), among other mediators, potently stimulates interstitial collagen production by smooth-muscle cells. These mediators may arise not only from neighboring vascular cells or leukocytes (a "paracrine" pathway), but also, in some instances, may arise from the same cell that responds to the factor (an "autocrine" pathway). Together, these alterations in smooth-muscle cells, signaled by these mediators acting at short distances, can hasten transformation of the fatty streak into a more fibrous smooth-muscle cell and extracellular matrix-rich lesion.

In addition to locally produced mediators, products of blood coagulation and thrombosis likely contribute to atheroma evolution and complication. This involvement justifies the use of the term *atherothrombosis* to convey the inextricable links between atherosclerosis and thrombosis. Fatty streak formation begins beneath a morphologically intact endothelium. In advanced fatty streaks,

however, microscopic breaches in endothelial integrity may occur. Microthrombi rich in platelets can form at such sites of limited endothelial denudation, owing to exposure of the thrombogenic extracellular matrix of the underlying basement membrane. Activated platelets release numerous factors that can promote the fibrotic response, including PDGF and TGF-β. Thrombin not only generates fibrin during coagulation, but also stimulates protease-activated receptors that can signal smooth-muscle migration, proliferation, and extracellular matrix production. Many arterial mural microthrombi resolve without clinical manifestation by a process of local fibrinolysis, resorption, and endothelial repair, yet can lead to lesion progression by stimulating these profibrotic functions of smooth-muscle cells (**Fig. 30-2D**).

Microvessels

As atherosclerotic lesions advance, abundant plexuses of microvessels develop in connection with the artery's vasa vasorum. Newly developing microvascular networks may contribute to lesion complications in several ways. These blood vessels provide an abundant surface area for leukocyte trafficking and may serve as the portal for entry and exit of white blood cells from the established atheroma. Microvessels in the plaques may also furnish foci for intraplaque hemorrhage. Like the neovessels in the diabetic retina, microvessels in the atheroma may be friable and prone to rupture and can produce focal hemorrhage. Such a vascular leak can provoke thrombosis in situ, yielding local thrombin generation, which in turn can activate smooth-muscle and endothelial cells through ligation of protease-activated receptors. Atherosclerotic plaques often contain fibrin and hemosiderin, an indication that episodes of intraplaque hemorrhage contribute to plaque complications.

Calcification

As they advance, atherosclerotic plaques also accumulate *calcium*. Proteins usually found in bone also localize in atherosclerotic lesions (e.g., osteocalcin, osteopontin, and bone morphogenetic proteins). Mineralization of the atherosclerotic plaque recapitulates many aspects of bone formation, including the regulatory participation of transcription factors such as Runx2.

Plaque evolution

Although atherosclerosis research has focused much attention on proliferation of smooth-muscle cells, as in the case of macrophages, smooth-muscle cells also can undergo apoptosis in the atherosclerotic plaque. Indeed, complex atheromata often have a mostly fibrous character and lack the cellularity of less advanced lesions. This relative paucity of smooth-muscle cells in advanced atheromata may result from the predominance of cytostatic mediators such as TGF-β and IFN-γ (which can inhibit smooth-muscle cell proliferation), and also from smooth-muscle cell apoptosis. Some of the same proinflammatory cytokines that activate atherogenic functions of vascular wall cells can also sensitize these cells to undergo apoptosis.

Thus, during the evolution of the atherosclerotic plaque, a complex balance between entry and egress of lipoproteins and leukocytes, cell proliferation and cell death, extracellular matrix production, and remodeling, as well as calcification and neovascularization, contribute to lesion formation. Multiple and often competing signals regulate these various cellular events. Many mediators related to atherogenic risk factors, including those derived from lipoproteins, cigarette smoking, and angiotensin II, provoke the production of proinflammatory cytokines and alter the behavior of the intrinsic vascular wall cells and infiltrating leukocytes that underlie the complex pathogenesis of these lesions. Thus, advances in vascular biology have led to increased understanding of the mechanisms that link risk factors to the pathogenesis of atherosclerosis and its complications.

CLINICAL SYNDROMES OF ATHEROSCLEROSIS

Atherosclerotic lesions occur ubiquitously in Western societies. Most atheromata produce no symptoms, and many never cause clinical manifestations. Numerous patients with diffuse atherosclerosis may succumb to unrelated illnesses without ever having experienced a clinically significant manifestation of atherosclerosis. What accounts for this variability in the clinical expression of atherosclerotic disease?

Arterial remodeling during atheroma formation (Fig. 30-2A) represents a frequently overlooked but clinically important feature of lesion evolution. During the initial phases of atheroma development, the plaque usually grows outward, in an abluminal direction. Vessels affected by atherogenesis tend to increase in diameter, a phenomenon known as *compensatory enlargement*, a type of vascular remodeling. The growing atheroma does not encroach on the arterial lumen until the burden of atherosclerotic plaque exceeds ~40% of the area encompassed by the internal elastic lamina. Thus, during much of its life history, an atheroma will not cause stenosis that can limit tissue perfusion.

Flow-limiting stenoses commonly form later in the history of the plaque. Many such plaques cause stable syndromes such as demand-induced angina pectoris or intermittent claudication in the extremities. In the coronary circulation and other circulations, even total vascular occlusion by an atheroma does not invariably lead to infarction. The hypoxic stimulus of repeated bouts of ischemia characteristically induces formation of collateral vessels in the myocardium, mitigating the consequences of an acute occlusion of an epicardial coronary artery. By contrast, many lesions that cause acute or unstable atherosclerotic syndromes, particularly in the coronary circulation, may arise from atherosclerotic plaques that do not produce a flow-limiting stenosis. Such lesions may produce only minimal luminal irregularities on traditional angiograms and often do not meet the traditional criteria for "significance" by arteriography. Thrombi arising from such nonocclusive stenoses may explain the frequency of MI as an initial manifestation of coronary artery disease (CAD) (in at least one-third of cases) in patients who report no prior history of angina pectoris, a syndrome usually caused by flow-limiting stenoses.

Plaque instability and rupture

Postmortem studies afford considerable insight into the microanatomic substrate underlying the "instability" of plaques that do not cause critical stenoses. A superficial erosion of the endothelium or a frank plaque rupture or fissure usually produces the thrombus that causes episodes of unstable angina pectoris or the occlusive and relatively persistent thrombus that causes acute MI (Fig. 30-2B). In the case of carotid atheromata, a deeper ulceration that provides a nidus for the formation of platelet thrombi may cause transient cerebral ischemic attacks.

Rupture of the plaque's fibrous cap (Fig. 30-2C) permits contact between coagulation factors in the blood and highly thrombogenic tissue factor expressed by macrophage foam cells in the plaque's lipid-rich core. If the ensuing thrombus is nonocclusive or transient, the episode of plaque disruption may not cause symptoms or may result in episodic ischemic symptoms such as rest angina. Occlusive thrombi that endure often cause acute MI, particularly in the absence of a well-developed collateral circulation that supplies the affected territory. Repetitive episodes of plaque disruption and healing provide one likely mechanism of transition of the fatty streak to a more complex fibrous lesion (Fig. 30-2D). The healing process in arteries, as in skin wounds, involves the laying down of new extracellular matrix and fibrosis.

Not all atheromata exhibit the same propensity to rupture. Pathologic studies of culprit lesions that have caused acute MI reveal several characteristic features. Plaques that have caused fatal thromboses tend to have thin fibrous caps, relatively large lipid cores, and a high content of macrophages. Morphometric studies of such culprit lesions show that at sites of plaque rupture, macrophages and T lymphocytes predominate and contain relatively few smooth-muscle cells. The cells that

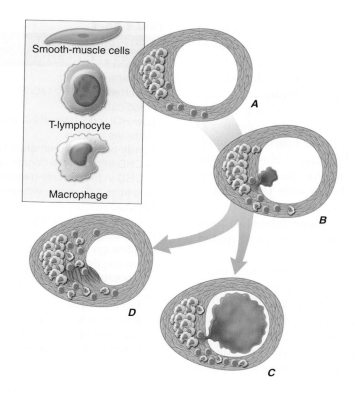

FIGURE 30-2

Plaque rupture, thrombosis, and healing. A. Arterial remodeling during atherogenesis. During the initial part of the life history of an atheroma, growth is often outward, preserving the caliber of the lumen. This phenomenon of "compensatory enlargement" accounts in part for the tendency of coronary arteriography to underestimate the degree of atherosclerosis. **B.** Rupture of the plaque's fibrous cap causes thrombosis. Physical disruption of the atherosclerotic plaque commonly causes arterial thrombosis by allowing blood coagulant factors to contact thrombogenic collagen found in the arterial extracellular matrix and tissue factor produced by macrophage-derived foam cells in the lipid core of lesions. In this manner, sites of plaque rupture form the nidus for thrombi. The normal artery wall has several fibrinolytic or antithrombotic mechanisms that tend to resist thrombosis and lyse clots that begin to form in situ. Such antithrombotic or thrombolytic molecules include thrombomodulin, tissue- and urokinase-type plasminogen activators, heparan sulfate proteoglycans, prostacyclin, and nitric oxide. **C.** When the clot overwhelms the endogenous fibrinolytic mechanisms, it may propagate and lead to arterial occlusion. The consequences of this occlusion depend on the degree of existing collateral vessels. In a patient with chronic multivessel occlusive coronary artery disease (CAD), collateral channels have often formed.

In such circumstances, even a total arterial occlusion may not lead to myocardial infarction (MI), or it may produce an unexpectedly modest or a non-ST-segment elevation infarct because of collateral flow. In a patient with less advanced disease and without substantial stenotic lesions to provide a stimulus for collateral vessel formation, sudden plaque rupture and arterial occlusion commonly produces an ST-segment elevation infarction. These are the types of patients who may present with MI or sudden death as a first manifestation of coronary atherosclerosis. In some cases, the thrombus may lyse or organize into a mural thrombus without occluding the vessel. Such instances may be clinically silent. **D.** The subsequent thrombin-induced fibrosis and healing causes a fibroproliferative response that can lead to a more fibrous lesion that can produce an eccentric plaque that causes a hemodynamically significant stenosis. In this way, a nonocclusive mural thrombus, even if clinically silent or causing unstable angina rather than infarction, can provoke a healing response that can promote lesion fibrosis and luminal encroachment. Such a sequence of events may convert a "vulnerable" atheroma with a thin fibrous cap that is prone to rupture into a more "stable" fibrous plaque with a reinforced cap. Angioplasty of unstable coronary lesions may "stabilize" the lesions by a similar mechanism, producing a wound followed by healing.

concentrate at sites of plaque rupture bear markers of inflammatory activation. In addition, patients with active atherosclerosis and acute coronary syndromes display signs of disseminated inflammation. For example, atherosclerotic plaques and even microvascular endothelial cells at sites remote from the "culprit" lesion

of an acute coronary syndrome can exhibit markers of inflammatory activation.

Inflammatory mediators regulate processes that govern the integrity of the plaque's fibrous cap and, hence, its propensity to rupture. For example, the T cell-derived cytokine IFN-γ, which is found in atherosclerotic plaques, can inhibit growth and collagen synthesis of smooth-muscle cells, as noted earlier. Cytokines derived from activated macrophages and lesional T cells can boost production of proteolytic enzymes that can degrade the extracellular matrix of the plaque's fibrous cap. Thus, inflammatory mediators can impair the collagen synthesis required for maintenance and repair of the fibrous cap and trigger degradation of extracellular matrix macromolecules, processes that weaken the plaque's fibrous cap and enhance its susceptibility to rupture (so-called vulnerable plaques). In contrast to plaques with these features of vulnerability, those with a dense extracellular matrix and relatively thick fibrous cap without substantial tissue factor–rich lipid cores seem generally resistant to rupture and unlikely to provoke thrombosis.

Features of the biology of the atheromatous plaque, in addition to its degree of luminal encroachment, influence the clinical manifestations of this disease. This enhanced understanding of plaque biology provides insight into the diverse ways in which atherosclerosis can present clinically and the reasons why the disease may remain silent or stable for prolonged periods, punctuated by acute complications at certain times. Increased understanding of atherogenesis provides new insight into the mechanisms linking it to the risk factors discussed later, indicates the ways in which current therapies may improve outcomes, and suggests new targets for future intervention.

PREVENTION AND TREATMENT

THE CONCEPT OF ATHEROSCLEROTIC RISK FACTORS

The systematic study of risk factors for atherosclerosis emerged from a coalescence of experimental results, as well as from cross-sectional and ultimately longitudinal studies in humans. The prospective, community-based Framingham Heart Study provided rigorous support for the concept that hypercholesterolemia, hypertension, and other factors correlate with cardiovascular risk. Similar observational studies performed worldwide bolstered the concept of "risk factors" for cardiovascular disease.

From a practical viewpoint, the cardiovascular risk factors that have emerged from such studies fall into two categories: those modifiable by lifestyle and/or pharmacotherapy, and those that are immutable, such as age and sex. The weight of evidence supporting various risk factors differs. For example, hypercholesterolemia and hypertension certainly predict coronary risk, but the magnitude of the contributions of other so-called nontraditional risk factors, such as levels of homocysteine, levels of lipoprotein (a) (Lp[a]), and infection,

TABLE 30-1

MAJOR RISK FACTORS (EXCLUSIVE OF LDL CHOLESTEROL) THAT MODIFY LDL GOALS

Cigarette smoking
Hypertension (BP ≥140/90 mmHg or on antihypertensive medication)
Low HDL cholesterol[a] (<1.0 mmol/L [<40 mg/dL])
Diabetes mellitus
Family history of premature CHD
    CHD in male first-degree relative <55 years
    CHD in female first-degree relative <65 years
Age (men ≥45 years; women ≥55 years)
Lifestyle risk factors
    Obesity (BMI ≥30 kg/m^2)
    Physical inactivity
    Atherogenic diet
Emerging risk factors
    Lipoprotein(a)
    Homocysteine
    Prothrombotic factors
    Proinflammatory factors
    Impaired fasting glucose
    Subclinical atherosclerosis

[a]HDL cholesterol ≥1.6 mmol/L (≥60 mg/dL) counts as a "negative" risk factor; its presence removes one risk factor from the total count.
Abbreviations: BMI, body mass index; BP, blood pressure; CHD, coronary heart disease; HDL, high-density lipoprotein; LDL, low-density lipoprotein.
Source: Modified from Third Report of the National Cholesterol Education Program (NCEP) Expert Panel on Detection, Evaluation, and Treatment of High Blood Cholesterol in Adults (Adult Treatment Panel III), Executive Summary. (Bethesda, MD: National Heart, Lung and Blood Institute, National Institutes of Health, 2001. NIH Publication No. 01-3670.)

remains controversial. Moreover, some biomarkers that predict cardiovascular risk may not participate in the causal pathway for the disease or its complications. For example, recent genetic studies suggest that C-reactive protein (CRP) does not itself mediate atherogenesis, despite its ability to predict risk. Table 30-1 lists the risk factors recognized by the current National Cholesterol Education Project Adult Treatment Panel III (ATP III). The later sections will consider some of these risk factors and approaches to their modification.

Lipid disorders

Abnormalities in plasma lipoproteins and derangements in lipid metabolism rank among the most firmly established and best understood risk factors for atherosclerosis. Chapter 31 describes the lipoprotein classes and provides a detailed discussion of lipoprotein metabolism. Current ATP III guidelines recommend lipid screening in all adults >20 years of age. The screen should include a fasting lipid profile (total cholesterol, triglycerides, LDL cholesterol, and HDL cholesterol) repeated every 5 years.

TABLE 30-2

LDL CHOLESTEROL GOALS AND CUT POINTS FOR THERAPEUTIC LIFESTYLE CHANGES (TLC) AND DRUG THERAPY IN DIFFERENT RISK CATEGORIES

RISK CATEGORY	LDL LEVEL, mmol/L (mg/dL)		
	GOAL	INITIATE TLC	CONSIDER DRUG THERAPY
Very high ACS, or CHD w/DM, or multiple CRFs	<1.8 (<70)	≥1.8 (≥70)	≥1.8 (≥70)
High CHD or CHD risk equivalents (10-year risk >20%) If LDL <2.6 (<100)	<2.6 (<100) (optional goal: <1.8 [<70]) <1.8 (<70)	≥2.6 (≥100)	≥2.6 (≥100) (<2.6 [<100]: consider drug Rx)
Moderately high 2 + risk factors (10-year risk, 10–20%)	<2.6 (<100)	≥3.4 (≥130)	≥3.4 (≥130) (2.6–3.3 [100–129]: consider drug Rx)
Moderate 2 + risk factors (risk <10%)	<3.4 (<130)	≥3.4 (≥130)	≥4.1 (≥160)
Lower 0–1 risk factor	<4.1 (<160)	≥4.1 (≥160)	≥4.9 (≥190)

Abbreviations: ACS, acute coronary syndrome; CHD, coronary heart disease; CRFs, coronary risk factors; DM, diabetes mellitus; LDL, low-density lipoprotein.

Source: Adapted from S Grundy et al: Circulation 110:227, 2004.

ATP III guidelines strive to match the intensity of treatment to an individual's risk. A quantitative estimate of risk places individuals in one of three treatment strata (Table 30-2). The first step in applying these guidelines involves counting an individual's risk factors (Table 30-1). Individuals with fewer than two risk factors fall into the lowest treatment intensity stratum (LDL goal <4.1 mmol/L [<160 mg/dL]). In those with two or more risk factors, the next step involves a simple calculation that estimates the 10-year risk of developing coronary heart disease (CHD) (Table 30-2); see *http://www.nhlbi.nih.gov/guidelines/cholesterol/* for the algorithm and a downloadable risk calculator. Those with a 10-year risk ≤20% fall into the intermediate stratum (LDL goal <3.4 mmol/L [<130 mg/dL]). Those with a calculated 10-year CHD risk of >20%, any evidence of established atherosclerosis, or diabetes (now considered a CHD risk equivalent) fall into the most intensive treatment group (LDL goal <2.6 mmol/L [<100 mg/dL]). Members of the ATP III panel recently suggested <1.8 mmol/L (<70 mg/dL) as a goal for very high-risk patients and an optional goal for high-risk patients based on recent clinical trial data (Table 30-2). Beyond the Framingham algorithm, there are multiple risk calculators for various countries or regions. Risk calculators that incorporate family history of premature (CAD) and a marker of inflammation (CRP) have been validated for U.S. women and men.

The first maneuver to achieve the LDL goal involves therapeutic lifestyle changes (TLC), including specific diet and exercise recommendations established by the guidelines. According to ATP III criteria, those with LDL levels exceeding goal for their risk group by >0.8 mmol/L (>30 mg/dL) merit consideration for drug therapy. In patients with triglycerides >2.6 mmol/L (>200 mg/dL), ATP III guidelines specify a secondary goal for therapy: "non-HDL cholesterol" (simply, the HDL cholesterol level subtracted from the total cholesterol). Cut points for the therapeutic decision for non-HDL cholesterol are 0.8 mmol/L (30 mg/dL) more than those for LDL.

An extensive and growing body of rigorous evidence now supports the effectiveness of aggressive management of LDL. Addition of drug therapy to dietary and other nonpharmacologic measures reduces cardiovascular risk in patients with established coronary atherosclerosis and also in individuals who have not previously experienced CHD events (Fig. 30-3). As guidelines often lag the emerging clinical trial evidence base, the practitioner may elect to exercise clinical judgment in making therapeutic decisions in individual patients.

LDL-lowering therapies do not appear to exert their beneficial effect on cardiovascular events by causing a marked "regression" of stenoses. Angiographically monitored studies of lipid lowering have shown at best a modest reduction in coronary artery stenoses over the duration of study, despite abundant evidence of event reduction. These results suggest that the beneficial mechanism of lipid lowering does not require a substantial reduction in the fixed stenoses. Rather, the benefit may derive from "stabilization" of atherosclerotic lesions without decreased stenosis. Such stabilization

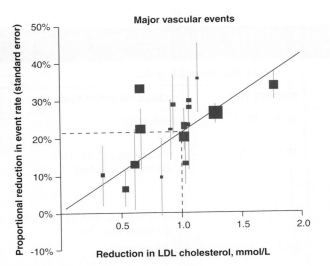

FIGURE 30-3

Lipid lowering reduces coronary events, as reflected on this graph showing the reduction in major cardiovascular events as a function of low-density lipoprotein level in a compendium of clinical trials with statins. (*Adapted from CTT Collaborators, Lancet 366:1267, 2005.*) The Management of Elevated Cholesterol in the Primary Prevention Group of Adult Japanese (MEGA), Treating to New Targets (TNT), and Incremental Decrease in Endpoints through Aggressive Lipid Lowering (IDEAL) studies have been added.

of atherosclerotic lesions and the attendant decrease in coronary events may result from the egress of lipids or from favorably influencing aspects of the biology of atherogenesis discussed earlier. In addition, as sizable lesions may protrude abluminally rather than into the lumen due to complementary enlargement, shrinkage of such plaques may not be apparent on angiograms. The consistent benefit of LDL lowering by 3-hydroxy-3-methylglutaryl coenzyme A (HMG-CoA) reductase inhibitors (statins) observed in many risk groups may depend not only on their salutary effects on the lipid profile but also on direct modulation of plaque biology independent of lipid lowering.

A new class of LDL-lowering medications reduces cholesterol absorption from the proximal small bowel by targeting an enterocyte cholesterol transporter denoted Niemann-Pick C1-like 1 protein (NPC1L1). The NPC1L1 inhibitor ezetimibe provides a useful adjunct to current therapies to achieve LDL goals; however, no clinical trial evidence has yet demonstrated that ezetimibe improves CHD outcomes.

As the mechanism by which elevated LDL levels promote atherogenesis probably involves oxidative modification, several trials have tested the possibility that antioxidant vitamin therapy might reduce CHD events. Rigorous and well-controlled clinical trials have failed to demonstrate that antioxidant vitamin therapy improves CHD outcomes. Therefore, the current evidence base does *not* support the use of antioxidant vitamins for this indication.

The clinical use of effective pharmacologic strategies for lowering LDL has reduced cardiovascular events markedly, but even their optimal utilization in clinical trials prevents only a minority of these endpoints. Hence, other aspects of the lipid profile have become tempting targets for addressing the residual burden of cardiovascular disease that persists despite aggressive LDL lowering. Indeed, in the "poststatin" era, patients with LDL levels at or below target not infrequently present with acute coronary syndromes. Low levels of HDL present a growing problem in patients with CAD as the prevalence of metabolic syndrome and diabetes increases. Blood HDL levels vary inversely with those of triglycerides, and the independent role of triglycerides as a cardiovascular risk factor remains unsettled. For these reasons, approaches to raising HDL have emerged as a prominent next hurdle in the management of dyslipidemia. Weight loss and physical activity can raise HDL. Nicotinic acid, particularly in combination with statins, can robustly raise HDL. Some clinical trial data support the effectiveness of nicotinic acid in cardiovascular risk reduction. However, flushing and pruritus remain a challenge to patient acceptance, even with improved dosage forms of nicotinic acid. A combination of nicotinic acid with an inhibitor of prostaglandin D receptor, a mediator of flushing, may limit this unwanted effect of nicotinic acid and is currently in clinical trials, but it has not received regulatory approval.

Agonists of nuclear receptors provide another potential avenue for raising HDL levels. Yet patients treated with peroxisome proliferator–activated receptors alpha and gamma (PPAR-α and -γ) agonists have not consistently shown improved cardiovascular outcomes, and at least some PPAR-agonists have been associated with worsened cardiovascular outcomes. Other agents in clinical development raise HDL levels by inhibiting cholesteryl ester transfer protein (CETP). The first of these agents to undergo large-scale clinical evaluation showed increased adverse events, leading to cessation of its development. Clinical studies currently underway will assess the effectiveness of other CETP inhibitors that lack some of the adverse off-target actions encountered with the first agent.

Hypertension

(See also Chap. 37) A wealth of epidemiologic data support a relationship between hypertension and atherosclerotic risk, and extensive clinical trial evidence has established that pharmacologic treatment of hypertension can reduce the risk of stroke, heart failure, and CHD events.

Diabetes mellitus, insulin resistance, and the metabolic syndrome

Most patients with diabetes mellitus die of atherosclerosis and its complications. Aging and rampant obesity underlie a current epidemic of type 2 diabetes mellitus. The abnormal lipoprotein profile associated with insulin resistance, known as *diabetic dyslipidemia*, accounts for part of the elevated cardiovascular risk in patients with type 2 diabetes. Although diabetic individuals often have LDL cholesterol levels near the average, the LDL particles tend to be smaller and denser and, therefore, more atherogenic. Other features of diabetic dyslipidemia include low HDL and elevated triglyceride levels. Hypertension also frequently accompanies obesity, insulin resistance, and dyslipidemia. Indeed, the ATP III guidelines now recognize this cluster of risk factors and provide criteria for diagnosis of the "metabolic syndrome" (Table 30-3). Despite legitimate concerns about whether clustered components confer more risk than an individual component, the metabolic syndrome concept may offer clinical utility.

Therapeutic objectives for intervention in these patients include addressing the underlying causes, including obesity and low physical activity, by initiating TLC. The ATP III guidelines provide an explicit step-by-step plan for implementing TLC, and treatment of the component risk factors should accompany TLC. Establishing that strict glycemic control reduces the risk of macrovascular complications of diabetes has proved much more elusive than the established beneficial effects on microvascular complications such as retinopathy and renal disease. Indeed, "tight" glycemic control may increase adverse events in patients with type 2 diabetes, lending even greater importance to aggressive control of other aspects of risk in this patient population. In this regard, multiple clinical trials, including the Collaborative Atorvastatin Diabetes Study (CARDS) that addressed specifically the diabetic population, have demonstrated unequivocal benefit of HMG-CoA reductase inhibitor therapy in diabetic patients over all ranges of LDL cholesterol levels (but not those with end-stage renal disease). In view of the consistent benefit of statin treatment for diabetic populations and the thus far equivocal results with PPAR agonists, the current stance of the American Diabetic Association that statins be considered for persons with diabetes older than age 40 who have a total cholesterol level ≥135 appears amply justified. Among the oral hypoglycemic agents, metformin possesses the best evidence base for cardiovascular event reduction.

Diabetic populations appear to derive particular benefit from antihypertensive strategies that block the action of angiotensin II. Thus, the antihypertensive regimen for patients with the metabolic syndrome should include angiotensin converting-enzyme inhibitors or angiotensin receptor blockers when possible. Most of these individuals will require more than one antihypertensive agent to achieve the recently updated American Diabetes Association blood pressure goal of 130/80 mmHg.

TABLE 30-3

CLINICAL IDENTIFICATION OF THE METABOLIC SYNDROME—ANY THREE RISK FACTORS	
RISK FACTOR	**DEFINING LEVEL**
Abdominal obesity[a]	
Men (waist circumference)[b]	>102 cm (>40 in.)
Women	>88 cm (>35 in.)
Triglycerides	>1.7 mmol/L (>150 mg/dL)
HDL cholesterol	
Men	<1 mmol/L (<40 mg/dL)
Women	<1.3 mmol/L (<50 mg/dL)
Blood pressure	≥130/≥85 mmHg
Fasting glucose	>6.1 mmol/L (>110 mg/dL)

[a]Overweight and obesity are associated with insulin resistance and the metabolic syndrome. However, the presence of abdominal obesity is more highly correlated with the metabolic risk factors than is an elevated body mass index (BMI). Therefore, the simple measure of waist circumference is recommended to identify the BMI component of the metabolic syndrome.

[b]Some male patients can develop multiple metabolic risk factors when the waist circumference is only marginally increased (e.g., 94–102 cm [37–39 in.]). Such patients may have a strong genetic contribution to insulin resistance. They should benefit from lifestyle changes, similarly to men with categorical increases in waist circumference.

Male sex/postmenopausal state

Decades of observational studies have verified excess coronary risk in men compared with premenopausal women. After menopause, however, coronary risk accelerates in women. At least part of the apparent protection against CHD in premenopausal women derives from their relatively higher HDL levels compared with those of men. After menopause, HDL values fall in concert with increased coronary risk. Estrogen therapy lowers LDL cholesterol and raises HDL cholesterol, changes that should decrease coronary risk.

Multiple observational and experimental studies have suggested that estrogen therapy reduces coronary risk. However, a spate of clinical trials has failed to demonstrate a net benefit of estrogen with or without progestins on CHD outcomes. In the Heart and Estrogen/Progestin Replacement Study (HERS), postmenopausal female survivors of acute MI were randomized to an estrogen/progestin combination or to placebo. This study showed no overall reduction in recurrent coronary events in the active treatment arm. Indeed, early in the 5-year course of this trial, there was a trend toward an actual increase in vascular events in the treated women. Extended follow-up of this cohort did not disclose an accrual of benefit in the treatment group. The Women's Health Initiative (WHI) study arm, using a similar estrogen plus progesterone regimen, was halted due to a small but significant hazard of cardiovascular events, stroke, and breast cancer. The estrogen without progestin arm of WHI (conducted in women without a uterus) was stopped early due to an increase in strokes, and failed to afford protection from MI or CHD death during observation over 7 years. The excess cardiovascular events in these trials may result from an increase in thromboembolism. Physicians should work with women to provide information and help weigh the small but evident CHD risk of estrogen ± progestin versus the benefits for postmenopausal symptoms and osteoporosis, taking personal preferences into account. Post hoc analyses of observational studies suggest that estrogen therapy in women younger than or closer to menopause than the women enrolled in WHI might confer cardiovascular benefit. Thus, the timing in relation to menopause or the age at which estrogen therapy begins may influence its risk/benefit balance.

The lack of efficacy of estrogen therapy in cardiovascular risk reduction highlights the need for redoubled attention to known modifiable risk factors in women. The recent JUPITER trials randomized over 6000 women over age 65 without known cardiovascular disease with LDL <130 mg/dL and high-sensitivity (hs) CRP >2 mg/L to a statin or placebo. The statin-treated women had a striking reduction in cardiovascular events, as did the men. This trial, which included more women than any prior statin study, provides strong evidence supporting the efficacy of statins in women who meet those entry criteria.

Dysregulated coagulation or fibrinolysis

Thrombosis ultimately causes the gravest complications of atherosclerosis. The propensity to form thrombi and/or lyse clots once they form clearly influences the manifestations of atherosclerosis. Thrombosis provoked by atheroma rupture and subsequent healing may promote plaque growth. Certain individual characteristics can influence thrombosis or fibrinolysis and have received attention as potential coronary risk factors. For example, fibrinogen levels correlate with coronary risk and provide information about coronary risk independent of the lipoprotein profile.

The stability of an arterial thrombus depends on the balance between fibrinolytic factors such as plasmin, and inhibitors of the fibrinolytic system such as plasminogen activator inhibitor 1 (PAI-1). Individuals with diabetes mellitus or the metabolic syndrome have elevated levels of PAI-1 in plasma, and this probably contributes to the increased risk of thrombotic events. Lp(a) (Chap. 31) may modulate fibrinolysis, and individuals with elevated Lp(a) levels have increased CHD risk.

Aspirin reduces CHD events in several contexts. Chapter 33 discusses aspirin therapy in stable ischemic heart disease and Chap. 34 reviews recommendations for aspirin treatment in acute coronary syndromes. In primary prevention, pooled trial data show that low-dose aspirin treatment (81 mg/d to 325 mg on alternate days) can reduce the risk of a first MI in men. Although the recent Women's Health Study (WHS) showed that aspirin (100 mg on alternate days) reduced strokes by 17%, it did not prevent MI in women. Current American Heart Association (AHA) guidelines recommend the use of low-dose aspirin (75–160 mg/d) for women with high cardiovascular risk (≥20% 10-year risk), for men with a ≥10% 10-year risk of CHD, and for all aspirin-tolerant patients with established cardiovascular disease who lack contraindications.

Homocysteine

A large body of literature suggests a relationship between hyperhomocysteinemia and coronary events. Several mutations in the enzymes involved in homocysteine accumulation correlate with thrombosis and, in some studies, with coronary risk. Prospective studies have not shown a robust utility of hyperhomocysteinemia in CHD risk stratification. Clinical trials have not shown that intervention to lower homocysteine levels reduces CHD events. Fortification of the U.S. diet with folic acid to reduce neural tube defects has lowered homocysteine levels in the population at large. Measurement of homocysteine levels should be reserved for individuals with atherosclerosis at a young age or out of proportion to established risk factors. Physicians who advise consumption of supplements containing folic acid should consider that this treatment may mask pernicious anemia.

Inflammation

An accumulation of clinical evidence shows that markers of inflammation correlate with coronary risk. For example, plasma levels of CRP, as measured by a high-sensitivity assay (hsCRP), prospectively predict the risk of MI. CRP levels also correlate with the outcome in patients with acute coronary syndromes. In contrast to several other novel risk factors, CRP adds predictive information to that derived from established risk factors, such as those included in the Framingham

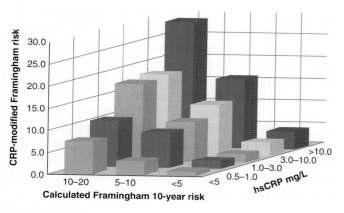

FIGURE 30-4

C-reactive protein (CRP) level adds to the predictive value of the Framingham score. hsCRP, high-sensitivity measurement of CRP. (*Adapted from PM Ridker et al: Circulation 109:2818, 2004.*)

score (**Fig. 30-4**). Recent Mendelian randomization studies do not support a causal role for CRP in cardiovascular disease. Thus, CRP serves as a validated biomarker of risk but probably not as a direct contributor to pathogenesis.

Elevations in acute-phase reactants such as fibrinogen and CRP reflect the overall inflammatory burden, not just vascular foci of inflammation. Visceral adipose tissue releases proinflammatory cytokines that drive CRP production and may represent a major extravascular stimulus to elevation of inflammatory markers in obese and overweight individuals. Indeed, CRP levels rise with body mass index (BMI), and weight reduction lowers CRP levels. Infectious agents might also furnish inflammatory stimuli related to cardiovascular risk. To date, randomized clinical trials have not supported the use of antibiotics to reduce CHD risk.

Intriguing evidence suggests that lipid-lowering therapy reduces coronary events in part by muting the inflammatory aspects of the pathogenesis of atherosclerosis. For example, in the JUPITER trial, a prespecified analysis showed that those who achieved lower levels of both LDL and CRP had better clinical outcomes than did those who only reached the lower level of either the inflammatory marker or the atherogenic lipoprotein (**Fig. 30-5**). Similar analyses of studies of statin

treatment in patients after acute coronary syndromes showed the same pattern. The anti-inflammatory effect of statins appears independent of LDL lowering, as these two variables correlated very poorly in individual subjects in multiple clinical trials.

Lifestyle modification

The prevention of atherosclerosis presents a long-term challenge to all health care professionals and for public health policy. Both individual practitioners and organizations providing health care should strive to help patients optimize their risk factor profiles long before atherosclerotic disease becomes manifest. The current accumulation of cardiovascular risk in youth and in certain minority populations presents a particularly vexing concern from a public health perspective.

The care plan for all patients seen by internists should include measures to assess and minimize cardiovascular risk. Physicians must counsel patients about the health risks of tobacco use and provide guidance and resources regarding smoking cessation. Similarly, physicians should advise all patients about prudent dietary and physical activity habits for maintaining ideal body weight. Both National Institutes of Health (NIH) and AHA statements recommend at least 30 min of moderate-intensity physical activity per day. Obesity, particularly the male pattern of centripetal or visceral fat accumulation, can contribute to the elements of the metabolic syndrome (Table 30-3). Physicians should encourage their patients to take personal responsibility for behavior related to modifiable risk factors for the development of premature atherosclerotic disease. Conscientious counseling and patient education may forestall the need for pharmacologic measures intended to reduce coronary risk.

Issues in risk assessment

A growing panel of markers of coronary risk presents a perplexing array to the practitioner. Markers measured in peripheral blood include size fractions of LDL particles and concentrations of homocysteine, Lp(a), fibrinogen, CRP, PAI-1, myeloperoxidase, and lipoprotein-associated phospholipase A_2, among many others. In general, such specialized tests add little to the information available

Group	N	Rate
Placebo	7832	1.11
LDL ≥ 70 mg/dL, hsCRP ≥ 2 mg/L	1384	1.11
LDL < 70 mg/dL, hsCRP ≥ 2 mg/L	2921	0.62
LDL ≥ 70 mg/dL, hsCRP < 2 mg/L	726	0.54
LDL < 70 mg/dL, hsCRP < 2 mg/L	2685	0.38

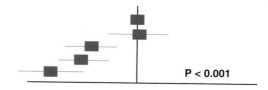

P < 0.001

FIGURE 30-5

Evidence from the JUPITER study that both LDL-lowering and anti-inflammatory actions contribute to the benefit of statin therapy in primary prevention. See text for explanation.

hsCRP, high-sensitivity measurement of C-reactive protein (CRP). (*Adapted from PM Ridker et al: Lancet 373:1175, 2009.*)

from a careful history and physical examination combined with measurement of a plasma lipoprotein profile and fasting blood glucose. The high-sensitivity CRP measurement may well prove an exception in view of its robustness in risk prediction, ease of reproducible and standardized measurement, relative stability in individuals over time, and, most important, ability to add to the risk information disclosed by standard measurements such as the components of the Framingham risk score (Fig. 30-4). The addition of information regarding a family history of premature atherosclerosis in parents (a simply obtained indicator of genetic susceptibility), together with the marker of inflammation hsCRP, permits correct reclassification of risk in individuals—especially those whose Framingham scores place them at intermediate risk. Current advisories, however, recommend the use of the hsCRP test only in individuals in this CHD event risk group (10–20%, 10-year risk).

Available data do not support the use of imaging studies to screen for subclinical disease (e.g., measurement of carotid-intima/media thickness, coronary artery calcification, and use of computed tomographic coronary angiograms). Inappropriate use of such imaging modalities may promote excessive alarm in asymptomatic individuals and prompt invasive diagnostic and therapeutic procedures of unproven value. Widespread application of such modalities for screening should await proof that clinical benefit derives from their application.

Progress in human genetics holds considerable promise for risk prediction and for individualization of cardiovascular therapy. Many reports have identified single-nucleotide polymorphisms (SNPs) in candidate genes as predictors of cardiovascular risk. To date, the validation of such genetic markers of risk and drug responsiveness in multiple populations has often proved disappointing. The advent of technology that permits relatively rapid and inexpensive genome-wide screens, in contrast to most SNP studies, has led to identification of sites of genetic variation that do reproducibly indicate heightened cardiovascular risk (e.g., chromosome 9p21). The results of genetic studies should identify new potential therapeutic targets (e.g., the enzyme mutated in autosomal dominant hypercholesterolemia, abbreviated *PCSK9*) and may lead to genetic tests that help refine cardiovascular risk assessment in the future.

THE CHALLENGE OF IMPLEMENTATION: CHANGING PHYSICIAN AND PATIENT BEHAVIOR

Despite declining age-adjusted rates of coronary death, cardiovascular mortality worldwide is rising due to the aging of the population, and the subsiding of communicable diseases and increased prevalence of risk factors in developing countries. Enormous challenges remain regarding translation of the current evidence base into practice. Physicians must learn how to help individuals adopt a healthy lifestyle in a culturally appropriate manner and to deploy their increasingly powerful pharmacologic tools most economically and effectively. The obstacles to implementation of current evidence-based prevention and treatment of atherosclerosis involve economics, education, physician awareness, and patient adherence to recommended regimens. Future goals in the treatment of atherosclerosis should include more widespread implementation of the current evidence-based guidelines regarding risk factor management and, when appropriate, drug therapy.

CHAPTER 31

DISORDERS OF LIPOPROTEIN METABOLISM

Daniel J. Rader ■ Helen H. Hobbs

Lipoproteins are complexes of lipids and proteins that are essential for the transport of cholesterol, triglycerides, and fat-soluble vitamins. Previously, lipoprotein disorders were the purview of specialized lipidologists, but the demonstration that lipid-lowering therapy significantly reduces the clinical complications of atherosclerotic cardiovascular disease (ASCVD) has brought the diagnosis and treatment of these disorders into the domain of the internist. The number of individuals who are candidates for lipid-lowering therapy has continued to increase. The development of safe, effective, and well-tolerated pharmacologic agents has greatly expanded the therapeutic armamentarium available to the physician to treat disorders of lipid metabolism. Therefore, the appropriate diagnosis and management of lipoprotein disorders is of critical importance in the practice of medicine. This chapter will review normal lipoprotein physiology, the pathophysiology of primary (inherited) disorders of lipoprotein metabolism, the diseases and environmental factors that cause secondary disorders of lipoprotein metabolism, and the practical approaches to their diagnosis and management.

LIPOPROTEIN METABOLISM

LIPOPROTEIN CLASSIFICATION AND COMPOSITION

Lipoproteins are large macromolecular complexes that transport hydrophobic lipids (primarily triglycerides, cholesterol, and fat-soluble vitamins) through body fluids (plasma, interstitial fluid, and lymph) to and from tissues. Lipoproteins play an essential role in the absorption of dietary cholesterol, long-chain fatty acids, and fat-soluble vitamins; the transport of triglycerides, cholesterol, and fat-soluble vitamins from the liver to peripheral tissues; and the transport of cholesterol from peripheral tissues to the liver.

Lipoproteins contain a core of hydrophobic lipids (triglycerides and cholesteryl esters) surrounded by hydrophilic lipids (phospholipids, unesterified cholesterol) and proteins that interact with body fluids. The plasma lipoproteins are divided into five major classes based on their relative density (**Fig. 31-1** and **Table 31-1**): chylomicrons, very low–density lipoproteins (VLDLs), intermediate-density lipoproteins (IDLs), low-density lipoproteins (LDLs), and high-density lipoproteins (HDLs). Each lipoprotein class comprises a family of particles that vary slightly in density, size, and protein composition. The density of a lipoprotein is determined by the amount of lipid per particle. HDL is the smallest and most dense lipoprotein, whereas chylomicrons and VLDLs are the largest and least dense lipoprotein particles. Most plasma triglyceride is transported in chylomicrons or VLDLs, and most plasma cholesterol is carried as cholesteryl esters in LDLs and HDLs.

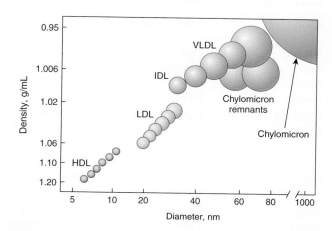

FIGURE 31-1

The density and size distribution of the major classes of lipoprotein particles. Lipoproteins are classified by density and size, which are inversely related. VLDL, very low-density lipoprotein; IDL, intermediate-density lipoprotein; LDL, low-density lipoprotein; HDL, high-density lipoprotein.

TABLE 31-1

MAJOR LIPOPROTEIN CLASSES

LIPOPROTEIN	DENSITY, g/mL[a]	SIZE, nm[b]	ELECTROPHORETIC MOBILITY[c]	ApoLIPOPROTEINS MAJOR	ApoLIPOPROTEINS OTHER	OTHER CONSTITUENTS
Chylomicrons	0.930	75–1200	Origin	ApoB-48	A-I, A-IV, C-I, C-II, C-III, E	Retinyl esters
Chylomicron remnants	0.930–1.006	30–80	Slow pre-β	ApoB-48	A-I, A-IV, C-I, C-II, C-III, E	Retinyl esters
VLDL	0.930–1.006	30–80	Pre-β	ApoB-100	A-I, A-II, A-V, C-I, C-II, C-III, E	Vitamin E
IDL	1.006–1.019	25–35	Slow pre-β	ApoB-100	C-I, C-II, C-III, E	Vitamin E
LDL	1.019–1.063	18–25	β	ApoB-100		Vitamin E
HDL	1.063–1.210	5–12	α	ApoA-I	A-II, A-IV, A-V, C-III, E	LCAT, CETP paroxonase
Lp(a)	1.050–1.120	25	Pre-β	ApoB-100	Apo(a)	

[a]The density of the particle is determined by ultracentrifugation.
[b]The size of the particle is measured using gel electrophoresis.
[c]The electrophoretic mobility of the particle on agarose gel electrophores reflects the size and surface charge of the particle, with β being the position of LDL and α being the position of HDL.
Note: All of the lipoprotein classes contain phospholipids, esterified and unesterified cholesterol, and triglycerides to varying degrees.
Abbreviations: CETP, cholesteryl ester transfer protein; HDL, high-density lipoprotein; IDL, intermediate-density lipoprotein; LCAT, lecithin-cholesterol acyltransferase; LDL, low-density lipoprotein; Lp(a), lipoprotein A; VLDL, very low-density lipoprotein.

The proteins associated with lipoproteins, called *apolipoproteins* (Table 31-2), are required for the assembly, structure, and function of lipoproteins. Apolipoproteins activate enzymes important in lipoprotein metabolism and act as ligands for cell surface receptors. ApoA-I, which is synthesized in the liver and intestine, is found on virtually all HDL particles. ApoA-II is the second most abundant HDL apolipoprotein and is on approximately two-thirds of the HDL particles. ApoB is the major structural protein of chylomicrons, VLDLs, IDLs, and LDLs; one molecule of apoB, either apoB-48 (chylomicron) or apoB-100 (VLDL, IDL, or LDL), is present on each lipoprotein particle. The human liver synthesizes apoB-100, and the intestine makes apoB-48, which is derived from the same gene by mRNA editing. ApoE is present in multiple copies on chylomicrons,

TABLE 31-2

MAJOR ApoLIPOPROTEINS

ApoLIPOPROTEIN	PRIMARY SOURCE	LIPOPROTEIN ASSOCIATION	FUNCTION
ApoA-I	Intestine, liver	HDL, chylomicrons	Structural protein for HDL Activates LCAT
ApoA-II	Liver	HDL, chylomicrons	Structural protein for HDL
ApoA-IV	Intestine	HDL, chylomicrons	Unknown
ApoA-V	Liver	VLDL, chylomicrons	Promotes LPL-mediated triglyceride lipolysis
Apo(a)	Liver	Lp(a)	Unknown
ApoB-48	Intestine	Chylomicrons	Structural protein for chylomicrons
ApoB-100	Liver	VLDL, IDL, LDL, Lp(a)	Structural protein for VLDL, LDL, IDL, Lp(a) Ligand for binding to LDL receptor
ApoC-I	Liver	Chylomicrons, VLDL, HDL	Unknown
ApoC-II	Liver	Chylomicrons, VLDL, HDL	Cofactor for LPL
ApoC-III	Liver	Chylomicrons, VLDL, HDL	Inhibits lipoprotein binding to receptors
ApoE	Liver	Chylomicron remnants, IDL, HDL	Ligand for binding to LDL receptor
ApoH	Liver	Chylomicrons, VLDL, LDL, HDL	B₂ glycoprotein I
ApoJ	Liver	HDL	Unknown
ApoL	Unknown	HDL	Unknown
ApoM	Liver	HDL	Unknown

Abbreviations: HDL, high-density lipoprotein; IDL, intermediate-density lipoprotein; LCAT, lecithin-cholesterol acyltransferase; LDL, low-density lipoprotein; Lp(a), lipoprotein A; LPL, lipoprotein lipase; VLDL, very low-density lipoprotein.

VLDL, and IDL, and it plays a critical role in the metabolism and clearance of triglyceride-rich particles. Three apolipoproteins of the C-series (apoC-I, apoC-II, and apoC-III) also participate in the metabolism of triglyceride-rich lipoproteins. ApoB is the only major apolipoprotein that does not transfer between lipoprotein particles. Some of the minor apolipoproteins are listed in Table 31-2.

TRANSPORT OF DIETARY LIPIDS (EXOGENOUS PATHWAY)

The exogenous pathway of lipoprotein metabolism permits efficient transport of dietary lipids (Fig. 31-2). Dietary triglycerides are hydrolyzed by lipases within the intestinal lumen and emulsified with bile acids to form micelles. Dietary cholesterol, fatty acids, and fat-soluble vitamins are absorbed in the proximal small intestine. Cholesterol and retinol are esterified (by the addition of a fatty acid) in the enterocyte to form cholesteryl esters and retinyl esters, respectively. Longer-chain fatty acids (>12 carbons) are incorporated into triglycerides and packaged with apoB-48, cholesteryl esters, retinyl esters, phospholipids, and cholesterol to form chylomicrons.

Nascent chylomicrons are secreted into the intestinal lymph and delivered via the thoracic duct directly to the systemic circulation, where they are extensively processed by peripheral tissues before reaching the liver. The particles encounter lipoprotein lipase (LPL), which is anchored to a glycosylphosphatidylinositol-anchored protein, GPIHBP1, that is attached to the endothelial surfaces of capillaries in adipose tissue, heart, and skeletal muscle (Fig. 31-2). The triglycerides of chylomicrons are hydrolyzed by LPL, and free fatty acids are released. ApoC-II, which is transferred to circulating chylomicrons from HDL, acts as a required cofactor for LPL in this reaction. The released free fatty acids are taken up by adjacent myocytes or adipocytes and either oxidized to generate energy or reesterified and stored as triglyceride. Some of the released free fatty acids bind albumin before entering cells and are transported to other tissues, especially the liver. The chylomicron particle progressively shrinks in size as the hydrophobic core is hydrolyzed and the hydrophilic lipids (cholesterol and phospholipids) and apolipoproteins on the particle surface are transferred to HDL, creating chylomicron remnants. Chylomicron remnants are rapidly removed from the circulation by the liver through a process that requires

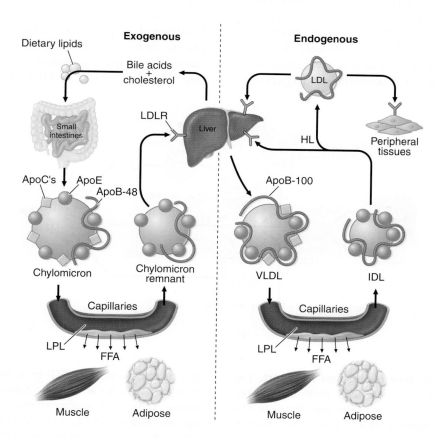

FIGURE 31-2

The exogenous and endogenous lipoprotein metabolic pathways. The exogenous pathway transports dietary lipids to the periphery and the liver. The endogenous pathway transports hepatic lipids to the periphery. LPL, lipoprotein lipase; FFA, free fatty acid; VLDL, very low-density lipoprotein; IDL, intermediate-density lipoprotein; LDL, low-density lipoprotein; LDLR, low-density lipoprotein receptor; HL, hepatic lipase.

apoE as a ligand for receptors in the liver. Consequently, few, if any, chylomicrons or chylomicron remnants are present in the blood after a 12-h fast, except in patients with disorders of chylomicron metabolism.

TRANSPORT OF HEPATIC LIPIDS (ENDOGENOUS PATHWAY)

The endogenous pathway of lipoprotein metabolism refers to the secretion of apoB-containing lipoproteins from the liver and the metabolism of these triglyceride-rich particles in peripheral tissues (Fig. 31-2). VLDL particles resemble chylomicrons in protein composition but contain apoB-100 rather than apoB-48 and have a higher ratio of cholesterol to triglyceride (~1 mg of cholesterol for every 5 mg of triglyceride). The triglycerides of VLDL are derived predominantly from the esterification of long-chain fatty acids in the liver. The packaging of hepatic triglycerides with the other major components of the nascent VLDL particle (apoB-100, cholesteryl esters, phospholipids, and vitamin E) requires the action of the enzyme microsomal triglyceride transfer protein (MTP). After secretion into the plasma, VLDL acquires multiple copies of apoE and apolipoproteins of the C series by transfer from HDL. As with chylomicrons, the triglycerides of VLDL are hydrolyzed by LPL, especially in muscle, heart, and adipose tissue. After the VLDL remnants dissociate from LPL, they are referred to as IDLs, which contain roughly similar amounts of cholesterol and triglyceride.

The liver removes approximately 40–60% of IDL by LDL receptor–mediated endocytosis via binding to apoE. The remainder of IDL is remodeled by hepatic lipase (HL) to form LDL. During this process, most of the triglyceride in the particle hydrolyzed, and all apolipoproteins except apoB-100 are transferred to other lipoproteins. The cholesterol in LDL accounts for more than one-half of the plasma cholesterol in most individuals. Approximately 70% of circulating LDL is cleared by LDL receptor–mediated endocytosis in the liver. *Lipoprotein(a)* [Lp(a)] is a lipoprotein similar to LDL in lipid and protein composition, but it contains an additional protein called *apolipoprotein(a)* [apo(a)]. Apo(a) is synthesized in the liver and attached to apoB-100 by a disulfide linkage. The major site of clearance of Lp(a) is the liver, but the uptake pathway is not known.

HDL METABOLISM AND REVERSE CHOLESTEROL TRANSPORT

All nucleated cells synthesize cholesterol, but only hepatocytes and enterocytes can effectively excrete cholesterol from the body, into either the bile or the gut lumen. In the liver, cholesterol is secreted into the bile, either directly or after conversion to bile acids. Cholesterol in peripheral cells is transported from the plasma membranes of peripheral cells to the liver and intestine by a process termed "reverse cholesterol transport" that is facilitated by HDL (**Fig. 31-3**).

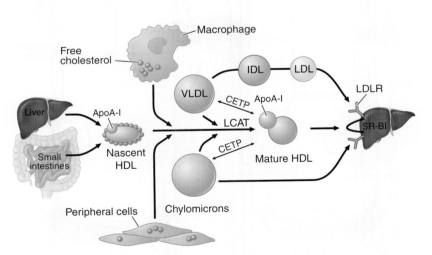

FIGURE 31-3

HDL metabolism and reverse cholesterol transport. This pathway transports excess cholesterol from the periphery back to the liver for excretion in the bile. The liver and the intestine produce nascent HDLs. Free cholesterol is acquired from macrophages and other peripheral cells and esterified by LCAT, forming mature HDLs. HDL cholesterol can be selectively taken up by the liver via SR-BI (scavenger receptor class BI). Alternatively, HDL cholesteryl ester can be transferred by CETP from HDLs to VLDLs and chylomicrons, which can then be taken up by the liver. LCAT, lecithin-cholesterol acyltransferase; CETP, cholesteryl ester transfer protein; VLDL, very low-density lipoprotein; IDL, intermediate-density lipoprotein; LDL, low-density lipoprotein; HDL, high-density lipoprotein; LDLR, low-density lipoprotein receptor.

Nascent HDL particles are synthesized by the intestine and the liver. Newly secreted apoA-I rapidly acquires phospholipids and unesterified cholesterol from its site of synthesis (intestine or liver) via efflux promoted by the membrane protein ATP-binding cassette protein A1 (ABCA1). This process results in the formation of discoidal HDL particles, which then recruit additional unesterified cholesterol from the periphery. Within the HDL particle, the cholesterol is esterified by lecithin-cholesterol acyltransferase (LCAT), a plasma enzyme associated with HDL, and the more hydrophobic cholesteryl ester moves to the core of the HDL particle. As HDL acquires more cholesteryl ester it becomes spherical, and additional apolipoproteins and lipids are transferred to the particles from the surfaces of chylomicrons and VLDLs during lipolysis.

HDL cholesterol is transported to hepatocytes by both an indirect and a direct pathway. HDL cholesteryl esters can be transferred to apoB-containing lipoproteins in exchange for triglyceride by the cholesteryl ester transfer protein (CETP). The cholesteryl esters are then removed from the circulation by LDL receptor–mediated endocytosis. HDL cholesterol can also be taken up directly by hepatocytes via the scavenger receptor class B1 (SR-B1), a cell surface receptor that mediates the selective transfer of lipids to cells.

HDL particles undergo extensive remodeling within the plasma compartment by a variety of lipid transfer proteins and lipases. The phospholipid transfer protein (PLTP) has the net effect of transferring phospholipids from other lipoproteins to HDL or among different classes of HDL particles. After CETP- and PLTP-mediated lipid exchange, the triglyceride-enriched HDL becomes a much better substrate for HL, which hydrolyzes the triglycerides and phospholipids to generate smaller HDL particles. A related enzyme called *endothelial lipase* hydrolyzes HDL phospholipids, generating smaller HDL particles that are catabolized faster. Remodeling of HDL influences the metabolism, function, and plasma concentrations of HDL.

DISORDERS OF LIPOPROTEIN METABOLISM

Fredrickson and Levy classified hyperlipoproteinemias according to the type of lipoprotein particles that accumulate in the blood (Type I to Type V) **(Table 31-3)**. A classification scheme based on the molecular etiology and pathophysiology of the lipoprotein disorders complements this system and forms the basis for this chapter. The identification and characterization of genes

TABLE 31-3

FREDRICKSON CLASSIFICATION OF HYPERLIPOPROTEINEMIAS

PHENOTYPE	I	IIa	IIb	III	IV	V
Lipoprotein, elevated	Chylomicrons	LDL	LDL and VLDL	Chylomicron and VLDL remnants	VLDL	Chylomicrons and VLDL
Triglycerides	↑↑↑	N	↑	↑↑	↑↑	↑↑↑
Cholesterol (total)	↑	↑↑↑	↑↑	↑↑	N/↑	↑↑
LDL-cholesterol	↓	↑↑↑	↑↑	↓	↓	↓
HDL-cholesterol	↓↓↓	N/↓	↓	N	↓↓	↓↓↓
Plasma appearance	Lactescent	Clear	Clear	Turbid	Turbid	Lactescent
Xanthomas	Eruptive	Tendon, tuberous	None	Palmar, tuberoeruptive	None	Eruptive
Pancreatitis	+++	0	0	0	0	+++
Coronary atherosclerosis	0	+++	+++	+++	+/−	+/−
Peripheral atherosclerosis	0	+	+	++	+/−	+/−
Molecular defects	LPL and ApoC-II	LDL receptor, ApoB-100, PCSK9, LDLRAP, ABCG5, and ABCG8		ApoE	ApoA-V	ApoA-V and GPIHBP1
Genetic nomenclature	FCS	FH, FDB, ADH, ARH, sitosterolemia	FCHL	FDBL	FHTG	FHTG

Abbreviations: ADH, autosomal dominant hypercholesterolemia; Apo, apolipoprotein; ARH, autosomal recessive hypercholesterolemia; FCHL, familial combined hyperlipidemia; FCS, familial chylomicronemia syndrome; FDB, familial defective ApoB; FDBL, familial dysbetalipoproteinemia; FH, familial hypercholesterolemia; FHTG, familial hypertriglyceridemia; LPL, lipoprotein lipase; LDLRAP, LDL receptor associated protein; GPIHBP1, glycosylphosphatidylinositol-anchored high-density lipoprotein binding protein1; N, normal.

responsible for the genetic forms of hyperlipidemia have provided important molecular insights into the critical roles of structural apolipoproteins, enzymes, and receptors in lipid metabolism (Table 31-4).

PRIMARY DISORDERS OF ELEVATED ApoB-CONTAINING LIPOPROTEINS

A variety of genetic conditions are associated with the accumulation in plasma of specific classes of lipoprotein particles. In general, these can be divided into those causing elevated LDL-cholesterol (LDL-C) with normal triglycerides and those causing elevated triglycerides (Table 31-4).

Lipid disorders associated with elevated LDL-C and normal triglycerides

■ Familial hypercholesterolemia (FH)

FH is an autosomal codominant disorder characterized by elevated plasma levels of LDL-C with normal triglycerides, tendon xanthomas, and premature coronary

atherosclerosis. FH is caused by a large number (>1000) mutations in the LDL receptor gene. It has a higher incidence in certain founder populations, such as Afrikaners, Christian Lebanese, and French Canadians. The elevated levels of LDL-C in FH are due to an increase in the production of LDL from IDL (since a portion of IDL is normally cleared by LDL receptor–mediated endocytosis) and a delayed removal of LDL from the blood. Individuals with two mutated LDL receptor alleles (FH homozygotes) have much higher LDL-C levels than those with one mutant allele (FH heterozygotes).

Homozygous FH occurs in approximately 1 in 1 million persons worldwide. Patients with homozygous FH can be classified into one of two groups based on the amount of LDL receptor activity measured in their skin fibroblasts: those patients with <2% of normal LDL receptor activity (receptor negative) and those patients with 2–25% of normal LDL receptor activity (receptor defective). Most patients with homozygous FH present in childhood with cutaneous xanthomas on the hands, wrists, elbows, knees, heels, or buttocks. Total cholesterol levels are usually >500 mg/dL and can be higher

TABLE 31-4

PRIMARY HYPERLIPOPROTEINEMIAS CAUSED BY KNOWN SINGLE GENE MUTATIONS

GENETIC DISORDER	PROTEIN (GENE) DEFECT	LIPOPROTEINS ELEVATED	CLINICAL FINDINGS	GENETIC TRANSMISSION	ESTIMATED INCIDENCE
Lipoprotein lipase deficiency	LPL (*LPL*)	Chylomicrons	Eruptive xanthomas, hepatosplenomegaly, pancreatitis	AR	1/1,000,000
Familial apolipoprotein C-II deficiency	ApoC-II (*APOC2*)	Chylomicrons	Eruptive xanthomas, hepatosplenomegaly, pancreatitis	AR	<1/1,000,000
ApoA-V deficiency	ApoA-V (*APOA5*)	Chylomicrons, VLDL	Eruptive xanthomas, hepatosplenomegaly, pancreatitis	AD	<1/1,000,000
GPIHBP1 deficiency	*GDIHBP1*	Chylomicrons	Eruptive xanthomas, pancreatitis	AD	<1/1,000,000
Familial hepatic lipase deficiency	Hepatic lipase (*LIPC*)	VLDL remnants	Pancreatitis, CHD	AR	<1/1,000,000
Familial dysbetalipoproteinemia	ApoE (*APOE*)	Chylomicron and VLDL remnants	Palmar and tuberoeruptive xanthomas, CHD, PVD	AR AD	1/10,000
Familial hypercholesterolemia	LDL receptor (*LDLR*)	LDL	Tendon xanthomas, CHD	AD	1/500
Familial defective apoB-100	ApoB-100 (*APOB*)	LDL	Tendon xanthomas, CHD	AD	<1/1000
Autosomal dominant hypercholesterolemia	PCSK9 (*PCSK9*)	LDL	Tendon xanthomas, CHD	AD	<1/1,000,000
Autosomal recessive hypercholesterolemia	*LDLRAP*	LDL	Tendon xanthomas, CHD	AR	<1/1,000,000
Sitosterolemia	*ABCG5 or ABCG8*	LDL	Tendon xanthomas, CHD	AR	<1/1,000,000

Abbreviations: AD, autosomal dominant; AR, autosomal recessive; ARH, autosomal recessive hypercholesterolemia; CHD, coronary heart disease; LDL, low-density lipoprotein; LPL, lipoprotein lipase; PVD, peripheral vascular disease; VLDL, very-low density lipoprotein.

than 1000 mg/dL. The devastating complication of homozygous FH is accelerated atherosclerosis, which can result in disability and death in childhood. Atherosclerosis often develops first in the aortic root, where it can cause aortic valvular or supravalvular stenosis, and typically extends into the coronary ostia, which become stenotic. Children with homozygous FH often develop symptomatic coronary atherosclerosis before puberty; symptoms can be atypical, and sudden death is not uncommon. Untreated, receptor-negative patients with homozygous FH rarely survive beyond the second decade; patients with receptor-defective LDL receptor defects have a better prognosis but almost invariably develop clinically apparent atherosclerotic vascular disease by age 30, and often much sooner. Carotid and femoral disease develops later in life and is usually not clinically significant.

A careful family history should be taken, and plasma lipid levels should be measured in the parents and other first-degree relatives of patients with homozygous FH. The disease has >90% penetrance so both parents of FH homozygotes usually have hypercholesterolemia. The diagnosis of homozygous FH can be confirmed by obtaining a skin biopsy and measuring LDL receptor activity in cultured skin fibroblasts, or by quantifying the number of LDL receptors on the surfaces of lymphocytes using cell sorting technology. Molecular assays are also available to define the mutations in the LDL receptor by DNA sequencing. In selected populations where particular mutations predominate (e.g., Africaners and French Canadians), the common mutations can be screened for directly. Alternatively, the entire coding region needs to be sequenced for mutation detection because a large number of different LDL receptor mutations can cause disease. Ten to 15% of LDL receptor mutations are large deletions or insertions, which may be missed by routine DNA sequencing.

Combination therapy with an HMG-CoA reductase inhibitor and a second drug (cholesterol absorption inhibitor or bile acid sequestrant) sometimes reduces plasma LDL-C in those FH homozygotes who have residual LDL receptor activity, but patients with homozygous FH invariably require additional lipid-lowering therapy. Since the liver is quantitatively the most important tissue for removing circulating LDLs via the LDL receptor, liver transplantation is effective in decreasing plasma LDL-C levels in this disorder. Liver transplantation, however, is associated with substantial risks, including the requirement for long-term immunosuppression. The current treatment of choice for homozygous FH is LDL apheresis (a process by which the LDL particles are selectively removed from the circulation), which can promote regression of xanthomas and may slow the progression of atherosclerosis. Initiation of LDL apheresis

should generally be delayed until approximately 5 years of age, except when evidence of atherosclerotic vascular disease is present.

Heterozygous FH is caused by the inheritance of one mutant LDL receptor allele and occurs in approximately 1 in 500 persons worldwide, making it one of the most common single-gene disorders. It is characterized by elevated plasma levels of LDL-C (usually 200–400 mg/dL) and normal levels of triglyceride. Patients with heterozygous FH have hypercholesterolemia from birth, and disease recognition is usually based on detection of hypercholesterolemia on routine screening, the appearance of tendon xanthomas, or the development of symptomatic ASCVD. Since the disease is codominant in inheritance, one parent and ~50% of the patient's siblings usually also have hypercholesterolemia. The family history is frequently positive for premature ASCVD on one side of the family. Corneal arcus is common, and tendon xanthomas involving the dorsum of the hands, elbows, knees, and especially the Achilles tendons are present in ~75% of patients. The age of onset of ASCVD is highly variable and depends in part on the molecular defect in the LDL receptor gene and also on coexisting cardiac risk factors. FH heterozygotes with elevated plasma levels of Lp(a) appear to be at greater risk for cardiovascular complications. Untreated men with heterozygous FH have an ~50% chance of having a myocardial infarction before age 60 years. Although the age of onset of atherosclerotic heart disease is later in women with FH, coronary heart disease (CHD) is significantly more common in women with FH than in the general female population.

No definitive diagnostic test for heterozygous FH is available. Although FH heterozygotes tend to have reduced levels of LDL receptor function in skin fibroblasts, significant overlap with the LDL receptor activity levels in normal fibroblasts exists. Molecular assays are now available to identify mutations in the LDL receptor gene by DNA sequencing, but the clinical utility of pinpointing the mutation has not been demonstrated. The clinical diagnosis is usually not problematic, but it is critical that hypothyroidism, nephrotic syndrome, and obstructive liver disease be excluded before initiating therapy.

FH patients should be aggressively treated to lower plasma levels of LDL-C. Initiation of a low-cholesterol, low-fat diet is recommended, but heterozygous FH patients require lipid-lowering drug therapy. Statins are effective in heterozygous FH, but combination drug therapy with the addition of a cholesterol absorption inhibitor and/or bile acid sequestrant is frequently required, and the addition of nicotinic acid is sometimes needed. Heterozygous FH patients who cannot be adequately controlled on combination drug therapy are candidates for LDL apheresis.

Familial defective ApoB-100 (FDB)

FDB is a dominantly inherited disorder that clinically resembles heterozygous FH. The disease is rare in most populations except individuals of German descent, where the frequency can be as high as 1 in 1000. FDB is characterized by elevated plasma LDL-C levels with normal triglycerides, tendon xanthomas, and an increased incidence of premature ASCVD. FDB is caused by mutations in the LDL receptor–binding domain of apoB-100, most commonly due to a substitution of glutamine for arginine at position 3500. As a consequence of the mutation in apoB-100, LDL binds the LDL receptor with reduced affinity, and LDL is removed from the circulation at a reduced rate. Patients with FDB cannot be clinically distinguished from patients with heterozygous FH, although patients with FDB tend to have lower plasma levels of LDL-C than FH heterozygotes. The apoB-100 gene mutation can be detected directly, but genetic diagnosis is not currently encouraged since the recommended management of FDB and heterozygous FH is identical.

Autosomal dominant hypercholesterolemia due to mutations in PCSK9 (ADH-PCSK9 or ADH3)

ADH-PCSK9 is a rare autosomal dominant disorder caused by gain-of-function mutations in proprotein convertase subtilisin/kexin type 9 (PCSK9). PCSK9 is a secreted protein that binds to the LDL receptor, resulting in its degradation. Normally, after LDL binds to the receptor it is internalized along with the receptor. In the low pH of the endosome, LDL dissociates from the receptor and returns to the cell surface. The LDL is delivered to the lysosome. When PCSK9 binds the receptor, the complex is internalized and the receptor is redirected to the lysosome rather than to the cell surface. The missense mutations in PCSK9 that cause hypercholesterolemia enhance the activity of PCSK9. As a consequence, the number of hepatic LDL receptors is reduced. Patients with ADH-PCSK9 are indistinguishable clinically from patients with FH. Interestingly, loss-of-function mutations in PCSK9 cause low LDL-C levels (see later).

Autosomal recessive hypercholesterolemia (ARH)

ARH is a rare disorder (except in Sardinia, Italy) due to mutations in a protein (ARH, also called LDLR adaptor protein, LDLRAP) involved in LDL receptor–mediated endocytosis in the liver. In the absence of LDLRAP, LDL binds to the LDL receptor but the lipoprotein-receptor complex fails to be internalized. ARH, like homozygous FH, is characterized by hypercholesterolemia, tendon xanthomas, and premature coronary artery disease (CAD). The levels of plasma LDL-C tend to be intermediate between the levels present in FH homozygotes and FH heterozygotes, and CAD is not usually symptomatic until at least the third decade. LDL

receptor function in cultured fibroblasts is normal or only modestly reduced in ARH, whereas LDL receptor function in lymphocytes and the liver is negligible. Unlike FH homozygotes, the hyperlipidemia responds partially to treatment with HMG-CoA reductase inhibitors, but these patients usually require LDL apheresis to lower plasma LDL-C to recommended levels.

Sitosterolemia

Sitosterolemia is another rare autosomal recessive disease that can result in severe hypercholesterolemia, tendon xanthomas, and premature ASCVD. Sitosterolemia is caused by mutations in either of two members of the ATP-binding cassette (ABC) half transporter family, ABCG5 and ABCG8. These genes are expressed in enterocytes and hepatocytes. The proteins heterodimerize to form a functional complex that pumps plant sterols such as sitosterol and campesterol, and animal sterols, predominantly cholesterol, into the gut lumen and into the bile. In normal individuals, <5% of dietary plant sterols are absorbed by the proximal small intestine and delivered to the liver. Absorbed plant sterols are preferentially secreted into the bile and are maintained at very low levels. In sitosterolemia, the intestinal absorption of sterols is increased and biliary excretion of the sterols is reduced, resulting in increased plasma and tissue levels of both plant sterols and cholesterol.

Incorporation of plant sterols into cell membranes results in misshapen red blood cells and megathrombocytes that are visible on blood smear. Episodes of hemolysis are a distinctive clinical feature of this disease compared to other genetic forms of hypercholesterolemia.

Sitosterolemia is diagnosed by demonstrating an increase in the plasma level of sitosterol using gas chromatography. The hypercholesterolemia is unusually responsive to reductions in dietary cholesterol content and should be suspected in individuals who have a >40% reduction in plasma cholesterol level on a low-cholesterol diet. The hypercholesterolemia does not respond to HMG-CoA reductase inhibitors, whereas bile acid sequestrants and cholesterol-absorption inhibitors such as ezetimibe, are effective in reducing plasma sterol levels in these patients.

Polygenic hypercholesterolemia

This condition is characterized by hypercholesterolemia due to elevated LDL-C with a normal plasma level of triglyceride in the absence of secondary causes of hypercholesterolemia. Plasma LDL-C levels are generally not as elevated as they are in FH and FDB. Family studies are useful to differentiate polygenic hypercholesterolemia from the single-gene disorders described above; one-half of the first-degree relatives of patients with FH and FDB are hypercholesterolemic, whereas <10% of first-degree relatives of patients with polygenic hypercholesterolemia have hypercholesterolemia. Treatment of polygenic hypercholesterolemia is identical to that of other forms of hypercholesterolemia.

Elevated plasma levels of lipoprotein(a)

Unlike the other major classes of lipoproteins, that have a normal distribution in the population, plasma levels of Lp(a) have a highly skewed distribution with levels varying over a 1000-fold range. Levels are strongly influenced by genetic factors, with individuals of African and South Asian descent having higher levels than those of European descent. Although it has been well documented that elevated levels of Lp(a) are associated with an increase in ASCVD, lowering plasma levels of Lp(a) has not been demonstrated to reduce cardiovascular risk.

Lipid disorders associated with elevated triglycerides

▇ Familial chylomicronemia syndrome (Type I hyperlipoproteinemia; lipoprotein lipase, and ApoC-II deficiency)

As noted above, LPL is required for the hydrolysis of triglycerides in chylomicrons and VLDLs, and apoC-II is a cofactor for LPL (Fig. 31-2). Genetic deficiency or inactivity of either protein results in impaired lipolysis and profound elevations in plasma chylomicrons. These patients can also have elevated plasma levels of VLDL, but chylomicronemia predominates. The fasting plasma is turbid, and if left at 4°C (39.2°F) for a few hours, the chylomicrons float to the top and form a creamy supernatant. In these disorders, called *familial chylomicronemia syndromes*, fasting triglyceride levels are almost invariably >1000 mg/dL. Fasting cholesterol levels are also elevated but to a lesser degree.

LPL deficiency has autosomal recessive inheritance and has a frequency of approximately 1 in 1 million in the population. *ApoC-II deficiency* is also recessive in inheritance pattern and is even less common than LPL deficiency. Multiple different mutations in the LPL and apoC-II genes cause these diseases. Obligate LPL heterozygotes have normal or mild-to-moderate elevations in plasma triglyceride levels, whereas individuals heterozygous for mutation in apoC-II do not have hypertriglyceridemia.

Both LPL and apoC-II deficiency usually present in childhood with recurrent episodes of severe abdominal pain due to acute pancreatitis. On funduscopic examination, the retinal blood vessels are opalescent (lipemia retinalis). Eruptive xanthomas, which are small, yellowish-white papules, often appear in clusters on the back, buttocks, and extensor surfaces of the arms and legs. These typically painless skin lesions may become pruritic. Hepatosplenomegaly results from the uptake of circulating chylomicrons by reticuloendothelial cells in the liver and spleen. For unknown reasons, some patients with persistent and pronounced chylomicronemia never develop pancreatitis, eruptive xanthomas, or hepatosplenomegaly. Premature CHD is not generally a feature of familial chylomicronemia syndromes.

The diagnoses of LPL and apoC-II deficiency are established enzymatically in specialized laboratories by assaying triglyceride lipolytic activity in postheparin plasma. Blood is sampled after an IV heparin injection to release the endothelial-bound LPL. LPL activity is profoundly reduced in both LPL and apoC-II deficiency; in patients with apoC-II deficiency, it normalizes after the addition of normal plasma (providing a source of apoC-II). Molecular sequencing of the genes can be used to confirm the diagnosis.

The major therapeutic intervention in familial chylomicronemia syndromes is dietary fat restriction (to as little as 15 g/d) with fat-soluble vitamin supplementation. Consultation with a registered dietician familiar with this disorder is essential. Caloric supplementation with medium-chain triglycerides, which are absorbed directly into the portal circulation, can be useful but may be associated with hepatic fibrosis if used for prolonged periods. If dietary fat restriction alone is not successful in resolving the chylomicronemia, fish oils have been effective in some patients. In patients with apoC-II deficiency, apoC-II can be provided by infusing fresh-frozen plasma to resolve the chylomicronemia in the acute setting. Management of patients with familial chylomicronemia syndrome is particularly challenging during pregnancy when VLDL production is increased and may require plasmapheresis to remove the circulating chylomicrons.

▇ ApoA-V deficiency

Another apolipoprotein, apoA-V, circulates at much lower concentrations than the other major apolipoproteins. Individuals harboring mutations in both apoA-V alleles can present as adults with chylomicronemia. The exact mechanism of action of apoA-V is not known, but it appears to be required for the association of VLDL and chylomicrons with LPL.

▇ GPIHBP1 deficiency

After LPL is synthesized in adipocytes, myocytes, or other cells, it is transported across the vascular endothelium and is attached to a protein on the endothelial surface of capillaries called GPIHBP1. Homozygosity for mutations that interfere with GPIHBP1 synthesis or folding cause severe hypertriglyceridemia. The frequency of chylomicronemia due to mutations in GHIHBP1 has not been established but appears to be very rare.

▇ Hepatic lipase deficiency

HL is a member of the same gene family as LPL and hydrolyzes triglycerides and phospholipids in remnant lipoproteins and HDLs. HL deficiency is a very rare autosomal recessive disorder characterized by elevated plasma levels of cholesterol and triglycerides (mixed hyperlipidemia) due to the accumulation of circulating lipoprotein remnants and either a normal or elevated plasma level of HDL-C. The diagnosis is confirmed by measuring HL activity in postheparin plasma. Due to the small number of patients with HL deficiency, the association of this genetic defect with ASCVD is not clearly known, but lipid-lowering therapy is recommended.

Familial dysbetalipoproteinemia (Type III hyperlipoproteinemia)

Like HL deficiency, familial dysbetalipoproteinemia (FDBL) (also known as *Type III hyperlipoproteinemia* or *familial broad β disease*) is characterized by a mixed hyperlipidemia due to the accumulation of remnant lipoprotein particles. ApoE is present in multiple copies on chylomicron and VLDL remnants and mediates their removal via hepatic lipoprotein receptors (Fig. 31-2). FDBL is due to genetic variations in apoE that interfere with its ability to bind lipoprotein receptors. The *APOE* gene is polymorphic in sequence, resulting in the expression of three common isoforms: apoE3, which is the most common; and apoE2 and apoE4, which both differ from apoE3 by a single amino acid. Although associated with slightly higher LDL-C levels and increased CHD risk, the apoE4 allele is not associated with FDBL. Patients with apoE4 have an increased incidence of late-onset Alzheimer's disease. ApoE2 has a lower affinity for the LDL receptor; therefore, chylomicron and VLDL remnants containing apoE2 are removed from plasma at a slower rate. Individuals who are homozygous for the E2 allele (the E2/E2 genotype) comprise the most common subset of patients with FDBL.

Approximately 0.5% of the general population are apoE2/E2 homozygotes, but only a small minority of these individuals develop FDBL. In most cases, an additional, identifiable factor precipitates the development of hyperlipoproteinemia. The most common precipitating factors are a high-fat diet, diabetes mellitus, obesity, hypothyroidism, renal disease, HIV infection, estrogen deficiency, alcohol use, or certain drugs. Other mutations in apoE can cause a dominant form of FDBL where the hyperlipidemia is fully manifest in the heterozygous state, but these mutations are rare.

Patients with FDBL usually present in adulthood with incidental hyperlipidemia, xanthomas, premature coronary disease, or peripheral vascular disease. The disease seldom presents in women before menopause. Two distinctive types of xanthomas, tuberoeruptive and palmar, are seen in FDBL patients. Tuberoeruptive xanthomas begin as clusters of small papules on the elbows, knees, or buttocks and can grow to the size of small grapes. Palmar xanthomas (alternatively called *xanthomata striata palmaris*) are orange-yellow discolorations of the creases in the palms and wrists. In FDBL, in contrast to other disorders of elevated triglycerides, the plasma levels of cholesterol and triglyceride are often elevated to a similar degree and the level of HDL-C is usually normal rather than being low.

The traditional approaches to diagnosis of this disorder are lipoprotein electrophoresis (broad β band) or ultracentrifugation (ratio of VLDL-C to total plasma triglyceride >0.30). Protein methods (apoE phenotyping) or DNA-based methods (apoE genotyping) can be performed to confirm homozygosity for apoE2. However, absence of the apoE2/E2 genotype does not rule out the diagnosis of FDBL, since other mutations in apoE can cause this condition.

Since FDBL is associated with increased risk of premature ASCVD, it should be treated aggressively. Subjects with FDBL tend to have more peripheral vascular disease than is typically seen in FH. Other metabolic conditions that can worsen the hyperlipidemia (see earlier) should be aggressively treated. Patients with FDBL are typically very diet responsive and can respond favorably to weight reduction and to low-cholesterol, low-fat diets. Alcohol intake should be curtailed. HMG-CoA reductase inhibitors, fibrates, and niacin are all generally effective in the treatment of FDBL, and sometimes combination drug therapy is required.

Familial hypertriglyceridemia (FHTG)

FHTG is a relatively common (~1 in 500) autosomal dominant disorder of unknown etiology characterized by moderately elevated plasma triglycerides accompanied by more modest elevations in cholesterol. Since the major class of lipoproteins elevated in this disorder is VLDL, patients with this disorder are often referred to as having *Type IV hyperlipoproteinemia* (Fredrickson classification, Table 31-3). The elevated plasma levels of VLDL are due to increased production of VLDL, impaired catabolism of VLDL, or a combination of these mechanisms. Some patients with FHTG have a more severe form of hyperlipidemia in which both VLDLs and chylomicrons are elevated (*Type V hyperlipidemia*), since these two classes of lipoproteins compete for the same lipolytic pathway. Increased intake of simple carbohydrates, obesity, insulin resistance, alcohol use, and estrogen treatment, all of which increase VLDL synthesis, can exacerbate this syndrome. FHTG appears not to be associated with increased risk of ASCVD in many families.

The diagnosis of FHTG is suggested by the triad of elevated levels of plasma triglycerides (250–1000 mg/dL), normal or only mildly increased cholesterol levels (<250 mg/dL), and reduced plasma levels of HDL-C. Plasma LDL-C levels are generally not increased and are often reduced due to defective metabolism of the triglyceride-rich particles. The identification of other first-degree relatives with hypertriglyceridemia is useful in making the diagnosis. FDBL and familial combined hyperlipidemia (FCHL) should also be ruled out since these two conditions are associated with a significantly increased risk of ASCVD. The plasma apoB levels are lower and the ratio of plasma triglyceride to cholesterol is higher in FHTG than in either FDBL or FCHL.

It is important to consider and rule out secondary causes of hypertriglyceridemia (Table 31-5) before making the diagnosis of FHTG. Lipid-lowering drug therapy can frequently be avoided with appropriate dietary and lifestyle changes. Patients with plasma triglyceride levels >500 mg/dL after a trial of diet and exercise should be considered for drug therapy to avoid the development of chylomicronemia and pancreatitis. Fibrate drugs or fish oils (omega 3 fatty acids) are reasonable first-line approaches for FHTG, and niacin can also be considered in this condition. For more moderate elevations in triglyceride levels (250–500 mg/dL), statins are effective at lowering triglyceride levels.

Familial combined hyperlipidemia (FCHL)

FCHL is generally characterized by moderate elevations in plasma levels of triglycerides (VLDL) and cholesterol (LDL) and reduced plasma levels of HDL-C. Approximately 20% of patients who develop CHD under age 60 have FCHL. The disease appears to be autosomal dominant with incomplete penetrance and affected family members typically have one of three possible phenotypes: (1) elevated plasma levels of LDL-C, (2) elevated plasma levels of triglycerides due to elevation in VLDL, or (3) elevated plasma levels of both LDL-C and triglyceride. A classic feature of FCHL is that the lipoprotein profile can switch among these three phenotypes in the same individual over time and may depend on factors such as diet, exercise, and weight. FCHL can manifest in childhood but is usually not fully expressed until adulthood. A cluster of other metabolic risk factors are often found in association with this hyperlipidemia, including obesity, glucose intolerance, insulin resistance, and hypertension (the so-called metabolic syndrome, Chap. 32). These patients do not develop xanthomas.

Patients with FCHL almost always have significantly elevated plasma levels of apoB. The levels of apoB are disproportionately high relative to the plasma LDL-C concentration, indicating the presence of small, dense LDL particles, which are characteristic of this syndrome. *Hyperapobetalipoproteinemia*, which has been used to describe the state of elevated plasma levels of apoB with normal plasma LDL-C levels, is probably a form of FCHL. Individuals with FCHL generally share the same metabolic defect, which is overproduction of VLDL by the liver. The molecular etiology of FCHL remains poorly understood, and it is likely that defects in several different genes can cause the phenotype of FCHL.

The presence of a mixed dyslipidemia (plasma triglyceride levels between 200 and 800 mg/dL and total cholesterol levels between 200 and 400 mg/dL, usually with HDL-C levels <40 mg/dL in men and <50 mg/dL in women) and a family history of hyperlipidemia and/or premature CHD strongly suggests the diagnosis of FCHL.

Individuals with FCHL should be treated aggressively due to significantly increased risk of premature CHD. Decreased dietary intake of saturated fat and simple carbohydrates, aerobic exercise, and weight loss can all have beneficial effects on the lipid profile. Patients with diabetes should be aggressively treated to maintain good glucose control. Most patients with FCHL require lipid-lowering drug therapy to reduce lipoprotein levels to the recommended range and reduce the high risk of ASCVD. Statins are effective in this condition, but many patients will require a second drug (cholesterol absorption inhibitor, niacin, fibrate, or fish oils) for optimal control of lipoprotein levels.

INHERITED CAUSES OF LOW LEVELS OF ApoB-CONTAINING LIPOPROTEINS

Familial hypobetalipoproteinemia (FHB)

Low plasma levels of LDL-C (the "β-lipoprotein") with a genetic or inherited basis are referred to generically as *familial hypobetalipoproteinemia*. Traditionally, this term has been used to refer to the condition of low total cholesterol and LDL-C due to mutations in apoB, which represents the most common inherited form of hypocholesterolemia. Most of the mutations causing FHB interfere with the production of apoB, resulting in reduced secretion and/or accelerated catabolism of the protein. Individuals heterozygous for these mutations usually have LDL-C levels <80 mg/dL and may enjoy protection from ASCVD, though this has not been rigorously demonstrated. Some heterozygotes have elevated levels of hepatic triglycerides.

Mutations in both apoB alleles cause homozygous FHB, a disorder resembling abetalipoproteinemia (see later), although the neurologic findings tend to be less severe. Patients with homozygous hypobetalipoproteinemia can be distinguished from individuals with abetalipoproteinemia by measuring the levels of LDL-C in the parents, which are low in hypobetalipoproteinemia and normal in abetalipoproteinemia.

PCSK9 deficiency

A phenocopy of FHB results from loss-of-function mutations in PCSK9. As reviewed earlier, PCSK9 normally promotes the degradation of the LDL receptor. Mutations that interfere with the synthesis of PCSK9, which are more common in individuals of African descent, result in

TABLE 31-5

SECONDARY FORMS OF HYPERLIPIDEMIA

LDL		HDL		VLDL ELEVATED	IDL ELEVATED	CHYLOMICRONS ELEVATED	LP(a) ELEVATED
ELEVATED	**REDUCED**	**ELEVATED**	**REDUCED**				
Hypothyroidism	Severe liver disease	Alcohol	Smoking	Obesity	Multiple myeloma	Autoimmune disease	Renal insufficiency
Nephrotic syndrome	Malabsorption Malnutrition	Exercise Exposure to chlorinated hydrocarbons	DM type 2 Obesity	DM type 2 Glycogen storage disease	Monoclonal gammopathy	DM type 2	Inflammation
Cholestasis	Gaucher's disease	Drugs: estrogen	Malnutrition	Hepatitis Alcohol	Autoimmune disease		Menopause
Acute intermittent porphyria	Chronic infectious disease		Gaucher's disease	Renal failure Sepsis Stress Cushing's syndrome Pregnancy Acromegaly Lipodystrophy Drugs: estrogen, beta blockers, glucocorticoids, bile acid binding resins, retinoic acid	Hypothyroidism		Orchidectomy
Anorexia nervosa Hepatoma Drugs: thiazides, cyclosporin, tegretol	Hyperthyroidism Drugs: niacin toxicity		Drugs: anabolic steroids, beta blockers				Hypothyroidism Acromegaly Nephrosis Drugs: growth hormone, isotretinoin

Abbreviations: DM, diabetes mellitus; HDL, high-density lipoprotein; IDL, intermediate-density lipoprotein; LDL, low-density lipoprotein; Lp(a), lipoprotein A; VLDL, very low-density lipoprotein.

increased LDL receptor activity and ~40% reduction in plasma level of LDL-C. A sequence variation of higher frequency (R46L) is found predominantly in individuals of European descent and is associated with a 15% reduction in LDL-C. Individuals with inactivating mutations are protected from developing CHD relative to those without these sequence variations, presumably due to having lower plasma cholesterol levels since birth.

Abetalipoproteinemia

The synthesis and secretion of apoB-containing lipoproteins in the enterocytes of the proximal small bowel and in the hepatocytes of the liver involve a complex series of events that coordinate the coupling of various lipids with apoB-48 and apoB-100, respectively. Abetalipoproteinemia is a rare autosomal recessive disease caused by loss-of-function mutations in the gene encoding microsomal triglyceride transfer protein (MTP), a protein that transfers lipids to nascent chylomicrons and VLDLs in the intestine and liver, respectively. Plasma levels of cholesterol and triglyceride are extremely low in this disorder, and chylomicrons, VLDLs, LDLs, and apoB are undetectable in plasma. The parents of patients with abetalipoproteinemia (obligate heterozygotes) have normal plasma lipid and apoB levels. Abetalipoproteinemia usually presents in early childhood with diarrhea and failure to thrive due to fat malabsorption. The initial neurologic manifestations are loss of deep-tendon reflexes, followed by decreased distal lower extremity vibratory and proprioceptive sense, dysmetria, ataxia, and the development of a spastic gait, often by the third or fourth decade. Patients with abetalipoproteinemia also develop a progressive pigmented retinopathy presenting with decreased night and color vision, followed by reductions in daytime visual acuity and ultimately progressing to near-blindness. The presence of spinocerebellar degeneration and pigmented retinopathy in this disease has resulted in some patients with abetalipoproteinemia being misdiagnosed as having Friedreich's ataxia.

Most clinical manifestations of abetalipoproteinemia result from defects in the absorption and transport of fat-soluble vitamins. Vitamin E and retinyl esters are normally transported from enterocytes to the liver by chylomicrons, and vitamin E is dependent on VLDL for transport out of the liver and into the circulation. As a consequence of the inability of these patients to secrete apoB-containing particles, patients with abetalipoproteinemia are markedly deficient in vitamin E and are also mildly to moderately deficient in vitamins A and K. Patients with abetalipoproteinemia should be referred to specialized centers for confirmation of the diagnosis and appropriate therapy. Treatment consists of a low-fat, high-caloric, vitamin-enriched diet accompanied by large supplemental doses of vitamin E. It is imperative that treatment be initiated as soon as possible to help forestall development of neurologic sequelae, which can progress even with appropriate therapy. New therapies for this serious disease are needed.

GENETIC DISORDERS OF HDL METABOLISM

Mutations in genes encoding proteins that play critical roles in HDL synthesis and catabolism can result in both reductions and elevations in plasma levels of HDL-C. Unlike the genetic forms of hypercholesterolemia, which are invariably associated with premature coronary atherosclerosis, genetic forms of hypoalphalipoproteinemia (low HDL-C) are not always associated with accelerated atherosclerosis.

INHERITED CAUSES OF LOW LEVELS OF HDL-C

Gene deletions in the ApoAV-AI-CIII-AIV locus and coding mutations in ApoA-I

Complete genetic deficiency of apoA-I due to deletion of the apoA-I gene results in the virtual absence of HDL from the plasma. The genes encoding apoA-I, apoC-III, apoA-IV, and apoA-V are clustered together on chromosome 11, and some patients with no apoA-I have genomic deletions that include other genes in the cluster. ApoA-I is required for LCAT activity. In the absence of LCAT, free cholesterol levels increase in both plasma (not HDL) and in tissues. The free cholesterol can form deposits in the cornea and in the skin, resulting in corneal opacities and planar xanthomas. Premature CHD is a common feature of apoA-I deficiency, especially when additional genes in the complex are also deleted.

Missense and nonsense mutations in the apoA-I gene have been identified in some patients with low plasma levels of HDL-C (usually 15–30 mg/dL), but these are very rare causes of low HDL-C levels. Patients heterozygous for an Arg173Cys substitution in APOAI (so-called apoA-I$_{Milano}$) have very low plasma levels of HDL due to impaired LCAT activation and rapid catabolism of the mutant apolipoprotein and yet have no increased risk of premature CHD. Most other individuals with low plasma HDL-C levels due to missense mutations in apoA-I do not appear to have premature CHD. A few selected missense mutations in apoA-I and apoA-II promote the formation of amyloid fibrils causing systemic amyloidosis.

Tangier disease (ABCA1 deficiency)

Tangier disease is a very rare autosomal codominant form of extremely low plasma HDL-C caused by mutations in the gene encoding ABCA1, a cellular transporter that facilitates efflux of unesterified cholesterol and phospholipids from cells to apoA-I (Fig. 31-3). ABCA1 in the liver and intestine rapidly lipidates the apoA-I secreted from these tissues. In the absence of ABCA1, the nascent, poorly lipidated apoA-I is immediately cleared from the circulation. Thus, patients with Tangier disease have extremely low circulating plasma levels of HDL-C (<5 mg/dL) and apoA-I (<5 mg/dL). Cholesterol accumulates in the reticuloendothelial system of these patients, resulting in hepatosplenomegaly and pathognomonic enlarged, grayish yellow or orange tonsils. An intermittent peripheral neuropathy (mononeuritis multiplex) or a sphingomyelia-like neurologic disorder can also be seen in this disorder. Tangier disease is probably associated with some increased risk of premature atherosclerotic disease, although the association is not as robust as might be anticipated, given the very low levels of HDL-C and apoA-I in these patients. Patients with Tangier disease also have low plasma levels of LDL-C, which may attenuate the atherosclerotic risk. Obligate heterozygotes for ABCA1 mutations have moderately reduced plasma HDL-C levels (15–30 mg/dL) but their risk of premature CHD remains uncertain. ABCA1 mutations appear to be the cause of low HDL-C in a minority of individuals.

LCAT deficiency

This very rare autosomal recessive disorder is caused by mutations in LCAT, an enzyme synthesized in the liver and secreted into the plasma, where it circulates associated with lipoproteins (Fig. 31-3). As reviewed earlier, the enzyme is activated by apoA-I and mediates the esterification of cholesterol to form cholesteryl esters. Consequently, in LCAT deficiency the proportion of free cholesterol in circulating lipoproteins is greatly increased (from ~25% to >70% of total plasma cholesterol). Lack of normal cholesterol esterification impairs formation of mature HDL particles, resulting in the rapid catabolism of circulating apoA-I. Two genetic forms of LCAT deficiency have been described in humans: complete deficiency (also called *classic LCAT deficiency*) and partial deficiency (also called *fish-eye disease*). Progressive corneal opacification due to the deposition of free cholesterol in the cornea, very low plasma levels of HDL-C (usually <10 mg/dL), and variable hypertriglyceridemia are characteristic of both disorders. In partial LCAT deficiency, there are no other known clinical sequelae. In contrast, patients with complete LCAT deficiency have hemolytic anemia and progressive renal insufficiency that eventually leads to end-stage renal disease (ESRD). Remarkably, despite the extremely low plasma levels of HDL-C and apoA-I, premature ASCVD is not a consistent feature of either LCAT deficiency or fish-eye disease. The diagnosis can be confirmed in a specialized laboratory by assaying plasma LCAT activity or by sequencing the LCAT gene.

Primary hypoalphalipoproteinemia

Low plasma levels of HDL-C (the "alpha lipoprotein") is referred to as *hypoalphalipoproteinemia*. Primary hypoalphalipoproteinemia is defined as a plasma HDL-C level below the tenth percentile in the setting of relatively normal cholesterol and triglyceride levels, no apparent secondary causes of low plasma HDL-C, and no clinical signs of LCAT deficiency or Tangier disease. This syndrome is often referred to as *isolated low HDL*. A family history of low HDL-C facilitates the diagnosis of an inherited condition, which usually follows an autosomal dominant pattern. The metabolic etiology of this disease appears to be primarily accelerated catabolism of HDL and its apolipoproteins. Some of these patients may have ABCA1 mutations and therefore technically have heterozygous Tangier disease. Several kindreds with primary hypoalphalipoproteinemia have been described in association with an increased incidence of premature CHD, although this is not an invariant association. Association of hypoalphalipoproteinemia with premature CHD may depend on the specific nature of the gene defect or the underlying metabolic defect responsible for the low plasma HDL-C level.

INHERITED CAUSES OF HIGH LEVELS OF HDL-C

CETP deficiency

Loss-of-function mutations in both alleles of the gene encoding CETP cause substantially elevated HDL-C levels (usually >150 mg/dL). As noted earlier, CETP facilitates the transfer of cholesteryl esters from HDL to apoB-containing lipoproteins (Fig. 31-3). The absence of this transfer results in an increase in the cholesteryl ester content of HDL and a reduction in plasma levels of LDL-C. The large, cholesterol-rich HDL particles circulating in these patients are cleared at a reduced rate. CETP deficiency was first diagnosed in Japanese persons and is rare outside of Japan. The relationship of CETP deficiency to ASCVD remains unresolved. Heterozygotes for CETP deficiency have only modestly elevated HDL-C levels. Based on the phenotype of high HDL-C in CETP deficiency, pharmacologic inhibition of CETP is under development as a new therapeutic approach to both raise HDL-C levels and lower LDL-C levels, but whether it will reduce risk of ASCVD remains to be determined.

Familial hyperalphalipoproteinemia

The condition of high plasma levels of HDL-C is referred to as *hyperalphalipoproteinemia* and is defined as a plasma HDL-C level above the ninetieth percentile. This trait runs in families, and outside of Japan it is unlikely to be due to CETP deficiency. Most, but not all, persons with this condition appear to have a reduced risk of CHD and increased longevity. Recent evidence is consistent with mutations in endothelial lipase contributing to this phenotype in some cases.

SECONDARY DISORDERS OF LIPOPROTEIN METABOLISM

Significant changes in plasma levels of lipoproteins are seen in a variety of diseases. It is crucial that secondary causes of dyslipidemias (Table 31-5) are considered prior to initiation of lipid-lowering therapy.

Obesity

Obesity is frequently accompanied by dyslipidemia. The increase in adipocyte mass and accompanying decreased insulin sensitivity associated with obesity has multiple effects on lipid metabolism. More free fatty acids are delivered from the expanded adipose tissue to the liver, where they are reesterified in hepatocytes to form triglycerides, which are packaged into VLDLs for secretion into the circulation. The increased insulin levels promote fatty acid synthesis in the liver. Increased dietary intake of simple carbohydrates also drives hepatic production of VLDLs, resulting in elevations in VLDL and/or LDL in some obese subjects. Plasma levels of HDL-C tend to be low in obesity, due in part to reduced lipolysis. Weight loss is often associated with reductions in plasma levels of circulating apoB-containing lipoproteins and increases in the plasma levels of HDL-C.

Diabetes mellitus

Patients with type I diabetes mellitus generally do not have hyperlipidemia if they remain under good glycemic control. Diabetic ketoacidosis is frequently accompanied by hypertriglyceridemia due to an increased hepatic influx of free fatty acids from adipose tissue. Patients with type II diabetes mellitus are usually dyslipidemic, even when under relatively good glycemic control. The high levels of insulin and insulin resistance associated with type II diabetes has multiple effects on fat metabolism: (1) a decrease in LPL activity resulting in reduced catabolism of chylomicrons and VLDLs, (2) an increase in the release of free fatty acid from the adipose tissue, (3) an increase in fatty acid synthesis in the liver, and (4) an increase in hepatic VLDL production. Patients with type II diabetes mellitus have several lipid abnormalities, including elevated plasma triglycerides (due to increased VLDL and lipoprotein remnants), elevated levels of dense LDL, and decreased plasma levels of HDL-C. In some diabetic patients, especially those with a genetic defect in lipid metabolism, the triglycerides can be extremely elevated, resulting in the development of pancreatitis. Elevated plasma

LDL-C levels usually are not a feature of diabetes mellitus and suggest the presence of an underlying lipoprotein abnormality or may indicate the development of diabetic nephropathy.

Lipodystrophy is associated with profound insulin resistance and elevated plasma levels of VLDL and chylomicrons that can be especially difficult to control. Those with congenital generalized lipodystrophy have absence of subcutaneous fat associated with muscle hypertrophy and hepatic steatosis; some of these patients have been treated successfully with leptin. Partial lipodystrophy can present with dyslipidemia and the diagnosis should be entertained in patients with variations in body fat distribution, particularly increased truncal fat accompanied by reduced fat in the buttocks and extremities.

Thyroid disease

Hypothyroidism is associated with elevated plasma LDL-C levels due primarily to a reduction in hepatic LDL receptor function and delayed clearance of LDL. Conversely, plasma levels of LDL-C are often reduced in the hyperthyroid patient. Hypothyroid patients also frequently have increased levels of circulating IDL, and some patients with hypothyroidism also have mild hypertriglyceridemia. Because hypothyroidism is often subtle and therefore easily overlooked, all patients presenting with elevated plasma levels of LDL-C, IDL, or triglycerides should be screened for hypothyroidism. Thyroid replacement therapy usually ameliorates the hypercholesterolemia; if not, the patient probably has a primary lipoprotein disorder and may require lipid-lowering drug therapy.

Renal disorders

Nephrotic syndrome is often associated with pronounced hyperlipoproteinemia, which is usually mixed but can manifest as hypercholesterolemia or hypertriglyceridemia. The hyperlipidemia of nephrotic syndrome appears to be due to a combination of increased hepatic production and decreased clearance of VLDLs, with increased LDL production. Effective treatment of the underlying renal disease normalizes the lipid profile, but most patients with chronic nephrotic syndrome require lipid-lowering drug therapy.

ESRD is often associated with mild hypertriglyceridemia (<300 mg/dL) due to the accumulation of VLDLs and remnant lipoproteins in the circulation. Triglyceride lipolysis and remnant clearance are both reduced in patients with renal failure. Because the risk of ASCVD is increased in ESRD subjects with hyperlipidemia, they should probably be aggressively treated with lipid-lowering agents, even though there is inadequate data at present to indicate that this population benefits from LDL-lowering therapy.

Patients with renal transplants usually have increased lipid levels due to the effect of the drugs required for immunosuppression (cyclosporine and glucocorticoids) and present a difficult management problem since HMG-CoA reductase inhibitors must be used cautiously in these patients.

Liver disorders

Because the liver is the principal site of formation and clearance of lipoproteins, it is not surprising that liver diseases can affect plasma lipid levels in a variety of ways. Hepatitis due to infection, drugs, or alcohol is often associated with increased VLDL synthesis and mild to moderate hypertriglyceridemia. Severe hepatitis and liver failure are associated with dramatic reductions in plasma cholesterol and triglycerides due to reduced lipoprotein biosynthetic capacity. Cholestasis is associated with hypercholesterolemia, which can be very severe. A major pathway by which cholesterol is excreted from the body is via secretion into bile, either directly or after conversion to bile acids, and cholestasis blocks this critical excretory pathway. In cholestasis, free cholesterol, coupled with phospholipids, is secreted into the plasma as a constituent of a lamellar particle called *LP-X*. The particles can deposit in skinfolds, producing lesions resembling those seen in patients with FDBL (xanthomata strata palmaris). Planar and eruptive xanthomas can also be seen in patients with cholestasis.

Alcohol

Regular alcohol consumption has a variable effect on plasma lipid levels. The most common effect of alcohol is to increase plasma triglyceride levels. Alcohol consumption stimulates hepatic secretion of VLDL, possibly by inhibiting the hepatic oxidation of free fatty acids, which then promote hepatic triglyceride synthesis and VLDL secretion. The usual lipoprotein pattern seen with alcohol consumption is Type IV (increased VLDLs), but persons with an underlying primary lipid disorder may develop severe hypertriglyceridemia (Type V) if they drink alcohol. Regular alcohol use also raises plasma levels of HDL-C.

Estrogen

Estrogen administration is associated with increased VLDL and HDL synthesis, resulting in elevated plasma levels of both triglycerides and HDL-C. This lipoprotein pattern is distinctive since the levels of plasma triglyceride and HDL-C are typically inversely related. Plasma triglyceride levels should be monitored when birth control pills or postmenopausal estrogen therapy is initiated to ensure that the increase in VLDL

production does not lead to severe hypertriglyceridemia. Use of low-dose preparations of estrogen or the estrogen patch can minimize the effect of exogenous estrogen on lipids.

Lysosomal storage diseases

Cholesteryl ester storage disease (due to deficiency in lysosomal acid lipase) and glycogen storage diseases such as von Gierke's disease (caused by mutations in glucose-6-phosphatase) are rare causes of secondary hyperlipidemias.

Cushing's syndrome

Glucocorticoid excess is associated with increased VLDL synthesis and hypertriglyceridemia. Patients with Cushing's syndrome can also have mild elevations in plasma levels of LDL-C.

Drugs

Many drugs have an impact on lipid metabolism and can result in significant alterations in the lipoprotein profile (Table 31-5).

SCREENING

(See also Chaps. 2 and 32) Guidelines for the screening and management of lipid disorders have been provided by an expert Adult Treatment Panel (ATP) convened by the National Cholesterol Education Program (NCEP) of the National Heart, Lung, and Blood Institute. The NCEP ATPIII guidelines published in 2001 recommend that all adults older than age 20 years should have plasma levels of cholesterol, triglyceride, LDL-C, and HDL-C measured after a 12-h overnight fast. In most clinical laboratories, the total cholesterol and triglycerides in the plasma are measured enzymatically, and then the cholesterol in the supernatant is measured after precipitation of apoB-containing lipoproteins to determine the HDL-C. The LDL-C is estimated using the following equation:

$$LDL\text{-}C = total\ cholesterol - (triglycerides/5) - HDL\text{-}C$$

(The VLDL-C is estimated by dividing the plasma triglyceride by 5, reflecting the ratio of cholesterol to triglyceride in VLDL particles.) This formula is reasonably accurate if test results are obtained on fasting plasma and if the triglyceride level does not exceed ~200 mg/dL; by convention it cannot be used if the triglyceride level is >400 mg/dL. The accurate determination of LDL-C levels in patients with triglyceride levels >200 mg/dL requires application of ultracentrifugation techniques or other direct assays for LDL-C.

If the triglyceride level is >200 mg/dL, the guidelines recommend that the "non-HDL-C" be calculated by simple subtraction of HDL-C from the total cholesterol and that this be considered a secondary target of therapy. Further evaluation and treatment is based primarily on the plasma LDL-C and non-HDL-C levels as well as assessment of overall cardiovascular risk.

DIAGNOSIS

The critical first step in managing a lipid disorder is to determine the class or classes of lipoproteins that are increased or decreased in the patient. The Fredrickson classification scheme for hyperlipoproteinemias (Table 31-3), though less commonly used now than in the past, can be helpful in this regard. Once the hyperlipidemia is accurately classified, efforts should be directed to rule out any possible secondary causes of the hyperlipidemia (Table 31-5). Although many patients with hyperlipidemia have a primary or genetic cause of their lipid disorder, secondary factors frequently contribute to the hyperlipidemia. A fasting glucose should be obtained in the initial workup of all subjects with an elevated triglyceride level. Nephrotic syndrome and chronic renal insufficiency should be excluded by obtaining urine protein and serum creatinine. Liver function tests should be performed to rule out hepatitis and cholestasis. Hypothyroidism should be ruled out by measuring serum TSH. Patients with hyperlipidemia, especially hypertriglyceridemia, who drink alcohol should be encouraged to decrease their intake. Sedentary lifestyle, obesity, and smoking are all associated with low HDL-C levels, and patients should be counseled about these issues.

Once secondary causes for the elevated lipoprotein levels have been ruled out, attempts should be made to diagnose the primary lipid disorder since the underlying etiology has a significant effect on the risk of developing CHD, on the response to drug therapy, and on the management of other family members. Often, determining the correct diagnosis requires a detailed family medical history and, in some cases, lipid analyses in family members.

If the fasting plasma triglyceride level is >1000 mg/dL, the patient almost always has chylomicronemia and either has Type I or Type V hyperlipoproteinemia (Table 31-3). The plasma triglyceride to cholesterol ratio helps distinguish between these two possibilities and is higher in Type I than Type V hyperlipoproteinemia. If the patient has Type I hyperlipoproteinemia, a postheparin lipolytic assay should be performed to determine if the patient has LPL or apoC-II deficiency. Type V is a much more frequent form of chylomicronemia in the adult patient. Often treatment of secondary factors contributing to the hyperlipidemia (diet, obesity, glucose intolerance, alcohol ingestion, estrogen therapy) will change a Type V into a Type IV pattern, reducing the risk of developing acute pancreatitis.

If the levels of LDL-C are very high (greater than a 95th percentile), it is likely the patient has a genetic form of hyperlipidemia. The presence of severe hypercholesterolemia, tendon xanthomas, and an autosomal dominant pattern of inheritance are consistent with the diagnosis of either FH, FDB, or ADH-PCSK9. At the present time, there is no compelling reason to perform molecular studies to further refine the molecular diagnosis, since the treatment of FH and FDB is identical. Recessive forms of severe hypercholesterolemia are rare and if the patient with severe hypercholesterolemia has parents with normal cholesterol levels, sitosterolemia should be considered; a clue to the diagnosis of sitosterolemia is the greater than expected response of the hypercholesterolemia to reductions in dietary cholesterol content or to treatment with either a cholesterol absorption inhibitor (ezetimibe) or to bile acid resins. Patients with more moderate hypercholesterolemia that does not segregate in families as a monogenic trait are likely to have polygenic hypercholesterolemia.

The most common error in the diagnosis and treatment of lipid disorders is in patients with a mixed hyperlipidemia without chylomicronemia. Elevations in the plasma levels of both cholesterol and triglycerides are seen in patients with increased plasma levels of IDL (Type III) and of LDL and VLDL (Type IIB) and in patients with increased levels of VLDL (Type IV). The ratio of triglyceride to cholesterol is higher in Type IV than the other two disorders. The plasma levels of apoB are highest in Type IIB. A beta quantification to determine the VLDL-C/triglyceride ratio in plasma (see discussion of FDBL) or a direct measurement of the plasma LDL-C should be performed at least once prior to initiation of lipid-lowering therapy to determine if the hyperlipidemia is due to the accumulation of remnants or to an increase in both LDL and VLDL.

TREATMENT   Lipoprotein Disorders

CLINICAL EVIDENCE THAT TREATMENT OF DYSLIPIDEMIA REDUCES RISK OF CHD

Observational Data   Multiple epidemiologic studies have demonstrated a strong relationship between plasma levels of LDL-C and CHD. A direct connection between plasma cholesterol levels and the atherosclerotic process was made in humans when aortic fatty streaks in young persons were shown to be strongly correlated with serum cholesterol levels. The elucidation of homozygous familial hypercholesterolemia was proof that high plasma levels of LDL-C alone are sufficient to cause CAD. Moreover, PCSK9 deficiency proves that having a lifelong reduction in plasma level of LDL-C is associated with a marked reduction in cardiovascular risk.

Clinical Trials: LDL-C Reduction Early clinical trials of cholesterol (mostly LDL-C) reduction utilized niacin, bile acid sequestrants, and even the surgical approach of partial ileal bypass to reduce serum cholesterol levels. Although most of these early studies found a small but significant reduction in cardiac events, no decrease in total mortality was seen. The discovery of more potent and well-tolerated cholesterol-lowering agents, namely HMG-CoA reductase inhibitors (statins), ushered in a series of large cholesterol reduction trials that unequivocally established the benefit of cholesterol reduction. The first of these studies was the Scandinavian Simvastatin Survival Study (4S) in which hypercholesterolemic men with CHD who were treated with simvastatin had a reduction in major coronary events of 44% and a reduction in total mortality of 30%. These impressive results were followed by additional studies using statins. The consistency of results of these studies is remarkable. They demonstrated statins to be effective in primary as well as secondary prevention, in women as well as men, in elderly as well as middle-aged individuals, and in patients with only modestly elevated LDL-C levels as well as those with severe hypercholesterolemia. In general, these studies demonstrated that a 1% reduction in LDL-C level is associated with a reduction in coronary events of a similar magnitude, and an ~40 mg/dL reduction in LDL-C is associated with an ~22% reduction in coronary events.

More recent studies have enrolled subjects with average or subaverage plasma LDL-C levels and have involved targeting the on-treatment LDL-C to even lower levels. For example, the Heart Protection Study (HPS) included 20,536 men and women, ages 40–80 years, who had either established ASCVD or were at high risk for the development of CHD (primarily diabetes); the only lipid entry criterion was a total plasma cholesterol level of >135 mg/dL. Treatment with simvastatin for an average of 5 years resulted in a 24% reduction in major coronary events and a highly significant 13% reduction in all-cause mortality. Importantly, the relative benefit of statin therapy was similar across tertiles of baseline LDL-C, and even the large subgroup of individuals with an LDL-C <100 mg/dL at baseline experienced significant benefit from therapy. This study demonstrated that statin therapy is beneficial in high-risk subjects, even if the baseline LDL-C level is below the currently recommended targeted goal; it also helped to shift the emphasis from simply treating elevated cholesterol to treating patients at high risk of CHD. Additional large-scale clinical trials have expanded on these findings and confirmed that individuals with other cardiovascular risk factors (hypertension, diabetes) benefit from LDL-lowering therapy even when the initial LDL-C level is only modestly elevated. The JUPITER trial was a primary prevention trial in subjects without CHD and with LDL-C <130 mg/dL but with an elevated plasma level of C-reactive protein (CRP). Treatment with rosuvastatin reduced LDL-C by an average of 50% and significantly reduced cardiovascular events, further extending the indication for statin therapy in primary prevention.

Further studies have compared different statin regimens to show that greater reductions in LDL-C levels with treatment are associated with a greater reduction in major cardiovascular events. Based on several of these studies, a white paper was issued by the NCEP in 2004 establishing an "optional" LDL-C goal of <70 mg/dL in high-risk patients with CHD and of <100 mg/dL in very-high-risk patients without known CHD. These optional targets have been widely embraced, and clinical practice is clearly evolving to treating CHD and high-risk patients more aggressively for LDL reduction.

Clinical Trials: The Triglyceride-HDL Axis Abnormalities of the triglyceride high-density lipoprotein (TG-HDL) axis are common in patients with CHD, although data supporting pharmacologic intervention in the TG-HDL axis is less compelling than data supporting LDL-C reduction. Fibric acid derivatives (fibrates), nicotinic acid (niacin), and omega 3 fatty acids (fish oils) are the primary agents currently available to lower plasma triglyceride levels and increase plasma levels of HDL-C. Fibrates have been used as lipid-lowering drugs for several decades and are more effective in reducing plasma triglyceride levels and relatively less effective in increasing plasma HDL-C levels. The results of clinical trials using fibrates have been mixed. Some studies such as the Helsinki Heart Study (HHS) and the Veteran Affairs High-Density Lipoprotein Cholesterol Intervention Trial (VA-HIT) demonstrated a significant reduction in nonfatal myocardial infarction and coronary death with gemfibrozil therapy. However, the Bezafibrate Infarction Prevention (BIP) trial of bezafibrate vs. placebo in CHD patients with low HDL-C failed to demonstrate a statistically significant reduction in coronary events, the Fenofibrate Intervention and Event Lowering in Diabetes (FIELD) trial of fenofibrate in patients with type 2 diabetes failed to show a significant reduction in its primary endpoint of nonfatal myocardial infarction and coronary death, and the Action to Control Cardiovascular Risk in Diabetes (ACCORD) study of fenofibrate vs. placebo added to simvastatin in patients with type 2 diabetes failed to show a significant reduction in its primary endpoint of major acute cardiovascular events. In each of these studies, the subgroup with elevated baseline triglycerides suggested benefit.

While niacin is the most effective HDL-raising drug currently available, it has not been tested for its ability to reduce cardiovascular risk in subjects with low plasma levels of HDL-C. The AIM-HIGH and HPS2-THRIVE trials are ongoing studies of the effect of niacin added to baseline statin therapy in patients with CHD and low HDL-C. Finally, while low-dose fish oils have been shown to reduce cardiovascular events, higher doses that reduce triglyceride levels have not been tested for their ability to reduce cardiovascular events. Definitive proof that treating the TG-HDL axis reduces cardiovascular events is likely to come from new therapies that are more effective at specifically targeting VLDL and/or HDL particles.

CLINICAL APPROACH TO LIPID-MODIFYING THERAPY
The major goal of lipid-modifying therapy in most patients with disorders of lipid metabolism is to prevent ASCVD and its complications. Management of lipid disorders should be based on clinical trial data demonstrating that treatment reduces cardiovascular morbidity and mortality, although reasonable extrapolation of these data to specific subgroups is sometimes required. Clearly, elevated plasma levels of LDL-C are strongly associated with increased risk of ASCVD, and treatment to lower the levels of plasma LDL-C decreases the risk of clinical cardiovascular events in both secondary and primary prevention. Although the proportional benefit accrued from reducing plasma LDL-C appears to be similar over the entire range of LDL-C values, the absolute risk reduction depends on the baseline level of cardiovascular risk. The treatment guidelines developed by NCEP ATPIII and the 2004 white paper incorporate these principles. As noted above, abnormalities in the TG-HDL axis (elevated triglyceride, low HDL-C, or both) are commonly seen in patients with CHD or who are at high risk for developing it, but clinical trial data supporting the treatment of these abnormalities is much less compelling, and the pharmacologic tools for their management are more limited. Importantly, the NCEP ATPIII guidelines promote the use of the "non-HDL-C" as a secondary target of therapy in patients with triglyceride levels >200 mg/dL. The goals for non-HDL-C are 30 mg/dL higher than the goals for LDL-C. Thus, many patients with abnormalities of the TG-HDL axis require additional therapy for reduction of non-HDL-C to recommended goals.

NONPHARMACOLOGIC TREATMENT
Diet Dietary modification is an important component in the management of dyslipidemia. The physician should assess the content of the patient's diet and provide suggestions for dietary modifications. In the patient with elevated LDL-C, dietary saturated fat and cholesterol should be restricted. For individuals with hypertriglyceridemia, the intake of simple carbohydrates should be curtailed. For severe hypertriglyceridemia (>1000 mg/dL), restriction of total fat intake is critical. The most widely used diet to lower the LDL-C level is the "Step I diet" developed by the American Heart Association. Most patients have a relatively modest (<10%) decrease in plasma levels of LDL-C on a Step I diet in the absence of any associated weight loss. Almost all persons experience a decrease in plasma HDL-C levels with a reduction in the amount of total and saturated fat in their diet.

Foods and Additives Certain foods and dietary additives are associated with modest reductions in plasma cholesterol levels. Plant stanol and sterol esters are available in a variety of foods, such as spreads, salad dressings, and snack bars. Plant sterol and sterol esters interfere with cholesterol absorption and reduce plasma LDL-C levels by ~10% when taken three times per day. The addition to the diet of psyllium, soy protein, or Chinese red yeast rice (which contains lovastatin) can have modest cholesterol-lowering effects. No controlled studies have been performed in which several of these nonpharmacologic options have been combined to address their additive or synergistic effects.

Weight Loss and Exercise The treatment of obesity, if present, can have a favorable impact on plasma lipid levels and should be actively encouraged. Plasma triglyceride and LDL-C levels tend to fall and HDL-C levels tend to increase in obese subjects after weight reduction. Regular aerobic exercise can also have a positive effect on lipids, in large measure due to the associated weight reduction. Aerobic exercise has a very modest elevating effect on plasma levels of HDL-C in most individuals but also has cardiovascular benefits that extend beyond the effects on plasma lipid levels.

PHARMACOLOGIC TREATMENT
The decision to use drug therapy depends on the level of cardiovascular risk. Drug therapy for hypercholesterolemia in patients with established CHD is well supported by clinical trial data, as reviewed above. Even patients with CHD or risk factors who have "average" LDL-C levels benefit from treatment. Drug treatment to lower LDL-C levels in patients with CHD is also highly cost-effective. Patients with diabetes mellitus without known CHD have similar cardiovascular risk to those without diabetes but with preexisting CHD. The NCEP ATPIII guidelines recommended estimating absolute risk of a cardiovascular event over 10 years using a scoring system based on the Framingham Heart Study database. Patients with a 10-year absolute CHD risk of >20% are considered "CHD risk equivalents" to be treated as aggressively as patients with existing CHD. Current NCEP ATPIII guidelines call for drug therapy to reduce LDL-C to <100 mg/dL in patients with established CHD, other ASCVD (aortic aneurysm, peripheral vascular disease, or cerebrovascular disease), diabetes mellitus, or CHD risk equivalents; and "optionally" to reduce LDL-C to <70 mg/dL in high-risk CHD patients. Based on these guidelines, virtually all CHD

and CHD risk-equivalent patients require cholesterol-lowering drug therapy. Moderate-risk patients with two or more risk factors and a 10-year absolute risk of 10–20% should be treated to a goal LDL-C of <130 mg/dL or "optionally" to LDL-C <100 mg/dL.

Although helpful to consider 10-year absolute risk in making clinical decisions about lipid-altering drug therapy, there are situations where 10-year risk is low but lifetime risk is very high and therefore treatment is indicated. A typical example would be a young adult with heterozygous FH and an LDL-C >220 mg/dL. Despite a very low 10-year absolute risk, every such patient should be treated with drug therapy to reduce lifetime risk. Indeed, all patients with markedly elevated plasma levels of LDL-C levels (>190 mg/dL) should be strongly considered for drug therapy even if their 10-year absolute CHD risk is not elevated. The decision of whether to initiate drug treatment in individuals with plasma LDL-C levels between 130 and 190 mg/dL remains controversial and depends on both 10-year and lifetime risk. Although it is desirable to avoid drug treatment in patients who are unlikely to develop CHD, a high proportion of patients who eventually develop CHD have plasma LDL-C levels within this range. The presence of other risk factors such as a low plasma level of HDL-C (<40 mg/dL) or the diagnosis of the metabolic syndrome would argue in favor of drug therapy (Chap. 32). Other laboratory tests such as an elevated plasma level of apoB, Lp(a), or high-sensitivity C-reactive protein, may assist in the identification of high-risk individuals who should be considered for drug therapy when their LDL-C is in a "gray zone."

Drug treatment is also indicated in patients with triglycerides >500 mg/dL who have been screened and treated for secondary causes of hypertriglyceridemia. The goal is to reduce fasting plasma triglycerides to below 500 mg/dL to prevent the risk of acute pancreatitis. When triglycerides are 200–500 mg/dL, the decision to use drug therapy depends on the risk of the patient developing chylomicronemia and an assessment of cardiovascular risk. Most major clinical endpoint trials with statins have excluded persons with triglyceride levels >350–450 mg/dL, and there are therefore few data regarding the effectiveness of statins in reducing cardiovascular risk in persons with hypertriglyceridemia. More data are needed regarding the relative effectiveness of statins, fibrates, niacin, and fish oils for reducing cardiovascular risk in this setting. Combination therapy is often required for optimal control of mixed dyslipidemia.

HMG-CoA Reductase Inhibitors (Statins)

HMG-CoA reductase is a key enzyme in cholesterol biosynthesis, and inhibition of this enzyme decreases cholesterol synthesis. By inhibiting cholesterol biosynthesis, statins lead to increased hepatic LDL receptor activity as a counterregulatory mechanism and thus accelerated clearance of circulating LDL, resulting in a dose-dependent reduction in plasma levels of LDL-C. The magnitude of LDL lowering associated with statin treatment varies widely among individuals, but once a patient is on a statin, the doubling of the statin dose produces an ~6% further reduction in the level of plasma LDL-C. The statins currently available differ in their LDL-C reducing potency (Table 31-6). Currently, there is no convincing evidence that any of the different statins confer an advantage that is independent of the effect on LDL-C. Statins also reduce plasma triglycerides in a dose-dependent fashion, which is roughly proportional to their LDL-C–lowering effects (if the triglycerides are <400 mg/dL). Statins have a modest HDL-raising effect (5–10%) that is not generally dose-dependent.

Statins are well tolerated and can be taken in tablet form once a day. Potential side effects include dyspepsia, headaches, fatigue, and muscle or joint pains. Severe myopathy and even rhabdomyolysis occur rarely with statin treatment. The risk of statin-associated myopathy is increased by the presence of older age, frailty, renal insufficiency, and coadministration of drugs that interfere with the metabolism of statins such as erythromycin and related antibiotics, antifungal agents, immunosuppressive drugs, and fibric acid derivatives (particularly gemfibrozil). Severe myopathy can usually be avoided by careful patient selection, avoidance of interacting drugs, and instructing the patient to contact the physician immediately in the event of unexplained muscle pain. In the event of muscle symptoms, the plasma creatine kinase (CK) level should be obtained to document the myopathy. Serum CK levels need not be monitored on a routine basis in patients taking statins, as an elevated CK in the absence of symptoms does not predict the development of myopathy and does not necessarily suggest the need for discontinuing the drug.

Another consequence of statin therapy can be elevation in liver transaminases (alanine [ALT] and aspartate [AST]). They should be checked before starting therapy, at 2–3 months, and then annually. Substantial (greater than three times the upper limit of normal) elevation in transaminases is relatively rare and mild-to-moderate (one to three times normal) elevation in transaminases in the absence of symptoms need not mandate discontinuing the medication. Severe clinical hepatitis associated with statins is exceedingly rare, and the trend is toward less frequent monitoring of transaminases in patients taking statins. The statin-associated elevation in liver enzymes resolves upon discontinuation of the medication.

Statins appear to be remarkably safe. Meta-analyses of large randomized controlled clinical trials with statins do not suggest an increase in any major noncardiac diseases. Statins are the drug class of choice for LDL-C reduction and are by far the most widely used class of lipid-lowering drugs.

TABLE 31-6

SUMMARY OF THE MAJOR DRUGS USED FOR THE TREATMENT OF HYPERLIPIDEMIA

DRUG	MAJOR INDICATIONS	STARTING DOSE	MAXIMAL DOSE	MECHANISM	COMMON SIDE EFFECTS
HMG-CoA reductase inhibitors (statins)	Elevated LDL-C			↓ Cholesterol synthesis, ↑ hepatic LDL receptors, ↓ VLDL production	Myalgias, arthralgias, elevated transaminases, dyspepsia
Lovastatin		20 mg daily	80 mg daily		
Pravastatin		40 mg qhs	80 mg qhs		
Simvastatin		20 mg qhs	80 mg qhs		
Fluvastatin		20 mg qhs	80 mg qhs		
Atorvastatin		10 mg qhs	80 mg qhs		
Rosuvastatin		10 mg qhs	40 mg qhs		
Cholesterol absorption inhibitors				↓ Intestinal cholesterol absorption	Elevated transaminases
Ezetimibe	Elevated LDL-C	10 mg daily	10 mg daily	LDL receptors	
Bile acid sequestrants	Elevated LDL-C			↑ Bile acid excretion and ↑ LDL receptors	Bloating, constipation, elevated triglycerides
Cholestyramine		4 g daily	32 g daily		
Colestipol		5 g daily	40 g daily		
Colesevelam		3750 mg daily	4375 mg daily		
Nicotinic acid	Elevated LDL-C, low HDL-C, elevated TG			↓ VLDL production	Cutaneous flushing, GI upset, elevated glucose, uric acid, and liver function tests
Immediate-release		100 mg tid	1 g tid		
Sustained-release		250 mg bid	1.5 g bid		
Extended-release		500 mg qhs	2 g qhs		
Fibric acid derivatives	Elevated TG, elevated remnants			↑ LPL, ↓ VLDL synthesis	Dyspepsia, myalgia, gallstones, elevated transaminases
Gemfibrozil		600 mg bid	600 mg bid		
Fenofibrate		145 mg qd	145 mg qd		
Omega 3 fatty acids	Elevated TG	3 g daily	6 g daily	↑ TG catabolism	Dyspepsia, diarrhea, fishy odor to breath

Abbreviations: GI, gastrointestinal; HDL-C, HDL-cholesterol; LDL, low-density lipoprotein; LDL-C, LDL-cholesterol; LPL, lipoprotein lipase; TG, triglyceride; VLDL, very low-density lipoprotein.

Cholesterol Absorption Inhibitors Cholesterol within the lumen of the small intestine is derived from the diet (about one-third) and the bile (about two-thirds) and is actively absorbed by the enterocyte through a process that involves the protein NPC1L1. Ezetimibe (Table 31-6) is a cholesterol absorption inhibitor that binds directly to and inhibits NPC1L1 and blocks the intestinal absorption of cholesterol. Ezetimibe (10 mg) inhibits cholesterol absorption by almost 60%, resulting in a reduction in delivery of dietary sterols in the liver and an increase in hepatic LDL receptor expression. The mean reduction in plasma LDL-C on ezetimibe (10 mg) is 18%, and the effect is additive when used in combination with a statin. Effects on triglyceride and HDL-C levels are negligible, and no cardiovascular outcome data have been reported. When used in combination with a statin, monitoring of liver transaminases is recommended. The only role for ezetimibe in monotherapy is in patients who do not tolerate statins; the drug is often added to a statin in patients who require further LDL-C reduction.

Bile Acid Sequestrants (Resins) Bile acid sequestrants bind bile acids in the intestine and promote their excretion rather than reabsorption in the ileum. To maintain the bile acid pool size, the liver diverts cholesterol to bile acid synthesis. The decreased hepatic intracellular cholesterol content results in upregulation of the LDL receptor and enhanced LDL clearance from the plasma. Bile acid sequestrants, including cholestyramine, colestipol, and colesevelam (Table 31-6), primarily reduce plasma LDL-C levels but can cause an increase in plasma triglycerides. Therefore, patients with hypertriglyceridemia should not be treated with bile acid–binding resins. Cholestyramine and colestipol are insoluble resins that must be suspended in liquids. Colesevelam is available as tablets but generally requires up to six to seven tablets per day for effective LDL-C lowering. Most side effects of resins are limited to the gastrointestinal tract and include bloating and constipation. Since bile acid sequestrants are not systemically absorbed, they are very safe and the cholesterol-lowering drug of choice in children and in women of childbearing age who are lactating, pregnant, or could become pregnant. They are effective in combination with statins as well as in combination with ezetimibe and are particularly useful with one or both of these drugs for difficult-to-treat patients or those with statin intolerance.

Nicotinic Acid (Niacin) Nicotinic acid, or niacin, is a B-complex vitamin that has been used as a lipid-modifying agent for more than five decades. Niacin reduces the flux of nonesterified fatty acids (NEFAs) to the liver, which is thought to be the mechanism for reduced hepatic triglyceride synthesis and VLDL secretion. Recently, a nicotinic acid receptor (GPR109A) was discovered that suppresses release of NEFA by adipose tissue, thus mediating the effect of niacin on NEFA suppression. Niacin reduces plasma triglyceride and LDL-C levels and raises the plasma concentration of HDL-C (Table 31-6), but it appears that these effects may not be mediated solely by GPR109A. Niacin is also the only currently available lipid-lowering drug that significantly reduces plasma levels of Lp(a) (up to 40%). If properly prescribed and monitored, niacin is a safe and effective lipid-lowering agent.

The most frequent side effect of niacin is cutaneous flushing, which is mediated by activating GPR109A in the skin, leading to local generation of prostaglandin D2 (PGD2) and prostaglandin E2. Flushing can be reduced by formulations that slow the absorption and by taking aspirin prior to dosing. A product is available in Europe that blocks the receptor for PGD2 and attenuates

flushing. There is rapid tachyphylaxis to the flushing. Niacin therapy is generally started at lower doses and gradually titrated up to higher doses. Immediate-release crystalline niacin is generally administered three times per day, over-the-counter sustained-release niacin is taken twice a day, and a prescription form of extended-release niacin is taken once a day. Mild elevations in transaminases occur in up to 15% of patients treated with any form of niacin, and on occasion these elevations may require stopping the medication. Niacin potentiates the effect of warfarin, and these two drugs should be prescribed together with caution. Acanthosis nigricans, a dark-colored coarse skin lesion, and maculopathy are infrequent side effects of niacin. Niacin is contraindicated in patients with peptic ulcer disease and can exacerbate the symptoms of esophageal reflux. It can also raise plasma levels of uric acid and precipitate gouty attacks in susceptible patients.

Niacin can raise fasting plasma glucose levels. A study in type 2 diabetics found only a slight increase in fasting glucose and no significant change in HbA1c level with niacin treatment. Low-dose niacin can be used effectively to reduce plasma triglyceride levels and increase HDL-C without adversely impacting on glycemic control. Thus, niacin can be used in diabetic patients, but every effort should be made to optimize the diabetes management before initiating niacin. Glucose should be carefully monitored in nondiabetic patients with impaired fasting glucose after initiation of niacin therapy.

Successful therapy with niacin requires careful education and motivation on the part of the patient. Its advantages are its low cost and long-term safety. It is the most effective drug currently available for raising HDL-C levels. It is particularly useful in patients with combined hyperlipidemia and low plasma levels of HDL-C and is effective in combination with statins. Outcome data are somewhat limited with niacin, but two clinical trials assessing the benefits of adding niacin to a statin in high-risk patients with low HDL-C are currently ongoing.

Fibric Acid Derivatives (Fibrates) Fibric acid derivatives are agonists of PPARα, a nuclear receptor involved in the regulation of lipid metabolism. Fibrates stimulate LPL activity (enhancing triglyceride hydrolysis), reduce apoC-III synthesis (enhancing lipoprotein remnant clearance), promote beta-oxidation of fatty acids, and may reduce VLDL triglyceride production. Fibrates are the most effective drugs available for reducing triglyceride levels and also raise HDL-C levels modestly (Table 31-6). They have variable effects on LDL-C and in hypertriglyceridemic patients can sometimes be associated with increases in plasma LDL-C levels.

Fibrates are generally very well tolerated. The most common side effect is dyspepsia. Myopathy and hepatitis occur rarely in the absence of other lipid-lowering agents. Fibrates promote cholesterol secretion into bile and are associated with an increased risk of gallstones. Fibrates can raise creatinine and should be used with caution in patients with chronic kidney disease. Importantly, fibrates can potentiate the effect of warfarin and certain oral hypoglycemic agents, so the anticoagulation status and plasma glucose levels should be closely monitored in patients on these agents.

Fibrates are useful and are a reasonable consideration for first-line therapy in patients with severe hypertriglyceridemia (>500 mg/dL) to prevent pancreatitis. Their role in patients with moderate hypertriglyceridemia (200–500 mg/dL) is to promote reduction in non-HDL-C levels, but outcome data regarding their effects on coronary events in this setting remains mixed. In patients with a triglyceride level <500 mg/dL, the role of fibrates is primarily in combination with statins in selected patients with mixed dyslipidemia. In this setting, the risk of myopathy can be minimized with appropriate patient and drug selection and must be carefully weighed against the clinical benefit of the therapy.

Omega 3 Fatty Acids (Fish Oils) N-3 poly-unsaturated fatty acids (n-3 PUFAs) are present in high concentration in fish and in flaxseeds. The most widely used n-3 PUFAs for the treatment of hyperlipidemias are the two active molecules in fish oil: eicosapentaenoic acid (EPA) and decohexanoic acid (DHA). N-3 PUFAs have been concentrated into tablets and in doses of 3–4 g/d are effective at lowering fasting triglyceride levels. Fish oils can cause an increase in plasma LDL-C levels in some patients. Fish oil supplements can be used in combination with fibrates, niacin, or statins to treat hypertriglyceridemia. In general, fish oils are well tolerated and appear to be safe, at least at doses up to 3–4 g. Although fish oil administration is associated with a prolongation in the bleeding time, no increase in bleeding has been seen in clinical trials. A lower dose of omega 3 (about 1 g) has been associated with reduction in cardiovascular events in CHD patients and is used by some clinicians for this purpose.

Combination Drug Therapy Combination drug therapy is frequently used for (1) patients unable to reach LDL-C and non-HDL-C goals on statin monotherapy, (2) patients with combined elevated LDL-C and abnormalities of the TG-HDL axis, and (3) patients with severe hypertriglyceridemia who do not achieve non-HDL-C goal on a fibrate or on fish oils alone. When LDL-C and non-HDL-C goals are not achieved on statin monotherapy, a cholesterol absorption inhibitor or bile acid sequestrant can be added to the drug regimen. Combination of niacin with a statin is an attractive option for high-risk patients who do not attain their target LDL-C level on statin monotherapy and have a low HDL-C level.

Conversely, in high-risk patients on statin therapy who have an elevated plasma triglyceride level, addition of a fibrate or fish oils is a reasonable consideration.

Severely hypertriglyceridemic patients treated first with a fibrate often fail to reach LDL-C and non-HDL-C goals and are therefore candidates for addition of a statin. Coadministration of statins and fibrates has obvious appeal in patients with combined hyperlipidemia, but no clinical trial has assessed the effectiveness of a statin-fibrate combination compared with either a statin or a fibrate alone in reducing cardiovascular events. The long-term safety of the statin-fibrate combination is not known. Since coadministration of statins and fibrates is associated with an increased incidence of severe myopathy and rhabdomyolysis, patients treated with this combination must be carefully counseled and monitored. This combination of drugs should be used cautiously in patients with underlying renal or hepatic insufficiency; in the elderly, frail, and chronically ill; and in those on multiple medications.

OTHER APPROACHES Occasionally, patients cannot tolerate any of the existing lipid-lowering drugs at doses required for adequate control of their lipid levels. A larger group of patients, most of whom have genetic lipid disorders, remain significantly hypercholesterolemic despite combination drug therapy. These patients are at high risk for the development or progression of CHD and clinical CHD events. The preferred option for management of patients with severe refractory hypercholesterolemia is LDL apheresis. In this process, the patient's plasma is passed over a column that selectively removes the LDL, and the LDL-depleted plasma is returned to the patient. Patients on maximally tolerated combination drug therapy who have CHD and a plasma LDL-C level >200 mg/dL or no CHD and a plasma LDL-C level >300 mg/dL are candidates for every-other-week LDL apheresis and should be referred to a specialized lipid center.

MANAGEMENT OF LOW HDL-C Severely reduced plasma levels of HDL-C (<20 mg/dL) accompanied by triglycerides <400 mg/dL usually indicate the presence of a genetic disorder such as a mutation in apoA-I, LCAT deficiency, or Tangier disease. HDL-C levels <20 mg/dL are common in the setting of severe hypertriglyceridemia, in which case the primary focus should be on the management of the triglycerides. HDL-C levels <20 mg/dL also occur in individuals using anabolic steroids. Secondary causes of more moderate reductions in plasma HDL (20–40 mg/dL) should be considered (Table 31-5). Smoking should be discontinued, obese persons should be encouraged to lose weight, sedentary persons should be encouraged to exercise, and diabetes should be optimally controlled. When possible, medications associated with reduced plasma levels of HDL-C should be discontinued. The presence of an isolated low plasma level of HDL-C in a patient with a borderline plasma level of LDL-C should prompt consideration of LDL-lowering drug therapy in high-risk individuals. Statins increase plasma levels of HDL-C only modestly (~5–10%). Fibrates also have only a modest effect on plasma HDL-C levels (increasing levels ~5–15%), except in patients with coexisting hypertriglyceridemia, where the effect on HDL levels can be greater. Niacin is the most effective HDL-C–raising therapeutic agent available and can increase plasma HDL-C by up to ~30%, although some patients fail to achieve clinically important increases in HDL-C levels from niacin therapy.

The issue of whether pharmacologic intervention should be used to specifically raise HDL-C levels has not been adequately addressed in clinical trials. In persons with established CHD and low HDL-C levels whose plasma LDL-C levels are at or below the goal, it may be reasonable to initiate therapy (with a fibrate or niacin) directed specifically at reducing plasma triglyceride levels and raising the level of plasma HDL-C. More data are required before broad recommendations are made to use drug therapy to specifically raise HDL-C levels to prevent cardiovascular events. New HDL-raising approaches are under development that may help to address this important issue.

Management of Elevated Levels of Lp(a)
High levels of Lp(a) are associated with increased risk of ASCVD. Genetic studies suggest that this association is causal, but there is no evidence that reducing plasma Lp(a) levels reduces cardiovascular risk. Until such studies are performed, the major therapeutic approach to patients with high plasma levels of Lp(a) and established CAD is to aggressively lower plasma levels of LDL-C. Niacin is the only drug currently available that lowers Lp(a), and might be considered as an addition to a statin in a very-high-risk patient with elevated Lp(a).

CHAPTER 32

THE METABOLIC SYNDROME

Robert H. Eckel

The metabolic syndrome (syndrome X, insulin resistance syndrome) consists of a constellation of metabolic abnormalities that confer increased risk of cardiovascular disease (CVD) and diabetes mellitus (DM). The criteria for the metabolic syndrome have evolved since the original definition by the World Health Organization in 1998, reflecting growing clinical evidence and analysis by a variety of consensus conferences and professional organizations. The major features of the metabolic syndrome include central obesity, hypertriglyceridemia, low high-density lipoprotein (HDL) cholesterol, hyperglycemia, and hypertension (Table 32-1).

EPIDEMIOLOGY

The prevalence of metabolic syndrome varies around the world, in part reflecting the age and ethnicity of the populations studied and the diagnostic criteria applied. In general, the prevalence of metabolic syndrome increases with age. The highest recorded prevalence worldwide is in Native Americans, with nearly 60% of women ages 45–49 and 45% of men ages 45–49 meeting National Cholesterol Education Program and Adult Treatment Panel III (NCEP:ATPIII) criteria. In the United States,

TABLE 32-1

NCEP:ATPIII 2001 AND IDF CRITERIA FOR THE METABOLIC SYNDROME

NCEP:ATPIII 2001	IDF CRITERIA FOR CENTRAL ADIPOSITY[a]		
Three or more of the following:	**Waist circumference**		
Central obesity: Waist circumference >102 cm (M), >88 cm (F)	**MEN**	**WOMEN**	**ETHNICITY**
Hypertriglyceridemia: Triglycerides ≥150 mg/dL or specific medication	≥94 cm	≥80 cm	Europid, Sub-Saharan African, Eastern and Middle Eastern
Low HDL cholesterol: <40 mg/dL and <50 mg/dL, respectively, or specific medication	≥90 cm	≥80 cm	South Asian, Chinese, and ethnic South and Central American
Hypertension: Blood pressure ≥130 mm systolic or ≥85 mm diastolic or specific medication	≥85 cm	≥90 cm	Japanese
Fasting plasma glucose ≥100 mg/dL or specific medication or previously diagnosed type 2 diabetes	**Two or more of the following:**		
	Fasting triglycerides >150 mg/dL or specific medication		
	HDL cholesterol <40 mg/dL and <50 mg/dL for men and women, respectively, or specific medication		
	Blood pressure >130 mm systolic or >85 mm diastolic or previous diagnosis or specific medication		
	Fasting plasma glucose ≥100 mg/dL or previously diagnosed type 2 diabetes		

[a]In this analysis, the following thresholds for waist circumference were used: white men, ≥94 cm; African-American men, ≥94 cm; Mexican-American men, ≥90 cm; white women, ≥80 cm; African-American women, ≥80 cm; Mexican-American women, ≥80 cm. For participants whose designation was "other race—including multiracial," thresholds that were once based on Europid cut points (≥94 cm for men and ≥80 cm for women) and once based on South Asian cut points (≥90 cm for men and ≥80 cm for women) were used. For participants who were considered "other Hispanic," the IDF thresholds for ethnic South and Central Americans were used.

Abbreviations: HDL, high-density lipoprotein; IDF, International Diabetes Foundation; NCEP:ATPIII, National Cholesterol Education Program, Adult Treatment Panel III.

metabolic syndrome is less common in African-American men and more common in Mexican-American women. Based on data from the National Health and Nutrition Examination Survey (NHANES) 1999–2000, the age-adjusted prevalence of the metabolic syndrome in U.S. adults who did not have diabetes is 28% for men and 30% for women. In France, a cohort 30 to 60 years old has shown a <10% prevalence for each sex, although 17.5% are affected in the age range 60–64. Greater industrialization worldwide is associated with rising rates of obesity, which is anticipated to increase prevalence of the metabolic syndrome dramatically, especially as the population ages. Moreover, the rising prevalence and severity of obesity in children is initiating features of the metabolic syndrome in a younger population.

The frequency distribution of the five components of the syndrome for the U.S. population (NHANES III) is summarized in **Fig. 32-1**. Increases in waist circumference predominate in women, whereas fasting triglycerides >150 mg/dL and hypertension are more likely in men.

RISK FACTORS

Overweight/obesity

Although the first description of the metabolic syndrome occurred in the early twentieth century, the worldwide overweight/obesity epidemic has been the driving force for more recent recognition of the syndrome. Central adiposity is a key feature of the syndrome, reflecting the fact that the syndrome's prevalence is driven by the strong relationship between waist circumference and increasing adiposity. However, despite the importance of obesity, patients who are

normal weight may also be insulin-resistant and have the syndrome.

Sedentary lifestyle

Physical inactivity is a predictor of CVD events and related mortality rate. Many components of the metabolic syndrome are associated with a sedentary lifestyle, including increased adipose tissue (predominantly central), reduced HDL cholesterol, and a trend toward increased triglycerides, high blood pressure, and increased glucose in the genetically susceptible. Compared with individuals who watched television or videos or used the computer <1 h daily, those who carried out those behaviors for >4 h daily had a twofold increased risk of the metabolic syndrome.

Aging

The metabolic syndrome affects 44% of the U.S. population older than age 50. A greater percentage of women over age 50 have the syndrome than men. The age dependency of the syndrome's prevalence is seen in most populations around the world.

Diabetes mellitus

DM is included in both the NCEP and International Diabetes Foundation (IDF) definitions of the metabolic syndrome. It is estimated that the great majority (~75%) of patients with type 2 diabetes or impaired glucose tolerance (IGT) have the metabolic syndrome. The presence of the metabolic syndrome in these populations relates to a higher prevalence of CVD compared with patients with type 2 diabetes or IGT without the syndrome.

Coronary heart disease

The approximate prevalence of the metabolic syndrome in patients with coronary heart disease (CHD) is 50%, with a prevalence of 37% in patients with premature coronary artery disease (≤age 45), particularly in women. With appropriate cardiac rehabilitation and changes in lifestyle (e.g., nutrition, physical activity, weight reduction, and, in some cases, pharmacologic agents), the prevalence of the syndrome can be reduced.

Lipodystrophy

Lipodystrophic disorders in general are associated with the metabolic syndrome. Both genetic (e.g., Berardinelli-Seip congenital lipodystrophy, Dunnigan familial partial lipodystrophy) and acquired (e.g., HIV-related lipodystrophy in patients treated with highly active antiretroviral therapy) forms of lipodystrophy may give rise to

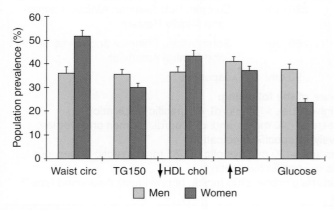

FIGURE 32-1
Prevalence of the metabolic syndrome components, from NHANES III. NHANES, National Health and Nutrition Examination Survey; TG, triglyceride; HDL, high-density lipoprotein; BP, blood pressure. The prevalence of elevated glucose includes individuals with known diabetes mellitus. (*Created from data in ES Ford et al: Diabetes Care 27:2444, 2004.*)

severe insulin resistance and many of the components of the metabolic syndrome.

ETIOLOGY

Insulin resistance

The most accepted and unifying hypothesis to describe the pathophysiology of the metabolic syndrome is insulin resistance, which is caused by an incompletely understood defect in insulin action. The onset of insulin resistance is heralded by postprandial hyperinsulinemia, followed by fasting hyperinsulinemia and, ultimately, hyperglycemia.

An early major contributor to the development of insulin resistance is an overabundance of circulating fatty acids (Fig. 32-2). Plasma albumin-bound free fatty acids (FFAs) are derived predominantly from adipose tissue triglyceride stores released by lipolytic enzymes lipase. Fatty acids are also derived from the lipolysis of triglyceride-rich lipoproteins in tissues by lipoprotein lipase (LPL). Insulin mediates both antilipolysis and the stimulation of LPL in adipose tissue. Of note, the inhibition of lipolysis in adipose tissue is the most sensitive pathway of insulin action. Thus, when insulin resistance develops, increased lipolysis produces more fatty acids, which further decrease the antilipolytic effect of insulin. Excessive fatty acids enhance substrate availability and create insulin resistance by modifying downstream signaling. Fatty acids impair insulin-mediated glucose uptake and accumulate as triglycerides in both skeletal and cardiac muscle, whereas increased glucose production and triglyceride accumulation are seen in the liver.

The oxidative stress hypothesis provides a unifying theory for aging and the predisposition to the metabolic

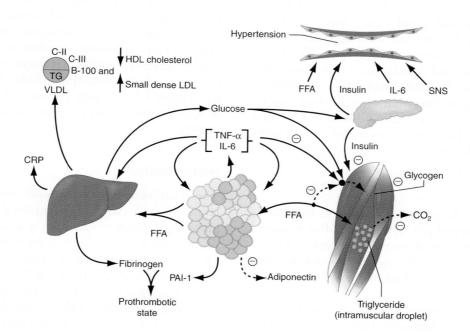

FIGURE 32-2

Pathophysiology of the metabolic syndrome. Free fatty acids (FFAs) are released in abundance from an expanded adipose tissue mass. In the liver, FFAs result in an increased production of glucose and triglycerides and secretion of very low-density lipoproteins (VLDLs). Associated lipid/lipoprotein abnormalities include reductions in high-density lipoprotein (HDL) cholesterol and an increased density of low-density lipoproteins (LDLs). FFAs also reduce insulin sensitivity in muscle by inhibiting insulin-mediated glucose uptake. Associated defects include a reduction in glucose partitioning to glycogen and increased lipid accumulation in triglyceride (TG). Increases in circulating glucose, and to some extent FFA, increase pancreatic insulin secretion, resulting in hyperinsulinemia. Hyperinsulinemia may result in enhanced sodium reabsorption and increased sympathetic nervous system (SNS) activity and contribute to the hypertension, as might increased levels of circulating FFAs. The proinflammatory state is superimposed and contributory to the insulin resistance produced by excessive FFAs. The enhanced secretion of interleukin 6 (IL-6) and tumor necrosis factor α (TNF-α) produced by adipocytes and monocyte-derived macrophages results in more insulin resistance and lipolysis of adipose tissue triglyceride stores to circulating FFAs. IL-6 and other cytokines also enhance hepatic glucose production, VLDL production by the liver, and insulin resistance in muscle. Cytokines and FFAs also increase the hepatic production of fibrinogen and adipocyte production of plasminogen activator inhibitor 1 (PAI-1), resulting in a prothrombotic state. Higher levels of circulating cytokines also stimulate the hepatic production of C-reactive protein (CRP). Reduced production of the anti-inflammatory and insulin-sensitizing cytokine adiponectin is also associated with the metabolic syndrome. (*Reprinted from RH Eckel et al: Lancet 365:1415, 2005, with permission from Elsevier.*)

syndrome. In studies carried out in insulin-resistant subjects with obesity or type 2 diabetes, the offspring of patients with type 2 diabetes, and the elderly, a defect has been identified in mitochondrial oxidative phosphorylation, leading to the accumulation of triglycerides and related lipid molecules in muscle. The accumulation of lipids in muscle is associated with insulin resistance.

Increased waist circumference

Waist circumference is an important component of the most recent and frequently applied diagnostic criteria for the metabolic syndrome. However, measuring waist circumference does not reliably distinguish increases in subcutaneous adipose tissue vs. visceral fat; this distinction requires CT or MRI. With increases in visceral adipose tissue, adipose tissue–derived FFAs are directed to the liver. In contrast, increases in abdominal subcutaneous fat release lipolysis products into the systemic circulation and avoid more direct effects on hepatic metabolism. Relative increases in visceral versus subcutaneous adipose tissue with increasing waist circumference in Asians and Asian Indians may explain the greater prevalence of the syndrome in those populations compared with African-American men in whom subcutaneous fat predominates. It is also possible that visceral fat is a marker for, but not the source of, excess postprandial FFAs in obesity.

Dyslipidemia

(See also Chap. 31) In general, FFA flux to the liver is associated with increased production of apoB-containing, triglyceride-rich very low-density lipoproteins (VLDLs). The effect of insulin on this process is complex, but *hypertriglyceridemia* is an excellent marker of the insulin-resistant condition.

The other major lipoprotein disturbance in the metabolic syndrome is a *reduction in HDL cholesterol*. This reduction is a consequence of changes in HDL composition and metabolism. In the presence of hypertriglyceridemia, a decrease in the cholesterol content of HDL is a consequence of reduced cholesteryl ester content of the lipoprotein core in combination with cholesteryl ester transfer protein–mediated alterations in triglyceride, making the particle small and dense. This change in lipoprotein composition also results in increased clearance of HDL from the circulation. The relationships of these changes in HDL to insulin resistance are probably indirect, occurring in concert with the changes in triglyceride-rich lipoprotein metabolism.

In addition to HDL, low-density lipoproteins (LDLs) are modified in composition. With fasting serum triglycerides >2.0 mM (~180 mg/dL), there is almost always a predominance of small dense LDLs. Small dense LDLs are thought to be more atherogenic. They

may be toxic to the endothelium, and they are able to transit through the endothelial basement membrane and adhere to glycosaminoglycans. They also have increased susceptibility to oxidation and are selectively bound to scavenger receptors on monocyte-derived macrophages. Subjects with increased small dense LDL particles and hypertriglyceridemia also have increased cholesterol content of both VLDL1 and VLDL2 subfractions. This relatively cholesterol-rich VLDL particle may contribute to the atherogenic risk in patients with metabolic syndrome.

Glucose intolerance

The defects in insulin action lead to impaired suppression of glucose production by the liver and kidney and reduced glucose uptake and metabolism in insulin-sensitive tissues, i.e., muscle and adipose tissue. The relationship between impaired fasting glucose (IFG) or impaired glucose tolerance (IGT) and insulin resistance is well supported by human, nonhuman primate, and rodent studies. To compensate for defects in insulin action, insulin secretion and/or clearance must be modified to sustain euglycemia. Ultimately, this compensatory mechanism fails, usually because of defects in insulin secretion, resulting in progress from IFG and/or IGT to DM.

Hypertension

The relationship between insulin resistance and hypertension is well established. Paradoxically, under normal physiologic conditions, insulin is a vasodilator with secondary effects on sodium reabsorption in the kidney. However, in the setting of insulin resistance, the vasodilatory effect of insulin is lost but the renal effect on sodium reabsorption is preserved. Sodium reabsorption is increased in whites with the metabolic syndrome but not in Africans or Asians. Insulin also increases the activity of the sympathetic nervous system, an effect that also may be preserved in the setting of the insulin resistance. Finally, insulin resistance is characterized by pathway-specific impairment in phosphatidylinositol-3-kinase signaling. In the endothelium, this may cause an imbalance between the production of nitric oxide and the secretion of endothelin 1, leading to decreased blood flow. Although these mechanisms are provocative, when insulin action is assessed by levels of fasting insulin or by the Homeostasis Model Assessment (HOMA), insulin resistance contributes only modestly to the increased prevalence of hypertension in the metabolic syndrome.

Proinflammatory cytokines

The increases in proinflammatory cytokines, including interleukin (IL)-1, IL-6, IL-18, resistin, tumor necrosis factor (TNF) α, and C-reactive protein (CRP), reflect overproduction by the expanded adipose tissue mass (Fig. 32-2). Adipose tissue-derived macrophages may be the primary source of proinflammatory cytokines locally and in the systemic circulation. It remains unclear, however, how much of the insulin resistance is caused by the paracrine vs. endocrine effects of these cytokines.

Adiponectin

Adiponectin is an anti-inflammatory cytokine produced exclusively by adipocytes. Adiponectin enhances insulin sensitivity and inhibits many steps in the inflammatory process. In the liver, adiponectin inhibits the expression of gluconeogenic enzymes and the rate of glucose production. In muscle, adiponectin increases glucose transport and enhances fatty acid oxidation, partially due to activation of adenosine monophosphate (AMP) kinase. Adiponectin is reduced in the metabolic syndrome. The relative contribution of adiponectin deficiency versus overabundance of the proinflammatory cytokines is unclear.

CLINICAL FEATURES

Symptoms and signs

The metabolic syndrome is typically not associated with symptoms. On physical examination, waist circumference may be expanded and blood pressure elevated. The presence of one or either of these signs should alert the clinician to search for other biochemical abnormalities that may be associated with the metabolic syndrome. Less frequently, lipoatrophy or acanthosis nigricans is found on examination. Because these physical findings typically are associated with severe insulin resistance, other components of the metabolic syndrome should be expected.

Associated diseases

Cardiovascular disease
The relative risk for new-onset CVD in patients with the metabolic syndrome, in the absence of diabetes, averages between 1.5-fold and threefold. However, in an 8-year follow-up of middle-aged men and women in the Framingham Offspring Study (FOS), the population-attributable risk for patients with the metabolic syndrome to develop CVD was 34% in men and only 16% in women. In the same study, both the metabolic syndrome and diabetes predicted ischemic stroke, with greater risk for patients with the metabolic syndrome than for those with diabetes alone (19% vs 7%), particularly in women (27% vs 5%). Patients with metabolic syndrome are also at increased risk for peripheral vascular disease.

Type 2 diabetes
Overall, the risk for type 2 diabetes in patients with the metabolic syndrome is increased three- to fivefold. In the FOS's 8-year follow-up of middle-aged men and women, the population-attributable risk for developing type 2 diabetes was 62% in men and 47% in women.

Other associated conditions

In addition to the features specifically associated with metabolic syndrome, insulin resistance is accompanied by other metabolic alterations. Those alterations include increases in apoB and apoC-III, uric acid, prothrombotic factors (fibrinogen, plasminogen activator inhibitor 1), serum viscosity, asymmetric dimethylarginine, homocysteine, white blood cell count, proinflammatory cytokines, CRP, microalbuminuria, nonalcoholic fatty liver disease (NAFLD) and/or nonalcoholic steatohepatitis (NASH), polycystic ovarian disease (PCOS), and obstructive sleep apnea (OSA).

Nonalcoholic fatty liver disease
Fatty liver is relatively common. However, in NASH, both triglyceride accumulation and inflammation coexist. NASH is now present in 2–3% of the population in the United States and other Western countries. As the prevalence of overweight/obesity and the metabolic syndrome increases, NASH may become one of the more common causes of end-stage liver disease and hepatocellular carcinoma.

Hyperuricemia
Hyperuricemia reflects defects in insulin action on the renal tubular reabsorption of uric acid, whereas the increase in asymmetric dimethylarginine, an endogenous inhibitor of nitric oxide synthase, relates to endothelial dysfunction. Microalbuminuria also may be caused by altered endothelial pathophysiology in the insulin-resistant state.

Polycystic ovary syndrome
PCOS is highly associated with the metabolic syndrome, with a prevalence between 40% and 50%. Women with PCOS are two to four times more likely to have the metabolic syndrome than are women without PCOS.

Obstructive sleep apnea
OSA is commonly associated with obesity, hypertension, increased circulating cytokines, IGT, and insulin resistance. With these associations, it is not surprising that the metabolic syndrome is frequently present. Moreover, when biomarkers of insulin resistance are compared between patients with OSA and weight-matched controls, insulin resistance is more severe in patients with OSA. Continuous positive airway pressure (CPAP) treatment in OSA patients improves insulin sensitivity.

DIAGNOSIS

The diagnosis of the metabolic syndrome relies on satisfying the criteria listed in Table 32-1 by using tools at the bedside and in the laboratory. The medical history should include evaluation of symptoms for OSA in all patients and PCOS in premenopausal women. Family history will help determine risk for CVD and DM. Blood pressure and waist circumference measurements provide information necessary for the diagnosis.

Laboratory tests

Fasting lipids and glucose are needed to determine if the metabolic syndrome is present. The measurement of additional biomarkers associated with insulin resistance can be individualized. Such tests might include apoB, high-sensitivity CRP, fibrinogen, uric acid, urinary microalbumin, and liver function tests. A sleep study should be performed if symptoms of OSA are present. If PCOS is suspected on the basis of clinical features and anovulation, testosterone, luteinizing hormone, and follicle-stimulating hormone should be measured.

TREATMENT   The Metabolic Syndrome

LIFESTYLE Obesity is the driving force behind the metabolic syndrome. Thus, weight reduction is the primary approach to the disorder. With weight reduction, the improvement in insulin sensitivity is often accompanied by favorable modifications in many components of the metabolic syndrome. In general, recommendations for weight loss include a combination of caloric restriction, increased physical activity, and behavior modification. For weight reduction, caloric restriction is the most important component, whereas increases in physical activity are important for maintenance of weight loss. Some, but not all, evidence suggests that the addition of exercise to caloric restriction may promote relatively greater weight loss from the visceral depot. The tendency for weight regain after successful weight reduction underscores the need for long-lasting behavioral changes.

Diet Before prescribing a weight-loss diet, it is important to emphasize that it takes a long time for a patient to achieve an expanded fat mass; thus, the correction need not occur quickly. On the basis of ~3500 kcal = 1 lb of fat, ~500 kcal restriction daily equates to weight reduction of 1 lb per week. Diets restricted in carbohydrate typically provide a rapid initial weight loss. However, after 1 year, the amount of weight reduction is usually unchanged. Thus, adherence to the diet is more important than which diet is chosen. Moreover, there

is concern about diets enriched in saturated fat, particularly for patients at risk for CVD. Therefore, a high-quality diet—i.e., enriched in fruits, vegetables, whole grains, lean poultry, and fish—should be encouraged to provide the maximum overall health benefit.

Physical Activity Before a physical activity recommendation is provided to patients with the metabolic syndrome, it is important to ensure that the increased activity does not incur risk. Some high-risk patients should undergo formal cardiovascular evaluation before initiating an exercise program. For an inactive participant, gradual increases in physical activity should be encouraged to enhance adherence and avoid injury. Although increases in physical activity can lead to modest weight reduction, 60–90 min of daily activity is required to achieve this goal. Even if an overweight or obese adult is unable to achieve this level of activity, he or she will still derive a significant health benefit from at least 30 min of moderate-intensity daily activity. The caloric value of 30 min of a variety of activities can be found at *http://www.americanheart.org/presenter .jhtml?identifier=3040364*. Of note, a variety of routine activities, such as gardening, walking, and housecleaning, require moderate caloric expenditure. Thus, physical activity need not be defined solely in terms of formal exercise such as jogging, swimming, or tennis.

Obesity In some patients with the metabolic syndrome, treatment options need to extend beyond lifestyle intervention. Weight-loss drugs come in two major classes: appetite suppressants and absorption inhibitors. Appetite suppressants approved by the U.S. Food and Drug Administration include phentermine (for short-term use only, 3 months) and sibutramine. Orlistat inhibits fat absorption by ~30% and is moderately effective compared to placebo (~5% weight loss). Orlistat has been shown to reduce the incidence of type 2 diabetes, an effect that was especially evident in patients with baseline IGT.

Bariatric surgery is an option for patients with the metabolic syndrome who have a body mass index (BMI) >40 kg/m^2 or >35 kg/m^2 with comorbidities. Gastric bypass results in a dramatic weight reduction and improvement in the features of metabolic syndrome. A survival benefit has also been realized.

LDL CHOLESTEROL (See also Chap. 31) The rationale for the NCEP:ATPIII panel to develop criteria for the metabolic syndrome was to go beyond LDL cholesterol in identifying and reducing risk for CVD. The working assumption by the panel was that LDL cholesterol goals had already been achieved, and increasing evidence supports a linear reduction in CVD events with progressive lowering of LDL cholesterol. For patients with the metabolic syndrome and diabetes,

LDL cholesterol should be reduced to <100 mg/dL and perhaps further in patients with a history of CVD events. For patients with the metabolic syndrome without diabetes, the Framingham risk score may predict a 10-year CVD risk that exceeds 20%. In these subjects, LDL cholesterol should also be reduced to <100 mg/dL. With a 10-year risk of <20%, however, the targeted LDL cholesterol goal is <130 mg/dL.

Diets restricted in saturated fats (<7% of calories), *trans*-fats (as few as possible), and cholesterol (<200 mg daily) should be applied aggressively. If LDL cholesterol remains above goal, pharmacologic intervention is needed. Statins (HMG-CoA reductase inhibitors), which produce a 20–60% lowering of LDL cholesterol, are generally the first choice for medication intervention. Of note, for each doubling of the statin dose, there is only ~6% additional lowering of LDL cholesterol. Side effects are rare and include an increase in hepatic transaminases and/or myopathy. The cholesterol absorption inhibitor ezetimibe is well tolerated and should be the second choice. Ezetimibe typically reduces LDL cholesterol by 15–20%. The bile acid sequestrants cholestyramine and colestipol are more effective than ezetimibe but must be used with caution in patients with the metabolic syndrome because they can increase triglycerides. In general, bile sequestrants should not be administered when fasting triglycerides are >200 mg/dL. Side effects include gastrointestinal symptoms (palatability, bloating, belching, constipation, anal irritation). Nicotinic acid has modest LDL cholesterol–lowering capabilities (<20%). Fibrates are best employed to lower LDL cholesterol when both LDL cholesterol and triglycerides are elevated. Fenofibrate may be more effective than gemfibrozil in this group.

TRIGLYCERIDES The NCEP:ATPIII has focused on non-HDL cholesterol rather than triglycerides. However, a fasting triglyceride value of <150 mg/dL is recommended. In general, the response of fasting triglycerides relates to the amount of weight reduction achieved. A weight reduction of >10% is necessary to lower fasting triglycerides.

A fibrate (gemfibrozil or fenofibrate) is the drug of choice to lower fasting triglycerides and typically achieve a 35–50% reduction. Concomitant administration with drugs metabolized by the 3A4 cytochrome P450 system (including some statins) greatly increases the risk of myopathy. In these cases, fenofibrate may be preferable to gemfibrozil. In the Veterans Affairs HDL Intervention Trial (VA-HIT), gemfibrozil was administered to men with known CHD and levels of HDL cholesterol <40 mg/dL. A coronary disease event and mortality rate benefit was experienced predominantly in men with hyperinsulinemia and/or diabetes, many of whom retrospectively were identified as having the metabolic syndrome. Of note, the amount of triglyceride lowering in the VA-HIT did not predict benefit. Although levels of LDL cholesterol did not change, a decrease in LDL particle number correlated with benefit. Although several additional clinical trials have been performed, they have not shown clear evidence that fibrates reduce CVD risk as a consequence of triglyceride lowering.

Other drugs that lower triglycerides include statins, nicotinic acid, and high doses of omega 3 fatty acids. In choosing a statin for this purpose, the dose must be high for the "less potent" statins (lovastatin, pravastatin, fluvastatin) or intermediate for the "more potent" statins (simvastatin, atorvastatin, rosuvastatin). The effect of nicotinic acid on fasting triglycerides is dose-related and less than that of fibrates (~20–40%). In patients with the metabolic syndrome and diabetes, nicotinic acid may increase fasting glucose. Omega 3 fatty acid preparations that include high doses of docosahexaenoic acid and eicosapentaenoic acid (~3.0–4.5 g daily) lower fasting triglycerides by ~40%. No interactions with fibrates or statins occur, and the main side effect is eructation with a fishy taste. This can be partially blocked by ingestion of the nutraceutical after freezing. Clinical trials of nicotinic acid or high-dose omega 3 fatty acids in patients with the metabolic syndrome have not been reported.

HDL CHOLESTEROL Beyond weight reduction, there are very few lipid-modifying compounds that increase HDL cholesterol. Statins, fibrates, and bile acid sequestrants have modest effects (5–10%), and there is no effect on HDL cholesterol with ezetimibe or omega 3 fatty acids. Nicotinic acid is the only currently available drug with predictable HDL cholesterol-raising properties. The response is dose-related and can increase HDL cholesterol ~30% above baseline. There is limited evidence at present that raising HDL has a benefit on CVD events independent of lowering LDL cholesterol, particularly in patients with the metabolic syndrome.

BLOOD PRESSURE (See also Chap. 37) The direct relationship between blood pressure and all-cause mortality rate has been well established, including patients with hypertension (>140/90) versus prehypertension (>120/80 but <140/90) versus individuals with normal blood pressure (<120/80). In patients with the metabolic syndrome without diabetes, the best choice for the first antihypertensive should usually be an angiotensin-converting enzyme (ACE) inhibitor or an angiotensin II receptor blocker, as these two classes of drugs appear to reduce the incidence of new-onset type 2 diabetes. In all patients with hypertension, a sodium-restricted diet enriched in fruits and vegetables and low-fat dairy products should be advocated. Home monitoring of blood pressure may assist in maintaining good blood pressure control.

IMPAIRED FASTING GLUCOSE In patients with the metabolic syndrome and type 2 diabetes, aggressive glycemic control may favorably modify fasting triglycerides and/or HDL cholesterol. In patients with IFG without a diagnosis of diabetes, a lifestyle intervention that includes weight reduction, dietary fat restriction, and increased physical activity has been shown to reduce the incidence of type 2 diabetes. Metformin has also been shown to reduce the incidence of diabetes, although the effect was less than that seen with lifestyle intervention.

INSULIN RESISTANCE Several drug classes (biguanides, thiazolidinediones [TZDs]) increase insulin sensitivity. Because insulin resistance is the primary pathophysiologic mechanism for the metabolic syndrome, representative drugs in these classes reduce its prevalence. Both metformin and TZDs enhance insulin action in the liver and suppress endogenous glucose production. TZDs, but not metformin, also improve insulin-mediated glucose uptake in muscle and adipose tissue. Benefits of both drugs have also been seen in patients with NAFLD and PCOS, and the drugs have been shown to reduce markers of inflammation and small dense LDL.

CHAPTER 33

ISCHEMIC HEART DISEASE

Elliott M. Antman ■ **Andrew P. Selwyn** ■ **Joseph Loscalzo**

Ischemic heart disease (IHD) is a condition in which there is an inadequate supply of blood and oxygen to a portion of the myocardium; it typically occurs when there is an imbalance between myocardial oxygen supply and demand. The most common cause of myocardial ischemia is atherosclerotic disease of an epicardial coronary artery (or arteries) sufficient to cause a regional reduction in myocardial blood flow and inadequate perfusion of the myocardium supplied by the involved coronary artery. Chapter 30 deals with the development and treatment of atherosclerosis. This chapter focuses on the chronic manifestations and treatment of ischemic heart disease. The following chapters address the acute phases of this disease.

EPIDEMIOLOGY

IHD causes more deaths and disability and incurs greater economic costs than any other illness in the developed world. IHD is the most common, serious, chronic, life-threatening illness in the United States, where 13 million persons have IHD, >6 million have angina pectoris, and >7 million have sustained a myocardial infarction. Genetic factors, a high-fat and energy-rich diet, smoking, and a sedentary lifestyle are associated with the emergence of IHD (Chap. 30). In the United States and Western Europe, it is growing among low-income groups, but primary prevention has delayed the disease to later in life in all socioeconomic groups. Despite these sobering statistics, it is worth noting that epidemiologic data show a decline in the rate of deaths due to IHD, about half of which is attributable to treatments and half to prevention by risk factor modification.

Obesity, insulin resistance, and type 2 diabetes mellitus are increasing and are powerful risk factors for IHD. With urbanization in countries with emerging economies and a growing middle class, elements of the energy-rich Western diet are being adopted. As a result, the prevalence of risk factors for and of IHD itself are both increasing rapidly in those regions such that a majority of the global burden of IHD occurs there. Population subgroups that appear to be particularly affected are men in South Asian countries, especially India and the Middle East. In light of the projection of large increases in IHD throughout the world, IHD is likely to become the most common cause of death worldwide by 2020.

PATHOPHYSIOLOGY

Central to an understanding of the pathophysiology of myocardial ischemia is the concept of myocardial supply and demand. In normal conditions, for any given level of a demand for oxygen, the myocardium will control the supply of oxygen-rich blood to prevent underperfusion of myocytes and the subsequent development of ischemia and infarction. The major determinants of myocardial oxygen demand (MVO_2) are heart rate, myocardial contractility, and myocardial wall tension (stress). An adequate supply of oxygen to the myocardium requires a satisfactory level of oxygen-carrying capacity of the blood (determined by the inspired level of oxygen, pulmonary function, and hemoglobin concentration and function) and an adequate level of coronary blood flow. Blood flows through the coronary arteries in a phasic fashion, with the majority occurring during diastole. About 75% of the total coronary resistance to flow occurs across three sets of arteries: (1) large epicardial arteries (Resistance 1 = R_1), (2) prearteriolar vessels (R_2), and (3) arteriolar and intramyocardial capillary vessels (R_3). In the absence of significant flow-limiting atherosclerotic obstructions, R_1 is trivial; the major determinant of coronary resistance is found in R_2 and R_3.

The normal coronary circulation is dominated and controlled by the heart's requirements for oxygen. This need is met by the ability of the coronary vascular bed to vary its resistance (and, therefore, blood flow) considerably while the myocardium extracts a high and relatively fixed percentage of oxygen. Normally, intramyocardial resistance vessels demonstrate an immense capacity for dilation (R_2 and R_3 decrease). For example, the changing oxygen needs of the heart with exercise and emotional stress affect coronary vascular resistance and in this manner regulate the supply of oxygen and substrate to the myocardium (*metabolic regulation*). The coronary resistance vessels also adapt to physiologic alterations in blood pressure to maintain coronary blood flow at levels appropriate to myocardial needs (*autoregulation*).

By reducing the lumen of the coronary arteries, atherosclerosis limits appropriate increases in perfusion when the demand for flow is augmented, as occurs during exertion or excitement. When the luminal reduction is severe, myocardial perfusion in the basal state is reduced. Coronary blood flow also can be limited by spasm (see Prinzmetal's angina in Chap. 34), arterial thrombi, and, rarely, coronary emboli as well as by ostial narrowing due to aortitis. Congenital abnormalities such as the origin of the left anterior descending coronary artery from the pulmonary artery may cause myocardial ischemia and infarction in infancy, but this cause is very rare in adults.

Myocardial ischemia also can occur if myocardial oxygen demands are markedly increased and particularly when coronary blood flow may be limited, as occurs in severe left ventricular hypertrophy due to aortic stenosis. The latter can present with angina that is indistinguishable from that caused by coronary atherosclerosis largely owing to subendocardial ischemia (Chap. 20). A reduction in the oxygen-carrying capacity of the blood, as in extremely severe anemia or in the presence of carboxyhemoglobin, rarely causes myocardial ischemia by itself but may lower the threshold for ischemia in patients with moderate coronary obstruction.

Not infrequently, two or more causes of ischemia coexist in a patient, such as an increase in oxygen demand due to left ventricular hypertrophy secondary to hypertension and a reduction in oxygen supply secondary to coronary atherosclerosis and anemia. Abnormal constriction or failure of normal dilation of the coronary resistance vessels also can cause ischemia. When it causes angina, this condition is referred to as *microvascular angina*.

CORONARY ATHEROSCLEROSIS

Epicardial coronary arteries are the major site of atherosclerotic disease. The major risk factors for atherosclerosis (high levels of plasma low-density lipoprotein [LDL], low plasma high-density lipoprotein [HDL], cigarette smoking, hypertension, and diabetes mellitus [Chap. 30]) disturb the normal functions of the vascular endothelium. These functions include local control of vascular tone, maintenance of an antithrombotic surface, and control of inflammatory cell adhesion and diapedesis. The loss of these defenses leads to inappropriate constriction, luminal thrombus formation, and abnormal interactions between blood cells, especially monocytes and platelets, and the activated vascular endothelium. Functional changes in the vascular milieu ultimately result in the subintimal collections of fat, smooth-muscle cells, fibroblasts, and intercellular matrix that define the atherosclerotic plaque. This process develops at irregular rates in different segments of the epicardial coronary tree and leads eventually to segmental reductions in cross-sectional area, i.e., plaque formation.

There is also a predilection for atherosclerotic plaques to develop at sites of increased turbulence in coronary flow, such as at branch points in the epicardial arteries. When a stenosis reduces the diameter of an epicardial artery by 50%, there is a limitation of the ability to increase flow to meet increased myocardial demand. When the diameter is reduced by ~80%, blood flow at rest may be reduced, and further minor decreases in the stenotic orifice area can reduce coronary flow dramatically to cause myocardial ischemia at rest or with minimal stress.

Segmental atherosclerotic narrowing of epicardial coronary arteries is caused most commonly by the formation of a plaque, which is subject to rupture or erosion of the cap separating the plaque from the bloodstream. Upon exposure of the plaque contents to blood, two important and interrelated processes are set in motion: (1) platelets are activated and aggregate, and (2) the coagulation cascade is activated, leading to deposition of fibrin strands. A thrombus composed of platelet aggregates and fibrin strands traps red blood cells and can reduce coronary blood flow, leading to the clinical manifestations of myocardial ischemia.

The location of the obstruction influences the quantity of myocardium rendered ischemic and determines the severity of the clinical manifestations. Thus, critical obstructions in vessels, such as the left main coronary artery and the proximal left anterior descending coronary artery, are particularly hazardous. Chronic severe coronary narrowing and myocardial ischemia frequently are accompanied by the development of collateral vessels, especially when the narrowing develops gradually. When well developed, such vessels can by themselves provide sufficient blood flow to sustain the viability of the myocardium at rest but not during conditions of increased demand.

With progressive worsening of a stenosis in a proximal epicardial artery, the distal resistance vessels (when they function normally) dilate to reduce vascular resistance and maintain coronary blood flow. A pressure gradient develops across the proximal stenosis, and poststenotic pressure falls. When the resistance vessels are maximally dilated, myocardial blood flow becomes dependent on the pressure in the coronary artery distal to the obstruction. In these circumstances, ischemia, manifest clinically by angina or electrocardiographically by ST-segment deviation, can be precipitated by increases in myocardial oxygen demand caused by physical activity, emotional stress, and/or tachycardia. Changes in the caliber of the stenosed coronary artery due to physiologic vasomotion, loss of endothelial control of dilation (as occurs in atherosclerosis), pathologic spasm (Prinzmetal's angina), or small platelet-rich plugs also can upset the critical balance between oxygen supply and demand and thereby precipitate myocardial ischemia.

EFFECTS OF ISCHEMIA

During episodes of inadequate perfusion caused by coronary atherosclerosis, myocardial tissue oxygen tension falls and may cause transient disturbances of the mechanical, biochemical, and electrical functions of the myocardium. Coronary atherosclerosis is a focal process that usually causes nonuniform ischemia. During ischemia, regional disturbances of ventricular contractility cause segmental hypokinesia, akinesia, or, in severe cases, bulging (dyskinesia), which can reduce myocardial pump function.

The abrupt development of severe ischemia, as occurs with total or subtotal coronary occlusion, is associated with almost instantaneous failure of normal muscle relaxation and then contraction. The relatively poor perfusion of the subendocardium causes more intense ischemia of this portion of the wall (compared with the subepicardial region). Ischemia of large portions of the ventricle causes transient left ventricular failure, and if the papillary muscle apparatus is involved, mitral regurgitation can occur. When ischemia is transient, it may be associated with angina pectoris; when it is prolonged, it can lead to myocardial necrosis and scarring with or without the clinical picture of acute myocardial infarction (Chap. 35).

A wide range of abnormalities in cell metabolism, function, and structure underlie these mechanical disturbances during ischemia. The normal myocardium metabolizes fatty acids and glucose to carbon dioxide and water. With severe oxygen deprivation, fatty acids cannot be oxidized, and glucose is converted to lactate; intracellular pH is reduced, as are the myocardial stores of high-energy phosphates, i.e., ATP and creatine phosphate. Impaired cell membrane function leads to the leakage of potassium and the uptake of sodium by myocytes as well as an increase in cytosolic calcium. The severity and duration of the imbalance between myocardial oxygen supply and demand determine whether the damage is reversible (≤20 min for total occlusion in the absence of collaterals) or permanent, with subsequent myocardial necrosis (>20 min).

Ischemia also causes characteristic changes in the electrocardiogram (ECG) such as repolarization abnormalities, as evidenced by inversion of T waves and, when more severe, displacement of ST segments (Chap. 11). Transient T-wave inversion probably reflects nontransmural, intramyocardial ischemia; transient ST-segment depression often reflects patchy subendocardial ischemia; and ST-segment elevation is thought to be caused by more severe transmural ischemia. Another important consequence of myocardial ischemia is electrical instability, which may lead to isolated ventricular premature beats or even ventricular tachycardia or ventricular fibrillation (Chap. 16). Most patients who die suddenly from IHD do so as a result of ischemia-induced ventricular tachyarrhythmias (Chap. 29).

ASYMPTOMATIC VERSUS SYMPTOMATIC IHD

Postmortem studies of accident victims and military casualties in Western countries have shown that coronary atherosclerosis often begins to develop before age 20 and is widespread even among adults who were asymptomatic during life. Exercise stress tests in asymptomatic persons may show evidence of silent myocardial ischemia, i.e., exercise-induced ECG changes not accompanied by angina pectoris; coronary angiographic studies of such persons may reveal coronary artery plaques and previously unrecognized obstructions (Chap. 13). Postmortem examination of patients with such obstructions without a history of clinical manifestations of myocardial ischemia often shows macroscopic scars secondary to myocardial infarction in regions supplied by diseased coronary arteries, with or without collateral circulation. According to population studies, ~25% of patients who survive acute myocardial infarction may not come to medical attention, and these patients have the same adverse prognosis as do those who present with the classic clinical picture of acute myocardial infarction (Chap. 35). Sudden death may be unheralded and is a common presenting manifestation of IHD (Chap. 29).

Patients with IHD also can present with cardiomegaly and heart failure secondary to ischemic damage of the left ventricular myocardium that may have caused no symptoms before the development of heart failure; this condition is referred to as *ischemic cardiomyopathy*. In contrast to the asymptomatic phase of IHD, the symptomatic phase is characterized by chest discomfort due to either angina pectoris or acute myocardial infarction (Chap. 35). Having entered the symptomatic phase, the patient may exhibit a stable or progressive course, revert to the asymptomatic stage, or die suddenly.

STABLE ANGINA PECTORIS

This episodic clinical syndrome is due to transient myocardial ischemia. Various diseases that cause myocardial ischemia as well as the numerous forms of discomfort with which it may be confused are discussed in Chap. 4. Males constitute ~70% of all patients with angina pectoris and an even greater proportion of those less than 50 years of age. It is, however, important to note that angina pectoris in women is often atypical in presentation (see later).

HISTORY

The typical patient with angina is a man >50 years or a woman >60 years of age who complains of episodes of chest discomfort, usually described as heaviness, pressure, squeezing, smothering, or choking and only rarely as frank pain. When the patient is asked to localize the sensation, he or she typically places a hand over the sternum, sometimes with a clenched fist, to indicate a squeezing, central, substernal discomfort (Levine's sign). Angina is usually crescendo-decrescendo in nature, typically lasts 2 to 5 min, and can radiate to either shoulder and to both arms (especially the ulnar surfaces of the forearm and hand). It also can arise in or radiate to the back, interscapular region, root of the neck, jaw, teeth, and epigastrium. Angina is rarely localized below the umbilicus or above the mandible. A useful finding in assessing a patient with chest discomfort is the fact that myocardial ischemic discomfort does not radiate to the trapezius muscles; that radiation pattern is more typical of pericarditis.

Although episodes of angina typically are caused by exertion (e.g., exercise, hurrying, or sexual activity) or emotion (e.g., stress, anger, fright, or frustration) and are relieved by rest, they also may occur at rest (see "Unstable Angina Pectoris," [Chap. 34]) and while the patient is recumbent (angina decubitus). The patient may be awakened at night by typical chest discomfort and dyspnea. Nocturnal angina may be due to episodic tachycardia, diminished oxygenation as the respiratory pattern changes during sleep, or expansion of the intrathoracic blood volume that occurs with recumbency; the latter causes an increase in cardiac size (end-diastolic volume), wall tension, and myocardial oxygen demand that can lead to ischemia and transient left ventricular failure.

The threshold for the development of angina pectoris may vary by time of day and emotional state. Many patients report a fixed threshold for angina, which occurs predictably at a certain level of activity, such as climbing two flights of stairs at a normal pace. In these patients, coronary stenosis and myocardial oxygen supply are fixed, and ischemia is precipitated by an increase in myocardial oxygen demand; they are said to have stable exertional angina. In other patients, the threshold for angina may vary considerably within any particular day and from day to day. In such patients, variations in myocardial oxygen supply, most likely due to changes in coronary vasomotor tone, may play an important role in defining the pattern of angina. A patient may report symptoms upon minor exertion in the morning (a short walk or shaving) yet by midday be capable of much greater effort without symptoms. Angina may also be precipitated by unfamiliar tasks, a heavy meal, exposure to cold, or a combination of these factors.

Exertional angina typically is relieved in 1 to 5 min by slowing or ceasing activities and even more rapidly by rest and sublingual nitroglycerin (see later). Indeed, the diagnosis of angina should be suspect if it does not respond to the combination of these measures. The severity of angina can be conveniently summarized by the Canadian Cardiac Society functional classification (Table 33-1). Its impact on the patient's functional capacity can be described by using the New York Heart Association functional classification (Table 33-1).

Sharp, fleeting chest pain or a prolonged, dull ache localized to the left submammary area is rarely due to myocardial ischemia. However, especially in women and diabetic patients, angina pectoris may be atypical in location and not strictly related to provoking factors. In addition, this symptom may exacerbate and remit over days, weeks, or months. Its occurrence can be seasonal, occurring more frequently in the winter in temperate climates. Anginal "equivalents" are symptoms of myocardial ischemia other than angina. They include dyspnea, nausea, fatigue, and faintness and are more common in the elderly and in diabetic patients.

Systematic questioning of a patient with suspected IHD is important to uncover the features of an unstable syndrome associated with increased risk, such as angina occurring with less exertion than in the past, occurring at rest, or awakening the patient from sleep. Since coronary atherosclerosis often is accompanied by similar lesions in other arteries, a patient with angina should be questioned and examined for peripheral arterial disease (intermittent claudication [Chap. 39]), stroke, or transient ischemic attacks. It is also important to uncover a family history of premature IHD (<55 years in first-degree male relatives and <65 in female relatives) and the presence of diabetes mellitus, hyperlipidemia, hypertension, cigarette smoking, and other risk factors for coronary atherosclerosis (Chap. 30).

TABLE 33-1

CARDIOVASCULAR DISEASE CLASSIFICATION CHART

CLASS	NEW YORK HEART ASSOCIATION FUNCTIONAL CLASSIFICATION	CANADIAN CARDIOVASCULAR SOCIETY FUNCTIONAL CLASSIFICATION
I	Patients have cardiac disease but *without* the resulting *limitations* of physical activity. Ordinary physical activity does not cause undue fatigue, palpitation, dyspnea, or anginal pain.	Ordinary physical activity, such as walking and climbing stairs, *does not cause angina*. Angina present with strenuous or rapid or prolonged exertion at work or recreation.
II	Patients have cardiac disease resulting in *slight limitation* of physical activity. They are comfortable at rest. Ordinary physical activity results in fatigue, palpitation, dyspnea, or anginal pain.	*Slight limitation* of ordinary activity. Walking or climbing stairs rapidly, walking uphill, walking or stair climbing after meals, in cold, or when under emotional stress or only during the few hours after awakening. Walking more than two blocks on the level and climbing more than one flight of stairs at a normal pace and in normal conditions.
III	Patients have cardiac disease resulting in *marked limitation* of physical activity. They are comfortable at rest. Less than ordinary physical activity causes fatigue, palpitation, dyspnea, or anginal pain.	*Marked limitation* of ordinary physical activity. Walking one to two blocks on the level and climbing more than one flight of stairs in normal conditions.
IV	Patients have cardiac disease resulting in *inability* to carry on any physical activity without discomfort. Symptoms of cardiac insufficiency or of the anginal syndrome may be present even at rest. If any physical activity is undertaken, discomfort is increased.	*Inability* to carry on any physical activity without discomfort—anginal syndrome *may* be present at rest.

Source: Modified from L Goldman et al: Circulation 64:1227, 1981.

The history of typical angina pectoris establishes the diagnosis of IHD until proven otherwise. In patients with atypical angina (Chap. 4), the coexistence of advanced age, male sex, the postmenopausal state, and risk factors for atherosclerosis increase the likelihood of hemodynamically significant coronary disease. A particularly challenging problem is the evaluation and management of patients with persistent ischemic-type chest discomfort but no flow-limiting obstructions in their epicardial coronary arteries. This situation arises more often in women than in men. Potential etiologies include microvascular coronary disease (detectable on coronary reactivity testing in response to vasoactive agents such as intracoronary adenosine, acetylcholine, and nitroglycerin) and abnormal cardiac nociception. Treatment of microvascular coronary disease should focus on efforts to improve endothelial function, including nitrates, beta blockers, calcium antagonists, statins, and angiotensin-converting enzyme (ACE) inhibitors. Abnormal cardiac nociception is more difficult to manage and may be ameliorated in some cases by imipramine.

PHYSICAL EXAMINATION

The physical examination is often normal in patients with stable angina when they are asymptomatic. However, because of the increased likelihood of ischemic heart disease in patients with diabetes and/or peripheral arterial disease, clinicians should search for evidence of atherosclerotic disease at other sites, such as an abdominal aortic aneurysm, carotid arterial bruits, and diminished arterial pulses in the lower extremities. The physical examination also should include a search for evidence of risk factors for atherosclerosis such as xanthelasmas and xanthomas (Chap. 30). Evidence for peripheral arterial disease should be sought by evaluating the pulse contour at multiple locations and comparing the blood pressure between the arms and between the arms and the legs (ankle-brachial index). Examination of the fundi may reveal an increased light reflex and arteriovenous nicking as evidence of hypertension. There also may be signs of anemia, thyroid disease, and nicotine stains on the fingertips from cigarette smoking.

Palpation may reveal cardiac enlargement and abnormal contraction of the cardiac impulse (left ventricular dyskinesia). Auscultation can uncover arterial bruits, a third and/or fourth heart sound, and, if acute ischemia or previous infarction has impaired papillary muscle function, an apical systolic murmur due to mitral regurgitation. These auscultatory signs are best appreciated with the patient in the left lateral decubitus position. Aortic stenosis, aortic regurgitation (Chap. 20), pulmonary hypertension (Chap. 40), and hypertrophic cardiomyopathy (Chap. 21) must be excluded, since these disorders may cause angina in the absence of coronary atherosclerosis. Examination during an anginal attack is useful, since ischemia can cause transient left ventricular failure with the appearance of a third and/or fourth heart sound, a dyskinetic cardiac apex, mitral regurgitation, and even pulmonary edema. Tenderness of the chest wall, localization of the discomfort with a single fingertip on the chest, or reproduction of the pain with palpation of the chest makes it unlikely that the pain is caused by myocardial ischemia. A protuberant abdomen may indicate that the patient has the metabolic syndrome and is at increased risk for atherosclerosis.

LABORATORY EXAMINATION

Although the diagnosis of IHD can be made with a high degree of confidence from the history and physical examination, a number of simple laboratory tests can be helpful. The urine should be examined for evidence of diabetes mellitus and renal disease (including microalbuminuria) since these conditions accelerate atherosclerosis. Similarly, examination of the blood should include measurements of lipids (cholesterol—total, LDL, HDL—and triglycerides), glucose (hemoglobin A_{1C}), creatinine, hematocrit, and, if indicated based on the physical examination, thyroid function. A chest x-ray is important as it may show the consequences of IHD, i.e., cardiac enlargement, ventricular aneurysm, or signs of heart failure. These signs can support the diagnosis of IHD and are important in assessing the degree of cardiac damage. Evidence exists that an elevated level of high-sensitivity C-reactive protein (CRP) (specifically, between 0 and 3 mg/dL) is an independent risk factor for IHD and may be useful in therapeutic decision making about the initiation of hypolipidemic treatment. The major benefit of high-sensitivity CRP is in reclassifying the risk of IHD in patients in the "intermediate" risk category on the basis of traditional risk factors.

ELECTROCARDIOGRAM

A 12-lead ECG recorded at rest may be normal in patients with typical angina pectoris, but there may also be signs of an old myocardial infarction (Chap. 11). Although repolarization abnormalities, i.e., ST-segment and T-wave changes, as well as left ventricular hypertrophy and disturbances of cardiac rhythm or intraventricular conduction are suggestive of IHD, they are nonspecific, since they also can occur in pericardial, myocardial, and valvular heart disease or, in the case of the former, transiently with anxiety, changes in posture, drugs, or esophageal disease. The presence of left ventricular hypertrophy (LVH) is a significant indication of increased risk of adverse outcomes from ischemic heart disease. Of note, even though LVH and cardiac rhythm

disturbances are nonspecific indicators of the development of IHD, they may be contributing factors to episodes of angina in patients in whom IHD has developed as a consequence of conventional risk factors. Dynamic ST-segment and T-wave changes that accompany episodes of angina pectoris and disappear thereafter are more specific.

STRESS TESTING

Electrocardiographic

The most widely used test for both the diagnosis of IHD and the estimation of risk and prognosis involves recording the 12-lead ECG before, during, and after exercise, usually on a treadmill (Fig. 33-1). The test consists of a standardized incremental increase in external workload (Table 33-2) while symptoms, the ECG, and arm blood pressure are monitored. Exercise duration is usually symptom-limited, and the test is discontinued upon evidence of chest discomfort, severe shortness of breath, dizziness, severe fatigue, ST-segment depression >0.2 mV (2 mm), a fall in systolic blood pressure >10 mmHg, or the development of a ventricular tachyarrhythmia. This test is used to discover any limitation in exercise performance, detect typical ECG signs of myocardial ischemia, and establish their relationship to chest discomfort. The ischemic ST-segment response generally is defined as a flat or downsloping depression of the ST segment >0.1 mV below baseline (i.e., the PR segment) and lasting longer than 0.08 s (Fig. 33-1). Upsloping or junctional ST-segment changes are not considered characteristic of ischemia and do not constitute a positive test. Although T-wave abnormalities, conduction disturbances, and ventricular arrhythmias that develop during exercise should be noted, they are also not diagnostic. Negative exercise tests in which the target heart rate (85% of maximal predicted heart rate for age and sex) is not achieved are considered nondiagnostic.

In interpreting ECG stress tests, the probability that coronary artery disease (CAD) exists in the patient or population under study (i.e., pretest probability) should be considered. Overall, false-positive or false-negative results occur in one-third of cases. However, a positive result on exercise indicates that the likelihood of CAD is 98% in males who are >50 years with a history of typical angina pectoris and who develop chest discomfort during the test. The likelihood decreases if the patient has atypical or no chest pain by history and/or during the test.

The incidence of false-positive tests is significantly increased in patients with low probabilities of IHD, such as asymptomatic men <age 40 or premenopausal women with no risk factors for premature

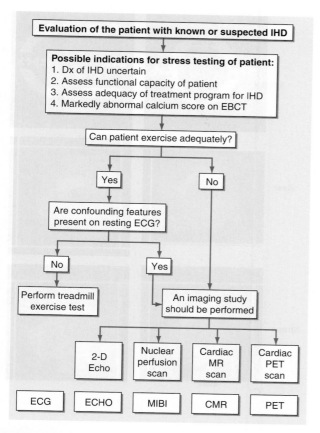

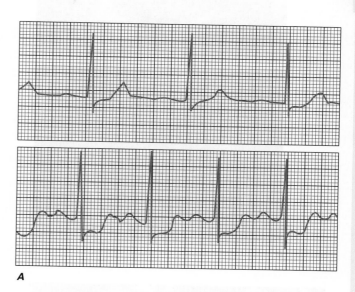

A

FIGURE 33-1

Evaluation of the patient with known or suspected ischemic heart disease. At the top of the figure is an algorithm for identifying patients who should be referred for stress testing and the decision pathway for determining whether a standard treadmill exercise with ECG monitoring alone is adequate. A specialized imaging study is necessary if the patient cannot exercise adequately (pharmacologic challenge is given) or if there are confounding features on the resting ECG (symptom-limited treadmill exercise may be used to stress the coronary circulation). At the bottom of the figure are examples of the data obtained with ECG monitoring and specialized imaging procedures. CMR, cardiac magnetic resonance; EBCT, electron beam computed tomography; ECG, electrocardiogram; ECHO, echocardiography; IHD, ischemic heart disease; MIBI, methoxyisobutyl isonitrite; MR, magnetic resonance; PET, positron emission tomography.

A. Lead V_4 at rest (*top*) and after 4½ min of exercise (*bottom*). There is 3 mm (0.3 mV) of horizontal ST-segment depression, indicating a positive test for ischemia. (*Modified from BR Chaitman, in E Braunwald et al [eds]: Heart Disease, 6th ed, Philadelphia, Saunders, 2001.*)

B. 45-year-old avid jogger who began experiencing classic substernal chest pressure underwent an exercise echo study. With exercise the patient's heart rate increased from 52 to 153 bpm. The left ventricular chamber dilated with exercise, and the septal and apical portions became akinetic to dyskinetic (*red arrow*). These findings are strongly suggestive of a significant flow-limiting stenosis in the proximal left anterior descending artery, which was confirmed at coronary angiography. (*Modified*

from SD Solomon, in E. Braunwald et al [eds]: Primary Cardiology, 2nd ed, Philadelphia, Saunders, 2003.)

C. Stress and rest myocardial perfusion SPECT images obtained with 99m-technetium sestamibi in a patient with chest pain and dyspnea on exertion. The images demonstrate a medium-size and severe stress perfusion defect involving the inferolateral and basal inferior walls, showing nearly complete reversibility, consistent with moderate ischemia in the right coronary artery territory (*red arrows*). (*Images provided by Dr. Marcello Di Carli, Nuclear Medicine Division, Brigham and Women's Hospital, Boston, MA.*)

D. A patient with a prior myocardial infarction presented with recurrent chest discomfort. On cardiac magnetic resonance (CMR) cine imaging, a large area of anterior akinesia was noted (marked by the arrows in the top left and right images, systolic frame only). This area of akinesia was matched by a larger extent of late gadolinium-DTPA enhancements consistent with a large transmural myocardial infarction (marked by arrows in the middle left and right images). Resting (*bottom left*) and adenosine vasodilating stress (*bottom right*) first-pass perfusion images revealed reversible perfusion abnormality that extended to the inferior septum. This patient was found to have an occluded proximal left anterior descending coronary artery with extensive collateral formation. This case illustrates the utility of different modalities in a CMR examination in characterizing ischemic and infarcted myocardium. DTPA, diethylenetriamine penta-acetic acid. (*Images provided by Dr. Raymond Kwong, Cardiovascular Division, Brigham and Women's Hospital, Boston, MA.*)

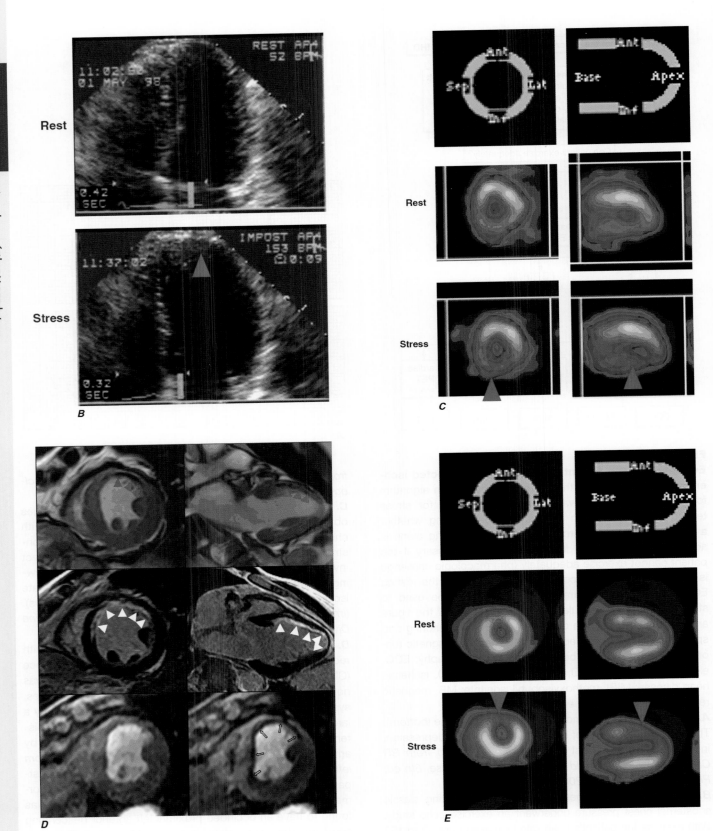

FIGURE 33-1 (*Continued*)

E. Stress and rest myocardial perfusion PET images obtained with rubidium-82 in a patient with chest pain on exertion. The images demonstrate a large and severe stress perfusion defect involving the mid and apical anterior, anterolateral, and anteroseptal walls and the LV apex, showing complete reversibility, consistent with extensive and severe ischemia in the mid-left anterior descending coronary artery territory (*red arrows*). (*Images provided by Dr. Marcello Di Carli, Nuclear Medicine Division, Brigham and Women's Hospital, Boston, MA.*)

TABLE 33-2

RELATION OF METABOLIC EQUIVALENT TASKS (METs) TO STAGES IN VARIOUS TESTING PROTOCOLS

FUNCTIONAL CLASS	CLINICAL STATUS	O₂ COST mL/kg/min	METS	BRUCE Modified 3 min Stage MPH	%GR	BRUCE 3 min Stages MPH	%GR
				6.0	22	6.0	22
				5.5	20	5.2	20
				5.0	18	5.0	18
NORMAL		56.0	16				
		52.5	15				
AND		49.0	14				
		45.5	13	4.2	16	4.2	16
I		42.0	12				
		38.5	11	3.4	14	3.4	14
		35.0	10				
		31.5	9				
		28.0	8				
		24.5	7	2.5	12	2.5	12
II		21.0	6				
		17.5	5	1.7	10	1.7	10
III		14.0	4				
		10.5	3	1.7	5		
		7.0	2	1.7	0		
IV		3.5	1				

(Functional class left margin labels: HEALTHY, DEPENDENT ON AGE, ACTIVITY; Clinical status vertical labels: SEDENTARY HEALTHY; LIMITED; SYMPTOMATIC)

Source: Modified from GF Fletcher et al: Circulation 104:1694, 2001.

atherosclerosis. It is also increased in patients taking cardioactive drugs, such as digitalis and antiarrhythmic agents, and in those with intraventricular conduction disturbances, resting ST-segment and T-wave abnormalities, ventricular hypertrophy, or abnormal serum potassium levels. Obstructive disease limited to the circumflex coronary artery may result in a false-negative stress test since the lateral portion of the heart that this vessel supplies is not well represented on the surface 12-lead ECG. Since the overall sensitivity of exercise stress electrocardiography is only ~75%, a negative result does not exclude CAD, although it makes the likelihood of three-vessel or left main CAD extremely unlikely.

The physician should be present throughout the exercise test. It is important to measure total duration of exercise, the times to the onset of ischemic ST-segment change and chest discomfort, the external work performed (generally expressed as the stage of exercise), and the internal cardiac work performed, i.e., by the heart rate–blood pressure product. The depth of the ST-segment depression and the time needed for recovery of these ECG changes are also important. Because the risks of exercise testing are small but real—estimated at one fatality and two nonfatal complications per 10,000 tests—equipment for resuscitation should be available. Modified (heart rate–limited rather than symptom-limited) exercise tests can be performed safely in patients as early as 6 days after uncomplicated myocardial infarction (Table 33-2). Contraindications to exercise stress testing include rest angina within 48 h, unstable rhythm, severe aortic stenosis, acute myocarditis, uncontrolled heart failure, severe pulmonary hypertension, and active infective endocarditis.

The normal response to graded exercise includes progressive increases in heart rate and blood pressure. Failure of the blood pressure to increase or an actual decrease with signs of ischemia during the test is an important adverse prognostic sign, since it may reflect ischemia-induced global left ventricular dysfunction. The development of angina and/or severe (>0.2 mV) ST-segment depression at a low workload, i.e., before completion of stage II of the Bruce protocol, and/or ST-segment depression that persists >5 min after the termination of exercise increases the specificity of the test and suggests severe IHD and a high risk of future adverse events.

Cardiac imaging

(See also Chap. 12) When the resting ECG is abnormal (e.g., preexcitation syndrome, >1 mm of resting ST-segment depression, left bundle branch block, paced ventricular rhythm), information gained from an exercise test can be enhanced by stress myocardial radionuclide perfusion imaging after the intravenous administration of thallium-201 or 99m-technetium sestamibi during exercise (or with pharmacologic) stress. Contemporary data also suggest positron emission tomography (PET) imaging (with exercise or pharmacologic stress) using N-13 ammonia or rubidium-82 nuclide as another technique for assessing perfusion. Images obtained immediately after cessation of exercise to detect regional ischemia are compared with those obtained at rest to confirm reversible ischemia and regions of persistently absent uptake that signify infarction.

A sizable fraction of patients who need noninvasive stress testing to identify myocardial ischemia and increased risk of coronary events cannot exercise because of peripheral vascular or musculoskeletal disease, exertional dyspnea, or deconditioning. In these circumstances, an intravenous pharmacologic challenge is used in place of exercise. For example, dipyridamole or adenosine can be given to create a coronary "steal" by temporarily increasing flow in nondiseased segments of the coronary vasculature at the expense of diseased segments. Alternatively, a graded incremental infusion of dobutamine may be administered to increase MVO_2. A variety of imaging options are available to accompany these pharmacologic stressors (Fig. 33-1). The development of a transient perfusion defect with a tracer such as thallium-201 or 99m-technetium sestamibi is used to detect myocardial ischemia.

Echocardiography is used to assess left ventricular function in patients with chronic stable angina and patients with a history of a prior myocardial infarction, pathologic Q waves, or clinical evidence of heart failure. Two-dimensional echocardiography can assess both global and regional wall motion abnormalities of the left ventricle that are transient when due to ischemia. Stress (exercise or dobutamine) echocardiography may cause the emergence of regions of akinesis or dyskinesis that are not present at rest. Stress echocardiography, like stress myocardial perfusion imaging, is more sensitive than exercise electrocardiography in the diagnosis of IHD. Cardiac magnetic resonance (CMR) stress testing is also evolving as an alternative to radionuclide, PET, or echocardiographic stress imaging. CMR stress testing performed with dobutamine infusion can be used to assess wall motion abnormalities accompanying ischemia, as well as myocardial perfusion. CMR can be used to provide more complete ventricular evaluation using multislice MR imaging (MRI) studies.

Atherosclerotic plaques become progressively calcified over time, and coronary calcification in general increases with age. For this reason, methods for detecting coronary calcium have been developed as a measure of the presence of coronary atherosclerosis. These methods involve computed tomography (CT) applications that achieve rapid acquisition of images (electron beam [EBCT], and multidetector [MDCT] detection). Coronary calcium detected by these imaging techniques most commonly is quantified by using the Agatston score, which is based on the area and density of calcification. Although the diagnostic accuracy of this imaging method is high (sensitivity, 90–94%; specificity, 95–97%; negative predictive value, 93–99%), its prognostic utility has not been defined. Thus, its role in CT, EBCT, and MDCT scans for the detection and management of patients with IHD has not been clarified.

CORONARY ARTERIOGRAPHY

(See also Chap. 13) This diagnostic method outlines the lumina of the coronary arteries and can be used to detect or exclude serious coronary obstruction. However, coronary arteriography provides no information about the arterial wall, and severe atherosclerosis that does not encroach on the lumen may go undetected. Of note, atherosclerotic plaques characteristically are scattered throughout the coronary tree, tend to occur more frequently at branch points, and grow progressively in the intima and media of an epicardial coronary artery at first without encroaching on the lumen, causing an outward bulging of the artery—a process referred to as remodeling (Chap. 30). Later in the course of the disease, further growth causes luminal narrowing.

Indications

Coronary arteriography is indicated in (1) patients with chronic stable angina pectoris who are severely symptomatic despite medical therapy and are being considered for revascularization, i.e., a percutaneous coronary intervention (PCI) or coronary artery bypass grafting (CABG), (2) patients with troublesome symptoms that present diagnostic difficulties in whom there is a need to confirm or rule out the diagnosis of IHD, (3) patients with known or possible angina pectoris who have survived cardiac arrest, (4) patients with angina or evidence of ischemia on noninvasive testing with clinical or laboratory evidence of ventricular dysfunction, and (5) patients judged to be at high risk of sustaining coronary events based on signs of severe ischemia on noninvasive testing, regardless of the presence or severity of symptoms (see later).

Examples of other indications for coronary arteriography include the following:

1. Patients with chest discomfort suggestive of angina pectoris but a negative or nondiagnostic stress test who require a definitive diagnosis for guiding medical management, alleviating psychological stress, career or family planning, or insurance purposes.
2. Patients who have been admitted repeatedly to the hospital for a suspected acute coronary syndrome (Chaps. 34 and 35) but in whom this diagnosis has not been established and in whom the presence or absence of CAD should be determined.
3. Patients with careers that involve the safety of others (e.g., pilots, firefighters, police) who have questionable symptoms or suspicious or positive noninvasive tests and in whom there are reasonable doubts about the state of the coronary arteries.
4. Patients with aortic stenosis or hypertrophic cardiomyopathy and angina in whom the chest pain could be due to IHD.
5. Male patients >45 years and females >55 years who are to undergo a cardiac operation such as valve replacement or repair and who may or may not have clinical evidence of myocardial ischemia.
6. Patients after myocardial infarction, especially those who are at high risk after myocardial infarction because of the recurrence of angina or the presence of heart failure, frequent ventricular premature contractions, or signs of ischemia on the stress test.
7. Patients with angina pectoris, regardless of severity, in whom noninvasive testing indicates a high risk of coronary events (poor exercise performance or severe ischemia).
8. Patients in whom coronary spasm or another nonatherosclerotic cause of myocardial ischemia (e.g., coronary artery anomaly, Kawasaki disease) is suspected.

Noninvasive alternatives to diagnostic coronary arteriography include CT angiography and cardiac MR angiography (Chap. 12). Although these new imaging techniques can provide information about obstructive lesions in the epicardial coronary arteries, their exact role in clinical practice has not been rigorously defined. Important aspects of their use that should be noted include the substantially higher radiation exposure with CT angiography compared to conventional diagnostic arteriography and the limitations on cardiac MR imposed by cardiac movement during the cardiac cycle, especially at high heart rates.

PROGNOSIS

The principal prognostic indicators in patients known to have IHD are age, the functional state of the left ventricle, the location(s) and severity of coronary artery narrowing, and the severity or activity of myocardial ischemia. Angina pectoris of recent onset, unstable angina (Chap. 34), early postmyocardial infarction angina, angina that is unresponsive or poorly responsive to medical therapy, and angina accompanied by symptoms of congestive heart failure all indicate an increased risk for adverse coronary events. The same is true for the physical signs of heart failure, episodes of pulmonary edema, transient third heart sounds, and mitral regurgitation and for echocardiographic or radioisotopic (or roentgenographic) evidence of cardiac enlargement and reduced (<0.40) ejection fraction.

Most important, any of the following signs during noninvasive testing indicates a high risk for coronary events: inability to exercise for 6 min, i.e., stage II (Bruce protocol) of the exercise test; a strongly positive exercise test showing onset of myocardial ischemia at low workloads (≥ 0.1 mV ST-segment depression before completion of stage II, ≥ 0.2 mV ST depression at any stage, ST depression for >5 min after the cessation of exercise, a decline in systolic pressure >10 mmHg during exercise, the development of ventricular tachyarrhythmias during exercise); the development of large or multiple perfusion defects or increased lung uptake during stress radioisotope perfusion imaging; and a decrease in left ventricular ejection fraction during exercise on radionuclide ventriculography or during stress echocardiography. Conversely, patients who can complete stage III of the Bruce exercise protocol and have a normal stress perfusion scan or negative stress echocardiographic evaluation are at very low risk for future coronary events. The finding of frequent episodes of ST-segment deviation on ambulatory ECG monitoring (even in the absence of symptoms) is also an adverse prognostic finding.

On cardiac catheterization, elevations of left ventricular end-diastolic pressure and ventricular volume and reduced ejection fraction are the most important signs of left ventricular dysfunction and are associated with a poor prognosis. Patients with chest discomfort but normal left ventricular function and normal coronary arteries have an excellent prognosis. Obstructive lesions of the left main (>50% luminal diameter) or left anterior descending coronary artery proximal to the origin of the first septal artery are associated with a greater risk than are lesions of the right or left circumflex coronary artery because of the greater quantity of myocardium at risk. Atherosclerotic plaques in epicardial arteries with fissuring or filling defects indicate increased risk. These lesions go through phases of inflammatory cellular activity, degeneration, endothelial dysfunction, abnormal vasomotion, platelet aggregation, and fissuring or hemorrhage. These factors can temporarily worsen the stenosis and cause thrombosis and/or abnormal reactivity of the vessel wall, thus exacerbating the manifestations of ischemia. The recent onset of symptoms, the development of severe ischemia during stress testing (see earlier), and unstable angina pectoris (Chap. 34) all reflect episodes of rapid progression in coronary lesions.

With any degree of obstructive CAD, mortality is greatly increased when left ventricular function is impaired; conversely, at any level of left ventricular function, the prognosis is influenced importantly by the quantity of myocardium perfused by critically obstructed vessels. Therefore, it is essential to collect all the evidence substantiating past myocardial damage (evidence of myocardial infarction on ECG, echocardiography, radioisotope imaging, or left ventriculography), residual left ventricular function (ejection fraction and wall motion), and risk of future damage from coronary events (extent of coronary disease and severity of ischemia defined by noninvasive stress testing). The larger the quantity of established myocardial necrosis is, the less the heart is able to withstand additional damage and the poorer the prognosis is. Risk estimation must include age, presenting symptoms, all risk factors, signs of arterial disease, existing cardiac damage, and signs of impending damage (i.e., ischemia).

The greater the number and severity of risk factors for coronary atherosclerosis (advanced age [>75 years], hypertension, dyslipidemia, diabetes, morbid obesity, accompanying peripheral and/or cerebrovascular disease, previous myocardial infarction), the worse the prognosis of an angina patient. Evidence exists that elevated levels of C-reactive protein in the plasma, extensive coronary calcification on electron beam CT (see earlier), and increased carotid intimal thickening on ultrasound examination also indicate an increased risk of coronary events.

TREATMENT Stable Angina Pectoris

Once the diagnosis of ischemic heart disease has been made, each patient must be evaluated individually with respect to his or her level of understanding, expectations and goals, control of symptoms, and prevention of adverse clinical outcomes such as myocardial infarction and premature death. The degree of disability as well as the physical and emotional stress that precipitates angina must be recorded carefully to set treatment goals. The management plan should include the following components: (1) explanation of the problem and reassurance about the ability to formulate a treatment plan, (2) identification and treatment of aggravating

conditions, (3) recommendations for adaptation of activity as needed, (4) treatment of risk factors that will decrease the occurrence of adverse coronary outcomes, (5) drug therapy for angina, and (6) consideration of revascularization.

EXPLANATION AND REASSURANCE Patients with IHD need to understand their condition and realize that a long and productive life is possible even though they have angina pectoris or have experienced and recovered from an acute myocardial infarction. Offering results of clinical trials showing improved outcomes can be of great value in encouraging patients to resume or maintain activity and return to work. A planned program of rehabilitation can encourage patients to lose weight, improve exercise tolerance, and control risk factors with more confidence.

IDENTIFICATION AND TREATMENT OF AGGRAVATING CONDITIONS A number of conditions may increase oxygen demand or decrease oxygen supply to the myocardium and may precipitate or exacerbate angina in patients with IHD. Left ventricular hypertrophy, aortic valve disease, and hypertrophic cardiomyopathy may cause or contribute to angina and should be excluded or treated. Obesity, hypertension, and hyperthyroidism should be treated aggressively to reduce the frequency and severity of anginal episodes. Decreased myocardial oxygen supply may be due to reduced oxygenation of the arterial blood (e.g., in pulmonary disease or, when carboxyhemoglobin is present, due to cigarette or cigar smoking) or decreased oxygen-carrying capacity (e.g., in anemia). Correction of these abnormalities, if present, may reduce or even eliminate angina pectoris.

ADAPTATION OF ACTIVITY Myocardial ischemia is caused by a discrepancy between the demand of the heart muscle for oxygen and the ability of the coronary circulation to meet that demand. Most patients can be helped to understand this concept and utilize it in the rational programming of activity. Many tasks that ordinarily evoke angina may be accomplished without symptoms simply by reducing the speed at which they are performed. Patients must appreciate the diurnal variation in their tolerance of certain activities and should reduce their energy requirements in the morning, immediately after meals, and in cold or inclement weather. On occasion, it may be necessary to recommend a change in employment or residence to avoid physical stress.

Physical conditioning usually improves the exercise tolerance of patients with angina and has substantial psychological benefits. A regular program of isotonic exercise that is within the limits of the individual patient's threshold for the development of angina pectoris and that does not exceed 80% of the heart rate associated with ischemia on exercise testing should be strongly encouraged. Based on the results of an exercise test, the number of metabolic equivalent tasks (METs) performed at the onset of ischemia can be estimated (Table 33-2) and a practical exercise prescription can be formulated to permit daily activities that will fall below the ischemic threshold (Table 33-3).

TREATMENT OF RISK FACTORS A *family history* of premature IHD is an important indicator of increased risk and should trigger a search for treatable risk factors such as hyperlipidemia, hypertension, and diabetes

mellitus. *Obesity* impairs the treatment of other risk factors and increases the risk of adverse coronary events. In addition, obesity often is accompanied by three other risk factors: diabetes mellitus, hypertension, and hyperlipidemia. The treatment of obesity and these accompanying risk factors is an important component of any management plan. A diet low in saturated and *trans*-unsaturated fatty acids and a reduced caloric intake to achieve optimal body weight are a cornerstone in the management of chronic IHD. It is especially important to emphasize weight loss and regular exercise in patients with the metabolic syndrome or overt diabetes mellitus.

TABLE 33-3

ENERGY REQUIREMENTS FOR SOME COMMON ACTIVITIES

LESS THAN 3 METs	3–5 METs	5–7 METs	7–9 METs	MORE THAN 9 METs
Self-care				
Washing/shaving	Cleaning windows	Easy digging in garden	Heavy shoveling	Carrying loads upstairs (objects more than 90 lb)
Dressing	Raking	Level hand lawn mowing	Carrying objects (60–90 lb)	Climbing stairs (quickly)
Light housekeeping	Power lawn mowing	Carrying objects (30–60 lb)		Shoveling heavy snow
Desk work	Bed making/stripping			
Driving auto	Carrying objects (15–30 lb)			
Occupational				
Sitting (clerical/assembly)	Stocking shelves (light objects)	Carpentry (exterior)	Digging ditches (pick and shovel)	Heavy labor
Desk work	Light welding/carpentry	Shoveling dirt		
Standing (store clerk)		Sawing wood		
Recreational				
Golf (cart)	Dancing (social)	Tennis (singles)	Canoeing	Squash
Knitting	Golf (walking)	Snow skiing (downhill)	Mountain climbing	Ski touring
	Sailing	Light backpacking		Vigorous basketball
	Tennis (doubles)	Basketball		
		Stream fishing		
Physical conditioning				
Walking (2 mph)	Level walking (3–4 mph)	Level walking (4.5–5.0 mph)	Level jogging (5 mph)	Running more than 6 mph
Stationary bike	Level biking (6–8 mph)	Bicycling (9–10 mph)	Swimming (crawl stroke)	Bicycling (more than 13 mph)
Very light calisthenics	Light calisthenics	Swimming, breast stroke	Rowing machine Heavy calisthenics Bicycling (12 mph)	Rope jumping Walking uphill (5 mph)

Abbreviation: METs, metabolic equivalent tasks.
Source: Modified from WL Haskell: Rehabilitation of the coronary patient, in NK Wenger, HK Hellerstein (eds): *Design and Implementation of Cardiac Conditioning Program*. New York, Churchill Livingstone, 1978.

Cigarette smoking accelerates coronary atherosclerosis in both sexes and at all ages and increases the risk of thrombosis, plaque instability, myocardial infarction, and death (Chap. 30). In addition, by increasing myocardial oxygen needs and reducing oxygen supply, it aggravates angina. Smoking cessation studies have demonstrated important benefits with a significant decline in the occurrence of these adverse outcomes. The physician's message must be clear and strong and supported by programs that achieve and monitor abstinence. *Hypertension* (Chap. 37) is associated with an increased risk of adverse clinical events from coronary atherosclerosis as well as stroke. In addition, the left ventricular hypertrophy that results from sustained hypertension aggravates ischemia. There is evidence that long-term effective treatment of hypertension can decrease the occurrence of adverse coronary events.

Diabetes mellitus accelerates coronary and peripheral atherosclerosis and is frequently associated with dyslipidemias and increases in the risk of angina, myocardial infarction, and sudden coronary death. Aggressive control of the dyslipidemia (target LDL cholesterol <70 mg/dL) and hypertension (target BP 120/80) that are frequently found in diabetic patients is highly effective and therefore essential, as described later.

DYSLIPIDEMIA The treatment of dyslipidemia is central in aiming for long-term relief from angina, reduced need for revascularization, and reduction in myocardial infarction and death. The control of lipids can be achieved by the combination of a diet low in saturated and *trans*-unsaturated fatty acids, exercise, and weight loss. Nearly always, HMG-CoA reductase inhibitors (statins) are required and can lower LDL cholesterol (25–50%), raise HDL cholesterol (5–9%), and lower triglycerides (5–30%). A powerful treatment effect of statins on atherosclerosis, IHD, and outcomes is seen regardless of the pretreatment LDL cholesterol level. Fibrates or niacin can be used to raise HDL cholesterol and lower triglycerides (Chaps. 30 and 31). Controlled trials with lipid-regulating regimens have shown equal proportional benefit for men, women, the elderly, diabetic patients, and even smokers.

Compliance with the health-promoting behaviors listed above is generally very poor, and a conscientious physician must not underestimate the major effort required to meet this challenge. Fewer than one-half of patients in the United States discharged from the hospital with proven coronary disease receive treatment for dyslipidemia. In light of the proof that treating dyslipidemia brings major benefits, physicians need to establish treatment pathways, monitor compliance, and follow up regularly.

RISK REDUCTION IN WOMEN WITH IHD

The incidence of clinical IHD in premenopausal women is very low; however, after menopause, the atherogenic risk factors increase (e.g., increased LDL, reduced HDL) and the rate of clinical coronary events accelerates to the levels observed in men. Women have not given up cigarette smoking as effectively as have men. Diabetes mellitus, which is more common in women, greatly increases the occurrence of clinical IHD and amplifies the deleterious effects of hypertension, hyperlipidemia, and smoking. Cardiac catheterization and coronary revascularization are underused in women and are performed at a later and more severe stage of the disease than in men. When cholesterol lowering, beta blockers after myocardial infarction, and coronary artery bypass grafting are applied in the appropriate patient groups, women receive the same benefits of improved outcome as do men.

DRUG THERAPY The commonly used drugs for the treatment of angina pectoris are summarized in **Tables 33-4** through **33-6**. Pharmacotherapy for IHD is designed to reduce the frequency of anginal episodes, myocardial infarction, and coronary death. There is a wealth of positive trial data to emphasize how important this medical management is when added to the health-promoting behaviors discussed earlier. To achieve maximum benefit from medical therapy for IHD, it is frequently necessary to combine agents from different classes and titrate the doses as guided by the individual profile of risk factors, symptoms, hemodynamic responses, and side effects.

NITRATES The organic nitrates are a valuable class of drugs in the management of angina pectoris (Table 33-4). Their major mechanisms of action include systemic venodilation with concomitant reduction in left ventricular end-diastolic volume and pressure, thereby reducing myocardial wall tension and oxygen requirements; dilation of epicardial coronary vessels; and increased blood flow in collateral vessels. When metabolized, organic nitrates release nitric oxide (NO) that binds to guanylyl cyclase in vascular smooth-muscle cells, leading to an increase in cyclic guanosine monophosphate, which causes relaxation of vascular smooth muscle. Nitrates also exert antithrombotic activity by NO-dependent activation of platelet guanylyl cyclase, impairment of intraplatelet calcium flux, and platelet activation.

The absorption of these agents is most rapid and complete through the mucous membranes. For this reason, nitroglycerin is most commonly administered sublingually in tablets of 0.4 or 0.6 mg. Patients with angina should be instructed to take the medication both to relieve angina and also approximately 5 min before

TABLE 33-4

NITROGLYCERIN AND NITRATES FOR PATIENTS WITH ISCHEMIC HEART DISEASE

COMPOUND	ROUTE	DOSE	DURATION OF EFFECT
Nitroglycerin	Sublingual tablets	0.3–0.6 mg up to 1.5 mg	Approximately 10 min
	Spray	0.4 mg as needed	Similar to sublingual tablets
	Ointment	2% 6 × 6 in. 15 ×15 cm 7.5–40 mg	Effect up to 7 h
	Transdermal	0.2–0.8 mg/h every 12 h	8–12 h during intermittent therapy
	Oral sustained release	2.5–13 mg	4–8 h
	Intravenous	5–200 mcg/min	Tolerance may be seen in 7–8 h
Isosorbide dinitrate	Sublingual	2.5–10 mg	Up to 60 min
	Oral	5–80 mg, 2–3 times daily	Up to 8 h
	Spray	1.25 mg daily	2–3 min
	Chewable	5 mg	2–2½ h
	Oral slow release	40 mg 1–2 daily	Up to 8 h
	Intravenous	1.25–5.0 mg/h	Tolerance in 7–8 h
	Ointment	100 mg/24 h	Not effective
Isosorbide mononitrate	Oral	20 mg twice daily 60–240 mg once daily	12–24 h
Pentaerythritol tetranitrate	Sublingual	10 mg as needed	Not known

Source: Modified from RJ Gibbons et al: J Am Coll Cardiol 41:159, 2002.

TABLE 33-5

PROPERTIES OF BETA BLOCKERS IN CLINICAL USE FOR ISCHEMIC HEART DISEASE

DRUGS	SELECTIVITY	PARTIAL AGONIST ACTIVITY	USUAL DOSE FOR ANGINA
Acebutolol	β1	Yes	200–600 mg twice daily
Atenolol	β1	No	50–200 mg/d
Betaxolol	β1	No	10–20 mg/d
Bisoprolol	β1	No	10 mg/d
Esmolol (intravenous)[a]	β1	No	50–300 mcg/kg/min
Labetalol[b]	None	Yes	200–600 mg twice daily
Metoprolol	β1	No	50–200 mg twice daily
Nadolol	None	No	40–80 mg/day
Nebivolol	β1 (at low doses)	No	5–40 mg/day
Pindolol	None	Yes	2.5–7.5 mg 3 times daily
Propranolol	None	No	80–120 mg twice daily
Timolol	None	No	10 mg twice daily

[a]Esmolol is an ultra-short-acting beta blocker that is administered as a continuous intravenous infusion. Its rapid offset of action makes esmolol an attractive agent to use in patients with relative contraindications to beta blockade.
[b]Labetalol is a combined alpha and beta blocker.
Note: This list of beta blockers that may be used to treat patients with angina pectoris is arranged alphabetically. The agents for which there is the greatest clinical experience include atenolol, metoprolol, and propranolol. It is preferable to use a sustained-release formulation that may be taken once daily to improve the patient's compliance with the regimen.
Source: Modified from RJ Gibbons et al: J Am Coll Cardiol 41:159, 2002.

TABLE 33-6

CALCIUM CHANNEL BLOCKERS IN CLINICAL USE FOR ISCHEMIC HEART DISEASE

DRUGS	USUAL DOSE	DURATION OF ACTION	SIDE EFFECTS
Dihydropyridines			
Amlodipine	5–10 mg qd	Long	Headache, edema
Felodipine	5–10 mg qd	Long	Headache, edema
Isradipine	2.5–10 mg bid	Medium	Headache, fatigue
Nicardipine	20–40 mg tid	Short	Headache, dizziness, flushing, edema
Nifedipine	Immediate release:[a] 30–90 mg daily orally	Short	Hypotension, dizziness, flushing, nausea, constipation, edema
Nisoldipine	Slow release: 30–180 mg orally 20–40 mg qd	Short	Similar to nifedipine
Nondihydropyridines			
Diltiazem	Immediate release: 30–80 mg 4 times daily	Short	Hypotension, dizziness, flushing, bradycardia, edema
	Slow release: 120–320 mg qd	Long	
Verapamil	Immediate release: 80–160 mg tid	Short	Hypotension, myocardial depression, heart failure, edema, bradycardia
	Slow release: 120–480 mg qd	Long	

[a]May be associated with increased risk of mortality if administered during acute myocardial infarction.
Note: This list of calcium channel blockers that may be used to treat patients with angina pectoris is divided into two broad classes, dihydropyridines and nondihydropyridines, and arranged alphabetically within each class. Among the dihydropyridines, the greatest clinical experience has been obtained with amlodipine and nifedipine. After the initial period of dose titration with a short-acting formulation, it is preferable to switch to a sustained-release formulation that may be taken once daily to improve patient compliance with the regimen.
Source: Modified from RJ Gibbons et al: J Am Coll Cardiol 41:159, 2002.

stress that is likely to induce an episode. The value of this prophylactic use of the drug cannot be overemphasized.

Nitrates improve exercise tolerance in patients with chronic angina and relieve ischemia in patients with unstable angina as well as patients with Prinzmetal's variant angina (Chap. 34). A diary of angina and nitroglycerin use may be valuable for detecting changes in the frequency, severity, or threshold for discomfort that may signify the development of unstable angina pectoris and/or herald an impending myocardial infarction.

Long-Acting Nitrates None of the long-acting nitrates are as effective as sublingual nitroglycerin for the acute relief of angina. These organic nitrate preparations can be swallowed, chewed, or administered as a patch or paste by the transdermal route (Table 33-4). They can provide effective plasma levels for up to 24 h, but the therapeutic response is highly variable. Different preparations and/or administration during the daytime should be tried only to prevent discomfort while avoiding side effects such as headache and dizziness. Individual dose titration is important to prevent side effects. To minimize the effects of tolerance, the minimum effective dose should be used and a minimum of 8 h each day kept free of the drug to restore any useful response(s).

β-Adrenergic Blockers These drugs represent an important component of the pharmacologic treatment of angina pectoris (Table 33-5). They reduce myocardial oxygen demand by inhibiting the increases in heart rate, arterial pressure, and myocardial contractility caused by adrenergic activation. Beta blockade reduces these variables most strikingly during exercise but causes only small reductions at rest. Long-acting beta-blocking drugs or sustained-release formulations offer the advantage of once-daily dosing (Table 33-5). The therapeutic aims include relief of angina and ischemia. These drugs also can reduce mortality and reinfarction rates in patients after myocardial infarction and are moderately effective antihypertensive agents.

Relative contraindications include asthma and reversible airway obstruction in patients with chronic lung disease, atrioventricular conduction disturbances, severe bradycardia, Raynaud's phenomenon, and a history of mental depression. Side effects include fatigue, reduced exercise tolerance, nightmares, impotence, cold extremities, intermittent claudication, bradycardia (sometimes severe), impaired atrioventricular conduction, left ventricular failure, bronchial asthma, worsening claudication, and intensification of the hypoglycemia produced by oral hypoglycemic agents and insulin. Reducing the dose or even discontinuation may be necessary if these side effects develop and persist. Since sudden discontinuation can intensify ischemia, the doses should be tapered over 2 weeks. Beta blockers with relative β_1-receptor specificity such as metoprolol and atenolol may be preferable in patients with mild bronchial obstruction and insulin-requiring diabetes mellitus.

Calcium Channel Blockers Calcium channel blockers (Table 33-6) are coronary vasodilators that produce variable and dose-dependent reductions in myocardial oxygen demand, contractility, and arterial pressure. These combined pharmacologic effects are advantageous and make these agents as effective as beta blockers in the treatment of angina pectoris. They are indicated when beta blockers are contraindicated, poorly tolerated, or ineffective. Verapamil and diltiazem may produce symptomatic disturbances in cardiac conduction and bradyarrhythmias. They also exert negative inotropic actions and are more likely to aggravate left ventricular failure, particularly when used in patients with left ventricular dysfunction, especially if the patients are also receiving beta blockers. Although useful effects usually are achieved when calcium channel blockers are combined with beta blockers and nitrates, individual titration of the doses is essential with these combinations. Variant (Prinzmetal's) angina responds particularly well to calcium channel blockers (especially members of the dihydropyridine class), supplemented when necessary by nitrates (Chap. 34).

Verapamil ordinarily should not be combined with beta blockers because of the combined adverse effects on heart rate and contractility. Diltiazem can be combined with beta blockers in patients with normal ventricular function and no conduction disturbances. Amlodipine and beta blockers have complementary actions on coronary blood supply and myocardial oxygen demands. Whereas the former decreases blood pressure and dilates coronary arteries, the latter slows heart rate and decreases contractility. Amlodipine and the other second-generation dihydropyridine calcium antagonists (nicardipine, isradipine, long-acting nifedipine, and felodipine) are potent vasodilators and are useful in the simultaneous treatment of angina and hypertension. Short-acting dihydropyridines should be avoided because of the risk of precipitating infarction, particularly in the absence of concomitant beta-blocker therapy.

Choice between Beta Blockers and Calcium Channel Blockers for Initial Therapy Since beta blockers have been shown to improve life expectancy after acute myocardial infarction (Chaps. 34 and 35) and calcium channel blockers have not, the former may also be preferable in patients with angina and a damaged left ventricle. However, calcium channel blockers are indicated in patients with the following: (1) inadequate responsiveness to the combination of beta blockers and nitrates; many of these patients do well with a combination of a beta blocker and a dihydropyridine calcium channel blocker, (2) adverse reactions to beta blockers such as depression, sexual disturbances, and fatigue, (3) angina and a history of asthma or chronic obstructive pulmonary disease, (4) sick-sinus syndrome or significant atrioventricular conduction disturbances, (5) Prinzmetal's angina, or (6) symptomatic peripheral arterial disease.

Antiplatelet Drugs Aspirin is an irreversible inhibitor of platelet cyclooxygenase and thereby interferes with platelet activation. Chronic administration of 75–325 mg orally per day has been shown to reduce coronary events in asymptomatic adult men over age 50, patients with chronic stable angina, and patients who have or have survived unstable angina and myocardial infarction. There is a dose-dependent increase in bleeding when aspirin is used chronically. It is preferable to use an enteric-coated formulation in the range of 81–162 mg/d. Administration of this drug should be considered in all patients with IHD in the absence of gastrointestinal bleeding, allergy, or dyspepsia. Clopidogrel (300–600 mg loading and 75 mg/d) is an oral agent that blocks P2Y12 ADP receptor–mediated platelet aggregation. It provides benefits similar to those of aspirin in patients with stable chronic IHD and may be substituted for aspirin if aspirin causes the side effects listed above. Clopidogrel combined with aspirin reduces death and coronary ischemic events in patients with an acute coronary syndrome (Chap. 34) and also reduces the risk of thrombus formation in patients undergoing implantation of a stent in a coronary artery (Chap. 36). Alternative antiplatelet agents that block the P2Y12 platelet receptor such as prasugrel have been shown to be more effective than clopidogrel for prevention of ischemic events after placement of a stent for an acute coronary syndrome but are associated with an increased risk of bleeding. Although combined treatment with clopidogrel and aspirin for at least a year is recommended in patients with an acute coronary syndrome treated with implantation of a drug-eluting stent, studies have not shown any benefit from the routine addition of clopidogrel to aspirin in patients with chronic stable IHD.

OTHER THERAPIES The angiotensin-converting enzyme (ACE) inhibitors are widely used in the treatment of survivors of myocardial infarction, patients with hypertension or chronic IHD including angina pectoris, and those at high risk of vascular diseases such as diabetes. The benefits of ACE inhibitors are most evident in IHD patients at increased risk, especially if diabetes mellitus or LV dysfunction is present, and those who have not achieved adequate control of blood pressure and LDL cholesterol on beta blockers and statins. However, the routine administration of ACE inhibitors to IHD patients who have normal LV function and have achieved blood pressure and LDL goals on other therapies does not reduce the incidence of events and therefore is not cost-effective.

Despite treatment with nitrates, beta blockers, or calcium channel blockers, some patients with IHD continue to experience angina, and additional medical therapy is now available to alleviate their symptoms. Ranolazine, a piperazine derivative, may be useful for patients with chronic angina despite standard medical therapy. Its antianginal action is believed to occur via inhibition of the late inward sodium current (I_{Na}). The benefits of I_{Na} inhibition include limitation of the Na overload of ischemic myocytes and prevention of Ca^{2+} overload via the Na^+–Ca^{2+} exchanger. A dose of 500–1000 mg orally twice daily is usually well tolerated. Ranolazine is contraindicated in patients with hepatic impairment or with conditions or drugs associated with QT_c prolongation and when drugs that inhibit the CYP3A metabolic system (e.g., ketoconazole, diltiazem, verapamil, macrolide antibiotics, HIV protease inhibitors, and large quantities of grapefruit juice) are being used.

Nonsteroidal anti-inflammatory drug (NSAID) use in patients with IHD may be associated with a small but finite increased risk of MI and mortality. For this reason, they generally should be avoided in IHD patients. If they are required for symptom relief, it is advisable to coadminister aspirin and strive to use the lowest NSAID dose required for the shortest period of time.

Another class of agents open ATP-sensitive potassium channels in myocytes, leading to a reduction of free intracellular calcium ions. The major drug in this class is nicorandil, which typically is administered orally in a dose of 20 mg twice daily for prevention of angina. (Nicorandil is not available for use in the United States but is used in several other countries.)

Angina and Heart Failure Transient left ventricular failure with angina can be controlled by the use of nitrates. For patients with established congestive heart failure the increased left ventricular wall tension raises myocardial oxygen demand. Treatment of congestive heart failure with an angiotensin-converting enzyme inhibitor, a diuretic, and digoxin (Chap. 17) reduces heart size, wall tension, and myocardial oxygen demand, which helps control angina and ischemia. If the symptoms and signs of heart failure are controlled, an effort should be made to use beta blockers not only for angina but because trials in heart failure have shown significant improvement in survival. A trial of the intravenous ultra-short-acting beta blocker esmolol may be useful to

establish the safety of beta blockade in selected patients. Nocturnal angina often can be relieved by the treatment of heart failure.

The combination of congestive heart failure and angina in patients with IHD usually indicates a poor prognosis and warrants serious consideration of cardiac catheterization and coronary revascularization.

CORONARY REVASCULARIZATION

Clinical trials have confirmed that with the initial diagnosis of stable IHD, it is first appropriate to initiate a thorough medical regimen as described earlier. Revascularization should be considered in the presence of unstable phases of the disease, intractable symptoms, severe ischemia or high-risk coronary anatomy, diabetes, and impaired LV function. *Revascularization should be employed in conjunction with but not replace the continuing need to modify risk factors and assess medical therapy.* An algorithm for integrating medical therapy and revascularization options in patients with IHD is shown in **Fig. 33-2.**

PERCUTANEOUS CORONARY INTERVENTION

(See also Chap. 36) Percutaneous coronary intervention (PCI) involving balloon dilatation usually accompanied by coronary stenting is widely used to achieve revascularization of the myocardium in patients with symptomatic IHD and suitable stenoses of epicardial coronary arteries. Whereas patients with stenosis of the left main coronary artery and those with three-vessel IHD (especially with diabetes and/or impaired left ventricular function) who require revascularization are best treated with CABG. PCI is widely employed in patients with symptoms and evidence of ischemia due to stenoses of one or two vessels and even in selected patients with three-vessel disease (and, perhaps, in some patients with left main disease) and may offer many advantages over surgery.

Indications and patient selection

The most common clinical indication for PCI is symptom-limiting angina pectoris, despite medical therapy, accompanied by evidence of ischemia during a stress test. PCI is more effective than medical therapy for the relief of angina. PCI improves outcomes in patients with unstable angina or when used early in the course of myocardial infarction with and without cardiogenic shock. However, in patients with stable exertional angina, clinical trials have confirmed that PCI does not reduce the occurrence of death or myocardial infarction

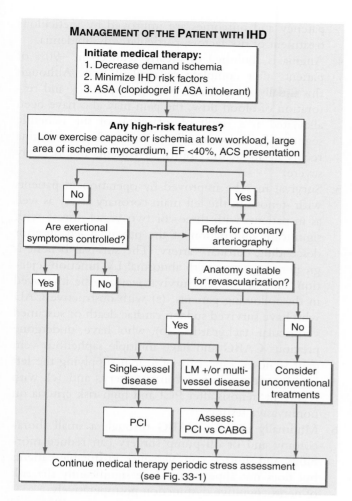

MANAGEMENT OF THE PATIENT WITH IHD

Initiate medical therapy:
1. Decrease demand ischemia
2. Minimize IHD risk factors
3. ASA (clopidogrel if ASA intolerant)

Any high-risk features?
Low exercise capacity or ischemia at low workload, large area of ischemic myocardium, EF <40%, ACS presentation

No → Are exertional symptoms controlled?

Yes → Refer for coronary arteriography

Are exertional symptoms controlled? → Yes / No

Anatomy suitable for revascularization?

Yes / No

Single-vessel disease → PCI

LM +/or multi-vessel disease → Assess: PCI vs CABG

Consider unconventional treatments

Continue medical therapy periodic stress assessment (see Fig. 33-1)

FIGURE 33-2

Algorithm for management of a patient with ischemic heart disease. All patients should receive the core elements of medical therapy as shown at the top of the algorithm. If high-risk features are present, as established by the clinical history, exercise test data, and imaging studies, the patient should be referred for coronary arteriography. Based on the number and location of the diseased vessels and their suitability for revascularization, the patient is treated with a percutaneous coronary intervention (PCI) or coronary artery bypass graft (CABG) surgery or should be considered for unconventional treatments. See text for further discussion. IHD, ischemic heart disease; ASA, aspirin; EF, ejection fraction; ACS, acute coronary syndrome; LM, left main.

compared to optimum medical therapy. PCI can be used to treat stenoses in native coronary arteries as well as in bypass grafts in patients who have recurrent angina after CABG.

Risks

When coronary stenoses are discrete and symmetric, two and even three vessels can be treated in sequence. However, case selection is essential to avoid

a prohibitive risk of complications, which are usually due to dissection or thrombosis with vessel occlusion, uncontrolled ischemia, and ventricular failure (Chap. 36). Oral aspirin, a thienopyridine, and an antithrombin agent are given to reduce coronary thrombus formation. Left main coronary artery stenosis generally is regarded as a contraindication to PCI; such patients should be treated with CABG. In selected cases such as patients with prohibitive surgical risks, PCI of an unprotected left main can be considered, but such a procedure should be performed only by a highly skilled operator; importantly, there are regional differences in the use of this approach internationally.

Efficacy

Primary success, i.e., adequate dilation (an increase in luminal diameter >20% to a residual diameter obstruction <50%) with relief of angina, is achieved in >95% of cases. Recurrent stenosis of the dilated vessels occurs in ~20% of cases within 6 months of PCI with bare metal stents, and angina will recur within 6 months in 10% of cases. Restenosis is more common in patients with diabetes mellitus, arteries with small caliber, incomplete dilation of the stenosis, long stents, occluded vessels, obstructed vein grafts, dilation of the left anterior descending coronary artery, and stenoses containing thrombi. In diseased vein grafts, procedural success has been improved by the use of capture devices or filters that prevent embolization, ischemia, and infarction.

It is usual clinical practice to administer aspirin indefinitely and a thienopyridine for 1–3 months after the implantation of a bare metal stent. Although aspirin in combination with a thienopyridine may help prevent coronary thrombosis during and shortly after PCI with stenting, there is no evidence that these medications reduce the incidence of restenosis.

The use of drug-eluting stents that locally deliver antiproliferative drugs can reduce restenosis to less than 10%. Advances in PCI, especially the availability of drug-eluting stents, have vastly extended the use of this revascularization option in patients with IHD. Of note, however, the delayed endothelial healing in the region of a drug-eluting stent also extends the period during which the patient is at risk for subacute stent thrombosis. Current recommendations are to administer aspirin indefinitely and a thienopyridine daily for at least 1 year after implantation of a drug-eluting stent. When a situation arises in which temporary discontinuation of antiplatelet therapy is necessary, the clinical circumstances should be reviewed with the operator who performed the PCI and a coordinated plan should be established for minimizing the risk of late stent thrombus; central to this plan is the discontinuation of antiplatelet therapy for the shortest acceptable period.

The risk of stent thrombosis is dependent on stent size and length, complexity of the lesions, age, diabetes, and technique. However, compliance with dual antiplatelet therapy and individual responsiveness to platelet inhibition are very important factors as well.

Successful PCI produces effective relief of angina in >95% of cases. More than one-half of patients with symptomatic IHD who require revascularization can be treated initially by PCI. Successful PCI is less invasive and expensive than CABG and permits savings in the *initial* cost of care. Successful PCI avoids the risk of stroke associated with CABG surgery, allows earlier return to work, and allows the resumption of an active life. However, the early health-related and economic benefit of PCI is reduced over time because of the greater need for follow-up and the increased need for repeat procedures. When directly compared in patients with diabetes or three-vessel or left main coronary artery disease, CABG was superior to PCI in preventing major adverse cardiac or cerebrovascular events over a 12-month follow-up.

CORONARY ARTERY BYPASS GRAFTING

Anastomosis of one or both of the internal mammary arteries or a radial artery to the coronary artery distal to the obstructive lesion is the preferred procedure. For additional obstructions that cannot be bypassed by an artery, a section of a vein (usually the saphenous) is used to form a connection between the aorta and the coronary artery distal to the obstructive lesion.

Although some indications for CABG are controversial, certain areas of agreement exist:

1. The operation is relatively safe, with mortality rates <1% in patients without serious comorbid disease and normal left ventricular function and when the procedure is performed by an experienced surgical team.

2. Intraoperative and postoperative mortality rates increase with the severity of ventricular dysfunction, comorbidities, age >80 years, and lack of surgical experience. The effectiveness and risk of CABG vary widely depending on case selection and the skill and experience of the surgical team.

3. Occlusion of *venous* grafts is observed in 10% to 20% of patients during the first postoperative year and in approximately 2% per year during 5- to 7-year follow-up and 4% per year thereafter. Long-term patency rates are considerably higher for internal mammary and radial artery implantations than for saphenous vein grafts. In patients with left anterior descending coronary artery obstruction, survival is better when coronary bypass involves the internal mammary artery rather than a saphenous vein. Graft patency and outcomes are improved by meticulous treatment of risk factors, particularly dyslipidemia.

4. Angina is abolished or greatly reduced in ~90% of patients after complete revascularization. Although this usually is associated with graft patency and restoration of blood flow, the pain may also have been alleviated as a result of infarction of the ischemic segment or a placebo effect. Within 3 years, angina recurs in about one-fourth of patients but is rarely severe.

5. Survival may be improved by operation in patients with stenosis of the left main coronary artery as well as in patients with three- or two-vessel disease with significant obstruction of the proximal left anterior descending coronary artery. The survival benefit is greater in patients with abnormal LV function (ejection fraction <50%). Survival *may* also be improved in the following patients: (a) with obstructive CAD who have survived sudden cardiac death or sustained ventricular tachycardia, (b) who have undergone previous CABG and have multiple saphenous vein graft stenoses, especially of a graft supplying the left anterior descending coronary artery, and (c) with recurrent stenosis after PCI and high-risk criteria on noninvasive testing.

6. Minimally invasive CABG through a small thoracotomy and/or off-pump surgery can reduce morbidity and shorten convalescence in suitable patients but does not appear to reduce significantly the risk of neurocognitive dysfunction postoperatively.

7. Among patients with type 2 diabetes mellitus and multivessel coronary disease, CABG surgery plus optimal medical therapy is superior to optimal medical therapy alone in preventing major cardiovascular events, a benefit mediated largely by a significant reduction in nonfatal MI. The benefits of CABG are especially evident in diabetic patients treated with an insulin-sensitizing strategy as opposed to an insulin-providing strategy.

Indications for CABG usually are based on the severity of symptoms, coronary anatomy, and ventricular function. The ideal candidate is male, is <80 years of age, has no other complicating disease, and has troublesome or disabling angina that is not adequately controlled by medical therapy or does not tolerate medical therapy. The patient wishes to lead a more active life and has severe stenoses of two or three epicardial coronary arteries with objective evidence of myocardial ischemia as a cause of the chest discomfort. Great symptomatic benefit can be anticipated in such patients. Congestive heart failure and/or left ventricular dysfunction, advanced age (>80 years), reoperation, urgent need for surgery, and the presence of diabetes mellitus are all associated with a higher perioperative mortality rate.

Left ventricular dysfunction can be due to noncontractile or hypocontractile segments that are viable but are chronically ischemic (hibernating myocardium). As a consequence of chronic reduction in myocardial blood flow, these segments downregulate their contractile function. They can be detected by using radionuclide scans of myocardial perfusion and metabolism, PET, cardiac MRI, or delayed scanning with thallium-201 or by improvement of regional functional impairment provoked by low-dose dobutamine. In such patients, revascularization improves myocardial blood flow, can return function, and can improve survival.

The choice between PCI and CABG

All the clinical characteristics of each individual patient must be used to decide on the method of revascularization (LV function, diabetes, lesion complexity, etc.). A number of randomized clinical trials have compared PCI and CABG in patients with multivessel CAD who were suitable technically for both procedures. The redevelopment of angina requiring repeat coronary angiography and repeat revascularization is higher with PCI. This is a result of restenosis in the stented segment (a problem largely solved with drug-eluting stents) and the development of new stenoses in unstented portions of the coronary vasculature. It has been argued that PCI with stenting focuses on culprit lesions whereas a bypass

graft to the target vessel also provides a conduit around future culprit lesions proximal to the anastomosis of the graft to the native vessel **(Fig. 33-3)**. By contrast, stroke rates are lower with PCI.

Comparison of mortality rates in patients treated with CABG versus PCI is a complex issue. There is an early increased risk of mortality with CABG, but mortality rates appear similar in the two revascularization strategies over the long term.

Based on available evidence, it is now recommended that patients with an unacceptable level of angina despite optimal medical management be considered for coronary revascularization. Patients with single- or two-vessel disease with normal LV function and anatomically suitable lesions ordinarily are advised to undergo PCI (Chap. 36). Patients with three-vessel disease (or two-vessel disease that includes the proximal left descending coronary artery) and impaired global LV function (LV ejection fraction <50%) or diabetes mellitus and those with left main coronary artery disease or other lesions unsuitable for catheter-based procedures should be considered for CABG as the initial method of revascularization. In light of the complexity of the decision making, it is desirable to have a multidisciplinary team, including a cardiologist and a cardiac surgeon in conjunction with the patient's primary care physician, provide input in conjunction with ascertaining the patient's preferences before committing to a particular revascularization option.

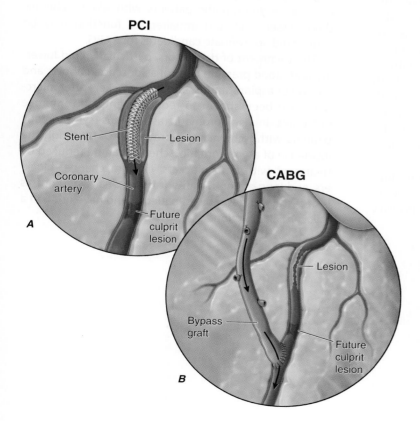

FIGURE 33-3

Difference in the approach to the lesion with percutaneous coronary intervention (PCI) and coronary artery bypass grafting (CABG). PCI is targeted at the "culprit" lesion or lesions, whereas CABG is directed at the epicardial vessel, including the culprit lesion or lesions and future culprits, proximal to the insertion of the vein graft, a difference that may account for the superiority of CABG, at least in the intermediate term, in patients with multivessel disease. (*Reproduced from BJ Gersh et al: N Engl J Med 352:2235, 2005.*)

UNCONVENTIONAL TREATMENTS FOR IHD

On occasion, clinicians will encounter a patient who has persistent disabling angina despite maximally tolerated medical therapy and for whom revascularization is not an option (e.g., small diffusely diseased vessels not amenable to stent implantation or acceptable targets for bypass grafting). In such situations unconventional treatments should be considered.

Enhanced external counterpulsation utilizes pneumatic cuffs on the lower extremities to provide diastolic augmentation and systolic unloading of blood pressure to decrease cardiac work and oxygen consumption while enhancing coronary blood flow. Clinical trials have shown that regular application improves angina, exercise capacity, and regional myocardial perfusion. Experimental approaches such as gene and stem cell therapies are also under active study.

ASYMPTOMATIC (SILENT) ISCHEMIA

Obstructive CAD, acute myocardial infarction, and transient myocardial ischemia are frequently asymptomatic. During continuous ambulatory ECG monitoring, the majority of ambulatory patients with typical chronic stable angina are found to have objective evidence of myocardial ischemia (ST-segment depression) during episodes of chest discomfort while they are active outside the hospital. In addition, many of these patients also have more frequent episodes of asymptomatic ischemia. Frequent episodes of ischemia (symptomatic and asymptomatic) during daily life appear to be associated with an increased likelihood of adverse coronary events (death and myocardial infarction). In addition, patients with asymptomatic ischemia after a myocardial infarction are at greater risk for a second coronary event. The widespread use of exercise ECG during routine examinations has also identified some of these previously unrecognized patients with asymptomatic CAD. Longitudinal studies have demonstrated an increased incidence of coronary events in asymptomatic patients with positive exercise tests.

TREATMENT   Asymptomatic Ischemia

The management of patients with asymptomatic ischemia must be individualized. When coronary disease has been confirmed, the aggressive treatment of hypertension and dyslipidemia is essential and will decrease the risk of infarction and death. In addition, the physician should consider the following: (1) the degree of positivity of the stress test, particularly the stage of exercise at which ECG signs of ischemia appear; the magnitude and number of the ischemic zones of myocardium on imaging; and the change in LV ejection fraction that occurs on radionuclide ventriculography or echocardiography during ischemia and/or during exercise, (2) the ECG leads showing a positive response, with changes in the anterior precordial leads indicating a less favorable prognosis than changes in the inferior leads, and (3) the patient's age, occupation, and general medical condition.

Most would agree that an asymptomatic 45-year-old commercial airline pilot with significant (0.4-mV) ST-segment depression in leads V_1 to V_4 during mild exercise should undergo coronary arteriography, whereas an asymptomatic, sedentary 85-year-old retiree with 0.1-mV ST-segment depression in leads II and III during maximal activity need not. However, there is no consensus about the most appropriate approach in the large majority of patients for whom the situation is less extreme. Asymptomatic patients with silent ischemia, three-vessel CAD, and impaired LV function may be considered appropriate candidates for CABG.

The treatment of risk factors, particularly lipid lowering and blood pressure control as described above, and the use of aspirin, statins, and beta blockers after infarction have been shown to reduce events and improve outcomes in asymptomatic as well as symptomatic patients with ischemia and proven CAD. Although the incidence of asymptomatic ischemia can be reduced by treatment with beta blockers, calcium channel blockers, and long-acting nitrates, it is not clear whether this is necessary or desirable in patients who have not had a myocardial infarction.

CHAPTER 34

UNSTABLE ANGINA AND NON-ST-SEGMENT ELEVATION MYOCARDIAL INFARCTION

Christopher P. Cannon ■ Eugene Braunwald

Patients with ischemic heart disease fall into two large groups: patients with chronic coronary artery disease (CAD) who most commonly present with stable angina (Chap. 33) and patients with acute coronary syndromes (ACSs). The latter group, in turn, is composed of patients with acute myocardial infarction (MI) with ST-segment elevation on their presenting electrocardiogram (ECG) (STEMI; Chap. 35) and those with unstable angina (UA) and non-ST-segment elevation MI (UA/NSTEMI; Fig. 35-1). Every year in the United States, approximately 1 million patients are admitted to hospitals with UA/NSTEMI as compared with ~300,000 patients with acute STEMI. The relative incidence of UA/NSTEMI compared to STEMI appears to be increasing. More than one-third of patients with UA/NSTEMI are women, while less than one-fourth of patients with STEMI are women.

DEFINITION

The diagnosis of UA is based largely on the clinical presentation. *Stable* angina pectoris is characterized by chest or arm discomfort that may not be described as pain but is reproducibly associated with physical exertion or stress and is relieved within 5–10 min by rest and/or sublingual nitroglycerin (Chap. 4). UA is defined as angina pectoris or equivalent ischemic discomfort with at least one of three features: (1) it occurs at rest (or with minimal exertion), usually lasting >10 min; (2) it is severe and of new onset (i.e., within the prior 4–6 weeks); and/or (3) it occurs with a crescendo pattern (i.e., distinctly more severe, prolonged, or frequent than previously). The diagnosis of NSTEMI is established if a patient with the clinical features of UA develops evidence of myocardial necrosis, as reflected in elevated cardiac biomarkers.

PATHOPHYSIOLOGY

UA/NSTEMI is most commonly caused by a reduction in oxygen supply and/or by an increase in myocardial oxygen demand superimposed on a lesion that causes coronary arterial obstruction, usually an atherothrombotic coronary plaque. Four pathophysiologic processes that may contribute to the development of UA/NSTEMI have been identified: (1) plaque rupture or erosion with a superimposed nonocclusive thrombus, believed to be the most common cause; in such patients, NSTEMI may occur with downstream embolization of platelet aggregates and/or atherosclerotic debris; (2) dynamic obstruction (e.g., coronary spasm, as in Prinzmetal's variant angina [PVA]); (3) progressive mechanical obstruction (e.g., rapidly advancing coronary atherosclerosis or restenosis following percutaneous coronary intervention [PCI]); and (4) UA secondary to increased myocardial oxygen demand and/or decreased supply (e.g., tachycardia, anemia). More than one of these processes may be involved.

Among patients with UA/NSTEMI studied at angiography, approximately 5% have stenosis of the left main coronary artery, 15% have three-vessel CAD, 30% have two-vessel disease, 40% have single-vessel disease, and 10% have no apparent critical epicardial coronary artery stenosis; some of the latter may have obstruction of the coronary microcirculation. The "culprit lesion" may show an eccentric stenosis with scalloped or overhanging edges and a narrow neck on angiography. Angioscopy has been reported to show "white" (platelet-rich) thrombi, as opposed to "red" (fibrin- and cell-rich) thrombi; the latter are more often seen in patients with acute STEMI. Patients with UA/NSTEMI frequently have multiple plaques at risk of disruption (vulnerable plaques).

CLINICAL PRESENTATION

History and physical examination

The clinical hallmark of UA/NSTEMI is chest pain, typically located in the substernal region or sometimes in the epigastrium, that radiates to the neck, left shoulder, and/or the left arm (Chap. 4). This discomfort is usually severe enough to be described as frank pain. Anginal "equivalents" such as dyspnea and epigastric discomfort may also occur, and these appear to be more frequent in women. The physical examination resembles that in patients with stable angina (Chap. 33) and may be unremarkable. If the patient has a large area of myocardial ischemia or a large NSTEMI, the physical findings can include diaphoresis; pale, cool skin; sinus tachycardia; a third and/or fourth heart sound; basilar rales; and, sometimes, hypotension, resembling the findings of large STEMI.

Electrocardiogram

In UA, ST-segment depression, transient ST-segment elevation, and/or T-wave inversion occur in 30% to 50% of patients. In patients with the clinical features of UA, the presence of new ST-segment deviation, even of only 0.05 mV, is an important predictor of adverse outcome. T-wave changes are sensitive for ischemia but less specific, unless they are new, deep T-wave inversions (≥0.3 mV).

Cardiac biomarkers

Patients with UA/NSTEMI who have elevated biomarkers of necrosis, such as CK-MB and troponin (a much more specific and sensitive marker of myocardial necrosis), are at increased risk for death or recurrent MI. Elevated levels of these markers distinguish patients with NSTEMI from those with UA. There is a direct relationship between the degree of troponin elevation and mortality. However, in patients *without* a clear clinical history of myocardial ischemia, minor troponin elevations have been reported and can be caused by congestive heart failure (CHF), myocarditis, or pulmonary embolism, or they may be false-positive readings. Thus, in patients with an *unclear* history, small troponin elevations may not be diagnostic of an ACS.

DIAGNOSTIC EVALUATION

(See also Chap. 4) Approximately 6 million persons per year in the United States present to hospital emergency departments (EDs) with a complaint of chest pain or other symptoms suggestive of ACS. A diagnosis of an ACS is established in 20% to 25% of such patients.

The first step in evaluating patients with possible UA/NSTEMI is to determine the *likelihood* that CAD is the cause of the presenting symptoms. The American College of Cardiology/American Heart Association (ACC/AHA) guidelines include, among the factors associated with a high likelihood of ACS, a prior history typical of stable angina, a history of established CAD by angiography, prior MI, CHF, new ECG changes, or elevated cardiac biomarkers.

Diagnostic pathways

Four major diagnostic tools are used in the diagnosis of UA/NSTEMI in the ED: clinical history, the ECG, cardiac markers, and stress testing (coronary imaging is an emerging option). The goals are to: (1) recognize or exclude MI (using cardiac markers), (2) evaluate for rest ischemia (using serial or continuous ECGs), and (3) evaluate for significant CAD (using provocative stress testing). Patients with a low likelihood of ischemia are usually managed with an ED-based critical pathway (which, in some institutions, is carried out in a "chest-pain unit" **Fig. 34-1**). Evaluation of such patients includes clinical monitoring for recurrent ischemic discomfort, serial ECGs, and cardiac markers, typically obtained at baseline and at 4–6 h and 12 h after presentation. If new elevations in cardiac markers or ECG changes are noted, the patient should be admitted to the hospital. If the patient remains pain free and the markers are negative, the patient may proceed to stress testing. CT angiography is used with increasing frequency to exclude obstructive CAD (Chap. 12).

RISK STRATIFICATION AND PROGNOSIS

Patients with documented UA/NSTEMI exhibit a wide spectrum of early (30 days) risk of death, ranging from 1% to 10%, and of new or recurrent infarction of 3–5% or recurrent ACS (5–15%). Assessment of risk can be accomplished by clinical risk scoring systems such as that developed from the Thrombolysis in Myocardial Infarction (TIMI) Trials, which includes seven independent risk factors: age ≥65 years, three or more risk factors for CAD, documented CAD at catheterization, development of UA/NSTEMI while on aspirin, more than two episodes of angina within the preceding 24 h, ST deviation ≥0.5 mm, and an elevated cardiac marker **(Fig. 34-2)**. Other risk factors include diabetes mellitus, left ventricular dysfunction, renal dysfunction and elevated levels of brain natriuretic peptides and C-reactive protein. Multimarker strategies involving several biomarkers are now gaining favor, both to define more fully the pathophysiologic mechanisms underlying a given patient's presentation and to stratify the patient's

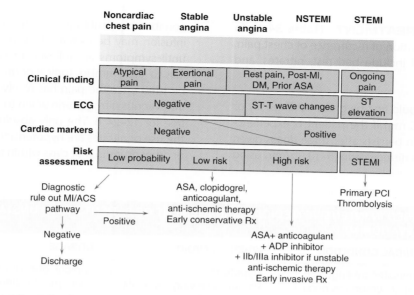

FIGURE 34-1

Algorithm for risk stratification and treatment of patients with suspected coronary artery disease. Using the clinical history of the type of pain and medical history, the ECG, and cardiac markers, one can identify patients who have a low likelihood of UA/NSTEMI, for whom a diagnostic "ruleout myocardial infarction (MI) or acute coronary syndrome (ACS)" is warranted. If this is negative, the patient may be discharged, but if positive, the patient is admitted and treated for UA/NSTEMI. On the other end of the spectrum, patients with acute ongoing pain and ST-segment elevation are treated with percutaneous coronary intervention (PCI) or fibrinolysis (Chap. 35). For those with UA/NSTEMI, risk stratification is used to identify patients at medium to high risk, for whom an early invasive

strategy is warranted. Antithrombotic therapy should include aspirin, an anticoagulant, an ADP antagonist (clopidogrel or prasugrel), with GP IIb/IIIa inhibition considered for use during PCI. For patients at low risk, treatment with aspirin, clopidogrel, an anticoagulant such as unfractionated or low molecular–weight heparin (LMWH) or fondaparinux and anti-ischemic therapy with beta blockers and nitrates, and a conservative strategy are indicated. ASA, aspirin; DM, diabetes mellitus; ECG, electrocardiogram; MI, myocardial infarction; Rx, treatment; STEMI, ST-segment elevation myocardial infarction. (*Adapted from CP Cannon, E Braunwald, in Braunwald's Heart Disease: A Textbook of Cardiovascular Medicine, 9th ed, R Bonow et al [eds]. Philadelphia, Saunders, 2011.*)

risk further. Early risk assessment (especially using troponin, ST-segment changes, and/or a global risk-scoring system) is useful both in predicting the risk of recurrent cardiac events and in identifying those patients

who would derive the greatest benefit from antithrombotic therapies more potent than unfractionated heparin, such as low molecular–weight heparin (LMWH) and glycoprotein IIb/IIIa inhibitors, and from an early invasive strategy. For example, in the TACTICS-TIMI 18 Trial, an early invasive strategy conferred a 40% reduction in recurrent cardiac events in patients with a positive troponin level, whereas no benefit was observed in those without detectable troponin.

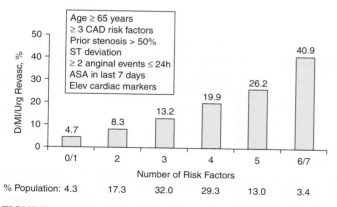

FIGURE 34-2

The TIMI Risk Score for UA/NSTEMI, a simple but comprehensive clinical risk stratification score to identify increasing risk of death, myocardial infarction, or urgent revascularization to day 14. CAD, coronary artery disease; ASA, aspirin. (*Adapted from EM Antman et al: JAMA 284:835, 2000.*)

TREATMENT Unstable Angina and Non-ST-Segment Elevation Myocardial Infarction

MEDICAL TREATMENT Patients with UA/NSTEMI should be placed at bed rest with continuous ECG monitoring for ST-segment deviation and cardiac arrhythmias. Ambulation is permitted if the patient shows no recurrence of ischemia (discomfort or ECG changes) and does not develop a biomarker of necrosis for 12–24 h. Medical therapy involves simultaneous anti-ischemic treatment and antithrombotic treatment.

ANTI-ISCHEMIC TREATMENT (Table 34-1) To provide relief and prevention of recurrence of chest pain, initial treatment should include bed rest, nitrates, and beta blockers.

Nitrates Nitrates should first be given sublingually or by buccal spray (0.3–0.6 mg) if the patient is experiencing ischemic pain. If pain persists after three doses given 5 min apart, intravenous nitroglycerin (5–10 μg/min using nonabsorbing tubing) is recommended. The rate of the infusion may be increased by 10 μg/min every 3–5 min until symptoms are relieved or systolic arterial pressure falls to <100 mmHg. Topical or oral nitrates (Chap. 33) can be used once the pain has resolved or they may replace intravenous nitroglycerin when the patient has been pain-free for 12–24 h. The only absolute contraindications to the use of nitrates are hypotension or the use of sildenafil or other drugs in that class within the previous 24–48 h.

TABLE 34-1

DRUGS COMMONLY USED IN INTENSIVE MEDICAL MANAGEMENT OF PATIENTS WITH UNSTABLE ANGINA AND NON-ST-SEGMENT ELEVATION MI

DRUG CATEGORY	CLINICAL CONDITION	WHEN TO AVOID[a]	DOSAGE
Nitrates	Administer sublingually, and, if symptoms persist, intravenously	Hypotension Patient receiving sildenafil or other PDE-5 inhibitor	Topical, oral, or buccal nitrates are acceptable alternatives for patients without ongoing or refractory symptoms 5–10 μg/min by continuous infusion titrated up to 75–100 μg/min until relief of symptoms or limiting side effects (headache or hypotension with a systolic blood pressure <90 mmHg or more than 30% below starting mean arterial pressure levels if significant hypertension is present)
Beta blockers[b]	Unstable angina	PR interval (ECG) >0.24 s 2° or 3° atrioventricular block Heart rate <60 beats/min Systolic pressure <90 mmHg Shock Left ventricular failure Severe reactive airway disease	Metoprolol 25–50 mg by mouth every 6 h If needed, and no heart failure, 5-mg increments by slow (over 1–2 min) IV administration
Calcium channel blockers	Patients whose symptoms are not relieved by adequate doses of nitrates and beta blockers, or in patients unable to tolerate adequate doses of one or both of these agents, or in patients with variant angina	Pulmonary edema Evidence of left ventricular dysfunction (for diltiazem or verapamil)	Dependent on specific agent
Morphine sulfate	Patients whose symptoms are not relieved after three serial sublingual nitroglycerin tablets or whose symptoms recur with adequate anti-ischemic therapy	Hypotension Respiratory depression Confusion Obtundation	2–5 mg IV dose May be repeated every 5–30 min as needed to relieve symptoms and maintain patient comfort

[a]Allergy or prior intolerance is a contraindication for all categories of drugs listed in this chart.
[b]Choice of the specific agent is not as important as ensuring that appropriate candidates receive this therapy. If there are concerns about patient intolerance owing to existing pulmonary disease, especially asthma, left ventricular dysfunction, risk of hypotension or severe bradycardia, initial selection should favor a short-acting agent, such as propranolol or metoprolol or the ultra-short-acting agent esmolol. Mild wheezing or a history of chronic obstructive pulmonary disease should prompt a trial of a short-acting agent at a reduced dose (e.g., 2.5 mg IV metoprolol, 12.5 mg oral metoprolol, or 25 μg/kg per min esmolol as initial doses) rather than complete avoidance of beta-blocker therapy.
Note: Some of the recommendations in this guide suggest the use of agents for purposes or in doses other than those specified by the U.S. Food and Drug Administration. Such recommendations are made after consideration of concerns regarding nonapproved indications. Where made, such recommendations are based on more recent clinical trials or expert consensus. IV, intravenous; ECG, electrocardiogram; 2°, second-degree; 3°, third-degree.
Source: Modified from E Braunwald et al: Circulation 90:613, 1994.

Beta Adrenergic Blockers and Other Agents Beta blockers are the other mainstay of anti-ischemic treatment. Oral beta blockade targeted to a heart rate of 50–60 beats/min is recommended as first-line treatment. A caution has been raised in the new ACC/AHA guidelines for use of intravenous beta blockade in patients with any evidence of acute heart failure, where they could increase the risk of cardiogenic shock. Heart rate–slowing calcium channel blockers, e.g., verapamil or diltiazem, are recommended for patients who have persistent or recurrent symptoms after treatment with full-dose nitrates and beta blockers and in patients with contraindications to beta blockade. Additional medical therapy includes angiotensin-converting enzyme (ACE) inhibition and HMG-CoA reductase inhibitors (statins) for long-term secondary prevention. Early administration of intensive statin therapy (e.g., atorvastatin 80 mg) prior to percutaneous coronary intervention (PCI) has been shown to reduce complications, suggesting that high-dose statin therapy should be started at the time of admission.

ANTITHROMBOTIC THERAPY (Table 34-2)

This is the other main component of treatment for UA/NSTEMI. Initial treatment should begin with the platelet cyclooxygenase inhibitor aspirin (Fig. 34-3). The typical initial dose is 325 mg/d, with lower doses (75–162 mg/d) recommended for long-term therapy. The OASIS-7 trial randomized 25,087 ACS patients to receive high-dose (300–325 mg/d) vs. low-dose (75–100 mg/d) aspirin for 30 days and reported no differences in the risk of major bleeding or in efficacy over this period of time. "Aspirin resistance" has been noted in 5–10% of patients and more frequently in patients treated with lower doses of aspirin, but frequently has been related to noncompliance.

The thienopyridine, clopidogrel, an inactive prodrug that is converted into an active metabolite, which blocks the platelet $P2Y_{12}$ component or the adenosine diphosphate receptor, in combination with aspirin, was shown in the CURE trial to confer a 20% relative reduction in cardiovascular death, MI, or stroke, compared with aspirin alone in both low- and high-risk patients, but to be associated with a moderate (absolute 1%) increase in major bleeding. Pretreatment with clopidogrel (a 300 or 600 mg loading dose, followed by 75 mg qd) is recommended prior to PCI. The OASIS-7 trial reported that 1 week of a higher dose of clopidogrel (600 mg loading dose and 150 mg/d for 1 week) did not result in an overall improvement in outcomes in ACS patients, but did so in patients receiving 325 mg of aspirin, especially those who underwent PCI.

Continued benefit of 1 year of treatment with the combination of clopidogrel and aspirin has been

TABLE 34-2

CLINICAL USE OF ANTITHROMBOTIC THERAPY

Oral Antiplatelet Therapy

Aspirin	Initial dose of 162–325 mg nonenteric formulation followed by 75–162 mg/d of an enteric or a nonenteric formulation
Clopidogrel	Loading dose of 300–600 mg followed by 75 mg/d
Prasugrel	Pre-PCI: Loading dose 60 mg followed by 10 mg/d

Intravenous Antiplatelet Therapy

Abciximab	0.25 mg/kg bolus followed by infusion of 0.125 µg/kg per min (maximum 10 µg/min) for 12 to 24 h
Eptifibatide	180 µg/kg bolus followed by infusion of 2.0 µg/kg per min for 72 to 96 h
Tirofiban	0.4 µg/kg per min for 30 min followed by infusion of 0.1 µg/kg per min for 48 to 96 h

Heparins[a]

Unfractionated Heparin (UFH)	Bolus 60–70 U/kg (maximum 5000 U) IV followed by infusion of 12–15 U/kg per h (initial maximum 1000 U/h) titrated to a PTT 50–70 s
Enoxaparin	1 mg/kg SC every 12 h; the first dose may be preceded by a 30-mg IV bolus; renal adjustment to 1 mg/kg once daily if creatine Cl <30 cc/min
Fondaparinux	2.5 mg SC qd
Bivalirudin	Initial bolus intravenous bolus of 0.1 mg/kg and an infusion of 0.25 mg/kg per hour. Before PCI, an additional intravenous bolus of 0.5 mg/kg was administered, and the infusion was increased to 1.75 mg/kg per hour.

[a]Other LMWH exist beyond those listed.
Abbreviations: IV, intravenous; SC, subcutaneously.
Source: Modified from J Anderson et al: JACO 50:e1, 2007.

observed both in patients treated conservatively and in those who underwent PCI and should certainly continue for at least 1 year in patients with a drug-eluting stent. Up to one-third of patients have low response to clopidogrel, and a substantial proportion of these are related to a genetic variant of the cytochrome P450

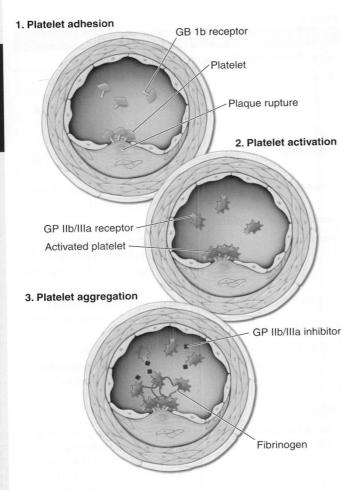

1. Platelet adhesion

- GB 1b receptor
- Platelet
- Plaque rupture

2. Platelet activation

- GP IIb/IIIa receptor
- Activated platelet

3. Platelet aggregation

- GP IIb/IIIa inhibitor
- Fibrinogen

FIGURE 34-3

Platelets initiate thrombosis at the site of a ruptured plaque with denuded endothelium: *platelet adhesion* occurs via (1) the GP 1b receptor in conjunction with von Willebrand factor. This is followed by *platelet activation* (2), which leads to a shape change of the platelet, degranulation of the alpha and dense granules, and expression of glycoprotein IIb/IIIa receptors on the platelet surface with activation of the receptor, such that it can bind fibrinogen. The final step is *platelet aggregation* (3), in which fibrinogen (or von Willebrand factor) binds to the activated GP IIb/IIIa receptors. Aspirin (ASA) and clopidogrel act to decrease platelet activation, whereas the GP IIb/IIIa inhibitors inhibit the final step of platelet aggregation. GP, glycoprotein. (*Modified from CP Cannon, E Braunwald, in Braunwald's Heart Disease: A Textbook of Cardiovascular Medicine, 8th ed, R Bonow et al [eds]. Philadelphia, Saunders, 2008.*)

system. A variant of the 2C19 gene leads to reduced conversion of clopidogrel into its active metabolite, which, in turn, causes lower platelet inhibition and a higher risk of cardiovascular events. Alternate agents, such as prasugrel, should be considered for ACS patients who are hyporesponsive to clopidogrel as identified by platelet and/or genetic testing, although such testing is not yet widespread.

A recently approved thienopyridine, prasugrel, has been shown to achieve a more rapid onset, and higher level of platelet inhibition than clopidogrel. It has been used in ACS patients following angiography in whom PCI is planned at a dose of 60 mg load followed by 10 mg/d for up to 15 months. The TRITON-TIMI 38 trial showed that relative to clopidogrel, prasugrel reduced the risk of cardiovascular death, MI, or stroke significantly by 19%, albeit with an increase in major bleeding. Stent thrombosis was also reduced by 52%. This agent is contraindicated in patients with prior stroke or transient ischemic attack. Ticagrelor is a novel, *reversible* ADP inhibitor that has recently been reported to reduce the risk of cardiovascular death, MI, or stroke by 16% compared with clopidogrel in a broad population of ACS patients. This agent also reduced mortality and did not increase the risk of total bleeding; it is not yet FDA approved at the time of this writing.

Four options are available for anticoagulant therapy to be added to aspirin and clopidogrel. Unfractionated heparin (UFH) is the mainstay of therapy. The low-molecular-weight heparin (LMWH), enoxaparin, has been shown in several studies to be superior to UFH in reducing recurrent cardiac events, especially in conservatively managed patients. The indirect Factor Xa inhibitor, fondaparinux, is equivalent for early efficacy compared with enoxaparin but appears to have a lower risk of major bleeding. Bivalirudin, a direct thrombin inhibitor, is similar in efficacy to either UFH or LMWH among patients treated with a GP IIb/IIIa inhibitor, but use of bivalirudin alone causes less bleeding than the combination of heparin and a GP IIb/IIIa inhibitor in patients with UA/NSTEMI undergoing catheterization and/or PCI.

Prior to the advent of clopidogrel, many trials had shown the benefit of intravenous GP IIb/IIIa inhibitors. The benefit, however, has been small, i.e., only a 9% reduction in death or MI, with a significant increase in major bleeding. Two recent studies also failed to show a benefit for early initiation compared with use only for PCI. The use of these agents may be reserved for unstable patients with recurrent rest pain and ECG changes who undergo PCI.

Excessive bleeding is the most important adverse effect of all antithrombotic agents, including anticoagulants and antiplatelet agents. Therefore, attention must be directed to the doses of antithrombotic agents, accounting for weight, creatinine clearance, and a previous history of excessive bleeding, as a means of reducing the risk of bleeding.

INVASIVE VERSUS CONSERVATIVE STRATEGY Multiple clinical trials have demonstrated the benefit of an early invasive strategy in high-risk patients, i.e., patients with multiple clinical risk factors, ST-segment

TABLE 34-3

CLASS I RECOMMENDATIONS FOR USE OF AN EARLY INVASIVE STRATEGY^a

CLASS I (LEVEL OF EVIDENCE: A) INDICATIONS

Recurrent angina at rest/low-level activity despite Rx
Elevated TnT or TnI
New ST-segment depression
Rec. angina/ischemia with CHF symptoms, rales, MR
Positive stress test
EF <0.40
Decreased BP
Sustained VT
PCI <6 months, prior CABG
High-risk score

^aAny one of the high-risk indicators.
Abbreviations: BP, blood pressure; CABG, coronary artery bypass grafting; CHF, congestive heart failure; EF, ejection fraction; MR, mitral regurgitation; PCI, percutaneous coronary intervention; Rec, recurrent; TnI, troponin I; TnT, troponin T; VT, ventricular tachycardia.
Source: J Anderson et al: JACO 50:e1, 2007.

deviation, and/or positive biomarkers (Table 34-3). In this strategy, following treatment with anti-ischemic and antithrombotic agents, coronary arteriography is carried out within ~48 h of admission, followed by coronary revascularization (PCI or coronary artery bypass grafting), depending on the coronary anatomy.

In low-risk patients, the outcomes from an invasive strategy are similar to those obtained from a conservative strategy, which consists of anti-ischemic and antithrombotic therapy followed by "watchful waiting," and in which coronary arteriography is carried out only if rest pain or ST-segment changes recur or there is evidence of ischemia on a stress test.

LONG-TERM MANAGEMENT

The time of hospital discharge is a "teachable moment" for the patient with UA/NSTEMI, when the physician can review and optimize the medical regimen. Risk-factor modification is key, and the caregiver should discuss with the patient the importance of smoking cessation, achieving optimal weight, daily exercise following an appropriate diet, blood-pressure control, tight control of hyperglycemia (for diabetic patients), and lipid management, as recommended for patients with chronic stable angina (Chap. 33).

There is evidence of benefit with long-term therapy with five classes of drugs that are directed at different components of the atherothrombotic process. Beta blockers, statins (at a high dose, e.g., atorvastatin 80 mg/d), and ACE inhibitors or angiotensin receptor blockers are recommended for long-term plaque stabilization. Antiplatelet therapy, now recommended to be the combination of aspirin and clopidogrel (or prasugrel in post PCS patients) for 1 year, with aspirin continued thereafter, prevents or reduces the severity of any thrombosis that would occur if a plaque were to rupture.

Observational registries have shown that patients with UA/NSTEMI at high risk, including women and the elderly as well as racial minorities, are less likely to receive evidence-based pharmacologic and interventional therapies with resultant poorer clinical outcomes and quality of life.

PRINZMETAL'S VARIANT ANGINA

In 1959, Prinzmetal et al. described a syndrome of severe ischemic pain that occurs at rest but not usually with exertion and is associated with transient ST-segment elevation. This syndrome is due to focal spasm of an epicardial coronary artery, leading to severe myocardial ischemia. The cause of the spasm is not well defined, but it may be related to hypercontractility of vascular smooth muscle due to vasoconstrictor mitogens, leukotrienes, or serotonin.

Clinical and angiographic manifestations

Patients with Prinzmetal's variant angina (PVA) are generally younger and have fewer coronary risk factors (with the exception of cigarette smoking) than patients with UA secondary to coronary atherosclerosis. Cardiac examination is usually unremarkable in the absence of ischemia. The clinical diagnosis of variant angina is made with the detection of transient ST-segment *elevation* with rest pain. Many patients also exhibit multiple episodes of asymptomatic ST-segment elevation (*silent ischemia*). Small elevations of troponin may occur in patients with prolonged attacks of variant angina.

Coronary angiography demonstrates transient coronary spasm as the diagnostic hallmark of PVA. Atherosclerotic plaques, which do not usually cause critical obstruction, in at least one proximal coronary artery occur in the majority of patients, and in them spasm usually occurs within 1 cm of the plaque. Focal spasm is most common in the right coronary artery, and it may occur at one or more sites in one artery or in multiple arteries simultaneously. Ergonovine, acetylcholine, other vasoconstrictor medications, and hyperventilation have been used to provoke focal coronary stenosis on angiography to establish the diagnosis. Hyperventilation has also been used to provoke rest angina, ST-segment elevation, and spasm on coronary arteriography.

TREATMENT   Prinzmetal's Variant Angina

Nitrates and calcium channel blockers are the main agents used to treat acute episodes and to abolish recurrent episodes of PVA. Aspirin may actually increase the severity of ischemic episodes, possibly as a result of the exquisite sensitivity of coronary tone to modest changes in the synthesis of prostacyclin. The response to beta blockers is variable. Coronary revascularization may be helpful in patients who also have discrete, proximal fixed obstructive lesions.

Prognosis

Many patients with PVA pass through an acute, active phase, with frequent episodes of angina and cardiac events during the first 6 months after presentation. Long-term survival at 5 years is excellent (~90–95%). Patients with no or mild fixed coronary obstruction tend to experience a more benign course than do patients with associated severe obstructive lesions. Nonfatal MI occurs in up to 20% of patients by 5 years. Patients with PVA who develop serious arrhythmias during spontaneous episodes of pain are at a higher risk for sudden cardiac death. In most patients who survive an infarction or the initial 3- to 6-month period of frequent episodes, the condition stabilizes, and there is a tendency for symptoms and cardiac events to diminish over time.

CHAPTER 35

ST-SEGMENT ELEVATION MYOCARDIAL INFARCTION

Elliott M. Antman ■ Joseph Loscalzo

Acute myocardial infarction (AMI) is one of the most common diagnoses in hospitalized patients in industrialized countries. In the United States, approximately 650,000 patients experience a new AMI and 450,000 experience a recurrent AMI each year. The early (30-day) mortality rate from AMI is ~30%, with more than half of these deaths occurring before the stricken individual reaches the hospital. Although the mortality rate after admission for AMI has declined by ~30% over the past two decades, approximately 1 of every 25 patients who survives the initial hospitalization dies in the first year after AMI. Mortality is approximately fourfold higher in elderly patients (over age 75) as compared with younger patients.

When patients with prolonged ischemic discomfort at rest are first seen, the working clinical diagnosis is that they are suffering from an acute coronary syndrome (Fig. 35-1). The 12-lead electrocardiogram (ECG) is a pivotal diagnostic and triage tool because it is at the center of the decision pathway for management; it permits distinction of those patients presenting with ST-segment elevation from those presenting without ST-segment elevation. Serum cardiac biomarkers are obtained to distinguish unstable angina (UA) from non–ST-segment MI (NSTEMI) and to assess the magnitude of an ST-segment elevation MI (STEMI). This chapter focuses on the evaluation and management of patients with STEMI, while Chap. 34 discusses UA/NSTEMI.

PATHOPHYSIOLOGY: ROLE OF ACUTE PLAQUE RUPTURE

STEMI usually occurs when coronary blood flow decreases abruptly after a thrombotic occlusion of a coronary artery previously affected by atherosclerosis.

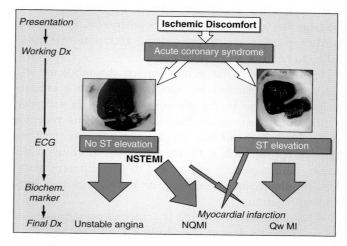

FIGURE 35-1

Acute coronary syndromes. Following disruption of a vulnerable plaque, patients experience ischemic discomfort resulting from a reduction of flow through the affected epicardial coronary artery. The flow reduction may be caused by a completely occlusive thrombus (***right***) or subtotally occlusive thrombus (***left***). Patients with ischemic discomfort may present with or without ST-segment elevation. Of patients with ST-segment elevation, the majority (*wide red arrow*) ultimately develop a Q wave on the ECG (QwMI), while a minority (*thin red arrow*) do not develop Q wave and, in older literature, were said to have sustained a non-Q-wave MI (NQMI). Patients who present without ST-segment elevation are suffering from either unstable angina or a non-ST-segment elevation MI (NSTEMI) (*wide green arrows*), a distinction that is ultimately made on the presence or absence of a serum cardiac marker such as CKMB or a cardiac troponin detected in the blood. The majority of patients presenting with NSTEMI do not develop a Q wave on the ECG; a minority develop a QwMI (*thin green arrow*). (*Adapted from CW Hamm et al: Lancet 358:1533, 2001, and MJ Davies: Heart 83:361, 2000; with permission from the BMJ Publishing Group.*)

Slowly developing, high-grade coronary artery stenoses do not typically precipitate STEMI because of the development of a rich collateral network over time. Instead, STEMI occurs when a coronary artery thrombus develops rapidly at a site of vascular injury. This injury is produced or facilitated by factors such as cigarette smoking, hypertension, and lipid accumulation. In most cases, STEMI occurs when the surface of an atherosclerotic plaque becomes disrupted (exposing its contents to the blood) and conditions (local or systemic) favor thrombogenesis. A mural thrombus forms at the site of plaque disruption, and the involved coronary artery becomes occluded. Histologic studies indicate that the coronary plaques prone to disruption are those with a rich lipid core and a thin fibrous cap (Chap. 30). After an initial platelet monolayer forms at the site of the disrupted plaque, various agonists (collagen, ADP, epinephrine, serotonin) promote platelet activation. After agonist stimulation of platelets, thromboxane A_2 (a potent local vasoconstrictor) is released, further platelet activation occurs, and potential resistance to fibrinolysis develops.

In addition to the generation of thromboxane A_2, activation of platelets by agonists promotes a conformational change in the glycoprotein IIb/IIIa receptor. Once converted to its functional state, this receptor develops a high affinity for soluble adhesive proteins (i.e., integrins) such as fibrinogen. Since fibrinogen is a multivalent molecule, it can bind to two different platelets simultaneously, resulting in platelet cross-linking and aggregation.

The coagulation cascade is activated on exposure of tissue factor in damaged endothelial cells at the site of the disrupted plaque. Factors VII and X are activated, ultimately leading to the conversion of prothrombin to thrombin, which then converts fibrinogen to fibrin. Fluid-phase and clot-bound thrombin participate in an autoamplification reaction leading to further activation of the coagulation cascade. The culprit coronary artery eventually becomes occluded by a thrombus containing platelet aggregates and fibrin strands.

In rare cases, STEMI may be due to coronary artery occlusion caused by coronary emboli, congenital abnormalities, coronary spasm, and a wide variety of systemic—particularly inflammatory—diseases. The amount of myocardial damage caused by coronary occlusion depends on (1) the territory supplied by the affected vessel, (2) whether or not the vessel becomes totally occluded, (3) the duration of coronary occlusion, (4) the quantity of blood supplied by collateral vessels to the affected tissue, (5) the demand for oxygen of the myocardium whose blood supply has been suddenly limited, (6) endogenous factors that can produce early spontaneous lysis of the occlusive thrombus, and (7) the adequacy of myocardial perfusion in the infarct zone when flow is restored in the occluded epicardial coronary artery.

Patients at increased risk for developing STEMI include those with multiple coronary risk factors (Chap. 30) and those with unstable angina (Chap. 34). Less common underlying medical conditions predisposing patients to STEMI include hypercoagulability, collagen vascular disease, cocaine abuse, and intracardiac thrombi or masses that can produce coronary emboli.

There have been major advances in the management of STEMI with recognition that the "chain of survival" involves a highly integrated system starting with prehospital care and extending to early hospital management so as to provide expeditious implementation of a reperfusion strategy.

CLINICAL PRESENTATION

In up to one-half of cases, a precipitating factor appears to be present before STEMI, such as vigorous physical exercise, emotional stress, or a medical or surgical illness. Although STEMI may commence at any time of the day or night, circadian variations have been reported such that clusters are seen in the morning within a few hours of awakening.

Pain is the most common presenting complaint in patients with STEMI. The pain is deep and visceral; adjectives commonly used to describe it are *heavy*, *squeezing*, and *crushing*, although, occasionally, it is described as stabbing or burning (Chap. 4). It is similar in character to the discomfort of angina pectoris (Chap. 33) but commonly occurs at rest, is usually more severe, and lasts longer. Typically, the pain involves the central portion of the chest and/or the epigastrium, and, on occasion, it radiates to the arms. Less common sites of radiation include the abdomen, back, lower jaw, and neck. The frequent location of the pain beneath the xiphoid and epigastrium and the patients' denial that they may be suffering a heart attack are chiefly responsible for the common mistaken impression of indigestion. The pain of STEMI may radiate as high as the occipital area but not below the umbilicus. It is often accompanied by weakness, sweating, nausea, vomiting, anxiety, and a sense of impending doom. The pain may commence when the patient is at rest, but when it begins during a period of exertion, it does not usually subside with cessation of activity, in contrast to angina pectoris.

The pain of STEMI can simulate pain from acute pericarditis (Chap. 22), pulmonary embolism, acute aortic dissection (Chap. 38), costochondritis, and gastrointestinal disorders. These conditions should therefore be considered in the differential diagnosis. Radiation of discomfort to the trapezius is not seen in patients with STEMI and may be a useful distinguishing feature that suggests pericarditis is the correct diagnosis. However, *pain is not uniformly present in patients with STEMI.* The proportion of painless STEMIs is greater in patients with diabetes mellitus, and it increases with age. In the elderly, STEMI may present as sudden-onset breathlessness, which may progress to pulmonary edema. Other less common presentations, with or without pain, include sudden loss of consciousness, a confusional state, a sensation of profound weakness, the appearance of an arrhythmia, evidence of peripheral embolism, or merely an unexplained drop in arterial pressure.

PHYSICAL FINDINGS

Most patients are anxious and restless, attempting unsuccessfully to relieve the pain by moving about in bed, altering their position, and stretching. Pallor associated with perspiration and coolness of the extremities occurs commonly. The combination of substernal chest pain persisting for >30 min and diaphoresis strongly suggests STEMI. Although many patients have a normal pulse rate and blood pressure within the first hour of STEMI, about one-fourth of patients with anterior infarction have manifestations of sympathetic nervous system hyperactivity (tachycardia and/or hypertension), and up to one-half with inferior infarction show evidence of parasympathetic hyperactivity (bradycardia and/or hypotension).

The precordium is usually quiet, and the apical impulse may be difficult to palpate. In patients with anterior wall infarction, an abnormal systolic pulsation caused by dyskinetic bulging of infarcted myocardium may develop in the periapical area within the first days of the illness and then may resolve. Other physical signs of ventricular dysfunction include fourth and third heart sounds, decreased intensity of the first heart sound, and paradoxical splitting of the second heart sound (Chap. 9). A transient mid-systolic or late systolic apical systolic murmur due to dysfunction of the mitral valve apparatus may be present. A pericardial friction rub is heard in many patients with transmural STEMI at some time in the course of the disease, if the patients are examined frequently. The carotid pulse is often decreased in volume, reflecting reduced stroke volume. Temperature elevations up to 38°C may be observed during the first week after STEMI. The arterial pressure is variable; in most patients with transmural infarction, systolic pressure declines by approximately 10–15 mmHg from the preinfarction state.

LABORATORY FINDINGS

Myocardial infarction (MI) progresses through the following temporal stages: (1) acute (first few hours–7 days), (2) healing (7–28 days), and (3) healed (29 days). When evaluating the results of diagnostic tests for STEMI, the temporal phase of the infarction must be considered.

The laboratory tests of value in confirming the diagnosis may be divided into four groups: (1) ECG, (2) serum cardiac biomarkers, (3) cardiac imaging, and (4) nonspecific indices of tissue necrosis and inflammation.

ELECTROCARDIOGRAM

The electrocardiographic manifestations of STEMI are described in Chap. 11. During the initial stage, total occlusion of an epicardial coronary artery produces ST-segment elevation. Most patients initially presenting with ST-segment elevation ultimately evolve Q waves on the ECG. However, Q waves in the leads overlying the infarct zone may vary in magnitude and even appear only transiently, depending on the reperfusion status of the ischemic myocardium and restoration of transmembrane potentials over time. A small proportion of patients initially presenting with ST-segment elevation will not develop Q waves when the obstructing thrombus is not totally occlusive, obstruction is transient, or if a rich collateral network is present. Among patients presenting with ischemic discomfort but *without* ST-segment elevation, if a serum cardiac biomarker of necrosis (see later) is detected, the diagnosis of NSTEMI is ultimately made (Fig. 35-1). A minority of patients who present initially without ST-segment elevation may develop a Q-wave MI. Previously, it was believed that transmural MI is present if the ECG demonstrates Q waves or loss of R waves, and nontransmural MI may be present if the ECG shows only transient ST-segment and T-wave changes. However, electrocardiographic-pathologic correlations are far from perfect and terms such as *Q-wave MI*, *non-Q-wave MI*, *transmural MI*, and *nontransmural MI*, have been replaced by STEMI and NSTEMI (Fig. 35-1). Contemporary studies using MRI suggest that the development of a Q wave on the ECG is more dependent on the volume of infarcted tissue rather than the transmurality of infarction.

SERUM CARDIAC BIOMARKERS

Certain proteins, called serum cardiac biomarkers, are released from necrotic heart muscle after STEMI. The rate of liberation of specific proteins differs depending on their intracellular location, their molecular weight, and the local blood and lymphatic flow. Cardiac biomarkers become detectable in the peripheral blood once the capacity of the cardiac lymphatics to clear the interstitium of the infarct zone is exceeded and spillover into the venous circulation occurs. The temporal pattern of protein release is of diagnostic importance, but contemporary urgent reperfusion strategies necessitate making a decision (based largely on a combination of clinical and ECG findings) before the results of blood tests have returned from the laboratory. Rapid whole-blood bedside assays for serum cardiac markers are now available and may facilitate management decisions, particularly in patients with nondiagnostic ECGs.

Cardiac-specific troponin T (cTnT) and *cardiac-specific troponin I* (cTnI) have amino-acid sequences different from those of the skeletal muscle forms of these proteins. These differences permitted the development of quantitative assays for cTnT and cTnI with highly specific monoclonal antibodies. Since cTnT and cTnI are not normally detectable in the blood of healthy individuals but may increase after STEMI to levels >20 times higher than the upper reference limit (the highest value seen in 99% of a reference population not suffering from MI), the measurement of cTnT or cTnI is of considerable diagnostic usefulness, and they are now the preferred biochemical markers for MI (**Fig. 35-2**). The cardiac troponins are particularly valuable when there is clinical suspicion of either skeletal muscle injury or a small MI that may be below the detection limit for creatine phosphokinase (CK) and its MB isoenzyme (CKMB) measurements, and they are, therefore, of particular value in distinguishing UA from NSTEMI. Levels of cTnI and cTnT may remain elevated for 7–10 days after STEMI.

CK rises within 4–8 h and generally returns to normal by 48–72 h (Fig. 35-2). An important drawback of total CK measurement is its lack of specificity for STEMI, as CK may be elevated with skeletal muscle disease or trauma, including intramuscular injection.

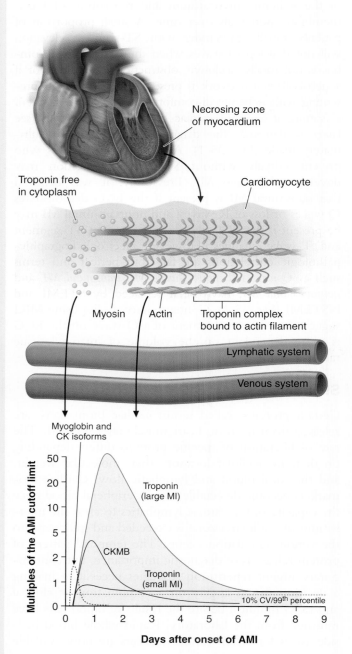

FIGURE 35-2

The zone of necrosing myocardium is shown at the top of the figure, followed in the middle portion of the figure by a diagram of a cardiomyocyte that is in the process of releasing biomarkers. The biomarkers that are released into the interstitium are first cleared by lymphatics followed subsequently by spillover into the venous system. After disruption of the sarcolemmal membrane of the cardiomyocyte, the cytoplasmic pool of biomarkers is released first (left-most arrow in bottom portion of figure). Markers such as myoglobin and CK isoforms are rapidly released, and blood levels rise quickly above the cutoff limit; this is then followed by a more protracted release of biomarkers from the disintegrating myofilaments that may continue for several days. Cardiac troponin levels rise to about 20 to 50 times the upper reference limit (the 99th percentile of values in a reference control group) in patients who have a "classic" acute myocardial infarction (MI) and sustain sufficient myocardial necrosis to result in abnormally elevated levels of the MB fraction of creatine kinase (CKMB). Clinicians can now diagnose episodes of microinfarction by sensitive assays that detect cardiac troponin elevations above the upper reference limit, even though CKMB levels may still be in the normal reference range (not shown). CV = coefficient of variation. (*Modified from EM Antman: Decision making with cardiac troponin tests. N Engl J Med 346:2079, 2002 and AS Jaffe et al: Biomarkers in acute cardiac disease: The present and the future. J Am Coll Cardiol 48:1, 2006.*)

The MB isoenzyme of CK has the advantage over total CK that it is not present in significant concentrations in extracardiac tissue and, therefore, is considerably more specific. However, cardiac surgery, myocarditis, and electrical cardioversion often result in elevated serum levels of the MB isoenzyme. A ratio (relative index) of CKMB mass: CK activity ≥2.5 suggests but is not diagnostic of a myocardial rather than a skeletal muscle source for the CKMB elevation.

Many hospitals are using cTnT or cTnI rather than CKMB as the routine serum cardiac marker for diagnosis of STEMI, although any of these analytes remain clinically acceptable. It is *not* cost-effective to measure both a cardiac-specific troponin and CKMB at all time points in every patient.

While it has long been recognized that the total quantity of protein released correlates with the size of the infarct, the peak protein concentration correlates only weakly with infarct size. Recanalization of a coronary artery occlusion (either spontaneously or by mechanical or pharmacologic means) in the early hours of STEMI causes earlier peaking of biomarker measurements (Fig. 35-2) because of a rapid washout from the interstitium of the infarct zone, quickly overwhelming lymphatic clearance of the proteins.

The *nonspecific reaction* to myocardial injury is associated with polymorphonuclear leukocytosis, which appears within a few hours after the onset of pain and persists for 3–7 days; the white blood cell count often reaches levels of 12,000–15,000/μL. The erythrocyte sedimentation rate rises more slowly than the white blood cell count, peaking during the first week and sometimes remaining elevated for 1 or 2 weeks.

CARDIAC IMAGING

Abnormalities of wall motion on *two-dimensional echocardiography* (Chap. 12) are almost universally present. Although acute STEMI cannot be distinguished from an old myocardial scar or from acute severe ischemia by echocardiography, the ease and safety of the procedure make its use appealing as a screening tool in the emergency department setting. When the ECG is not diagnostic of STEMI, early detection of the presence or absence of wall motion abnormalities by echocardiography can aid in management decisions, such as whether the patient should receive reperfusion therapy (e.g., fibrinolysis or a percutaneous coronary intervention [PCI]). Echocardiographic estimation of left ventricular (LV) function is useful prognostically; detection of reduced function serves as an indication for therapy with an inhibitor of the renin-angiotensin-aldosterone system. Echocardiography may also identify the presence of right ventricular (RV) infarction, ventricular aneurysm, pericardial effusion, and LV thrombus. In addition, Doppler echocardiography is useful in the detection and quantitation of a ventricular septal defect and mitral regurgitation, two serious complications of STEMI.

Several *radionuclide imaging techniques* (Chap. 12) are available for evaluating patients with suspected STEMI. However, these imaging modalities are used less often than echocardiography because they are more cumbersome and lack sensitivity and specificity in many clinical circumstances. Myocardial perfusion imaging with [^{201}Tl] or [^{99m}Tc]-sestamibi, which are distributed in proportion to myocardial blood flow and concentrated by viable myocardium (Chap. 33), reveal a defect ("cold spot") in most patients during the first few hours after development of a transmural infarct. Although perfusion scanning is extremely sensitive, it cannot distinguish acute infarcts from chronic scars and, thus, is not specific for the diagnosis of *acute* MI. Radionuclide ventriculography, carried out with [^{99m}Tc]-labeled red blood cells, frequently demonstrates wall motion disorders and reduction in the ventricular ejection fraction in patients with STEMI. While of value in assessing the hemodynamic consequences of infarction and in aiding in the diagnosis of RV infarction when the RV ejection fraction is depressed, this technique is nonspecific, as many cardiac abnormalities other than MI alter the radionuclide ventriculogram.

Myocardial infarction can be detected accurately with high-resolution cardiac MRI (Chap. 12) using a technique referred to as late enhancement. A standard imaging agent (gadolinium) is administered and images are obtained after a 10-min delay. Since little gadolinium enters normal myocardium, where there are tightly packed myocytes, but does percolate into the expanded intercellular region of the infarct zone, there is a bright signal in areas of infarction that appears in stark contrast to the dark areas of normal myocardium.

INITIAL MANAGEMENT

PREHOSPITAL CARE

The prognosis in STEMI is largely related to the occurrence of two general classes of complications: (1) electrical complications (arrhythmias) and (2) mechanical complications ("pump failure"). Most out-of-hospital deaths from STEMI are due to the sudden development of ventricular fibrillation. The vast majority of deaths due to ventricular fibrillation occur within the first 24 h of the onset of symptoms, and of these, over half occur in the first hour. Therefore, the major elements of prehospital care of patients with suspected STEMI include (1) recognition of symptoms by the patient and prompt seeking of medical attention; (2) rapid deployment of an emergency medical team capable of performing resuscitative maneuvers, including defibrillation;

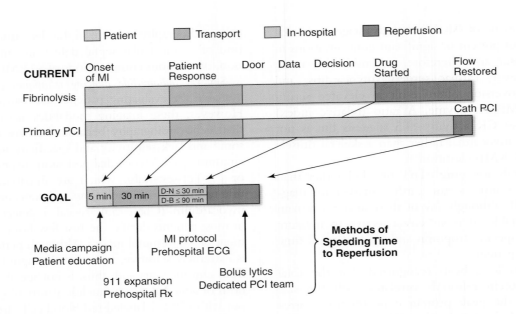

FIGURE 35-3

Major components of time delay between onset of symptoms from STEMI and restoration of flow in the infarct-related artery. Plotted sequentially from left to right are the times for patients to recognize symptoms and seek medical attention, transportation to the hospital, in-hospital decision making, implementation of reperfusion strategy, and restoration of flow once the reperfusion strategy has been initiated. The time to initiate fibrinolytic therapy is the "door-to-needle" (D-N) time; this is followed by the period of time required for pharmacologic restoration of flow. More time is required to move the patient to the catheterization laboratory for a percutaneous coronary interventional (PCI) procedure, referred to as the "door-to-balloon" (D-B) time, but restoration of flow in the epicardial infarct–related artery occurs promptly after PCI. At the bottom is a variety of methods for speeding the time to reperfusion along with the goals for the time intervals for the various components of the time delay. (*Adapted from CP Cannon et al: J Thromb Thrombol 1:27, 1994.*)

(3) expeditious transportation of the patient to a hospital facility that is continuously staffed by physicians and nurses skilled in managing arrhythmias and providing advanced cardiac life support; and (4) expeditious implementation of reperfusion therapy (**Fig. 35–3**). The greatest delay usually occurs not during transportation to the hospital but, rather, between the onset of pain and the patient's decision to call for help. This delay can best be reduced by health care professionals educating the public concerning the significance of chest discomfort and the importance of seeking early medical attention. Regular office visits with patients having a history of or who are at risk for ischemic heart disease are important "teachable moments" for clinicians to review the symptoms of STEMI and the appropriate action plan.

Increasingly, monitoring and treatment are carried out by trained personnel in the ambulance, further shortening the time between the onset of the infarction and appropriate treatment. General guidelines for initiation of fibrinolysis in the prehospital setting include the ability to transmit 12-lead ECGs to confirm the diagnosis, the presence of paramedics in the ambulance, training of paramedics in the interpretation of ECGs and management of STEMI, and online medical command and control that can authorize the initiation of treatment in the field.

MANAGEMENT IN THE EMERGENCY DEPARTMENT

In the emergency department, the goals for the management of patients with suspected STEMI include control of cardiac discomfort, rapid identification of patients who are candidates for urgent reperfusion therapy, triage of lower-risk patients to the appropriate location in the hospital, and avoidance of inappropriate discharge of patients with STEMI. Many aspects of the treatment of STEMI are initiated in the emergency department and then continued during the in-hospital phase of management.

Aspirin is essential in the management of patients with suspected STEMI and is effective across the entire spectrum of acute coronary syndromes (Fig. 35-1). Rapid inhibition of cyclooxygenase-1 in platelets followed by a reduction of thromboxane A_2 levels is achieved by buccal absorption of a chewed 160–325-mg tablet in the emergency department. This measure should be followed by daily oral administration of aspirin in a dose of 75–162 mg.

In patients whose arterial O_2 saturation is normal, supplemental O_2 is of limited if any clinical benefit and therefore is not cost-effective. However, when hypoxemia is present, O_2 should be administered by nasal prongs or face mask (2–4 L/min) for the first 6–12 h after infarction; the patient should then be reassessed to determine if there is a continued need for such treatment.

CONTROL OF DISCOMFORT

Sublingual *nitroglycerin* can be given safely to most patients with STEMI. Up to three doses of 0.4 mg should be administered at about 5-min intervals. In addition to diminishing or abolishing chest discomfort, nitroglycerin may be capable of both decreasing myocardial oxygen demand (by lowering preload) and increasing myocardial oxygen supply (by dilating infarct-related coronary vessels or collateral vessels). In patients whose initially favorable response to sublingual nitroglycerin is followed by the return of chest discomfort, particularly if accompanied by other evidence of ongoing ischemia such as further ST-segment or T-wave shifts, the use of intravenous nitroglycerin should be considered. Therapy with nitrates should be avoided in patients who present with low systolic arterial pressure (<90 mmHg) or in whom there is clinical suspicion of right ventricular infarction (inferior infarction on ECG, elevated jugular venous pressure, clear lungs, and hypotension). Nitrates should not be administered to patients who have taken the phosphodiesterase-5 inhibitor sildenafil for erectile dysfunction within the preceding 24 h, because it may potentiate the hypotensive effects of nitrates. An idiosyncratic reaction to nitrates, consisting of sudden marked hypotension, sometimes occurs but can usually be reversed promptly by the rapid administration of intravenous atropine.

Morphine is a very effective analgesic for the pain associated with STEMI. However, it may reduce sympathetically mediated arteriolar and venous constriction, and the resulting venous pooling may reduce cardiac output and arterial pressure. These hemodynamic disturbances usually respond promptly to elevation of the legs, but in some patients volume expansion with intravenous saline is required. The patient may experience diaphoresis and nausea, but these events usually pass and are replaced by a feeling of well-being associated with the relief of pain. Morphine also has a vagotonic effect and may cause bradycardia or advanced degrees of heart block, particularly in patients with inferior infarction. These side effects usually respond to atropine (0.5 mg intravenously). Morphine is routinely administered by repetitive (every 5 min) intravenous injection of small doses (2–4 mg), rather than by the subcutaneous administration of a larger quantity, because absorption may be unpredictable by the latter route.

Intravenous *beta blockers* are also useful in the control of the pain of STEMI. These drugs control pain effectively in some patients, presumably by diminishing myocardial O$_2$ demand and hence ischemia. More important, there is evidence that intravenous beta blockers reduce the risks of reinfarction and ventricular fibrillation (see "Beta-Adrenoceptor Blockers," later). However, patient selection is important when considering beta blockers for STEMI. Oral beta-blocker therapy should be initiated in the first 24 h for patients who do not have any of the following: (1) signs of heart failure, (2) evidence of a low-output state, (3) increased risk for cardiogenic shock, or (4) other relative contraindications to beta blockade (PR interval greater than 0.24 s, second- or third-degree heart block, active asthma, or reactive airway disease). A commonly employed regimen is metoprolol, 5 mg every 2–5 min for a total of 3 doses, provided the patient has a heart rate >60 beats per minute (bpm), systolic pressure >100 mmHg, a PR interval <0.24 s, and rales that are no higher than 10 cm up from the diaphragm. Fifteen min after the last intravenous dose, an oral regimen is initiated of 50 mg every 6 h for 48 h, followed by 100 mg every 12 h.

Unlike beta blockers, calcium antagonists are of little value in the acute setting, and there is evidence that short-acting dihydropyridines may be associated with an increased mortality risk.

MANAGEMENT STRATEGIES

The primary tool for screening patients and making triage decisions is the initial 12-lead ECG. When ST-segment elevation of at least 2 mm in two contiguous precordial leads and 1 mm in two adjacent limb leads is present, a patient should be considered a candidate for *reperfusion therapy* (Fig. 35-4). The process of selecting patients for fibrinolysis versus primary PCI (angioplasty, or stenting; Chap. 36) is discussed later. In the absence of ST-segment elevation, fibrinolysis is not helpful, and evidence exists suggesting that it may be harmful.

LIMITATION OF INFARCT SIZE

The quantity of myocardium that becomes necrotic as a consequence of a coronary artery occlusion is determined by factors other than just the site of occlusion. While the central zone of the infarct contains necrotic tissue that is irretrievably lost, the fate of the surrounding ischemic myocardium (ischemic penumbra) may be improved by timely restoration of coronary perfusion, reduction of myocardial O$_2$ demands, prevention of the accumulation of noxious metabolites, and blunting of the impact of mediators of reperfusion injury (e.g., calcium overload and oxygen-derived free radicals). Up to one-third of patients with STEMI may achieve *spontaneous* reperfusion of the infarct-related coronary artery within 24 h and experience improved healing of infarcted tissue. Reperfusion, either pharmacologically (by fibrinolysis) or by PCI, accelerates the opening of infarct-related arteries in those patients in whom spontaneous fibrinolysis ultimately would have occurred and also greatly increases the number of patients in whom

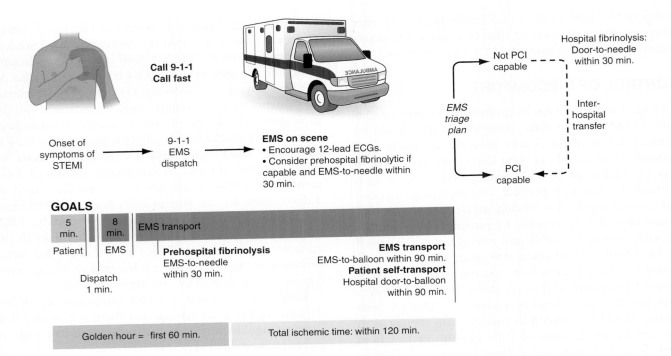

FIGURE 35-4

Options for transportation of patients with STEMI and initial reperfusion treatment. Patient transported by EMS after calling 911: Reperfusion in patients with STEMI can be accomplished by the pharmacologic (fibrinolysis) or catheter-based (primary PCI) approaches. Implementation of these strategies varies based on the mode of transportation of the patient and capabilities at the receiving hospital. Transport time to the hospital is variable from case to case, but the goal is to keep total ischemic time within 120 min. There are three possible scenarios: (1) If EMS has fibrinolytic capability and the patient qualifies for therapy, prehospital fibrinolysis should be started within 30 min of EMS arrival on scene. (2) If EMS is not capable of administering prehospital fibrinolysis and the patient is transported to a non-PCI-capable hospital, the hospital door-to-needle time should be within 30 min for patients in whom fibrinolysis is indicated. (3) If EMS is not capable of administering prehospital fibrinolysis and the patient is transported to a PCI-capable hospital, the hospital door-to-balloon time should be within 90 min. *Interhospital transfer*: It is also appropriate to consider emergency interhospital transfer of the patient to a PCI-capable hospital for mechanical revascularization if: (1) there is a contraindication to fibrinolysis, (2) PCI can be initiated promptly (within 90 min after the patient presented to the initial receiving hospital or within 60 min compared to when fibrinolysis with a fibrin-specific agent could be initiated at the initial receiving hospital), (3) fibrinolysis is administered and is unsuccessful (i.e., "rescue PCI"). Secondary nonemergency interhospital transfer can be considered for recurrent ischemia. *Patient self-transport*: Patient self-transportation is discouraged. If the patient arrives at a non-PCI-capable hospital, the door-to-needle time should be within 30 min. If the patient arrives at a PCI-capable hospital, the door-to-balloon time should be within 90 min. The treatment options and time recommended after first hospital arrival are the same. (*Adapted with permission from Antman et al: ACC/AHA guidelines for the management of patients with ST-elevation myocardial infarction: A report of the American College of Cardiology/American Heart Association Task Force on Practice Guidelines [Committee to Revise the 1999 Guidelines for the Management of Patients with Acute Myocardial Infarction]. Circulation 110:e82, 2004.*)

restoration of flow in the infarct–related artery is accomplished. Timely restoration of flow in the epicardial infarct–related artery combined with improved perfusion of the downstream zone of infarcted myocardium results in a limitation of infarct size. Protection of the ischemic myocardium by the maintenance of an optimal balance between myocardial O_2 supply and demand through pain control, treatment of congestive heart failure (CHF), and minimization of tachycardia and hypertension extends the "window" of time for the salvage of myocardium by reperfusion strategies.

Glucocorticoids and nonsteroidal anti–inflammatory agents, with the exception of aspirin, should be avoided in patients with STEMI. They can impair infarct healing and increase the risk of myocardial rupture, and their use may result in a larger infarct scar. In addition, they can increase coronary vascular resistance, thereby potentially reducing flow to ischemic myocardium.

Primary percutaneous coronary intervention

(See also Chap. 36) PCI, usually angioplasty and/or stenting without preceding fibrinolysis, referred to as *primary PCI*, is effective in restoring perfusion in STEMI when carried out on an emergency basis in the first few hours of MI. It has the advantage of being applicable to patients who have contraindications to fibrinolytic therapy (see later) but otherwise are considered appropriate candidates for reperfusion. It appears to be more effective than fibrinolysis in opening occluded coronary arteries and, *when performed by experienced operators [≥75 PCI cases (not necessarily primary) per year] in dedicated medical centers (≥36 primary PCI cases per year)*, is associated with better short-term and long-term clinical outcomes. Compared with fibrinolysis, primary PCI is generally preferred when the diagnosis is in doubt, cardiogenic shock is present, bleeding risk is increased, or symptoms have been present for at least 2–3 h when the clot is more mature and less easily lysed by fibrinolytic drugs. However, PCI is expensive in terms of personnel and facilities, and its applicability is limited by its availability, around the clock, in only a minority of hospitals.

Fibrinolysis

If no contraindications are present (see later), fibrinolytic therapy should ideally be initiated within 30 min of presentation (i.e., door-to-needle time ≤30 min). The principal goal of fibrinolysis is prompt restoration of full coronary arterial patency. The fibrinolytic agents tissue plasminogen activator (tPA), streptokinase, tenecteplase (TNK), and reteplase (rPA) have been approved by the U.S. Food and Drug Administration for intravenous use in patients with STEMI. These drugs all act by promoting the conversion of plasminogen to plasmin, which subsequently lyses fibrin thrombi. Although considerable emphasis was first placed on a distinction between more fibrin-specific agents, such as tPA, and non-fibrin-specific agents, such as streptokinase, it is now recognized that these differences are only relative, as some degree of systemic fibrinolysis occurs with the former agents. TNK and rPA are referred to as *bolus fibrinolytics* since their administration does not require a prolonged intravenous infusion.

When assessed angiographically, flow in the culprit coronary artery is described by a simple qualitative scale called the *thrombolysis in myocardial infarction (TIMI) grading system*: grade 0 indicates complete occlusion of the infarct-related artery; grade 1 indicates some penetration of the contrast material beyond the point of obstruction but without perfusion of the distal coronary bed; grade 2 indicates perfusion of the entire infarct vessel into the distal bed, but with flow that is delayed compared with that of a normal artery; and grade 3 indicates full perfusion of the infarct vessel with normal flow. The latter is the goal of reperfusion therapy, because full perfusion of the infarct-related coronary artery yields far better results in terms of limiting infarct size, maintenance of LV function, and reduction of both short- and long-term mortality rates. Additional methods of angiographic assessment of the efficacy of fibrinolysis include counting the number of frames on the cine film required for dye to flow from the origin of the infarct-related artery to a landmark in the distal vascular bed (*TIMI frame count*) and determining the rate of entry and exit of contrast dye from the microvasculature in the myocardial infarct zone (*TIMI myocardial perfusion grade*). These methods have an even tighter correlation with outcomes after STEMI than the more commonly employed TIMI flow grade.

Fibrinolytic therapy can reduce the relative risk of in-hospital death by up to 50% when administered within the first hour of the onset of symptoms of STEMI, and much of this benefit is maintained for at least 10 years. When appropriately used, fibrinolytic therapy appears to reduce infarct size, limit LV dysfunction, and reduce the incidence of serious complications such as septal rupture, cardiogenic shock, and malignant ventricular arrhythmias. Since myocardium can be salvaged only before it has been irreversibly injured, the timing of reperfusion therapy, by fibrinolysis or a catheter-based approach, is of extreme importance in achieving maximum benefit. While the upper time limit depends on specific factors in individual patients, it is clear that every minute counts and that patients treated within 1–3 h of the onset of symptoms generally benefit most. Although reduction of the mortality rate is more modest, the therapy remains of benefit for many patients seen 3–6 h after the onset of infarction, and some benefit appears to be possible up to 12 h, especially if chest discomfort is still present and ST segments remain elevated. Compared with PCI for STEMI (primary PCI), fibrinolysis is generally the preferred reperfusion strategy for patients presenting in the first hour of symptoms, if there are logistical concerns about transportation of the patient to a suitable PCI center (experienced operator and team with a track record for a "door-to-balloon" time of <2 h), or there is an anticipated delay of at least 1 h between the time that fibrinolysis could be started versus implementation of PCI. Although patients <75 years achieve a greater relative reduction in the mortality rate with fibrinolytic therapy than do older patients, the higher *absolute* mortality rate (15–25%) in the latter results in similar absolute reductions in the mortality rates for both age groups.

tPA and the other relatively fibrin-specific plasminogen activators, rPA and TNK, are more effective than streptokinase at restoring full perfusion—i.e., TIMI grade 3 coronary flow—and have a small edge in improving survival as well. The current recommended regimen of tPA consists of a 15-mg bolus followed by 50 mg intravenously over the first 30 min, followed by

35 mg over the next 60 min. Streptokinase is administered as 1.5 million units (MU) intravenously over 1 h. rPA is administered in a double-bolus regimen consisting of a 10-MU bolus given over 2–3 min, followed by a second 10-MU bolus 30 min later. TNK is given as a single weight-based intravenous bolus of 0.53 mg/kg over 10 s. In addition to the fibrinolytic agents discussed earlier, pharmacologic reperfusion typically involves adjunctive antiplatelet and antithrombotic drugs, as discussed later.

Alternative pharmacologic regimens for reperfusion combine an intravenous glycoprotein IIb/IIIa inhibitor with a reduced dose of a fibrinolytic agent. Compared with fibrinolytic agents that involve a prolonged infusion (e.g., tPA), such combination reperfusion regimens facilitate the rate and extent of fibrinolysis by inhibiting platelet aggregation, weakening the clot structure, and allowing penetration of the fibrinolytic agent deeper into the clot. However, combination reperfusion regimens have similar efficacy as compared with bolus fibrinolytics and are associated with an increased risk of bleeding, especially in patients >75 years. Therefore, combination reperfusion regimens are not recommended for routine use. Glycoprotein IIb/IIIa inhibitors, given alone or in combination with a reduced dose of a fibrinolytic agent as part of a preparatory regimen before planned immediate PCI (facilitated PCI), have not been shown to reduce infarct size or improve outcomes and, furthermore, are associated with increased bleeding. Facilitated PCI is, therefore, also not a strategy that is recommended for routine use.

Integrated reperfusion strategy

Evidence has emerged that suggests PCI plays an increasingly important role in the management of STEMI. Prior approaches that segregated the pharmacologic and catheter-based approaches to reperfusion have now been replaced with an integrated approach to triage and transfer of STEMI patients to receive PCI (Fig. 35-5).

Contraindications and complications

Clear contraindications to the use of fibrinolytic agents include a history of cerebrovascular hemorrhage at any time, a nonhemorrhagic stroke or other cerebrovascular event within the past year, marked hypertension (a reliably determined systolic arterial pressure >180 mmHg and/or a diastolic pressure >110 mmHg) at any time during the acute presentation, suspicion of aortic dissection, and active internal bleeding (excluding menses). While advanced age is associated with an increase in hemorrhagic complications, the benefit of fibrinolytic therapy in the elderly appears to justify its use if no other contraindications are present and the amount of myocardium in jeopardy appears to be substantial.

Relative contraindications to fibrinolytic therapy, which require assessment of the risk:benefit ratio, include current use of anticoagulants (international normalized ratio ≥2), a recent (<2 weeks) invasive or surgical procedure or prolonged (>10 min) cardiopulmonary resuscitation, known bleeding diathesis, pregnancy, a hemorrhagic ophthalmic condition (e.g., hemorrhagic diabetic retinopathy), active peptic ulcer disease, and a history of severe hypertension that is currently adequately controlled. Because of the risk of an allergic reaction, patients should not receive streptokinase if that agent had been received within the preceding 5 days to 2 years.

Allergic reactions to streptokinase occur in ~2% of patients who receive it. While a minor degree of hypotension occurs in 4–10% of patients given this agent, marked hypotension occurs, although rarely, in association with severe allergic reactions.

Hemorrhage is the most frequent and potentially the most serious complication. Because bleeding episodes that require transfusion are more common when patients require invasive procedures, unnecessary venous or arterial interventions should be avoided in patients receiving fibrinolytic agents. Hemorrhagic stroke is the most serious complication and occurs in ~0.5–0.9% of patients being treated with these agents. This rate increases with advancing age, with patients >70 years experiencing roughly twice the rate of intracranial hemorrhage as those <65 years. Large-scale trials have suggested that the rate of intracranial hemorrhage with tPA or rPA is slightly higher than with streptokinase.

Cardiac catheterization and coronary angiography should be carried out after fibrinolytic therapy if there is evidence of either (1) failure of reperfusion (persistent chest pain and ST-segment elevation >90 min), in which case a *rescue PCI* should be considered; or (2) coronary artery reocclusion (re-elevation of ST segments and/or recurrent chest pain) or the development of recurrent ischemia (such as recurrent angina in the early hospital course or a positive exercise stress test before discharge), in which case an *urgent PCI* should be considered. The potential benefits of routine angiography and *elective* PCI even in asymptomatic patients following administration of fibrinolytic therapy are controversial, but such an approach may have merit given the numerous technological advances that have occurred in the catheterization laboratory and the increasing number of skilled interventionalists. Coronary artery bypass surgery should be reserved for patients whose coronary anatomy is unsuited to PCI but in whom revascularization appears to be advisable because of extensive jeopardized myocardium or recurrent ischemia.

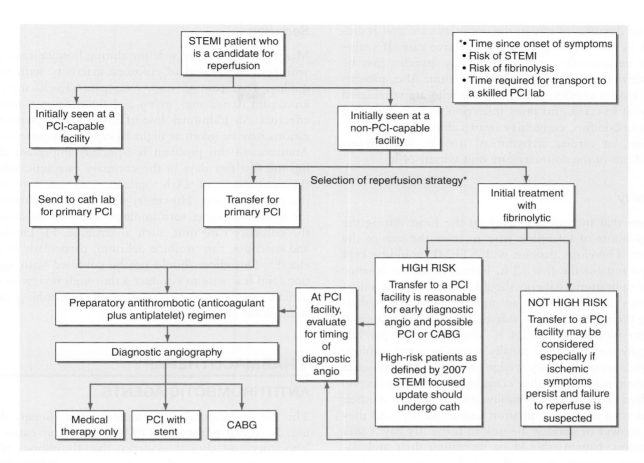

FIGURE 35-5

Each community and each facility in that community should have an agreed-upon plan for how STEMI patients are to be treated that includes which hospitals should receive STEMI patients from EMS units capable of obtaining diagnostic ECGs, management at the initial receiving hospital, and written criteria and agreements for expeditious transfer of patients from non-PCI-capable facilities. Patients initially seen at a PCI-capable facility (left side of diagram) should be sent promptly to the cardiac catheterization laboratory with the intent to perform primary PCI. Patients initially seen at a non-PCI-capable facility (right side of diagram) should rapidly be assessed for the optimum reperfusion therapy (see box in top right corner for assessment criteria). This may include transfer for primary PCI or initial treatment with a fibrinolytic. Following administration of a fibrinolytic, management is dictated by the patient's overall risk for death/serious complications of STEMI, and whether or not they experience recurrent ischemic symptoms or left-ventricular failure (see the two boxes at the bottom right of diagram). (*Adapted from FG Kushner et al: 2009 focused update of the ACC/AHA Guidelines for the Management of Patients with ST-Elevation Myocardial Infarction [updating the 2004 guideline and 2007 focused update]: a report of the American College of Cardiology Foundation/American Heart Association Task Force on Practice Guidelines. Circulation 120:2271, 2009.*)

HOSPITAL PHASE MANAGEMENT

CORONARY CARE UNITS

These units are routinely equipped with a system that permits continuous monitoring of the cardiac rhythm of each patient and hemodynamic monitoring in selected patients. Defibrillators, respirators, noninvasive transthoracic pacemakers, and facilities for introducing pacing catheters and flow-directed balloon-tipped catheters are also usually available. Equally important is the organization of a highly trained team of nurses who can recognize arrhythmias; adjust the dosage of antiarrhythmic, vasoactive, and anticoagulant drugs; and perform cardiac resuscitation, including electroshock, when necessary.

Patients should be admitted to a coronary care unit early in their illness when it is expected that they will derive benefit from the sophisticated and expensive care provided. The availability of electrocardiographic monitoring and trained personnel outside the coronary care unit has made it possible to admit lower-risk patients (e.g., those not hemodynamically compromised and without active arrhythmias) to "intermediate care units."

The duration of stay in the coronary care unit is dictated by the ongoing need for intensive care. If symptoms are controlled with oral therapy, patients may be transferred out of the coronary care unit. Also, patients who have a confirmed STEMI but who are considered to be at low risk (no prior infarction and no persistent chest discomfort, congestive heart failure [CHF], hypotension, or cardiac arrhythmias) may be safely transferred out of the coronary care unit within 24 h.

Activity

Factors that increase the work of the heart during the initial hours of infarction may increase the size of the infarct. Therefore, patients with STEMI should be kept at bed rest for the first 12 h. However, in the absence of complications, patients should be encouraged, under supervision, to resume an upright posture by dangling their feet over the side of the bed and sitting in a chair within the first 24 h. This practice is psychologically beneficial and usually results in a reduction in the pulmonary capillary wedge pressure. In the absence of hypotension and other complications, by the second or third day, patients typically are ambulating in their room with increasing duration and frequency, and they may shower or stand at the sink to bathe. By day 3 after infarction, patients should be increasing their ambulation progressively to a goal of 185 m (600 ft) at least three times a day.

Diet

Because of the risk of emesis and aspiration soon after STEMI, patients should receive either nothing or only clear liquids by mouth for the first 4–12 h. The typical coronary care unit diet should provide ≤30% of total calories as fat and have a cholesterol content of ≤300 mg/d. Complex carbohydrates should make up 50–55% of total calories. Portions should not be unusually large, and the menu should be enriched with foods that are high in potassium, magnesium, and fiber, but low in sodium. Diabetes mellitus and hypertriglyceridemia are managed by restriction of concentrated sweets in the diet.

Bowel management

Bed rest and the effect of the narcotics used for the relief of pain often lead to constipation. A bedside commode rather than a bedpan, a diet rich in bulk, and the routine use of a stool softener such as dioctyl sodium sulfosuccinate (200 mg/d) are recommended. If the patient remains constipated despite these measures, a laxative can be prescribed. Contrary to prior belief, it is safe to perform a gentle rectal examination on patients with STEMI.

Sedation

Many patients require sedation during hospitalization to withstand the period of enforced inactivity with tranquillity. Diazepam (5 mg), oxazepam (15–30 mg), or lorazepam (0.5–2 mg), given 3–4 times daily, is usually effective. An additional dose of any of the above medications may be given at night to ensure adequate sleep. Attention to this problem is especially important during the first few days in the coronary care unit, where the atmosphere of 24-h vigilance may interfere with the patient's sleep. However, sedation is no substitute for reassuring, quiet surroundings. Many drugs used in the coronary care unit, such as atropine, H_2 blockers, and narcotics, can produce delirium, particularly in the elderly. This effect should not be confused with agitation, and it is wise to conduct a thorough review of the patient's medications before arbitrarily prescribing additional doses of anxiolytics.

PHARMACOTHERAPY

ANTITHROMBOTIC AGENTS

The use of antiplatelet and anticoagulant therapy during the initial phase of STEMI is based on extensive laboratory and clinical evidence that thrombosis plays an important role in the pathogenesis of this condition. The primary goal of treatment with antiplatelet and anticoagulant agents is to maintain patency of the infarct-related artery, in conjunction with reperfusion strategies. A secondary goal is to reduce the patient's tendency to thrombosis and, thus, the likelihood of mural thrombus formation or deep venous thrombosis, either of which could result in pulmonary embolization. The degree to which antiplatelet and anticoagulant therapy achieves these goals partly determines how effectively it reduces the risk of mortality from STEMI.

As noted previously (see "Management in the Emergency Department" above), aspirin is the standard antiplatelet agent for patients with STEMI. The most compelling evidence for the benefits of antiplatelet therapy (mainly with aspirin) in STEMI is found in the comprehensive overview by the Antiplatelet Trialists' Collaboration. Data from nearly 20,000 patients with MI enrolled in 15 randomized trials were pooled and revealed a relative reduction of 27% in the mortality rate, from 14.2% in control patients to 10.4% in patients receiving antiplatelet agents.

Inhibitors of the P2Y12 ADP receptor prevent activation and aggregation of platelets. The addition of the P2Y12 inhibitor clopidogrel to background treatment with aspirin to STEMI patients reduces the risk of clinical events (death, reinfarction, stroke) and, in patients receiving fibrinolytic therapy, has been shown to prevent reocclusion of a successfully reperfused infarct artery. New P2Y12 ADP receptor antagonists, such as prasugrel and ticagrelor, are more effective than clopidogrel in preventing ischemic complications in STEMI patients undergoing PCI, but are associated with an increased risk of bleeding. Glycoprotein IIb/IIIa receptor inhibitors appear useful for preventing thrombotic complications in patients with STEMI undergoing PCI.

The standard anticoagulant agent used in clinical practice is unfractionated heparin (UFH). The available data suggest that when UFH is added to a regimen of aspirin and a non–fibrin-specific thrombolytic agent such as streptokinase, additional mortality benefit occurs (about 5 lives saved per 1000 patients treated). It appears that the immediate administration of intravenous UFH, in addition to a regimen of aspirin and relatively fibrin-specific fibrinolytic agents (tPA, rPA, or TNK), helps to maintain patency of the infarct-related artery. This effect is achieved at the cost of a small increased risk of bleeding. The recommended dose of UFH is an initial bolus of 60 U/kg (maximum 4000 U) followed by an initial infusion of 12 U/kg per hour (maximum 1000 U/h). The activated partial thromboplastin time during maintenance therapy should be 1.5–2 times the control value.

Alternatives to UFH for anticoagulation of patients with STEMI are the low-molecular-weight heparin (LMWH) preparations, a synthetic version of the critical pentasaccharide sequence (fondaparinux), and the direct antithrombin bivalirudin. Advantages of LMWHs include high bioavailability permitting administration subcutaneously, reliable anticoagulation without monitoring, and greater antiXa:IIa activity. Enoxaparin has been shown to reduce significantly the composite endpoints of death/nonfatal reinfarction and death/nonfatal reinfarction/urgent revascularization compared with UFH in STEMI patients who receive fibrinolysis. Treatment with enoxaparin is associated with higher rates of serious bleeding, but net clinical benefit—a composite endpoint that combines efficacy and safety—still favors enoxaparin over UFH. Interpretation of the data on fondaparinux is difficult because of the complex nature of the pivotal clinical trial evaluating it in STEMI (OASIS-6). Fondaparinux appears superior to placebo in STEMI patients not receiving reperfusion therapy, but its relative efficacy and safety compared with UFH is less certain. Owing to the risk of catheter thrombosis, fondaparinux should not be used alone at the time of coronary angiography and PCI but should be combined with another anticoagulant with antithrombin activity such as UFH or bivalirudin. Contemporary trials of bivalirudin used an open-label design to evaluate its efficacy and safety compared with UFH plus a glycoprotein IIb/IIIa inhibitor. Bivalirudin was associated with a lower rate of bleeding, largely driven by reductions in vascular access site hematomas ≥5 cm or the administration of blood transfusions.

Patients with an anterior location of the infarction, severe LV dysfunction, heart failure, a history of embolism, two-dimensional echocardiographic evidence of mural thrombus, or atrial fibrillation are at increased risk of systemic or pulmonary thromboembolism. Such individuals should receive full therapeutic levels of anticoagulant therapy (LMWH or UFH) while hospitalized, followed by at least 3 months of warfarin therapy.

BETA-ADRENOCEPTOR BLOCKERS

The benefits of beta blockers in patients with STEMI can be divided into those that occur immediately when the drug is given acutely and those that accrue over the long term when the drug is given for secondary prevention after an infarction. Acute intravenous beta blockade improves the myocardial O_2 supply-demand relationship, decreases pain, reduces infarct size, and decreases the incidence of serious ventricular arrhythmias. In patients who undergo fibrinolysis soon after the onset of chest pain, no incremental reduction in mortality rate is seen with beta blockers, but recurrent ischemia and reinfarction are reduced.

Thus, beta-blocker therapy after STEMI is useful for most patients (including those treated with an angiotensin-converting enzyme [ACE] inhibitor) except those in whom it is specifically contraindicated (patients with heart failure or severely compromised LV function, heart block, orthostatic hypotension, or a history of asthma) and perhaps those whose excellent long-term prognosis (defined as an expected mortality rate of <1% per year, patients <55 years, no previous MI, with normal ventricular function, no complex ventricular ectopy, and no angina) markedly diminishes any potential benefit.

INHIBITION OF THE RENIN-ANGIOTENSIN-ALDOSTERONE SYSTEM

ACE inhibitors reduce the mortality rate after STEMI, and the mortality benefits are additive to those achieved with aspirin and beta blockers. The maximum benefit is seen in high-risk patients (those who are elderly or who have an anterior infarction, a prior infarction, and/or globally depressed LV function), but evidence suggests that a short-term benefit occurs when ACE inhibitors are prescribed unselectively to all hemodynamically stable patients with STEMI (i.e., those with a systolic pressure >100 mmHg). The mechanism involves a reduction in ventricular remodeling after infarction (see "Ventricular Dysfunction," later) with a subsequent reduction in the risk of CHF. The rate of recurrent infarction may also be lower in patients treated chronically with ACE inhibitors after infarction.

Before hospital discharge, LV function should be assessed with an imaging study. ACE inhibitors should be continued indefinitely in patients who have clinically evident CHF, in patients in whom an imaging study shows a reduction in global LV function or a large regional wall motion abnormality, or in those who are hypertensive.

Angiotensin receptor blockers (ARBs) should be administered to STEMI patients who are intolerant of ACE inhibitors and who have either clinical or radiological signs of heart failure. Long-term aldosterone blockade should be prescribed for STEMI patients without significant renal dysfunction (creatinine ≥2.5 mg/dL in men and ≥2.0 mg/dL in women) or hyperkalemia (potassium ≥5.0 mEq/L) who are already receiving therapeutic doses of an ACE inhibitor, an LV ejection fraction ≤40 percent, and either symptomatic heart failure or diabetes mellitus. A multidrug regimen for inhibiting the renin-angiotensin-aldosterone system has been shown to reduce both heart failure–related and sudden cardiac death–related cardiovascular mortality after STEMI, but has not been as thoroughly explored as ACE inhibitors in STEMI patients.

OTHER AGENTS

Favorable effects on the ischemic process and ventricular remodeling (see later) previously led many physicians to routinely use *intravenous nitroglycerin* (5–10 μg/min initial dose and up to 200 μg/min as long as hemodynamic stability is maintained) for the first 24–48 h after the onset of infarction. However, the benefits of routine use of intravenous nitroglycerin are less in the contemporary era where beta-adrenoceptor blockers and ACE inhibitors are routinely prescribed for patients with STEMI.

Results of multiple trials of different calcium antagonists have failed to establish a role for these agents in the treatment of most patients with STEMI. Therefore, the routine use of calcium antagonists cannot be recommended. Strict control of blood glucose in diabetic patients with STEMI has been shown to reduce the mortality rate. Serum magnesium should be measured in all patients on admission, and any demonstrated deficits should be corrected to minimize the risk of arrhythmias.

COMPLICATIONS AND THEIR MANAGEMENT

VENTRICULAR DYSFUNCTION

After STEMI, the left ventricle undergoes a series of changes in shape, size, and thickness in both the infarcted and noninfarcted segments. This process is referred to as *ventricular remodeling* and generally precedes the development of clinically evident CHF in

the months to years after infarction. Soon after STEMI, the left ventricle begins to dilate. Acutely, this results from expansion of the infarct, i.e., slippage of muscle bundles, disruption of normal myocardial cells, and tissue loss within the necrotic zone, resulting in disproportionate thinning and elongation of the infarct zone. Later, lengthening of the noninfarcted segments occurs as well. The overall chamber enlargement that occurs is related to the size and location of the infarct, with greater dilation following infarction of the anterior wall and apex of the left ventricle and causing more marked hemodynamic impairment, more frequent heart failure, and a poorer prognosis. Progressive dilation and its clinical consequences may be ameliorated by therapy with ACE inhibitors and other vasodilators (e.g., nitrates). In patients with an ejection fraction <40%, regardless of whether or not heart failure is present, ACE inhibitors or ARBs should be prescribed (see "Inhibition of the Renin-Angiotensin-Aldosterone System," earlier).

HEMODYNAMIC ASSESSMENT

Pump failure is now the primary cause of in-hospital death from STEMI. The extent of infarction correlates well with the degree of pump failure and with mortality, both early (within 10 days of infarction) and later. The most common clinical signs are pulmonary rales and S₃ and S₄ gallop sounds. Pulmonary congestion is also frequently seen on the chest roentgenogram. Elevated LV filling pressure and elevated pulmonary artery pressure are the characteristic hemodynamic findings, but these findings may result from a reduction of ventricular compliance (diastolic failure) and/or a reduction of stroke volume with secondary cardiac dilation (systolic failure) (Chap. 17).

A classification originally proposed by Killip divides patients into four groups: class I, no signs of pulmonary or venous congestion; class II, moderate heart failure as evidenced by rales at the lung bases, S₃ gallop, tachypnea, or signs of failure of the right side of the heart, including venous and hepatic congestion; class III, severe heart failure, pulmonary edema; and class IV, shock with systolic pressure <90 mmHg and evidence of peripheral vasoconstriction, peripheral cyanosis, mental confusion, and oliguria. When this classification was established in 1967, the expected hospital mortality rate of patients in these classes was as follows: class I, 0–5%; class II, 10–20%; class III, 35–45%; and class IV, 85–95%. With advances in management, the mortality rate in each class has fallen, perhaps by as much as one-third to one-half.

Hemodynamic evidence of abnormal global LV function appears when contraction is seriously impaired in 20–25% of the left ventricle. Infarction of ≥40% of the left ventricle usually results in cardiogenic shock

(Chap. 28). Positioning of a balloon flotation (Swan-Ganz) catheter in the pulmonary artery permits monitoring of LV filling pressure; this technique is useful in patients who exhibit hypotension and/or clinical evidence of CHF. Cardiac output can also be determined with a pulmonary artery catheter. With the addition of intraarterial pressure monitoring, systemic vascular resistance can be calculated as a guide to adjusting vasopressor and vasodilator therapy. Some patients with STEMI have markedly elevated LV filling pressures (>22 mmHg) and normal cardiac indices (2.6–3.6 L/[min/m^2]), while others have relatively low LV filling pressures (<15 mmHg) and reduced cardiac indices. The former patients usually benefit from diuresis, while the latter may respond to volume expansion.

HYPOVOLEMIA

This is an easily corrected condition that may contribute to the hypotension and vascular collapse associated with STEMI in some patients. It may be secondary to previous diuretic use, to reduced fluid intake during the early stages of the illness, and/or to vomiting associated with pain or medications. Consequently, hypovolemia should be identified and corrected in patients with STEMI and hypotension before more vigorous forms of therapy are begun. Central venous pressure reflects RV rather than LV filling pressure and is an inadequate guide for adjustment of blood volume, because LV function is almost always affected much more adversely than RV function in patients with STEMI. The optimal LV filling or pulmonary artery wedge pressure may vary considerably among patients. Each patient's ideal level (generally ~20 mmHg) is reached by cautious fluid administration during careful monitoring of oxygenation and cardiac output. Eventually, the cardiac output level plateaus, and further increases in LV filling pressure only increase congestive symptoms and decrease systemic oxygenation without raising arterial pressure.

TREATMENT	Congestive Heart Failure

The management of CHF in association with STEMI is similar to that of acute heart failure secondary to other forms of heart disease (avoidance of hypoxemia, diuresis, afterload reduction, inotropic support) (Chap. 17), except that the benefits of digitalis administration to patients with STEMI are unimpressive. By contrast, diuretic agents are extremely effective, as they diminish pulmonary congestion in the presence of systolic and/or diastolic heart failure. LV filling pressure falls and orthopnea and dyspnea improve after the intravenous administration of furosemide or other loop diuretics. These drugs should be used with caution, however, as they can result in a massive diuresis with associated decreases in plasma volume, cardiac output, systemic blood pressure, and, hence, coronary perfusion. Nitrates in various forms may be used to decrease preload and congestive symptoms. Oral isosorbide dinitrate, topical nitroglycerin ointment, or intravenous nitroglycerin all have the advantage over a diuretic of lowering preload through venodilation without decreasing the total plasma volume. In addition, nitrates may improve ventricular compliance if ischemia is present, as ischemia causes an elevation of LV filling pressure. Vasodilators must be used with caution to prevent serious hypotension. As noted earlier, ACE inhibitors are an ideal class of drugs for management of ventricular dysfunction after STEMI, especially for the long term. (See "Inhibition of the Renin-Angiotensin-Aldosterone System," earlier.)

CARDIOGENIC SHOCK

Prompt reperfusion, efforts to reduce infarct size and treatment of ongoing ischemia and other complications of MI appear to have reduced the incidence of cardiogenic shock from 20% to about 7%. Only 10% of patients with this condition present with it on admission, while 90% develop it during hospitalization. Typically, patients who develop cardiogenic shock have severe multivessel coronary artery disease with evidence of "piecemeal" necrosis extending outward from the original infarct zone. The evaluation and management of cardiogenic shock and severe power failure after STEMI are discussed in detail in Chap. 28.

RIGHT VENTRICULAR INFARCTION

Approximately one-third of patients with inferior infarction demonstrate at least a minor degree of RV necrosis. An occasional patient with inferoposterior LV infarction also has extensive RV infarction, and rare patients present with infarction limited primarily to the RV. Clinically significant RV infarction causes signs of severe RV failure (jugular venous distention, Kussmaul's sign, hepatomegaly [Chap. 9]) with or without hypotension. ST-segment elevations of right-sided precordial ECG leads, particularly lead V$_4$R, are frequently present in the first 24 h in patients with RV infarction. Two-dimensional echocardiography is helpful in determining the degree of RV dysfunction. Catheterization of the right side of the heart often reveals a distinctive hemodynamic pattern resembling constrictive pericarditis (steep right atrial "y" descent and an early diastolic dip and plateau in RV waveforms) (Chap. 22). Therapy consists of volume expansion to maintain adequate RV preload and efforts to improve LV performance with attendant reduction in pulmonary capillary wedge and pulmonary arterial pressures.

ARRHYTHMIAS

(See also Chaps. 15 and 16) The incidence of arrhythmias after STEMI is higher in patients seen early after the onset of symptoms. The mechanisms responsible for infarction-related arrhythmias include autonomic nervous system imbalance, electrolyte disturbances, ischemia, and slowed conduction in zones of ischemic myocardium. An arrhythmia can usually be managed successfully if trained personnel and appropriate equipment are available when it develops. Since most deaths from arrhythmia occur during the first few hours after infarction, the effectiveness of treatment relates directly to the speed with which patients come under medical observation. The prompt management of arrhythmias constitutes a significant advance in the treatment of STEMI.

Ventricular premature beats

Infrequent, sporadic ventricular premature depolarizations occur in almost all patients with STEMI and do not require therapy. Whereas in the past, frequent, multifocal, or early diastolic ventricular extrasystoles (so-called warning arrhythmias) were routinely treated with antiarrhythmic drugs to reduce the risk of development of ventricular tachycardia and ventricular fibrillation, pharmacologic therapy is now reserved for patients with sustained ventricular arrhythmias. Prophylactic antiarrhythmic therapy (either intravenous lidocaine early or oral agents later) is contraindicated for ventricular premature beats in the absence of clinically important ventricular tachyarrhythmias, as such therapy may actually increase the mortality rate. Beta-adrenoceptor blocking agents are effective in abolishing ventricular ectopic activity in patients with STEMI and in the prevention of ventricular fibrillation. As described earlier (see "Beta-Adrenoceptor Blockers"), they should be used routinely in patients without contraindications. In addition, hypokalemia and hypomagnesemia are risk factors for ventricular fibrillation in patients with STEMI; to reduce the risk, the serum potassium concentration should be adjusted to approximately 4.5 mmol/L and magnesium to about 2.0 mmol/L.

Ventricular tachycardia and fibrillation

Within the first 24 h of STEMI, ventricular tachycardia and fibrillation can occur without prior warning arrhythmias. The occurrence of ventricular fibrillation can be reduced by prophylactic administration of intravenous lidocaine. However, prophylactic use of lidocaine has not been shown to reduce overall mortality from STEMI. In fact, in addition to causing possible noncardiac complications, lidocaine may predispose to an excess risk of bradycardia and asystole. For these reasons, and with earlier treatment of active ischemia, more frequent use of beta-blocking agents, and the nearly universal success of electrical cardioversion or defibrillation, routine prophylactic antiarrhythmic drug therapy *is no longer recommended*.

Sustained ventricular tachycardia that is well tolerated hemodynamically should be treated with an intravenous regimen of amiodarone (bolus of 150 mg over 10 min, followed by infusion of 1.0 mg/min for 6 h and then 0.5 mg/min) or procainamide (bolus of 15 mg/kg over 20–30 min; infusion of 1–4 mg/min); if it does not stop promptly, electroversion should be used (Chap. 16). An unsynchronized discharge of 200–300 J (monophasic waveform; approximately 50% of these energies with biphasic waveforms) is used immediately in patients with ventricular fibrillation or when ventricular tachycardia causes hemodynamic deterioration. Ventricular tachycardia or fibrillation that is refractory to electroshock may be more responsive after the patient is treated with epinephrine (1 mg intravenously or 10 mL of a 1:10,000 solution via the intracardiac route) or amiodarone (a 75–150-mg bolus).

Ventricular arrhythmias, including the unusual form of ventricular tachycardia known as torsades des pointes (Chap. 16), may occur in patients with STEMI as a consequence of other concurrent problems (such as hypoxia, hypokalemia, or other electrolyte disturbances) or of the toxic effects of an agent being administered to the patient (such as digoxin or quinidine). A search for such secondary causes should always be undertaken.

Although the in-hospital mortality rate is increased, the long-term survival is excellent in patients who survive to hospital discharge after *primary* ventricular fibrillation; i.e., ventricular fibrillation that is a primary response to acute ischemia that occurs during the first 48 h and is not associated with predisposing factors such as CHF, shock, bundle branch block, or ventricular aneurysm. This result is in sharp contrast to the poor prognosis for patients who develop ventricular fibrillation *secondary* to severe pump failure. For patients who develop ventricular tachycardia or ventricular fibrillation late in their hospital course (i.e., after the first 48 h), the mortality rate is increased both in-hospital and during long-term follow-up. Such patients should be considered for electrophysiologic study and implantation of a cardioverter/defibrillator (ICD) (Chap. 16). A more challenging issue is the prevention of sudden cardiac death from ventricular fibrillation late after STEMI in patients who have not exhibited sustained ventricular tachyarrhythmias during their index hospitalization. An algorithm for selection of patients who warrant prophylactic implantation of an ICD is shown in **Fig. 35-6**.

Accelerated idioventricular rhythm

Accelerated idioventricular rhythm (AIVR, "slow ventricular tachycardia"), a ventricular rhythm with a rate of 60–100 bpm, often occurs transiently during fibrinolytic therapy at the time of reperfusion. For the most part, AIVR, whether it occurs in association with fibrinolytic

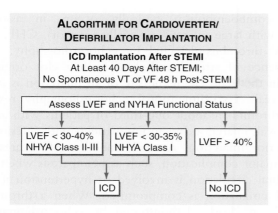

FIGURE 35-6

Algorithm for assessment of need for implantation of a cardioverter/defibrillator. The appropriate management is selected based upon measurement of left ventricular ejection fraction and assessment of the NYHA functional class. Patients with depressed left ventricular function at least 40 days post-STEMI are referred for insertion of an implantable cardioverter/defibrillator (ICD) if the LVEF is <30–40% and they are in NYHA class II–III or if the LVEF is <30–35% and they are in NYHA class I functional status. Patients with preserved left ventricular function (LVEF >40%) do not receive an ICD regardless of NYHA functional class. All patients are treated with medical therapy post-STEMI. (*Adapted from data contained in DP Zipes et al: ACC/AHA/ESC 2006 guidelines for management of patients with ventricular arrhythmias and the prevention of sudden cardiac death; a report of the American College of Cardiology/American Heart Association Task Force and the European Society of Cardiology Committee for Practice Guidelines [Writing Committee to Develop Guidelines for Management of Patients with Ventricular Arrhythmias and the Prevention of Sudden Cardiac Death]. J Am Coll Cardiol 48:1064, 2006.*)

therapy or spontaneously, is benign and does not presage the development of classic ventricular tachycardia. Most episodes of AIVR do not require treatment if the patient is monitored carefully, as degeneration into a more serious arrhythmia is rare.

Supraventricular arrhythmias

Sinus tachycardia is the most common supraventricular arrhythmia. If it occurs secondary to another cause (such as anemia, fever, heart failure, or a metabolic derangement), the primary problem should be treated first. However, if it appears to be due to sympathetic overstimulation (e.g., as part of a hyperdynamic state), then treatment with a beta blocker is indicated. Other common arrhythmias in this group are atrial flutter and atrial fibrillation, which are often secondary to LV failure. Digoxin is usually the treatment of choice for supraventricular arrhythmias if heart failure is present. If heart failure is absent, beta blockers, verapamil, or diltiazem are suitable alternatives for controlling the ventricular rate, as they may also help to control ischemia. If

the abnormal rhythm persists for >2 h with a ventricular rate >120 bpm, or if tachycardia induces heart failure, shock, or ischemia (as manifested by recurrent pain or ECG changes), a synchronized electroshock (100–200 J monophasic waveform) should be used.

Accelerated junctional rhythms have diverse causes but may occur in patients with inferoposterior infarction. Digitalis excess must be ruled out. In some patients with severely compromised LV function, the loss of appropriately timed atrial systole results in a marked reduction of cardiac output. Right atrial or coronary sinus pacing is indicated in such instances.

Sinus bradycardia

Treatment of sinus bradycardia is indicated if hemodynamic compromise results from the slow heart rate. Atropine is the most useful drug for increasing heart rate and should be given intravenously in doses of 0.5 mg initially. If the rate remains <50–60 bpm, additional doses of 0.2 mg, up to a total of 2.0 mg, may be given. Persistent bradycardia (<40 bpm) despite atropine may be treated with electrical pacing. Isoproterenol should be avoided.

Atrioventricular and intraventricular conduction disturbances

(See also Chap. 15) Both the in-hospital mortality rate and the post-discharge mortality rate of patients who have complete atrioventricular (AV) block in association with anterior infarction are markedly higher than those of patients who develop AV block with inferior infarction. This difference is related to the fact that heart block in inferior infarction is commonly a result of increased vagal tone and/or the release of adenosine and therefore is transient. In anterior wall infarction, however, heart block is usually related to ischemic malfunction of the conduction system, which is commonly associated with extensive myocardial necrosis.

Temporary electrical pacing provides an effective means of increasing the heart rate of patients with bradycardia due to AV block. However, acceleration of the heart rate may have only a limited impact on prognosis in patients with anterior wall infarction and complete heart block in whom the large size of the infarct is the major factor determining outcome. It should be carried out if it improves hemodynamics. Pacing does appear to be beneficial in patients with inferoposterior infarction who have complete heart block associated with heart failure, hypotension, marked bradycardia, or significant ventricular ectopic activity. A subgroup of these patients, those with RV infarction, often respond poorly to ventricular pacing because of the loss of the atrial contribution to ventricular filling. In such patients, dual-chamber AV sequential pacing may be required.

External noninvasive pacing electrodes should be positioned in a "demand" mode for patients with sinus bradycardia (rate <50 bpm) that is unresponsive to drug therapy, Mobitz II second-degree AV block, third-degree heart block, or bilateral bundle branch block (e.g., right bundle branch block plus left anterior fascicular block). Retrospective studies suggest that permanent pacing may reduce the long-term risk of sudden death due to bradyarrhythmias in the rare patient who develops combined persistent bifascicular and transient third-degree heart block during the acute phase of MI.

OTHER COMPLICATIONS

Recurrent chest discomfort

Recurrent angina develops in ~25% of patients hospitalized for STEMI. This percentage is even higher in patients who undergo successful fibrinolysis. Because recurrent or persistent ischemia often heralds extension of the original infarct or reinfarction in a new myocardial zone and is associated with a near tripling of mortality after STEMI, patients with these symptoms should be referred for prompt coronary arteriography and mechanical revascularization. Repeat administration of a fibrinolytic agent is an alternative to early mechanical revascularization.

Pericarditis

(See also Chap. 22) Pericardial friction rubs and/or pericardial pain are frequently encountered in patients with STEMI involving the epicardium. This complication can usually be managed with aspirin (650 mg 4 times daily). It is important to diagnose the chest pain of pericarditis accurately, because failure to recognize it may lead to the erroneous diagnosis of recurrent ischemic pain and/or infarct extension, with resulting inappropriate use of anticoagulants, nitrates, beta blockers, or coronary arteriography. When it occurs, complaints of pain radiating to either trapezius muscle is helpful, because such a pattern of discomfort is typical of pericarditis but rarely occurs with ischemic discomfort. Anticoagulants potentially could cause tamponade in the presence of acute pericarditis (as manifested by either pain or persistent rub) and therefore should not be used unless there is a compelling indication.

Thromboembolism

Clinically apparent thromboembolism complicates STEMI in ~10% of cases, but embolic lesions are found in 20% of patients in necropsy series, suggesting that thromboembolism is often clinically silent. Thromboembolism is considered to be an important contributing cause of death in 25% of patients with STEMI who die after admission to the hospital. Arterial emboli originate from LV mural thrombi, while most pulmonary emboli arise in the leg veins.

Thromboembolism typically occurs in association with large infarcts (especially anterior), CHF, and a LV thrombus detected by echocardiography. The incidence of arterial embolism from a clot originating in the ventricle at the site of an infarction is small but real. Two-dimensional echocardiography reveals LV thrombi in about one-third of patients with anterior wall infarction but in few patients with inferior or posterior infarction. Arterial embolism often presents as a major complication, such as hemiparesis when the cerebral circulation is involved or hypertension if the renal circulation is compromised. When a thrombus has been clearly demonstrated by echocardiographic or other techniques or when a large area of regional wall motion abnormality is seen even in the absence of a detectable mural thrombus, systemic anticoagulation should be undertaken (in the absence of contraindications), as the incidence of embolic complications appears to be markedly lowered by such therapy. The appropriate duration of therapy is unknown, but 3–6 months is probably prudent.

Left ventricular aneurysm

The term *ventricular aneurysm* is usually used to describe *dyskinesis* or local expansile paradoxical wall motion. Normally functioning myocardial fibers must shorten more if stroke volume and cardiac output are to be maintained in patients with ventricular aneurysm; if they cannot, overall ventricular function is impaired. True aneurysms are composed of scar tissue and neither predispose to nor are associated with cardiac rupture.

The complications of LV aneurysm do not usually occur for weeks to months after STEMI; they include CHF, arterial embolism, and ventricular arrhythmias. Apical aneurysms are the most common and the most easily detected by clinical examination. The physical finding of greatest value is a double, diffuse, or displaced apical impulse. Ventricular aneurysms are readily detected by two-dimensional echocardiography, which may also reveal a mural thrombus in an aneurysm.

Rarely, myocardial rupture may be contained by a local area of pericardium, along with organizing thrombus and hematoma. Over time, this *pseudoaneurysm* enlarges, maintaining communication with the LV cavity through a narrow neck. Because a pseudoaneurysm often ruptures spontaneously, it should be surgically repaired if recognized.

POSTINFARCTION RISK STRATIFICATION AND MANAGEMENT

Many clinical and laboratory factors have been identified that are associated with an increase in cardiovascular risk after initial recovery from STEMI. Some of the most important factors include persistent ischemia (spontaneous or provoked), depressed LV ejection fraction (<40%), rales above the lung bases on physical examination or congestion on chest radiograph, and symptomatic ventricular arrhythmias. Other features associated with increased risk include a history of previous MI, age >75, diabetes mellitus, prolonged sinus tachycardia, hypotension, ST-segment changes at rest without angina ("silent ischemia"), an abnormal signal-averaged ECG, nonpatency of the infarct-related coronary artery (if angiography is undertaken), and persistent advanced heart block or a new intraventricular conduction abnormality on the ECG. Therapy must be individualized on the basis of the relative importance of the risk(s) present.

The goal of preventing reinfarction and death after recovery from STEMI has led to strategies to evaluate risk after infarction. In stable patients, submaximal exercise stress testing may be carried out before hospital discharge to detect residual ischemia and ventricular ectopy and to provide the patient with a guideline for exercise in the early recovery period. Alternatively, or in addition, a maximal (symptom-limited) exercise stress test may be carried out 4–6 weeks after infarction. Evaluation of LV function is usually warranted as well. Recognition of a depressed LV ejection fraction by echocardiography or radionuclide ventriculography identifies patients who should receive medications to inhibit the renin-angiotensin-aldosterone system. Patients in whom angina is induced at relatively low workloads, those who have a large reversible defect on perfusion imaging or a depressed ejection fraction, those with demonstrable ischemia, and those in whom exercise provokes symptomatic ventricular arrhythmias should be considered at high risk for recurrent MI or death from arrhythmia (Fig. 35-6). Cardiac catheterization with coronary angiography and/or invasive electrophysiologic evaluation is advised.

Exercise tests also aid in formulating an individualized exercise prescription, which can be much more vigorous in patients who tolerate exercise without any of the above-mentioned adverse signs. In addition, predischarge stress testing may provide an important psychological benefit, building the patient's confidence by demonstrating a reasonable exercise tolerance.

In many hospitals, a cardiac rehabilitation program with progressive exercise is initiated in the hospital and continued after discharge. Ideally, such programs should include an educational component that informs patients about their disease and its risk factors.

The usual duration of hospitalization for an uncomplicated STEMI is about 5 days. The remainder of the convalescent phase may be accomplished at home. During the first 1–2 weeks, the patient should be encouraged to increase activity by walking about the house and outdoors in good weather. Normal sexual activity may be resumed during this period. After 2 weeks, the physician must regulate the patient's activity on the basis of exercise tolerance. Most patients will be able to return to work within 2–4 weeks.

SECONDARY PREVENTION

Various secondary preventive measures are at least partly responsible for the improvement in the long-term mortality and morbidity rates after STEMI. Long-term treatment with an antiplatelet agent (usually aspirin) after STEMI is associated with a 25% reduction in the risk of recurrent infarction, stroke, or cardiovascular mortality (36 fewer events for every 1000 patients treated). An alternative antiplatelet agent that may be used for secondary prevention in patients intolerant of aspirin is clopidogrel (75 mg orally daily). ACE inhibitors or ARBs and, in appropriate patients, aldosterone antagonists should be used indefinitely by patients with clinically evident heart failure, a moderate decrease in global ejection fraction, or a large regional wall motion abnormality to prevent late ventricular remodeling and recurrent ischemic events.

The chronic routine use of oral beta-adrenoceptor blockers for at least 2 years after STEMI is supported by well-conducted, placebo-controlled trials.

Evidence suggests that warfarin lowers the risk of late mortality and the incidence of reinfarction after STEMI. Most physicians prescribe aspirin routinely for all patients without contraindications and add warfarin for patients at increased risk of embolism (see "Thromboembolism," earlier). Several studies suggest that in patients <75 years a low dose of aspirin (75–81 mg/d) in combination with warfarin administered to achieve an INR >2.0 is more effective than aspirin alone for preventing recurrent MI and embolic cerebrovascular accident. However, there is an increased risk of bleeding and a high rate of discontinuation of warfarin that has limited clinical acceptance of combination antithrombotic therapy. There is increased risk of bleeding when warfarin is added to dual antiplatelet therapy (aspirin and clopidogrel). However, patients who have had a stent implanted and have an indication for anticoagulation should receive dual antiplatelet therapies in combination with warfarin. Such patients should also receive a proton pump inhibitor to minimize the risk of gastrointestinal bleeding and should have regular monitoring of their hemoglobin levels and stool hematest while on combination antithrombotic therapy.

Finally, risk factors for *atherosclerosis* (Chap. 1) should be discussed with the patient, and, when possible, favorably modified.

CHAPTER 36

PERCUTANEOUS CORONARY INTERVENTIONS AND OTHER INTERVENTIONAL PROCEDURES

David P. Faxon ■ Deepak L. Bhatt

Percutaneous transluminal coronary angioplasty (PTCA) was first introduced by Andreas Gruentzig in 1977 as an alternative to coronary bypass surgery. The concept of percutaneous dilatation of the atherosclerotic peripheral vessels was initially demonstrated by Charles Dotter in 1964 in peripheral vessels where rigid catheters of graduated diameter were used to progressively enlarge the vessel lumen. The development of a small inelastic balloon catheter by Gruentzig allowed expansion of the technique into smaller peripheral and coronary vessels. Initial coronary experience was limited to the small percentage of patients who had single-vessel coronary disease and discrete proximal lesions due to the technical limitations of the equipment. Advances in technology and greater operator experience allowed the procedure to grow rapidly with expanded use in patients with more complex lesions and multivessel disease; by 1990, it was being performed in more than 300,000 patients annually. The addition of atherectomy devices that removed plaques aided in the growth of the procedure, but the introduction of coronary stents in 1994 was one of the major advances in the field. These devices reduced acute complications and reduced by half the significant problem of restenosis (or recurrence of the stenosis). Further reductions in restenosis were achieved by the introduction of drug-eluting stents in 2003. These stents have a polymer coating over the metal stent that is impregnated with antiproliferative agents that slowly release drugs directly into the plaque over a few months. Today, more than 1 million stents are placed in the United States per year and more than 4 million worldwide. Percutaneous coronary intervention (PCI) is the most common revascularization procedure in the United States and is performed nearly twice as often as coronary artery bypass surgery.

The field of interventional cardiology has matured to be recognized as a separate discipline in cardiology that requires specialized training. A dedicated 1-year interventional cardiology fellowship following a 3-year general cardiology fellowship and a separate board certification examination are now required to be certified in interventional cardiology. The discipline has also expanded to include interventions for structural heart disease including treatment of congenital heart disease, and valvular heart disease; it also includes interventions to treat peripheral vascular disease, including atherosclerotic and nonatherosclerotic lesions in the carotid, renal, aortic, and peripheral circulations.

TECHNIQUE

The initial procedure is performed in a similar manner as a diagnostic cardiac catheterization (Chap. 13). As is done with diagnostic catheterization, arterial access is obtained by percutaneous needle puncture into a peripheral artery. Most commonly, the arterial access site is the femoral artery, but radial artery access is gaining favor. To prevent thrombotic complications during the procedure, patients who are anticipated to need an angioplasty are given aspirin (325 mg) and clopidogrel (loading dose of 300–600 mg) before the procedure. During the procedure, anticoagulation is achieved by administration of unfractionated heparin, enoxaparin (a low-molecular-weight heparin), or bivalirudin (a direct thrombin inhibitor). In patients with ST-elevation myocardial infarction, high-risk acute coronary syndrome, or those with a large thrombus in the coronary artery, a glycoprotein IIb/IIIa inhibitor (abciximab, tirofiban, or eptifibatide) may also be given.

Following placement of an introducing sheath, preformed guiding catheters are used to cannulate selectively the origins of the coronary arteries. These catheters have larger internal diameters than diagnostic catheters in

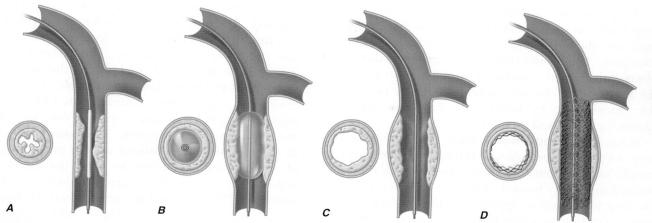

FIGURE 36-1

Schematic diagram of the primary mechanisms of balloon angioplasty and stenting. *A.* A balloon angioplasty catheter is positioned into the stenosis over a guidewire under fluoroscopic guidance. ***B.*** The balloon is inflated temporarily occluding the vessel. ***C.*** The lumen is enlarged primarily by stretching the vessel often resulting in small dissections in the neointima. ***D.*** A stent mounted on a deflated balloon is placed into the lesion and pressed against the vessel wall with balloon inflation (not shown). The balloon is deflated and removed leaving the stent permanently against the wall acting as a scaffold to hold the dissections against the wall and prevent vessel recoil. (*Adapted from EJ Topol: Textbook of Cardiovascular Medicine, 2nd ed. Philadelphia, Lippincott Williams & Wilkins, 2002.*)

order to allow passage of the balloon catheter and wires. Through the guiding catheter, a flexible, steerable guide-wire (diameter 0.4 mm) is negotiated down the coronary artery lumen using fluoroscopic guidance; it is then advanced through the stenosis and into the vessel beyond. This guidewire then serves as a "rail" over which angioplasty balloons, stents, or other therapeutic devices can be advanced to enlarge the narrowed segment of coronary artery. The artery is usually dilated with a balloon catheter and most often a stent is then placed with assessment of the final result by repeat angiography through the guiding catheter. The catheters and introducing sheath are removed and the artery manually held or closed using one of several arterial closure devices to achieve hemostasis. Because PCI is performed under local anesthesia and mild sedation, it requires only a short (1-day) hospitalization that decreases recovery time and hospital expense, as compared to coronary bypass surgery.

The inflated diameter of the angioplasty balloons range in size from 1.5 to 4.0 mm, and balloons are chosen to approximate the "normal" less diseased proximal or distal vessel without stenosis. The major advance introduced by Dr. Gruentzig was the use of inelastic balloons that do not overexpand the vessel beyond their predetermined size despite high pressures up to 10–20 atmospheres.

Angioplasty works by stretching the artery and compressing the plaque into the vessel wall, away from the lumen, enlarging the entire vessel (**Figs. 36-1** and **36-2**). The procedure rarely results in embolization of atherosclerotic material. Owing to inelastic elements

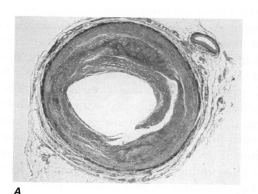

FIGURE 36-2

Pathology of acute effects of balloon angioplasty with intimal dissection and vessel stretching (*panel A*) (*From M Ueda et al: Eur Heart J 12:937, 1991; with permission*) and an example of neointimal hyperplasia and restenosis showing renarrowing of the vessel (*panel B*). (*From CE Essed et al: Br Heart J 49:393, 1983; with permission.*)

in the plaque, the stretching of the vessel by the balloon results in small localized dissections that can protrude into the lumen and be a nidus for acute thrombus formation. If the dissections are severe, then they can obstruct the lumen or induce a thrombotic occlusion of the artery (acute closure). Stents have largely prevented this complication by holding the dissection flaps up against the vessel wall (Fig. 36-1).

Stents are currently used in more than 90% of coronary angioplasty procedures. Stents are wire meshes (usually made of stainless steel) that are compressed over a deflated angioplasty balloon. When the balloon is inflated, the stent is enlarged to approximate the "normal" vessel lumen. The balloon is then deflated and removed, leaving the stent behind to provide a permanent scaffold in the artery. Owing to the design of the struts, these devices are flexible, allowing their passage through diseased and tortuous coronary vessels. Stents are rigid enough to prevent elastic recoil of the vessel and have dramatically improved the success and safety of the procedure as a result.

Drug-eluting stents were first introduced in 2003. Using a metal stent, an antiproliferative agent is attached to the stent by use of a thin polymer coating. The antiproliferative drug elutes from the stent over a 1- to 3-month period after implantation. Drug-eluting stents have been shown to reduce clinical restenosis by 50% so that in uncomplicated lesions symptomatic restenosis occurs in 5–12% of patients. Not surprisingly, this led to the rapid acceptance of these devices; currently 50–90% of all stents implanted are drug-eluting. The first-generation devices were coated with either sirolimus or paclitaxel. *Sirolimus* is an immunosuppressive agent that arrests cell proliferation in the G_1 phase. *Paclitaxel* is an inhibitor of microtubules that can arrest cell division at the M phase in high concentrations, but can have cytostatic G_1, antimigratory, and antiinflammatory effects on smooth-muscle cells at lower concentrations. Second-generation drug-eluting stents use newer agents such as everolimus, biolimus, and zotarolimus. These second-generation drug-eluting stents appear to be more effective with fewer complications than the first-generation devices. Preliminary data from long-term follow-up suggests that the second-generation drug-eluting stents have lower rates of stent thrombosis and myocardial infarction than the first-generation drug-eluting stents.

Other interventional devices include atherectomy devices, laser catheters, and thrombectomy catheters. These devices are designed to remove atherosclerotic plaque or thrombus and are used in conjunction with balloon dilatation and stent placement. Rotational atherectomy is the most commonly used adjunctive device for heavily calcified lesions and is modeled after a dentist's drill, with small round burrs of 1.5–2.5 mm at the tip of a flexible wire shaft. They are passed over the guidewire up to the stenosis and activated to rotate at 180,000 rpm in order to drill away atherosclerotic material. Because the atherosclerotic particles are <25 μm, they pass through the coronary microcirculation and rarely cause problems. The device is particularly useful in heavily calcified plaques that are resistant to balloon dilatation. Another available device is the directional atherectomy catheter. This catheter has a rigid housing at its tip that is open on one side, exposing a sliding rotating cutter. The catheter is placed in the stenosis, and a balloon on the noncutting side of the housing is inflated to push the housing up against the wall of the artery. When the cutter is rotated at 2500 rpm and advanced down the housing, it slices off atherosclerotic plaques into a distal collection chamber, allowing the plaque to be removed from the patient. Given the current advances in stents, neither rotational nor directional atherectomy is as frequently used today as in the past. Other devices include fiberoptic laser catheters that can vaporize atherosclerotic plaques. These are infrequently used today, as well. In acute myocardial infarction, specialized catheters without a balloon are used to aspirate thrombus in order to prevent embolization down the coronary vessel and to improve blood flow before angioplasty and stent placement. Data suggest that manual catheter thrombus aspiration may even reduce mortality rate in primary PCI.

PCI of degenerated saphenous vein graft lesions has been associated with a significant incidence of distal embolization of atherosclerotic material, unlike PCI of native vessel disease. A number of distal protection devices have been shown to significantly reduce embolization and myocardial infarction in this setting. Most devices work by using a collapsible wire mesh at the end of a guidewire that is expanded in the distal vessel before angioplasty. If atherosclerotic debris is dislodged, the basket captures the material, and at the end of the PCI, the basket is pulled into a delivery catheter and the debris safely removed from the patient.

SUCCESS AND COMPLICATIONS

The advances in the technology have greatly improved the success and reduced the complications of the procedure. Currently, a successful procedure (angiographic success), defined as a reduction of the stenosis to less than a 20% diameter narrowing, occurs in 95–99% of patients. The success is dependent upon the coronary anatomy, with lower success rates in patients with tortuous, small, or calcified vessels or chronic total occlusions. Chronic total occlusions have the lowest success rates and their recanalization is usually not attempted unless the occlusion is recent (within 3 months) or there are favorable anatomic features. Improvements in equipment and technique have increased the success rates of recanalization of chronic total occlusions.

Serious complications are rare but include a mortality rate of 0.1–0.3% for elective cases, a large myocardial infarction occurs in less than 3%, and stroke in less than 0.1%. Patients who are elderly (>65 years), undergoing an emergent or urgent procedure, have chronic kidney disease, present with an ST-segment elevation myocardial infarction (STEMI), or are in shock have a significantly higher risk. Scoring systems can help to estimate the risk of the procedure, although no perfect scoring system has yet been developed.

Myocardial infarction during PCI can occur for multiple reasons including an acute occluding thrombus, severe coronary dissection, embolization of thrombus or atherosclerotic material, or closure of a side branch vessel at the site of angioplasty. Most myocardial infarctions are small and only detected by a rise in the creatinine phosphokinase (CPK) or troponin level after the procedure. Only those with significant enzyme elevations (more than three times the upper limit of normal) are associated with a less favorable long-term outcome. Coronary stents have largely prevented coronary dissections due to the scaffolding effect of the stent. Metallic stents are also prone to thrombotic occlusion (1–3%), either acute (<24 h) or subacute (1–30 days), which can be ameliorated by greater attention to full initial stent deployment and the use of dual antiplatelet therapy (aspirin, plus a platelet P_2Y_{12}-receptor blocker [clopidogrel or prasugrel]). Late (30 days–1 year) and very late stent thromboses (>1 year) occur very infrequently with stents but are slightly more common with drug-eluting stents, necessitating dual antiplatelet therapy with these stents for up to 1 year or longer. Premature discontinuation of dual antiplatelet therapy particularly in the first month after implantation is associated with a significantly increased risk for stent thrombosis (three- to ninefold greater). Stent thrombosis results in death in 10–20% and a myocardial infarction in 30–70% of patients. Elective surgery that requires discontinuation of antiplatelet therapy after drug-eluting stent implantation should be postponed until after 6 months and preferably after 1 year, if at all possible.

Restenosis, or renarrowing of the dilated coronary stenosis, is the most common complication of angioplasty and occurs in 20–50% of patients with balloon angioplasty alone, 10–30% of patients with bare metal stents, and in 5–15% of patients with drug-eluting stents. The fact that stent placement provides a larger acute luminal area than balloon angioplasty alone reduces the incidence of subsequent restenosis. Drug-eluting stents further reduce restenosis through a reduction in excessive neointimal growth over the stent. If restenosis does not occur, the long-term outcome is excellent (**Fig. 36-3**). Clinical restenosis is recognized by recurrence of angina or symptoms within 9 months of the procedure. Most commonly, patients with clinical restenosis present with worsening angina (60–70%), but patients can present with non-ST-elevation

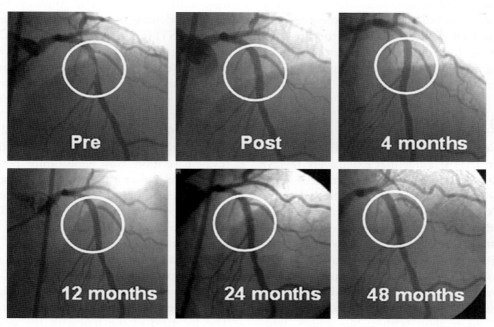

FIGURE 36-3

Long-term results from one of the first patients to receive a sirolimus-eluting stent from early Sao Paulo experience. (*From: GW Stone, in D Baim [ed]: Cardiac Catheterization,* *Angiography and Intervention, 7th ed, Philadelphia, Lippincott Williams & Wilkins, 2006; with permission.*)

myocardial infarction (10%) or ST-elevation myocardial infarction (5%) as well. Clinical restenosis requires confirmation of a significant stenosis at the site of the prior PCI, with repeat PCI or coronary artery bypass grafting (CABG). This is termed *target lesion revascularization* (TLR) or *target vessel revascularization* (TVR). By angiography, the incidence of restenosis is significantly higher than clinical restenosis (TLR or TVR) because many patients have mild restenosis that does not result in a recurrence of symptoms. The management of clinical restenosis is usually to repeat the PCI with balloon dilatation and, placement of a bare metal or a drug-eluting stent. Rarely, intracoronary brachytherapy using beta radiation is used. Once a patient has had restenosis, the risk of a second restenosis is further increased. The risk factors for restenosis are diabetes, long lesions, small-diameter vessels, and suboptimal initial PCI result.

The mechanism of restenosis is similar to that of wound healing, with inflammation and the migration and proliferation of smooth-muscle cells that create a thick neointima (scar) that narrows the lumen at the site of dilatation (Fig. 36-2). The neointima is covered with endothelium, but it remains dysfunctional. The primary cause of restenosis in balloon angioplasty is adverse vessel remodeling with constriction of the vessel relative to the adjacent nondilated vessel. This change in remodeling can be appreciated by intravascular ultrasound but not by angiography since the latter only shows the lumen and not the entire vessel size. In addition to remodeling, excessive growth of the neointima further narrows the lumen. Stents prevent this unfavorable constrictive remodeling, and drug-eluting stents not only prevent this constriction but reduce the excessive neointimal growth as well. Common risk factors for atherosclerosis such as hyperlipidemia, hypertension, or cigarette smoking do not increase the risk of restenosis, although diabetes mellitus does.

INDICATIONS

The American College of Cardiology (ACC)/American Heart Association (AHA) guidelines extensively review the indications for PCI in patients with stable angina, unstable angina, non-ST-elevation, and ST-elevation myocardial infarction and should be referred to for a comprehensive discussion of the indications. Briefly, the two principal indications for coronary revascularization in patients with *chronic stable angina* (Chap. 33) are (1) to improve anginal symptoms in patients who remain symptomatic despite adequate medical therapy and (2) to reduce mortality rates in patients with severe coronary disease. In patients with stable angina, who are well controlled on medical therapy, older studies and the more current Clinical Outcomes Utilizing Revascularization and Aggressive Drug Evaluation

(COURAGE) and Bypass Angioplasty Revascularization Investigation 2 Diabetes (BARI 2D) trials have shown that revascularization does not lead to better outcomes and can be safely delayed until symptoms worsen or evidence of severe ischemia on noninvasive testing occurs. Randomized trials done in the 1960s and 1970s showed that CABG reduced mortality rates in patients with severe three-vessel or left main coronary disease when compared with medical therapy alone regardless of the degree of symptoms. Whether PCI also confers the same degree of protection is not known as trials of PCI versus medical therapy in patients with three-vessel disease have not been conducted, but randomized trials comparing CABG and PCI have shown equal rates of death and myocardial infarction (MI) rates over 5–10 years of follow-up. Consistently these studies have also shown that PCI, despite the use of stents, is associated with a 10–30% need for repeat PCI during the first year after the procedure due largely to restenosis, although drug-eluting stents have decreased this rate. This contrasts with a need for PCI or repeat CABG in bypass patients of 2–5%.

When revascularization is indicated, the choice of PCI or CABG depends upon a number of clinical and anatomic factors (Fig. 36-4). A subgroup analysis from the Bypass Angioplasty Revascularization Investigation (BARI) randomized trial showed that patients with treated diabetes mellitus and multivessel disease fared better with CABG; however, registry experiences suggest that PCI can be done in selected diabetic patients with less-severe multivessel disease with good long-term outcome. The Synergy between Percutaneous Coronary Intervention with Taxus and Cardiac Surgery (SYNTAX) trial compared PCI with the paclitaxel drug-eluting stent to CABG in 1800 patients with three-vessel coronary disease or left main disease. The study found no difference in death or myocardial infarction at 1 year, but repeat revascularization was significantly higher in the stent-treated group (13.5% vs. 5.9%), while stroke was higher in the surgical group (2.2% vs. 0.6%). The primary endpoint of death, MI, stroke, or revascularization was significantly better with CABG due to the higher rate of revascularization in the drug-eluting stent group. Only 1 year of results are currently available and longer follow-up is needed to assess fully these two revascularization strategies in patients with severe coronary disease.

The choice of PCI versus CABG is also related to the anticipated procedural success and complications of PCI and the risks of CABG. For PCI, the characteristics of the coronary anatomy are critically important. The location of the lesion in the vessel (proximal or distal), the degree of tortuosity, and size of the vessel are considered. In addition, the lesion characteristics including the degree of the stenosis, the presence

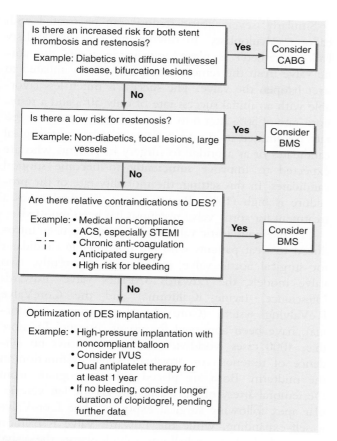

FIGURE 36-4

In patients requiring revascularization, several factors need to be considered in choosing between bare metal stents, drug-eluting stents, or coronary artery bypass surgery. ACS, acute coronary syndrome; BMS, bare metal stent; CABG, coronary artery bypass grafting; DES, drug-eluting stent; IVUS, intravascular ultrasound; STEMI, ST-segment elevation myocardial infarction. (*From AA Bavry, DL Bhatt: Circulation 116:696, 2007; with permission.*)

of calcium, lesion length, and presence of thrombus are assessed. The most common reason to decide not to do angioplasty is that the lesion felt to be responsible for the patient's symptoms is not treatable. This is most commonly due to the presence of a chronic total occlusion (>3 months in duration). In this setting, the historical success rate has been low (30–70%) and complications are more common. A lesion classification to characterize the likelihood of success or failure of PCI has been developed by the ACC/AHA. Lesions with the highest success are called type A lesions (such as proximal noncalcified subtotal lesion) and those with the lowest success or highest complication rate are type C lesions (such as chronic total occlusions). Intermediate lesions are classified as type B1 or B2 depending on the number of unfavorable characteristics. Approximately 25–30% of patients will not be candidates for PCI due to unfavorable anatomy,

whereas only 5% of CABG patients will not be candidates for surgery due to coronary anatomy. The primary reason for being considered inoperable is the presence of severe comorbidities such as advanced age, frailty, severe chronic obstructive pulmonary disease (COPD), or poor left ventricular function. Another consideration in choosing a revascularization strategy is the degree of revascularization. In patients with multivessel disease, bypass grafts can usually be placed in all vessels with significant stenosis, while PCI may be able to treat only some of the lesions due to the presence of unfavorable anatomy. The decision to do PCI versus CABG will then depend upon the importance of complete revascularization in the patient. Given the multiple factors that need to be considered in choosing the best revascularization for an individual patient with multivessel disease, it is optimal to have a discussion between the cardiac surgeon and interventional cardiologist and the physicians caring for the patient to properly weigh the choices.

Patients with acute coronary syndrome are at excess risk of short- and long-term mortality. Randomized clinical trials have shown that PCI is superior to intensive medical therapy in reducing mortality rate and myocardial infarction, with the benefit largely confined to those patients who are high risk. This includes patients with refractory ischemia, recurrent angina, positive cardiac-specific enzymes, new ST-segment depression, low ejection fraction, severe arrhythmias, or a recent PCI or CABG. PCI is preferred over surgical therapy in most high-risk patients with acute coronary syndromes unless they have severe multivessel disease or the culprit lesion responsible for the unstable presentation cannot be adequately treated. In STEMI, thrombolysis or PCI (primary PCI) are effective methods to restore coronary blood flow and salvage myocardium within the first 12 h after onset of chest pain. Because PCI is more effective than thrombolysis, it is preferred if readily available. PCI is also performed following thrombolysis to facilitate adequate reperfusion or as a rescue procedure in those who do not achieve reperfusion from thrombolysis or in those who develop cardiogenic shock.

OTHER INTERVENTIONAL TECHNIQUES
Structural heart disease

Interventional treatment for structural heart disease (adult congenital heart disease and valvular heart disease) is a significant component of the field of interventional cardiology.

The most common adult congenital lesion to be treated with percutaneous techniques is closure of atrial septal defects (Chap. 19). The procedure is done as in a diagnostic right heart catheterization with the passage of a catheter up the femoral vein into the right atrium. With echo and fluoroscopic guidance the size and location of the defect can be accurately defined, and closure is accomplished using one of several approved devices. All devices use a left atrial and right atrial wire mesh or covered disk that are pulled together to capture the atrial septum around the defect and seal it off. The Amplatzer Septal Occluder device (AGA Medical, Minneapolis, Minnesota) is the most commonly used in the United States. The success rate in selected patients is 85–95%, and the device complications are rare and include device embolization, infection, or erosion. Closure of patent foramen ovale (PFO) is done in a similar way. PFO closure is an approved procedure in patients who have had recurrent paradoxical stroke despite adequate medical therapy including anticoagulation. The use in the treatment of migraine is under clinical investigation and is not an approved indication.

Similar devices can also be used to close patent ductus arteriosus and ventricular septal defects. Other congenital diseases that can be treated percutaneously include coarctation of the aorta, pulmonic stenosis, peripheral pulmonary stenosis, and other abnormal communications between the cardiac chambers or vessels.

The treatment of valvular heart disease is the most rapidly growing area in interventional cardiology. Until recently the only available techniques were balloon valvuoplasty for the treatment of aortic, mitral, or pulmonic stenosis (Chap. 20). Mitral valvuloplasty is the preferred treatment for symptomatic patients with rheumatic mitral stenosis who have favorable anatomy. The outcome in these patients is equal to that of surgical commissurotomy. The success is highly related to the echocardiographic appearance of the valve. The most favorable setting is commissural fusion without calcification or subchordal fusion and the absence of significant mitral regurgitation. Access is obtained from the femoral vein using a transseptal technique where a long metal catheter with a needle tip is advanced from the femoral vein through the right atrium and atrial septum at the level of the foramen ovale into the left atrium. A guidewire is advanced into the left ventricle, and a balloon-dilatation catheter is negotiated across the mitral valve and inflated to a predetermined size to enlarge the valve. The most commonly used dilatation catheter is the Inoue balloon. The technique splits the commissural fusion and commonly results in a doubling of the mitral valve area. The success of the procedure in favorable anatomy is 95% and severe complications are rare (1–2%). The most common complications are tamponade due to puncture into the pericardium and the creation of severe mitral regurgitation.

Similarly, severe aortic stenosis can be treated with balloon valvuloplasty. In this setting, the valvuloplasty balloon catheter is placed retrograde across the aortic valve from the femoral artery and briefly inflated to stretch open the valve. The success is much less favorable with an initial success rate of only 50% and a restenosis rate of 50% after 6 to 12 months. This poor success rate has limited its use to patients who are not surgical candidates or as a bridge to surgery in patients who are expected to improve sufficiently to become surgical candidates. In this setting, the mortality rate of the procedure is high (10%). Repeat aortic valvuloplasty as a treatment for aortic valve restenosis has been reported.

Percutaneous aortic valve replacement has been introduced to treat patients who are not suitable candidates for surgical aortic valve replacement. Currently, two valve models, the Edwards SAPIEN valve (Edwards Lifescience, Irvine, California) and the CoreValve ReValving system (CoreValve Inc., Irvine, California), have been approved for use in Europe. In more than 4000 cases worldwide, follow-up shows no evidence of restenosis or prosthetic valve dysfunction in the midterm. Both are placed either retrograde from the femoral artery or can be placed via the left ventricular apex following surgical exposure. The CoreValve is self-expanding, while the Edwards valve is balloon expanded. Following balloon valvuloplasty, the valve is positioned across the valve and deployed with post-deployment balloon inflation to ensure full contact with the aortic annulus. The success rate is 80–90% and the 30-day mortality rate is 10–15%, not unexpectedly as only high-risk patients are undergoing the procedure currently. Both valves are undergoing clinical testing in the United States.

PERIPHERAL ARTERIAL INTERVENTIONS

The use of percutaneous interventions to treat symptomatic patients with arterial obstruction in the carotid, renal, aortic, and peripheral vessels is also part of the field of interventional cardiology. Randomized clinical trial data already support the use of carotid stenting in patients at high risk of complications from carotid endarterectomy (Fig. 36-5). Ongoing trials will determine whether carotid stenting should be used even more broadly. The success rate of peripheral interventional procedures has been improving, including for long segments of occlusive disease historically treated by peripheral bypass surgery (Fig. 36-6). Peripheral intervention is increasingly part of the training of an interventional cardiologist, and most programs now require an additional year of training after the interventional cardiology training year. The techniques and outcomes are described in detail in the chapter on peripheral vascular disease (Chap. 39).

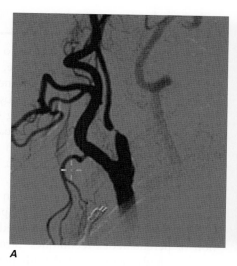
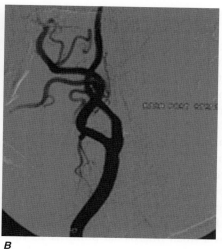

FIGURE 36-5

An example of a high-risk patient who requires carotid revascularization, but who is not a candidate for carotid endarterectomy. Carotid artery stenting resulted in an excellent angiographic result. (*From M Belkin, DL Bhatt: Circulation 119:2302, 2009; with permission.*)

Circulatory support techniques

The use of circulatory support techniques is occasionally needed in order to safely perform PCI on hemodynamically unstable patients. It also can be useful in helping to stabilize patients before surgical interventions. The most commonly used device is the percutaneous intraaortic balloon developed in the early 1960s. A 7-10 French 25- to 40-mL balloon catheter is placed retrograde from the femoral artery into the descending aorta between the aortic arch and the abdominal aortic bifurcation. It is connected to a helium gas inflation system that synchronizes the

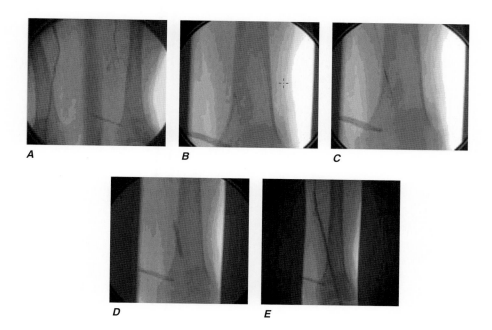

FIGURE 36-6

Peripheral interventional procedures have become highly effective at treating anatomic lesions previously amenable only to bypass surgery. A. Complete occlusion of the left superficial femoral artery. **B.** Wire and catheter advanced into subintimal space. **C.** Intravascular ultrasound positioned in the subintimal space to guide retrograde wire placement through the occluded vessel. **D.** Balloon dilation of the occlusion. **E.** Stent placement with excellent angiographic result. (*From A Al Mahameed, DL Bhatt: Cleve Clin J Med 73:S45, 2006; with permission.*)

inflation to coincide with early diastole with deflation by mid-diastole. As a result, it increases early diastolic pressure, lowers systolic pressure, and lowers late diastolic pressure through displacement of blood from the descending aorta (counterpulsation). This results in an increase in coronary blood flow and a decrease in afterload. It is contraindicated in patients with aortic regurgitation, aortic dissection, or severe peripheral vascular disease. The major complications are vascular and thrombotic. Intravenous heparin is given in order to reduce thrombotic complications.

Another useful tool is the Impella device (Abiomed, Danvers, Massachusetts). The catheter is placed percutaneously from the femoral artery into the left ventricle. The catheter has a small microaxial pump at its tip that can pump up to 2.5 liters per minute at a speed of 50,000 rpm from the left ventricle to the aorta. Other support devices include the hemopump and percutaneous cardiopulmonary bypass.

CONCLUSIONS

Interventional cardiology continues to expand its borders. Treatment for coronary artery disease, including complex anatomic subsets, continues to advance, encroaching on what has traditionally been treated by CABG. Technological advances such as drug-eluting stents, now already in their second generation, and manual aspiration devices are improving the results of PCI. In particular, the data for PCI preventing future ischemic events in unstable ischemic syndromes are substantial. For patients with stable coronary disease, PCI has an important role in symptom alleviation. Treatment of peripheral and cerebrovascular disease has also benefited from the application of percutaneous techniques. Structural heart disease is increasingly being treated with percutaneous options, with a high likelihood that interventional approaches will supplant open-heart surgery in a significant proportion of cases in years to come.

CHAPTER 37
HYPERTENSIVE VASCULAR DISEASE

Theodore A. Kotchen

Hypertension is one of the leading causes of the global burden of disease. Approximately 7.6 million deaths (13–15% of the total) and 92 million disability-adjusted life years worldwide were attributable to high blood pressure in 2001. Hypertension doubles the risk of cardiovascular diseases, including coronary heart disease (CHD), congestive heart failure (CHF), ischemic and hemorrhagic stroke, renal failure, and peripheral arterial disease. It often is associated with additional cardiovascular disease risk factors, and the risk of cardiovascular disease increases with the total burden of risk factors. Although antihypertensive therapy clearly reduces the risks of cardiovascular and renal disease, large segments of the hypertensive population are either untreated or inadequately treated.

EPIDEMIOLOGY

Blood pressure levels, the rate of age-related increases in blood pressure, and the prevalence of hypertension vary among countries and among subpopulations within a country. Hypertension is present in all populations except for a small number of individuals living in primitive, culturally isolated societies. In industrialized societies, blood pressure increases steadily during the first two decades of life. In children and adolescents, blood pressure is associated with growth and maturation. Blood pressure "tracks" over time in children and between adolescence and young adulthood. In the United States, average systolic blood pressure is higher for men than for women during early adulthood, although among older individuals the age-related rate of rise is steeper for women. Consequently, among individuals age 60 and older, systolic blood pressures of women are higher than those of men. Among adults, diastolic blood pressure also increases progressively with age until ~55 years, after which it tends to decrease. The consequence is a widening of pulse pressure (the difference between systolic and diastolic blood pressure) beyond age 60. The probability that a middle-aged or elderly individual will develop hypertension in his or her lifetime is 90%.

In the United States, based on results of the National Health and Nutrition Examination Survey (NHANES), approximately 30% (age-adjusted prevalence) of adults, or at least 65 million individuals, have hypertension (defined as any one of the following: systolic blood pressure ≥140 mmHg, diastolic blood pressure ≥90 mmHg, taking antihypertensive medications). Hypertension prevalence is 33.5% in non-Hispanic blacks, 28.9% in non-Hispanic whites, and 20.7% in Mexican Americans. The likelihood of hypertension increases with age, and among individuals age ≥60, the prevalence is 65.4%. Recent evidence suggests that the prevalence of hypertension in the United States may be increasing, possibly as a consequence of increasing obesity. The prevalence of hypertension and stroke mortality rates are higher in the southeastern United States than in other regions. In African Americans, hypertension appears earlier, is generally more severe, and results in higher rates of morbidity and mortality from stroke, left ventricular hypertrophy, CHF, and end-stage renal disease (ESRD) than in white Americans.

Both environmental and genetic factors may contribute to regional and racial variations in blood pressure and hypertension prevalence. Studies of societies undergoing "acculturation" and studies of migrants from a less to a more urbanized setting indicate a profound environmental contribution to blood pressure. Obesity and weight gain are strong, independent risk factors for hypertension. It has been estimated that 60% of hypertensives are >20% overweight. Among populations, hypertension prevalence is related to dietary NaCl intake, and the age-related increase in blood pressure may be augmented by a high NaCl intake. Low dietary intakes of calcium and potassium also may contribute to the risk of hypertension. The urine sodium-to-potassium ratio is a stronger correlate of blood pressure than is either sodium or potassium alone. Alcohol consumption, psychosocial stress, and low levels of physical activity also may contribute to hypertension.

Adoption, twin, and family studies document a significant heritable component to blood pressure levels and hypertension. Family studies controlling for a common environment indicate that blood pressure heritabilities are in the range 15–35%. In twin studies, heritability estimates of blood pressure are ~60% for males and 30–40% for females. High blood pressure before age 55 occurs 3.8 times more frequently among persons with a positive family history of hypertension.

GENETIC CONSIDERATIONS

Although specific genetic variants have been identified in rare Mendelian forms of hypertension (Table 37-5), these variants are not applicable to the vast majority (>98%) of patients with essential hypertension. For most individuals, it is likely that hypertension represents a polygenic disorder in which a combination of genes acts in concert with environmental exposures to make only a modest contribution to blood pressure. Further, different subsets of genes may lead to different phenotypes associated with hypertension, e.g., obesity, dyslipidemia, insulin resistance.

Several strategies are being utilized in the search for specific hypertension-related genes. Animal models (including selectively bred rats and congenic rat strains) provide a powerful approach for evaluating genetic loci and genes associated with hypertension. Comparative mapping strategies allow for the identification of syntenic genomic regions between the rat and human genomes that may be involved in blood pressure regulation. In association studies, different alleles (or combinations of alleles at different loci) of specific candidate genes or chromosomal regions are compared in hypertensive patients and normotensive control subjects. Current evidence suggests that genes that encode components of the renin-angiotensin-aldosterone system, along with angiotensinogen and angiotensin-converting enzyme (ACE) polymorphisms, may be related to hypertension and to blood pressure sensitivity to dietary NaCl. The alpha-adducin gene is thought to be associated with increased renal tubular absorption of sodium, and variants of this gene may be associated with hypertension and salt sensitivity of blood pressure. Other genes possibly related to hypertension include genes encoding the AT_1 receptor, aldosterone synthase, and the β_2 adrenoreceptor. Genomewide association studies involve rapidly scanning markers across the entire genome to identify loci (not specific genes) associated with an observable trait (e.g., blood pressure) or a particular disease. This strategy has been facilitated by the availability of dense genotyping chips and the International HapMap. To date, the results of candidate gene studies often have not been replicated, and in contrast to several other polygenic disorders, genomewide association studies have had limited success in identifying genetic determinants of hypertension.

Preliminary evidence suggests that there may also be genetic determinants of target organ damage attributed to hypertension. Family studies indicate significant heritability of left ventricular mass, and there is considerable individual variation in the responses of the heart to hypertension. Family studies and variations in candidate genes associated with renal damage suggest that genetic factors also may contribute to hypertensive nephropathy. Specific genetic variants have been linked to CHD and stroke.

In the future, it is possible that DNA analysis will predict individual risk for hypertension and target organ damage and will identify responders to specific classes of antihypertensive agents. However, with the exception of the rare, monogenic hypertensive diseases, the genetic variants associated with hypertension remain to be confirmed, and the intermediate steps by which these variants affect blood pressure remain to be determined.

MECHANISMS OF HYPERTENSION

To provide a framework for understanding the pathogenesis of and treatment options for hypertensive disorders, it is useful to understand factors involved in the regulation of both normal and elevated arterial pressure. Cardiac output and peripheral resistance are the two determinants of arterial pressure (Fig. 37-1). Cardiac output is determined by stroke volume and heart rate; stroke volume is related to myocardial contractility and to the size of the vascular compartment. Peripheral resistance is determined by functional and anatomic changes in small arteries (lumen diameter 100–400 μm) and arterioles.

INTRAVASCULAR VOLUME

Vascular volume is a primary determinant of arterial pressure over the long term. Sodium is predominantly an extracellular ion and is a primary determinant of the

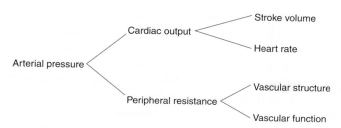

FIGURE 37-1
Determinants of arterial pressure.

extracellular fluid volume. When NaCl intake exceeds the capacity of the kidney to excrete sodium, vascular volume initially expands and cardiac output increases. However, many vascular beds (including kidney and brain) have the capacity to autoregulate blood flow, and if constant blood flow is to be maintained in the face of increased arterial pressure, resistance within that bed must increase, since

$$\text{Blood flow} = \frac{\text{pressure across the vascular bed}}{\text{vascular resistance}}.$$

The initial elevation of blood pressure in response to vascular volume expansion may be related to an increase of cardiac output; however, over time, peripheral resistance increases and cardiac output reverts toward normal. The effect of sodium on blood pressure is related to the provision of sodium with chloride; nonchloride salts of sodium have little or no effect on blood pressure. As arterial pressure increases in response to a high NaCl intake, urinary sodium excretion increases and sodium balance is maintained at the expense of an increase in arterial pressure. The mechanism for this "pressure-natriuresis" phenomenon may involve a subtle increase in the glomerular filtration rate, decreased absorbing capacity of the renal tubules, and possibly hormonal factors such as atrial natriuretic factor. In individuals with an impaired capacity to excrete sodium, greater increases in arterial pressure are required to achieve natriuresis and sodium balance.

NaCl-dependent hypertension may be a consequence of a decreased capacity of the kidney to excrete sodium, due either to intrinsic renal disease or to increased production of a salt-retaining hormone (mineralocorticoid) resulting in increased renal tubular reabsorption of sodium. Renal tubular sodium reabsorption also may be augmented by increased neural activity to the kidney. In each of these situations, a higher arterial pressure may be required to achieve sodium balance. Conversely, salt-wasting disorders are associated with low blood pressure levels. ESRD is an extreme example of volume-dependent hypertension. In ~80% of these patients, vascular volume and hypertension can be controlled with adequate dialysis; in the

other 20%, the mechanism of hypertension is related to increased activity of the renin-angiotensin system and is likely to be responsive to pharmacologic blockade of renin-angiotensin.

AUTONOMIC NERVOUS SYSTEM

The autonomic nervous system maintains cardiovascular homeostasis via pressure, volume, and chemoreceptor signals. Adrenergic reflexes modulate blood pressure over the short term, and adrenergic function, in concert with hormonal and volume-related factors, contributes to the long-term regulation of arterial pressure. The three endogenous catecholamines are norepinephrine, epinephrine, and dopamine. All three play important roles in tonic and phasic cardiovascular regulation.

The activities of the adrenergic receptors are mediated by guanosine nucleotide-binding regulatory proteins (G proteins) and by intracellular concentrations of downstream second messengers. In addition to receptor affinity and density, physiologic responsiveness to catecholamines may be altered by the efficiency of receptor-effector coupling at a site "distal" to receptor binding. The receptor sites are relatively specific both for the transmitter substance and for the response that occupancy of the receptor site elicits. Norepinephrine and epinephrine are agonists for all adrenergic receptor subtypes, although with varying affinities. Based on their physiology and pharmacology, adrenergic receptors have been divided into two principal types: α and β. These types have been differentiated further into α_1, α_2, β_1, and β_2 receptors. Recent molecular cloning studies have identified several additional subtypes. α Receptors are occupied and activated more avidly by norepinephrine than by epinephrine, and the reverse is true for β receptors. α_1 Receptors are located on postsynaptic cells in smooth muscle and elicit vasoconstriction. α_2 Receptors are localized on presynaptic membranes of postganglionic nerve terminals that synthesize norepinephrine. When activated by catecholamines, α_2 receptors act as negative feedback controllers, inhibiting further norepinephrine release. In the kidney, activation of α_1-adrenergic receptors increases renal tubular reabsorption of sodium. Different classes of antihypertensive agents either inhibit α_1 receptors or act as agonists of α_2 receptors and reduce systemic sympathetic outflow. Activation of myocardial β_1 receptors stimulates the rate and strength of cardiac contraction and consequently increases cardiac output. β_1 Receptor activation also stimulates renin release from the kidney. Another class of antihypertensive agents acts by inhibiting β_1 receptors. Activation of β_2 receptors by epinephrine relaxes vascular smooth muscle and results in vasodilation.

Circulating catecholamine concentrations may affect the number of adrenoreceptors in various tissues. Downregulation of receptors may be a consequence of sustained high levels of catecholamines and provides an explanation for decreasing responsiveness, or tachyphylaxis, to catecholamines. For example, orthostatic hypotension frequently is observed in patients with pheochromocytoma, possibly due to the lack of norepinephrine-induced vasoconstriction with assumption of the upright posture. Conversely, with chronic reduction of neurotransmitter substances, adrenoreceptors may increase in number or be upregulated, resulting in increased responsiveness to the neurotransmitter. Chronic administration of agents that block adrenergic receptors may result in upregulation, and withdrawal of those agents may produce a condition of temporary hypersensitivity to sympathetic stimuli. For example, clonidine is an antihypertensive agent that is a centrally acting α_2 agonist that inhibits sympathetic outflow. Rebound hypertension may occur with the abrupt cessation of clonidine therapy, probably as a consequence of upregulation of α_1 receptors.

Several reflexes modulate blood pressure on a minute-to-minute basis. One arterial baroreflex is mediated by stretch-sensitive sensory nerve endings in the carotid sinuses and the aortic arch. The rate of firing of these baroreceptors increases with arterial pressure, and the net effect is a decrease in sympathetic outflow, resulting in decreases in arterial pressure and heart rate. This is a primary mechanism for rapid buffering of acute fluctuations of arterial pressure that may occur during postural changes, behavioral or physiologic stress, and changes in blood volume. However, the activity of the baroreflex declines or adapts to sustained increases in arterial pressure such that the baroreceptors are reset to higher pressures. Patients with autonomic neuropathy and impaired baroreflex function may have extremely labile blood pressures with difficult-to-control episodic blood pressure spikes associated with tachycardia.

In both normal-weight and obese individuals, hypertension often is associated with increased sympathetic outflow. Based on recordings of postganglionic muscle nerve activity (detected by a microelectrode inserted in a peroneal nerve in the leg), sympathetic outflow tends to be higher in hypertensive than in normotensive individuals. Sympathetic outflow is increased in obesity-related hypertension and in hypertension associated with obstructive sleep apnea. Baroreceptor activation via electrical stimulation of carotid sinus afferent nerves has been shown to lower blood pressure in patients with "resistant" hypertension. Drugs that block the sympathetic nervous system are potent antihypertensive agents, indicating that the sympathetic nervous system plays a permissive, although not necessarily a causative, role in the maintenance of increased arterial pressure.

Pheochromocytoma is the most blatant example of hypertension related to increased catecholamine production, in this instance by a tumor. Blood pressure can be reduced by surgical excision of the tumor or by pharmacologic treatment with an α_1 receptor antagonist or with an inhibitor of tyrosine hydroxylase, the rate-limiting step in catecholamine biosynthesis.

RENIN-ANGIOTENSIN-ALDOSTERONE

The renin-angiotensin-aldosterone system contributes to the regulation of arterial pressure primarily via the vasoconstrictor properties of angiotensin II and the sodium-retaining properties of aldosterone. Renin is an aspartyl protease that is synthesized as an enzymatically inactive precursor, prorenin. Most renin in the circulation is synthesized in the renal afferent renal arteriole. Prorenin may be secreted directly into the circulation or may be activated within secretory cells and released as active renin. Although human plasma contains two to five times more prorenin than renin, there is no evidence that prorenin contributes to the physiologic activity of this system. There are three primary stimuli for renin secretion: (1) decreased NaCl transport in the distal portion of the thick ascending limb of the loop of Henle that abuts the corresponding afferent arteriole (macula densa), (2) decreased pressure or stretch within the renal afferent arteriole (baroreceptor mechanism), and (3) sympathetic nervous system stimulation of renin-secreting cells via β_1 adrenoreceptors. Conversely, renin secretion is inhibited by increased NaCl transport in the thick ascending limb of the loop of Henle, by increased stretch within the renal afferent arteriole, and by β_1 receptor blockade. In addition, angiotensin II directly inhibits renin secretion due to angiotensin II type 1 receptors on juxtaglomerular cells, and renin secretion increases in response to pharmacologic blockade of either ACE or angiotensin II receptors.

Once released into the circulation, active renin cleaves a substrate, angiotensinogen, to form an inactive decapeptide, angiotensin I (Fig. 37-2). A converting enzyme, located primarily but not exclusively in the pulmonary circulation, converts angiotensin I to the active octapeptide, angiotensin II, by releasing the C-terminal histidyl-leucine dipeptide. The same converting enzyme cleaves a number of other peptides, including and thereby inactivating the vasodilator bradykinin. Acting primarily through angiotensin II type 1 (AT_1) receptors on cell membranes, angiotensin II is a potent pressor substance, the primary tropic factor for the secretion of aldosterone by the adrenal zona glomerulosa, and a potent mitogen that stimulates vascular smooth-muscle cell and myocyte growth. Independent of its hemodynamic effects, angiotensin II may play a role in the pathogenesis of atherosclerosis through

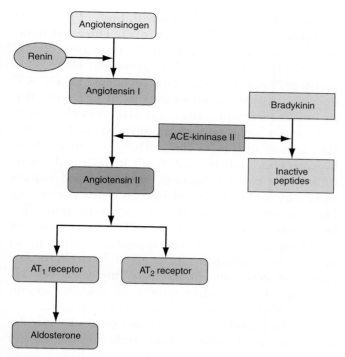

FIGURE 37-2
Renin-angiotensin-aldosterone axis.

a direct cellular action on the vessel wall. An angiotensin II type 2 (AT$_2$) receptor has been characterized. It is widely distributed in the kidney and has the opposite functional effects of the AT$_1$ receptor. The AT$_2$ receptor induces vasodilation, sodium excretion, and inhibition of cell growth and matrix formation. Experimental evidence suggests that the AT$_2$ receptor improves vascular remodeling by stimulating smooth-muscle cell apoptosis and contributes to the regulation of glomerular filtration rate. AT$_1$ receptor blockade induces an increase in AT$_2$ receptor activity.

Renin-secreting tumors are clear examples of renin-dependent hypertension. In the kidney, these tumors include benign hemangiopericytomas of the juxtaglomerular apparatus and, infrequently, renal carcinomas, including Wilms' tumors. Renin-producing carcinomas also have been described in the lung, liver, pancreas, colon, and adrenals. In these instances, in addition to excision and/or ablation of the tumor, treatment of hypertension includes pharmacologic therapies targeted to inhibit angiotensin II production or action. Renovascular hypertension is another renin-mediated form of hypertension. Obstruction of the renal artery leads to decreased renal perfusion pressure, thereby stimulating renin secretion. Over time, as a consequence of secondary renal damage, this form of hypertension may become less renin dependent.

Angiotensinogen, renin, and angiotensin II are also synthesized locally in many tissues, including the brain, pituitary, aorta, arteries, heart, adrenal glands, kidneys,

adipocytes, leukocytes, ovaries, testes, uterus, spleen, and skin. Angiotensin II in tissues may be formed by the enzymatic activity of renin or by other proteases, e.g., tonin, chymase, and cathepsins. In addition to regulating local blood flow, tissue angiotensin II is a mitogen that stimulates growth and contributes to modeling and repair. Excess tissue angiotensin II may contribute to atherosclerosis, cardiac hypertrophy, and renal failure and consequently may be a target for pharmacologic therapy to prevent target organ damage.

Angiotensin II is the primary tropic factor regulating the synthesis and secretion of aldosterone by the zona glomerulosa of the adrenal cortex. Aldosterone synthesis is also dependent on potassium, and aldosterone secretion may be decreased in potassium-depleted individuals. Although acute elevations of adrenocorticotropic hormone (ACTH) levels also increase aldosterone secretion, ACTH is not an important tropic factor for the chronic regulation of aldosterone.

Aldosterone is a potent mineralocorticoid that increases sodium reabsorption by amiloride-sensitive epithelial sodium channels (ENaC) on the apical surface of the principal cells of the renal cortical collecting duct. Electric neutrality is maintained by exchanging sodium for potassium and hydrogen ions. Consequently, increased aldosterone secretion may result in hypokalemia and alkalosis. Because potassium depletion may inhibit aldosterone synthesis, clinically, hypokalemia should be corrected before a patient is evaluated for hyperaldosteronism.

Mineralocorticoid receptors also are expressed in the colon, salivary glands, and sweat glands. Cortisol also binds to these receptors but normally functions as a less potent mineralocorticoid than aldosterone because cortisol is converted to cortisone by the enzyme 11 β-hydroxysteroid dehydrogenase type 2. Cortisone has no affinity for the mineralocorticoid receptor. Primary aldosteronism is a compelling example of mineralocorticoid-mediated hypertension. In this disorder, adrenal aldosterone synthesis and release are independent of renin-angiotensin, and renin release is suppressed by the resulting volume expansion.

Aldosterone also has effects on nonepithelial targets. Aldosterone and/or mineralocorticoid receptor activation induces structural and functional alterations in the heart, kidney, and blood vessels, leading to myocardial fibrosis, nephrosclerosis, and vascular inflammation and remodeling, perhaps as a consequence of oxidative stress. These effects are amplified by a high salt intake. In animal models, high circulating aldosterone levels stimulate cardiac fibrosis and left ventricular hypertrophy, and spironolactone (an aldosterone antagonist) prevents aldosterone-induced myocardial fibrosis. Pathologic patterns of left ventricular geometry also have been associated with elevations of plasma aldosterone concentration in patients with essential hypertension as well as in patients with primary aldosteronism. In patients with CHF, low-dose spironolactone reduces the risk of progressive heart failure and sudden death from cardiac causes by 30%. Owing to a renal hemodynamic effect, in patients with primary aldosteronism, high circulating levels of aldosterone also may cause glomerular hyperfiltration and albuminuria. These renal effects are reversible after removal of the effects of excess aldosterone by adrenalectomy or spironolactone.

Increased activity of the renin-angiotensin-aldosterone axis is not invariably associated with hypertension. In response to a low-NaCl diet or to volume contraction, arterial pressure and volume homeostasis may be maintained by increased activity of the renin-angiotensin-aldosterone axis. Secondary aldosteronism (i.e., increased aldosterone secondary to increased renin-angiotensin), but not hypertension, also is observed in edematous states such as CHF and liver disease.

VASCULAR MECHANISMS

Vascular radius and compliance of resistance arteries are also important determinants of arterial pressure. Resistance to flow varies inversely with the fourth power of the radius, and consequently, small decreases in lumen size significantly increase resistance. In hypertensive patients, structural, mechanical, or functional changes may reduce the lumen diameter of small arteries and arterioles. Remodeling refers to geometric alterations in the vessel wall without a change in vessel volume. Hypertrophic (increased cell size, and increased deposition of intercellular matrix) or eutrophic vascular remodeling results in decreased lumen size and hence contributes to increased peripheral resistance. Apoptosis, low-grade inflammation, and vascular fibrosis also contribute to remodeling. Lumen diameter also is related to elasticity of the vessel. Vessels with a high degree of elasticity can accommodate an increase of volume with relatively little change in pressure, whereas in a semirigid vascular system, a small increment in volume induces a relatively large increment of pressure.

Hypertensive patients have stiffer arteries, and arteriosclerotic patients may have particularly high systolic blood pressures and wide pulse pressures as a consequence of decreased vascular compliance due to structural changes in the vascular wall. Recent evidence suggests that arterial stiffness has independent predictive value for cardiovascular events. Clinically, a number of devices are available to evaluate arterial stiffness or compliance, including ultrasound and magnetic resonance imaging (MRI).

Ion transport by vascular smooth-muscle cells may contribute to hypertension-associated abnormalities of vascular tone and vascular growth, both of which are modulated by intracellular pH (pH_i). Three ion transport mechanisms participate in the regulation of pH_i: (1) Na^+-H^+ exchange, (2) Na^+-dependent HCO_3^--Cl^- exchange, and (3) cation-independent HCO_3^--Cl^- exchange. Based on measurements in cell types that are more accessible than vascular smooth muscle (e.g., leukocytes, erythrocytes, platelets, skeletal muscle), activity of the Na^+-H^+ exchanger is increased in hypertension, and this may result in increased vascular tone by two mechanisms. First, increased sodium entry may lead to increased vascular tone by activating Na^+-Ca^{2+} exchange and thereby increasing intracellular calcium. Second, increased pH_i enhances calcium sensitivity of the contractile apparatus, leading to an increase in contractility for a given intracellular calcium concentration. Additionally, increased Na^+-H^+ exchange may stimulate growth of vascular smooth muscle cells by enhancing sensitivity to mitogens.

Vascular endothelial function also modulates vascular tone. The vascular endothelium synthesizes and releases a spectrum of vasoactive substances, including nitric oxide, a potent vasodilator. Endothelium-dependent vasodilation is impaired in hypertensive patients. This impairment often is assessed with high-resolution ultrasonography before and after the hyperemic phase of reperfusion that follows 5 min of forearm ischemia. Alternatively, endothelium-dependent vasodilation may be assessed in response to an intraarterially infused endothelium-dependent vasodilator, e.g., acetylcholine. Endothelin is a vasoconstrictor peptide produced by the endothelium, and orally active endothelin antagonists may lower blood pressure in patients with resistant hypertension.

Currently, it is not known if the hypertension-related vascular abnormalities of ion transport and endothelial function are primary alterations or secondary consequences of elevated arterial pressure. Limited evidence suggests that vascular compliance and endothelium-dependent vasodilation may be improved by aerobic exercise, weight loss, and antihypertensive agents. It remains to be determined whether these interventions affect arterial structure and stiffness via a blood pressure–independent mechanism and whether different classes of antihypertensive agents preferentially affect vascular structure and function.

PATHOLOGIC CONSEQUENCES OF HYPERTENSION

Hypertension is an independent predisposing factor for heart failure, coronary artery disease, stroke, renal disease, and peripheral arterial disease (PAD).

HEART

Heart disease is the most common cause of death in hypertensive patients. Hypertensive heart disease is the result of structural and functional adaptations leading to left ventricular hypertrophy, CHF, abnormalities of blood flow due to atherosclerotic coronary artery disease and microvascular disease, and cardiac arrhythmias.

Both genetic and hemodynamic factors contribute to left ventricular hypertrophy. Clinically, left ventricular hypertrophy can be diagnosed by electrocardiography, although echocardiography provides a more sensitive measure of left ventricular wall thickness. Individuals with left ventricular hypertrophy are at increased risk for CHD, stroke, CHF, and sudden death. Aggressive control of hypertension can regress or reverse left ventricular hypertrophy and reduce the risk of cardiovascular disease. It is not clear whether different classes of antihypertensive agents have an added impact on reducing left ventricular mass, independent of their blood pressure–lowering effect.

CHF may be related to systolic dysfunction, diastolic dysfunction, or a combination of the two. Abnormalities of diastolic function that range from asymptomatic heart disease to overt heart failure are common in hypertensive patients. Patients with diastolic heart failure have a preserved ejection fraction, which is a measure of systolic function. Approximately one-third of patients with CHF have normal systolic function but abnormal diastolic function. Diastolic dysfunction is an early consequence of hypertension-related heart disease and is exacerbated by left ventricular hypertrophy and ischemia. Cardiac catheterization provides the most accurate assessment of diastolic function. Alternatively, diastolic function can be evaluated by several noninvasive methods, including echocardiography and radionuclide angiography.

BRAIN

Stroke is the second most frequent cause of death in the world; it accounts for 5 million deaths each year, with an additional 15 million persons having nonfatal strokes. Elevated blood pressure is the strongest risk factor for stroke. Approximately 85% of strokes are due to infarction, and the remainder are due to either intracerebral or subarachnoid hemorrhage. The incidence of stroke rises progressively with increasing blood pressure levels, particularly systolic blood pressure in individuals >65 years. Treatment of hypertension convincingly decreases the incidence of both ischemic and hemorrhagic strokes.

Hypertension also is associated with impaired cognition in an aging population, and longitudinal studies support an association between midlife hypertension and late-life cognitive decline. Hypertension-related cognitive impairment and dementia may be a consequence of a single infarct due to occlusion of a "strategic" larger vessel or multiple lacunar infarcts due to occlusive small vessel disease resulting in subcortical white matter ischemia. Several clinical trials suggest that antihypertensive therapy has a beneficial effect on cognitive function, although this remains an active area of investigation.

Cerebral blood flow remains unchanged over a wide range of arterial pressures (mean arterial pressure of 50–150 mmHg) through a process termed *autoregulation* of blood flow. In patients with the clinical syndrome of malignant hypertension, encephalopathy is related to failure of autoregulation of cerebral blood flow at the upper pressure limit, resulting in vasodilation and hyperperfusion. Signs and symptoms of hypertensive encephalopathy may include severe headache, nausea and vomiting (often of a projectile nature), focal neurologic signs, and alterations in mental status. Untreated, hypertensive encephalopathy may progress to stupor, coma, seizures, and death within hours. It is important to distinguish hypertensive encephalopathy from other neurologic syndromes that may be associated with hypertension, e.g., cerebral ischemia, hemorrhagic or thrombotic stroke, seizure disorder, mass lesions, pseudotumor cerebri, delirium tremens, meningitis, acute intermittent porphyria, traumatic or chemical injury to the brain, and uremic encephalopathy.

KIDNEY

The kidney is both a target and a cause of hypertension. Primary renal disease is the most common etiology of secondary hypertension. Mechanisms of kidney-related hypertension include a diminished capacity to excrete sodium, excessive renin secretion in relation to volume status, and sympathetic nervous system overactivity. Conversely, hypertension is a risk factor for renal injury and end-stage renal disease. The increased risk associated with high blood pressure is graded, continuous, and present throughout the distribution of blood pressure above optimal pressure. Renal risk appears to be more closely related to systolic than to diastolic blood pressure, and black men are at greater risk than white men for developing ESRD at every level of blood pressure. Proteinuria is a reliable marker of the severity of chronic kidney disease and is a predictor of its progression. Patients with high urine protein excretion (>3 g/24 h) have a more rapid rate of progression than do those with lower protein excretion rates.

Atherosclerotic, hypertension-related vascular lesions in the kidney primarily affect preglomerular arterioles, resulting in ischemic changes in the glomeruli and postglomerular structures. Glomerular injury also may be a consequence of direct damage to the glomerular capillaries due to glomerular hyperperfusion. Studies of hypertension-related renal damage, primarily in experimental animals, suggest that loss of autoregulation of renal blood flow at the afferent arteriole results in transmission of elevated pressures to an unprotected glomerulus with ensuing hyperfiltration, hypertrophy, and eventual focal segmental glomerular sclerosis. With progressive renal injury there is a loss of autoregulation of renal blood flow and glomerular filtration rate, resulting in a lower blood pressure threshold for renal damage and a steeper slope between blood pressure and renal damage. The result may be a vicious cycle of renal damage and nephron loss leading to more severe hypertension, glomerular hyperfiltration, and further renal damage. Glomerular pathology progresses to glomerulosclerosis, and eventually the renal tubules may also become ischemic and gradually atrophic. The renal lesion associated with malignant hypertension consists of fibrinoid necrosis of the afferent arterioles, sometimes extending into the glomerulus, and may result in focal necrosis of the glomerular tuft.

Clinically, macroalbuminuria (a random urine albumin/creatinine ratio >300 mg/g) or microalbuminuria (a random urine albumin/creatinine ratio 30–300 mg/g) are early markers of renal injury. These are also risk factors for renal disease progression and cardiovascular disease.

PERIPHERAL ARTERIES

In addition to contributing to the pathogenesis of hypertension, blood vessels may be a target organ for atherosclerotic disease secondary to long-standing elevated blood pressure. Hypertensive patients with arterial disease of the lower extremities are at increased risk for future cardiovascular disease. Although patients with stenotic lesions of the lower extremities may be asymptomatic, intermittent claudication is the classic symptom of PAD. This is characterized by aching pain in the calves or buttocks while walking that is relieved by rest. The ankle-brachial index is a useful approach for evaluating PAD and is defined as the ratio of noninvasively assessed ankle to brachial (arm) systolic blood pressure. An ankle-brachial index <0.90 is considered diagnostic of PAD and is associated with >50% stenosis in at least one major lower limb vessel. Several studies suggest that an ankle-brachial index <0.80 is associated with elevated blood pressure, particularly systolic blood pressure.

DEFINING HYPERTENSION

From an epidemiologic perspective, there is no obvious level of blood pressure that defines hypertension. In adults, there is a continuous, incremental risk of cardiovascular disease, stroke, and renal disease across levels of both systolic and diastolic blood pressure.

The Multiple Risk Factor Intervention Trial (MRFIT), which included >350,000 male participants, demonstrated a continuous and graded influence of both systolic and diastolic blood pressure on CHD mortality, extending down to systolic blood pressures of 120 mmHg. Similarly, results of a meta-analysis involving almost 1 million participants indicate that ischemic heart disease mortality, stroke mortality, and mortality from other vascular causes are directly related to the height of the blood pressure, beginning at 115/75 mmHg, without evidence of a threshold. Cardiovascular disease risk doubles for every 20-mmHg increase in systolic and 10-mmHg increase in diastolic pressure. Among older individuals, systolic blood pressure and pulse pressure are more powerful predictors of cardiovascular disease than is diastolic blood pressure.

Clinically, hypertension may be defined as that level of blood pressure at which the institution of therapy reduces blood pressure–related morbidity and mortality. Current clinical criteria for defining hypertension generally are based on the average of two or more seated blood pressure readings during each of two or more outpatient visits. A recent classification recommends blood pressure criteria for defining normal blood pressure, prehypertension, hypertension (stages I and II), and isolated systolic hypertension, which is a common occurrence among the elderly (Table 37-1). In children and adolescents, hypertension generally is defined as systolic and/or diastolic blood pressure consistently >95th percentile for age, sex, and height. Blood pressures between the 90th and 95th percentiles are considered prehypertensive and are an indication for lifestyle interventions.

Home blood pressure and average 24-h ambulatory blood pressure measurements are generally lower than clinic blood pressures. Because ambulatory blood pressure recordings yield multiple readings throughout the day and night, they provide a more comprehensive assessment of the vascular burden of hypertension than do a limited number of office readings. Increasing evidence suggests that home blood pressures, including

TABLE 37-1

BLOOD PRESSURE CLASSIFICATION		
BLOOD PRESSURE CLASSIFICATION	**SYSTOLIC, mmHg**	**DIASTOLIC, mmHg**
Normal	<120	*and* <80
Prehypertension	120–139	*or* 80–89
Stage 1 hypertension	140–159	*or* 90–99
Stage 2 hypertension	≥160	*or* ≥100
Isolated systolic hypertension	≥140	*and* <90

Source: Adapted from AV Chobanian et al: JAMA 289:2560, 2003.

24-h blood pressure recordings, more reliably predict target organ damage than do office blood pressures. Blood pressure tends to be higher in the early morning hours, soon after waking, than at other times of day. Myocardial infarction and stroke are more common in the early morning hours. Nighttime blood pressures are generally 10–20% lower than daytime blood pressures, and an attenuated nighttime blood pressure "dip" is associated with increased cardiovascular disease risk. Recommended criteria for a diagnosis of hypertension are average awake blood pressure ≥135/85 mmHg and asleep blood pressure ≥120/75 mmHg. These levels approximate a clinic blood pressure of 140/90 mmHg.

Approximately 15–20% of patients with stage 1 hypertension (as defined in Table 37-1) based on office blood pressures have average ambulatory readings <135/85 mmHg. This phenomenon, so-called white coat hypertension, also may be associated with an increased risk of target organ damage (e.g., left ventricular hypertrophy, carotid atherosclerosis, overall cardiovascular morbidity), although to a lesser extent than in individuals with elevated office and ambulatory readings. Individuals with white coat hypertension are also at increased risk for developing sustained hypertension.

CLINICAL DISORDERS OF HYPERTENSION

Depending on methods of patient ascertainment, ~80–95% of hypertensive patients are diagnosed as having "essential" hypertension (also referred to as primary or idiopathic hypertension). In the remaining 5–20% of hypertensive patients, a specific underlying disorder causing the elevation of blood pressure can be identified (Tables 37-2 and 37-3). In individuals with "secondary" hypertension, a specific mechanism for the blood pressure elevation is often more apparent.

TABLE 37-2

SYSTOLIC HYPERTENSION WITH WIDE PULSE PRESSURE

1. Decreased vascular compliance (arteriosclerosis)
2. Increased cardiac output
   a. Aortic regurgitation
   b. Thyrotoxicosis
   c. Hyperkinetic heart syndrome
   d. Fever
   e. Arteriovenous fistula
   f. Patent ductus arteriosus

ESSENTIAL HYPERTENSION

Essential hypertension tends to be familial and is likely to be the consequence of an interaction between environmental and genetic factors. The prevalence of essential hypertension increases with age, and individuals with relatively high blood pressures at younger ages are at increased risk for the subsequent development of hypertension. It is likely that essential hypertension represents a spectrum of disorders with different underlying pathophysiologies. In the majority of patients with established hypertension, peripheral resistance is increased and cardiac output is normal or decreased; however, in younger patients with mild or labile

TABLE 37-3

SECONDARY CAUSES OF SYSTOLIC AND DIASTOLIC HYPERTENSION	
Renal	Parenchymal diseases, renal cysts (including polycystic kidney disease), renal tumors (including renin-secreting tumors), obstructive uropathy
Renovascular	Arteriosclerotic, fibromuscular dysplasia
Adrenal	Primary aldosteronism, Cushing's syndrome, 17α-hydroxylase deficiency, 11β-hydroxylase deficiency, 11-hydroxysteroid dehydrogenase deficiency (licorice), pheochromocytoma
Aortic coarctation	
Obstructive sleep apnea	
Preeclampsia/eclampsia	
Neurogenic	Psychogenic, diencephalic syndrome, familial dysautonomia, polyneuritis (acute porphyria, lead poisoning), acute increased intracranial pressure, acute spinal cord section
Miscellaneous endocrine	Hypothyroidism, hyperthyroidism, hypercalcemia, acromegaly
Medications	High-dose estrogens, adrenal steroids, decongestants, appetite suppressants, cyclosporine, tricyclic antidepressants, monamine oxidase inhibitors, erythropoietin, nonsteroidal anti-inflammatory agents, cocaine
Mendelian forms of hypertension	See Table 37-4

hypertension, cardiac output may be increased and peripheral resistance may be normal.

When plasma renin activity (PRA) is plotted against 24-h sodium excretion, ~10–15% of hypertensive patients have high PRA and 25% have low PRA. High-renin patients may have a vasoconstrictor form of hypertension, whereas low-renin patients may have volume-dependent hypertension. Inconsistent associations between plasma aldosterone and blood pressure have been described in patients with essential hypertension. The association between aldosterone and blood pressure is more striking in African Americans, and PRA tends to be low in hypertensive African Americans. This raises the possibility that subtle increases in aldosterone may contribute to hypertension in at least some groups of patients who do not have overt primary aldosteronism. Furthermore, spironolactone, an aldosterone antagonist, may be a particularly effective antihypertensive agent for some patients with essential hypertension, including some patients with "drug-resistant" hypertension.

OBESITY AND THE METABOLIC SYNDROME

(See also Chap. 32) There is a well-documented association between obesity (body mass index >30 kg/m²) and hypertension. Further, cross-sectional studies indicate a direct linear correlation between body weight (or body mass index) and blood pressure. Centrally located body fat is a more important determinant of blood pressure elevation than is peripheral body fat. In longitudinal studies, a direct correlation exists between change in weight and change in blood pressure over time. Sixty percent of hypertensive adults are more than 20% overweight. It has been established that 60–70% of hypertension in adults may be directly attributable to adiposity.

Hypertension and dyslipidemia frequently occur together and in association with resistance to insulin-stimulated glucose uptake. This clustering of risk factors is often, but not invariably, associated with obesity, particularly abdominal obesity. Insulin resistance also is associated with an unfavorable imbalance in the endothelial production of mediators that regulate platelet aggregation, coagulation, fibrinolysis, and vessel tone. When these risk factors cluster, the risks for CHD, stroke, diabetes, and cardiovascular disease mortality are increased further.

Depending on the populations studied and the methodologies for defining insulin resistance, ~25–50% of nonobese, nondiabetic hypertensive persons are insulin resistant. The constellation of insulin resistance, abdominal obesity, hypertension, and dyslipidemia has been designated as the *metabolic syndrome*. As a group, first-degree relatives of patients with essential hypertension are also insulin resistant, and hyperinsulinemia

(a surrogate marker of insulin resistance) may predict the eventual development of hypertension and cardiovascular disease. Although the metabolic syndrome may in part be heritable as a polygenic condition, the expression of the syndrome is modified by environmental factors, such as degree of physical activity and diet. Insulin sensitivity increases and blood pressure decreases in response to weight loss. The recognition that cardiovascular disease risk factors tend to cluster within individuals has important implications for the evaluation and treatment of hypertension. Evaluation of both hypertensive patients and individuals at risk for developing hypertension should include assessment of overall cardiovascular disease risk. Similarly, introduction of lifestyle modification strategies and drug therapies should address overall risk and not simply focus on hypertension.

RENAL PARENCHYMAL DISEASES

Virtually all disorders of the kidney may cause hypertension (Table 37-3), and renal disease is the most common cause of secondary hypertension. Hypertension is present in >80% of patients with chronic renal failure. In general, hypertension is more severe in glomerular diseases than in interstitial diseases such as chronic pyelonephritis. Conversely, hypertension may cause nephrosclerosis, and in some instances it may be difficult to determine whether hypertension or renal disease was the initial disorder. Proteinuria >1000 mg/d and an active urine sediment are indicative of primary renal disease. In either instance, the goals are to control blood pressure and retard the rate of progression of renal dysfunction.

RENOVASCULAR HYPERTENSION

Hypertension due to an occlusive lesion of a renal artery, renovascular hypertension, is a potentially curable form of hypertension. In the initial stages, the mechanism of hypertension generally is related to activation of the renin-angiotensin system. However, renin activity and other components of the renin-angiotensin system may be elevated only transiently; over time, sodium retention and recruitment of other pressure mechanisms may contribute to elevated arterial pressure. Two groups of patients are at risk for this disorder: older arteriosclerotic patients who have a plaque obstructing the renal artery, frequently at its origin, and patients with fibromuscular dysplasia. Atherosclerosis accounts for the large majority of patients with renovascular hypertension. Although fibromuscular dysplasia may occur at any age, it has a strong predilection for young white women. The prevalence in females is eightfold than in males. There are several histologic variants of fibromuscular dysplasia, including medial fibroplasia, perimedial fibroplasia, medial hyperplasia, and intimal fibroplasia. Medial fibroplasia is the most common variant and accounts for approximately two-thirds of patients. The lesions of fibromuscular dysplasia are frequently bilateral and, in contrast to atherosclerotic renovascular disease, tend to affect more distal portions of the renal artery.

In addition to the age and sex of the patient, several clues from the history and physical examination suggest a diagnosis of renovascular hypertension. The diagnosis should be considered in patients with other evidence of atherosclerotic vascular disease. Although response to antihypertensive therapy does not exclude the diagnosis, severe or refractory hypertension, recent loss of hypertension control or recent onset of moderately severe hypertension, and unexplained deterioration of renal function or deterioration of renal function associated with an ACE inhibitor should raise the possibility of renovascular hypertension. Approximately 50% of patients with renovascular hypertension have an abdominal or flank bruit, and the bruit is more likely to be hemodynamically significant if it lateralizes or extends throughout systole into diastole.

If blood pressure is adequately controlled with a simple antihypertensive regimen and renal function remains stable, there may be little impetus to pursue an evaluation for renal artery stenosis, particularly in an older patient with atherosclerotic disease and comorbid conditions. Patients with long-standing hypertension, advanced renal insufficiency, or diabetes mellitus are less likely to benefit from renal vascular repair. The most effective medical therapies include an ACE inhibitor or an angiotensin II receptor blocker; however, these agents decrease glomerular filtration rate in a stenotic kidney owing to efferent renal arteriolar dilation. In the presence of bilateral renal artery stenosis or renal artery stenosis to a solitary kidney, progressive renal insufficiency may result from the use of these agents. Importantly, the renal insufficiency is generally reversible after discontinuation of the offending drug.

If renal artery stenosis is suspected and if the clinical condition warrants an intervention such as percutaneous transluminal renal angioplasty (PTRA), placement of a vascular endoprosthesis (stent), or surgical renal revascularization, imaging studies should be the next step in the evaluation. As a screening test, renal blood flow may be evaluated with a radionuclide [131I]-orthoiodohippurate (OIH) scan or glomerular filtration rate may be evaluated with a [99mTc]-diethylenetriamine pentaacetic acid (DTPA) scan before and after a single dose of captopril (or another ACE inhibitor). The following are consistent with a positive study: (1) decreased relative uptake by the involved kidney, which contributes <40% of total renal function, (2) delayed uptake on the affected side, and (3) delayed washout on the affected side. In patients with normal, or nearly normal, renal function,

a normal captopril renogram essentially excludes functionally significant renal artery stenosis; however, its usefulness is limited in patients with renal insufficiency (creatinine clearance <20 mL/min) or bilateral renal artery stenosis. Additional imaging studies are indicated if the scan is positive. Doppler ultrasound of the renal arteries produces reliable estimates of renal blood flow velocity and offers the opportunity to track a lesion over time. Positive studies usually are confirmed at angiography, whereas false-negative results occur frequently, particularly in obese patients. Gadolinium-contrast magnetic resonance angiography offers clear images of the proximal renal artery but may miss distal lesions. An advantage is the opportunity to image the renal arteries with an agent that is not nephrotoxic. Contrast arteriography remains the "gold standard" for evaluation and identification of renal artery lesions. Potential risks include nephrotoxicity, particularly in patients with diabetes mellitus or preexisting renal insufficiency.

Some degree of renal artery obstruction may be observed in almost 50% of patients with atherosclerotic disease, and there are several approaches for evaluating the functional significance of such a lesion to predict the effect of vascular repair on blood pressure control and renal function. Each approach has varying degrees of sensitivity and specificity, and no single test is sufficiently reliable to determine a causal relationship between a renal artery lesion and hypertension. Functionally significant lesions generally occlude more than 70% of the lumen of the affected renal artery. On angiography, the presence of collateral vessels to the ischemic kidney suggests a functionally significant lesion. A lateralizing renal vein renin ratio (ratio >1.5 of affected side/contralateral side) has a 90% predictive value for a lesion that would respond to vascular repair; however, the false-negative rate for blood pressure control is 50–60%. Measurement of the pressure gradient across a renal artery lesion does not reliably predict the response to vascular repair.

In the final analysis, a decision concerning vascular repair vs. medical therapy and the type of repair procedure should be individualized for each patient. Patients with fibromuscular disease have more favorable outcomes than do patients with atherosclerotic lesions, presumably owing to their younger age, shorter duration of hypertension, and less systemic disease. Because of its low risk-versus-benefit ratio and high success rate (improvement or cure of hypertension in 90% of patients and restenosis rate of 10%), PTRA is the initial treatment of choice for these patients. Surgical revascularization may be undertaken if PTRA is unsuccessful or if a branch lesion is present. In atherosclerotic patients, vascular repair should be considered if blood pressure cannot be controlled adequately despite optimal medical therapy or if renal function deteriorates. Surgery may be the preferred initial approach for younger atherosclerotic patients without comorbid conditions; however, for most atherosclerotic patients, depending on the location of the lesion, the initial approach may be PTRA and/or stenting. Surgical revascularization may be indicated if these approaches are unsuccessful, the vascular lesion is not amenable to PTRA or stenting, or concomitant aortic surgery is required, e.g., to repair an aneurysm. A National Institutes of Health–sponsored prospective, randomized clinical trial is in progress comparing medical therapy alone with medical therapy plus renal revascularization regarding Cardiovascular Outcomes for Renal Atherosclerotic Lesions (CORAL).

PRIMARY ALDOSTERONISM

Excess aldosterone production due to primary aldosteronism is a potentially curable form of hypertension. In patients with primary aldosteronism, increased aldosterone production is independent of the renin-angiotensin system, and the consequences are sodium retention, hypertension, hypokalemia, and low PRA. The reported prevalence of this disorder varies from <2% to ~15% of hypertensive individuals. In part, this variation is related to the intensity of screening and the criteria for establishing the diagnosis.

History and physical examination provide little information about the diagnosis. The age at the time of diagnosis is generally the third through fifth decade. Hypertension is usually mild to moderate but occasionally may be severe; primary aldosteronism should be considered in all patients with refractory hypertension. Hypertension in these patients may be associated with glucose intolerance. Most patients are asymptomatic, although, infrequently, polyuria, polydipsia, paresthesias, or muscle weakness may be present as a consequence of hypokalemic alkalosis. In a hypertensive patient with unprovoked hypokalemia (i.e., unrelated to diuretics, vomiting, or diarrhea), the prevalence of primary aldosteronism approaches 40–50%. In patients on diuretics, serum potassium <3.1 mmol/L (<3.1 meq/L) also raises the possibility of primary aldosteronism; however, serum potassium is an insensitive and nonspecific screening test. However, serum potassium is normal in ~25% of patients subsequently found to have an aldosterone-producing adenoma, and higher percentages of patients with other etiologies of primary aldosteronism are not hypokalemic. Additionally, hypokalemic hypertension may be a consequence of secondary aldosteronism, other mineralocorticoid- and glucocorticoid-induced hypertensive disorders, and pheochromocytoma.

The ratio of plasma aldosterone to plasma renin activity (PA/PRA) is a useful screening test. These measurements preferably are obtained in ambulatory patients in the morning. A ratio >30:1 in conjunction with a plasma aldosterone concentration >555 pmol/L (>20 ng/dL) reportedly has a sensitivity of 90% and a specificity of 91% for an aldosterone-producing adenoma. In a Mayo Clinic series, an aldosterone-producing adenoma subsequently was confirmed surgically in >90% of hypertensive patients with a PA/PRA ratio ≥20 and a plasma aldosterone concentration ≥415 pmol/L (≥15 ng/dL). There are, however, several caveats to interpreting the ratio. The cutoff for a "high" ratio is laboratory- and assay-dependent. Some antihypertensive agents may affect the ratio (e.g., aldosterone antagonists, angiotensin receptor antagonists, and ACE inhibitors may increase renin; aldosterone antagonists may increase aldosterone). Current recommendations are to withdraw aldosterone antagonists for at least 4 weeks before obtaining these measurements, with this caveat. The ratio has been reported to be useful as a screening test in measurements obtained with patients taking their usual antihypertensive medications. A high ratio in the absence of an elevated plasma aldosterone level is considerably less specific for primary aldosteronism since many patients with essential hypertension have low renin levels in this setting, particularly African Americans and elderly patients. In patients with renal insufficiency, the ratio may also be elevated because of decreased aldosterone clearance. In patients with an elevated PA/PRA ratio, the diagnosis of primary aldosteronism can be confirmed by demonstrating failure to suppress plasma aldosterone to <277 pmol/L (<10 ng/dL) after IV infusion of 2 L of isotonic saline over 4 h; post-saline infusion plasma aldosterone values between 138 and 277 pmol/L (5–10 ng/dL) are not determinant. Alternative confirmatory tests include failure to suppress aldosterone (based on test-specific criteria) in response to an oral NaCl load, fludrocortisone, or captopril.

Several adrenal abnormalities may culminate in the syndrome of primary aldosteronism, and appropriate therapy depends on the specific etiology. Some 60–70% of patients have an aldosterone-producing adrenal adenoma. The tumor is almost always unilateral, and most often measures <3 cm in diameter. Most of the remainder of these patients have bilateral adrenocortical hyperplasia (idiopathic hyperaldosteronism). Rarely, primary aldosteronism may be caused by an adrenal carcinoma or an ectopic malignancy, e.g., ovarian arrhenoblastoma. Most aldosterone-producing carcinomas, in contrast to adrenal adenomas and hyperplasia, produce excessive amounts of other adrenal steroids in addition to aldosterone. Functional differences in hormone secretion may assist in the differential diagnosis. Aldosterone biosynthesis is more responsive to adrenocorticotropic hormone (ACTH) in patients with adenoma and more responsive to angiotensin in patients with hyperplasia. Consequently, patients with adenoma tend to have higher plasma aldosterone in the early morning that decreases during the day, reflecting the diurnal rhythm of ACTH, whereas plasma aldosterone tends to increase with upright posture in patients with hyperplasia, reflecting the normal postural response of the renin-angiotensin-aldosterone axis. However, there is some overlap in the ability of these measurements to discriminate between adenoma and hyperplasia.

Adrenal computed tomography (CT) should be carried out in all patients diagnosed with primary aldosteronism. High-resolution CT may identify tumors as small as 0.3 cm and is positive for an adrenal tumor 90% of the time. If the CT is not diagnostic, an adenoma may be detected by adrenal scintigraphy with 6 β-[I^{131}]iodomethyl-19-norcholesterol after dexamethasone suppression (0.5 mg every 6 h for 7 days); however, this technique has decreased sensitivity for adenomas <1.5 cm.

When carried out by an experienced radiologist, bilateral adrenal venous sampling for measurement of plasma aldosterone is the most accurate means of differentiating unilateral from bilateral forms of primary aldosteronism. The sensitivity and specificity of adrenal venous sampling (95% and 100%, respectively) for detecting unilateral aldosterone hypersecretion are superior to those of adrenal CT; success rates are 90–96%, and complication rates are <2.5%. One frequently used protocol involves sampling for aldosterone and cortisol levels in response to ACTH stimulation. An ipsilateral/ contralateral aldosterone ratio >4, with symmetric ACTH-stimulated cortisol levels, is indicative of unilateral aldosterone production.

Hypertension generally is responsive to surgery in patients with adenoma but not in patients with bilateral adrenal hyperplasia. Unilateral adrenalectomy, often done via a laparoscopic approach, is curative in 40–70% of patients with an adenoma. Surgery should be undertaken after blood pressure has been controlled and hypokalemia corrected. Transient hypoaldosteronism may occur up to 3 months postoperatively, resulting in hyperkalemia. Potassium should be monitored during this time, and hyperkalemia should be treated with potassium-wasting diuretics and with fludrocortisone, if needed. Patients with bilateral hyperplasia should be treated medically. The drug regimen for these patients, as well as for patients with an adenoma who are poor surgical candidates, should include an aldosterone antagonist and, if necessary, other potassium-sparing diuretics.

Glucocorticoid-remediable hyperaldosteronism is a rare, monogenic autosomal dominant disorder characterized by moderate to severe hypertension, often occurring at an early age. These patients may have a family history of hemorrhagic stroke at a young age. Hypokalemia is usually mild or absent. Normally, angiotensin II stimulates aldosterone production by the adrenal zona glomerulosa, whereas ACTH stimulates cortisol production in the zona fasciculata. Owing to a chimeric gene on chromosome 8, ACTH also regulates aldosterone secretion by the zona fasciculata in patients with glucocorticoid-remediable hyperaldosteronism. The consequence is overproduction in the zona fasciculata of both aldosterone and hybrid steroids (18-hydroxycortisol and 18-oxocortisol) due to oxidation of cortisol. The diagnosis may be established by urine excretion rates of these hybrid steroids that are 20 to 30 times normal or by direct genetic testing. Therapeutically, suppression of ACTH with low-dose glucocorticoids corrects the hyperaldosteronism, hypertension, and hypokalemia. Spironolactone is also a therapeutic option.

CUSHING'S SYNDROME

Cushing's syndrome is related to excess cortisol production due either to excess ACTH secretion (from a pituitary tumor or an ectopic tumor) or to ACTH-independent adrenal production of cortisol. Hypertension occurs in 75–80% of patients with Cushing's syndrome. The mechanism of hypertension may be related to stimulation of mineralocorticoid receptors by cortisol and increased secretion of other adrenal steroids. If clinically suspected based on phenotypic characteristics, in patients not taking exogenous glucocorticoids, laboratory screening may be carried out with measurement of 24-h excretion rates of urine free cortisol or an overnight dexamethasone-suppression test. Recent evidence suggests that late night salivary cortisol is also a sensitive and convenient screening test. Further evaluation is required to confirm the diagnosis and identify the specific etiology of Cushing's syndrome. Appropriate therapy depends on the etiology.

PHEOCHROMOCYTOMA

Catecholamine-secreting tumors are located in the adrenal medulla (pheochromocytoma) or in extra-adrenal paraganglion tissue (paraganglioma) and account for hypertension in ~0.05% of patients. If unrecognized, pheochromocytoma may result in lethal cardiovascular consequences. Clinical manifestations, including hypertension, are primarily related to increased circulating catecholamines, although some of these tumors may secrete a number of other vasoactive substances. In a small percentage of patients, epinephrine is the predominant catecholamine secreted by the tumor, and these patients may present with hypotension rather than hypertension. The initial suspicion of the diagnosis is based on symptoms and/or the association of pheochromocytoma with other disorders (Table 37-4). Approximately 20% of pheochromocytomas are familial with

TABLE 37-4

RARE MENDELIAN FORMS OF HYPERTENSION

DISEASE	PHENOTYPE	GENETIC CAUSE
Glucocorticoid-remediable hyperaldosteronism	Autosomal dominant Absent or mild hypokalemia	Chimeric 11β-hydroxylase/aldosterone gene on chromosome 8
17α-hydroxylase deficiency	Autosomal recessive Males: pseudohermaphroditism Females: primary amenorrhea, absent secondary sexual characteristics	Random mutations of the CYP17 gene on chromosome 10
11β-hydroxylase deficiency	Autosomal recessive Masculinization	Mutations of the CYP11B1 gene on chromosome 8q21-q22
11β-hydroxysteroid dehydrogenase deficiency (apparent mineralocorticoid excess syndrome)	Autosomal recessive Hypokalemia, low renin, low aldosterone	Mutations in the 11β-hydroxysteroid dehydrogenase gene
Liddle's syndrome	Autosomal dominant Hypokalemia, low renin, low aldosterone	Mutation subunits of the epithelial sodium channel SCNN1B and SCNN1C genes
Pseudohypoaldosteronism type II (Gordon's syndrome)	Autosomal dominant Hyperkalemia, normal glomerular filtration rate	Linkage to chromosomes 1q31–q42 and 17p11–q21
Hypertension exacerbated in pregnancy	Autosomal dominant Severe hypertension in early pregnancy	Missense mutation with substitution of leucine for serine at codon 810 (MRL$_{810}$)
Polycystic kidney disease	Autosomal dominant Large cystic kidneys, renal failure, liver cysts, cerebral aneurysms, valvular heart disease	Mutations in the PKD1 gene on chromosome 16 and PKD2 gene on chromosome 4
Pheochromocytoma	Autosomal dominant (a) Multiple endocrine neoplasia, type 2A Medullary thyroid carcinoma, hyperparathyroidism	(a) Mutations in the RET protooncogene
	(b) Multiple endocrine neoplasia, type 2B Medullary thyroid carcinoma, mucosal neuromas, thickened corneal nerves, alimentary ganglioneuromatoses, marfanoid habitus	(b) Mutations in the RET protooncogene
	(c) von Hippel-Lindau disease Retinal angiomas, hemangioblastomas of the cerebellum and spinal cord, renal cell carcinoma	(c) Mutations in the VHL tumor-suppressor gene
	(d) Neurofibromatosis type 1 Multiple neurofibromas, café-au-lait spots	(d) Mutations in the NF1 tumor-suppressor gene

autosomal dominant inheritance. Inherited pheochromocytomas may be associated with multiple endocrine neoplasia (MEN) type 2A and type 2B, von Hippel-Lindau disease, and neurofibromatosis (Table 37-4). Each of these syndromes is related to specific, identifiable germ-line mutations. Additionally, mutations of succinate dehydrogenase genes are associated with paraganglioma syndromes, generally characterized by head and neck paragangliomas. Laboratory testing consists of measuring catecholamines in either urine or plasma. Genetic screening is available for evaluating patients and relatives suspected of harboring a pheochromocytoma

associated with a familial syndrome. Surgical excision is the definitive treatment of pheochromocytoma and results in cure in ~90% of patients.

MISCELLANEOUS CAUSES OF HYPERTENSION

Hypertension due to *obstructive sleep apnea* is being recognized with increasing frequency. Independent of obesity, hypertension occurs in >50% of individuals with obstructive sleep apnea. The severity of hypertension correlates with the severity of sleep apnea. Approximately 70% of patients with obstructive sleep apnea are obese. Hypertension related to obstructive sleep apnea also should be considered in patients with drug-resistant hypertension and patients with a history of snoring. The diagnosis can be confirmed by polysomnography. In obese patients, weight loss may alleviate or cure sleep apnea and related hypertension. Continuous positive airway pressure (CPAP) administered during sleep is an effective therapy for obstructive sleep apnea. With CPAP, patients with apparently drug-resistant hypertension may be more responsive to antihypertensive agents.

Coarctation of the aorta is the most common congenital cardiovascular cause of hypertension (Chap. 19). The incidence is 1–8 per 1000 live births. It is usually sporadic but occurs in 35% of children with Turner syndrome. Even when the anatomic lesion is surgically corrected in infancy, up to 30% of patients develop subsequent hypertension and are at risk of accelerated coronary artery disease and cerebrovascular events. Patients with less severe lesions may not be diagnosed until young adulthood. The physical findings are diagnostic and include diminished and delayed femoral pulses and a systolic pressure gradient between the right arm and the legs and, depending on the location of the coarctation, between the right and left arms. A blowing systolic murmur may be heard in the posterior left interscapular areas. The diagnosis may be confirmed by chest x-ray and transesophageal echocardiography. Therapeutic options include surgical repair and balloon angioplasty,

with or without placement of an intravascular stent. Subsequently, many patients do not have a normal life expectancy but may have persistent hypertension, with death due to ischemic heart disease, cerebral hemorrhage, or aortic aneurysm.

Several additional endocrine disorders, including *thyroid diseases* and *acromegaly*, cause hypertension. Mild diastolic hypertension may be a consequence of hypothyroidism, whereas hyperthyroidism may result in systolic hypertension. *Hypercalcemia* of any etiology, the most common being primary hyperparathyroidism, may result in hypertension. Hypertension also may be related to a number of prescribed or over-the-counter *medications*.

MONOGENIC HYPERTENSION

A number of rare forms of monogenic hypertension have been identified (Table 37-4). These disorders may be recognized by their characteristic phenotypes, and in many instances the diagnosis may be confirmed by genetic analysis. Several inherited defects in adrenal steroid biosynthesis and metabolism result in mineralocorticoid-induced hypertension and hypokalemia. In patients with a 17α-hydroxylase deficiency, synthesis of sex hormones and cortisol is decreased (Fig. 37-3). Consequently, these individuals do not mature sexually; males may present with pseudohermaphroditism and females with primary amenorrhea and absent secondary

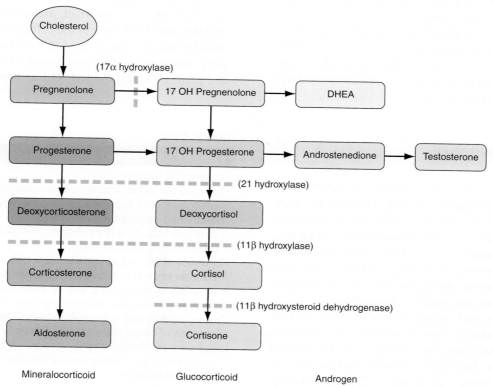

FIGURE 37-3
Adrenal enzymatic defects.

sexual characteristics. Because cortisol-induced negative feedback on pituitary ACTH production is diminished, ACTH-stimulated adrenal steroid synthesis proximal to the enzymatic block is increased. Hypertension and hypokalemia are consequences of increased synthesis of mineralocorticoids proximal to the enzymatic block, particularly desoxycorticosterone. Increased steroid production and, hence, hypertension may be treated with low-dose glucocorticoids. An 11β-hydroxylase deficiency results in a salt-retaining adrenogenital syndrome that occurs in 1 in 100,000 live births. This enzymatic defect results in decreased cortisol synthesis, increased synthesis of mineralocorticoids (e.g., desoxycorticosterone), and shunting of steroid biosynthesis into the androgen pathway. In the severe form, the syndrome may present early in life, including the newborn period, with virilization and ambiguous genitalia in females and penile enlargement in males, or in older children as precocious puberty and short stature. Acne, hirsutism, and menstrual irregularities may be the presenting features when the disorder is first recognized in adolescence or early adulthood. Hypertension is less common in the late-onset forms. Patients with an 11β-hydroxysteroid dehydrogenase deficiency have an impaired capacity to metabolize cortisol to its inactive metabolite, cortisone, and hypertension is related to activation of mineralocorticoid receptors by cortisol. This defect may be inherited or acquired, due to licorice-containing glycyrrhizin acid. The same substance is present in the paste of several brands of chewing tobacco. The defect in Liddle's syndrome results from constitutive activation of amiloride-sensitive epithelial sodium channels on the distal renal tubule, resulting in excess sodium reabsorption; the syndrome is ameliorated by amiloride. Hypertension exacerbated in pregnancy is due to activation of the mineralocorticoid receptor by progesterone.

is localized to the occipital region. Other nonspecific symptoms that may be related to elevated blood pressure include dizziness, palpitations, easy fatigability, and impotence. When symptoms are present, they are generally related to hypertensive cardiovascular disease or to manifestations of secondary hypertension. Table 37-5 lists salient features that should be addressed in obtaining a history from a hypertensive patient.

MEASUREMENT OF BLOOD PRESSURE Reliable measurements of blood pressure depend on attention to the details of the technique and conditions of the measurement. Proper training of observers, positioning of the patient, and selection of cuff size are essential. Owing to recent regulations preventing the use of mercury because of concerns about its potential toxicity, most office measurements are made with aneroid sphygmomanometers or with oscillometric devices. These instruments should be calibrated periodically, and their accuracy confirmed. Before the blood pressure measurement is taken, the individual should be seated quietly in a chair (not the exam table) with feet on the floor for 5 min in a private, quiet setting with a comfortable room temperature. At least two measurements should be made. The center of the cuff should be at heart level, and the width of the bladder cuff should equal at least 40% of the arm circumference; the length of the cuff bladder should be enough to encircle at least 80% of the arm circumference. It is important to pay attention to cuff placement, stethoscope placement, and the rate of deflation of the cuff (2 mmHg/s). Systolic blood pressure is the first of at least two regular "tapping" Korotkoff sounds, and diastolic blood pressure is the point at which the last regular Korotkoff sound is

APPROACH TO THE PATIENT | **Hypertension**

HISTORY The initial assessment of a hypertensive patient should include a complete history and physical examination to confirm a diagnosis of hypertension, screen for other cardiovascular disease risk factors, screen for secondary causes of hypertension, identify cardiovascular consequences of hypertension and other comorbidities, assess blood pressure–related lifestyles, and determine the potential for intervention.

Most patients with hypertension have no specific symptoms referable to their blood pressure elevation. Although popularly considered a symptom of elevated arterial pressure, headache generally occurs only in patients with severe hypertension. Characteristically, a "hypertensive headache" occurs in the morning and

TABLE 37-5

PATIENT'S RELEVANT HISTORY

Duration of hypertension
Previous therapies: responses and side effects
Family history of hypertension and cardiovascular disease
Dietary and psychosocial history
Other risk factors: weight change, dyslipidemia, smoking, diabetes, physical inactivity
Evidence of secondary hypertension: history of renal disease; change in appearance; muscle weakness; spells of sweating, palpitations, tremor; erratic sleep, snoring, daytime somnolence; symptoms of hypo- or hyperthyroidism; use of agents that may increase blood pressure
Evidence of target organ damage: history of TIA, stroke, transient blindness; angina, myocardial infarction, congestive heart failure; sexual function
Other comorbidities

Abbreviation: TIA, transient ischemic attack.

heard. In current practice, a diagnosis of hypertension generally is based on seated, office measurements.

Currently available ambulatory monitors are fully automated, use the oscillometric technique, and typically are programmed to take readings every 15–30 min. Twenty-four-hour ambulatory blood pressure monitoring more reliably predicts cardiovascular disease risk than do office measurements. However, ambulatory monitoring is not used routinely in clinical practice and generally is reserved for patients in whom white coat hypertension is suspected. The Seventh Report of the Joint National Committee on Prevention, Detection, Evaluation, and Treatment of High Blood Pressure (JNC 7) has also recommended ambulatory monitoring for treatment resistance, symptomatic hypotension, autonomic failure, and episodic hypertension.

PHYSICAL EXAMINATION Body habitus, including weight and height, should be noted. At the initial examination, blood pressure should be measured in both arms and preferably in the supine, sitting, and standing positions to evaluate for postural hypotension. Even if the femoral pulse is normal to palpation, arterial pressure should be measured at least once in the lower extremity in patients in whom hypertension is discovered before age 30. Heart rate also should be recorded. Hypertensive individuals have an increased prevalence of atrial fibrillation. The neck should be palpated for an enlarged thyroid gland, and patients should be assessed for signs of hypo- and hyperthyroidism. Examination of blood vessels may provide clues about underlying vascular disease and should include funduscopic examination, auscultation for bruits over the carotid and femoral arteries, and palpation of femoral and pedal pulses. The retina is the only tissue in which arteries and arterioles can be examined directly. With increasing severity of hypertension and atherosclerotic disease, progressive funduscopic changes include increased arteriolar light reflex, arteriovenous crossing defects, hemorrhages and exudates, and, in patients with malignant hypertension, papilledema. Examination of the heart may reveal a loud second heart sound due to closure of the aortic valve and an S_4 gallop attributed to atrial contraction against a noncompliant left ventricle. Left ventricular hypertrophy may be detected by an enlarged, sustained, and laterally displaced apical impulse. An abdominal bruit, particularly a bruit that lateralizes and extends throughout systole into diastole, raises the possibility of renovascular hypertension. Kidneys of patients with polycystic kidney disease may be palpable in the abdomen. The physical examination also should include evaluation for signs of CHF and a neurologic examination.

TABLE 37-6

BASIC LABORATORY TESTS FOR INITIAL EVALUATION

SYSTEM	TEST
Renal	Microscopic urinalysis, albumin excretion, serum BUN and/or creatinine
Endocrine	Serum sodium, potassium, calcium, ?TSH
Metabolic	Fasting blood glucose, total cholesterol, HDL and LDL (often computed) cholesterol, triglycerides
Other	Hematocrit, electrocardiogram

Abbreviations: BUN, blood urea nitrogen; HDL, LDL, high-/low-density lipoprotein; TSH, thyroid-stimulating hormone.

LABORATORY TESTING Table 37-6 lists recommended laboratory tests in the initial evaluation of hypertensive patients. Repeat measurements of renal function, serum electrolytes, fasting glucose, and lipids may be obtained after the introduction of a new antihypertensive agent and then annually or more frequently if clinically indicated. More extensive laboratory testing is appropriate for patients with apparent drug-resistant hypertension or when the clinical evaluation suggests a secondary form of hypertension.

TREATMENT Hypertension

LIFESTYLE INTERVENTIONS Implementation of lifestyles that favorably affect blood pressure has implications for both the prevention and the treatment of hypertension. Health-promoting lifestyle modifications are recommended for individuals with prehypertension and as an adjunct to drug therapy in hypertensive individuals. These interventions should address overall cardiovascular disease risk. Although the impact of lifestyle interventions on blood pressure is more pronounced in persons with hypertension, in short-term trials, weight loss and reduction of dietary NaCl have been shown to prevent the development of hypertension. In hypertensive individuals, even if these interventions do not produce a sufficient reduction in blood pressure to avoid drug therapy, the number of medications or doses required for blood pressure control may be reduced. Dietary modifications that effectively lower blood pressure are weight loss, reduced NaCl intake, increased potassium intake, moderation of alcohol consumption, and an overall healthy dietary pattern (Table 37-7).

Prevention and treatment of obesity are important for reducing blood pressure and cardiovascular disease risk. In short-term trials, even modest weight loss can

TABLE 37-7

LIFESTYLE MODIFICATIONS TO MANAGE HYPERTENSION

Weight reduction	Attain and maintain BMI <25 kg/m^2
Dietary salt reduction	<6 g NaCl/d
Adapt DASH-type dietary plan	Diet rich in fruits, vegetables, and low-fat dairy products with reduced content of saturated and total fat
Moderation of alcohol consumption	For those who drink alcohol, consume ≤2 drinks/day in men and ≤1 drink/day in women
Physical activity	Regular aerobic activity, e.g., brisk walking for 30 min/d

Abbreviations: BMI, body mass index; DASH, Dietary Approaches to Stop Hypertension (trial).

lead to a reduction of blood pressure and an increase in insulin sensitivity. Average blood pressure reductions of 6.3/3.1 mmHg have been observed with a reduction in mean body weight of 9.2 kg. Regular physical activity facilitates weight loss, decreases blood pressure, and reduces the overall risk of cardiovascular disease. Blood pressure may be lowered by 30 min of moderately intense physical activity, such as brisk walking, 6–7 days a week, or by more intense, less frequent workouts.

There is individual variability in the sensitivity of blood pressure to NaCl, and this variability may have a genetic basis. Based on results of meta-analyses, lowering of blood pressure by limiting daily NaCl intake to 4.4–7.4 g (75–125 meq) results in blood pressure reductions of 3.7–4.9/0.9–2.9 mmHg in hypertensive individuals and lesser reductions in normotensive individuals. Dietary NaCl reduction also has been shown to reduce the long-term risk of cardiovascular events in adults with "prehypertension." Potassium and calcium supplementation have inconsistent, modest antihypertensive effects, and, independent of blood pressure, potassium supplementation may be associated with reduced stroke mortality. Alcohol use in persons consuming three or more drinks per day (a standard drink contains ~14 g ethanol) is associated with higher blood pressures, and a reduction of alcohol consumption is associated with a reduction of blood pressure. In patients with advanced renal disease, dietary protein restriction may have a modest effect in mitigating renal damage by reducing the intrarenal transmission of systemic arterial pressure.

The DASH (Dietary Approaches to Stop Hypertension) trial convincingly demonstrated that over an 8-week period a diet high in fruits, vegetables, and low-fat dairy products lowers blood pressure in individuals with high-normal blood pressures or mild hypertension. Reduction of daily NaCl intake to <6 g (100 meq) augmented the effect of this diet on blood pressure. Fruits and vegetables are enriched sources of potassium, magnesium, and fiber, and dairy products are an important source of calcium.

PHARMACOLOGIC THERAPY Drug therapy is recommended for individuals with blood pressures ≥140/90 mmHg. The degree of benefit derived from antihypertensive agents is related to the magnitude of the blood pressure reduction. Lowering systolic blood pressure by 10–12 mmHg and diastolic blood pressure by 5–6 mmHg confers relative risk reductions of 35–40% for stroke and 12–16% for CHD within 5 years of the initiation of treatment. Risk of heart failure is reduced by >50%. Hypertension control is the single most effective intervention for slowing the rate of progression of hypertension-related chronic kidney disease.

There is considerable variation in individual responses to different classes of antihypertensive agents, and the magnitude of response to any single agent may be limited by activation of counterregulatory mechanisms that oppose the hypotensive effect of the agent. Most available agents reduce systolic blood pressure by 7–13 mmHg and diastolic blood pressure by 4–8 mmHg when corrected for placebo effect. More often than not, combinations of agents, with complementary antihypertensive mechanisms, are required to achieve goal blood pressure reductions. Selection of antihypertensive agents and combinations of agents should be individualized, taking into account age, severity of hypertension, other cardiovascular disease risk factors, comorbid conditions, and practical considerations related to cost, side effects, and frequency of dosing (Table 37-8).

Diuretics Low-dose thiazide diuretics often are used as first-line agents alone or in combination with other antihypertensive drugs. Thiazides inhibit the Na$^+$/Cl$^-$ pump in the distal convoluted tubule and hence increase sodium excretion. In the long term, they also may act as vasodilators. Thiazides are safe, efficacious, inexpensive, and reduce clinical events. They provide additive blood pressure–lowering effects when combined with beta blockers, angiotensin-converting enzyme inhibitors (ACEIs), or angiotensin receptor blockers (ARBs). In contrast, addition of a diuretic to a calcium channel blocker is less effective. Usual doses of hydrochlorothiazide range from 6.25–50 mg/d. Owing to an increased incidence of metabolic side effects (hypokalemia, insulin resistance, increased cholesterol), higher doses generally are not recommended. Two potassium-sparing diuretics, amiloride and triamterene, act by inhibiting epithelial sodium channels in the distal nephron. These agents are weak antihypertensive

TABLE 37-8

EXAMPLES OF ORAL DRUGS USED IN TREATMENT OF HYPERTENSION

DRUG CLASS	EXAMPLES	USUAL TOTAL DAILY DOSE[a] (DOSING FREQUENCY/DAY)	OTHER INDICATIONS	CONTRAINDICATIONS/ CAUTIONS
Diuretics				
Thiazides	Hydrochlorothiazide	6.25–50 mg (1–2)		Diabetes, dyslipidemia, hyperuricemia, gout, hypokalemia
	Chlorthalidone	25–50 mg (1)		
Loop diuretics	Furosemide	40–80 mg (2–3)	CHF due to systolic dysfunction, renal failure	Diabetes, dyslipidemia, hyperuricemia, gout, hypokalemia
	Ethacrynic acid	50–100 mg (2–3)		
Aldosterone antagonists	Spironolactone	25–100 mg (1–2)	CHF due to systolic dysfunction, primary aldosteronism	Renal failure, hyperkalemia
	Eplerenone	50–100 mg (1–2)		
K+ retaining	Amiloride	5–10 mg (1–2)		Renal failure, hyperkalemia
	Triamterene	50–100 mg (1–2)		
Beta blockers				
Cardioselective	Atenolol	25–100 mg (1)	Angina, CHF due to systolic dysfunction, post-MI, sinus tachycardia, ventricular tachyarrhythmias	Asthma, COPD, 2nd- or 3rd-degree heart block, sick-sinus syndrome
	Metoprolol	25–100 mg (1–2)		
Nonselective	Propranolol	40–160 mg (2)		
	Propranolol LA	60–180 (1)		
Combined alpha/ beta	Labetalol	200–800 mg (2)		
	Carvedilol	12.5–50 mg (2)	?Post-MI, CHF	
Alpha antagonists				
Selective	Prazosin	2–20 mg (2–3)	Prostatism	
	Doxazosin	1–16 mg (1)		
	Terazosin	1–10 mg (1–2)		
Nonselective	Phenoxybenzamine	20–120 mg (2–3)	Pheochromocytoma	
Sympatholytics				
Central	Clonidine	0.1–0.6 mg (2)		
	Clonidine patch	0.1–0.3 mg (1/week)		
	Methyldopa	250–1000 mg (2)		
	Reserpine	0.05–0.25 mg (1)		
	Guanfacine	0.5–2 mg (1)		
ACE inhibitors	Captopril	25–200 mg (2)	Post-MI, coronary syndromes, CHF with low ejection fraction, nephropathy	Acute renal failure, bilateral renal artery stenosis, pregnancy, hyperkalemia
	Lisinopril	10–40 mg (1)		
	Ramipril	2.5–20 mg (1–2)		
Angiotensin II antagonists	Losartan	25–100 mg (1–2)	CHF with low ejection fraction, nephropathy, ACE inhibitor cough	Renal failure, bilateral renal artery stenosis, pregnancy, hyperkalemia
	Valsartan	80–320 mg (1)		
	Candesartan	2–32 mg (1–2)		
Renin inhibitors	Aliskiren	150–300 mg (1)	Diabetic nephropathy	Pregnancy
Calcium antagonists				
Dihydropyridines	Nifedipine (long-acting)	30–60 mg (1)		
Nondihydropyridines	Verapamil (long-acting)	120–360 mg (1–2)	Post-MI, supraventricular tachycardias, angina	2nd- or 3rd-degree heart block
	Diltiazem (long-acting)	180–420 mg (1)		
Direct vasodilators	Hydralazine	25–100 mg (2)		Severe coronary artery disease
	Minoxidil	2.5–80 mg (1–2)		

[a]At the initiation of therapy, lower doses may be preferable for elderly patients and for select combinations of antihypertensive agents.
Abbreviations: ACE, angiotensin-converting enzyme; CHF, congestive heart failure; COPD, chronic obstructive pulmonary disease; MI, myocardial infarction.

agents but may be used in combination with a thiazide to protect against hypokalemia. The main pharmacologic target for loop diuretics is the Na^+-K^+-$2Cl^-$ cotransporter in the thick ascending limb of the loop of Henle. Loop diuretics generally are reserved for hypertensive patients with reduced glomerular filtration rates (reflected in serum creatinine >220 μmol/L [>2.5 mg/ dL]), CHF, or sodium retention and edema for some other reason, such as treatment with a potent vasodilator, e.g., minoxidil.

Blockers of the Renin-Angiotensin System

ACEIs decrease the production of angiotensin II, increase bradykinin levels, and reduce sympathetic nervous system activity. ARBs provide selective blockade of AT_1 receptors, and the effect of angiotensin II on unblocked AT_2 receptors may augment their hypotensive effect. Both classes of agents are effective antihypertensive agents that may be used as monotherapy or in combination with diuretics, calcium antagonists, and alpha blocking agents. ACEIs and ARBs have been shown to improve insulin action and ameliorate the adverse effects of diuretics on glucose metabolism. Although the overall impact on the incidence of diabetes is modest, compared with amlodipine (a calcium antagonist), valsartan (an ARB) has been shown to reduce the risk of developing diabetes in high-risk hypertensive patients. ACEI/ARB combinations are less effective in lowering blood pressure than is the case when either class of these agents is used in combination with other classes of agents. In patients with vascular disease or a high risk of diabetes, combination ACEI/ARB therapy has been associated with more adverse events (e.g., cardiovascular death, myocardial infarction, stroke, and hospitalization for heart failure) without increases in benefit. However, in hypertensive patients with proteinuria, preliminary data suggest that reduction of proteinuria with ACEI/ARB combination treatment may be more effective than treatment with either agent alone.

Side effects of ACEIs and ARBs include functional renal insufficiency due to efferent renal arteriolar dilation in a kidney with a stenotic lesion of the renal artery. Additional predisposing conditions to renal insufficiency induced by these agents include dehydration, CHF, and use of nonsteroidal anti-inflammatory drugs. Dry cough occurs in ~15% of patients, and angioedema occurs in <1% of patients taking ACEIs. Angioedema occurs most commonly in individuals of Asian origin and more commonly in African Americans than in whites. Hyperkalemia due to hypoaldosteronism is an occasional side effect of both ACEIs and ARBs.

A new approach to blocking the renin-angiotensin system has been introduced into clinical practice for the treatment of hypertension: direct renin inhibitors. Blockade of the renin-angiotensin system is more complete with renin inhibitors than with ACEIs or ARBs. Aliskiren is the first of a class of oral, nonpeptide competitive inhibitors of the enzymatic activity of renin. Monotherapy with aliskiren seems to be as effective as an ACEI or ARB for lowering blood pressure, but not more effective. Further blood reductions may be achieved when aliskiren is used in combination with a thiazide diuretic, an ACEI, an ARB, or calcium antagonists. Currently, aliskiren is not considered a first-line antihypertensive agent.

Aldosterone Antagonists

Spironolactone is a nonselective aldosterone antagonist that may be used alone or in combination with a thiazide diuretic. It may be a particularly effective agent in patients with low-renin essential hypertension, resistant hypertension, and primary aldosteronism. In patients with CHF, low-dose spironolactone reduces mortality and hospitalizations for heart failure when given in addition to conventional therapy with ACEIs, digoxin, and loop diuretics. Because spironolactone binds to progesterone and androgen receptors, side effects may include gynecomastia, impotence, and menstrual abnormalities. These side effects are circumvented by a newer agent, eplerenone, which is a selective aldosterone antagonist. Eplerenone has recently been approved in the United States for the treatment of hypertension.

Beta Blockers

β-Adrenergic receptor blockers lower blood pressure by decreasing cardiac output, due to a reduction of heart rate and contractility. Other proposed mechanisms by which beta blockers lower blood pressure include a central nervous system effect and inhibition of renin release. Beta blockers are particularly effective in hypertensive patients with tachycardia, and their hypotensive potency is enhanced by coadministration with a diuretic. In lower doses, some beta blockers selectively inhibit cardiac β_1 receptors and have less influence on β_2 receptors on bronchial and vascular smooth-muscle cells; however, there seems to be no difference in the antihypertensive potencies of cardioselective and nonselective beta blockers. Certain beta blockers have intrinsic sympathomimetic activity, and it is uncertain whether this constitutes an overall advantage or disadvantage in cardiac therapy. Beta blockers without intrinsic sympathomimetic activity decrease the rate of sudden death, overall mortality, and recurrent myocardial infarction. In patients with CHF, beta blockers have been shown to reduce the risks of hospitalization and mortality. Carvedilol and labetalol block both β receptors and peripheral α-adrenergic receptors. The potential advantages of combined β- and α-adrenergic blockade in treating hypertension remain to be determined.

α-Adrenergic Blockers

Postsynaptic, selective α-adrenoreceptor antagonists lower blood pressure by decreasing peripheral vascular resistance. They are effective antihypertensive agents used either as monotherapy or in combination with other agents. However, in clinical trials of hypertensive patients, alpha blockade has not been shown to reduce cardiovascular morbidity and mortality or to provide as much protection against CHF as other classes of antihypertensive agents. These agents are also effective in treating lower urinary tract symptoms in men with prostatic hypertrophy. Nonselective α-adrenoreceptor antagonists bind to postsynaptic and presynaptic receptors and are used primarily for the management of patients with pheochromocytoma.

Sympatholytic Agents Centrally acting α_2 sympathetic agonists decrease peripheral resistance by inhibiting sympathetic outflow. They may be particularly useful in patients with autonomic neuropathy who have wide variations in blood pressure due to baroreceptor denervation. Drawbacks include somnolence, dry mouth, and rebound hypertension on withdrawal. Peripheral sympatholytics decrease peripheral resistance and venous constriction by depleting nerve terminal norepinephrine. Although they are potentially effective antihypertensive agents, their usefulness is limited by orthostatic hypotension, sexual dysfunction, and numerous drug-drug interactions.

Calcium Channel Blockers Calcium antagonists reduce vascular resistance through L-channel blockade, which reduces intracellular calcium and blunts vasoconstriction. This is a heterogeneous group of agents that includes drugs in the following three classes: phenylalkylamines (verapamil), benzothiazepines (diltiazem), and 1,4-dihydropyridines (nifedipine-like). Used alone and in combination with other agents (ACEIs, beta blockers, α_1-adrenergic blockers), calcium antagonists effectively lower blood pressure; however, it is unclear if adding a diuretic to a calcium blocker results in a further lowering of blood pressure. Side effects of flushing, headache, and edema with dihydropyridine use are related to their potencies as arteriolar dilators; edema is due to an increase in transcapillary pressure gradients, not to net salt and water retention.

Direct Vasodilators Direct vasodilators decrease peripheral resistance and concomitantly activate mechanisms that defend arterial pressure, notably the sympathetic nervous system, the renin-angiotensin-aldosterone system, and sodium retention. Usually, they are not considered first-line agents but are most effective when added to a combination that includes a diuretic and a beta blocker. Hydralazine is a potent direct vasodilator that has antioxidant and nitric oxide–enhancing actions, and minoxidil is a particularly potent agent and is used most frequently in patients with renal insufficiency who are refractory to all other drugs. Hydralazine may induce a lupus-like syndrome, and side effects of minoxidil include hypertrichosis and pericardial effusion.

COMPARISONS OF ANTIHYPERTENSIVES

Based on pooling results from clinical trials, meta-analyses of the efficacy of different classes of antihypertensive agents suggest essentially equivalent blood pressure–lowering effects of the following six major classes of antihypertensive agents when used as monotherapy: thiazide diuretics, beta blockers, ACEIs, ARBs, calcium antagonists, and α_2 blockers. On average, standard doses of most antihypertensive agents reduce blood pressure by 8–10/4–7 mmHg; however, there may be subgroup differences in responsiveness. Younger patients may be more responsive to beta blockers and ACEIs, whereas patients over age 50 may be more responsive to diuretics and calcium antagonists. There is a limited relationship between plasma renin and blood pressure response. Patients with high-renin hypertension may be more responsive to ACEIs and ARBs than to other classes of agents, whereas patients with low-renin hypertension are more responsive to diuretics and calcium antagonists. Hypertensive African Americans tend to have low renin and may require higher doses of ACEIs and ARBs than whites for optimal blood pressure control, although this difference is abolished when these agents are combined with a diuretic. Beta blockers also appear to be less effective than thiazide diuretics in African Americans than in non-African Americans. Identification of genetic variants that influence blood pressure responsiveness would potentially provide a rational basis for the selection of a specific class of an antihypertensive agent in an individual patient. Early pharmacogenetic studies, utilizing either a candidate gene approach or genomewide scans, have shown associations of gene polymorphisms with blood pressure responsiveness to specific antihypertensive drugs. However, the reported effects have generally been too small to affect clinical decisions, and associated polymorphisms remain to be confirmed in subsequent studies. Currently, in practical terms, the presence of comorbidities often influences the selection of antihypertensive agents.

A recent meta-analysis of more than 30 randomized trials of blood pressure–lowering therapy indicates that for a given reduction in blood pressure, the major drug classes seem to produce similar overall net effects on total cardiovascular events. In both nondiabetic and diabetic hypertensive patients, most trials have failed to show significant differences in cardiovascular outcomes with different drug regimens as long as equivalent decreases in blood pressure were achieved. For example, the Antihypertensive and Lipid-Lowering Treatment to Prevent Heart Attack Trial (ALLHAT) demonstrated that the occurrence of coronary heart disease death and nonfatal myocardial infarction, as well as overall mortality, was virtually identical in hypertensive patients treated with either an ACEI (lisinopril), a diuretic (chlorthalidone), or a calcium antagonist (amlodipine).

However, in specific patient groups, ACEIs may have particular advantages, beyond that of blood pressure control, in reducing cardiovascular and renal outcomes. ACEIs and ARBs decrease intraglomerular pressure and proteinuria and may retard the rate of progression of renal insufficiency, not totally accounted for by their hypotensive effects, in both diabetic and nondiabetic renal diseases. Among African Americans with hypertension-related renal disease, ACEIs appear to be more effective than beta blockers or dihydropyridine calcium channel blockers in slowing, although not preventing, the decline of glomerular filtration rate. In experimental models of hypertension and diabetes, renal protection with aliskiren (a renin inhibitor) was comparable to that with ACEIs and ARBs. Independent of its blood pressure–lowering effect, aliskiren has renal protective effects in patients with hypertension, type 2 diabetes, and nephropathy. The renoprotective effect of these renin-angiotensin blockers, compared with other antihypertensive drugs, is less obvious at lower blood pressures. In most patients with hypertension and heart failure due to systolic and/or diastolic dysfunction, the use of diuretics, ACEIs or ARBs, and beta blockers is recommended to improve survival. Independent of blood pressure, in both hypertensive and normotensive individuals, ACEIs attenuate the development of left ventricular hypertrophy, improve symptomatology and risk of death from CHF, and reduce morbidity and mortality rates in post-myocardial infarction patients. Similar benefits in cardiovascular morbidity and mortality rates in patients with CHF have been observed with the use of ARBs. ACEIs provide better coronary protection than do calcium channel blockers, whereas calcium channel blockers provide more stroke protection than do either ACEIs or beta blockers. Results of a recent large, double-blind prospective clinical trial (Rationale and Design of the Avoiding Cardiovascular Events through Combination Therapy in Patients Living with Systolic Hypertension [ACCOMPLISH Trial]) indicated that combination treatment with an ACEI (benazepril) plus a calcium antagonist (amlodipine) was superior to treatment with the ACEI plus a diuretic (hydrochlorothiazide) in reducing the risk of cardiovascular events and death among high-risk patients with hypertension. However, the combination of an ACEI and a diuretic has recently been shown to produce major reductions in morbidity and mortality in the very elderly.

After a stroke, combination therapy with an ACEI and a diuretic, but not with an ARB, reduces the rate of recurrent stroke. Some of these apparent differences may reflect differences in trial design and/or patient groups.

BLOOD PRESSURE GOALS OF ANTIHYPERTENSIVE THERAPY

Based on clinical trial data, the maximum protection against combined cardiovascular endpoints is achieved with pressures <135–140 mmHg for systolic blood pressure and <80–85 mmHg for diastolic blood pressure; however, treatment has not reduced cardiovascular disease risk to the level in nonhypertensive individuals. More aggressive blood pressure targets for blood pressure control (e.g., office or clinic blood pressure <130/80 mmHg) are generally recommended for patients with diabetes, coronary heart disease, chronic kidney disease, or additional cardiovascular disease risk factors. An even lower goal blood pressure (systolic blood pressure ~120 mmHg) may be desirable for patients with proteinuria (>1 g/d) since the decline of glomerular filtration rate in these patients is particularly blood pressure–dependent. In diabetic patients, effective blood pressure control reduces the risk of cardiovascular events and death as well as the risk for microvascular disease (nephropathy, retinopathy). Risk reduction is greater in diabetic than in nondiabetic individuals. Although the optimal target blood pressure in patients with heart failure has not been established, a reasonable goal is the lowest blood pressure that is not associated with evidence of hypoperfusion.

To achieve recommended blood pressure goals, the majority of individuals with hypertension will require treatment with more than one drug. Three or more drugs frequently are needed in patients with diabetes and renal insufficiency. For most agents, reduction of blood pressure at half-standard doses is only ~20% less than at standard doses. Appropriate combinations of agents at these lower doses may have additive or almost additive effects on blood pressure with a lower incidence of side effects.

Despite theoretical concerns about decreasing cerebral, coronary, and renal blood flow by overly aggressive antihypertensive therapy, clinical trials have found no evidence for a "J-curve" phenomenon; i.e., at blood pressure reductions achieved in clinical practice, there does *not* appear to be a lower threshold for increasing cardiovascular risk. A small nonprogressive increase in the serum creatinine concentration with blood pressure reduction may occur in patients with chronic renal insufficiency. This generally reflects a hemodynamic response, not structural renal injury, indicating that intraglomerular pressure has been reduced. Blood pressure control should not be allowed to deteriorate in order to prevent a modest rise in creatinine. Even among older patients with isolated systolic hypertension, further lowering of diastolic blood pressure does not result in harm. However, relatively little information is available concerning the risk-versus-benefit ratio of antihypertensive therapy in individuals >80 years, and in this population, gradual blood pressure reduction to less aggressive target levels of control may be appropriate.

The term *resistant hypertension* refers to patients with blood pressures persistently >140/90 mmHg despite taking three or more antihypertensive agents, including a diuretic, in a reasonable combination and at full doses. Resistant or difficult-to-control hypertension is more common in patients >60 years than in younger patients. Resistant hypertension may be related to "pseudoresistance" (high office blood pressures and lower home blood pressures), nonadherence to therapy, identifiable causes of hypertension (including obesity and excessive alcohol intake), and the use of any of a number of nonprescription and prescription drugs (Table 37-3). Rarely, in older patients, pseudohypertension may be related to the inability to measure blood pressure accurately in severely sclerotic arteries. This condition is suggested if the radial pulse remains palpable despite occlusion of the brachial artery by the cuff (Osler maneuver). The actual blood pressure can be determined by direct intraarterial measurement. Evaluation of patients with resistant hypertension might include home blood pressure monitoring to determine if office blood pressures are representative of the usual blood pressure. A more extensive evaluation for a secondary form of hypertension should be undertaken if no other explanation for hypertension resistance becomes apparent.

HYPERTENSIVE EMERGENCIES Probably due to the widespread availability of antihypertensive therapy, in the United States there has been a decline in the numbers of patients presenting with "crisis levels" of blood pressure. Most patients who present with severe hypertension are chronically hypertensive, and in the absence of acute end-organ damage, precipitous lowering of blood pressure may be associated with significant morbidity and should be avoided. The key to successful management of severe hypertension is to differentiate hypertensive crises from hypertensive urgencies. The degree of target organ damage, rather than the level of blood pressure alone, determines the rapidity with which blood pressure should be lowered. Tables 37-9 and 37-10 list a number of hypertension-related emergencies and recommended therapies.

Malignant hypertension is a syndrome associated with an abrupt increase of blood pressure in a patient with underlying hypertension or related to the sudden onset of hypertension in a previously normotensive individual. The absolute level of blood pressure is not as important as its rate of rise. Pathologically, the syndrome is associated with diffuse necrotizing vasculitis, arteriolar thrombi, and fibrin deposition in arteriolar walls. Fibrinoid necrosis has been observed in arterioles of the kidney, brain, retina, and other organs. Clinically, the syndrome is recognized by progressive retinopathy (arteriolar spasm, hemorrhages, exudates, and papilledema), deteriorating renal function with proteinuria, microangiopathic hemolytic anemia, and encephalopathy. In these patients, historic inquiry should include questions about the use of monamine oxidase inhibitors and recreational drugs (e.g., cocaine, amphetamines).

Although blood pressure should be lowered rapidly in patients with hypertensive encephalopathy,

TABLE 37-9

PREFERRED PARENTERAL DRUGS FOR SELECTED HYPERTENSIVE EMERGENCIES

Hypertensive encephalopathy	Nitroprusside, nicardipine, labetalol
Malignant hypertension (when IV therapy is indicated)	Labetalol, nicardipine, nitroprusside, enalaprilat
Stroke	Nicardipine, labetalol, nitroprusside
Myocardial infarction/ unstable angina	Nitroglycerin, nicardipine, labetalol, esmolol
Acute left ventricular failure	Nitroglycerin, enalaprilat, loop diuretics
Aortic dissection	Nitroprusside, esmolol, labetalol
Adrenergic crisis	Phentolamine, nitroprusside
Postoperative hypertension	Nitroglycerin, nitroprusside, labetalol, nicardipine
Preeclampsia/eclampsia of pregnancy	Hydralazine, labetalol, nicardipine

Source: Adapted from DG Vidt, in S Oparil, MA Weber (eds): *Hypertension*, 2nd ed. Philadelphia, Elsevier Saunders, 2005.

TABLE 37-10

USUAL INTRAVENOUS DOSES OF ANTIHYPERTENSIVE AGENTS USED IN HYPERTENSIVE EMERGENCIES[a]

ANTIHYPERTENSIVE AGENT	INTRAVENOUS DOSE
Nitroprusside	Initial 0.3 (μg/kg)/min; usual 2–4 (μg/kg)/min; maximum 10 (μg/kg)/min for 10 min
Nicardipine	Initial 5 mg/h; titrate by 2.5 mg/h at 5–15 min intervals; max 15 mg/h
Labetalol	2 mg/min up to 300 mg or 20 mg over 2 min, then 40–80 mg at 10-min intervals up to 300 mg total
Enalaprilat	Usual 0.625–1.25 mg over 5 min every 6–8 h; maximum 5 mg/dose
Esmolol	Initial 80–500 μg/kg over 1 min, then 50–300 (μg/kg)/min
Phentolamine	5–15 mg bolus
Nitroglycerin	Initial 5 μg/min, then titrate by 5 μg/min at 3–5-min intervals; if no response is seen at 20 μg/min, incremental increases of 10–20 μg/min may be used
Hydralazine	10–50 mg at 30-min intervals

[a]Constant blood pressure monitoring is required. Start with the lowest dose. Subsequent doses and intervals of administration should be adjusted according to the blood pressure response and duration of action of the specific agent.

there are inherent risks of overly aggressive therapy. In hypertensive individuals, the upper and lower limits of autoregulation of cerebral blood flow are shifted to higher levels of arterial pressure, and rapid lowering of blood pressure to below the lower limit of autoregulation may precipitate cerebral ischemia or infarction as a consequence of decreased cerebral blood flow. Renal and coronary blood flows also may decrease with overly aggressive acute therapy. The initial goal of therapy is to reduce mean arterial blood pressure by no more than 25% within minutes to 2 h or to a blood pressure in the range of 160/100–110 mmHg. This may be accomplished with IV nitroprusside, a short-acting vasodilator with a rapid onset of action that allows for minute-to-minute control of blood pressure. Parenteral labetalol and nicardipine are also effective agents for the treatment of hypertensive encephalopathy.

In patients with malignant hypertension without encephalopathy or another catastrophic event, it is preferable to reduce blood pressure over hours or longer rather than minutes. This goal may effectively be achieved initially with frequent dosing of short-acting oral agents such as captopril, clonidine, and labetalol.

Acute, transient blood pressure elevations that last days to weeks frequently occur after thrombotic and hemorrhagic strokes. Autoregulation of cerebral blood flow is impaired in ischemic cerebral tissue, and higher arterial pressures may be required to maintain cerebral blood flow. Although specific blood pressure targets have not been defined for patients with acute cerebrovascular events, aggressive reductions of blood pressure are to be avoided. With the increasing availability of improved methods for measuring cerebral blood flow (using CT technology), studies are in progress to evaluate the effects of different classes of antihypertensive agents on both blood pressure and cerebral blood flow after an acute stroke. Currently, in the absence of other indications for acute therapy, for patients with cerebral infarction who are not candidates for thrombolytic therapy, one recommended guideline is to institute antihypertensive therapy only for patients with a systolic blood pressure >220 mmHg or a diastolic blood pressure >130 mmHg. If thrombolytic therapy is to be used, the recommended goal blood pressure is <185 mmHg systolic pressure and <110 mmHg diastolic pressure. In patients with hemorrhagic stroke, suggested guidelines for initiating antihypertensive therapy are systolic >180 mmHg or diastolic pressure >130 mmHg. The management of hypertension after subarachnoid hemorrhage is controversial. Cautious reduction of blood pressure is indicated if mean arterial pressure is >130 mmHg.

In addition to pheochromocytoma, an adrenergic crisis due to catecholamine excess may be related to cocaine or amphetamine overdose, clonidine withdrawal, acute spinal cord injuries, and an interaction of tyramine-containing compounds with monamine oxidase inhibitors. These patients may be treated with phentolamine or nitroprusside.

Treatment of hypertension in patients with acute aortic dissection is discussed in Chap. 38.

CHAPTER 38
DISEASES OF THE AORTA

Mark A. Creager ■ Joseph Loscalzo

The aorta is the conduit through which blood ejected from the left ventricle is delivered to the systemic arterial bed. In adults, its diameter is approximately 3 cm at the origin and in the ascending portion, 2.5 cm in the descending portion in the thorax, and 1.8–2 cm in the abdomen. The aortic wall consists of a thin intima composed of endothelium, subendothelial connective tissue, and an internal elastic lamina; a thick tunica media composed of smooth-muscle cells and extracellular matrix; and an adventitia composed primarily of connective tissue enclosing the vasa vasorum and nervi vascularis. In addition to the conduit function of the aorta, its viscoelastic and compliant properties serve a buffering function. The aorta is distended during systole to allow a portion of the stroke volume and elastic energy to be stored, and it recoils during diastole so that blood continues to flow to the periphery. Because of its continuous exposure to high pulsatile pressure and shear stress, the aorta is particularly prone to injury and disease resulting from mechanical trauma. The aorta is also more prone to rupture than is any other vessel, especially with the development of aneurysmal dilation, since its wall tension, as governed by Laplace's law (i.e., proportional to the product of pressure and radius), will be increased.

CONGENITAL ANOMALIES OF THE AORTA

Congenital anomalies of the aorta usually involve the aortic arch and its branches. Symptoms such as dysphagia, stridor, and cough may occur if an anomaly causes a ring around or otherwise compresses the esophagus or trachea. Anomalies associated with symptoms include double aortic arch, origin of the right subclavian artery distal to the left subclavian artery, and right-sided aortic arch with an aberrant left subclavian artery. A Kommerell's diverticulum is an anatomic remnant of a right aortic arch. Most congenital anomalies of the aorta do not cause symptoms and are detected during catheter-based procedures. The diagnosis of suspected congenital anomalies of the aorta typically is confirmed by computed tomographic (CT) or magnetic resonance (MR) angiography. Surgery is used to treat symptomatic anomalies.

AORTIC ANEURYSM

An *aneurysm* is defined as a pathologic dilation of a segment of a blood vessel. A *true aneurysm* involves all three layers of the vessel wall and is distinguished from a *pseudoaneurysm*, in which the intimal and medial layers are disrupted and the dilated segment of the aorta is lined by adventitia only and, at times, by perivascular clot. Aneurysms also may be classified according to their gross appearance. A *fusiform aneurysm* affects the entire circumference of a segment of the vessel, resulting in a diffusely dilated artery. In contrast, a *saccular aneurysm* involves only a portion of the circumference, resulting in an outpouching of the vessel wall. Aortic aneurysms also are classified according to location, i.e., abdominal versus thoracic. Aneurysms of the descending thoracic aorta are usually contiguous with infradiaphragmatic aneurysms and are referred to as *thoracoabdominal aortic aneurysms*.

ETIOLOGY

Aortic aneurysms result from conditions that cause degradation or abnormal production of the structural components of the aortic wall: elastin and collagen. The causes of aortic aneurysms may be broadly categorized as degenerative diseases, inherited or developmental diseases, infections, vasculitis, and trauma (Table 38-1). Inflammation, proteolysis, and biomechanical wall stress contribute to the degenerative processes that characterize most aneurysms of the abdominal and descending thoracic aorta. These are mediated by B-cell and T-cell lymphocytes, macrophages, inflammatory cytokines, and matrix metalloproteinases that degrade elastin and collagen and alter the tensile strength and ability of the aorta to accommodate pulsatile stretch. The associated histopathology demonstrates destruction of elastin and collagen, decreased vascular smooth muscle, in-growth of new blood vessels, and inflammation. Factors associated with degenerative aortic aneurysms include aging, cigarette smoking, hypercholesterolemia, male sex, and a family history of aortic aneurysms.

TABLE 38-1

DISEASES OF THE AORTA: ETIOLOGY AND ASSOCIATED FACTORS

Aortic aneurysm
  Degenerative/atherosclerosis
    Aging
    Cigarette smoking
    Male gender
    Family history
  Cystic medial necrosis
    Marfan syndrome
    Loeys-Dietz syndrome
    Ehlers-Danlos syndrome type IV
    Familial
    Bicuspid aortic valve
  Chronic aortic dissection
  Infective (see below)
  Trauma
Acute aortic syndromes (aortic dissection, acute intramural hematoma, penetrating atherosclerotic ulcer)
  Atherosclerosis
  Cystic medial necrosis (see above)
  Hypertension
  Vasculitis (see below)
  Pregnancy
  Trauma
Aortic occlusion
  Atherosclerosis
  Thromboembolism
Aortitis
  Vasculitis
    Takayasu's arteritis
    Giant cell arteritis
  Rheumatic
    HLA-B27–associated spondyloarthropathies
    Behçet's syndrome
    Cogan's syndrome
  Idiopathic aortitis
  Infective
    Syphilis
    Tuberculosis
  Mycotic (*Salmonella*, staphylococcal, streptococcal, fungal)

The most common pathologic condition associated with degenerative aortic aneurysms is *atherosclerosis*. Many patients with aortic aneurysms have coexisting risk factors for atherosclerosis (Chap. 30), as well as atherosclerosis in other blood vessels.

Cystic medial necrosis is the histopathologic term used to describe the degeneration of collagen and elastic fibers in the tunica media of the aorta as well as the loss of medial cells that are replaced by multiple clefts of mucoid material. Cystic medial necrosis characteristically affects the proximal aorta, results in circumferential weakness and dilation, and leads to the development of fusiform aneurysms involving the ascending aorta and the sinuses of Valsalva. This condition is particularly prevalent in patients with Marfan syndrome, Loeys-Dietz syndrome, Ehlers-Danlos syndrome type IV, hypertension, congenital bicuspid aortic valves, and familial thoracic aortic aneurysm syndromes; sometimes it appears as an isolated condition in patients without any other apparent disease.

Familial clusterings of aortic aneurysms occur in 20% of patients, suggesting a hereditary basis for the disease. Mutations of the gene that encodes fibrillin-1 are present in patients with Marfan syndrome. Fibrillin-1 is an important component of extracellular micofibrils, which support the architecture of elastic fibers and other connective tissue. Deficiency of fibrillin-1 in the extracellular matrix leads to excessive signaling by transforming growth factor β (TGF-β). Loeys-Dietz syndrome is caused by mutations in the genes that encode TGF-β receptors 1 (*TGFBR1*) and 2 (*TGFBR2*). Increased signaling by TGF-β and mutations of *TGFBR1* and *TGFBR2* may cause thoracic aortic aneurysms. Mutations of type III procollagen have been implicated in Ehlers-Danlos type IV syndrome. Linkage analysis has identified loci on chromosomes 5q13–14, 11q23.3–q24, and 3p24–25 in several families, although the specific alleles have not been described.

The infectious causes of aortic aneurysms include syphilis, tuberculosis, and other bacterial infections. *Syphilis* is a relatively uncommon cause of aortic aneurysm. Syphilitic periaortitis and mesoaortitis damage elastic fibers, resulting in thickening and weakening of the aortic wall. Approximately 90% of syphilitic aneurysms are located in the ascending aorta or aortic arch. *Tuberculous aneurysms* typically affect the thoracic aorta and result from direct extension of infection from hilar lymph nodes or contiguous abscesses as well as from bacterial seeding. Loss of aortic wall elasticity results from granulomatous destruction of the medial layer. A *mycotic aneurysm* is a rare condition that develops as a result of staphylococcal, streptococcal, *Salmonella*, or other bacterial or fungal infections of the aorta, usually at an atherosclerotic plaque. These aneurysms are usually saccular. Blood cultures are often positive and reveal the nature of the infective agent.

Vasculitides associated with aortic aneurysm include Takayasu's arteritis and giant cell arteritis, which may cause aneurysms of the aortic arch and descending thoracic aorta. Spondyloarthropathies such as ankylosing spondylitis, rheumatoid arthritis, psoriatic arthritis, relapsing polychondritis, and reactive arthritis (formerly known as Reiter's syndrome) are associated with dilation of the ascending aorta. Aortic aneurysms occur in patients with Behçet's syndrome and Cogan's syndrome. Aortic aneurysms also result from idiopathic aortitis. *Traumatic aneurysms* may occur after penetrating or nonpenetrating chest trauma and most commonly affect the descending thoracic aorta just beyond the site of insertion of the ligamentum arteriosum. Chronic aortic dissections are associated with weakening of the aortic wall that may lead to the development of aneurysmal dilatation.

THORACIC AORTIC ANEURYSMS

The clinical manifestations and natural history of thoracic aortic aneurysms depend on their location. Cystic medial necrosis is the most common pathology associated with ascending aortic aneurysms, whereas atherosclerosis is the condition most frequently associated with aneurysms of the aortic arch and descending thoracic aorta. The average growth rate of thoracic aneurysms is 0.1–0.2 cm per year. Thoracic aortic aneurysms associated with Marfan syndrome or aortic dissection may expand at a greater rate. The risk of rupture is related to the size of the aneurysm and the presence of symptoms, ranging approximately from 2–3% per year for thoracic aortic aneurysms <4.0 cm in diameter to 7% per year for those >6 cm in diameter. Most thoracic aortic aneurysms are asymptomatic; however, compression or erosion of adjacent tissue by aneurysms may cause symptoms such as chest pain, shortness of breath, cough, hoarseness, and dysphagia. Aneurysmal dilation of the ascending aorta may cause congestive heart failure as a consequence of aortic regurgitation, and compression of the superior vena cava may produce congestion of the head, neck, and upper extremities.

A chest x-ray may be the first test that suggests the diagnosis of a thoracic aortic aneurysm (**Fig. 38-1**). Findings include widening of the mediastinal shadow and displacement or compression of the trachea or left mainstem bronchus. Echocardiography, particularly transesophageal echocardiography, can be used to assess the proximal ascending aorta and descending thoracic aorta. Contrast-enhanced CT, magnetic resonance imaging (MRI), and conventional invasive aortography are sensitive and specific tests for assessment of aneurysms of the thoracic aorta and involvement of branch vessels (**Fig. 38-2**). In asymptomatic patients whose aneurysms are too small to justify surgery, noninvasive testing with

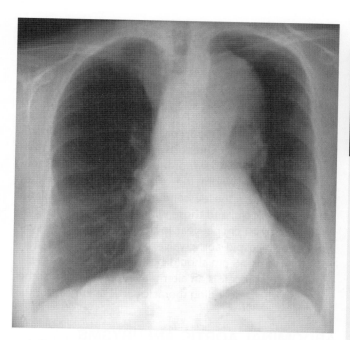

FIGURE 38-1
A chest x-ray of a patient with a thoracic aortic aneurysm.

either contrast-enhanced CT or MRI should be performed at least every 6–12 months to monitor expansion.

TREATMENT	Thoracic Aortic Aneurysms

β-Adrenergic blockers currently are recommended for patients with thoracic aortic aneurysms, particularly those with Marfan syndrome, who have evidence of aortic root dilatation to reduce the rate of further

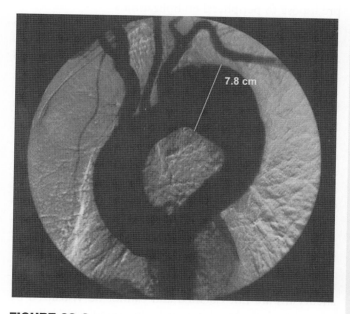

FIGURE 38-2
An aortogram demonstrating a large fusiform aneurysm of the descending thoracic aorta.

expansion. Additional medical therapy should be given as necessary to control hypertension. Recent preliminary studies indicate that angiotensin receptor antagonists and angiotensin-converting enzyme inhibitors will reduce the rate of aortic dilation in patients with Marfan syndrome by blocking TGF-β signaling; clinical outcome trials of this treatment approach are in progress. Operative repair with placement of a prosthetic graft is indicated in patients with symptomatic thoracic aortic aneurysms, those in whom the ascending aortic diameter is >5.5–6 cm or the descending thoracic aortic diameter is >6.5–7 cm, and those with an aneurysm that has increased by >1 cm per year. In patients with Marfan syndrome or bicuspid aortic valve, ascending thoracic aortic aneurysms >5 cm should be considered for surgery. Endovascular repair is an alternative treatment for some patients with descending thoracic aortic aneurysms.

ABDOMINAL AORTIC ANEURYSMS

Abdominal aortic aneurysms occur more frequently in males than in females, and the incidence increases with age. Abdominal aortic aneurysms ≥4.0 cm may affect 1–2% of men older than 50 years. At least 90% of all abdominal aortic aneurysms >4.0 cm are related to atherosclerotic disease, and most of these aneurysms are below the level of the renal arteries. Prognosis is related to both the size of the aneurysm and the severity of coexisting coronary artery and cerebrovascular disease. The risk of rupture increases with the size of the aneurysm: the 5-year risk for aneurysms <5 cm is 1–2%, whereas it is 20–40% for aneurysms >5 cm in diameter. The formation of mural thrombi within aneurysms may predispose to peripheral embolization.

An abdominal aortic aneurysm commonly produces no symptoms. It usually is detected on routine examination as a palpable, pulsatile, expansile, and nontender mass, or it is an incidental finding observed on an abdominal x-ray or ultrasound study performed for other reasons. As abdominal aortic aneurysms expand, however, they may become painful. Some patients complain of strong pulsations in the abdomen; others experience pain in the chest, lower back, or scrotum. Aneurysmal pain is usually a harbinger of rupture and represents a medical emergency. More often, acute rupture occurs without any prior warning, and this complication is always life threatening. Rarely, there is leakage of the aneurysm with severe pain and tenderness. Acute pain and hypotension occur with rupture of the aneurysm, which requires an emergency operation.

Abdominal radiography may demonstrate the calcified outline of the aneurysm; however, about 25% of aneurysms are not calcified and cannot be visualized by x-ray imaging. An abdominal ultrasound can delineate the transverse and longitudinal dimensions of an abdominal aortic aneurysm and may detect mural thrombus.

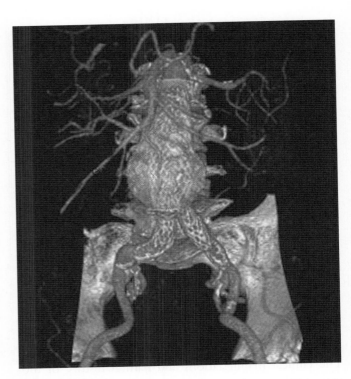

FIGURE 38-3

A computed tomographic angiogram (CTA) depicting a fusiform abdominal aortic aneurysm that has been treated with a bifurcated stent graft.

Abdominal ultrasound is useful for serial documentation of aneurysm size and can be used to screen patients at risk for developing an aortic aneurysm. In one large study, ultrasound screening of men age 65–74 years was associated with a risk reduction in aneurysm-related death of 42%. For this reason, screening by ultrasonography is recommended for men age 65–75 years who have ever smoked. In addition, siblings or offspring of persons with abdominal aortic aneurysms, as well as individuals with thoracic aortic or peripheral arterial aneurysms, should be considered for screening for abdominal aortic aneurysms. CT with contrast and MRI are accurate noninvasive tests to determine the location and size of abdominal aortic aneurysms and to plan endovascular or open surgical repair (**Fig. 38-3**). Contrast aortography may be used for the evaluation of patients with aneurysms, but the procedure carries a small risk of complications such as bleeding, allergic reactions, and atheroembolism. Since the presence of mural thrombi may reduce the luminal size, aortography may underestimate the diameter of an aneurysm.

| TREATMENT | Abdominal Aortic Aneurysms |

Operative repair of the aneurysm with insertion of a prosthetic graft or endovascular placement of an aortic stent graft (Fig. 38-3) is indicated for abdominal aortic aneurysms of any size that are expanding rapidly or are associated with symptoms. For asymptomatic aneurysms, abdominal aortic aneurysm repair is indicated if the diameter is >5.5 cm. In randomized trials of patients with abdominal aortic aneurysms <5.5 cm, there was no difference in the long-term (5- to 8-year) mortality rate between those followed with ultrasound surveillance and those undergoing elective surgical repair. Thus, serial noninvasive follow-up of smaller aneurysms (<5 cm) is an alternative to immediate repair. The decision to perform an open surgical operation or endovascular repair is based in part on the vascular anatomy and comorbid conditions. Endovascular repair of abdominal aortic aneurysms has a lower short-term morbidity rate but a comparable long-term mortality rate with open surgical reconstruction. Long-term surveillance with CT or MR aortography is indicated after endovascular repair to detect leaks and possible aneurysm expansion.

In surgical candidates, careful preoperative cardiac and general medical evaluations (followed by appropriate therapy for complicating conditions) are essential. Preexisting coronary artery disease, congestive heart failure, pulmonary disease, diabetes mellitus, and advanced age add to the risk of surgery. β-Adrenergic blockers decrease perioperative cardiovascular morbidity and mortality. With careful preoperative cardiac evaluation and postoperative care, the operative mortality rate approximates 1–2%. After acute rupture, the mortality rate of emergent operation is 45–50%. Endovascular repair with stent placement is an emerging approach but at the current time is associated with a mortality rate of approximately 40%.

ACUTE AORTIC SYNDROMES

The four major acute aortic syndromes are aortic rupture (discussed earlier), aortic dissection, intramural hematoma, and penetrating atherosclerotic ulcer. Aortic dissection is caused by a circumferential or, less frequently, transverse tear of the intima. It often occurs along the right lateral wall of the ascending aorta where the hydraulic shear stress is high. Another common site is the descending thoracic aorta just below the ligamentum arteriosum. The initiating event is either a primary intimal tear with secondary dissection into the media or a medial hemorrhage that dissects into and disrupts the intima. The pulsatile aortic flow then dissects along the elastic lamellar plates of the aorta and creates a false lumen. The dissection usually propagates distally down the descending aorta and into its major branches, but it may propagate proximally. Distal propagation may be limited by atherosclerotic plaque. In some cases, a secondary distal intimal disruption occurs, resulting in the reentry of blood from the false to the true lumen.

There are at least two important pathologic and radiologic variants of aortic dissection: intramural hematoma without an intimal flap and penetrating atherosclerotic ulcer. Acute intramural hematoma is thought to result from rupture of the vasa vasorum with hemorrhage into the wall of the aorta. Most of these hematomas occur in the descending thoracic aorta. Acute intramural hematomas may progress to dissection and rupture. Penetrating atherosclerotic ulcers are caused by erosion of a plaque into the aortic media, are usually localized, and are not associated with extensive propagation. They are found primarily in the middle and distal portions of the descending thoracic aorta and are associated with extensive atherosclerotic disease. The ulcer can erode beyond the internal elastic lamina, leading to medial hematoma, and may progress to false aneurysm formation or rupture.

Several classification schemes have been developed for thoracic aortic dissections. DeBakey and colleagues initially classified aortic dissections as type I, in which an intimal tear occurs in the ascending aorta but involves the descending aorta as well; type II, in which the dissection is limited to the ascending aorta; and type III, in which the intimal tear is located in the descending aorta with distal propagation of the dissection (Fig. 38-4). Another classification (Stanford) is that of type A, in which the dissection involves the ascending aorta (proximal dissection), and type B, in which it is limited to the descending aorta (distal dissection). From a management standpoint, classification of aortic dissections and intramural hematomas into type A or B is more practical and useful, since DeBakey types I and II are managed in a similar manner.

The factors that predispose to aortic dissection include systemic hypertension, a coexisting condition in 70% of patients, and cystic medial necrosis. Aortic dissection is the major cause of morbidity and mortality in patients with Marfan syndrome and similarly may affect patients with Ehlers-Danlos syndrome. The incidence also is increased in patients with inflammatory aortitis (i.e., Takayasu's arteritis, giant cell arteritis), congenital aortic valve anomalies (e.g., bicuspid valve), coarctation of the aorta, and a history of aortic trauma. In addition, the risk of dissection is increased in otherwise normal women during the third trimester of pregnancy.

CLINICAL MANIFESTATIONS

The peak incidence of aortic dissection is in the sixth and seventh decades. Men are more affected than women by a ratio of 2:1. The presentations of aortic dissection and its variants are the consequences of intimal tear, dissecting hematoma, occlusion of involved arteries, and compression of adjacent tissues. Acute aortic dissection presents with the sudden onset of pain (Chap. 4), which often is described as very severe

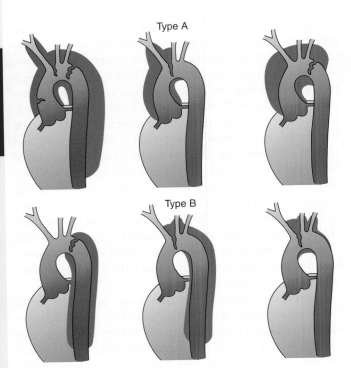

FIGURE 38-4
Classification of aortic dissections. Stanford classification: Type A dissections (*top panels*) involve the ascending aorta independent of site of tear and distal extension; type B dissections (*bottom panels*) involve transverse and/or descending aorta without involvement of the ascending aorta. DeBakey classification: Type I dissection involves ascending to descending aorta (*top left*); type II dissection is limited to ascending or transverse aorta, without descending aorta (*top center + top right*); type III dissection involves descending aorta only (*bottom left*). (*From DC Miller, in RM Doroghazi, EE Slater [eds]: Aortic Dissection. New York, McGraw-Hill, 1983; with permission.*)

and tearing and is associated with diaphoresis. The pain may be localized to the front or back of the chest, often the interscapular region, and typically migrates with propagation of the dissection. Other symptoms include syncope, dyspnea, and weakness. Physical findings may include hypertension or hypotension, loss of pulses, aortic regurgitation, pulmonary edema, and neurologic findings due to carotid artery obstruction (hemiplegia, hemianesthesia) or spinal cord ischemia (paraplegia). Bowel ischemia, hematuria, and myocardial ischemia have all been observed. These clinical manifestations reflect complications resulting from the dissection occluding the major arteries. Furthermore, clinical manifestations may result from the compression of adjacent structures (e.g., superior cervical ganglia, superior vena cava, bronchus, esophagus) by the expanding dissection, causing aneurysmal dilation, and include Horner's syndrome, superior vena cava syndrome, hoarseness, dysphagia, and airway compromise. Hemopericardium and cardiac tamponade may

complicate a type A lesion with retrograde dissection. Acute aortic regurgitation is an important and common (>50%) complication of proximal dissection. It is the outcome of either a circumferential tear that widens the aortic root or a disruption of the annulus by a dissecting hematoma that tears a leaflet(s) or displaces it, inferior to the line of closure. Signs of aortic regurgitation include bounding pulses, a wide pulse pressure, a diastolic murmur often radiating along the right sternal border, and evidence of congestive heart failure. The clinical manifestations depend on the severity of the regurgitation.

In dissections involving the ascending aorta, the chest x-ray often reveals a widened superior mediastinum. A pleural effusion (usually left-sided) also may be present. This effusion is typically serosanguineous and not indicative of rupture unless accompanied by hypotension and falling hematocrit. In dissections of the descending thoracic aorta, a widened mediastinum may be observed on chest x-ray. In addition, the descending aorta may appear to be wider than the ascending portion. An electrocardiogram that shows no evidence of myocardial ischemia is helpful in distinguishing aortic dissection from myocardial infarction. Rarely, the dissection involves the right or, less commonly, left coronary ostium and causes acute myocardial infarction.

The diagnosis of aortic dissection can be established by noninvasive techniques such as echocardiography, CT, and MRI. Aortography is used less commonly because of the accuracy of these noninvasive techniques. Transthoracic echocardiography can be performed simply and rapidly and has an overall sensitivity of 60–85% for aortic dissection. For diagnosing proximal ascending aortic dissections, its sensitivity exceeds 80%; it is less useful for detecting dissection of the arch and descending thoracic aorta. Transesophageal echocardiography requires greater skill and patient cooperation but is very accurate in identifying dissections of the ascending and descending thoracic aorta but not the arch, achieving 98% sensitivity and approximately 90% specificity. Echocardiography also provides important information regarding the presence and severity of aortic regurgitation and pericardial effusion. CT and MRI are both highly accurate in identifying the intimal flap and the extent of the dissection and involvement of major arteries; each has a sensitivity and specificity >90%. They are useful in recognizing intramural hemorrhage and penetrating ulcers. MRI also can detect blood flow, which may be useful in characterizing antegrade versus retrograde dissection. The relative utility of transesophageal echocardiography, CT, and MRI depends on the availability and expertise in individual institutions as well as on the hemodynamic stability of the patient, with CT and MRI obviously less suitable for unstable patients.

TREATMENT ▶ Aortic Dissection

Medical therapy should be initiated as soon as the diagnosis is considered. The patient should be admitted to an intensive care unit for hemodynamic monitoring. Unless hypotension is present, therapy should be aimed at reducing cardiac contractility and systemic arterial pressure, and thus shear stress. For acute dissection, unless contraindicated, β-adrenergic blockers should be administered parenterally, using intravenous propranolol, metoprolol, or the short-acting esmolol to achieve a heart rate of approximately 60 beats/min. This should be accompanied by sodium nitroprusside infusion to lower systolic blood pressure to ≤120 mmHg. Labetalol (Chap. 37), a drug with both β- and α-adrenergic blocking properties, also may be used as a parenteral agent in acute therapy for dissection.

The calcium channel antagonists verapamil and diltiazem may be used intravenously if nitroprusside or β-adrenergic blockers cannot be employed. The addition of a parenteral angiotensin-converting enzyme (ACE) inhibitor such as enalaprilat to a β-adrenergic blocker also may be considered. Isolated use of a direct vasodilator such as hydralazine is contraindicated because these agents can increase hydraulic shear and may propagate the dissection.

Emergent or urgent surgical correction is the preferred treatment for acute ascending aortic dissections and intramural hematomas (type A) and for complicated type B dissections, including those characterized by propagation, compromise of major aortic branches, impending rupture, or continued pain. Surgery involves excision of the intimal flap, obliteration of the false lumen, and placement of an interposition graft. A composite valve-graft conduit is used if the aortic valve is disrupted. The overall in-hospital mortality rate after surgical treatment of patients with aortic dissection is reported to be 15–25%. The major causes of perioperative mortality and morbidity include myocardial infarction, paraplegia, renal failure, tamponade, hemorrhage, and sepsis. Endoluminal stent grafts may be considered in selected patients. Other transcatheter techniques, such as fenestration of the intimal flaps and stenting of narrowed branch vessels to increase flow to compromised organs, are used in selected patients. For uncomplicated and stable distal dissections and intramural hematomas (type B), medical therapy is the preferred treatment. The in-hospital mortality rate of medically treated patients with type B dissection is 10–20%. Long-term therapy for patients with aortic dissection and intramural hematomas (with or without surgery) consists of control of hypertension and reduction of cardiac contractility with the use of beta blockers plus other antihypertensive agents, such as ACE inhibitors or calcium antagonists. Patients with chronic type B dissection and intramural hematomas should be followed on an outpatient basis every 6–12 months with contrast-enhanced CT or MRI to detect propagation or expansion. Patients with Marfan syndrome are at high risk for postdissection complications. The long-term prognosis for patients with treated dissections is generally good with careful follow-up; the 10-year survival rate is approximately 60%.

CHRONIC ATHEROSCLEROTIC OCCLUSIVE DISEASE

Atherosclerosis may affect the thoracic and abdominal aorta. Occlusive aortic disease caused by atherosclerosis usually is confined to the distal abdominal aorta below the renal arteries. Frequently, the disease extends to the iliac arteries (Chap. 39). Claudication characteristically involves the buttocks, thighs, and calves and may be associated with impotence in males (Leriche syndrome). The severity of the symptoms depends on the adequacy of collaterals. With sufficient collateral blood flow, a complete occlusion of the abdominal aorta may occur without the development of ischemic symptoms. The physical findings include the absence of femoral and other distal pulses bilaterally and the detection of an audible bruit over the abdomen (usually at or below the umbilicus) and the common femoral arteries. Atrophic skin, loss of hair, and coolness of the lower extremities usually are observed. In advanced ischemia, rubor on dependency and pallor on elevation can be seen.

The diagnosis usually is established by physical examination and noninvasive testing, including leg pressure measurements, Doppler velocity analysis, pulse volume recordings, and duplex ultrasonography. The anatomy may be defined by MRI, CT, or conventional aortography, typically performed when one is considering revascularization. Catheter-based endovascular or operative treatment is indicated in patients with lifestyle-limiting or debilitating symptoms of claudication and patients with critical limb ischemia.

ACUTE AORTIC OCCLUSION

Acute occlusion in the distal abdominal aorta constitutes a medical emergency because it threatens the viability of the lower extremities; it usually results from an occlusive (saddle) embolus that almost always originates from the heart. Rarely, acute occlusion may occur as the result of in situ thrombosis in a preexisting severely narrowed segment of the aorta.

The clinical picture is one of acute ischemia of the lower extremities. Severe rest pain, coolness, and pallor of the lower extremities and the absence of distal pulses bilaterally are the usual manifestations. Diagnosis should be established rapidly by MRI, CT, or aortography. Emergency thrombectomy or revascularization is indicated.

AORTITIS

Aortitis, a term referring to inflammatory disease of the aorta, may be caused by large vessel vasculitides such as Takayasu's arteritis and giant cell arteritis, rheumatic and HLA-B27–associated spondyloarthropathies, Behçet's syndrome, antineutrophil cytoplasmic antibodies (ANCA)-associated vasculitides, Cogan's syndrome, and infections such as syphilis, tuberculosis, and *Salmonella*, or may be associated with retroperitoneal fibrosis. Aortitis may result in aneurysmal dilation and aortic regurgitation, occlusion of the aorta and its branch vessels, or acute aortic syndromes.

TAKAYASU'S ARTERITIS

This inflammatory disease often affects the ascending aorta and aortic arch, causing obstruction of the aorta and its major arteries. Takayasu's arteritis is also termed *pulseless disease* because of the frequent occlusion of the large arteries originating from the aorta. It also may involve the descending thoracic and abdominal aorta and occlude large branches such as the renal arteries. Aortic aneurysms also may occur. The pathology is a panarteritis characterized by mononuclear cells and occasionally giant cells, with marked intimal hyperplasia, medial and adventitial thickening, and, in the chronic form, fibrotic occlusion. The disease is most prevalent in young females of Asian descent but does occur in women of other geographic and ethnic origins and also in young men. During the acute stage, fever, malaise, weight loss, and other systemic symptoms may be evident. Elevations of the erythrocyte sedimentation rate and C-reactive protein are common. The chronic stages of the disease, which is intermittently active, present with symptoms related to large artery occlusion, such as upper extremity claudication, cerebral ischemia, and syncope. The process is progressive, and there is no definitive therapy. Glucocorticoids and immunosuppressive agents have been reported to be effective in some patients during the acute phase. Surgical bypass or endovascular intervention of a critically stenotic artery may be necessary.

GIANT CELL ARTERITIS

This vasculitis occurs in older individuals and affects women more often than men. Primarily large and medium-size arteries are affected. The pathology is that of focal granulomatous lesions involving the entire arterial wall; it may be associated with polymyalgia rheumatica. Obstruction of medium-size arteries (e.g., temporal and ophthalmic arteries) and major branches of the aorta and the development of aortitis and aortic regurgitation are important complications of the disease.

High-dose glucocorticoid therapy may be effective when given early.

RHEUMATIC AORTITIS

Rheumatoid arthritis, ankylosing spondylitis, psoriatic arthritis, reactive arthritis (formerly known as Reiter's syndrome), relapsing polychondritis, and inflammatory bowel disorders may all be associated with aortitis involving the ascending aorta. The inflammatory lesions usually involve the ascending aorta and may extend to the sinuses of Valsalva, the mitral valve leaflets, and adjacent myocardium. The clinical manifestations are aneurysm, aortic regurgitation, and involvement of the cardiac conduction system.

IDIOPATHIC AORTITIS

Idiopathic abdominal aortitis is characterized by adventitial and periaortic inflammation with thickening of the aortic wall. It is associated with abdominal aortic aneurysms and idiopathic retroperitoneal fibrosis. Affected individuals may present with vague constitutional symptoms, fever, and abdominal pain. Retroperitoneal fibrosis can cause ureteral obstruction and hydronephrosis. Glucocorticoids and immunosuppressive agents may reduce the inflammation.

INFECTIVE AORTITIS

Infective aortitis may result from direct invasion of the aortic wall by bacterial pathogens such as *Staphylococcus*, *Streptococcus*, and *Salmonella* or by fungi. These bacteria cause aortitis by infecting the aorta at sites of atherosclerotic plaque. Bacterial proteases lead to degradation of collagen, and the ensuing destruction of the aortic wall leads to the formation of a saccular aneurysm referred to as a mycotic aneurysm. Mycotic aneurysms have a predilection for the suprarenal abdominal aorta. The pathologic characteristics of the aortic wall include acute and chronic inflammation, abscesses, hemorrhage, and necrosis. Mycotic aneurysms typically affect the elderly and occur in men three times more frequently than in women. Patients may present with fever, sepsis, and chest, back, or abdominal pain; there may have been a preceding diarrheal illness. Blood cultures are positive in the majority of patients. Both CT and MRI are useful to diagnose mycotic aneurysms. Treatment includes antibiotic therapy and surgical removal of the affected part of the aorta and revascularization of the lower extremities with grafts placed in uninfected tissue.

Syphilitic aortitis is a late manifestation of luetic infection that usually affects the proximal ascending aorta, particularly the aortic root, resulting in aortic dilation and aneurysm formation. Syphilitic aortitis occasionally may involve the aortic arch or the descending aorta. The aneurysms may be saccular or fusiform and are usually asymptomatic, but compression of and erosion into adjacent structures may result in symptoms; rupture also may occur.

The initial lesion is an obliterative endarteritis of the vasa vasorum, especially in the adventitia. This is an inflammatory response to the invasion of the adventitia by the spirochetes. Destruction of the aortic media occurs as the spirochetes spread into this layer, usually via the lymphatics accompanying the vasa vasorum. Destruction of collagen and elastic tissues leads to dilation of the aorta, scar formation, and calcification. These changes account for the characteristic radiographic appearance of linear calcification of the ascending aorta.

The disease typically presents as an incidental chest radiographic finding 15–30 years after initial infection. Symptoms may result from aortic regurgitation, narrowing of coronary ostia due to syphilitic aortitis, compression of adjacent structures (e.g., esophagus), or rupture. Diagnosis is established by a positive serologic test, i.e., rapid plasmin reagin (RPR) or fluorescent treponemal antibody. Treatment includes penicillin and surgical excision and repair.

CHAPTER 39

VASCULAR DISEASES OF THE EXTREMITIES

Mark A. Creager ■ Joseph Loscalzo

ARTERIAL DISORDERS

PERIPHERAL ARTERY DISEASE

Peripheral artery disease (PAD) is defined as a clinical disorder in which there is a stenosis or occlusion in the aorta or the arteries of the limbs. Atherosclerosis is the leading cause of PAD in patients >40 years old. Other causes include thrombosis, embolism, vasculitis, fibromuscular dysplasia, entrapment, cystic adventitial disease, and trauma. The highest prevalence of atherosclerotic PAD occurs in the sixth and seventh decades of life. As in patients with atherosclerosis of the coronary and cerebral vasculature, there is an increased risk of developing PAD in cigarette smokers and in persons with diabetes mellitus, hypercholesterolemia, hypertension, or hyperhomocysteinemia.

Pathology

(See also Chap. 30) Segmental lesions that cause stenosis or occlusion are usually localized to large and medium-size vessels. The pathology of the lesions includes atherosclerotic plaques with calcium deposition, thinning of the media, patchy destruction of muscle and elastic fibers, fragmentation of the internal elastic lamina, and thrombi composed of platelets and fibrin. The primary sites of involvement are the abdominal aorta and iliac arteries (30% of symptomatic patients), the femoral and popliteal arteries (80–90% of patients), and the more distal vessels, including the tibial and peroneal arteries (40–50% of patients). Atherosclerotic lesions occur preferentially at arterial branch points, which are sites of increased turbulence, altered shear stress, and intimal injury. Involvement of the distal vasculature is most common in elderly individuals and patients with diabetes mellitus.

Clinical evaluation

Fewer than 50% of patients with PAD are symptomatic, although many have a slow or impaired gait. The most common *symptom* is intermittent claudication, which is defined as a pain, ache, cramp, numbness, or a sense of fatigue in the muscles; it occurs during exercise and is relieved by rest. The site of claudication is distal to the location of the occlusive lesion. For example, buttock, hip, and thigh discomfort occurs in patients with aortoiliac disease, whereas calf claudication develops in patients with femoral-popliteal disease. Symptoms are far more common in the lower than in the upper extremities because of the higher incidence of obstructive lesions in the former region. In patients with severe arterial occlusive disease in whom resting blood flow cannot accommodate basal nutritional needs of the tissues, critical limb ischemia may develop. Patients complain of rest pain or a feeling of cold or numbness in the foot and toes. Frequently, these symptoms occur at night when the legs are horizontal and improve when the legs are in a dependent position. With severe ischemia, rest pain may be persistent.

Important *physical findings* of PAD include decreased or absent pulses distal to the obstruction, the presence of bruits over the narrowed artery, and muscle atrophy. With more severe disease, hair loss, thickened nails, smooth and shiny skin, reduced skin temperature, and pallor or cyanosis are common physical signs. In patients with critical limb ischemia, ulcers or gangrene may occur. Elevation of the legs and repeated flexing of the calf muscles produce pallor of the soles of the feet, whereas rubor, secondary to reactive hyperemia, may develop when the legs are dependent. The time required for rubor to develop or for the veins in the foot to fill when the patient's legs are transferred from an elevated to a dependent position is related to the severity of the ischemia and the presence of collateral vessels.

Patients with severe ischemia may develop peripheral edema because they keep their legs in a dependent position much of the time. Ischemic neuropathy can result in numbness and hyporeflexia.

Noninvasive testing

The history and physical examination are often sufficient to establish the diagnosis of PAD. An objective assessment of the presence and severity of disease is obtained by noninvasive techniques. Arterial pressure can be recorded noninvasively in the legs by placement of sphygmomanometric cuffs at the ankles and the use of a Doppler device to auscultate or record blood flow from the dorsalis pedis and posterior tibial arteries. Normally, systolic blood pressure in the legs and arms is similar. Indeed, ankle pressure may be slightly higher than arm pressure due to pulse-wave amplification. In the presence of hemodynamically significant stenoses, the systolic blood pressure in the leg is decreased. Thus, the ratio of the ankle and brachial artery pressures (termed the *ankle:brachial index*, or ABI) is ≥1.0 in normal individuals and <1.0 in patients with PAD; a ratio of <0.5 is consistent with severe ischemia.

Other noninvasive tests include segmental pressure measurements, segmental pulse volume recordings, duplex ultrasonography (which combines B-mode imaging and Doppler flow velocity waveform analysis

examination), transcutaneous oximetry, and stress testing (usually using a treadmill). Placement of pneumatic cuffs enables assessment of systolic pressure along the legs. The presence of pressure gradients between sequential cuffs provides evidence of the presence and location of hemodynamically significant stenoses. In addition, the amplitude of the pulse volume contour becomes blunted in the presence of significant PAD. Duplex ultrasonography is used to image and detect stenotic lesions in native arteries and bypass grafts.

Treadmill testing allows the physician to assess functional limitations objectively. Decline of the ABI immediately after exercise provides further support for the diagnosis of PAD in patients with equivocal symptoms and findings on examination.

Magnetic resonance angiography (MRA), computed tomographic angiography (CTA), and conventional contrast angiography should not be used for routine diagnostic testing but are performed before potential revascularization **(Fig. 39-1)**. Each test is useful in defining the anatomy to assist planning for catheter-based and surgical revascularization procedures.

Prognosis

The natural history of patients with PAD is influenced primarily by the extent of coexisting coronary artery and cerebrovascular disease. Approximately one-third to

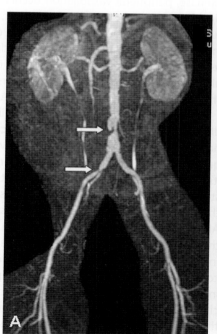
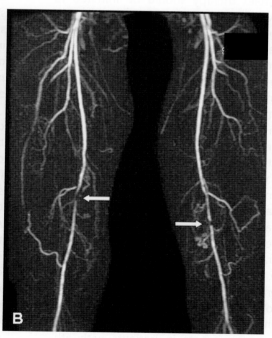

FIGURE 39-1

Magnetic resonance angiography of a patient with intermittent claudication, showing stenoses of the distal abdominal aorta and right iliac common iliac artery (**A**) and stenoses of the right and left superficial femoral arteries (**B**). (*Courtesy of Dr. Edwin Gravereaux; with permission.*)

one-half of patients with symptomatic PAD have evidence of coronary artery disease (CAD) based on clinical presentation and electrocardiogram, and over one-half have significant CAD by coronary angiography. Patients with PAD have a 15–30% 5-year mortality rate and a two- to sixfold increased risk of death from coronary heart disease. Mortality rates are highest in those with the most severe PAD. Measurement of ABI is useful for detecting PAD and identifying persons at risk for future atherothrombotic events. The likelihood of symptomatic progression of PAD is lower than the chance of succumbing to CAD. Approximately 75–80% of nondiabetic patients who present with mild to moderate claudication remain symptomatically stable. Deterioration is likely to occur in the remainder, with approximately 1–2% of the group ultimately developing critical limb ischemia each year. Approximately 25–30% of patients with critical limb ischemia undergo amputation within 1 year. The prognosis is worse in patients who continue to smoke cigarettes or have diabetes mellitus.

TREATMENT   Peripheral Artery Disease

Patients with PAD should receive therapies to reduce the risk of associated cardiovascular events, such as myocardial infarction and death, and to improve limb symptoms, prevent progression to critical limb ischemia, and preserve limb viability. Risk factor modification and antiplatelet therapy should be initiated to improve cardiovascular outcomes. The importance of discontinuing cigarette smoking cannot be overemphasized. The physician must assume a major role in this lifestyle modification. Counseling and adjunctive drug therapy with the nicotine patch, bupropion, or varenicline increase smoking cessation rates and reduce recidivism. It is important to control blood pressure in hypertensive patients. Angiotensin converting-enzyme inhibitors may reduce the risk of cardiovascular events in patients with symptomatic PAD. β-adrenergic blockers do not worsen claudication and may be used to treat hypertension, especially in patients with coexistent CAD. Treatment of hypercholesterolemia with statins is advocated to reduce the risk of myocardial infarction, stroke, and death. The National Cholesterol Education Program Adult Treatment Panel considers PAD a coronary heart disease equivalent and recommends treatment to reduce low-density lipoprotein (LDL) cholesterol to <100 mg/dL. Platelet inhibitors, including aspirin and clopidogrel, reduce the risk of adverse cardiovascular events in patients with atherosclerosis and are recommended for patients with PAD. Dual antiplatelet therapy with both aspirin and clopidogrel is not more effective than aspirin alone in reducing cardiovascular morbidity and mortality rates in patients with PAD. The anticoagulant warfarin is as effective as antiplatelet therapy in preventing adverse cardiovascular events but causes more major bleeding; therefore, it is not indicated to improve outcomes in patients with chronic PAD.

Therapies for intermittent claudication and critical limb ischemia include supportive measures, medications, nonoperative interventions, and surgery. Supportive measures include meticulous care of the feet, which should be kept clean and protected against excessive drying with moisturizing creams. Well-fitting and protective shoes are advised to reduce trauma. Elastic support hose should be avoided, as it reduces blood flow to the skin. In patients with critical limb ischemia, shock blocks under the head of the bed together with a canopy over the feet may improve perfusion pressure and ameliorate some of the rest pain.

Patients with claudication should be encouraged to exercise regularly and at progressively more strenuous levels. Supervised exercise training programs for 30- to 45-min sessions, three to five times per week for at least 12 weeks, prolong walking distance. Patients also should be advised to walk until nearly maximum claudication discomfort occurs and then rest until the symptoms resolve before resuming ambulation. Pharmacologic treatment of PAD has not been as successful as the medical treatment of CAD (Chap. 33). In particular, vasodilators as a class have not proved to be beneficial. During exercise, peripheral vasodilation occurs distal to sites of significant arterial stenoses. As a result, perfusion pressure falls, often to levels lower than that generated in the interstitial tissue by the exercising muscle. Drugs such as α-adrenergic blocking agents, calcium channel antagonists, papaverine, and other vasodilators have not been shown to be effective in patients with PAD.

Cilostazol, a phosphodiesterase inhibitor with vasodilator and antiplatelet properties, increases claudication distance by 40–60% and improves measures of quality of life. The mechanism of action accounting for its beneficial effects is not known. Pentoxifylline, a substituted xanthine derivative, increases blood flow to the microcirculation and enhances tissue oxygenation. Although several placebo-controlled studies have found that pentoxifylline increases the duration of exercise in patients with claudication, its efficacy has not been confirmed in all clinical trials. Statins appeared promising for treatment of intermittent claudication in initial clinical trials, but more studies are needed to confirm their efficacy. There is no definitive medical therapy for critical limb ischemia, although several studies have suggested that long-term parenteral administration of vasodilator prostaglandins decreases pain and facilitates healing of ulcers. Clinical trials of angiogenic growth factors are proceeding. Intramuscular gene transfer of DNA encoding vascular endothelial growth factor, fibroblast growth factor, hepatocyte growth factor, or hypoxia-inducible factor 1α, as well as administration of endothelial progenitor cells, may promote collateral blood vessel growth in patients with critical limb ischemia. Some trial results have been negative, and others encouraging. The outcome of ongoing studies will further elucidate the potential role of therapeutic angiogenesis for PAD.

REVASCULARIZATION Revascularization procedures, including catheter-based and surgical interventions, are usually indicated for patients with disabling, progressive, or severe symptoms of intermittent claudication despite medical therapy and for those with critical limb ischemia. MRA, CTA, or conventional contrast angiography should be performed to assess vascular anatomy in patients who are being considered for revascularization. Nonoperative interventions include percutaneous transluminal angiography (PTA), stent placement, and atherectomy (Chap. 36). PTA and stenting of the iliac artery are associated with higher success rates than are PTA and stenting of the femoral and popliteal arteries. Approximately 90–95% of iliac PTAs are initially successful, and the 3-year patency rate is >75%. Patency rates may be higher if a stent is placed in the iliac artery. The initial success rates for femoral-popliteal PTA and stenting are approximately 80%, with 60% 3-year patency rates. Patency rates are influenced by the severity of pretreatment stenoses; the prognosis of occlusive lesions is worse than that of nonocclusive stenotic lesions. The role of drug-eluting stents in PAD is under investigation.

Several operative procedures are available for treating patients with aortoiliac and femoral-popliteal artery disease. The preferred operative procedure depends on the location and extent of the obstruction(s) and the general medical condition of the patient. Operative procedures for aortoiliac disease include aortobifemoral bypass, axillofemoral bypass, femoro-femoral bypass, and aortoiliac endarterectomy. The most frequently used procedure is the aortobifemoral bypass using knitted Dacron grafts. Immediate graft patency approaches 99%, and 5- and 10-year graft patency in survivors is >90% and 80%, respectively. Operative complications include myocardial infarction and stroke, infection of the graft, peripheral embolization, and sexual dysfunction from interruption of autonomic nerves in the pelvis. The operative mortality rate ranges from 1–3%, mostly due to ischemic heart disease.

Operative therapy for femoral-popliteal artery disease includes in situ and reverse autogenous saphenous vein bypass grafts, placement of polytetrafluoroethylene (PTFE) or other synthetic grafts, and thromboendarterectomy. The operative mortality rate ranges from

1–3%. The long-term patency rate depends on the type of graft used, the location of the distal anastomosis, and the patency of runoff vessels beyond the anastomosis. Patency rates of femoral-popliteal saphenous vein bypass grafts approach 90% at 1 year and 70–80% at 5 years. Five-year patency rates of infrapopliteal saphenous vein bypass grafts are 60–70%. In contrast, 5-year patency rates of infrapopliteal PTFE grafts are <30%. Lumbar sympathectomy alone or as an adjunct to aortofemoral reconstruction has fallen into disfavor.

Preoperative cardiac risk assessment may identify individuals who are especially likely to experience an adverse cardiac event during the perioperative period. Patients with angina, prior myocardial infarction, ventricular ectopy, heart failure, or diabetes are among those at increased risk. Stress testing with treadmill exercise (if feasible), radionuclide myocardial perfusion imaging, or echocardiography permits further stratification of patient risk (Chap. 36). Patients with abnormal test results require close supervision and adjunctive management with anti-ischemic medications. β-adrenergic blockers and statins reduce the risk of postoperative cardiovascular complications. Coronary angiography and coronary artery revascularization compared with optimal medical therapy do not improve outcomes in most patients undergoing peripheral vascular surgery, but cardiac catheterization should be considered in patients with unstable angina and angina refractory to medical therapy as well as those suspected of having left main or three-vessel CAD.

FIBROMUSCULAR DYSPLASIA

Fibromuscular dysplasia is a hyperplastic disorder that affects medium-size and small arteries. It occurs predominantly in females and usually involves the renal and carotid arteries but can affect extremity vessels such as the iliac and subclavian arteries. The histologic classification includes intimal fibroplasia, medial dysplasia, and adventitial hyperplasia. Medial dysplasia is subdivided into medial fibroplasia, perimedial fibroplasia, and medial hyperplasia. Medial fibroplasia is the most common type and is characterized by alternating areas of thinned media and fibromuscular ridges. The internal elastic lamina usually is preserved. The iliac arteries are the limb arteries most likely to be affected by fibromuscular dysplasia. It is identified angiographically by a "string of beads" appearance caused by thickened fibromuscular ridges contiguous with thin, less-involved portions of the arterial wall. When limb vessels are involved, clinical manifestations are similar to those for atherosclerosis, including claudication and rest pain. PTA and surgical reconstruction have been beneficial in patients with debilitating symptoms or threatened limbs.

THROMBOANGIITIS OBLITERANS

Thromboangiitis obliterans (Buerger's disease) is an inflammatory occlusive vascular disorder involving small and medium-size arteries and veins in the distal upper and lower extremities. Cerebral, visceral, and coronary vessels may be affected rarely. This disorder develops most frequently in men <40 years of age. The prevalence is higher in Asians and individuals of Eastern European descent. Although the cause of thromboangiitis obliterans is not known, there is a definite relationship to cigarette smoking in patients with this disorder.

In the initial stages of thromboangiitis obliterans, polymorphonuclear leukocytes infiltrate the walls of the small and medium-size arteries and veins. The internal elastic lamina is preserved, and a cellular, inflammatory thrombus develops in the vascular lumen. As the disease progresses, mononuclear cells, fibroblasts, and giant cells replace the neutrophils. Later stages are characterized by perivascular fibrosis, organized thrombus, and recanalization.

The clinical features of thromboangiitis obliterans often include a triad of claudication of the affected extremity, Raynaud's phenomenon, and migratory superficial vein thrombophlebitis. Claudication usually is confined to the calves and feet or the forearms and hands because this disorder primarily affects distal vessels. In the presence of severe digital ischemia, trophic nail changes, painful ulcerations, and gangrene may develop at the tips of the fingers or toes. The physical examination shows normal brachial and popliteal pulses but reduced or absent radial, ulnar, and/or tibial pulses. Arteriography is helpful in making the diagnosis. Smooth, tapering segmental lesions in the distal vessels are characteristic, as are collateral vessels at sites of vascular occlusion. Proximal atherosclerotic disease is usually absent. The diagnosis can be confirmed by excisional biopsy and pathologic examination of an involved vessel.

There is no specific treatment except abstention from tobacco. The prognosis is worse in individuals who continue to smoke, but results are discouraging even in those who stop smoking. Arterial bypass of the larger vessels may be used in selected instances, as well as local debridement, depending on the symptoms and severity of ischemia. Antibiotics may be useful; anticoagulants and glucocorticoids are not helpful. If these measures fail, amputation may be required.

VASCULITIS

Other vasculitides may affect the arteries that supply the upper and lower extremities.

ACUTE ARTERIAL OCCLUSION

Acute arterial occlusion results in the sudden cessation of blood flow to an extremity. The severity of ischemia and the viability of the extremity depend on the location and extent of the occlusion and the presence and subsequent development of collateral blood vessels. There are two principal causes of acute arterial occlusion: embolism and thrombus in situ.

The most common sources of arterial emboli are the heart, aorta, and large arteries. Cardiac disorders that cause thromboembolism include atrial fibrillation, both chronic and paroxysmal; acute myocardial infarction; ventricular aneurysm; cardiomyopathy; infectious and marantic endocarditis; thrombi associated with prosthetic heart valves; and atrial myxoma. Emboli to the distal vessels may also originate from proximal sites of atherosclerosis and aneurysms of the aorta and large vessels. Less frequently, an arterial occlusion results paradoxically from a venous thrombus that has entered the systemic circulation via a patent foramen ovale or another septal defect. Arterial emboli tend to lodge at vessel bifurcations because the vessel caliber decreases at those sites; in the lower extremities, emboli lodge most frequently in the femoral artery, followed by the iliac artery, aorta, and popliteal and tibioperoneal arteries.

Acute arterial thrombosis in situ occurs most frequently in atherosclerotic vessels at the site of an atherosclerotic plaque or aneurysm and in arterial bypass grafts. Trauma to an artery may also result in the formation of an acute arterial thrombus. Arterial occlusion may complicate arterial punctures and placement of catheters; it also may result from arterial dissection if the intimal flap obstructs the artery. Less common causes include thoracic outlet compression syndrome, which causes subclavian artery occlusion, and entrapment of the popliteal artery by abnormal placement of the medial head of the gastrocnemius muscle. Polycythemia and hypercoagulable disorders are also associated with acute arterial thrombosis.

Clinical features

The symptoms of an acute arterial occlusion depend on the location, duration, and severity of the obstruction. Often, severe pain, paresthesia, numbness, and coldness develop in the involved extremity within 1 h. Paralysis may occur with severe and persistent ischemia. Physical findings include loss of pulses distal to the occlusion, cyanosis or pallor, mottling, decreased skin temperature, muscle stiffening, loss of sensation, weakness, and/or absent deep tendon reflexes. If acute arterial occlusion occurs in the presence of an adequate collateral circulation, as is often the case in acute graft occlusion, the symptoms and findings may be less impressive. In this situation, the patient complains about an abrupt decrease in the distance walked before claudication occurs or of modest pain and paresthesia. Pallor and coolness are evident, but sensory and motor functions generally are preserved. The diagnosis of acute arterial occlusion is usually apparent from the clinical presentation. In most circumstances, MRA, CTA, or catheter-based arteriography is used to confirm the diagnosis and demonstrate the location and extent of occlusion.

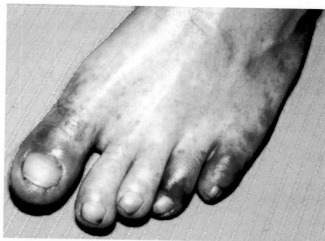

FIGURE 39-2
Atheroembolism causing cyanotic discoloration and impending necrosis of the toes ("blue toe" syndrome).

TREATMENT   Acute Arterial Occlusion

Once the diagnosis is made, the patient should be anti-coagulated with intravenous heparin to prevent propagation of the clot. In cases of severe ischemia of recent onset, particularly when limb viability is jeopardized, immediate intervention to ensure reperfusion is indicated. Endovascular or surgical thromboembolectomy or arterial bypass procedures are used to restore blood flow to the ischemic extremity promptly, particularly when a large proximal vessel is occluded.

Intraarterial thrombolytic therapy with recombinant tissue plasminogen activator, reteplase, or tenecteplase is often effective when acute arterial occlusion is caused by a thrombus in an atherosclerotic vessel or arterial bypass graft. Thrombolytic therapy may also be indicated when the patient's overall condition contra-indicates surgical intervention or when smaller distal vessels are occluded, thus preventing surgical access. Meticulous observation for hemorrhagic complications is required during intraarterial thrombolytic therapy. Another endovascular approach to thrombus removal is percutaneous mechanical thrombectomy using devices that employ hydrodynamic forces or rotating baskets to fragment and remove the clot. These treatments may be used alone but usually are used in conjunction with pharmacologic thrombolysis. Amputation is performed when the limb is not viable, as characterized by loss of sensation, paralysis, and the absence of Doppler-detected blood flow in both arteries and veins.

If the limb is not in jeopardy, a more conservative approach that includes observation and administration of anticoagulants may be taken. Anticoagulation prevents recurrent embolism and reduces the likelihood of thrombus propagation; it can be initiated with intravenous heparin and followed by oral warfarin. Recommended doses are the same as those used for deep vein thrombosis. Emboli resulting from infective endocarditis, the presence of prosthetic heart valves, or atrial myxoma often require surgical intervention to remove the cause.

ATHEROEMBOLISM

Atheroembolism constitutes a subset of acute arterial occlusion. In this condition, multiple small deposits of fibrin, platelets, and cholesterol debris embolize from proximal atherosclerotic lesions or aneurysmal sites. Large protruding aortic atheromas are a source of emboli that may lead to stroke and renal insufficiency as well as limb ischemia. Atheroembolism may occur after intraarterial procedures. Since the emboli tend to lodge in the small vessels of the muscle and skin and may not occlude the large vessels, distal pulses usually remain palpable. Patients complain of acute pain and tenderness at the site of embolization. Digital vascular occlusion may result in ischemia and the "blue toe" syndrome; digital necrosis and gangrene may develop (**Fig. 39-2**). Localized areas of tenderness, pallor, and livedo reticularis (see later) occur at sites of emboli. Skin or muscle biopsy may demonstrate cholesterol crystals.

Ischemia resulting from atheroemboli is notoriously difficult to treat. Usually, neither surgical revascularization procedures nor thrombolytic therapy is helpful because of the multiplicity, composition, and distal location of the emboli. Some evidence suggests that platelet inhibitors prevent atheroembolism. Surgical intervention to remove or bypass the atherosclerotic vessel or aneurysm that causes the recurrent atheroemboli may be necessary.

THORACIC OUTLET COMPRESSION SYNDROME

This is a symptom complex resulting from compression of the neurovascular bundle (artery, vein, or nerves) at the thoracic outlet as it courses through the neck and shoulder. Cervical ribs, abnormalities of the scalenus anticus muscle, proximity of the clavicle to the first rib, or abnormal insertion of the pectoralis minor muscle may compress the subclavian artery, subclavian vein, and brachial plexus as these structures pass from the thorax to the arm. Depending on the structures affected, thoracic outlet compression syndrome is divided into arterial, venous, and neurogenic forms. Patients with neurogenic thoracic outlet compression may develop shoulder and arm pain, weakness, and paresthesias. Patients with arterial compression may experience claudication, Raynaud's phenomenon, and even ischemic tissue loss and gangrene. Venous compression may cause thrombosis of the subclavian and axillary veins; this is often associated with effort and is referred to as *Paget-Schroetter syndrome.*

APPROACH TO THE PATIENT | **Thoracic Outlet Compression Syndrome**

Examination of a patient with thoracic outlet compression syndrome is often normal unless provocative maneuvers are performed. Occasionally, distal pulses are decreased or absent and digital cyanosis and ischemia may be evident. Tenderness may be present in the supraclavicular fossa. In patients with axillo-subclavian venous thrombosis, the affected extremity typically is swollen. Dilated collateral veins may be apparent around the shoulder and upper arm.

Several maneuvers that support the diagnosis of thoracic outlet compression syndrome may be used to precipitate symptoms, cause a subclavian artery bruit, and diminish arm pulses. These maneuvers include the abduction and external rotation test, in which the affected arm is abducted by 90° and the shoulder is externally rotated; the scalene maneuver (extension of the neck and rotation of the head to the side of the symptoms); the costoclavicular maneuver (posterior rotation of shoulders); and the hyperabduction maneuver (raising the arm 180°). A chest x-ray will indicate the presence of cervical ribs. Duplex ultrasonography, MRA, and contrast angiography can be performed during provocative maneuvers to demonstrate thoracic outlet compression of the subclavian artery. Duplex ultrasography, magnetic resonance venography, or contrast venography can be used to diagnose axillo-subclavian vein thrombosis. Neurophysiologic tests such as the electromyogram, nerve conduction studies, and somatosensory evoked potentials may be abnormal if the brachial plexus is involved, but the diagnosis of neurogenic thoracic outlet syndrome is not necessarily excluded if these tests are normal owing to their low sensitivity.

Most patients can be managed conservatively. They should be advised to avoid the positions that cause symptoms. Many patients benefit from shoulder girdle exercises. Surgical procedures such as removal of the first rib and resection of the scalenus anticus muscle are necessary occasionally for relief of symptoms or treatment of ischemia.

POPLITEAL ARTERY ENTRAPMENT

Popliteal artery entrapment typically affects young athletic men and women when the gastrocnemius or popliteus muscle compresses the popliteal artery and causes intermittent claudication. Thrombosis, embolism, or popliteal artery aneurysm may occur. The pulse examination may be normal unless provocative maneuvers such as ankle dorsiflexion and plantar flexion are performed. The diagnosis is confirmed by duplex ultrasound, CTA, MRA, or conventional angiography. Treatment involves surgical release of the popliteal artery or vascular reconstruction.

POPLITEAL ARTERY ANEURYSM

Popliteal artery aneurysms are the most common peripheral artery aneurysms. Approximately 50% are bilateral. Patients with popliteal artery aneurysms often have aneurysms of other arteries, especially the aorta. The most common clinical presentation is limb ischemia secondary to thrombosis or embolism. Rupture occurs less frequently. Other complications include compression of the adjacent popliteal vein or peroneal nerve. Popliteal artery aneurysm can be detected by palpation and confirmed by duplex ultrasonography. Repair is indicated for symptomatic aneurysms or when the diameter exceeds 2–3 cm, owing to the risk of thrombosis, embolism, or rupture.

ARTERIOVENOUS FISTULA

Abnormal communications between an artery and a vein, bypassing the capillary bed, may be congenital or acquired. Congenital arteriovenous fistulas are a result of persistent embryonic vessels that fail to differentiate into arteries and veins; they may be associated with birthmarks, can be located in almost any organ of the body, and frequently occur in the extremities. Acquired arteriovenous fistulas either are created to provide vascular access for hemodialysis or occur as a result of a penetrating injury such as a gunshot or knife wound or as complications of arterial catheterization or surgical dissection. An uncommon cause of arteriovenous fistula is rupture of an arterial aneurysm into a vein.

The clinical features depend on the location and size of the fistula. Frequently, a pulsatile mass is palpable, and a thrill and a bruit lasting throughout systole and diastole are present over the fistula. With long-standing fistulas, clinical manifestations of chronic venous insufficiency, including peripheral edema; large, tortuous varicose veins; and stasis pigmentation become apparent because of the high venous pressure. Evidence of ischemia may occur in the distal portion of the extremity. Skin temperature is higher over the arteriovenous fistula. Large arteriovenous fistulas may result in an increased cardiac output with consequent cardiomegaly and high-output heart failure (Chap. 17).

The diagnosis is often evident from the physical examination. Compression of a large arteriovenous fistula may cause reflex slowing of the heart rate (Nicoladoni-Branham sign). Duplex ultrasonography may detect an arteriovenous fistula, especially one that affects the femoral artery and vein at the site of catheter access. Computed tomographic and conventional angiography can confirm the diagnosis and are useful in demonstrating the site and size of the arteriovenous fistula.

Management of arteriovenous fistulas may involve surgery, radiotherapy, or embolization. Congenital arteriovenous fistulas are often difficult to treat because the communications may be numerous and extensive, and new communications frequently develop after ligation of the most obvious ones. Many of these lesions are best treated conservatively using elastic support hose to reduce the consequences of venous hypertension. Occasionally, embolization with autologous material, such as fat or muscle, or with hemostatic agents, such as gelatin sponges or silicon spheres, is used to obliterate the fistula. Acquired arteriovenous fistulas are usually amenable to surgical treatment that involves division or excision of the fistula. Occasionally, autogenous or synthetic grafting is necessary to reestablish continuity of the artery and vein.

RAYNAUD'S PHENOMENON

Raynaud's phenomenon is characterized by episodic digital ischemia, manifested clinically by the sequential development of digital blanching, cyanosis, and rubor of the fingers or toes after cold exposure and subsequent rewarming. Emotional stress may also precipitate Raynaud's phenomenon. The color changes are usually well demarcated and are confined to the fingers or toes. Typically, one or more digits will appear white when the patient is exposed to a cold environment or touches a cold object. The blanching, or pallor, represents the ischemic phase of the phenomenon and results from vasospasm of digital arteries. During the ischemic phase, capillaries and venules dilate, and cyanosis results from the deoxygenated blood that is present in these vessels. A sensation of cold or numbness or paresthesia of the digits often accompanies the phases of pallor and cyanosis.

With rewarming, the digital vasospasm resolves, and blood flow into the dilated arterioles and capillaries increases dramatically. This "reactive hyperemia" imparts a bright red color to the digits. In addition to rubor and warmth, patients often experience a throbbing, painful sensation during the hyperemic phase. Although the triphasic color response is typical of

TABLE 39-1

CLASSIFICATION OF RAYNAUD'S PHENOMENON
Primary or idiopathic Raynaud's phenomenon: Raynaud's disease
Secondary Raynaud's phenomenon
Collagen vascular diseases: scleroderma, systemic lupus erythematosus, rheumatoid arthritis, dermatomyositis, polymyositis
Arterial occlusive diseases: atherosclerosis of the extremities, thromboangiitis obliterans, acute arterial occlusion, thoracic outlet syndrome
Pulmonary hypertension
Neurologic disorders: intervertebral disk disease, syringomyelia, spinal cord tumors, stroke, poliomyelitis, carpal tunnel syndrome
Blood dyscrasias: cold agglutinins, cryoglobulinemia, cryofibrinogenemia, myeloproliferative disorders, Waldenström's macroglobulinemia
Trauma: vibration injury, hammer hand syndrome, electric shock, cold injury, typing, piano playing
Drugs: ergot derivatives, methysergide, β-adrenergic receptor blockers, bleomycin, vinblastine, cisplatin

Raynaud's phenomenon, some patients may develop only pallor and cyanosis; others may experience only cyanosis.

Raynaud's phenomenon is broadly separated into two categories: the idiopathic variety, termed *Raynaud's disease*, and the secondary variety, which is associated with other disease states or known causes of vasospasm **(Table 39-1)**.

Raynaud's disease

This appellation is applied when the secondary causes of Raynaud's phenomenon have been excluded. Over 50% of patients with Raynaud's phenomenon have Raynaud's disease. Women are affected about five times more often than men, and the age of presentation is usually between 20 and 40 years. The fingers are involved more frequently than the toes. Initial episodes may involve only one or two fingertips, but subsequent attacks may involve the entire finger and may include all the fingers. The toes are affected in 40% of patients. Although vasospasm of the toes usually occurs in patients with symptoms in the fingers, it may happen alone. Rarely, the earlobes, the tip of the nose, and the penis are involved. Raynaud's phenomenon occurs frequently in patients who also have migraine headaches or variant angina. These associations suggest that there may be a common predisposing cause for the vasospasm.

Results of physical examination are often entirely normal; the radial, ulnar, and pedal pulses are normal. The fingers and toes may be cool between attacks and may perspire excessively. Thickening and tightening of the digital subcutaneous tissue (*sclerodactyly*) develop in 10% of patients. Angiography of the digits for diagnostic purposes is not indicated.

In general, patients with Raynaud's disease have milder forms of Raynaud's phenomenon. Fewer than 1% of these patients lose a part of a digit. After the diagnosis is made, the disease improves spontaneously in approximately 15% of patients and progresses in about 30%.

Secondary causes of Raynaud's phenomenon

Raynaud's phenomenon occurs in 80–90% of patients with systemic sclerosis (scleroderma) and is the presenting symptom in 30%. It may be the only symptom of scleroderma for many years. Abnormalities of the digital vessels may contribute to the development of Raynaud's phenomenon in this disorder. Ischemic fingertip ulcers may develop and progress to gangrene and autoamputation. About 20% of patients with systemic lupus erythematosus (SLE) have Raynaud's phenomenon. Occasionally, persistent digital ischemia develops and may result in ulcers or gangrene. In most severe cases, the small vessels are occluded by a proliferative endarteritis. Raynaud's phenomenon occurs in about 30% of patients with dermatomyositis or polymyositis. It frequently develops in patients with rheumatoid arthritis and may be related to the intimal proliferation that occurs in the digital arteries.

Atherosclerosis of the extremities is a common cause of Raynaud's phenomenon in men >50 years. Thromboangiitis obliterans is an uncommon cause of Raynaud's phenomenon but should be considered in young men, particularly those who are cigarette smokers. The development of cold-induced pallor in these disorders may be confined to one or two digits of the involved extremity. Occasionally, Raynaud's phenomenon may follow acute occlusion of large and medium-size arteries by a thrombus or embolus. Embolization of atheroembolic debris may cause digital ischemia. The latter situation often involves one or two digits and should not be confused with Raynaud's phenomenon. In patients with thoracic outlet compression syndrome, Raynaud's phenomenon may result from diminished intravascular pressure, stimulation of sympathetic fibers in the brachial plexus, or a combination of both. Raynaud's phenomenon occurs in patients with primary pulmonary hypertension (Chap. 40); this is more than coincidental and may reflect a neurohumoral abnormality that affects both the pulmonary and digital circulations.

A variety of blood dyscrasias may be associated with Raynaud's phenomenon. Cold-induced precipitation of plasma proteins, hyperviscosity, and aggregation of red cells and platelets may occur in patients with cold agglutinins, cryoglobulinemia, or cryofibrinogenemia.

Hyperviscosity syndromes that accompany myeloproliferative disorders and Waldenström macroglobulinemia should also be considered in the initial evaluation of patients with Raynaud's phenomenon.

Raynaud's phenomenon occurs often in patients whose vocations require the use of vibrating hand tools, such as chain saws or jackhammers. The frequency of Raynaud's phenomenon also seems to be increased in pianists and keyboard operators. Electric shock injury to the hands or frostbite may lead to the later development of Raynaud's phenomenon.

Several drugs have been causally implicated in Raynaud's phenomenon. They include ergot preparations, methysergide, β-adrenergic receptor antagonists, and the chemotherapeutic agents bleomycin, vinblastine, and cisplatin.

TREATMENT Raynaud's Phenomenon

Most patients with Raynaud's phenomenon experience only mild and infrequent episodes. These patients need reassurance and should be instructed to dress warmly and avoid unnecessary cold exposure. In addition to gloves and mittens, patients should protect the trunk, head, and feet with warm clothing to prevent cold-induced reflex vasoconstriction. Tobacco use is contraindicated.

Drug treatment should be reserved for severe cases. Dihydropyridine calcium channel antagonists such as nifedipine, isradipine, felodipine, and amlodipine decrease the frequency and severity of Raynaud's phenomenon. Diltiazem may be considered but is less effective. The postsynaptic α_1-adrenergic antagonist prazosin has been used with favorable responses; doxazosin and terazosin may also be effective. Topical glyceryl trinitrate may be useful in some patients. Digital sympathectomy is helpful in some patients who are unresponsive to medical therapy.

ACROCYANOSIS

In this condition, there is arterial vasoconstriction and secondary dilation of the capillaries and venules with resulting persistent cyanosis of the hands and, less frequently, the feet. Cyanosis may be intensified by exposure to a cold environment. Acrocyanosis may be categorized as primary or secondary to an underlying condition. In primary acrocyanosis, women are affected much more frequently than men, and the age of onset is usually <30 years. Generally, patients are asymptomatic but seek medical attention because of the discoloration. The prognosis is favorable, and pain, ulcers, and gangrene do not occur. Examination reveals normal pulses, peripheral cyanosis, and moist palms. Trophic skin changes and ulcerations do *not* occur. The disorder can be distinguished from Raynaud's phenomenon because it is persistent and not episodic, the discoloration extends proximally from the digits, and blanching does not occur. Ischemia secondary to arterial occlusive disease can usually be excluded by the presence of normal pulses. Central cyanosis and decreased arterial oxygen saturation are not present. Patients should be reassured and advised to dress warmly and avoid cold exposure. Pharmacologic intervention is not indicated.

Secondary acrocyanosis may result from hypoxemia, connective tissue diseases, atheroembolism, antiphospholipid antibodies, cold agglutinins, or cryoglobulins and is associated with anorexia nervosa and orthostatic tachycardia syndrome. Treatment should be directed at the underlying disorder.

LIVEDO RETICULARIS

In this condition, localized areas of the extremities develop a mottled or rete (netlike) appearance of reddish to blue discoloration. The mottled appearance may be more prominent after cold exposure. There are primary and secondary forms of livedo reticularis. The primary, or idiopathic, form of this disorder may be benign or associated with ulcerations. The benign form occurs more frequently in women than in men, and the most common age of onset is the third decade. Patients with the benign form are usually asymptomatic and seek attention for cosmetic reasons. These patients should be reassured and advised to avoid cold environments. No drug treatment is indicated. Primary livedo reticularis with ulceration is also called *atrophie blanche en plaque*. The ulcers are painful and may take months to heal. Secondary livedo reticularis can occur with atheroembolism (see earlier), SLE and other vasculitides, anticardiolipin antibodies, hyperviscosity, cryoglobulinemia, and Sneddon's syndrome (ischemic stroke and livedo reticularis). Rarely, skin ulcerations develop.

PERNIO (CHILBLAINS)

Pernio is a vasculitic disorder associated with exposure to cold; acute forms have been described. Raised erythematous lesions develop on the lower part of the legs and feet in cold weather. They are associated with pruritus and a burning sensation, and they may blister and ulcerate. Pathologic examination demonstrates angiitis characterized by intimal proliferation and perivascular infiltration of mononuclear and polymorphonuclear leukocytes. Giant cells may be present in the subcutaneous tissue. Patients should avoid exposure to cold, and ulcers should be kept clean and protected with sterile dressings. Sympatholytic drugs and dihydropyridine calcium channel antagonists may be effective in some patients.

ERYTHROMELALGIA

This disorder is characterized by burning pain and erythema of the extremities. The feet are involved more frequently than the hands, and males are affected more frequently than females. Erythromelalgia may occur at any age but is most common in middle age. It may be primary (also termed erythermalgia) or secondary. The most common causes of secondary erythromelalgia are myeloproliferative disorders such as polycythemia vera and essential thrombocytosis. Less common causes include drugs, such as calcium channel blockers, bromocriptine, and pergolide; neuropathies; connective tissue diseases such as SLE; and paraneoplastic syndromes. Patients complain of burning in the extremities that is precipitated by exposure to a warm environment and aggravated by a dependent position. The symptoms are relieved by exposing the affected area to cool air or water or by elevation. Erythromelalgia can be distinguished from ischemia secondary to peripheral arterial disorders and peripheral neuropathy because the peripheral pulses are present and the neurologic examination is normal. There is no specific treatment; aspirin may produce relief in patients with erythromelalgia secondary to myeloproliferative disease. Treatment of associated disorders in secondary erythromelalgia may be helpful.

FROSTBITE

In this condition, tissue damage results from severe environmental cold exposure or from direct contact with a very cold object. Tissue injury results from both freezing and vasoconstriction. Frostbite usually affects the distal aspects of the extremities or exposed parts of the face, such as the ears, nose, chin, and cheeks. Superficial frostbite involves the skin and subcutaneous tissue. Patients experience pain or paresthesia, and the skin appears white and waxy. After rewarming, there is cyanosis and erythema, wheal-and-flare formation, edema, and superficial blisters. Deep frostbite involves muscle, nerves, and deeper blood vessels. It may result in edema of the hand or foot, vesicles and bullae, tissue necrosis, and gangrene.

Initial treatment is rewarming, performed in an environment where reexposure to freezing conditions will not occur. Rewarming is accomplished by immersion of the affected part in a water bath at temperatures of 40°–44°C (104°–111°F). Massage, application of ice water, and extreme heat are contraindicated. The injured area should be cleansed with soap or antiseptic, and sterile dressings should be applied. Analgesics are often required during rewarming. Antibiotics are used if there is evidence of infection. The efficacy of sympathetic blocking drugs is not established. After recovery, the affected extremity may exhibit increased sensitivity to cold.

DISORDERS OF THE VEINS AND LYMPHATICS

VENOUS DISORDERS

Veins in the extremities can be broadly classified as either superficial or deep. In the lower extremity, the superficial venous system includes the greater and lesser saphenous veins and their tributaries. The deep veins of the leg accompany the major arteries. Perforating veins connect the superficial and deep systems at multiple locations. Bicuspid valves are present throughout the venous system to direct the flow of venous blood centrally.

Venous thrombosis

The presence of thrombus within a superficial or deep vein, along with the accompanying inflammatory response in the vessel wall, is termed *venous thrombosis* or *thrombophlebitis*. Initially the thrombus is composed principally of platelets and fibrin. Red cells become interspersed with fibrin, and the thrombus tends to propagate in the direction of blood flow. The inflammatory response in the vessel wall may be minimal or characterized by granulocyte infiltration, loss of endothelium, and edema.

The factors that predispose to venous thrombosis were initially described by Virchow in 1856 and include stasis, vascular damage, and hypercoagulability. Accordingly, a variety of clinical situations are associated with increased risk of venous thrombosis **(Table 39-2)**. Venous thrombosis may occur in >50% of patients having orthopedic surgical procedures, particularly those involving the hip or knee, and in 10–40% of patients who undergo abdominal or thoracic operations. The prevalence of venous thrombosis is particularly high in patients with cancer of the pancreas, lungs, genitourinary tract, stomach, and breast. Approximately 10–20% of patients with idiopathic deep vein thrombosis have or develop clinically overt cancer; there is no consensus on whether these individuals should be subjected to intensive diagnostic workup to search for occult malignancy.

The risk of thrombosis is increased after trauma such as fractures of the spine, pelvis, femur, and tibia. Immobilization, regardless of the underlying disease, is a major predisposing cause of venous thrombosis. This may account for the relatively high incidence in patients with acute myocardial infarction or congestive heart failure. The incidence of venous thrombosis is increased during pregnancy, particularly in the third trimester, and in the first month postpartum, as well as in individuals who use oral contraceptives, postmenopausal hormone replacement therapy, or selective estrogen receptor modulators. A variety of inherited and acquired disorders that produce systemic hypercoagulability, including resistance to activated protein C (factor V Leiden); prothrombin G20210A gene mutation; antithrombin III,

TABLE 39-2

CONDITIONS ASSOCIATED WITH AN INCREASED RISK FOR DEVELOPMENT OF VENOUS THROMBOSIS

Surgery
  Orthopedic, thoracic, abdominal, and genitourinary procedures
Neoplasms
  Pancreas, lung, ovary, testes, urinary tract, breast, stomach
Trauma
  Fractures of spine, pelvis, femur, or tibia; spinal cord injuries
Immobilization
  Acute myocardial infarction, congestive heart failure, stroke, postoperative convalescence
Pregnancy
Estrogen for replacement or contraception
  Selective estrogen replacement modulators
Hypercoagulable states
  Resistance to activated protein C; prothrombin 20210A gene mutation deficiencies of antithrombin III, protein C, or protein S; antiphospholipid antibodies; myeloproliferative diseases; dysfibrinogenemia; disseminated intravascular coagulation
Venulitis
  Thromboangiitis obliterans, Behçet's disease, homocysteinuria
Previous deep vein thrombosis

protein C, and protein S deficiencies; antiphospholipid syndrome; hyperhomocysteinemia; SLE; myeloproliferative diseases; dysfibrinogenemia; heparin–induced thrombocytopenia; and disseminated intravascular coagulation, are associated with venous thrombosis. Venulitis occurring in thromboangiitis obliterans, Behçet's syndrome, and homocystinuria may also cause venous thrombosis.

Superficial vein thrombosis

Thrombosis of the greater or lesser saphenous veins or their tributaries (i.e., superficial vein thrombosis) does not result in pulmonary embolism. It is associated with intravenous catheters and infusions, occurs in varicose veins, and may develop in association with deep venous thrombosis (DVT). Migrating superficial vein thrombosis is often a marker for a carcinoma and may also occur in patients with vasculitides, such as thromboangiitis obliterans. The clinical features of superficial vein thrombosis are easily distinguished from those of DVT. Patients complain of pain localized to the site of the thrombus. Examination reveals a reddened, warm, and tender cord extending along a superficial vein. The surrounding area may be red and edematous.

TREATMENT   Superficial Vein Thrombosis

Treatment is primarily supportive. Initially, patients can be placed at bed rest with leg elevation and application of warm compresses. Nonsteroidal anti-inflammatory drugs may provide analgesia but may also obscure clinical evidence of thrombus propagation. If a thrombosis of the greater saphenous vein develops in the thigh and extends toward the saphenofemoral vein junction, it is reasonable to consider anticoagulant therapy to prevent extension of the thrombus into the deep system and a possible pulmonary embolism.

Varicose veins

Varicose veins are dilated, tortuous superficial veins that result from defective structure and function of the valves of the saphenous veins, intrinsic weakness of the vein wall, high intraluminal pressure, or, rarely, arteriovenous fistulas. Varicose veins can be categorized as primary or secondary. Primary varicose veins originate in the superficial system and occur two to three times as frequently in women as in men. Approximately one-half of these patients have a family history of varicose veins. Secondary varicose veins result from deep venous insufficiency and incompetent perforating veins or from deep venous occlusion that causes enlargement of superficial veins that are serving as collaterals.

Patients with venous varicosities are often concerned about the cosmetic appearance of their legs. Symptoms consist of a dull ache or pressure sensation in the legs after prolonged standing; this is relieved with leg elevation. The legs feel heavy, and mild ankle edema develops occasionally. Extensive venous varicosities may cause skin ulcerations near the ankle. Superficial venous thrombosis may be a recurring problem, and, rarely, a varicosity ruptures and bleeds. Visual inspection of the legs in the dependent position usually confirms the presence of varicose veins.

Varicose veins usually can be treated with conservative measures. Symptoms often decrease when the legs are elevated periodically, prolonged standing is avoided, and elastic support hose are worn. External compression stockings provide a counterbalance to the hydrostatic pressure in the veins. Ablative procedures, including sclerotherapy, endovenous radio frequency or laser ablation, and surgery, may be considered to treat varicose veins in selected patients who have persistent symptoms, have recurrent superficial vein thrombosis, and/or develop skin ulceration. Ablative therapy may also be indicated for cosmetic reasons. Small, symptomatic varicose veins can be treated with sclerotherapy, in which a sclerosing solution is injected into the involved varicose vein and a compression bandage is applied. Percutaneous, endovenous delivery of radio frequency or laser energy can be used to treat incompetent great saphenous veins. Surgical therapy usually involves ligation and stripping of the great and small saphenous veins.

Chronic venous insufficiency

Chronic venous insufficiency may result from DVT and/or valvular incompetence. After DVT, the delicate valve leaflets become thickened and contracted so that they cannot prevent retrograde flow of blood; the vein becomes rigid and thick walled. Although most veins recanalize after an episode of thrombosis, the large proximal veins may remain occluded. Secondary incompetence develops in distal valves because high pressures distend the vein and separate the leaflets. Primary deep venous valvular dysfunction may also occur without previous thrombosis. Patients with venous insufficiency often complain of a dull ache in the leg that worsens with prolonged standing and resolves with leg elevation. Examination demonstrates increased leg circumference, edema, and superficial varicose veins. Erythema, dermatitis, and hyperpigmentation develop along the distal aspect of the leg, and skin ulceration may occur near the medial and lateral malleoli **(Fig. 39-3)**. Cellulitis may be a recurring problem. The CEAP (clinical, etiologic, anatomic, pathophysiologic) classification schema incorporates the range of symptoms and signs of chronic venous insufficiency to characterize its severity **(Table 39-3)**.

Patients should be advised to avoid prolonged standing or sitting; frequent leg elevation is helpful. Graduated compression stockings should be worn during the day.

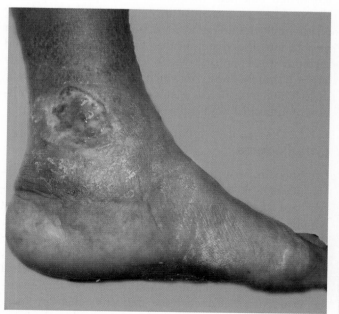

FIGURE 39-3

Venous insufficiency with active venous ulcer near the medial malleolus. (*Courtesy of Dr. Steven Dean, with permission.*)

TABLE 39-3

CEAP (CLINICAL, ETIOLOGIC, ANATOMIC, PATHOPHYSIOLOGIC) CLASSIFICATION

C0 No visible or palpable signs of venous disease
C1 Telangiectases, reticular veins
C2 Varicose veins
C3 Edema without skin changes
C4 Skin changes, including pigmentation, eczema, lipodermatosclerosis, and *atrophie blanche*
C5 Healed venous ulcer
C6 Active venous ulcer

TABLE 39-4

CAUSES OF LYMPHEDEMA

Primary	Secondary
Congenital (includes Milroy's disease)	Recurrent lymphangitis
	Filariasis
Lymphedema praecox (includes Nonne-Milroy-Meige [or chronic familial lymphedema of the limbs] disease)	Tuberculosis
	Neoplasm
	Surgery
	Radiation therapy
Lymphedema tarda	

These efforts should be intensified if skin ulcers develop. Ulcers should be treated with applications of wet to dry dressings or occlusive hydrocolloid dressings. Commercially available compressive dressings that consist of paste with zinc oxide, calamine, glycerin, and gelatin may be applied and should be changed weekly until healing occurs. Recurrent ulceration and severe edema may be treated by surgical interruption of incompetent communicating veins. Subfascial endoscopic perforator surgery (SEPS) is a minimally invasive technique to interrupt incompetent communicating veins. Rarely, surgical valvuloplasty and bypass of venous occlusions are employed.

LYMPHATIC DISORDERS

Lymphatic capillaries are blind-ended tubes formed by a single layer of endothelial cells. The absent or widely fenestrated basement membrane of lymphatic capillaries allows access to interstitial proteins and particles. Lymphatic capillaries merge to form larger vessels that contain smooth muscle and are capable of vasomotion. Small- and medium-size lymphatic vessels empty into progressively larger channels, most of which drain into the thoracic duct. The lymphatic circulation is involved in the absorption of interstitial fluid and in the response to infection.

Lymphedema

Lymphedema may be categorized as primary or secondary (Table 39-4). The prevalence of primary lymphedema is approximately 1 per 10,000 individuals. Primary lymphedema may be secondary to agenesis, hypoplasia, or obstruction of the lymphatic vessels. It may be associated with Turner's syndrome, Klinefelter's syndrome, Noonan's syndrome, yellow nail syndrome, intestinal lymphangiectasia syndrome, and lymphangiomyomatosis. Women are affected more frequently than are men. There are three clinical subtypes: congenital lymphedema, which appears shortly after birth; lymphedema praecox,

which has its onset at the time of puberty; and lymphedema tarda, which usually begins after age 35. Familial forms of congenital lymphedema (Milroy's disease) and lymphedema praecox (Meige's disease) may be inherited in an autosomal dominant manner with variable penetrance; autosomal or sex-linked recessive forms are less common.

Secondary lymphedema is an acquired condition that results from damage to or obstruction of previously normal lymphatic channels (Table 39-4). Recurrent episodes of bacterial lymphangitis, usually caused by streptococci, are a very common cause of lymphedema. The most common cause of secondary lymphedema worldwide is filariasis. Tumors, such as prostate cancer and lymphoma, can also obstruct lymphatic vessels. Both surgery and radiation therapy for breast carcinoma may cause lymphedema of the upper extremity. Less common causes include tuberculosis, contact dermatitis, lymphogranuloma venereum, rheumatoid arthritis, pregnancy, and self-induced or factitious lymphedema after application of tourniquets.

Lymphedema is generally a painless condition, but patients may experience a chronic dull, heavy sensation in the leg, and most often they are concerned about the appearance of the leg. Lymphedema of the lower extremity, initially involving the foot, gradually progresses up the leg so that the entire limb becomes edematous. In the early stages, the edema is soft and pits easily with pressure. In the chronic stages, the limb has a woody texture, and the tissues become indurated and fibrotic. At this point the edema may no longer be pitting. The limb loses its normal contour, and the toes appear square. Lymphedema should be distinguished from other disorders that cause unilateral leg swelling, such as DVT and chronic venous insufficiency. In the latter condition, the edema is softer, and there is often evidence of a stasis dermatitis, hyperpigmentation, and superficial venous varicosities. Other causes of leg swelling that resemble lymphedema are pretibial myxedema and lipedema. Pretibial myxedema occurs in patients with hyperthyroidism, especially Graves' disease, and is caused by deposition of hyaluronic acid-rich protein in the dermis. Lipedema usually occurs in women and is caused by accumulation of adipose tissue in the leg from the thigh to the ankle with sparing of the feet. The evaluation of patients with lymphedema should include diagnostic studies to clarify the cause. Abdominal and pelvic ultrasound and CT can be used to detect obstructing lesions such as neoplasms. MRI may reveal edema in the epifascial compartment and identify lymph nodes and enlarged lymphatic channels. Lymphoscintigraphy and lymphangiography are rarely indicated, but either can be used to confirm the diagnosis or differentiate primary from secondary lymphedema. Lymphoscintigraphy involves the injection of radioactively labeled technetium-containing colloid into the distal subcutaneous tissue of the affected extremity. In lymphangiography, contrast material is injected into a distal lymphatic vessel that has been isolated and cannulated. In primary lymphedema, lymphatic channels are absent, hypoplastic, or ectatic. In secondary lymphedema, lymphatic channels are usually dilated, and it may be possible to determine the level of obstruction.

TREATMENT | Lymphedema

Patients with lymphedema of the lower extremities must be instructed to take meticulous care of their feet to prevent recurrent lymphangitis. Skin hygiene is important, and emollients can be used to prevent drying. Prophylactic antibiotics are often helpful, and fungal infection should be treated aggressively. Patients should be encouraged to participate in physical activity; frequent leg elevation can reduce the amount of edema. Physical therapy, including massage to facilitate lymphatic drainage, may be helpful. Patients can be fitted with graduated compression hose to reduce the amount of lymphedema that develops with upright posture. Occasionally, intermittent pneumatic compression devices can be applied at home to facilitate reduction of the edema. Diuretics are contraindicated and may cause depletion of intravascular volume and metabolic abnormalities. Microsurgical lymphaticovenous anastomotic procedures have been performed to rechannel lymph flow from obstructed lymphatic vessels into the venous system.

CHAPTER 40

PULMONARY HYPERTENSION

Stuart Rich

Pulmonary hypertension, an abnormal elevation in pulmonary artery pressure, may be the result of left heart failure, pulmonary parenchymal or vascular disease, thromboembolism, or a combination of these factors. Whether the pulmonary hypertension arises from cardiac, pulmonary, or intrinsic vascular disease, it generally is a feature of advanced disease. Because the causes of pulmonary hypertension are so diverse, it is essential that the etiology underlying the pulmonary hypertension be clearly determined before beginning treatment.

PATHOPHYSIOLOGY

The right ventricle responds to an increase in pulmonary vascular resistance by increasing right ventricular (RV) systolic pressure to preserve cardiac output. In some patients, chronic changes occur in the pulmonary circulation, resulting in progressive remodeling of the vasculature, which can sustain or promote pulmonary hypertension even if the initiating factor is removed.

The ability of the RV to adapt to increased vascular resistance is influenced by several factors, including age and the rapidity of the development of pulmonary hypertension. For example, a large acute pulmonary thromboembolism can result in RV failure and shock, whereas chronic thromboembolic disease of equal severity may result in only mild exercise intolerance. Coexisting hypoxemia can impair the ability of the ventricle to compensate. Studies support the concept that RV failure occurs in pulmonary hypertension when the RV myocardium becomes ischemic as a result of excessive demands and inadequate RV coronary blood flow. The onset of RV failure, often manifest by peripheral edema, is associated with a poor outcome.

DIAGNOSIS

The most common symptom attributable to pulmonary hypertension is exertional dyspnea. Other common symptoms are fatigue, angina pectoris, syncope, near syncope, and peripheral edema.

The physical examination typically reveals increased jugular venous pressure, a reduced carotid pulse, and a palpable RV impulse. Most patients have an increased pulmonic component of the second heart sound, a right-sided fourth heart sound, and tricuspid regurgitation (Chap. 9). Peripheral cyanosis and/or edema tend to occur in later stages of the disease.

Laboratory findings

(Fig. 40-1) The chest x-ray generally shows enlarged central pulmonary arteries. The lung fields may reveal other pathology. The electrocardiogram usually shows right axis deviation and RV hypertrophy. The echocardiogram commonly demonstrates RV and right atrial enlargement, a reduction in left ventricular (LV) cavity size, and a tricuspid regurgitant jet that can be used to estimate RV systolic pressure by Doppler. Pulmonary function tests are helpful in documenting underlying obstructive airways disease, whereas high-resolution chest computed tomography (CT) is preferred to diagnose restrictive lung disease. Hypoxemia and an abnormal diffusing capacity for carbon monoxide occur with pulmonary hypertension of many causes. A perfusion lung scan is almost always abnormal in patients with thromboembolic pulmonary hypertension. However, diffuse defects of a nonsegmental nature often can be seen in long-standing pulmonary hypertension in the absence of thromboemboli. Laboratory tests should include antinuclear antibody and HIV testing. Because of the high frequency of thyroid abnormalities in patients with idiopathic pulmonary hypertension, it is recommended that the thyroid-stimulating hormone level be determined periodically.

Cardiac catheterization

Cardiac catheterization is mandatory for accurate measurement of pulmonary artery pressure, cardiac output,

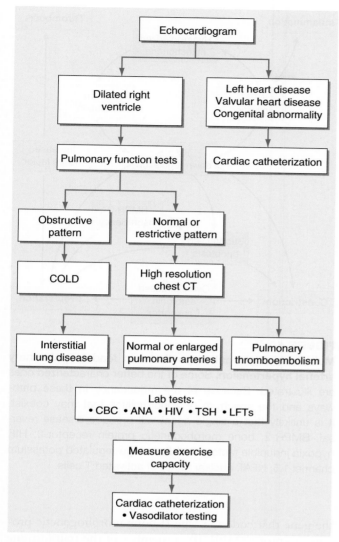

FIGURE 40-1

An algorithm for the workup of a patient with unexplained pulmonary hypertension. All potential etiologies and associated conditions must be investigated in a patient with clinical findings consistent with pulmonary hypertension. COLD, chronic obstructive lung disease; CBC, complete blood count; ANA, antinuclear antibodies; HIV, human immunodeficiency virus; TSH, thyroid-stimulating hormone; LFTs, liver function tests.

and LV filling pressure as well as documentation of an underlying cardiac shunt. Care should be taken to record pressures only at end expiration. It is recommended that patients with pulmonary arterial hypertension undergo drug testing with a short-acting pulmonary vasodilator to determine the extent of pulmonary vasodilator reactivity. Inhaled nitric oxide, intravenous adenosine, and intravenous epoprostenol have comparable effects in reducing pulmonary artery pressure acutely. Nitric oxide is administered via inhalation in 10–20 parts per million. Adenosine is given in doses

of 50 μg/kg per min and increased every 2 min until side effects develop. Epoprostenol is given in doses of 2 ng/kg per min and increased every 30 min until side effects develop. Patients who respond usually can be treated with calcium channel blockers and have a more favorable prognosis.

PULMONARY ARTERIAL HYPERTENSION

Pulmonary arterial hypertension (PAH) refers to a variety of diseases that include idiopathic PAH, as noted in **Table 40-1**. Patients with PAH have a common histopathology characterized by medial hypertrophy, eccentric and concentric intimal fibrosis, recanalized thrombi appearing as fibrous webs, and plexiform lesions.

PATHOBIOLOGY

Vasoconstriction, vascular proliferation, thrombosis, and inflammation appear to underlie the development of PAH **(Fig. 40-2)**. Abnormalities in multiple molecular pathways and genes that regulate the pulmonary vascular endothelial and smooth-muscle cells have been identified. These abnormalities include decreased expression of the voltage-regulated potassium channel, mutations in the bone morphogenetic protein-2 receptor, increased tissue factor expression, overactivation of the serotonin transporter, transcription factor activation of hypoxia-inducible factor-1 alpha, and activation of nuclear factor of activated T cells. As a result, there appears to be loss of apoptosis of the smooth-muscle cells that allows their proliferation and the emergence of apoptosis-resistant endothelial cells that can obliterate the vascular lumen. In addition, thrombin deposition in the pulmonary vasculature from a procoagulant state that develops as an independent abnormality or as a result of endothelial dysfunction may amplify the vascular proliferation.

IDIOPATHIC PULMONARY ARTERIAL HYPERTENSION

Idiopathic pulmonary arterial hypertension (IPAH), formerly referred to as primary pulmonary hypertension, is uncommon, with an estimated incidence of two cases per million. There is a female predominance, with most patients presenting in the fourth and fifth decades, although the age range is from infancy to >60 years.

Familial IPAH accounts for up to 20% of cases of IPAH and is characterized by autosomal dominant inheritance and incomplete penetrance. The clinical and pathologic features of familial and sporadic IPAH are identical. Heterozygous germ-line mutations involving

TABLE 40-1

A CLINICAL CLASSIFICATION OF PULMONARY HYPERTENSION

Category 1. Pulmonary arterial hypertension (PAH)

Key feature: elevation in pulmonary arterial pressure (PAP) with normal pulmonary capillary wedge pressure (pcwp)

Includes:

Idiopathic (IPAH)
- Sporadic
- Familial
- Exposure to drugs or toxins
- Persistent pulmonary hypertension of the newborn
- Pulmonary capillary hemangiomatosis (PCH)

Associated with other active conditions
- Collagen vascular disease
- Congenital systemic-to-pulmonary shunts
- Portal hypertension
- HIV infection

Category 2. Pulmonary venous hypertension

Key feature: elevation in PAP with elevation in pcwp

Includes:
- Left-sided atrial or ventricular heart disease
- Left-sided valvular heart disease
- Pulmonary venous obstruction
- Pulmonary venoocclusive disease (PVOD)

Category 3. Pulmonary hypertension associated with hypoxemic lung disease

Key feature: chronic hypoxia with mild elevation of PAP

Includes:
- Chronic obstructive lung disease
- Interstitial lung disease
- Sleep-disordered breathing
- Alveolar hypoventilation disorders
- Chronic exposure to high altitude
- Developmental abnormalities

Category 4. Pulmonary hypertension due to chronic thromboembolic disease

Key feature: elevation of PA pressure with documentation of pulmonary arterial obstruction for >3 months

Includes:
- Chronic pulmonary thromboembolism
- Nonthrombotic pulmonary embolism (tumor, foreign material)

Category 5. Miscellaneous

Key feature: elevation in PAP in association with a systemic disease where a causal relationship is not clearly understood

Includes:
- Sarcoidosis
- Chronic anemias
- Histiocytosis X
- Lymphangiomatosis
- Schistosomiasis

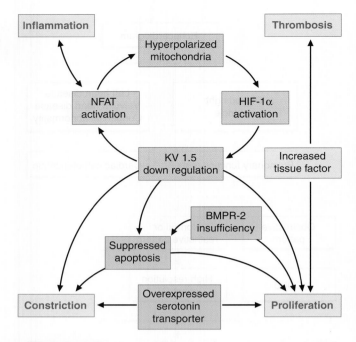

FIGURE 40-2

Multiple biologic pathways that can lead to pulmonary arterial hypertension. Some of the better-characterized ones are illustrated. Because of the redundancy in these pathways and the spectrum of abnormalities that may coexist, it is unlikely that a single agent will produce disease reversal. BMPR-2, bone morphogenetic protein receptor-2; HIF, hypoxia inducible factor; KV 1.5, voltage-regulated potassium channel 1.5; NFAT, nuclear factor of activated T cells.

the gene that code the type II bone morphogenetic protein receptor (BMPR II), a member of the transforming growth factor (TGF) β superfamily, appear to account for most cases of familial IPAH. The TGF-β superfamilies include multifunctional proteins that initiate diverse cellular responses by binding to and activating serine/threonine kinase receptors. The low gene penetrance indicates that other risk factors or abnormalities are necessary to manifest clinical disease. Germ-line mutations in the activin-like kinase gene and endoglin gene, which have been linked to hereditary hemorrhagic telangiectasia, coexist in some patients with familial IPAH.

NATURAL HISTORY

The natural history of IPAH is uncertain, but the disease typically is diagnosed late in its course. Before current therapies, a mean survival of 2–3 years from the time of diagnosis was reported. Functional class remains a strong predictor of survival, with patients who are in New York Heart Association (NYHA) functional class IV having a mean survival of <6 months. The cause of death is usually RV failure, which is manifest by progressive hypoxemia, tachycardia, hypotension, and edema.

TREATMENT ▸ Pulmonary Arterial Hypertension

Because the pulmonary artery pressure in PAH increases with exercise, patients should be cautioned against participating in activities that impose physical stress. Diuretic therapy relieves peripheral edema and may be useful in reducing RV volume overload. Pulse oximetry should be monitored, as O_2 supplementation helps alleviate dyspnea and RV ischemia in patients whose arterial O_2 saturation is reduced. Anticoagulant therapy is advocated for all patients with PAH based on studies demonstrating that warfarin increases survival of patients with PAH. The dose of warfarin generally is titrated to achieve an international normalized ratio (INR) of 2–3 times control.

Several treatments are approved for PAH; they are reviewed below without making a distinction among the different types. However, the efficacy and side effects of these drugs may not be the same in all types of PAH. Other than calcium channel blockers, none of the drugs produce a significant lowering of the pulmonary arterial pressure, and their long-term effects on survival are undefined. The principles for the selection and use of the approved drug treatments are reviewed in **Table 40-2**.

CALCIUM CHANNEL BLOCKERS Patients who respond to short-acting vasodilators at the time of cardiac catheterization (a fall in mean pulmonary arterial pressure ≥10 mmHg and a final mean pressure <40 mmHg) should be treated with calcium channel blockers. Typically, these patients require high doses (e.g., nifedipine, 240 mg/d, or amlodipine, 20 mg/d). Patients may have dramatic reductions in pulmonary artery pressure and pulmonary vascular resistance associated with improved symptoms, regression of RV hypertrophy, and improved survival now documented to exceed 20 years. However, <20% of patients respond to calcium channel blockers in the long term. These drugs are not effective in patients who are not vasoreactive. They also have not been approved for the treatment of PAH by the U.S. Food and Drug Administration.

ENDOTHELIN RECEPTOR ANTAGONISTS The endothelin receptor antagonists *bosentan* and *ambrisentan* are approved treatments of PAH. In randomized clinical trials, both improved exercise tolerance as measured by an increase in 6-min walking distance. Therapy with bosentan is initiated at 62.5 mg bid for the first month and increased to 125 mg bid thereafter. Ambrisentan is initiated as 5 mg once daily and can be increased to 10 mg daily. Because of the high frequency of abnormal hepatic function tests associated with these drugs, primarily an increase in transaminases, it is recommended that liver function be monitored monthly throughout the duration of use. Bosentan is contraindicated in patients who are on cyclosporine or glyburide concurrently.

TABLE 40-2

PRINCIPLES OF DRUG TREATMENT OF PULMONARY ARTERIAL HYPERTENSION

- Establish a correct diagnosis:
  Patients should undergo cardiac catheterization before initiating therapy.
- Obtain baseline assessments of the disease:
  Tests should be obtained to monitor the patient's response to therapy to know whether the treatments are effective.
- Test vasoreactivity:
  Patients should be tested at the time of diagnosis so that reactive patients are not missed.
- Reactive patients should be treated with calcium channel blockers:
  Calcium blockers in high doses are the drugs of choice.
- Nonreactive patients should be offered other therapies:
  No specific treatment has been established as first-line therapy.
- Periodic follow-up assessment of drug efficacy is essential:
  Repeat assessments should be performed within 8 weeks of initiating a new drug, as patients who do not respond initially are not likely to respond with longer exposure.
  Therapies can lose efficacy over time.
- Ineffective treatments should be replaced:
  A different treatment should be substituted rather than added.
  Patients who fail all treatments should be considered for lung transplantation.
- Benefits and risks of combination therapies are largely unknown:
  Only the addition of sildenafil to epoprostenol has been shown to be efficacious.

PHOSPHODIESTERASE-5 INHIBITORS *Sildenafil* and *tadalafil*, phosphodiesterase-5 inhibitors, are approved for the treatment of PAH. Phosphodiesterase-5 is responsible for the hydrolysis of cyclic GMP in pulmonary vascular smooth muscle, the mediator through which nitric oxide lowers pulmonary artery pressure and inhibits pulmonary vascular growth. Clinical trials have shown that both drugs improve exercise tolerance in patients with PAH. The effective dose for sildenafil is 20–80 mg tid. The effective dose for tadalafil is 40 mg once daily. The most common side effect is headache. Neither drug should be given to patients who are taking nitrovasodilators.

PROSTACYCLINS *Iloprost,* a prostacyclin analogue, is approved via inhalation for PAH. It has been shown to improve a composite measure of symptoms and exercise tolerance by 10%. Therapy can be given at either 2.5 or 5 µg per inhalation treatment via a dedicated nebulizer. The most common side effects are flushing and cough. Because of the very short half-life (<30 min) it is recommended that treatments be administered as often as every 2 h.

Epoprostenol is approved as a chronic IV treatment of PAH. Clinical trials have demonstrated an improvement in symptoms, exercise tolerance, and survival even if no acute hemodynamic response to drug challenge occurs. Drug administration requires placement of a permanent central venous catheter and infusion through an ambulatory infusion pump system. Side effects include flushing, jaw pain, and diarrhea, which are tolerated by most patients.

Treprostinil, an analogue of epoprostenol, is approved for PAH and may be given intravenously, subcutaneously, or via inhalation. Clinical trials have demonstrated an improvement in symptoms with exercise. Local pain at the infusion site with subcutaneous administration has caused most patients to switch to another therapy. Side effects are similar to those seen with epoprostenol.

The intravenous prostacyclins have the greatest efficacy as treatments for PAH and are often effective in patients who have failed all other treatments. Favorable properties include vasodilation, platelet inhibition, inhibition of vascular smooth muscle growth, and inotropic effects. It generally takes several months to titrate the dose of epoprostenol or treprostinil upward to achieve optimal clinical efficacy, which can be determined by symptoms, exercise testing, and catheterization. The optimal doses of these drugs have not been determined, but the typical doses of epoprostenol range from 25 to 40 ng/kg per min, and from 75 to 150 ng/kg per min for treprostinil. The major problem with intravenous therapy is infection related to the indwelling venous catheter, which requires close monitoring and diligence on the part of the patient. In addition, abrupt discontinuation of intravenous prostacyclins can lead to a rebound increase in pulmonary pressure.

It is recommended that every patient diagnosed with PAH be treated. Although no drug has been demonstrated to be superior as first-line therapy, many prefer to initiate treatment with an oral or inhaled form of therapy. Patients who fail to improve adequately within the first 2 months should be switched to a different treatment, as there is concern that delaying a more effective treatment may allow the disease to progress and become less responsive. The use of these drugs in combination has become popular, but the only randomized clinical trial demonstrating beneficial effects added sildenafil to patients treated with epoprostenol.

LUNG TRANSPLANTATION Lung transplantation is considered for patients who, while on an intravenous prostacyclin, continue to manifest right heart failure. Acceptable results have been achieved with heart-lung, bilateral lung, and single-lung transplantation. The availability of donor organs often influences the choice of procedure.

CONDITIONS ASSOCIATED WITH PULMONARY HYPERTENSION

COLLAGEN VASCULAR DISEASE

All the collagen vascular diseases may be associated with PAH. This complication occurs commonly with the CREST syndrome (calcinosis, Raynaud's phenomenon, esophageal involvement, sclerodactyly, and telangiectasia) and in scleroderma and less frequently in systemic lupus erythematosus, Sjögren's syndrome, dermatomyositis, polymyositis, and rheumatoid arthritis. Often these patients have coexistent interstitial pulmonary fibrosis even though it may not be apparent on chest x-ray, CT, or pulmonary function tests. Consequently, they tend to have hypoxemia as an important clinical feature, along with the other classic findings of pulmonary hypertension. A fall in diffusing capacity may precede the development of pulmonary hypertension. Treatment of these patients is identical to that of patients with IPAH (see earlier) but is less effective. The treatment of the pulmonary hypertension, however, does not affect the natural history of the underlying collagen vascular disease.

CONGENITAL SYSTEMIC TO PULMONARY SHUNTS

It is common for large post-tricuspid cardiac shunts (e.g., ventricular septal defect, patent ductus arteriosus) to produce severe PAH (Chap. 19). Although less common, this also may occur in pretricuspid shunts (e.g., atrial septal defect, anomalous pulmonary venous drainage). In patients with uncorrected shunts, the clinical features include those associated with right-to-left shunting, such as hypoxemia and peripheral cyanosis, which worsen dramatically with exertion (Chap. 6). PAH may also occur years or even decades after surgical correction in the absence of right-to-left shunting. These patients present similarly to patients with IPAH but tend to have better long-term survival. The treatments are similar to those for IPAH.

PORTAL HYPERTENSION

Portal hypertension is associated with PAH, but the mechanism is unknown. Patients with advanced cirrhosis can have the combined features of a high–output cardiac state in association with the features of pulmonary hypertension and RV failure. Thus, a normal cardiac output may actually reflect a marked impairment of RV function. The etiology of ascites and edema can be confusing in these patients because this condition can have both cardiac and hepatic causes. Overall, these patients have a worse prognosis than do patients with IPAH. Patients with mild pulmonary hypertension who have a favorable response to epoprostenol have undergone successful liver transplantation with improvement of the pulmonary vascular disease.

ANOREXIGENS

A causal relationship has been established between exposure to several anorexigens, including aminorex and the fenfluramines, and the development of PAH. Often the pulmonary hypertension will develop years after the last exposure. Although the clinical features are identical to those of IPAH, the patients appear to be less responsive to medical treatments.

PULMONARY CAPILLARY HEMANGIOMATOSIS

Pulmonary capillary hemangiomatosis is a very rare form of pulmonary hypertension. Histologically it is characterized by the presence of infiltrating thin-walled blood vessels throughout the pulmonary interstitium and walls of the pulmonary arteries and veins. The presenting symptoms are those of IPAH but often with hypoxemia or hemoptysis as a clinical feature. The diagnosis may be suggested by findings on chest CT. The clinical course is usually one of progressive deterioration leading to death. There is no established therapy.

PULMONARY VENOUS HYPERTENSION

Pulmonary hypertension occurs as a result of increased resistance to pulmonary venous drainage. It is associated with diastolic dysfunction of the left ventricle, diseases affecting the pericardium or mitral or aortic valves, and rare entities such as cor triatriatum, left atrial myxoma, extrinsic compression of the central pulmonary veins from fibrosing mediastinitis, and pulmonary venoocclusive disease. Pulmonary venous hypertension affects the pulmonary veins and venules, producing arterialization of the external elastic lamina, medial hypertrophy, and focal eccentric intimal fibrosis. Microcirculatory lesions include capillary congestion, focal alveolar edema, and dilation of the interstitial lymphatics. Although these lesions are potentially reversible, regression may take years after the underlying cause is removed. Pulmonary venous hypertension often triggers reactive vasoconstriction in the pulmonary arterial bed and results in proliferative changes of the intima and media that can produce severe elevations in pulmonary artery pressure. Clinically it may be confusing and appear as if two separate disease processes are occurring simultaneously. The distinction is important, however, as treatments that are effective in PAH may make patients with pulmonary venous hypertension worse.

LEFT VENTRICULAR DIASTOLIC DYSFUNCTION

Pulmonary hypertension as a result of LV diastolic failure is common but often unrecognized (Chap. 17). It can occur with or without LV systolic failure. The most common risk factors are hypertensive heart disease; coronary artery disease; and impaired LV compliance related to age, diabetes, obesity, and hypoxemia. Symptoms of orthopnea and paroxysmal nocturnal dyspnea are prominent. Many patients improve considerably if LV end-diastolic pressure is lowered, but current treatments are unsatisfactory.

MITRAL VALVE DISEASE

Mitral stenosis and mitral regurgitation represent important causes of pulmonary hypertension (Chap. 20) from reactive pulmonary vasoconstriction resulting in marked elevations in pulmonary artery pressures. An echocardiogram usually shows abnormalities such as thickened mitral valve leaflets with reduced mobility or severe mitral regurgitation documented by Doppler echocardiography (Chap. 12). At cardiac catheterization, a pressure gradient between the pulmonary capillary wedge pressure and LV end-diastolic pressure is diagnostic of mitral stenosis.

In patients with mitral stenosis, corrective surgery of the mitral valve or mitral balloon valvuloplasty predictably results in a reduction in pulmonary artery pressure and pulmonary vascular resistance. Patients with mitral regurgitation, however, may not have as dramatic a response to surgery because of persistent elevations in LV end-diastolic pressure.

PULMONARY VENOOCCLUSIVE DISEASE

Pulmonary venoocclusive disease is a rare and distinct pathologic entity found in <10% of patients who present with unexplained pulmonary hypertension. Histologically it is manifest by intimal proliferation and fibrosis of the intrapulmonary veins and venules, occasionally extending to the arteriolar bed. A CT scan may reveal septal thickening, diffuse or mosaic ground-glass opacities, multiple small nodules, or areas of alveolar consolidation. Advanced pulmonary venous obstruction explains the orthopnea that can mimic LV failure, pulmonary edema noted on chest x-ray, and the increase in pulmonary capillary wedge pressure at catheterization. Effective therapy for this condition has not been established.

PULMONARY HYPERTENSION ASSOCIATED WITH LUNG DISEASE AND HYPOXEMIA

The acute hypoxic response of the pulmonary arterial smooth-muscle cells involves inhibition of the potassium current, membrane depolarization, and calcium entry through L-type calcium channels. Hypoxia, acting through the small G protein RhoA, stimulates Rho kinase, which inhibits myosin vs. heavy chain in light chain phosphatase, thereby increasing phosphorylation of the light chain and augmenting contraction. Chronic hypoxia results in muscularization of the arterioles with minimal effects on the intima. When it occurs as an isolated entity, the changes produced are potentially reversible.

Although chronic hypoxia is an established cause of pulmonary hypertension, it rarely leads to an increase in the systolic pulmonary artery pressure >50 mmHg. Polycythemia in response to the hypoxemia is a characteristic finding. Hypoxia also may occur in conjunction with other causes of pulmonary hypertension associated with more extensive vascular changes. Clinically, the hypoxia has an added adverse effect. Patients with chronic hypoxia who have a marked elevation in pulmonary pressure should be evaluated for the other causes of the pulmonary hypertension.

CHRONIC OBSTRUCTIVE LUNG DISEASE

Chronic obstructive lung disease (COLD) is associated with mild pulmonary hypertension in the advanced stages. The factors leading to an increase in pulmonary vascular resistance are numerous, but alveolar hypoxia is considered the predominant one. The presence of pulmonary hypertension in patients with COLD confers a worse outcome. The only effective therapy is supplemental oxygen. Clinical trials have documented that continuous oxygen therapy relieves the pulmonary vasoconstriction, reverses chronic ischemia throughout the systemic and pulmonary vascular beds, and improves survival. Long-term oxygen therapy is indicated if the resting arterial Po_2 remains <55 mmHg. Pulmonary vasodilators can worsen gas exchange and should not be used.

INTERSTITIAL LUNG DISEASE

Pulmonary hypertension is common in interstitial lung disease that results from parenchymal and vascular remodeling. Coexisting hypoxemia occurs frequently and contributes to morbidity. Interstitial lung disease often is associated with the collagen vascular diseases. Many patients have pulmonary fibrosis of unknown etiology. Patients are commonly older than 50 years and report an insidious onset of progressive dyspnea and cough for months to years. It is uncommon for the mean pulmonary artery pressure to exceed 40 mmHg. The pulmonary vasodilators approved for PAH have not been shown to be helpful.

SLEEP-DISORDERED BREATHING

The incidence of pulmonary hypertension in the setting of *obstructive sleep apnea*, a common condition, is <20% and is generally mild. Some patients have severe pulmonary hypertension in conjunction with sleep apnea, which may be unrelated. It is recommended that the sleep apnea and the PAH be treated as coexisting problems.

ALVEOLAR HYPOVENTILATION

Pulmonary hypertension can occur in patients with chronic hypoventilation and hypoxia secondary to thoracovertebral deformities. Symptoms are slowly progressive and are related to hypoxemia. In patients with advanced disease, intermittent positive-pressure breathing and supplemental oxygen have been used successfully.

Pulmonary hypertension secondary to hypoxemia has been reported in patients with neuromuscular disease as a result of generalized weakness of the respiratory muscles and in patients with diaphragmatic paralysis, generally from trauma to the phrenic nerve. Patients with nontraumatic bilateral diaphragmatic paralysis may go unrecognized until they present with either respiratory failure or pulmonary hypertension.

PULMONARY HYPERTENSION DUE TO THROMBOEMBOLIC DISEASE

CHRONIC THROMBOEMBOLIC PULMONARY HYPERTENSION

Most patients treated for acute pulmonary thromboembolism with intravenous heparin and chronic oral warfarin do not develop chronic pulmonary hypertension. However, some patients have impaired fibrinolytic resolution of the thromboembolism, which leads to organization and incomplete recanalization and chronic obstruction of the pulmonary vascular bed. Because the initial pulmonary thromboembolism goes undetected or untreated, many patients are misdiagnosed as having IPAH. These patients may have underlying thrombophilic disorders, such as the lupus anticoagulant/anticardiolipin antibody syndrome, prothrombin gene mutation, or factor V Leiden.

Diagnosis

The physical examination is characteristic of pulmonary hypertension but may include bruits heard over areas of the lung, representing blood flow through vessels with partial occlusion. A perfusion lung scan or contrast-enhanced spiral CT scan should reveal multiple thromboemboli. High-resolution CT scanning is necessary to document the location and proximal extent of the thromboemboli and hence the potential for operability.

TREATMENT	Chronic Thromboembolic Pulmonary Hypertension

Pulmonary thromboendarterectomy is an established surgical treatment in patients whose thrombi are accessible to surgical removal. The operative mortality is <10% in experienced centers. Postoperative survivors can expect an improvement in functional class and exercise tolerance. Lifelong anticoagulation using warfarin is mandatory. Thrombolytic therapy is rarely helpful in patients with chronic thromboembolic pulmonary hypertension and may expose them to the increased risk of bleeding without potential benefit.

OTHER DISORDERS AFFECTING THE PULMONARY VASCULATURE

SARCOIDOSIS

Sarcoidosis can produce pulmonary hypertension as a result of fibrocystic lung involvement or direct cardiovascular involvement. Consequently, patients with sarcoidosis who present with progressive dyspnea and pulmonary hypertension require a thorough evaluation. There is a subset of patients with sarcoidosis and severe pulmonary hypertension who exhibit a favorable response to epoprostenol therapy.

SICKLE CELL DISEASE

Cardiovascular system abnormalities are prominent in the clinical spectrum of sickle cell disease, including pulmonary hypertension. The etiology is multifactorial, including hemolysis, hypoxemia, thromboembolism, chronic high cardiac output, and chronic liver disease. The presence of pulmonary hypertension in patients with sickle cell disease is associated with higher mortality. Intensification of sickle cell disease–specific therapy appears to reduce the morbidity. Clinical trials assessing drugs to treat pulmonary hypertension are ongoing, but the efficacy of those drugs is unknown.

SCHISTOSOMIASIS

 Although extremely rare in North America, schistosomiasis is one of the most common causes of pulmonary hypertension worldwide. The development of pulmonary hypertension occurs in the setting of hepatosplenic disease and portal hypertension. Studies suggest that inflammation from the infection triggers the pulmonary vascular changes that occur. The diagnosis is confirmed by finding the parasite ova in the urine or stools of patients with symptoms, which can be difficult. The efficacy of therapies directed toward pulmonary hypertension in these patients is unknown.

HIV INFECTION

The mechanism by which HIV infection produces pulmonary hypertension is unknown. Although the incidence is estimated at 1 per 200 cases, the marked rise in the prevalence of HIV infection worldwide could have a significant impact on the frequency with which these entities are seen in combination. The evaluation and treatments are identical to those for IPAH. Treatment of the HIV infection does not appear to affect the severity or natural history of the underlying pulmonary hypertension.

SECTION VI

CARDIOVASCULAR ATLASES

CHAPTER 41

ATLAS OF ELECTROCARDIOGRAPHY

Ary L. Goldberger

The electrocardiograms (ECGs) in this Atlas supplement those illustrated in Chap. 11. The interpretations emphasize findings of specific teaching value.

All of the figures are from ECG Wave-Maven, Copyright 2003, Beth Israel Deaconess Medical Center, *http://ecg.bidmc.harvard.edu.*

The abbreviations used in this chapter are as follows:

AF—atrial fibrillation
HCM—hypertrophic cardiomyopathy

LVH—left ventricular hypertrophy
MI—myocardial infarction
NSR—normal sinus rhythm
RBBB—right bundle branch block
RV—right ventricular
RVH—right ventricular hypertrophy

MYOCARDIAL ISCHEMIA AND INFARCTION

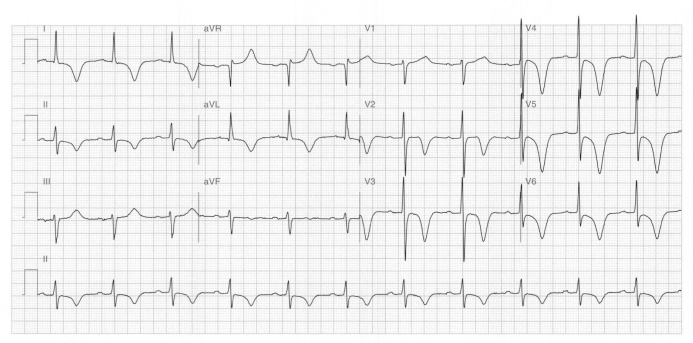

FIGURE 41-1

Anterior wall ischemia (deep T-wave inversions and ST-segment depressions in I, aVL, V$_3$–V$_6$) in a patient with **LVH** (increased voltage in V$_2$–V$_5$).

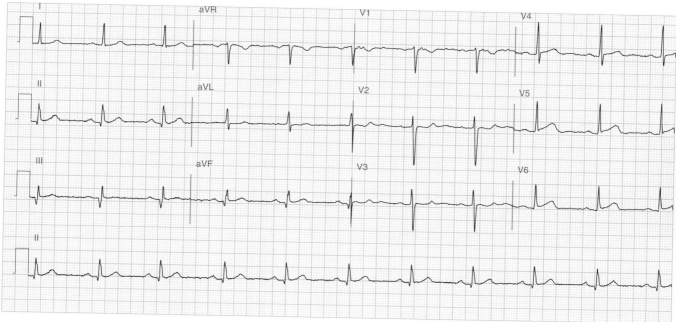

FIGURE 41-2

Acute anterolateral wall ischemia with ST elevations in V_4–V_6. Probable prior inferior MI with Q waves in leads II, III, and aVF.

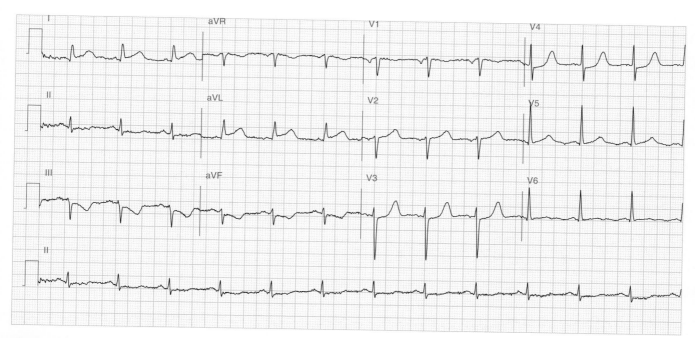

FIGURE 41-3

Acute lateral ischemia with ST elevations in I and aVL with probable reciprocal ST depressions inferiorly (II, III, and aVF). Ischemic ST depressions also in V_3 and V_4. **Left atrial abnormality**.

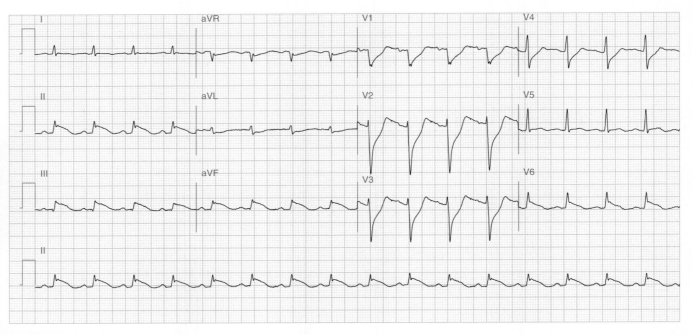

FIGURE 41-4

Sinus tachycardia. Marked ischemic ST-segment elevations in inferior limb leads (II, III, aVF) and laterally (V$_6$) suggestive of **acute inferolateral MI,** and prominent ST-segment depressions with upright T waves in V$_1$–V$_4$ are consistent with associated **acute posterior MI**.

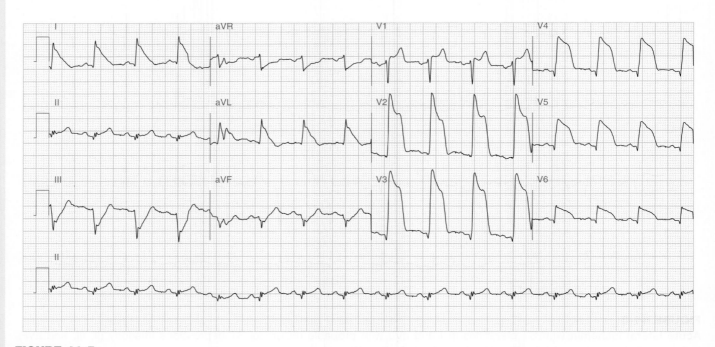

FIGURE 41-5

Acute, extensive anterior MI with marked ST elevations in I, aVL, V$_1$–V$_6$ and small pathologic Q waves in V$_3$–V$_6$. Marked reciprocal ST-segment depressions in III and aVF.

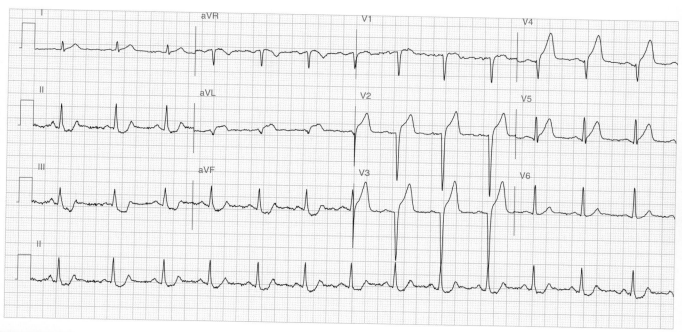

FIGURE 41-6

Acute anterior wall MI with ST elevations and Q waves in V_1–V_4 and aVL and reciprocal inferior ST depressions.

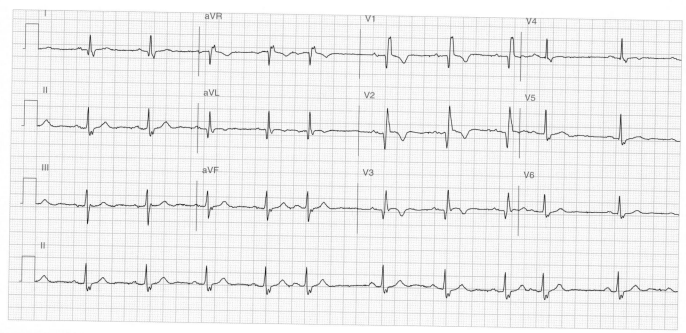

FIGURE 41-7

NSR with premature atrial complexes. **RBBB;** pathologic Q waves and ST elevation due to **acute anterior/septal MI** in V_1–V_3.

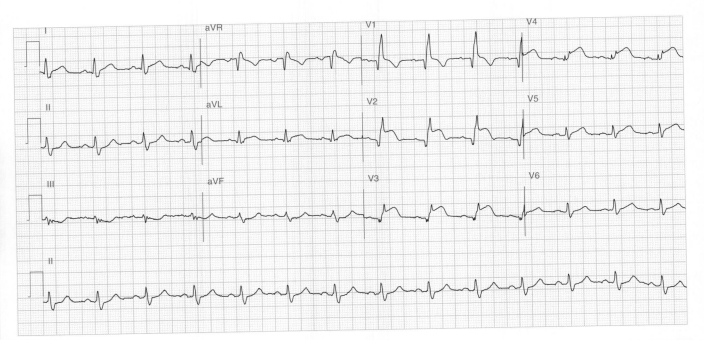

FIGURE 41-8
Acute anteroseptal MI (Q waves and ST elevations in V₁–V₄) with **RBBB** (note terminal R waves in V₁).

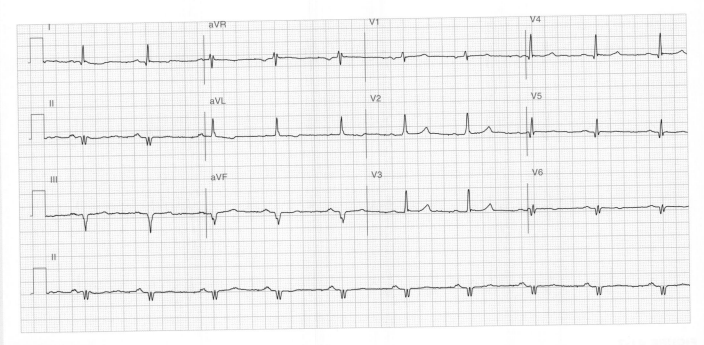

FIGURE 41-9
Extensive prior MI involving inferior-posterior-lateral wall (Q waves in leads II, III, aVF, tall R waves in V₁, V₂, and Q waves in V₅, V₆). T-wave abnormalities in leads I and aVL, V₅, and V₆.

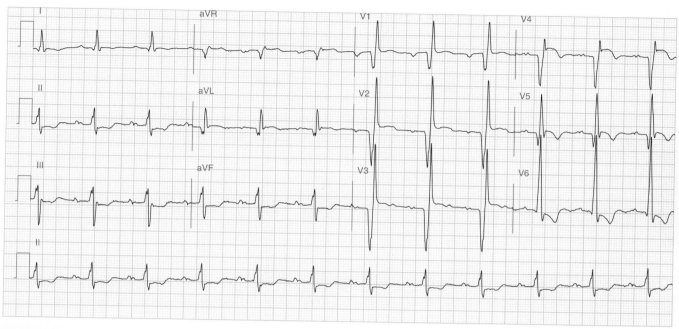

FIGURE 41-10

NSR with PR prolongation ("1st-degree AV block"), left atrial abnormality, LVH, and RBBB. Pathologic Q waves in V_1–V_5 and aVL with ST elevations (a chronic finding in this patient). Findings compatible with **prior anterolateral MI and LV aneurysm**.

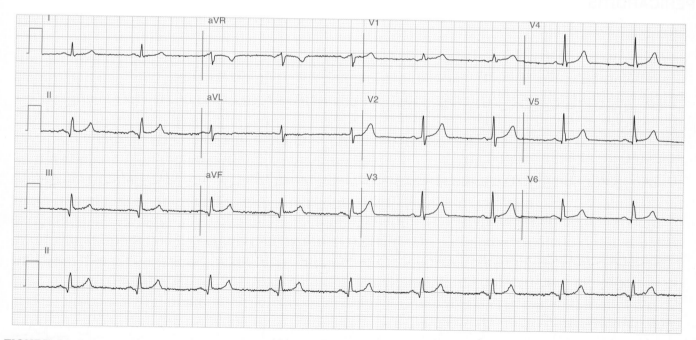

FIGURE 41-11

Prior inferior-posterior MI. Wide (0.04 s) Q waves in the inferior leads (II, III, aVF); broad R wave in V_1 (a Q wave "equivalent" here). Absence of right-axis deviation and the presence of upright T waves in V_1–V_2 are also against RVH.

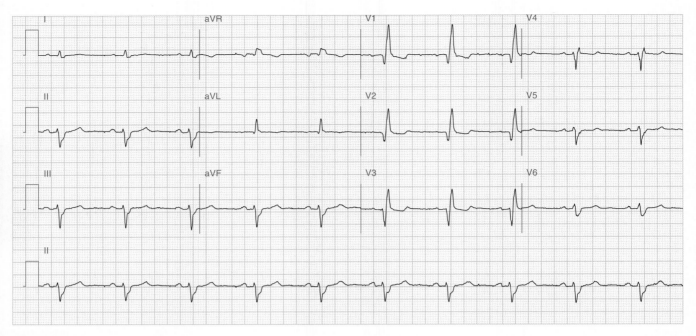

FIGURE 41-12

NSR with RBBB (broad terminal R wave in V_1) and left anterior fascicular block (hemiblock) and pathologic anterior Q waves in V_1–V_3. Patient had **severe multivessel coronary artery disease,** with echocardiogram showing septal dyskinesis and apical akinesis.

PERICARDITIS

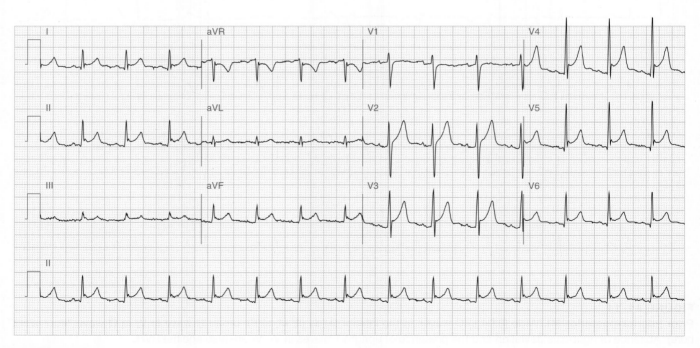

FIGURE 41-13

Acute pericarditis with diffuse ST elevations in I, II, III, aVF, V_3–V_6, without T-wave inversions. Also note concomitant PR-segment elevation in aVR and PR depression in the inferolateral leads.

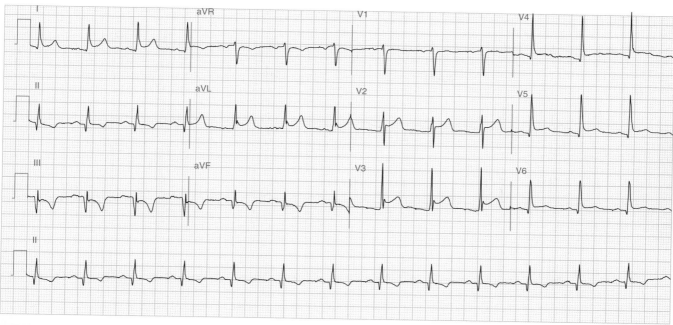

FIGURE 41-14

Sinus rhythm; diffuse ST elevations (I, II, aVL, aVF, V_2–V_6) with associated PR deviations (elevated PR in aVR; depressed in V_4–V_6); borderline low voltage. Q-wave and T-wave inversions in II, III, and aVF. Diagnosis: **acute pericarditis with inferior Q-wave MI**.

VALVULAR HEART DISEASE AND HYPERTROPHIC CARDIOMYOPATHY

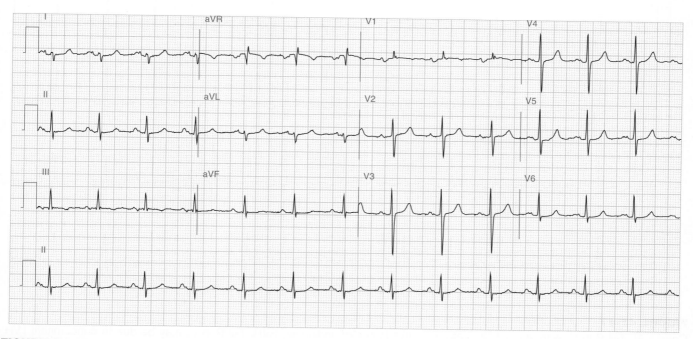

FIGURE 41-15

NSR, prominent left atrial abnormality (see I, II, V_1), right-axis deviation and **RVH** (tall, relatively narrow R wave in V_1) in a patient with **mitral stenosis**.

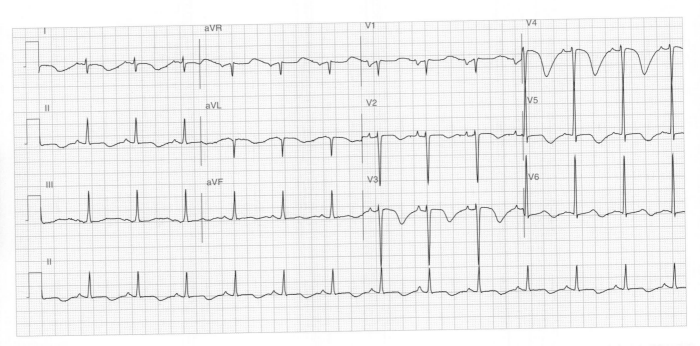

FIGURE 41-16

NSR, left atrial abnormality, and LVH by voltage criteria with borderline right-axis deviation in a patient with **mixed mitral stenosis** (left atrial abnormality and right-axis deviation) and **mitral regurgitation** (LVH). Prominent precordial T-wave inversions and QT prolongation also present.

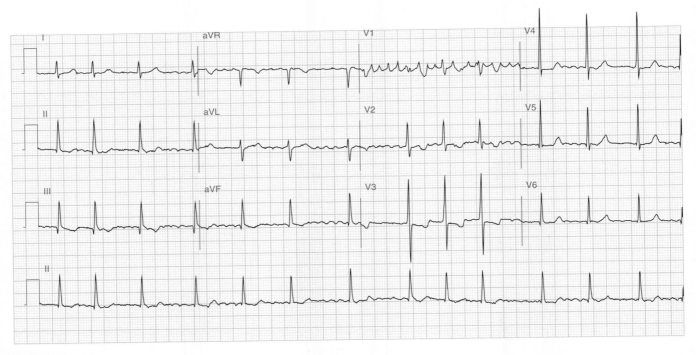

FIGURE 41-17

Coarse AF, tall R in V$_2$ with vertical QRS axis (positive R in aVF) indicating RVH. Tall R in V$_4$ may be due to concomitant LVH. Patient had **severe mitral stenosis with moderate mitral regurgitation**.

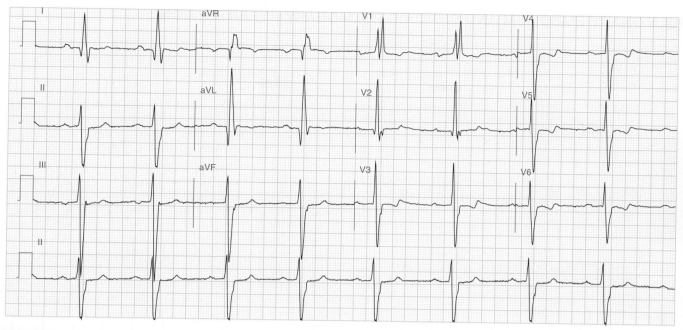

FIGURE 41-18

NSR; first-degree A-V "block" (P-R prolongation); LVH (tall R in aVL); RBBB (wide multiphasic R wave in V₁) and left anterior fascicular block in a patient with **HCM.** Deep Q waves in I and aVL are consistent with **septal hypertrophy**.

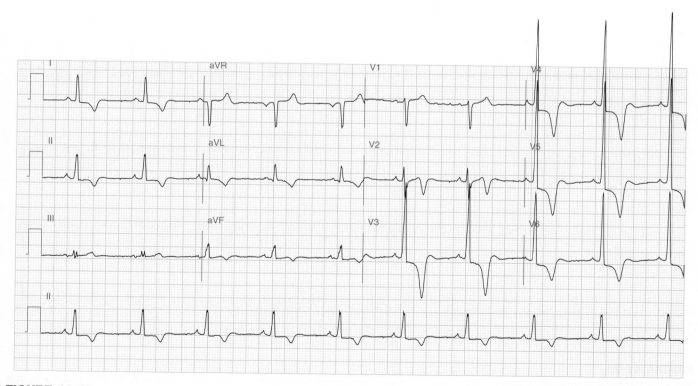

FIGURE 41-19

LVH with deep T-wave inversions in limb leads and precordial leads. Striking T-wave inversions in mid-precordial leads suggest **apical HCM** (Yamaguchi's syndrome).

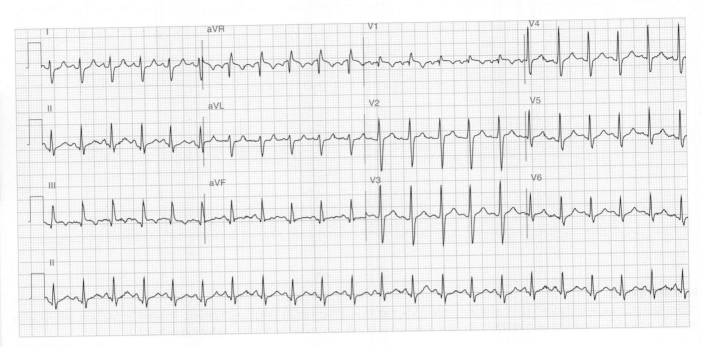

FIGURE 41-20

Sinus tachycardia with S1Q3T3 pattern (T-wave inversion in III), incomplete RBBB, and right precordial T-wave inversions consistent with acute RV overload in a patient with **pulmonary emboli**.

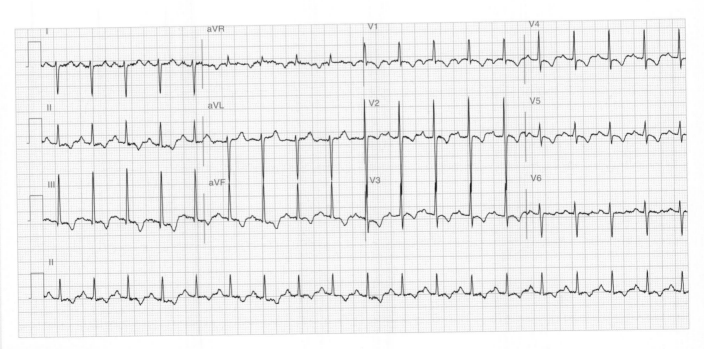

FIGURE 41-21

Sinus tachycardia, right-axis deviation, RVH with tall R in V_1 and deep S in V_6 and inverted T waves in II, III, aVF, and V_1–V_5 in a patient with **atrial septal defect and severe pulmonary hypertension**.

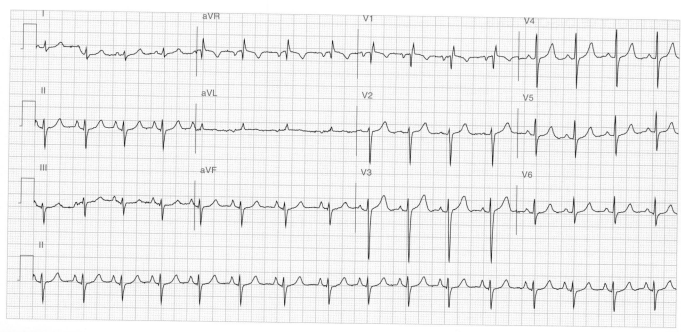

FIGURE 41-22

Signs of right atrial/RV overload in a patient with **chronic obstructive lung disease:** (1) peaked P waves in II; (2) QR in V_1 with narrow QRS; (3) delayed precordial transition, with terminal S waves in V_5/V_6; (4) superior axis deviation with an S_1-S_2-S_3 pattern.

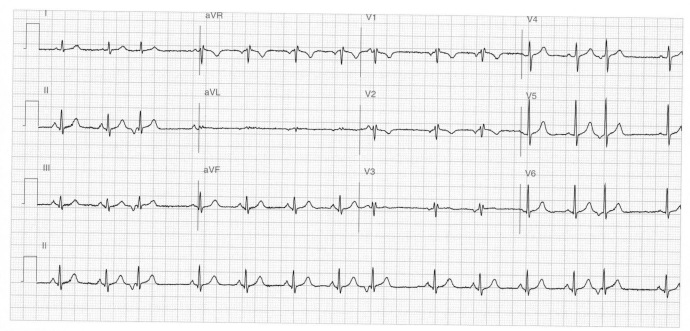

FIGURE 41-23

(1) Low voltage; (2) incomplete RBBB (rsr' in V_1–V_3); (3) borderline peaked P waves in lead II with vertical P-wave axis (probable right atrial overload); (4) slow R-wave progression in V_1–V_3; (5) prominent S waves in V_6; and (6) atrial premature beats. This combination is seen typically in **severe chronic obstructive lung disease**.

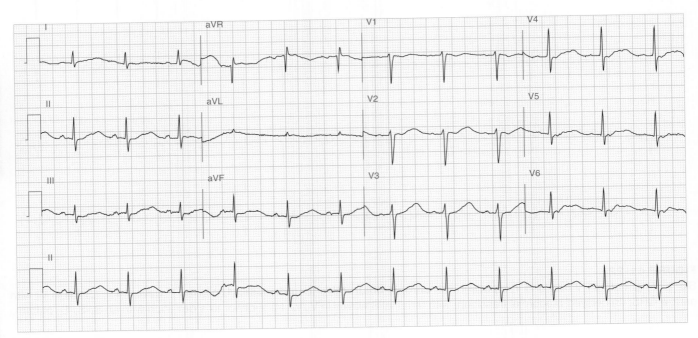

FIGURE 41-24

Prominent U waves (II, III, and V$_4$–V$_6$) with ventricular repolarization prolongation in a patient with **severe hypokalemia**.

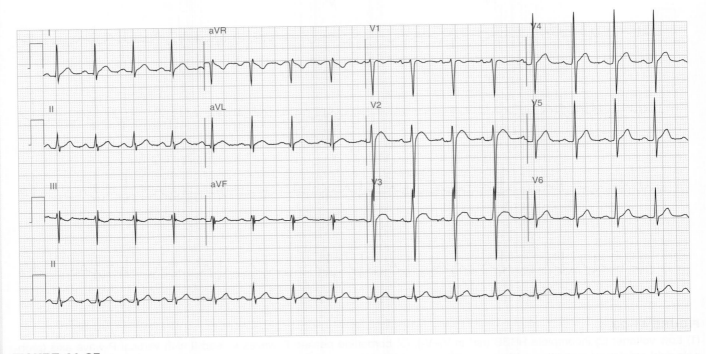

FIGURE 41-25

Abbreviated ST segment such that the T wave looks like it takes off directly from QRS in some leads (I, V$_4$, aVL, and V$_5$) in a patient with severe **hypercalcemia**. Note also high takeoff of ST segment in V$_2$/V$_3$ simulating acute ischemia.

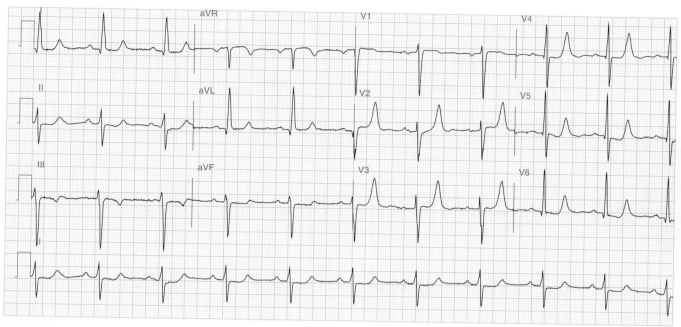

FIGURE 41-26

NSR with LVH, left atrial abnormality, and tall peaked T waves in the precordial leads with inferolateral ST depressions (II, III, aVF, and V_6); left anterior fascicular block and borderline prolonged QT interval in a patient with **renal failure, hypertension, and hyperkalemia;** prolonged QT is secondary to **associated hypocalcemia.**

MISCELLANEOUS

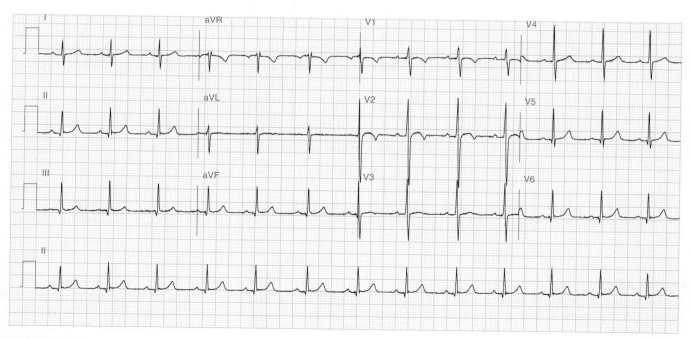

FIGURE 41-27

Normal ECG in an 11-year-old male. T-wave inversions in V_1–V_2. Vertical QRS axis ($+90°$) and early precordial transition between V_2 and V_3 are **normal findings in children.**

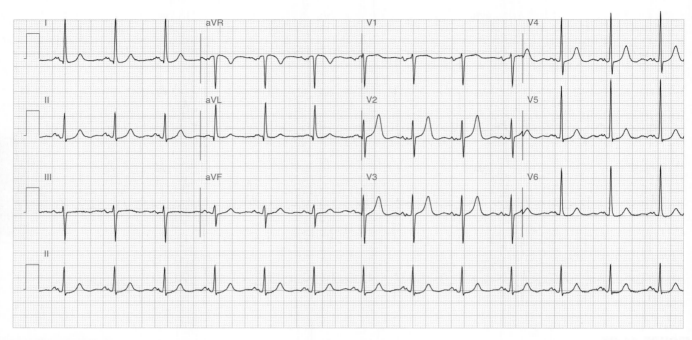

FIGURE 41-28

Left atrial abnormality and **LVH** in a patient with **long-standing hypertension**.

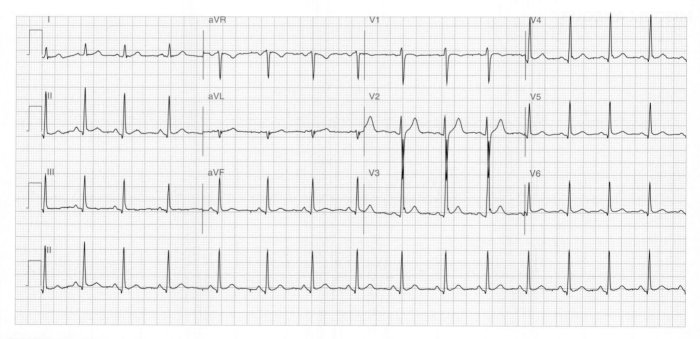

FIGURE 41-29

Normal variant ST-segment elevations in a healthy 21-year-old male (commonly referred to as *benign early repolarization pattern*). ST elevations exhibit upward concavity and are most apparent in V_3 and V_4, and less than 1 mm in the limb leads. Precordial QRS voltages are prominent, but within normal limits for a young adult. No evidence of left atrial abnormality or ST depression/T wave inversions to go along with **LVH**.

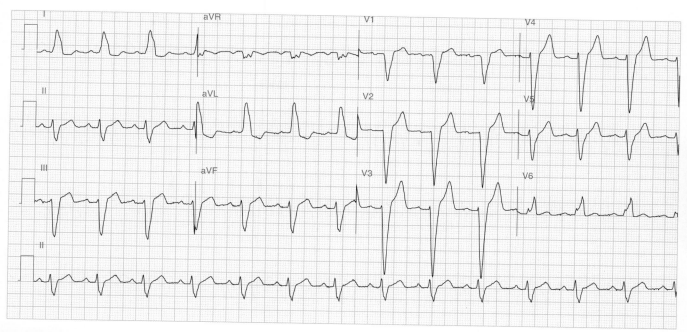

FIGURE 41-30
NSR with first-degree AV "block" (PR interval = 0.24 s) and complete **left bundle branch block**.

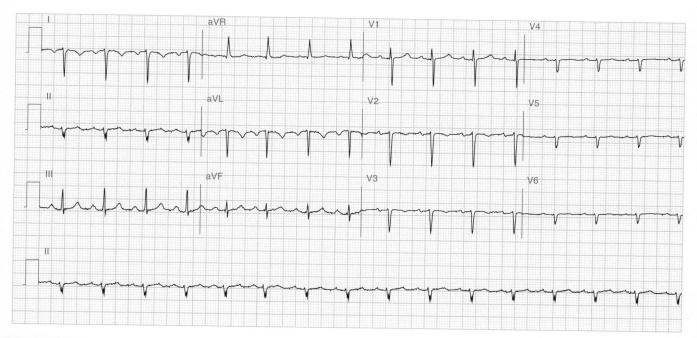

FIGURE 41-31
Dextrocardia with: (1) inverted P waves in I and aVL; (2) negative QRS complex and T wave in I; and (3) progressively decreasing voltage across the precordium.

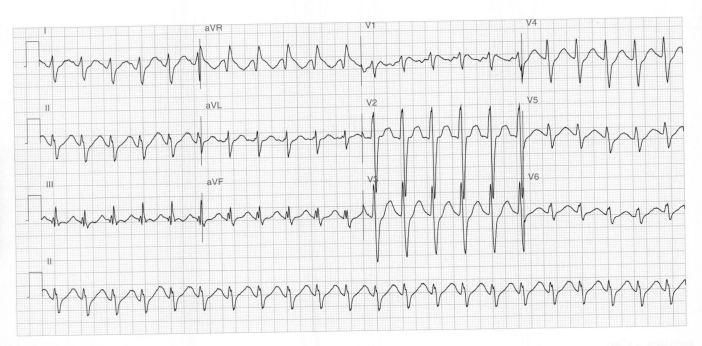

FIGURE 41-32

Sinus tachycardia; intraventricular conduction delay (IVCD) with a rightward QRS axis. QT interval is prolonged for the rate. The triad of sinus tachycardia, a wide QRS complex, and a long QT in appropriate clinical context suggests **tricyclic antidepressant overdose**. Terminal S wave (rS) in I, and terminal R wave (qR) in aVR are also noted as part of this IVCD variant.

CHAPTER 42
ATLAS OF NONINVASIVE CARDIAC IMAGING

Rick A Nishimura ■ Panithya Chareonthaitawee ■ Matthew Martinez

ECHOCARDIOGRAPHIC IMAGES

All videos can be accessed via the following link: http://www.mhprofessional.com/mediacenter/.

Video 42-1   Real-time two-dimensional echocardiographic images of a patient with a normal heart. **A.** Parasternal long-axis view. **B.** Parasternal short-axis view. There is symmetric contraction of the ventricles, evidenced by a decrease in cavity size and increase in wall thickness during systole. Echocardiographic imaging is performed in multiple acoustic windows with different transducer rotations so that the entire heart and great vessels can be displayed in various planes. Most information from a study is obtained from visual analysis of the two-dimensional images, although objective measurements of cardiac dimensions can be made.

Video 42-2   Real-time two-dimensional echocardiographic images of a patient with a severe decrease in left ventricular systolic function. The estimated ejection fraction is 20%. **A.** Parasternal long-axis view. **B.** Parasternal short-axis view.

Video 42-3   Real-time two-dimensional echocardiographic images of a patient with hypertrophic cardiomyopathy. There is a marked increase in left ventricular wall thickness with hyperdynamic systolic function. **A.** Parasternal long-axis view. **B.** Parasternal short-axis view.

Video 42-4   Real-time two-dimensional parasternal long-axis images from a patient with aortic stenosis. There is normal left ventricular cavity size with normal systolic function. The aortic valve is thickened and calcified, with restricted opening.

Video 42-5   Real-time two-dimensional echocardiographic images of a patient with mitral stenosis. There is diastolic doming and restricted leaflet opening secondary to fusion of the commissures. **A.** Parasternal long-axis view. **B.** Parasternal short-axis view.

Video 42-6   Real-time two-dimensional echocardiographic images from the parasternal long-axis view of a patient with mitral valve prolapse. During systole, both anterior and posterior leaflet of the mitral valve prolapse into the left atrium.

A. Gray-scale images demonstrate a leaflet morphology and motion. **B.** Color flow imaging demonstrating late systolic blue-colored jet of mitral regurgitation. Abnormalities of the valve apparatus such as annular dilatation, prolapse, flail leaflets, vegetation, and rheumatic involvement can be diagnosed by two-dimensional echocardiography. The left ventricular response to volume overload can be assessed by two-dimensional echocardiography.

Video 42-7   Real-time two-dimensional images with color flow Doppler imaging of a patient with mitral regurgitation due to ruptured chordae tendineae. **A.** Gray-scale image showing a thickened redundant posterior leaflet of the mitral valve with loss of coaptation during systole. **B.** Color flow imaging showing severe mitral regurgitation as high velocity turbulence (mosaic pattern) extending into the left atrium during systole.

Video 42-8   Real-time transesophageal echocardiographic images of a patient with severe mitral regurgitation due to a flail posterior leaflet. The posterior mitral valve leaflet is completely unsupported and moves into the left atrium during systole. Transesophageal echocardiography provides high-resolution images of posterior structure such as the left atrium, mitral valve, and aorta.

Video 42-9   Real-time two-dimensional echocardiographic images of a patient with a vegetation on the mitral valve. There is a mobile echo density attached directly to the mitral valve apparatus that intermittently appears in the left atrium.

Video 42-10   Real-time transesophageal echocardiographic images of a patient with a left atrial myxoma. There is a large echo-dense mass in the left atrium that is attached to the atrial septum. The mass moves across the mitral valve during diastole. Although an echocardiographic image cannot provide pathologic confirmation of the etiology of a mass, the diagnosis of atrial myxoma can be suspected from the appearance, mobility, and attachment to the atrial septum.

Video 42-11   Real-time two-dimensional echocardiographic images from the parasternal long-axis view of a patient with a large aneurysm of the ascending aorta.

Video 42-12   Real-time two-dimensional echocardiographic images of a patient with pericardial effusion. The effusion is shown as a black echo-free space surrounding the heart.

Video 42-13   Real-time two-dimensional echocardiographic images from a subcostal view showing a large secundum atrial septal defect. There is a "drop out" in the region of the mid atrial septum. The right ventricle is enlarged from right ventricular volume overload.

Video 42-14   Real-time two-dimensional echocardiographic images showing a close-up view of the atrial septum in a patient with the question of an atrial septal defect. *A.* Grayscale image showing a questionable "drop out" in the atrial septum. *B.* Color flow imaging confirms left to right flow across the atrial septum.

Video 42-15   Real-time two-dimensional stress echocardiogram in a normal subject. The studies at rest are shown on the left and the studies during peak exercise are shown on the right. *A.* Parasternal long-axis (*top*) and short-axis (*bottom*) views. *B.* Apical four-chamber (*top*) and two-chamber (*bottom*)

views. At rest, there is contraction of all segments of the myocardium. During exercise, there is an increase in contractility and in the thickening of all segments of the myocardium with a decrease in end-systolic volume.

Video 42-16   Real-time two-dimensional stress echocardiogram of a patient with coronary artery disease. The studies at rest are shown on the left and studies during peak exercise are shown on the right. *A.* Parasternal long-axis (*top*) and short-axis (*bottom*) views. *B.* Apical four-chamber (*top*) and two-chamber (*bottom*) views. The images during peak exercise show regional wall motion abnormalities in the anteroseptal distribution indicative of myocardial ischemia. This was subsequently found to be associated with a high-grade lesion on the left anterior descending artery.

NUCLEAR IMAGES

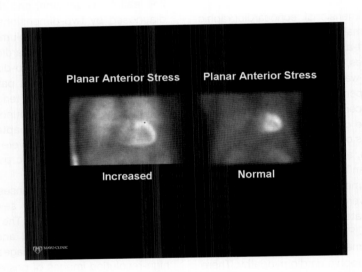

FIGURE 42-1

Anterior planar thallium images following stress, showing increased lung uptake on the left (count intensity in lung >50% of that in myocardium) and normal lung uptake on the right (count intensity in lung <50% of that in myocardium).

Increased lung uptake of thallium may be seen immediately after stress. It reflects increased pulmonary capillary wedge pressure and occurs in the presence of severe coronary artery disease and/or left ventricular systolic dysfunction. It provides important adverse prognostic information that is incremental to other clinical, stress, and coronary angiographic variables.

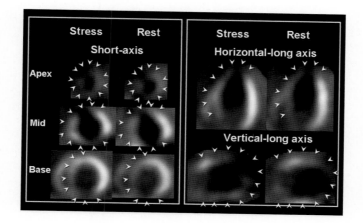

FIGURE 42-2

Exercise SPECT ^{99m}Tc sestamibi scan in a 64-year-old male patient with a previous infarct. The stress images (*left*) show a large defect involving the apex, anterior, septal, and inferior walls (*arrowheads*) with little change from the rest images (*right*), signifying a fixed defect consistent with infarction. There is also severe left ventricular enlargement and severely reduced left ventricular systolic function by gated images (*next image*). The relative advantage of ^{201}Tl and ^{99m}Tc are detailed in Table e20-1 of *Harrison's Principles of Internal Medicine*, 17th edition. The better image quality and assessment of ventricular function permitted by ^{99m}Tc compounds have contributed to their more common use for stress imaging, although both ^{201}Tl- and ^{99m}Tc-labeled compounds provide clinically useful myocardial perfusion images in the majority of patients. A "dual-isotope" protocol is employed in some centers. This uses ^{201}Tl for the initial rest image and a ^{99m}Tc-labeled compound for the subsequent stress image, primarily for patient and scheduling convenience. SPECT, single-photon emission computed tomography; ^{99m}Tc, technetium 99m.

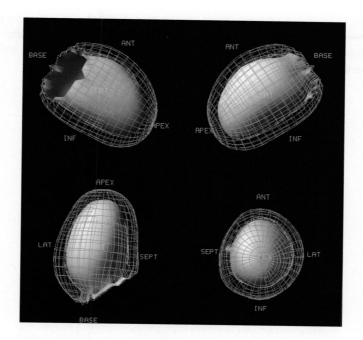

FIGURE 42-3

Mesh cinegraphic display of images obtained from electrocardiographic gating of a SPECT ^{99m}Tc sestamibi scan in a 64-year-old male patient with a previous infarct (same patient as in Fig. 42-2). Gated images are generally acquired about 30–45 min following stress. Electrocardiographic gating allows calculation of left ventricular volumes and global systolic function, as well as visual assessment of regional wall motion. In this patient, the calculated left ventricular ejection fraction was 13%. There was severe global hypokinesis.

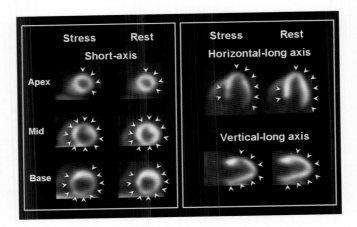

FIGURE 42-4

Adenosine PET N-13 ammonia in a 55-year-old obese male patient with typical angina. The stress images *(left)* show a large defect involving the apex, anterior, septal, inferior, and lateral walls *(arrowheads)* with normal or near-normal tracer uptake in the corresponding regions on the rest images *(arrowheads)*, signifying a reversible defect consistent with ischemia. The patient was found to have severe multivessel coronary artery disease on subsequent invasive angiography.

The robust methods for attenuation correction with PET improve the specificity, particularly in obese populations and women, while the superior resolution and higher extraction fraction of PET tracers increase the sensitivity of detection of coronary artery disease. The excellent image quality of PET has contributed to their emerging use for stress imaging. Additional advantages include assessment of left ventricular volumes and systolic function, shorter imaging protocols, and lower radiation exposure, particularly with N-13 ammonia.

PET, positron emission tomography; SPECT, single-photon emission computed tomography.

MRI/CT IMAGES

Video 42-17   MRI scan in real time of a patient with a large left ventricular apical aneurysm. The long-axis view demonstrates a thin dyskinetic apical aneurysm with a preserved systolic function of the basal anterior and basal inferior wall. MRI scanning allows excellent visualization of the endocardial border.

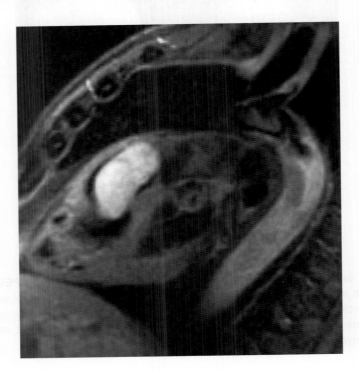

FIGURE 42-5

MR image of a patient with a right ventricular myxoma, which is shown as a bright oblong structure in the right ventricular out-flow tract.

Video 42-18 Cine MRI scan of a patient with a dilated ascending aorta (annulo-aortic ectasia). There is a central jet of aortic regurgitation entering the left ventricular outflow tract.

521

CHAPTER 42 Atlas of Noninvasive Cardiac Imaging

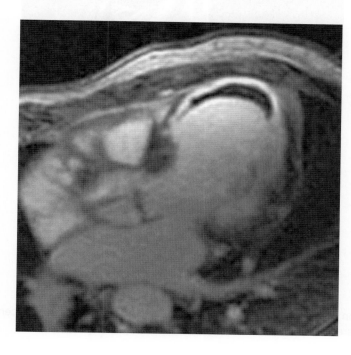

FIGURE 42-6

MR image with contrast enhancement of a patient with a large apical aneurysm and thrombus. Imaging the heart 10–20 min after gadolinium injection demonstrates enhancement of the infarcted tissue (visible as dense white image). The infarcted tissue retains contrast by virtual of its large extracellular volume. The left ventricular thrombus adherent to the infarcted myocardium is shown as a dark laminated area adjacent to the white myocardium.

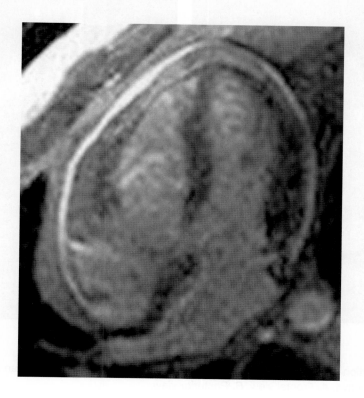

FIGURE 42-7

MR images with contrast enhancement in a patient with acute pericarditis. In the presence of pericardial inflammation, the gadolinium enhancement occurs, seen as a white layer in the pericardium.

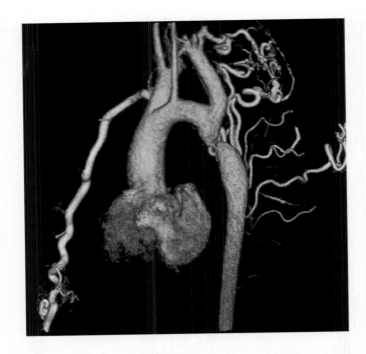

FIGURE 42-8

Three-dimensional reconstruction of a CT angiogram, showing a severe coarctation of the descending aorta. The large collateral vessels are the result of the severe stenosis of the distal thoracic aorta.

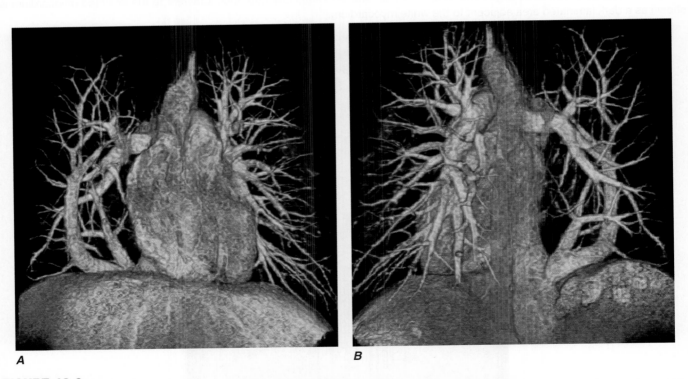

A   *B*

FIGURE 42-9

Three-dimensional reconstruction of a CT angiogram of the pulmonary veins, demonstrating an anomalous pulmonary venous drainage into the inferior vena cava. *A.* Frontal view. *B.* Posterior view.

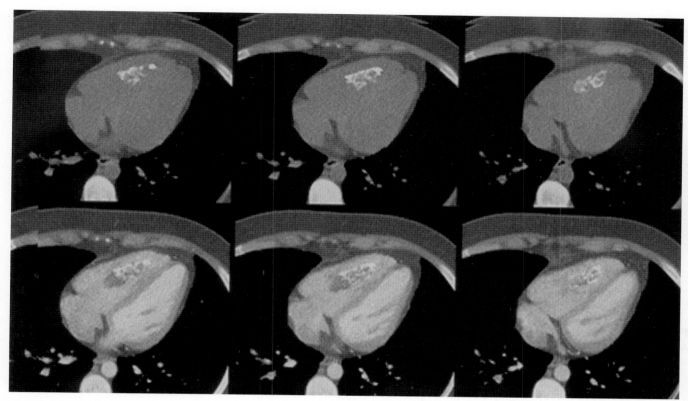

FIGURE 42-10
Cardiac CT images demonstrating a calcified mass in the right ventricle, which at pathologic examination was a chronic thrombus. Calcification is seen as a bright signal in both the noncontrast (*upper*) and contrast-enhanced (*lower*) images.

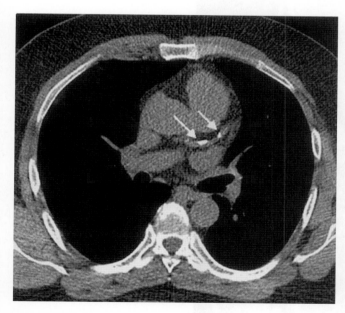

FIGURE 42-11
Noncontrast image from an electron beam CT revealing two small foci of calcification in the left anterior descending artery (*arrows*).

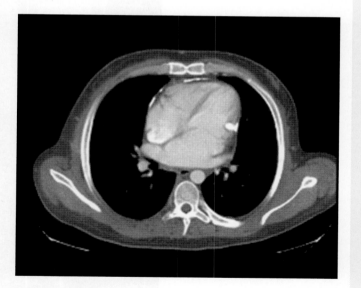

FIGURE 42-12
CT image from a patient with calcific constrictive pericarditis. Calcification is seen as a bright signal in the anterior pericardium as well as calcification extending into the lateral wall of the left ventricle.

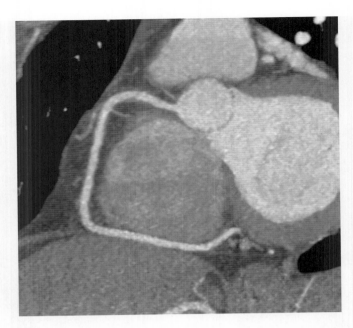

FIGURE 42-13

A reconstructed CT coronary angiogram showing a normal right coronary artery.

Video 42-19 CT coronary angiogram showing a normal right coronary artery. The video highlights multiple thin slices through the right coronary artery.

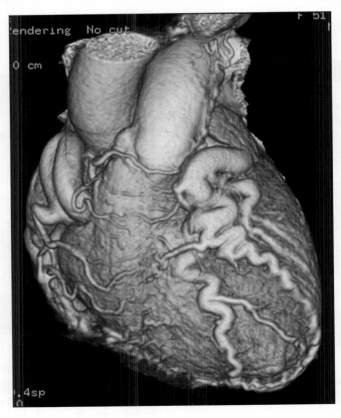

FIGURE 42-14

Three-dimensional reconstruction of a CT angiogram showing a large fistula of the left anterior descending artery.

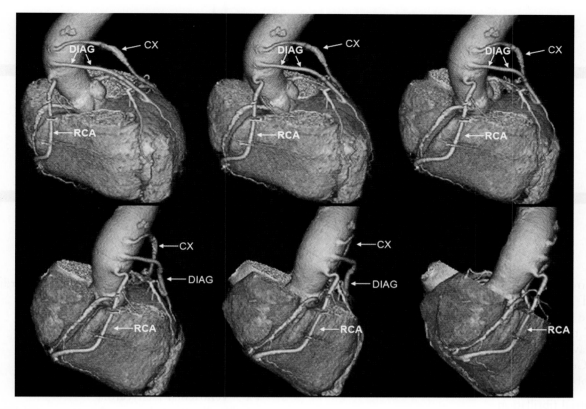

FIGURE 42-15

Three-dimensional reconstruction of a CT angiogram demonstrating three saphenous vein coronary artery bypass grafts in different views. In the upper left-hand panel is an anterior posterior view of the heart and grafts. The heart is sequentially rotated clockwise in the panels going from left to right to illustrate the ability of CT angiography to visualize the saphenous vein grafts. RCA, saphenous vein graft to the right coronary artery; CX, saphenous vein graft to the circumflex artery; DIAG, saphenous vein graft to the diagonal artery.

CHAPTER 43

ATLAS OF CARDIAC ARRHYTHMIAS

Ary L. Goldberger

The electrocardiograms in this Atlas supplement those illustrated in Chaps. 15 and 16. The interpretations emphasize findings of specific teaching value.

All of the figures are adapted from cases in ECG Wave-Maven, Copyright 2003, Beth Israel Deaconess Medical Center, *http://ecg.bidmc.harvard.edu.*

The abbreviations used in this chapter are as follows:

AF—atrial fibrillation
AV—atrioventricular

AVRT—atrioventricular reentrant tachycardia
LBBB—left bundle branch block
LV—left ventricular
LVH—left ventricular hypertrophy
MI—myocardial infarction
NSR—normal sinus rhythm
RBBB—right bundle branch block
VT—ventricular tachycardia
WPW—Wolff-Parkinson-White

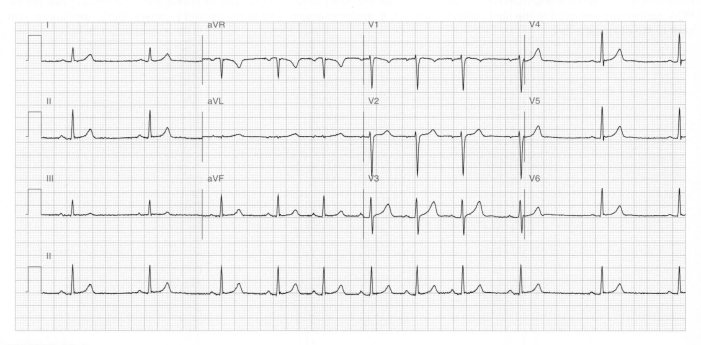

FIGURE 43-1

Respiratory sinus arrhythmia, a physiologic finding in a healthy young adult. The rate of the sinus pacemaker is relatively slow at the beginning of the strip during expiration, then accelerates during inspiration and slows again with expiration. Changes are due to cardiac vagal tone modulation with breathing.

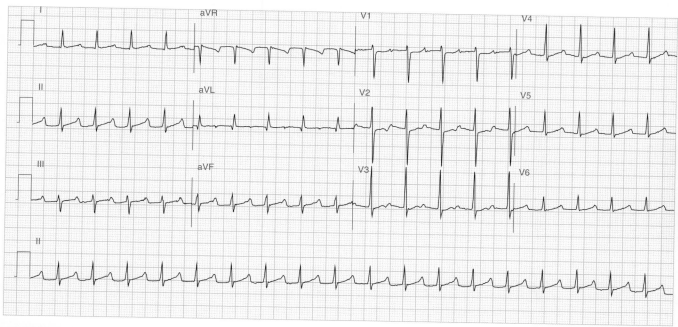

FIGURE 43-2

Sinus tachycardia (110/min) with first-degree AV "block" (conduction delay) with PR interval = 0.28 s. The P wave is visible after the ST-T wave in V_1–V_3 and superimposed on the T wave in other leads. Atrial (nonsinus) tachycardias may produce a similar pattern, but the rate is usually faster.

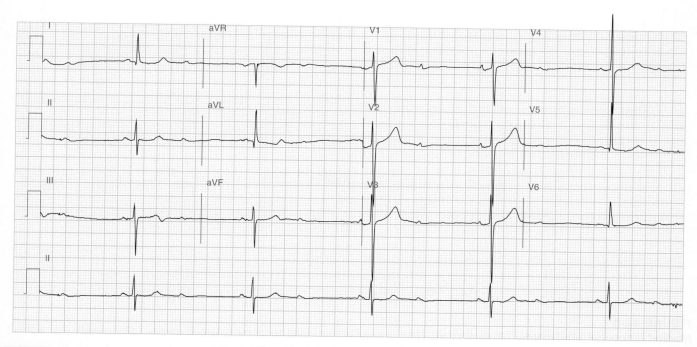

FIGURE 43-3

Sinus rhythm (P wave rate about 60/min) with **2:1 AV (second-degree) block** causing **marked bradycardia** (ventricular rate of about 30/min). **LVH** is also present.

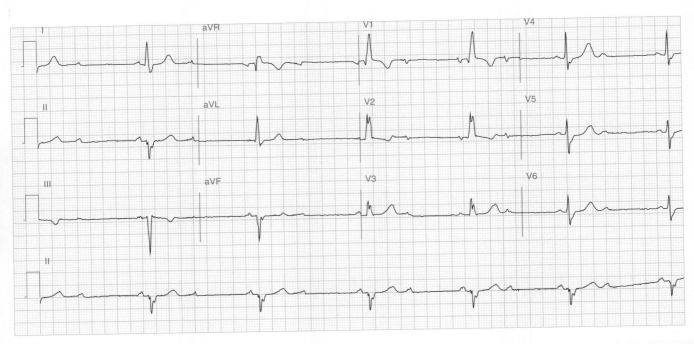

FIGURE 43-4

Sinus rhythm (P wave rate about 60/min) **with 2:1 (second-degree) AV block** yielding a ventricular (pulse) rate of about 30/min.
Left atrial abnormality. RBBB with **left anterior fascicular block.** Possible **inferior MI.**

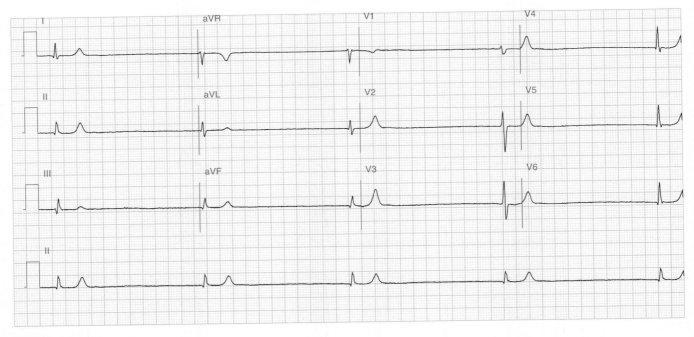

FIGURE 43-5

Marked junctional bradycardia (25 beats/min). Rate is regular with a flat baseline between narrow QRS complexes, without
evident P waves. Patient was on atenolol, with **possible underlying sick sinus syndrome.**

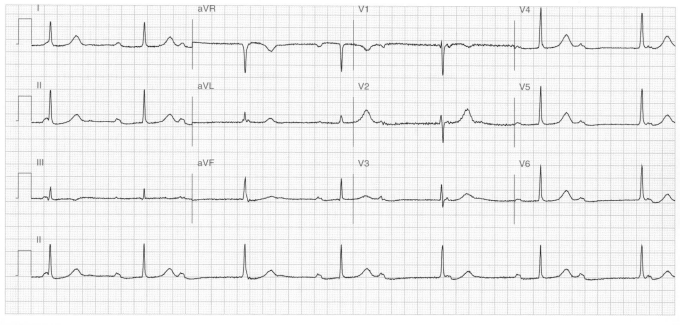

FIGURE 43-6

Sinus rhythm at a rate of 64/min (P wave rate) with **third-degree (complete) AV block** yielding an effective heart (pulse) rate of 40/min. The slow, narrow QRS complexes indicate an A-V junctional escape pacemaker. **Left atrial abnormality.**

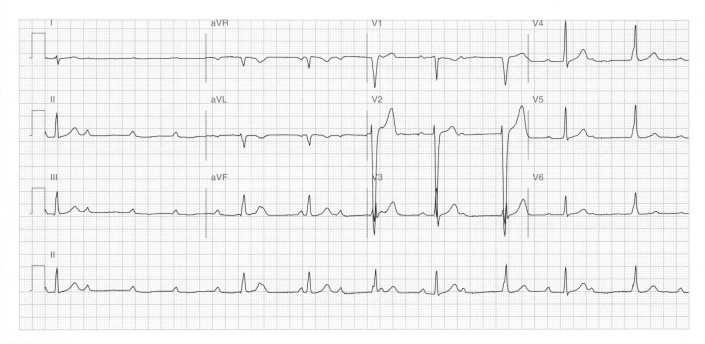

FIGURE 43-7

Sinus rhythm at a rate of 90/min with **advanced second-degree AV** block and **possible transient complete heart block** with **Lyme carditis.**

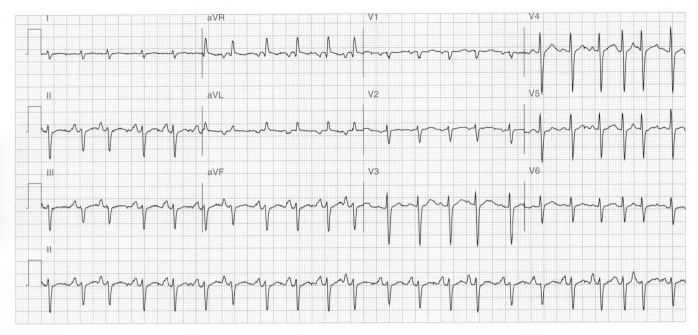

FIGURE 43-8

Multifocal atrial tachycardia with varying P-wave morphologies and P-P intervals; right atrial overload with peaked P waves in II, III, and aVF (with vertical P wave axis); superior QRS axis; slow R-wave progression with delayed transition in precordial leads in patient with **severe chronic obstructive lung disease.**

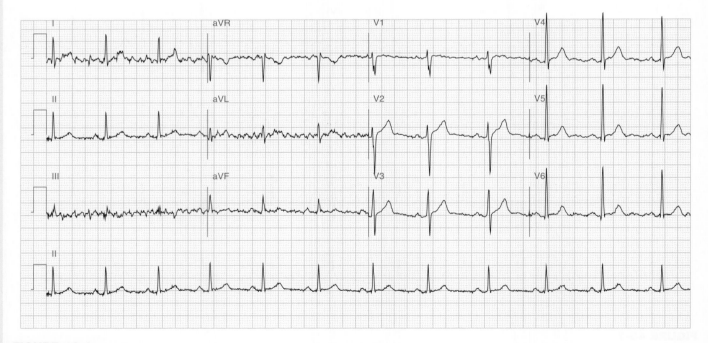

FIGURE 43-9

NSR in a patient with **Parkinson's disease.** Tremor artifact, best seen in limb leads. This **tremor artifact** may sometimes be confused with atrial flutter/fibrillation. Borderline voltage criteria for LVH are present.

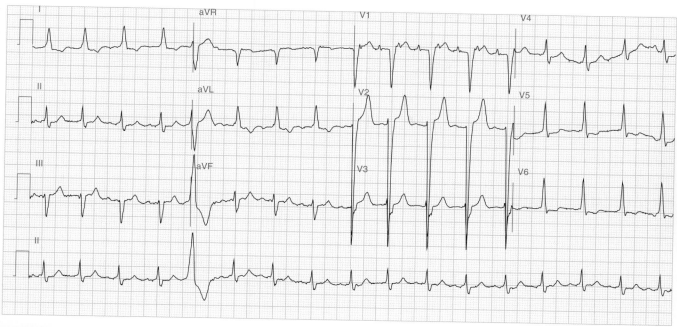

FIGURE 43-10

Atrial tachycardia with atrial rate of about 200/min (note lead V₁), **2:1 AV block (conduction),** and one premature ventricular complex. Also present: LVH with intraventricular conduction delay and slow precordial R-wave progression (cannot rule out prior anterior MI).

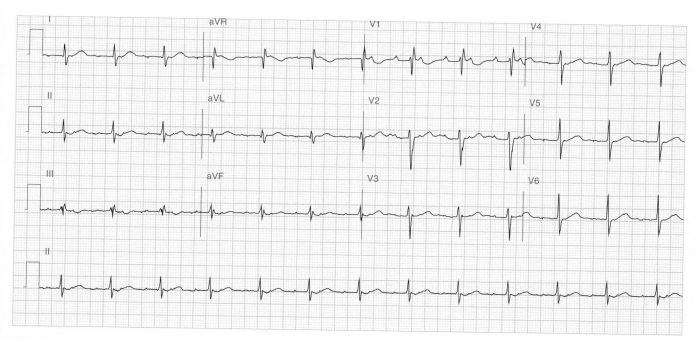

FIGURE 43-11

Atrial tachycardia with 2:1 block. P-wave rate is about 150/min, with ventricular (QRS) rate of about 75/min. The nonconducted ("extra") P waves just after the QRS complex are best seen in lead V₁. Also, note incomplete RBBB and borderline QT prolongation.

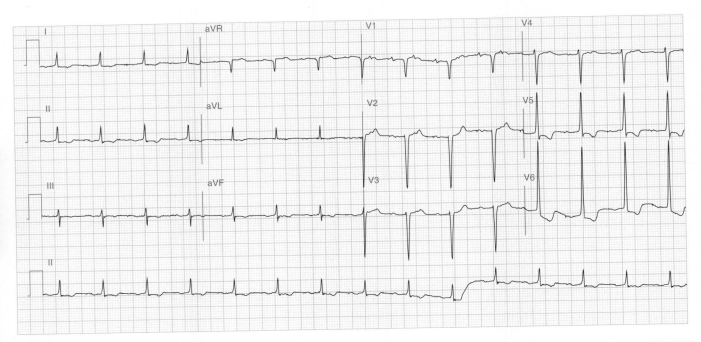

FIGURE 43-12
Atrial tachycardia (180/min with 2:1 AV block [see lead V₁]). **LVH** by precordial voltage and nonspecific ST-T changes. Slow R-wave progression (V₁–V₄) raises consideration of prior anterior MI.

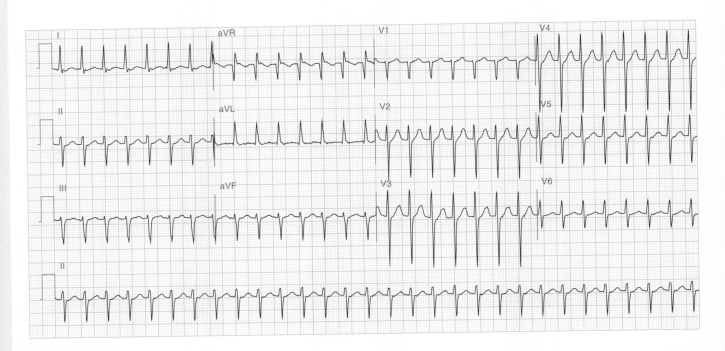

FIGURE 43-13
AV nodal reentrant tachycardia (AVNRT) at a rate of 150/min. Note subtle "pseudo" R waves in lead aVR due to retrograde atrial activation, which occurs nearly simultaneous with ventricles in AVNRT. Left-axis deviation consistent with left anterior fascicular block (hemiblock) is also present.

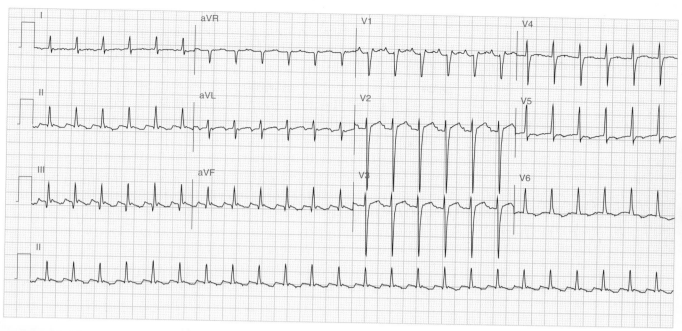

FIGURE 43-14

Atrial flutter with 2:1 AV conduction. Note atrial flutter waves, partly hidden in the early ST segment, seen, for example, in leads II and V$_1$.

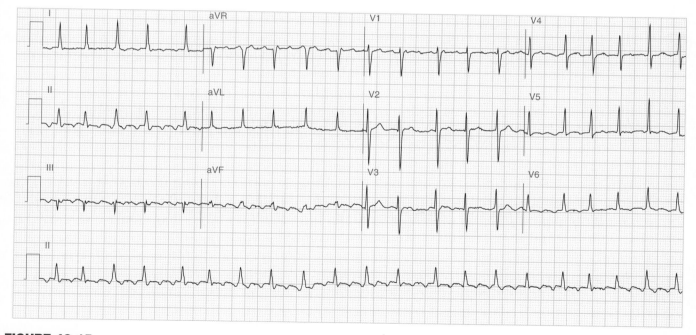

FIGURE 43-15

Atrial flutter with atrial rate 300/min and variable (predominant 2:1 and 3:1) AV conduction. Typical flutter waves best seen in lead II.

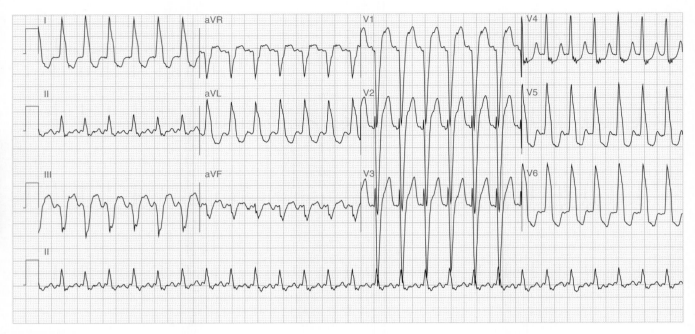

FIGURE 43-16

Wide complex tachycardia. Atrial flutter with 2:1 AV conduction (block) and **LBBB**, not to be mistaken for VT. Typical atrial flutter activity is clearly present in lead II at a cycle rate of about 320/min, with an effective ventricular rate of about 160/min.

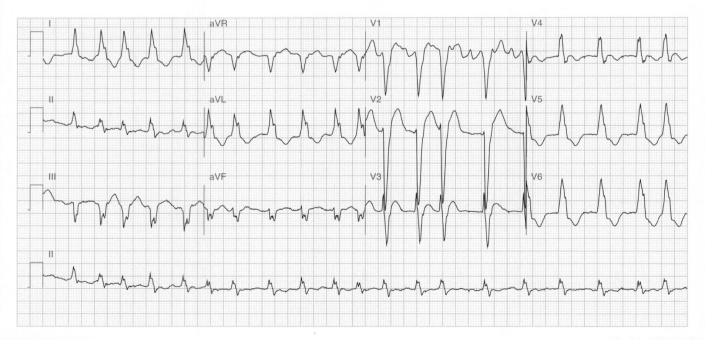

FIGURE 43-17

AF with LBBB. The ventricular rhythm is erratically irregular. Coarse fibrillatory waves are best seen in lead V_1, with a typical LBBB pattern.

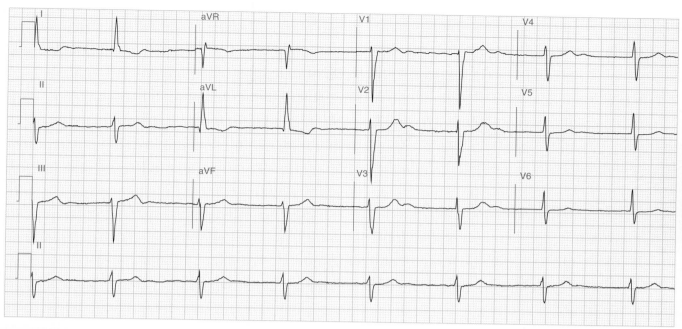

FIGURE 43-18

AF with complete heart block and a junctional escape mechanism causing a slow regular ventricular response (45/min). The QRS complexes show an intraventricular conduction delay with left-axis deviation and LVH. Q-T (U) prolongation is also present.

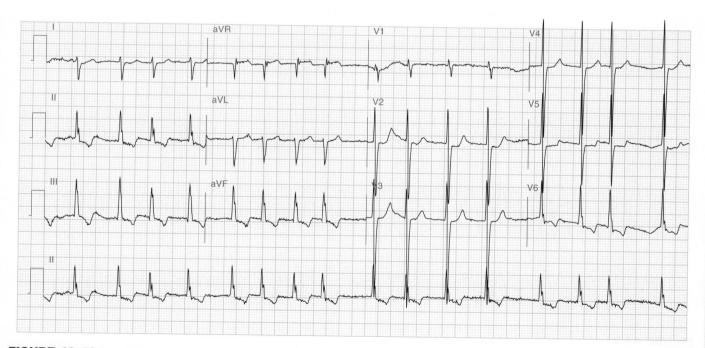

FIGURE 43-19

AF with right-axis deviation and LVH. Tracing suggests biventricular hypertrophy in a patient with **mitral stenosis and aortic valve disease.**

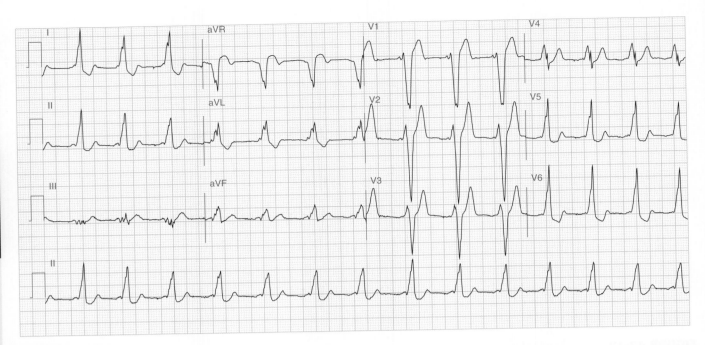

FIGURE 43-20

WPW pre-excitation pattern, with triad of short PR, wide QRS, and delta waves. Polarity of the delta waves (slightly positive in leads V_1 and V_2 and most positive in lead II and lateral chest leads) is consistent with a right-sided bypass tract.

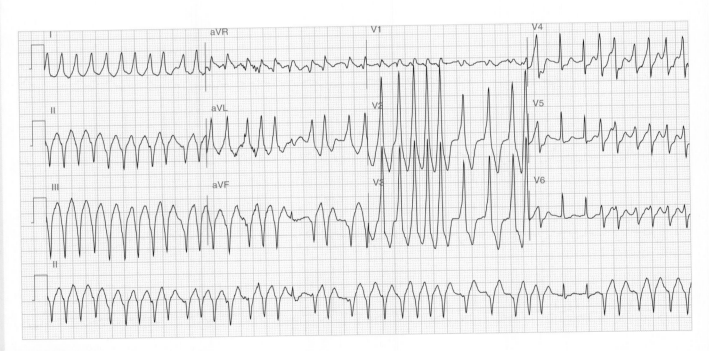

FIGURE 43-21

AF in patient with the WPW syndrome and antegrade conduction down the bypass tract leading to a wide complex tachycardia. Rhythm is "irregularly irregular" and rate is extremely rapid (about 230/min). Not all beats are pre-excited.

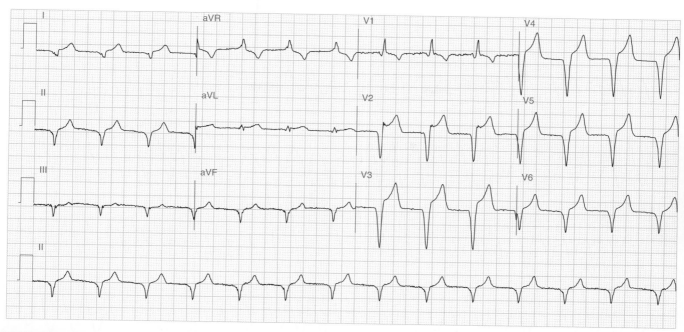

FIGURE 43-22
Accelerated idioventricular rhythm (AIVR) originating from the LV and accounting for RBBB morphology. ST elevations in the precordial leads from **underlying acute MI.**

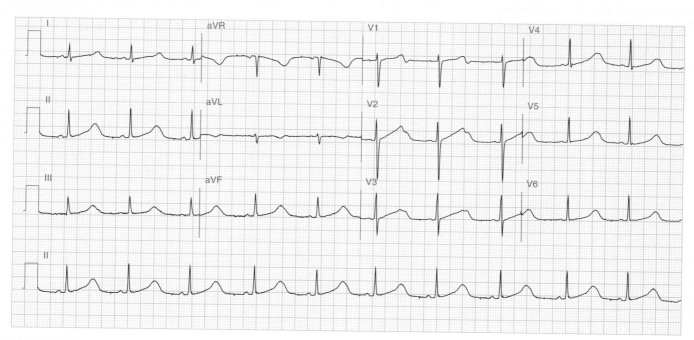

FIGURE 43-23
Prolonged (0.60 s) QT interval in a patient with **hereditary long-QT syndrome.**

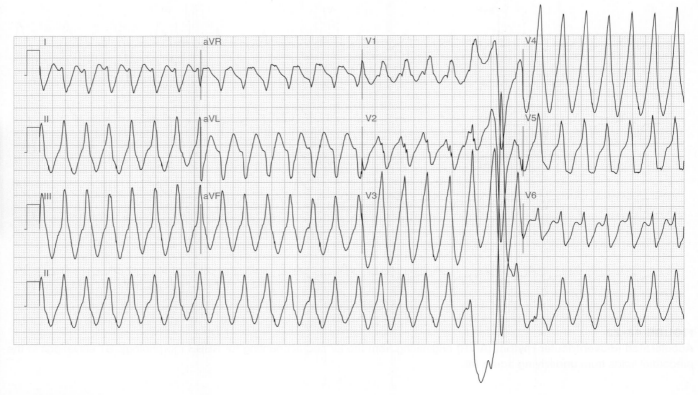

FIGURE 43-24

Monomorphic VT at rate of 170/min. The RBBB morphology in V_1 and the R:S ratio <1 in V_6 are both suggestive of VT. The morphology of the VT is suggestive of origin from the left side of the heart, near the base (RBBB with inferior/rightward axis). Baseline artifact is present in leads V_1–V_3.

CHAPTER 44

ATLAS OF PERCUTANEOUS REVASCULARIZATION

Jane A. Leopold ■ Deepak L. Bhatt ■ David P. Faxon

Percutaneous coronary intervention (PCI) is the most widely employed coronary revascularization procedure worldwide (Chap. 36). It is now applied to patients with stable angina, acute coronary syndromes, including unstable angina and non–ST-segment elevation myocardial infarction (NSTEMI), and as a primary treatment strategy in patients with ST-segment elevation myocardial infarction (STEMI). PCI is also applicable to patients with either single- or multivessel disease.

In this chapter, the use of PCI will be illustrated in a variety of commonly encountered clinical and anatomic situations such as chronic total occlusion of a coronary artery, bifurcation disease, acute STEMI, saphenous vein graft disease, left main coronary artery disease, multivessel disease, and stent thrombosis. In addition, the use of interventional techniques to treat structural heart disease will be shown, including closure of an atrial septal defect (ASD) and percutaneous aortic valve implantation; the latter is approved in Europe but is under active investigation in clinical trials in the United States and not yet approved for use.

CASE 1: CHRONIC TOTAL OCCLUSION

(Videos 44–1 to 44–7 can be accessed at the following link: http://www.mhprofessional.com/mediacenter/)

- An 81-year-old man with angina, NYHA class IV congestive heart failure and inferior-apical-posterior ischemia on an exercise technetium-99m scan.
- Diagnostic cardiac catheterization revealed a left dominant system with a totally occluded left circumflex (LCx) artery. The distal LCx filled via collaterals from the left anterior descending (LAD) artery, indicating chronicity of the total occlusion.

Video 44-1 Baseline left coronary angiogram shows an occluded LCx with left-to-left collaterals originating from LAD septal vessels.

Video 44-2 Attempts to cross the total occlusion in the LCx using a hydrophilic wire and an antegrade approach were not successful, with the wire tracking to the right of the trajectory.

Video 44-3 The LAD septal collateral is accessed with a guidewire and directed toward the distal LCx to cross the total occlusion retrograde.

Video 44-4 The total occlusion is crossed retrograde. The wire is snared in the guide, exteriorized, and used to provide antegrade access to the LCx.

Video 44-5 Antegrade flow in the LCx is restored after balloon inflation.

Video 44-6 Following stenting of the total occlusion, blood flow in the distal vessel is improved and a second significant stenosis is seen.

Video 44-7 Final result after LCx stenting.

SUMMARY

- Approximately 15–30% of all patients referred for cardiac catheterization will have a chronic total occlusion (CTO) of a coronary artery.
- CTO often leads to a surgical referral for complete revascularization.
- Incomplete revascularization due to an untreated CTO is associated with an increased mortality rate (Hazard Ratio = 1.36, 95% CI = 1.12–1.66, $p <$ 0.05).
- Successful PCI of a CTO leads to a 3.8–8.4% absolute reduction in mortality, symptom relief, and improved left ventricular function.

- Newer techniques, such as the retrograde approach to crossing total occlusions, are useful when the antegrade approach fails, or is not feasible, and there are well-developed collateral vessels.

(Case contributed with permission by Dr. Frederick G. P. Welt.)

CASE 2: BIFURCATION STENTING

(Fig. 44-1; Videos 44-8 to 44-16 can be accessed at the following link: http://www.mhprofessional.com/mediacenter/)

- A 52-year-old man with an acute coronary syndrome and a troponin I = 0.18 (upper limit normal ≥0.04).
- Diagnostic cardiac catheterization showed single-vessel coronary artery disease with a significant stenosis in the mid-LAD and a bifurcation lesion involving a large diagonal branch.

Video 44-8   Baseline angiogram of the left coronary circulation shows the significant stenosis in the mid-LAD and the bifurcation lesion involving a large diagonal branch.

Video 44-9   Both vessels are accessed with guidewires and pretreated with balloon angioplasty.

Video 44-10   Result after balloon angioplasty.

Video 44-11   Stent being positioned in the LAD.

Video 44-12   LAD post-stent result.

Video 44-13   Stent deployed in diagonal branch through the stent struts in the LAD using the "culotte" technique.

Video 44-14   Diagonal branch post-stent result.

Video 44-15   Simultaneous inflation of two 2.5-mm "kissing" balloons.

Video 44-16   Final postbifurcation stenting result.

SUMMARY

- Approximately 15–20% of PCIs will involve the treatment of bifurcation lesions.
- Bifurcation lesions require consideration of PCI strategies that protect side-branch patency.
- There are both one-stent and two-stent techniques to treat bifurcation lesions; the selection of technique depends upon anatomic considerations, including plaque burden, angle of side-branch take-off, plaque shift during angioplasty, and side-branch distribution.
- Rates of target lesion revascularization and stent thrombosis are similar between one-stent and two-stent procedures.

CASE 3: INFERIOR MYOCARDIAL INFARCTION—THROMBUS AND MANUAL THROMBECTOMY

(Figs. 44-2 to 44-4; Videos 44-17 to 44-22 can be accessed at the following link: http://www.mhprofessional.com/mediacenter/)

- A 59-year-old man presented to the emergency room with 2 h of severe midsternal chest pressure.

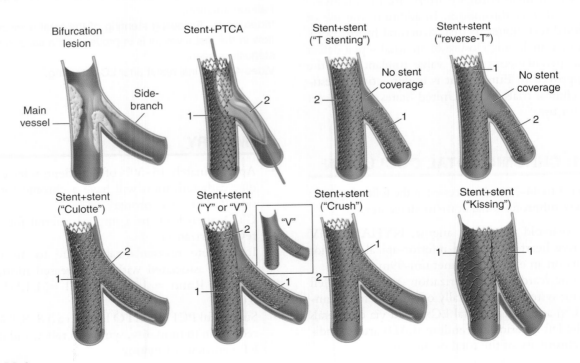

FIGURE 44-1

Schematic representation of 1-stent and 2-stent techniques to treat bifurcation lesions. PTCA, Percutaneous transluminal coronary angioplasty. (*Reprinted with permission from SK Sharma, A Kini: Cardiol Clin 24:233, 2006.*)

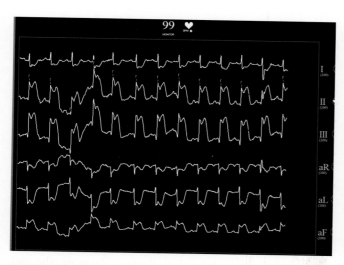

FIGURE 44-2

Preprocedure ECG showing inferior ST-segment elevations and lateral ST-segment depressions.

- His systolic blood pressure was 100 mmHg and he was tachycardic in sinus rhythm with a heart rate of 90–100 bpm.
- His initial ECG showed inferior ST-segment elevations with lateral ST-segment depressions.
- He was referred emergently to the cardiac catheterization laboratory for primary PCI.

Video 44-17   The right coronary artery (RCA) is totally occluded with filling defects in the vessel after contrast injection, indicating thrombus is present in the vessel.

Video 44-18   An angioplasty wire is threaded through the thrombotic lesion, but this does not restore blood flow to the distal vessel.

Video 44-19   Result after manual thrombectomy and thrombus extraction. The "culprit" ruptured plaque and residual thrombus are now apparent in the vessel.

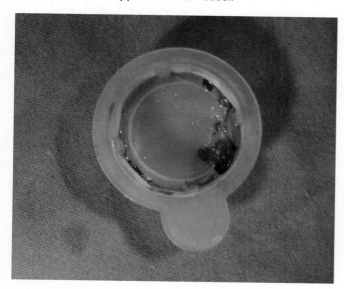

FIGURE 44-3

Example of an organized red thrombus retrieved by manual thrombectomy. (*Reprinted with permission from C Trani et al: J Invasive Cardiol 19:E317, 2007.*)

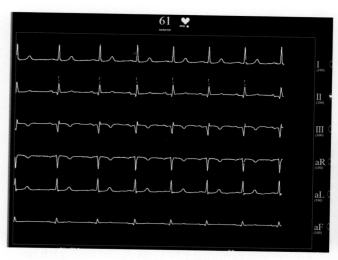

FIGURE 44-4

Postprocedure ECG showing resolution of ST-segment elevations.

Video 44-20   After balloon angioplasty and stenting, thrombus is still present.

Video 44-21   After repeat manual thrombectomy and expansion of the stent, the thrombus is no longer present.

Video 44-22   Final result.

SUMMARY

- An acute STEMI occurs following plaque rupture that promotes thrombotic occlusion of a coronary artery.
- Despite successful revascularization of the epicardial coronary artery, microemboli liberated during balloon angioplasty and stenting may lead to persistent microvascular dysfunction. When present, microvascular dysfunction is associated with a larger infarct size, heart failure, malignant ventricular arrhythmias, and death.
- Manual thrombectomy is used to aspirate or remove thrombus in the vessel and limit distal embolization during angioplasty and stenting.
- Manual thrombectomy in primary PCI is associated with improved myocardial perfusion and a reduction in mortality.
- Adjunctive antiplatelet and antithrombin agents are important to aid in the resolution of intracoronary thrombus.

CASE 4: SAPHENOUS VEIN GRAFT INTERVENTION WITH DISTAL PROTECTION

(Fig. 44-5; Videos 44-23 to 44-26 can be accessed at the following link: http://www.mhprofessional.com/mediacenter/)

- A 62-year-old man with a history of chronic stable angina.

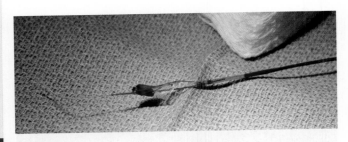

FIGURE 44-5

Distal protection device showing captured atherosclerotic debris liberated by initial balloon dilation. (*Reprinted with permission from RA Aqel et al: J Invasive Cardiol 19:E104, 2007.*)

- A four-vessel coronary artery bypass grafting (CABG) surgery was performed 17 years earlier with a left internal mammary artery graft to the LAD, a right internal mammary artery graft to the RCA, a saphenous vein graft to the first obtuse marginal branch, and a saphenous vein graft to the first diagonal branch.

- The patient had a recent increase in angina with exertion and was found to have lateral ischemia on an exercise technetium-99m scan.

- Diagnostic cardiac catheterization revealed a significant stenosis in the body of the saphenous vein graft to the first obtuse marginal branch.

Video 44-23 Saphenous vein graft to a first obtuse marginal branch with an 80% eccentric stenosis in the midgraft.

Video 44-24   A distal protection device is deployed past the lesion.

Video 44-25 Angioplasty balloon inflation with the distal protection device in place.

Video 44-26   Final result after stent placement.

SUMMARY

- Saphenous vein grafts have a failure rate of up to 20% after 1 year and as high as 50% by 5 years.

- Graft failure (>1 month) results from intimal hyperplasia and atherosclerosis.

- Saphenous vein graft PCI is associated with distal embolization of atherosclerotic debris and microthrombi, leading to microvascular occlusion, reduced antegrade blood flow (the "no-reflow" phenomenon), and myocardial infarction.

- Embolic distal protection devices decrease the risk of distal embolization, as well as the incidence of no-reflow and myocardial infarction associated with saphenous vein graft interventions.

CASE 5: UNPROTECTED LEFT MAIN PCI IN A HIGH-RISK PATIENT

(Figs. 44-6 and 44-7; Videos 44-27 to 44-34 can be accessed at the following link: http://www.mhprofessional.com/mediacenter/)

- An 89-year-old woman presented with an NSTEMI associated with 5-mm ST-segment depression in the apical leads occurring 2 weeks after hospitalization for an NSTEMI that was treated conservatively.

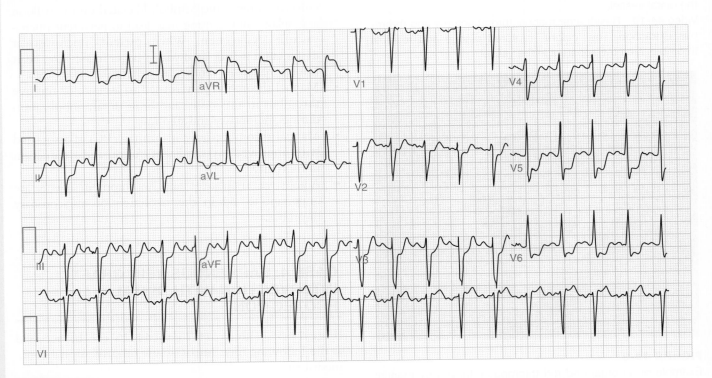

FIGURE 44-6

During chest pain, the ECG showed diffuse ST-segment depression of up to 5 mm in the inferior and lateral leads.

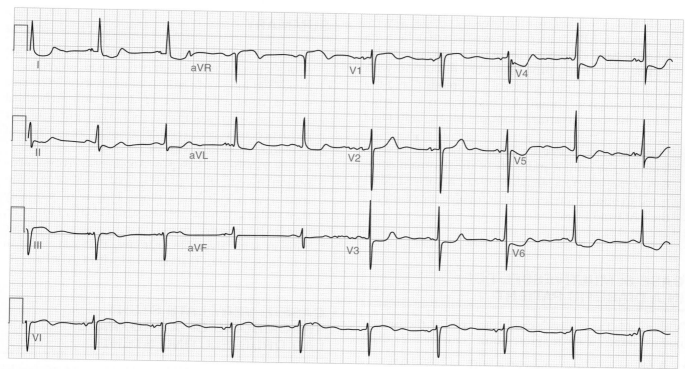

FIGURE 44-7
Following resolution of the chest pain, the ST-segment depression is less marked.

- Chronic obstructive lung disease, elderly age, and the patient's refusal to consider cardiac surgery restricted the choice of therapeutic options to medical and/or percutaneous interventions.
- Diagnostic catheterization revealed a left dominant circulation with a heavily calcified 80% distal left main coronary artery stenosis extending into the LAD and into the proximal LCx coronary arteries. A 70% proximal LAD lesion was also present.
- After consultation with the patient, family, and a cardiac surgeon, PCI was performed with intraaortic balloon pump support and a temporary pacemaker in the right ventricle.

Video 44-27 Baseline left coronary artery injection in right anterior oblique (RAO) cranial projection shows a high-grade calcified stenosis in the left main coronary artery and a significant stenosis in the proximal LAD.

Video 44-28 In the left anterior oblique (LAO) caudal view, the left main coronary artery lesion can be seen to extend into the ostia of both the LCx and the LAD.

Video 44-29 Guidewires were placed into both the LCx and LAD. After the left main coronary artery and LCx are dilated with balloon angioplasty, the proximal LAD is dilated and a long drug-eluting stent is placed to cover a lesion dissection that occurred with wiring of the vessel.

Video 44-30 The bifurcation lesion in the left main coronary artery extending into the LCx and LAD ostia is treated using a "culotte" technique. First, a drug-eluting stent is placed in the left main coronary artery and into the proximal LCx.

Video 44-31 Next, the LAD wire is removed and passed through the stent into the distal LAD. A second drug-eluting stent is deployed through the struts of the left main coronary artery/LCx stent.

Video 44-32 Following rewiring of the LCx, both stents are redilated simultaneously ("kissing" balloons).

Video 44-33 The final result in the LAO caudal view.

Video 44-34 The final result in the RAO cranial view showing patent left main, LCx, and LAD coronary arteries.

SUMMARY

- Left main coronary artery disease occurs in 5–10% of patients with symptomatic coronary artery disease.
- In patients with left main coronary artery disease, revascularization with CABG has been shown to decrease mortality significantly over 5–10 years of follow-up.
- PCI with drug-eluting stents in selected cases has been shown to have equal in-hospital and 1-year death and myocardial infarction rates as compared to CABG in the Synergy between PCI with Taxus and Cardiac Surgery (SYNTAX) trial. Long-term outcome differences between the two treatment strategies are not known.
- Indications for PCI of left main coronary artery lesions are high-risk surgical patients and patients

with protected left main coronary artery disease (i.e., prior CABG with patent bypass grafts). Patients who are good candidates for bypass surgery may also undergo a stenting procedure, but discussion with the patient, the interventional cardiologist, and the cardiac surgeon should be undertaken to determine the best treatment option in an individual case.

- Outcomes are better for patients with an isolated lesion in the ostium and body of the left main coronary artery where a single stent can be placed compared to bifurcation lesions that involve the ostium of the LAD and LCx.

CASE 6: MULTIVESSEL PCI IN A DIABETIC PATIENT

(Videos 44-35 to 44-42 can be accessed at the following link: http://www.mhprofessional.com/mediacenter/)

- A 58-year-old man presented with an NSTEMI.
- The patient has hyperlipidemia and type 2 diabetes mellitus treated with oral hypoglycemic agents.
- Diagnostic catheterization revealed two-vessel disease with a total occlusion of the second obtuse marginal branch that was felt to be responsible for the patient's symptoms (culprit lesion). In addition, there was a high-grade stenosis in a large ramus intermedius branch and the RCA had a significant stenosis in the midsegment of the vessel.

Video 44-35 Baseline angiogram of the left coronary circulation in the RAO view shows the total occlusion of the second obtuse marginal branch with delayed retrograde filling via collateral vessels and a high-grade stenosis in the ramus intermedius.

Video 44-36 A guidewire is passed through the total occlusion and the lesion is pretreated with balloon angioplasty.

Video 44-37 Following placement of a drug-eluting stent in the lesion, the vessel is widely patent. A third obtuse marginal vessel, not previously seen, now fills faintly (TIMI 1 flow) with contrast but was not treated.

Video 44-38 The ramus intermedius lesion was crossed with a guidewire and pretreated with balloon angioplasty.

Video 44-39 A drug-eluting stent is placed across the ramus lesion and deployed. The final result shows no residual stenosis in either the ramus or second obtuse marginal vessels.

Video 44-40 Baseline angiogram of the RCA shows a high-grade lesion in the midsegment of the vessel.

Video 44-41 The lesion was pretreated with balloon dilation followed by stent deployment.

Video 44-42 The final result shows no residual stenosis in the mid-RCA.

SUMMARY

- Multivessel PCI is performed commonly and may be done in one setting or staged with two or more procedures.
- Acute and long-term studies of multivessel PCI have shown comparable rates of death and myocardial infarction when compared to CABG but a higher incidence of repeat revascularization as a result of restenosis associated with PCI.
- In the randomized Bypass Angioplasty Revascularization Investigation (BARI) trial, diabetic patients treated with PCI had a worse long-term mortality than diabetic patients treated with CABG. However, the BARI registry found that in selected diabetic patients with favorable anatomy, PCI can result in outcomes equal to that observed with CABG.

CASE 7: VERY LATE STENT THROMBOSIS OF A PROXIMAL LAD DRUG-ELUTING STENT

(Figs. 44-8 and 44-9; Videos 44-43 to 44-46 can be accessed at the following link: http://www.mhprofessional.com/mediacenter/)

- A 62-year-old man had a drug-eluting stent placed in a proximal LAD lesion to treat severe angina. He received dual antiplatelet therapy with aspirin and

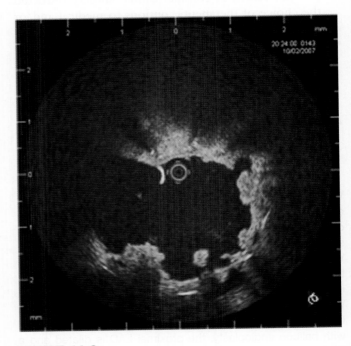

FIGURE 44-8
Optical coherence tomography image following initial balloon dilation. Residual thrombus that is adherent to the stent struts is seen. (*Reprinted with permission from AF Schinkel et al: JACC Cardiovasc Interv 1:449, 2008.*)

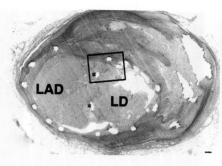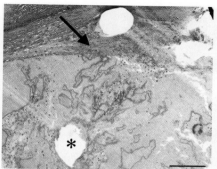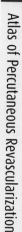

FIGURE 44-9

Pathologic specimen of late stent thrombosis obtained at autopsy. Thrombus is seen filling the LAD vessel lumen and extending into a diagonal branch (LD). Stent struts occupied the space denoted by asterisk (*) (*left*). A magnified view of the vessel reveals thrombus around the stent strut and neointima formation (*arrow*) (*right*). (*Reprinted with permission from A Farb et al: Circulation 108:1701, 2003.*)

clopidogrel for 1 year and then discontinued clopidogrel per protocol.

- He remained asymptomatic until 15 months after the initial stent placement, when he presented with severe chest pain due to an acute anterior STEMI.
- He was taken to the catheterization laboratory within 70 min of presentation and his initial angiogram showed a total occlusion of the proximal LAD stent.

Video 44-43 Baseline angiogram showing a total occlusion of the proximal LAD within the drug-eluting stent and a significant stenosis at the origin of the LCx.

Video 44-44 The LAO view shows the LCx stenosis with a filling defect, indicating that thrombus is present in the vessel lumen.

Video 44-45 The LAD lesion was crossed with a guidewire, which resulted in slow filling of the mid-LAD (TIMI 2 flow), and revealed thrombus filling the stent.

Video 44-46 The final result after LAD and LCx stenting. The LAD lesion was pretreated with balloon angioplasty and a bare metal stent was deployed to cover the proximal lesion. The LCx ostial lesion was dilated with balloon angioplasty and a bare metal stent was placed using a "V- stenting" technique.

SUMMARY

- Stent thrombosis is an infrequent (1–2%) but serious complication of stent placement. It occurs most commonly within the first month, but rarely, as late as 1 year (0.2–0.6%) with bare metal stents. Very late stent thrombosis (VLST), which occurs after 1 year, is very rare with bare metal stents but can occur with drug-eluting stents.

- Premature discontinuation of dual antiplatelet therapy is the most common cause of early and late stent thrombosis; however, the etiology of VLST is not clear.
- The majority of patients with stent thrombosis present with acute coronary syndromes or STEMI; this presentation is associated with a high mortality rate (10%).
- Treatment is immediate PCI with balloon angioplasty or restenting.

CASE 8: TRANSCATHETER AORTIC VALVE IMPLANTATION

(Figs. 44-10 to 44-14; Videos 44-47 to 44-50 can be accessed at the following link: http://www.mhprofessional.com/mediacenter/)

- A 75-year-old woman with symptomatic aortic stenosis and a valve area of 0.58 cm^2 by transthoracic echocardiogram.
- Chronic obstructive pulmonary disease (FEV$_1$ = .54) and other comorbidities contributed to an unacceptably high cardiac surgical risk (calculated logistic Euroscore = 29.57%) for aortic valve replacement.
- She was referred for transcatheter aortic valve implantation (TAVI) as part of a clinical trial.

Video 44-47 Aortogram shows patent coronary arteries and minimal aortic insufficiency.

Video 44-48 Balloon valvuloplasty is performed with rapid ventricular pacing at 180 bpm.

Video 44-49 A 26-mm Edwards-SAPIEN valve is positioned using fluoroscopic and transesophageal echo guidance and deployed.

Video 44-50 Aortogram after valve deployment shows a functional valve with mild aortic insufficiency and without impingement of the coronary ostia.

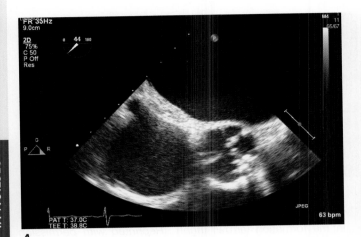

A

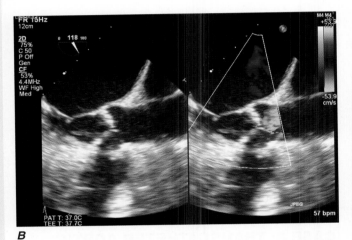

B

FIGURE 44-10

Transesophageal echocardiogram shows a calcified trileaf-let aortic valve (**A**) with reduced leaflet excursion and a narrowed orifice in peak systole (**B**).

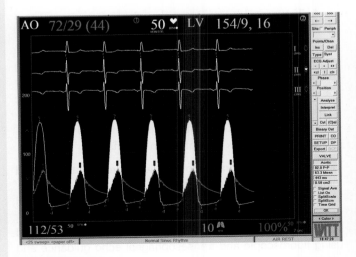

FIGURE 44-11

Hemodynamically significant aortic (AO) stenosis. Simultaneous recording of AO and left ventricle (LV) pressures shows an 82-mmHg peak-to-peak gradient and a 63.3-mmHg mean gradient between the LV (154/9 mmHg) and AO (72/29 mmHg) pressures. This is consistent with an aortic valve area of 0.58 cm^2.

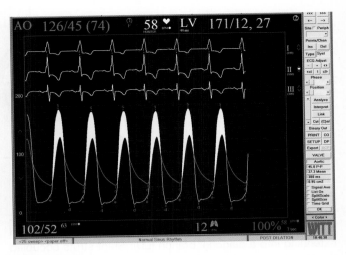

FIGURE 44-12

After balloon valvuloplasty, the LV–AO mean pressure gradient decreased to 37.3 mmHg, indicating that the aortic valve area increased to 0.95 cm^2.

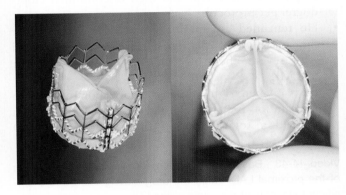

FIGURE 44-13

The Edwards SAPIEN Transcatheter Heart Valve. (*Reprinted with permission from A Zajarias and A Cribier: JACC 53:1829, 2009.*)

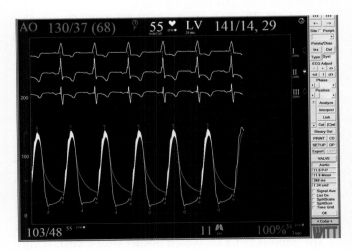

FIGURE 44-14

Once the valve was deployed, the pressure gradient between the LV and AO decreased to 11.6 mmHg and the functional valve area is 1.34 cm^2.

SUMMARY

- The prevalence of calcific aortic stenosis is 2–3% in individuals aged ≥75 years.
- Symptomatic aortic stenosis is associated with an average survival of 2–3 years and an increased risk of sudden death; aortic valve replacement improves both symptoms and survival.
- In high-risk patients with severe aortic stenosis who are not surgical candidates, 1-year and 5-year survival rates are ~62% and 38%, respectively.
- Transcatheter aortic valve implantation (TAVI) is approved in Europe and being evaluated in the United States in clinical trials as an alternative to surgical aortic valve replacement in high-risk patients.

(Case contributed with permission by Dr. Andrew C. Eisenhauer.)

CASE 9: ATRIAL SEPTAL DEFECT CLOSURE

(Figs. 44–15 to 44–19; Videos 44–51 to 44–53 can be accessed at the following link: http://www.mhprofessional.com/mediacenter/)

- A 48-year-old woman with increased shortness of breath, exercise intolerance, and an 18-mm secundum ASD.
- Echocardiogram showed a dilated right atrium (RA) and right ventricle (RV) with evidence of right ventricular volume overload.
- A shunt ratio (Qp/Qs) of 2.3:1 was determined at cardiac catheterization.
- Based on her symptoms, evidence of right-side chamber dilation, and a moderately sized atrial septal defect, the patient was referred for percutaneous closure of the ASD.

Video 44-51   A sizing balloon is placed across the ASD.

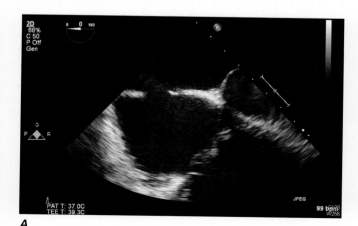

A

FIGURE 44-15

Transesophageal echocardiogram of a secundum ASD. The ASD is seen as "dropout" in the interatrial septum between

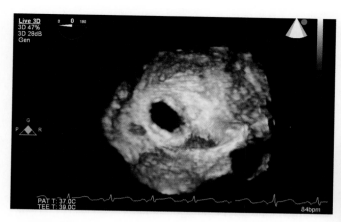

FIGURE 44-16

Three-dimensional echocardiographic reconstruction of the secundum ASD. The ASD is round and has an acceptable margin of tissue to seat a septal occluder device.

Video 44-52   An Amplatzer septal occluder is being positioned across the ASD.

Video 44-53   The two discs of the device in place across the ASD.

SUMMARY

- Unrepaired ASDs lead to signs and symptoms of increased pulmonary blood flow and right heart failure; dyspnea, exercise intolerance, fatigue, palpitations and atrial arrhythmias, and pulmonary infections.
- Percutaneous closure of an ASD may be recommended for individuals with a secundum ASD and evidence of RA and RV enlargement with or without symptoms.
- Percutaneous closure is contraindicated in patients with irreversible pulmonary arterial hypertension and no left-to-right shunt. It is not recommended for

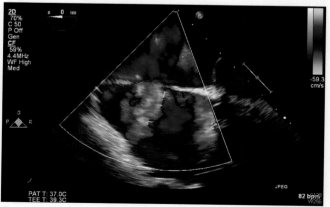

B

the left atrium (LA) and RA (**A**). Doppler color flow imaging shows blue in the RA consistent with left-to-right flow (**B**).

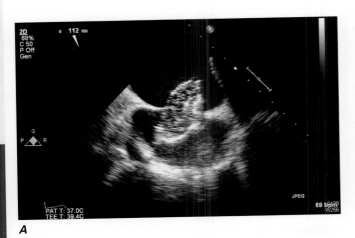

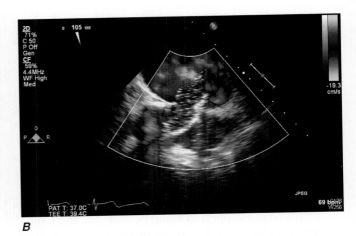

FIGURE 44-17

Transesophageal echocardiogram showing sizing balloon (**A**) and no flow (**B**) across the atrial septal defect.

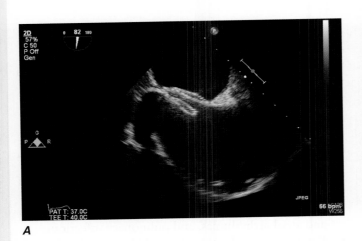

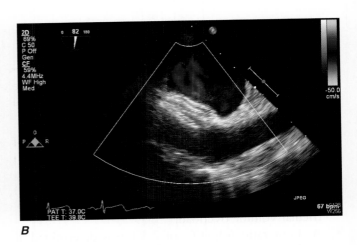

FIGURE 44-18

Amplatzer septal occluder in place (**A**). There is no blood flow across the device (**B**).

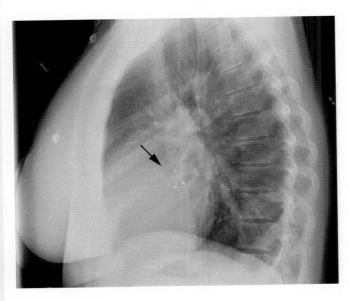

FIGURE 44-19

Postprocedure lateral chest x-ray showing the Amplatzer septal occluder in place.

closure of sinus venosus, coronary sinus, or primum ASDs.

- After the atrial septal occluder device is placed, patients are treated with antiplatelet agents and use antibiotic prophylaxis for certain procedures for 6 months. Follow-up echocardiograms to assess for device migration or erosion, residual shunting, thrombus or pericardial effusion are recommended at 1 day, 1 month, 6 months, 1 year, and periodically thereafter.

(Case contributed with permission by Dr. Andrew C. Eisenhauer.)

APPENDIX

LABORATORY VALUES OF CLINICAL IMPORTANCE

Alexander Kratz ■ Michael A. Pesce ■ Robert C. Basner ■ Andrew J. Einstein

This Appendix contains tables of reference values for laboratory tests, special analytes, and special function tests. A variety of factors can influence reference values. Such variables include the population studied, the duration and means of specimen transport, laboratory methods and instrumentation, and even the type of container used for the collection of the specimen. The reference or "normal" ranges given in this appendix may therefore not be appropriate for all laboratories, and these values should only be used as general guidelines. Whenever possible, reference values provided by the laboratory performing the testing should be utilized in the interpretation of laboratory data. Values supplied in this Appendix reflect typical reference ranges in adults. Pediatric reference ranges may vary significantly from adult values.

In preparing the Appendix, the authors have taken into account the fact that the system of international units (SI, système international d'unités) is used in most countries and in some medical journals. However, clinical laboratories may continue to report values in "traditional" or conventional units. Therefore, both systems are provided in the Appendix. The dual system is also used in the text except for (1) those instances in which the numbers remain the same but only the terminology is changed (mmol/L for meq/L or IU/L for mIU/mL), when only the SI units are given; and (2) most pressure measurements (e.g., blood and cerebrospinal fluid pressures), when the traditional units (mmHg, mmH$_2$O) are used. In all other instances in the text the SI unit is followed by the traditional unit in parentheses.

REFERENCE VALUES FOR LABORATORY TESTS

TABLE 1

HEMATOLOGY AND COAGULATION

ANALYTE	SPECIMEN	SI UNITS	CONVENTIONAL UNITS
Activated clotting time	WB	70–180 s	70–180 s
Activated protein C resistance (factor V Leiden)	P	Not applicable	Ratio >2.1
ADAMTS13 activity	P	≥0.67	≥67%
ADAMTS13 inhibitor activity	P	Not applicable	≤0.4 U
ADAMTS13 antibody	P	Not applicable	≤18 U
Alpha$_2$ antiplasmin	P	0.87–1.55	87–155%
Antiphospholipid antibody panel			
PTT-LA (lupus anticoagulant screen)	P	Negative	Negative
Platelet neutralization procedure	P	Negative	Negative
Dilute viper venom screen	P	Negative	Negative
Anticardiolipin antibody	S		
IgG		0–15 arbitrary units	0–15 GPL
IgM		0–15 arbitrary units	0–15 MPL

(continued)

TABLE 1

HEMATOLOGY AND COAGULATION (*CONTINUED*)

ANALYTE	SPECIMEN	SI UNITS	CONVENTIONAL UNITS
Antithrombin III	P		
Antigenic		220–390 mg/L	22–39 mg/dL
Functional		0.7–1.30 U/L	70–130%
Anti-Xa assay (heparin assay)	P		
Unfractionated heparin		0.3–0.7 kIU/L	0.3–0.7 IU/mL
Low-molecular-weight heparin		0.5–1.0 kIU/L	0.5–1.0 IU/mL
Danaparoid (Orgaran)		0.5–0.8 kIU/L	0.5–0.8 IU/mL
Autohemolysis test	WB	0.004–0.045	0.4–4.50%
Autohemolysis test with glucose	WB	0.003–0.007	0.3–0.7%
Bleeding time (adult)		<7.1 min	<7.1 min
Bone marrow: See Table 7			
Clot retraction	WB	0.50–1.00/2 h	50–100%/2 h
Cryofibrinogen	P	Negative	Negative
D-dimer	P	220–740 ng/mL FEU	220–740 ng/mL FEU
Differential blood count	WB		
Relative counts:			
Neutrophils		0.40–0.70	40–70%
Bands		0.0–0.05	0–5%
Lymphocytes		0.20–0.50	20–50%
Monocytes		0.04–0.08	4–8%
Eosinophils		0.0–0.6	0–6%
Basophils		0.0–0.02	0–2%
Absolute counts:			
Neutrophils		$1.42–6.34 \times 10^9$/L	1420–6340/mm^3
Bands		$0–0.45 \times 10^9$/L	0–450/mm^3
Lymphocytes		$0.71–4.53 \times 10^9$/L	710–4530/mm^3
Monocytes		$0.14–0.72 \times 10^9$/L	140–720/mm^3
Eosinophils		$0–0.54 \times 10^9$/L	0–540/mm^3
Basophils		$0–0.18 \times 10^9$/L	0–180/mm^3
Erythrocyte count	WB		
Adult males		$4.30–5.60 \times 10^{12}$/L	$4.30–5.60 \times 10^6$/mm^3
Adult females		$4.00–5.20 \times 10^{12}$/L	$4.00–5.20 \times 10^6$/mm^3
Erythrocyte life span	WB		
Normal survival		120 days	120 days
Chromium labeled, half-life ($t_{1/2}$)		25–35 days	25–35 days
Erythrocyte sedimentation rate	WB		
Females		0–20 mm/h	0–20 mm/h
Males		0–15 mm/h	0–15 mm/h
Euglobulin lysis time	P	7200–14,400 s	120–240 min
Factor II, prothrombin	P	0.50–1.50	50–150%
Factor V	P	0.50–1.50	50–150%
Factor VII	P	0.50–1.50	50–150%
Factor VIII	P	0.50–1.50	50–150%
Factor IX	P	0.50–1.50	50–150%
Factor X	P	0.50–1.50	50–150%
Factor XI	P	0.50–1.50	50–150%
Factor XII	P	0.50–1.50	50–150 %
Factor XIII screen	P	Not applicable	Present
Factor inhibitor assay	P	<0.5 Bethesda Units	<0.5 Bethesda Units
Fibrin(ogen) degradation products	P	0–1 mg/L	0–1 µg/mL
Fibrinogen	P	2.33–4.96 g/L	233–496 mg/dL
Glucose-6-phosphate dehydrogenase (erythrocyte)	WB	<2400 s	<40 min
Ham's test (acid serum)	WB	Negative	Negative

(continued)

TABLE 1

HEMATOLOGY AND COAGULATION (*CONTINUED*)

ANALYTE	SPECIMEN	SI UNITS	CONVENTIONAL UNITS
Hematocrit	WB		
Adult males		0.388–0.464	38.8–46.4
Adult females		0.354–0.444	35.4–44.4
Hemoglobin			
Plasma	P	6–50 mg/L	0.6–5.0 mg/dL
Whole blood:	WB		
Adult males		133–162 g/L	13.3–16.2 g/dL
Adult females		120–158 g/L	12.0–15.8 g/dL
Hemoglobin electrophoresis	WB		
Hemoglobin A		0.95–0.98	95–98%
Hemoglobin A_2		0.015–0.031	1.5–3.1%
Hemoglobin F		0–0.02	0–2.0%
Hemoglobins other than A, A_2, or F		Absent	Absent
Heparin-induced thrombocytopenia antibody	P	Negative	Negative
Immature platelet fraction (IPF)	WB	0.011–0.061	1.1–6.1%
Joint fluid crystal	JF	Not applicable	No crystals seen
Joint fluid mucin	JF	Not applicable	Only type I mucin present
Leukocytes			
Alkaline phosphatase (LAP)	WB	0.2–1.6 μkat/L	13–100 μ/L
Count (WBC)	WB	$3.54–9.06 \times 10^9$/L	$3.54–9.06 \times 10^3$/mm³
Mean corpuscular hemoglobin (MCH)	WB	26.7–31.9 pg/cell	26.7–31.9 pg/cell
Mean corpuscular hemoglobin concentration (MCHC)	WB	323–359 g/L	32.3–35.9 g/dL
Mean corpuscular hemoglobin of reticulocytes (CH)	WB	24–36 pg	24–36 pg
Mean corpuscular volume (MCV)	WB	79–93.3 fL	79–93.3 μm³
Mean platelet volume (MPV)	WB	9.00–12.95 fL	9.00–12.95
Osmotic fragility of erythrocytes	WB		
Direct		0.0035–0.0045	0.35–0.45%
Indirect		0.0030–0.0065	0.30–0.65%
Partial thromboplastin time, activated	P	26.3–39.4 s	26.3–39.4 s
Plasminogen	P		
Antigen		84–140 mg/L	8.4–14.0 mg/dL
Functional		0.70–1.30	70–130%
Plasminogen activator inhibitor 1	P	4–43 μg/L	4–43 ng/mL
Platelet aggregation	PRP	Not applicable	>65% aggregation in response to adenosine diphosphate, epinephrine, collagen, ristocetin, and arachidonic acid
Platelet count	WB	$165–415 \times 10^9$/L	$165–415 \times 10^3$/mm³
Platelet, mean volume	WB	6.4–11 fL	6.4–11.0 μm³
Prekallikrein assay	P	0.50–1.5	50–150%
Prekallikrein screen	P		No deficiency detected
Protein C	P		
Total antigen		0.70–1.40	70–140%
Functional		0.70–1.30	70–130%
Protein S	P		
Total antigen		0.70–1.40	70–140%
Functional		0.65–1.40	65–140%
Free antigen		0.70–1.40	70–140%
Prothrombin gene mutation G20210A	WB	Not applicable	Not present
Prothrombin time	P	12.7–15.4 s	12.7–15.4 s

(continued)

TABLE 1

HEMATOLOGY AND COAGULATION (*CONTINUED*)

ANALYTE	SPECIMEN	SI UNITS	CONVENTIONAL UNITS
Protoporphyrin, free erythrocyte	WB	0.28–0.64 µmol/L of red blood cells	16–36 µg/dL of red blood cells
Red cell distribution width	WB	<0.145	<14.5%
Reptilase time	P	16–23.6 s	16–23.6 s
Reticulocyte count	WB		
Adult males		0.008–0.023 red cells	0.8–2.3% red cells
Adult females		0.008–0.020 red cells	0.8–2.0% red cells
Reticulocyte hemoglobin content	WB	>26 pg/cell	>26 pg/cell
Ristocetin cofactor (functional von Willebrand factor)	P		
Blood group O		0.75 mean of normal	75% mean of normal
Blood group A		1.05 mean of normal	105% mean of normal
Blood group B		1.15 mean of normal	115% mean of normal
Blood group AB		1.25 mean of normal	125% mean of normal
Serotonin release assay	S	<0.2 release	<20% release
Sickle cell test	WB	Negative	Negative
Sucrose hemolysis	WB	<0.1	<10% hemolysis
Thrombin time	P	15.3–18.5 s	15.3–18.5 s
Total eosinophils	WB	$150–300 \times 10^6$/L	150–300/mm^3
Transferrin receptor	S, P	9.6–29.6 nmol/L	9.6–29.6 nmol/L
Viscosity			
Plasma	P	1.7–2.1	1.7–2.1
Serum	S	1.4–1.8	1.4–1.8
von Willebrand factor (vWF) antigen (factor VIII:R antigen)			
Blood group O		0.75 mean of normal	75% mean of normal
Blood group A		1.05 mean of normal	105% mean of normal
Blood group B		1.15 mean of normal	115% mean of normal
Blood group AB		1.25 mean of normal	125% mean of normal
von Willebrand factor multimers	P	Normal distribution	Normal distribution
White blood cells: see "Leukocytes"			

Abbreviations: JF, joint fluid; P, plasma; PRP, platelet-rich plasma; S, serum; WB, whole blood.

TABLE 2

CLINICAL CHEMISTRY AND IMMUNOLOGY

ANALYTE	SPECIMEN	SI UNITS	CONVENTIONAL UNITS
Acetoacetate	P	49–294 µmol/L	0.5–3.0 mg/dL
Adrenocorticotropin (ACTH)	P	1.3–16.7 pmol/L	6.0–76.0 pg/mL
Alanine aminotransferase (ALT, SGPT)	S	0.12–0.70 µkat/L	7–41 U/L
Albumin	S	40–50 g/L	4.0–5.0 mg/dL
Aldolase	S	26–138 nkat/L	1.5–8.1 U/L
Aldosterone (adult)			
Supine, normal sodium diet	S, P	<443 pmol/L	<16 ng/dL
Upright, normal	S, P	111–858 pmol/L	4–31 ng/dL
Alpha fetoprotein (adult)	S	0–8.5 µg/L	0–8.5 ng/mL
Alpha$_1$ antitrypsin	S	1.0–2.0 g/L	100–200 mg/dL
Ammonia, as NH$_3$	P	11–35 µmol/L	19–60 µg/dL
Amylase (method dependent)	S	0.34–1.6 µkat/L	20–96 U/L

(continued)

TABLE 2

CLINICAL CHEMISTRY AND IMMUNOLOGY (*CONTINUED*)

ANALYTE	SPECIMEN	SI UNITS	CONVENTIONAL UNITS
Androstendione (adult)	S		
Males		0.81–3.1 nmol/L	23–89 ng/dL
Females			
Premenopausal		0.91–7.5 nmol/L	26–214 ng/dL
Postmenopausal		0.46–2.9 nmol/L	13–82 ng/dL
Angiotensin-converting enzyme (ACE)	S	0.15–1.1 μkat/L	9–67 U/L
Anion gap	S	7–16 mmol/L	7–16 mmol/L
Apolipoprotein A-1	S		
Male		0.94–1.78 g/L	94–178 mg/dL
Female		1.01–1.99 g/L	101–199 mg/dL
Apolipoprotein B	S		
Male		0.55–1.40 g/L	55–140 mg/dL
Female		0.55–1.25 g/L	55–125 mg/dL
Arterial blood gases	WB		
[HCO_3^-]		22–30 mmol/L	22–30 meq/L
P_{CO_2}		4.3–6.0 kPa	32–45 mmHg
pH		7.35–7.45	7.35–7.45
P_{O_2}		9.6–13.8 kPa	72–104 mmHg
Aspartate aminotransferase (AST, SGOT)	S	0.20–0.65 μkat/L	12–38 U/L
Autoantibodies	S		
Anti-centromere antibody IgG		≤29 AU/mL	≤29 AU/mL
Anti-double-strand (native) DNA		<25 IU/L	<25 IU/L
Anti-glomerular basement membrane antibodies			
Qualitative IgG, IgA		Negative	Negative
Quantitative IgG antibody		≤19 AU/mL	≤19 AU/mL
Anti-histone antibodies		<1.0 U	<1.0 U
Anti-Jo-1 antibody		≤29 AU/mL	≤29 AU/mL
Anti-mitochondrial antibody		Not applicable	<20 Units
Anti-neutrophil cytoplasmic autoantibodies		Not applicable	<1:20
Serine proteinase 3 antibodies		≤19 AU/mL	≤19 AU/mL
Myeloperoxidase antibodies		≤19 AU/mL	≤19 AU/mL
Antinuclear antibody		Not applicable	Negative at 1:40
Anti-parietal cell antibody		Not applicable	None detected
Anti-RNP antibody		Not applicable	<1.0 U
Anti-Scl 70 antibody		Not applicable	<1.0 U
Anti-Smith antibody		Not applicable	<1.0 U
Anti-smooth muscle antibody		Not applicable	<1.0 U
Anti-SSA antibody		Not applicable	<1.0 U
Anti-SSB antibody		Not applicable	Negative
Anti-thyroglobulin antibody		<40 kIU/L	<40 IU/mL
Anti-thyroid peroxidase antibody		<35 kIU/L	<35 IU/mL
B-type natriuretic peptide (BNP)	P	Age and gender specific: <100 ng/L	Age and gender specific: <100 pg/mL
Bence Jones protein, serum qualitative	S	Not applicable	None detected
Bence Jones protein, serum quantitative	S		
Free kappa		3.3–19.4 mg/L	0.33–1.94 mg/dL
Free lambda		5.7–26.3 mg/L	0.57–2.63 mg/dL
K/L ratio		0.26–1.65	0.26–1.65
Beta-2-microglobulin	S	1.1–2.4 mg/L	1.1–2.4 mg/L
Bilirubin	S		
Total		5.1–22 μmol/L	0.3–1.3 mg/dL
Direct		1.7–6.8 μmol/L	0.1–0.4 mg/dL
Indirect		3.4–15.2 μmol/L	0.2–0.9 mg/dL

(continued)

TABLE 2

CLINICAL CHEMISTRY AND IMMUNOLOGY (*CONTINUED*)

ANALYTE	SPECIMEN	SI UNITS	CONVENTIONAL UNITS
C peptide	S	0.27–1.19 nmol/L	0.8–3.5 ng/mL
C1-esterase-inhibitor protein	S	210–390 mg/L	21–39 mg/dL
CA 125	S	<35 kU/L	<35 U/mL
CA 19-9	S	<37 kU/L	<37 U/mL
CA 15-3	S	<33 kU/L	<33 U/mL
CA 27-29	S	0–40 kU/L	0–40 U/mL

Calcitonin
  Male
  Female
	S	
		0–7.5 ng/L
		0–5.1 ng/L
			
			0–7.5 pg/mL
			0–5.1 pg/mL

Calcium	S	2.2–2.6 mmol/L	8.7–10.2 mg/dL
Calcium, ionized	WB	1.12–1.32 mmol/L	4.5–5.3 mg/dL
Carbon dioxide content (TCO$_2$)	P (sea level)	22–30 mmol/L	22–30 meq/L

Carboxyhemoglobin (carbon monoxide content)
  Nonsmokers
  Smokers
  Loss of consciousness and death
	WB	
		0.0–0.015
		0.04–0.09
		>0.50
			
			0–1.5%
			4–9%
			>50%

Carcinoembryonic antigen (CEA)
  Nonsmokers
  Smokers
	S	
		0.0–3.0 µg/L
		0.0–5.0 µg/L
			
			0.0–3.0 ng/mL
			0.0–5.0 ng/mL

Ceruloplasmin	S	250–630 mg/L	25–63 mg/dL
Chloride	S	102–109 mmol/L	102–109 meq/L
Cholesterol: see Table 5			
Cholinesterase	S	5–12 kU/L	5–12 U/mL
Chromogranin A	S	0–50 µg/L	0–50 ng/mL

Complement
  C3
  C4
  Complement total
	S	
		0.83–1.77 g/L
		0.16–0.47 g/L
		60–144 CAE units
			
			83–177 mg/dL
			16–47 mg/dL
			60–144 CAE units

Cortisol
  Fasting, 8 A.M.–12 noon
  12 noon–8 P.M.
  8 P.M.–8 A.M.
	S	
		138–690 nmol/L
		138–414 nmol/L
		0–276 nmol/L
			
			5–25 µg/dL
			5–15 µg/dL
			0–10 µg/dL

C-reactive protein	S	<10 mg/L	<10 mg/L

C-reactive protein, high sensitivity	S	Cardiac risk
		  Low: <1.0 mg/L
		  Average: 1.0–3.0 mg/L
		  High: >3.0 mg/L
			Cardiac risk
			  Low: <1.0 mg/L
			  Average: 1.0–3.0 mg/L
			  High: >3.0 mg/L

Creatine kinase (total)
  Females
  Males
	S	
		0.66–4.0 µkat/L
		0.875.0 µkat/L
			
			39–238 U/L
			51–294 U/L

Creatine kinase-MB
  Mass
  Fraction of total activity (by electrophoresis)
	S	
		0.0–5.5 µg/L
		0–0.04
			
			0.0–5.5 ng/mL
			0–4.0%

Creatinine
  Female
  Male
	S	
		44–80 µmol/L
		53–106 µmol/L
			
			0.5–0.9 mg/dL
			0.6–1.2 mg/dL

Cryoglobulins	S	Not applicable	None detected
Cystatin C	S	0.5–1.0 mg/L	0.5–1.0 mg/L

(continued)

TABLE 2

CLINICAL CHEMISTRY AND IMMUNOLOGY (*CONTINUED*)

ANALYTE	SPECIMEN	SI UNITS	CONVENTIONAL UNITS
Dehydroepiandrosterone (DHEA) (adult)			
Male	S	6.2–43.4 nmol/L	180–1250 ng/dL
Female		4.5–34.0 nmol/L	130–980 ng/dL
Dehydroepiandrosterone (DHEA) sulfate	S		
Male (adult)		100–6190 µg/L	10–619 µg/dL
Female (adult, premenopausal)		120–5350 µg/L	12–535 µg/dL
Female (adult, postmenopausal)		300–2600 µg/L	30–260 µg/dL
11-Deoxycortisol (adult) (compound S)	S	0.34–4.56 nmol/L	12–158 ng/dL
Dihydrotestosterone			
Male	S, P	1.03–2.92 nmol/L	30–85 ng/dL
Female		0.14–0.76 nmol/L	4–22 ng/dL
Dopamine	P	0–130 pmol/L	0–20 pg/mL
Epinephrine	P		
Supine (30 min)		<273 pmol/L	<50 pg/mL
Sitting		<328 pmol/L	<60 pg/mL
Standing (30 min)		<491 pmol/L	<90 pg/mL
Erythropoietin	S	4–27 U/L	4–27 U/L
Estradiol	S, P		
Female			
Menstruating:			
Follicular phase		74–532 pmol/L	<20–145 pg/mL
Midcycle peak		411–1626 pmol/L	112–443 pg/mL
Luteal phase		74–885 pmol/L	<20–241 pg/mL
Postmenopausal		217 pmol/L	<59 pg/mL
Male		74 pmol/L	<20 pg/mL
Estrone	S, P		
Female			
Menstruating:			
Follicular phase		<555 pmol/L	<150 pg/mL
Luteal phase		<740 pmol/L	<200 pg/mL
Postmenopausal		11–118 pmol/L	3–32 pg/mL
Male		33–133 pmol/L	9–36 pg/mL
Fatty acids, free (nonesterified)	P	0.1–0.6 mmol/L	2.8–16.8 mg/dL
Ferritin	S		
Female		10–150 µg/L	10–150 ng/mL
Male		29–248 µg/L	29–248 ng/mL
Follicle-stimulating hormone (FSH)	S, P		
Female			
Menstruating:			
Follicular phase		3.0–20.0 IU/L	3.0–20.0 mIU/mL
Ovulatory phase		9.0–26.0 IU/L	9.0–26.0 mIU/mL
Luteal phase		1.0–12.0 IU/L	1.0–12.0 mIU/mL
Postmenopausal		18.0–153.0 IU/L	18.0–153.0 mIU/mL
Male		1.0–12.0 IU/L	1.0–12.0 mIU/mL
Fructosamine	S	<285 umol/L	<285 umol/L
Gamma glutamyltransferase	S	0.15–0.99 µkat/L	9–58 U/L
Gastrin	S	<100 ng/L	<100 pg/mL
Glucagon	P	40–130 ng/L	40–130 pg/mL

(continued)

TABLE 2

CLINICAL CHEMISTRY AND IMMUNOLOGY (*CONTINUED*)

ANALYTE	SPECIMEN	SI UNITS	CONVENTIONAL UNITS
Glucose	WB	3.6–5.3 mmol/L	65–95 mg/dL
Glucose (fasting)	P		
Normal		4.2–5.6 mmol/L	75–100 mg/dL
Increased risk for diabetes		5.6–6.9 mmol/L	100–125 mg/dL
Diabetes mellitus		Fasting >7.0 mmol/L	Fasting >126 mg/dL
		A 2-hour level of >11.1 mmol/L during an oral glucose tolerance test	A 2-hour level of ≥200 mg/dL during an oral glucose tolerance test
		A random glucose level of ≥11.1 mmol/L in patients with symptoms of hyperglycemia	A random glucose level of ≥200 mg/dL in patients with symptoms of hyperglycemia
Growth hormone	S	0–5 µg/L	0–5 ng/mL
Hemoglobin A$_{1c}$	WB	0.04–0.06 HgB fraction	4.0–5.6%
Pre-diabetes		0.057–0.064 HgB fraction	5.7–6.4%
Diabetes mellitus		A hemoglobin A$_{1c}$ level of ≥0.065 Hgb fraction as suggested by the American Diabetes Association	A hemoglobin A$_{1c}$ level of ≥6.5% as suggested by the American Diabetes Association
Hemoglobin A$_{1c}$ with estimated average glucose (eAg)	WB	eAg mmoL/L = 1.59 × HbA$_{1c}$ − 2.59	eAg (mg/dL) = 28.7 × HbA$_{1c}$ − 46.7
High-density lipoprotein (HDL) (see Table 5)			
Homocysteine	P	4.4–10.8 µmol/L	4.4–10.8 µmol/L
Human chorionic gonadotropin (HCG)	S		
Nonpregnant female		<5 IU/L	<5 mIU/mL
1–2 weeks postconception		9–130 IU/L	9–130 mIU/mL
2–3 weeks postconception		75–2600 IU/L	75–2600 mIU/mL
3–4 weeks postconception		850–20,800 IU/L	850–20,800 mIU/mL
4–5 weeks postconception		4000–100,200 IU/L	4000–100,200 mIU/mL
5–10 weeks postconception		11,500–289,000 IU/L	11,500–289,000 mIU/mL
10–14 weeks post conception		18,300–137,000 IU/L	18,300–137,000 mIU/mL
Second trimester		1400–53,000 IU/L	1400–53,000 mIU/mL
Third trimester		940–60,000 IU/L	940–60,000 mIU/mL
β-Hydroxybutyrate	P	60–170 µmol/L	0.6–1.8 mg/dL
17-Hydroxyprogesterone (adult)	S		
Male		<4.17 nmol/L	<139 ng/dL
Female			
Follicular phase		0.45–2.1 nmol/L	15–70 ng/dL
Luteal phase		1.05–8.7 nmol/L	35–290 ng/dL
Immunofixation	S	Not applicable	No bands detected
Immunoglobulin, quantitation (adult)			
IgA	S	0.70–3.50 g/L	70–350 mg/dL
IgD	S	0–140 mg/L	0–14 mg/dL
IgE	S	1–87 kIU/L	1–87 IU/mL
IgG	S	7.0–17.0 g/L	700–1700 mg/dL
IgG$_1$	S	2.7–17.4 g/L	270–1740 mg/dL
IgG$_2$	S	0.3–6.3 g/L	30–630 mg/dL
IgG$_3$	S	0.13–3.2 g/L	13–320 mg/dL
IgG$_4$	S	0.11–6.2 g/L	11–620 mg/dL
IgM	S	0.50–3.0 g/L	50–300 mg/dL
Insulin	S, P	14.35–143.5 pmol/L	2–20 µU/mL
Iron	S	7–25 µmol/L	41–141 µg/dL

(continued)

TABLE 2

CLINICAL CHEMISTRY AND IMMUNOLOGY (CONTINUED)

ANALYTE	SPECIMEN	SI UNITS	CONVENTIONAL UNITS
Iron-binding capacity	S	45–73 µmol/L	251–406 µg/dL
Iron-binding capacity saturation	S	0.16–0.35	16–35%
Ischemia modified albumin	S	<85 kU/L	<85 U/mL
Joint fluid crystal	JF	Not applicable	No crystals seen
Joint fluid mucin	JF	Not applicable	Only type I mucin present
Ketone (acetone)	S	Negative	Negative
Lactate	P, arterial P, venous	0.5–1.6 mmol/L 0.5–2.2 mmol/L	4.5–14.4 mg/dL 4.5–19.8 mg/dL
Lactate dehydrogenase	S	2.0–3.8 µkat/L	115–221 U/L
Lipase	S	0.51–0.73 µkat/L	3–43 U/L
Lipids: see Table 5			
Lipoprotein (a)	S	0–300 mg/L	0–30 mg/dL
Low-density lipoprotein (LDL) (see Table 5)			
Luteinizing hormone (LH) 　Female 　　Menstruating: 　　　Follicular phase 　　　Ovulatory phase 　　　Luteal phase 　　Postmenopausal 　Male	S, P	 　 　 2.0–15.0 U/L 22.0–105.0 U/L 0.6–19.0 U/L 16.0–64.0 U/L 2.0–12.0 U/L	 　 　 2.0–15.0 mIU/mL 22.0–105.0 mIU/mL 0.6–19.0 mIU/mL 16.0–64.0 mIU/mL 2.0–12.0 mIU/mL
Magnesium	S	0.62–0.95 mmol/L	1.5–2.3 mg/dL
Metanephrine	P	<0.5 nmol/L	<100 pg/mL
Methemoglobin	WB	0.0–0.01	0–1%
Myoglobin 　Male 　Female	S	 20–71 µg/L 25–58 µg/L	 20–71 µg/L 25–58 µg/L
Norepinephrine 　Supine (30 min) 　Sitting 　Standing (30 min)	P	 650–2423 pmol/L 709–4019 pmol/L 739–4137 pmol/L	 110–410 pg/mL 120–680 pg/mL 125–700 pg/mL
N-telopeptide (cross-linked), NTx 　Female, premenopausal 　Male 　BCE = bone collagen equivalent	S	 6.2–19.0 nmol BCE 5.4–24.2 nmol BCE	 6.2–19.0 nmol BCE 5.4–24.2 nmol BCE
NT-Pro BNP	S, P	<125 ng/L up to 75 years <450 ng/L >75 years	<125 pg/mL up to 75 years <450 pg/mL >75 years
5′ Nucleotidase	S	0.00–0.19 µkat/L	0–11 U/L
Osmolality	P	275–295 mOsmol/kg 　serum water	275–295 mOsmol/kg serum 　water
Osteocalcin	S	11–50 µg/L	11–50 ng/mL
Oxygen content 　Arterial (sea level) 　Venous (sea level)	WB	 17–21 10–16	 17–21 vol% 10–16 vol%
Oxygen saturation (sea level) 　Arterial 　Venous, arm	WB	Fraction: 0.94–1.0 0.60–0.85	Percent: 94–100% 60–85%
Parathyroid hormone (intact)	S	8–51 ng/L	8–51 pg/mL

(continued)

TABLE 2

CLINICAL CHEMISTRY AND IMMUNOLOGY (*CONTINUED*)

ANALYTE	SPECIMEN	SI UNITS	CONVENTIONAL UNITS
Phosphatase, alkaline	S	0.56–1.63 µkat/L	33–96 U/L
Phosphorus, inorganic	S	0.81–1.4 mmol/L	2.5–4.3 mg/dL
Potassium	S	3.5–5.0 mmol/L	3.5–5.0 meq/L
Prealbumin	S	170–340 mg/L	17–34 mg/dL
Procalcitonin	S	<0.1 µg/L	<0.1 ng/mL
Progesterone Female: Follicular Midluteal Male	S, P	<3.18 nmol/L 9.54–63.6 nmol/L <3.18 nmol/L	<1.0 ng/mL 3–20 ng/mL <1.0 ng/mL
Prolactin Male Female	S	53–360 mg/L 40–530 mg/L	2.5–17 ng/mL 1.9–25 ng/mL
Prostate-specific antigen (PSA)	S	0.0–4.0 µg/L	0.0–4.0 ng/mL
Prostate-specific antigen, free	S	With total PSA between 4 and 10 µg/L and when the free PSA is: >0.25 decreased risk of prostate cancer <0.10 increased risk of prostate cancer	With total PSA between 4 and 10 ng/mL and when the free PSA is: >25% decreased risk of prostate cancer <10% increased risk of prostate cancer
Protein fractions: Albumin Globulin Alpha$_1$ Alpha$_2$ Beta Gamma	S	35–55 g/L 20–35 g/L 2–4 g/L 5–9 g/L 6–11 g/L 7–17 g/L	3.5–5.5 g/dL (50–60%) 2.0–3.5 g/dL (40–50%) 0.2–0.4 g/dL (4.2–7.2%) 0.5–0.9 g/dL (6.8–12%) 0.6–1.1 g/dL (9.3–15%) 0.7–1.7 g/dL (13–23%)
Protein, total	S	67–86 g/L	6.7–8.6 g/dL
Pyruvate	P	40–130 µmol/L	0.35–1.14 mg/dL
Rheumatoid factor	S	<15 kIU/L	<15 IU/mL
Serotonin	WB	0.28–1.14 umol/L	50–200 ng/mL
Serum protein electrophoresis	S	Not applicable	Normal pattern
Sex hormone–binding globulin (adult) Male Female	S	11–80 nmol/L 30–135 nmol/L	11–80 nmol/L 30–135 nmol/L
Sodium	S	136–146 mmol/L	136–146 meq/L
Somatomedin-C (IGF-1) (adult) 16 years 17 years 18 years 19 years 20 years 21–25 years 26–30 years 31–35 years 36–40 years 41–45 years 46–50 years 51–55 years 56–60 years 61–65 years	S	226–903 µg/L 193–731 µg/L 163–584 µg/L 141–483 µg/L 127–424 µg/L 116–358 µg/L 117–329 µg/L 115–307 µg/L 119–204 µg/L 101–267 µg/L 94–252 µg/L 87–238 µg/L 81–225 µg/L 75–212 µg/L	226–903 ng/mL 193–731 ng/mL 163–584 ng/mL 141–483 ng/mL 127–424 ng/mL 116–358 ng/mL 117–329 ng/mL 115–307 ng/mL 119–204 ng/mL 101–267 ng/mL 94–252 ng/mL 87–238 ng/mL 81–225 ng/mL 75–212 ng/mL

(*continued*)

TABLE 2

CLINICAL CHEMISTRY AND IMMUNOLOGY (CONTINUED)

ANALYTE	SPECIMEN	SI UNITS	CONVENTIONAL UNITS
66–70 years		69–200 μg/L	69–200 ng/mL
71–75 years		64–188 μg/L	64–188 ng/mL
76–80 years		59–177 μg/L	59–177 ng/mL
81–85 years		55–166 μg/L	55–166 ng/mL
Somatostatin	P	<25 ng/L	<25 pg/mL
Testosterone, free			
Female, adult	S	10.4–65.9 pmol/L	3–19 pg/mL
Male, adult		312–1041 pmol/L	90–300 pg/mL
Testosterone, total,	S		
Female		0.21–2.98 nmol/L	6–86 ng/dL
Male		9.36–37.10 nmol/L	270–1070 ng/dL
Thyroglobulin	S	1.3–31.8 μg/L	1.3–31.8 ng/mL
Thyroid-binding globulin	S	13–30 mg/L	1.3–3.0 mg/dL
Thyroid-stimulating hormone	S	0.34–4.25 mIU/L	0.34–4.25 μIU/mL
Thyroxine, free (fT4)	S	9.0–16 pmol/L	0.7–1.24 ng/dL
Thyroxine, total (T4)	S	70–151 nmol/L	5.4–11.7 μg/dL
Thyroxine index (free)	S	6.7–10.9	6.7–10.9
Transferrin	S	2.0–4.0 g/L	200–400 mg/dL
Triglycerides (see Table 5)	S	0.34–2.26 mmol/L	30–200 mg/dL
Triiodothyronine, free (fT3)	S	3.7–6.5 pmol/L	2.4–4.2 pg/mL
Triiodothyronine, total (T3)	S	1.2–2.1 nmol/L	77–135 ng/dL
Troponin I (method dependent)	S, P		
99th percentile of a healthy population		0–0.04 μg/L	0–0.04 ng/mL
Troponin T	S, P		
99th percentile of a healthy population		0–0.01 μg/L	0–0.01 ng/mL
Urea nitrogen	S	2.5–7.1 mmol/L	7–20 mg/dL
Uric acid	S		
Females		0.15–0.33 mmol/L	2.5–5.6 mg/dL
Males		0.18–0.41 mmol/L	3.1–7.0 mg/dL
Vasoactive intestinal polypeptide	P	0–60 ng/L	0–60 pg/mL
Zinc protoporphyrin	WB	0–400 μg/L	0–40 μg/dL
Zinc protoporphyrin (ZPP)-to-heme ratio	WB	0–69 μmol ZPP/mol heme	0–69 μmol ZPP/mol heme

Abbreviations: P, plasma; S, serum; WB, whole blood.

TABLE 3

TOXICOLOGY AND THERAPEUTIC DRUG MONITORING

DRUG	THERAPEUTIC RANGE		TOXIC LEVEL	
	SI UNITS	CONVENTIONAL UNITS	SI UNITS	CONVENTIONAL UNITS
Acetaminophen	66–199 µmol/L	10–30 µg/mL	>1320 µmol/L	>200 µg/mL
Amikacin				
Peak	34–51 µmol/L	20–30 µg/mL	>60 µmol/L	>35 µg/mL
Trough	0–17 µmol/L	0–10 µg/mL	>17 µmol/L	>10 µg/mL
Amitriptyline/nortriptyline (total drug)	430–900 nmol/L	120–250 ng/mL	>1800 nmol/L	>500 ng/mL
Amphetamine	150–220 nmol/L	20–30 ng/mL	>1500 nmol/L	>200 ng/mL
Bromide	9.4–18.7 mmol/L	75–150 mg/dL	>18.8 mmol/L	>150 mg/dL
Mild toxicity			6.4–18.8 mmol/L	51–150 mg/dL
Severe toxicity			>18.8 mmol/L	>150 mg/dL
Lethal			>37.5 mmol/L	>300 mg/dL
Caffeine	25.8–103 µmol/L	5–20 µg/mL	>206 µmol/L	>40 µg/mL
Carbamazepine	17–42 µmol/L	4–10 µg/mL	>85 µmol/L	>20 µg/mL
Chloramphenicol				
Peak	31–62 µmol/L	10–20 µg/mL	>77 µmol/L	>25 µg/mL
Trough	15–31 µmol/L	5–10 µg/mL	>46 µmol/L	>15 µg/mL
Chlordiazepoxide	1.7–10 µmol/L	0.5–3.0 µg/mL	>17 µmol/L	>5.0 µg/mL
Clonazepam	32–240 nmol/L	10–75 ng/mL	>320 nmol/L	>100 ng/mL
Clozapine	0.6–2.1 µmol/L	200–700 ng/mL	>3.7 µmol/L	>1200 ng/mL
Cocaine			>3.3 µmol/L	>1.0 µg/mL
Codeine	43–110 nmol/mL	13–33 ng/mL	>3700 nmol/mL	>1100 ng/mL (lethal)
Cyclosporine				
Renal transplant				
0–6 months	208–312 nmol/L	250–375 ng/mL	>312 nmol/L	>375 ng/mL
6–12 months after transplant	166–250 nmol/L	200–300 ng/mL	>250 nmol/L	>300 ng/mL
>12 months	83–125 nmol/L	100–150 ng/mL	>125 nmol/L	>150 ng/mL
Cardiac transplant				
0–6 months	208–291 nmol/L	250–350 ng/mL	>291 nmol/L	>350 ng/mL
6–12 months after transplant	125–208 nmol/L	150–250 ng/mL	>208 nmol/L	>250 ng/mL
>12 months	83–125 nmol/L	100–150 ng/mL	>125 nmol/L	150 ng/mL
Lung transplant				
0–6 months	250–374 nmol/L	300–450 ng/mL	>374 nmol/L	>450 ng/mL
Liver transplant				
Initiation	208–291 nmol/L	250–350 ng/mL	>291 nmol/L	>350 ng/mL
Maintenance	83–166 nmol/L	100–200 ng/mL	>166 nmol/L	>200 ng/mL
Desipramine	375–1130 nmol/L	100–300 ng/mL	>1880 nmol/L	>500 ng/mL
Diazepam (and metabolite)				
Diazepam	0.7–3.5 µmol/L	0.2–1.0 µg/mL	>7.0 µmol/L	>2.0 µg/mL
Nordiazepam	0.4–6.6 µmol/L	0.1–1.8 µg/mL	>9.2 µmol/L	>2.5 µg/mL
Digoxin	0.64–2.6 nmol/L	0.5–2.0 ng/mL	>5.0 nmol/L	>3.9 ng/mL
Disopyramide	5.3–14.7 µmol/L	2–5 µg/mL	>20.6 µmol/L	>7 µg/mL
Doxepin and nordoxepin				
Doxepin	0.36–0.98 µmol/L	101–274 ng/mL	>1.8 µmol/L	>503 ng/mL
Nordoxepin	0.38–1.04 µmol/L	106–291 ng/mL	>1.9 µmol/L	>531 ng/mL
Ethanol				
Behavioral changes			>4.3 mmol/L	>20 mg/dL
Legal limit			≥17 mmol/L	≥80 mg/dL
Critical with acute exposure			>54 mmol/L	>250 mg/dL
Ethylene glycol				
Toxic			>2 mmol/L	>12 mg/dL
Lethal			>20 mmol/L	>120 mg/dL

(continued)

TABLE 3

TOXICOLOGY AND THERAPEUTIC DRUG MONITORING (*CONTINUED*)

DRUG	THERAPEUTIC RANGE		TOXIC LEVEL	
	SI UNITS	CONVENTIONAL UNITS	SI UNITS	CONVENTIONAL UNITS
Ethosuximide	280–700 µmol/L	40–100 µg/mL	>700 µmol/L	>100 µg/mL
Everolimus	3.13–8.35 nmol/L	3–8 ng/mL	>12.5 nmol/L	>12 ng/mL
Flecainide	0.5–2.4 µmol/L	0.2–1.0 µg/mL	>3.6 µmol/L	>1.5 µg/mL
Gentamicin				
Peak	10–21 µmol/mL	5–10 µg/mL	>25 µmol/mL	>12 µg/mL
Trough	0–4.2 µmol/mL	0–2 µg/mL	>4.2 µmol/mL	>2 µg/mL
Heroin (diacetyl morphine)			>700 µmol/L	>200 ng/mL (as morphine)
Ibuprofen	49–243 µmol/L	10–50 µg/mL	>970 µmol/L	>200 µg/mL
Imipramine (and metabolite)				
Desimipramine	375–1130 nmol/L	100–300 ng/mL	>1880 nmol/L	>500 ng/mL
Total imipramine + desimipramine	563–1130 nmol/L	150–300 ng/mL	>1880 nmol/L	>500 ng/mL
Lamotrigine	11.7–54.7 µmol/L	3–14 µg/mL	>58.7 µmol/L	>15 µg/mL
Lidocaine	5.1–21.3 µmol/L	1.2–5.0 µg/mL	>38.4 µmol/L	>9.0 µg/mL
Lithium	0.5–1.3 mmol/L	0.5–1.3 meq/L	>2 mmol/L	>2 meq/L
Methadone	1.0–3.2 µmol/L	0.3–1.0 µg/mL	>6.5 µmol/L	>2 µg/mL
Methamphetamine	0.07–0.34 µmol/L	0.01–0.05 µg/mL	>3.35 µmol/L	>0.5 µg/mL
Methanol			>6 mmol/L	>20 mg/dL
Methotrexate				
Low-dose	0.01–0.1 µmol/L	0.01–0.1 µmol/L	>0.1 mmol/L	>0.1 mmol/L
High-dose (24 h)	<5.0 µmol/L	<5.0 µmol/L	>5.0 µmol/L	>5.0 µmol/L
High-dose (48 h)	<0.50 µmol/L	<0.50 µmol/L	>0.5 µmol/L	>0.5 µmol/L
High-dose (72 h)	<0.10 µmol/L	<0.10 µmol/L	>0.1 µmol/L	>0.1 µmol/L
Morphine	232–286 µmol/L	65–80 ng/mL	>720 µmol/L	>200 ng/mL
Mycophenolic acid	3.1–10.9 µmol/L	1.0–3.5 ng/mL	>37 µmol/L	>12 ng/mL
Nitroprusside (as thiocyanate)	103–499 µmol/L	6–29 µg/mL	860 µmol/L	>50 µg/mL
Nortriptyline	190–569 nmol/L	50–150 ng/mL	>1900 nmol/L	>500 ng/mL
Phenobarbital	65–172 µmol/L	15–40 µg/mL	>258 µmol/L	>60 µg/mL
Phenytoin	40–79 µmol/L	10–20 µg/mL	>158 µmol/L	>40 µg/mL
Phenytoin, free	4.0–7.9 µg/mL	1–2 µg/mL	>13.9 µg/mL	>3.5 µg/mL
% Free	0.08–0.14	8–14%		
Primidone and metabolite				
Primidone	23–55 µmol/L	5–12 µg/mL	>69 µmol/L	>15 µg/mL
Phenobarbital	65–172 µmol/L	15–40 µg/mL	>215 µmol/L	>50 µg/mL
Procainamide				
Procainamide	17–42 µmol/L	4–10 µg/mL	>43 µmol/L	>10 µg/mL
NAPA (*N*-acetylprocainamide)	22–72 µmol/L	6–20 µg/mL	>126 µmol/L	>35 µg/mL
Quinidine	6.2–15.4 µmol/L	2.0–5.0 µg/mL	>19 µmol/L	>6 µg/mL
Salicylates	145–2100 µmol/L	2–29 mg/dL	>2900 µmol/L	>40 mg/dL
Sirolimus (trough level)				
Kidney transplant	4.4–15.4 nmol/L	4–14 ng/mL	>16 nmol/L	>15 ng/mL
Tacrolimus (FK506) (trough)				
Kidney and liver				
Initiation	12–19 nmol/L	10–15 ng/mL	>25 nmol/L	>20 ng/mL
Maintenance	6–12 nmol/L	5–10 ng/mL	>25 nmol/L	>20 ng/mL
Heart				
Initiation	19–25 nmol/L	15–20 ng/mL		
Maintenance	6–12 nmol/L	5–10 ng/mL		

(continued)

APPENDIX

Laboratory Values of Clinical Importance

TABLE 3

TOXICOLOGY AND THERAPEUTIC DRUG MONITORING (*CONTINUED*)

DRUG	THERAPEUTIC RANGE		TOXIC LEVEL	
	SI UNITS	CONVENTIONAL UNITS	SI UNITS	CONVENTIONAL UNITS
Theophylline	56–111 µg/mL	10–20 µg/mL	>168 µg/mL	>30 µg/mL
Thiocyanate				
After nitroprusside infusion	103–499 µmol/L	6–29 µg/mL	860 µmol/L	>50 µg/mL
Nonsmoker	17–69 µmol/L	1–4 µg/mL		
Smoker	52–206 µmol/L	3–12 µg/mL		
Tobramycin				
Peak	11–22 µg/L	5–10 µg/mL	>26 µg/L	>12 µg/mL
Trough	0–4.3 µg/L	0–2 µg/mL	>4.3 µg/L	>2 µg/mL
Valproic acid	346–693 µmol/L	50–100 µg/mL	>693 µmol/L	>100 µg/mL
Vancomycin				
Peak	14–28 µmol/L	20–40 µg/mL	>55 µmol/L	>80 µg/mL
Trough	3.5–10.4 µmol/L	5–15 µg/mL	>14 µmol/L	>20 µg/mL

TABLE 4

VITAMINS AND SELECTED TRACE MINERALS

SPECIMEN	ANALYTE	REFERENCE RANGE	
		SI UNITS	CONVENTIONAL UNITS
Aluminum	S	<0.2 µmol/L	<5.41 µg/L
Arsenic	WB	0.03–0.31 µmol/L	2–23 µg/L
Cadmium	WB	<44.5 nmol/L	<5.0 µg/L
Coenzyme Q10 (ubiquinone)	P	433–1532 µg/L	433–1532 µg/L
β-Carotene	S	0.07–1.43 µmol/L	4–77 µg/dL
Copper	S	11–22 µmol/L	70–140 µg/dL
Folic acid	RC	340–1020 nmol/L cells	150–450 ng/mL cells
Folic acid	S	12.2–40.8 nmol/L	5.4–18.0 ng/mL
Lead (adult)	S	<0.5 µmol/L	<10 µg/dL
Mercury	WB	3.0–294 nmol/L	0.6–59 µg/L
Selenium	S	0.8–2.0 umol/L	63–160 µg/L
Vitamin A	S	0.7–3.5 µmol/L	20–100 µg/dL
Vitamin B$_1$ (thiamine)	S	0–75 nmol/L	0–2 µg/dL
Vitamin B$_2$ (riboflavin)	S	106–638 nmol/L	4–24 µg/dL
Vitamin B$_6$	P	20–121 nmol/L	5–30 ng/mL
Vitamin B$_{12}$	S	206–735 pmol/L	279–996 pg/mL
Vitamin C (ascorbic acid)	S	23–57 µmol/L	0.4–1.0 mg/dL
Vitamin D$_3$,1,25-dihydroxy, total	S, P	36–180 pmol/L	15–75 pg/mL
Vitamin D$_3$,25-hydroxy, total	P	75–250 nmol/L	30–100 ng/mL
Vitamin E	S	12–42 µmol/L	5–18 µg/mL
Vitamin K	S	0.29–2.64 nmol/L	0.13–1.19 ng/mL
Zinc	S	11.5–18.4 µmol/L	75–120 µg/dL

Abbreviations: P, plasma; RC, red cells; S, serum; WB, whole blood.

TABLE 5

CLASSIFICATION OF LDL, TOTAL, AND HDL CHOLESTEROL

LDL Cholesterol

<70 mg/dL	Therapeutic option for very high risk patients
<100 mg/dL	Optimal
100–129 mg/dL	Near optimal/above optimal
130–159 mg/dL	Borderline high
160–189 mg/dL	High
≥190 mg/dL	Very high

Total Cholesterol

<200 mg/dL	Desirable
200–239 mg/dL	Borderline high
≥240 mg/dL	High

HDL Cholesterol

<40 mg/dL	Low
≥60 mg/dL	High

Abbreviations: LDL, low-density lipoprotein; HDL, high-density lipoprotein.

Source: Executive summary of the third report of the National Cholesterol Education Program (NCEP) expert panel on detection, evaluation, and treatment of high blood cholesterol in adults (adult treatment panel III). JAMA 2001; 285:2486–97. Implications of Recent Clinical Trials for the National Cholesterol Education Program Adult Treatment Panel III Guidelines. SM Grundy et al for the Coordinating Committee of the National Cholesterol Education Program: Circulation 110:227, 2004.

REFERENCE VALUES FOR SPECIFIC ANALYTES

TABLE 6

CEREBROSPINAL FLUID[a]

CONSTITUENT	SI UNITS	CONVENTIONAL UNITS
	REFERENCE RANGE	
Osmolarity	292–297 mmol/kg water	292–297 mOsm/L
Electrolytes		
Sodium	137–145 mmol/L	137–145 meq/L
Potassium	2.7–3.9 mmol/L	2.7–3.9 meq/L
Calcium	1.0–1.5 mmol/L	2.1–3.0 meq/L
Magnesium	1.0–1.2 mmol/L	2.0–2.5 meq/L
Chloride	116–122 mmol/L	116–122 meq/L
CO_2 content	20–24 mmol/L	20–24 meq/L
P_{CO_2}	6–7 kPa	45–49 mmHg
pH	7.31–7.34	
Glucose	2.22–3.89 mmol/L	40–70 mg/dL
Lactate	1–2 mmol/L	10–20 mg/dL
Total protein:		
Lumbar	0.15–0.5 g/L	15–50 mg/dL
Cisternal	0.15–0.25 g/L	15–25 mg/dL
Ventricular	0.06–0.15 g/L	6–15 mg/dL
Albumin	0.066–0.442 g/L	6.6–44.2 mg/dL
IgG	0.009–0.057 g/L	0.9–5.7 mg/dL
IgG index[b]	0.29–0.59	
Oligoclonal bands (OGB)	<2 bands not present in matched serum sample	
Ammonia	15–47 µmol/L	25–80 µg/dL
Creatinine	44–168 µmol/L	0.5–1.9 mg/dL
Myelin basic protein	<4 µg/L	
CSF pressure		50–180 mmH$_2$O
CSF volume (adult)	~150 mL	
Red blood cells	0	0
Leukocytes		
Total	0–5 mononuclear cells per µL	
Differential		
Lymphocytes	60–70%	
Monocytes	30–50%	
Neutrophils	None	

[a]Since cerebrospinal fluid concentrations are equilibrium values, measurements of the same parameters in blood plasma obtained at the same time are recommended. However, there is a time lag in attainment of equilibrium, and cerebrospinal levels of plasma constituents that can fluctuate rapidly (such as plasma glucose) may not achieve stable values until after a significant lag phase.
[b]IgG index = CSF IgG (mg/dL) × serum albumin (g/dL)/serum IgG (g/dL) × CSF albumin (mg/dL).

TABLE 7A

DIFFERENTIAL NUCLEATED CELL COUNTS OF BONE MARROW ASPIRATES[a]

	OBSERVED RANGE (%)	95% RANGE (%)	MEAN (%)
Blast cells	0–3.2	0–3.0	1.4
Promyelocytes	3.6–13.2	3.2–12.4	7.8
Neutrophil myelocytes	4–21.4	3.7–10.0	7.6
Eosinophil myelocytes	0–5.0	0–2.8	1.3
Metamyelocytes	1–7.0	2.3–5.9	4.1
Neutrophils			
Males	21.0–45.6	21.9–42.3	32.1
Females	29.6–46.6	28.8–45.9	37.4
Eosinophils	0.4–4.2	0.3–4.2	2.2
Eosinophils plus eosinophil myelocytes	0.9–7.4	0.7–6.3	3.5
Basophils	0–0.8	0–0.4	0.1
Erythroblasts			
Male	18.0–39.4	16.2–40.1	28.1
Females	14.0–31.8	13.0–32.0	22.5
Lymphocytes	4.6–22.6	6.0–20.0	13.1
Plasma cells	0–1.4	0–1.2	0.6
Monocytes	0–3.2	0–2.6	1.3
Macrophages	0–1.8	0–1.3	0.4
M:E ratio			
Males	1.1–4.0	1.1–4.1	2.1
Females	1.6–5.4	1.6–5.2	2.8

[a]Based on bone marrow aspirate from 50 healthy volunteers (30 men, 20 women).
Abbreviation: M:E, myeloid to erythroid ratio.
Source: BJ Bain: Br J Haematol 94:206, 1996.

TABLE 7B

BONE MARROW CELLULARITY

AGE	OBSERVED RANGE	95% RANGE	MEAN
Under 10 years	59.0–95.1%	72.9–84.7%	78.8%
10–19 years	41.5–86.6%	59.2–69.4%	64.3%
20–29 years	32.0–83.7%	54.1–61.9%	58.0%
30–39 years	30.3–81.3%	41.1–54.1%	47.6%
40–49 years	16.3–75.1%	43.5–52.9%	48.2%
50–59 years	19.7–73.6%	41.2–51.4%	46.3%
60–69 years	16.3–65.7%	40.8–50.6%	45.7%
70–79 years	11.3–47.1%	22.6–35.2%	28.9%

Source: From RJ Hartsock et al: Am J Clin Pathol 1965; 43:326, 1965.

TABLE 8

STOOL ANALYSIS

	REFERENCE RANGE	
	SI UNITS	CONVENTIONAL UNITS
Alpha-1-antitrypsin	≤540 mg/L	≤54 mg/dL
Amount	0.1–0.2 kg/d	100–200 g/24 h
Coproporphyrin	611–1832 nmol/d	400–1200 µg/24 h
Fat		
Adult		<7 g/d
Adult on fat-free diet		<4 g/d
Fatty acids	0–21 mmol/d	0–6 g/24 h
Leukocytes	None	None
Nitrogen	<178 mmol/d	<2.5 g/24 h
pH	7.0–7.5	
Potassium	14–102 mmol/L	14–102 mmol/L
Occult blood	Negative	Negative
Osmolality	280–325 mOsmol/kg	280–325 mOsmol/kg
Sodium	7–72 mmol/L	7–72 mmol/L
Trypsin		20–95 U/g
Urobilinogen	85–510 µmol/d	50–300 mg/24 h
Uroporphyrins	12–48 nmol/d	10–40 µg/24 h
Water	<0.75	<75%

Source: Modified from: FT Fishbach, MB Dunning III: *A Manual of Laboratory and Diagnostic Tests*, 7th ed. Philadelphia, Lippincott Williams & Wilkins, 2004.

TABLE 9

URINE ANALYSIS AND RENAL FUNCTION TESTS

	REFERENCE RANGE	
	SI UNITS	CONVENTIONAL UNITS
Acidity, titratable	20–40 mmol/d	20–40 meq/d
Aldosterone	Normal diet: 6–25 μg/d Low-salt diet: 17–44 μg/d High-salt diet: 0–6 μg/d	Normal diet: 6–25 μg/d Low-salt diet: 17–44 μg/d High-salt diet: 0–6 μg/d
Aluminum	0.19–1.11 μmol/L	5–30 μg/L
Ammonia	30–50 mmol/d	30–50 meq/d
Amylase		4–400 U/L
Amylase/creatinine clearance ratio $[(Cl_{am}/Cl_{cr}) \times 100]$	1–5	1–5
Arsenic	0.07–0.67 μmol/d	5–50 μg/d
Bence Jones protein, urine, qualitative	Not applicable	None detected

Bence Jones protein, urine, quantitative
    Free Kappa
    Free Lambda
    K/L ratio
	
	1.4–24.2 mg/L
	0.2–6.7 mg/L
	2.04–10.37
		
		0.14–2.42 mg/dL
		0.02–0.67 mg/dL
		2.04–10.37

Calcium (10 meq/d or 200 mg/d dietary calcium)	<7.5 mmol/d	<300 mg/d
Chloride	140–250 mmol/d	140–250 mmol/d
Citrate	320–1240 mg/d	320–1240 mg/d
Copper	<0.95 μmol/d	<60 μg/d
Coproporphyrins (types I and III)	0–20 μmol/mol creatinine	0–20 μmol/mol creatinine
Cortisol, free	55–193 nmol/d	20–70 μg/d

Creatine, as creatinine
    Female
    Male
	
	<760 μmol/d
	<380 μmol/d
		
		<100 mg/d
		<50 mg/d

Creatinine	8.8–14 mmol/d	1.0–1.6 g/d
Dopamine	392–2876 nmol/d	60–440 μg/d
Eosinophils	<100 eosinophils/mL	<100 eosinophils/mL
Epinephrine	0–109 nmol/d	0–20 μg/d
Glomerular filtration rate	>60 mL/min/1.73 m^2 For African Americans multiply the result by 1.21	>60 mL/min/1.73 m^2 For African Americans multiply the result by 1.21
Glucose (glucose oxidase method)	0.3–1.7 mmol/d	50–300 mg/d
5-Hydroindoleacetic acid [5-HIAA]	0–78.8 μmol/d	0–15 mg/d
Hydroxyproline	53–328 μmol/d	53–328 μmol/d

Iodine, spot urine
  WHO classification of iodine deficiency:
    Not iodine deficient
    Mild iodine deficiency
    Moderate iodine deficiency
    Severe iodine deficiency
	
	>100 μg/L
	50–100 μg/L
	20–49 μg/L
	<20 μg/L
		
		>100 μg/L
		50–100 μg/L
		20–49 μg/L
		<20 μg/L

Ketone (acetone)	Negative	Negative
17 Ketosteroids	3–12 mg/d	3–12 mg/d

Metanephrines
    Metanephrine
    Normetanephrine
	
	30–350 μg/d
	50–650 μg/d
		
		30–350 μg/d
		50–650 μg/d

(continued)

TABLE 9

URINE ANALYSIS AND RENAL FUNCTION TESTS (*CONTINUED*)

	REFERENCE RANGE	
	SI UNITS	**CONVENTIONAL UNITS**
Microalbumin		
Normal	0.0–0.03 g/d	0–30 mg/d
Microalbuminuria	0.03–0.30 g/d	30–300 mg/d
Clinical albuminuria	>0.3 g/d	>300 mg/d
Microalbumin/creatinine ratio		
Normal	0–3.4 g/mol creatinine	0–30 µg/mg creatinine
Microalbuminuria	3.4–34 g/mol creatinine	30–300 µg/mg creatinine
Clinical albuminuria	>34 g/mol creatinine	>300 µg/mg creatinine
β_2-Microglobulin	0–160 µg/L	0–160 µg/L
Norepinephrine	89–473 nmol/d	15–80 µg/d
N-telopeptide (cross-linked), NTx		
Female, premenopausal	17–94 nmol BCE/mmol creatinine	17–94 nmol BCE/mmol creatinine
Female, postmenopausal	26–124 nmol BCE/mmol creatinine	26–124 nmol BCE/mmol creatinine
Male	21–83 nmol BCE/mmol creatinine	21–83 nmol BCE/mmol creatinine
BCE = bone collagen equivalent		
Osmolality	100–800 mOsm/kg	100–800 mOsm/kg
Oxalate		
Male	80–500 µmol/d	7–44 mg/d
Female	45–350 µmol/d	4–31 mg/d
pH	5.0–9.0	5.0–9.0
Phosphate (phosphorus) (varies with intake)	12.9–42.0 mmol/d	400–1300 mg/d
Porphobilinogen	None	None
Potassium (varies with intake)	25–100 mmol/d	25–100 meq/d
Protein	<0.15 g/d	<150 mg/d
Protein/creatinine ratio	Male: 15–68 mg/g Female: 10–107 mg/g	Male: 15–68 mg/g Female: 10–107 mg/g
Sediment		
Red blood cells	0–2/high-power field	
White blood cells	0–2/high-power field	
Bacteria	None	
Crystals	None	
Bladder cells	None	
Squamous cells	None	
Tubular cells	None	
Broad casts	None	
Epithelial cell casts	None	
Granular casts	None	
Hyaline casts	0–5/low-power field	
Red blood cell casts	None	
Waxy casts	None	
White cell casts	None	
Sodium (varies with intake)	100–260 mmol/d	100–260 meq/d
Specific gravity:		
After 12-h fluid restriction	>1.025	>1.025
After 12-h deliberate water intake	≤1.003	≤1.003
Tubular reabsorption, phosphorus	0.79–0.94 of filtered load	79–94% of filtered load
Urea nitrogen	214–607 mmol/d	6–17 g/d
Uric acid (normal diet)	1.49–4.76 mmol/d	250–800 mg/d
Vanillylmandelic acid (VMA)	<30 µmol/d	<6 mg/d

TABLE 10

NORMAL PRESSURES IN HEART AND GREAT VESSELS

PRESSURE (mmHg)	AVERAGE	RANGE
Right Atrium		
Mean	2.8	1–5
a wave	5.6	2.5–7
c wave	3.8	1.5–6
x wave	1.7	0–5
v wave	4.6	2–7.5
y wave	2.4	0–6
Right Ventricle		
Peak systolic	25	17–32
End-diastolic	4	1–7
Pulmonary Artery		
Mean	15	9–19
Peak systolic	25	17–32
End-diastolic	9	4–13
Pulmonary Artery Wedge		
Mean	9	4.5–13
Left Atrium		
Mean	7.9	2–12
a wave	10.4	4–16
v wave	12.8	6–21
Left Ventricle		
Peak systolic	130	90–140
End-diastolic	8.7	5–12
Brachial Artery		
Mean	85	70–105
Peak systolic	130	90–140
End-diastolic	70	60–90

Source: Reproduced from: MJ Kern *The Cardiac Catheterization Handbook*, 4th ed. Philadelphia, Mosby, 2003.

TABLE 11

CIRCULATORY FUNCTION TESTS

	RESULTS: REFERENCE RANGE	
TEST	SI UNITS (RANGE)	CONVENTIONAL UNITS (RANGE)
Arteriovenous oxygen difference	30–50 mL/L	30–50 mL/L
Cardiac output (Fick)	2.5–3.6 L/m^2 of body surface area per min	2.5–3.6 L/m^2 of body surface area per min
Contractility indexes		
Max. left ventricular dp/dt (dp/dt)	220 kPa/s (176–250 kPa/s)	1650 mmHg/s (1320–1880 mmHg/s)
DP when DP = 5.3 kPa	(37.6 ± 12.2)/s	(37.6 ± 12.2)/s
(40 mmHg) (DP, developed LV pressure)	3.32 ± 0.84 end-diastolic volumes per second	3.32 ± 0.84 end-diastolic volumes per second
Mean normalized systolic ejection rate (angiography)	1.83 ± 0.56 circumferences per second	1.83 ± 0.56 circumferences per second
Mean velocity of circumferential fiber shortening (angiography)		
Ejection fraction: stroke volume/ end-diastolic volume (SV/EDV)	0.67 ± 0.08 (0.55–0.78)	0.67 ± 0.08 (0.55–0.78)
End-diastolic volume	70 ± 20.0 mL/m^2 (60–88 mL/m^2)	70 ± 20.0 mL/m^2 (60–88 mL/m^2)
End-systolic volume	25 ± 5.0 mL/m^2 (20–33 mL/m^2)	25 ± 5.0 mL/m^2 (20–33 mL/m^2)
Left ventricular work		
Stroke work index	50 ± 20.0 (g·m)/m^2 (30–110)	50 ± 20.0 (g·m)/m^2 (30–110)
Left ventricular minute work index	1.8–6.6 [(kg·m)/m^2]/min	1.8–6.6 [(kg·m)/m^2]/min
Oxygen consumption index	110–150 mL	110–150 mL
Maximum oxygen uptake	35 mL/min (20–60 mL/min)	35 mL/min (20–60 mL/min)
Pulmonary vascular resistance	2–12 (kPa·s)/L	20–130 (dyn·s)/cm^5
Systemic vascular resistance	77–150 (kPa·s)/L	770–1600 (dyn·s)/cm^5

Source: E Braunwald et al: *Heart Disease*, 6th ed. Philadelphia, W.B. Saunders Co., 2001.

TABLE 12

NORMAL ECHOCARDIOGRAPHIC REFERENCE LIMITS AND PARTITION VALUES IN ADULTS

	WOMEN REFERENCE RANGE	MILDLY ABNORMAL	MODERATELY ABNORMAL	SEVERELY ABNORMAL	MEN REFERENCE RANGE	MILDLY ABNORMAL	MODERATELY ABNORMAL	SEVERELY ABNORMAL
Left ventricular dimensions								
Septal thickness, cm	0.6–0.9	1.0–1.2	1.3–1.5	≥1.6	0.6–1.0	1.1–1.3	1.4–1.6	≥1.7
Posterior wall thickness, cm	0.6–0.9	1.0–1.2	1.3–1.5	≥1.6	0.6–1.0	1.1–1.3	1.4–1.6	≥1.7
Diastolic diameter, cm	3.9–5.3	5.4–5.7	5.8–6.1	≥6.2	4.2–5.9	6.0–6.3	6.4–6.8	≥6.9
Diastolic diameter/BSA, cm/m²	2.4–3.2	3.3–3.4	3.5–3.7	≥3.8	2.2–3.1	3.2–3.4	3.5–3.6	≥3.7
Diastolic diameter/height, cm/m	2.5–3.2	3.3–3.4	3.5–3.6	≥3.7	2.4–3.3	3.4–3.5	3.6–3.7	≥3.8
Left ventricular volumes								
Diastolic, mL	56–104	105–117	118–130	≥131	67–155	156–178	179–201	≥202
Diastolic/BSA, mL/m²	35–75	76–86	87–96	≥97	35–75	76–86	87–96	≥97
Systolic, mL	19–49	50–59	60–69	≥70	22–58	59–70	71–82	≥83
Systolic/BSA, mL/m²	12–30	31–36	37–42	≥43	12–30	31–36	37–42	≥43
Left ventricular mass, 2D method								
Mass, g	66–150	151–171	172–182	≥183	96–200	201–227	228–254	≥255
Mass/BSA, g/m²	44–88	89–100	101–112	≥113	50–102	103–116	117–130	≥131
Left ventricular function								
Endocardial fractional shortening (%)	27–45	22–26	17–21	≤16	25–43	20–24	15–19	≤14
Midwall fractional shortening (%)	15–23	13–14	11–12	≤10	14–22	12–13	10–11	≤9
Ejection fraction, 2D method (%)	≥55	45–54	30–44	≤29	≥55	45–54	30–44	≤29
Right heart dimensions (cm)								
Basal RV diameter	2.0–2.8	2.9–3.3	3.4–3.8	≥3.9	2.0–2.8	2.9–3.3	3.4–3.8	≥3.9
Mid-RV diameter	2.7–3.3	3.4–3.7	3.8–4.1	≥4.2	2.7–3.3	3.4–3.7	3.8–4.1	≥4.2
Base-to-apex length	7.1–7.9	8.0–8.5	8.6–9.1	≥9.2	7.1–7.9	8.0–8.5	8.6–9.1	≥9.2
RVOT diameter above aortic valve	2.5–2.9	3.0–3.2	3.3–3.5	≥3.6	2.5–2.9	3.0–3.2	3.3–3.5	≥3.6
RVOT diameter above pulmonic valve	1.7–2.3	2.4–2.7	2.8–3.1	≥3.2	1.7–2.3	2.4–2.7	2.8–3.1	≥3.2
Pulmonary artery diameter below pulmonic valve	1.5–2.1	2.2–2.5	2.6–2.9	≥3.0	1.5–2.1	2.2–2.5	2.6–2.9	≥3.0
Right ventricular size and function in 4-chamber view								
Diastolic area, cm²	11–28	29–32	33–37	≥38	11–28	29–32	33–37	≥38
Systolic area, cm²	7.5–16	17–19	20–22	≥23	7.5–16	17–19	20–22	≥23
Fractional area change, %	32–60	25–31	18–24	≤17	32–60	25–31	18–24	≤17
Atrial sizes								
LA diameter, cm	2.7–3.8	3.9–4.2	4.3–4.6	≥4.7	3.0–4.0	4.1–4.6	4.7–5.2	≥5.3
LA diameter/BSA, cm/m²	1.5–2.3	2.4–2.6	2.7–2.9	≥3.0	1.5–2.3	2.4–2.6	2.7–2.9	≥3.0
RA minor axis, cm	2.9–4.5	4.6–4.9	5.0–5.4	≥5.5	2.9–4.5	4.6–4.9	5.0–5.4	≥5.5
RA minor axis/BSA, cm/m²	1.7–2.5	2.6–2.8	2.9–3.1	≥3.2	1.7–2.5	2.6–2.8	2.9–3.1	≥3.2

(continued)

APPENDIX

Laboratory Values of Clinical Importance

TABLE 12

NORMAL ECHOCARDIOGRAPHIC REFERENCE LIMITS AND PARTITION VALUES IN ADULTS (CONTINUED)

	WOMEN REFERENCE RANGE	MILDLY ABNORMAL	MODERATELY ABNORMAL	SEVERELY ABNORMAL	MEN REFERENCE RANGE	MILDLY ABNORMAL	MODERATELY ABNORMAL	SEVERELY ABNORMAL
LA area, cm²	<20	20–30	30–40	≥41	<20	20–30	30–40	≥41
LA volume, mL	22–52	53–62	63–72	≥73	18–58	59–68	69–78	≥79
LA volume/BSA, mL/m²	16–28	29–33	34–39	≥40	16–28	29–33	34–39	≥40
Aortic stenosis, classification of severity								
Aortic jet velocity, m/s		2.6–2.9	3.0–4.0	>4.0		2.6–2.9	3.0–4.0	>4.0
Mean gradient, mmHg		<20	20–40	>40		<20	20–40	>40
Valve area, cm²		>1.5	1.0–1.5	<1.0		>1.5	1.0–1.5	<1.0
Indexed valve area, cm²/m²		>0.85	0.60–0.85	<0.6		>0.85	0.60–0.85	<0.6
Velocity ratio		>0.50	0.25–0.50	<0.25		>0.50	0.25–0.50	<0.25
Mitral stenosis, classification of severity								
Valve area, cm²		>1.5	1.0–1.5	<1.0		>1.5	1.0–1.5	<1.0
Mean gradient, mmHg		<5	5–10	>10		<5	5–10	>10
Pulmonary artery pressure, mmHg		<30	30–50	>50		<30	30–50	>50
Aortic regurgitation, indices of severity								
Vena contracta width, cm		<0.30	0.30–0.60	≥0.60		<0.30	0.30–0.60	≥0.60
Jet width/LVOT width, %		<25	25–64	≥65		<25	25–64	≥65
Jet CSA/LVOT CSA, %		<5	5–59	≥60		<5	5–59	≥60
Regurgitant volume, mL/beat		<30	30–59	≥60		<30	30–59	≥60
Regurgitant fraction, %		<30	30–49	≥50		<30	30–49	≥50
Effective regurgitant orifice area, cm²		<0.10	0.10–0.29	≥0.30		<0.10	0.10–0.29	≥0.30
Mitral regurgitation, indices of severity								
Vena contracta width, cm		<0.30	0.30–0.69	≥0.70		<0.30	0.30–0.69	≥0.70
Regurgitant volume, mL/beat		<30	30–59	≥60		<30	30–59	≥60
Regurgitant fraction, %		<30	30–49	≥50		<30	30–49	≥50
Effective regurgitant orifice area, cm²		<0.20	0.20–0.39	≥0.40		<0.20	0.20–0.39	≥0.40

Abbreviations: BSA, body surface area; CSA, cross-sectional area; LA, left atrium; LVOT, left ventricular outflow tract; RA, right atrium; RV, right ventricle; RVOT, right ventricular outflow tract; 2D, 2-dimensional.

Source: Values adapted from: American Society of Echocardiography, Guidelines and Standards. *http://www.asecho.org/i4a/pages/index.cfm?pageid=3317.* Accessed Feb 23, 2010.

TABLE 13

SUMMARY OF VALUES USEFUL IN PULMONARY PHYSIOLOGY

	SYMBOL	TYPICAL VALUES	
		MAN AGED 40, 75 kg, 175 cm TALL	WOMAN AGED 40, 60 kg, 160 cm TALL
Pulmonary Mechanics			
Spirometry—volume-time curves			
Forced vital capacity	FVC	5.0 L	3.4 L
Forced expiratory volume in 1 s	FEV_1	4.0 L	2.8 L
FEV_1/FVC	$FEV_1\%$	80%	78%
Maximal midexpiratory flow rate	MMEF (FEF 25–75)	4.1 L/s	3.2 L/s
Maximal expiratory flow rate	MEFR (FEF 200–1200)	9.0 L/s	6.1 L/s
Spirometry—flow-volume curves			
Maximal expiratory flow at 50% of expired vital capacity	V_{max} 50 (FEF 50%)	5.0 L/s	4.0 L/s
Maximal expiratory flow at 75% of expired vital capacity	V_{max} 75 (FEF 75%)	2.1 L/s	2.0 L/s
Resistance to airflow:			
Pulmonary resistance	RL (R_L)	<3.0 $(cmH_2O/s)/L$	
Airway resistance	Raw	<2.5 $(cmH_2O/s)/L$	
Specific conductance	SGaw	>0.13 cmH_2O/s	
Pulmonary compliance			
Static recoil pressure at total lung capacity	Pst TLC	$25 \pm 5\ cmH_2O$	
Compliance of lungs (static)	CL	0.2 L cmH_2O	
Compliance of lungs and thorax	C(L + T)	0.1 L cmH_2O	
Dynamic compliance of 20 breaths per minute	C dyn 20	$0.25 \pm 0.05\ L/cmH_2O$	
Maximal static respiratory pressures:			
Maximal inspiratory pressure	MIP	>110 cmH_2O	>70 cmH_2O
Maximal expiratory pressure	MEP	>200 cmH_2O	>140 cmH_2O
Lung Volumes			
Total lung capacity	TLC	6.9 L	4.9 L
Functional residual capacity	FRC	3.3 L	2.6 L
Residual volume	RV	1.9 L	1.5 L
Inspiratory capacity	IC	3.7 L	2.3 L
Expiratory reserve volume	ERV	1.4 L	1.1 L
Vital capacity	VC	5.0 L	3.4 L
Gas Exchange (Sea Level)			
Arterial O_2 tension	Pa_{O_2}	12.7 ± 0.7 kPa (95 ± 5 mmHg)	
Arterial CO_2 tension	Pa_{CO_2}	5.3 ± 0.3 kPa (40 ± 2 mmHg)	
Arterial O_2 saturation	Sa_{O_2}	0.97 ± 0.02 ($97 \pm 2\%$)	
Arterial blood pH	pH	7.40 ± 0.02	
Arterial bicarbonate	HCO_3^-	24 + 2 meq/L	
Base excess	BE	0 ± 2 meq/L	
Diffusing capacity for carbon monoxide (single breath)	DL_{CO}	37 mL CO/min/mmHg 27 mL CO/min/mmHg	
Dead space volume	V_D	2 mL/kg body wt	
Physiologic dead space; dead space-tidal volume ratio	V_D/V_T		
Rest		≤35% V_T	
Exercise		≤20% V_T	
Alveolar-arterial difference for O_2	P(A − a)$_{O_2}$	≤2.7 kPa ≤20 kPa (≤24 mmHg)	

Source: Based on: AH Morris et al: *Clinical Pulmonary Function Testing. A Manual of Uniform Laboratory Procedures*, 2nd ed. Salt Lake City, Utah, Intermountain Thoracic Society, 1984.

TABLE 14

GASTROINTESTINAL TESTS

TEST	RESULTS	
	SI UNITS	CONVENTIONAL UNITS
Absorption tests		
D-Xylose: after overnight fast, 25 g xylose given in oral aqueous solution		
Urine, collected for following 5 h	25% of ingested dose	25% of ingested dose
Serum, 2 h after dose	2.0–3.5 mmol/L	30–52 mg/dL
Vitamin A: a fasting blood specimen is obtained and 200,000 units of vitamin A in oil is given orally	Serum level should rise to twice fasting level in 3–5 h	Serum level should rise to twice fasting level in 3–5 h
Bentiromide test (pancreatic function): 500 mg bentiromide (chymex) orally; *p*-aminobenzoic acid (PABA) measured		
Plasma		>3.6 (±1.1) µg/mL at 90 min
Urine	>50% recovered in 6 h	>50% recovered in 6 h
Gastric juice		
Volume		
24 h	2–3 L	2–3 L
Nocturnal	600–700 mL	600–700 mL
Basal, fasting	30–70 mL/h	30–70 mL/h
Reaction		
pH	1.6–1.8	1.6–1.8
Titratable acidity of fasting juice	4–9 µmol/s	15–35 meq/h
Acid output		
Basal		
Females (mean ± 1 SD)	0.6 ± 0.5 µmol/s	2.0 ± 1.8 meq/h
Males (mean ± 1 SD)	0.8 ± 0.6 µmol/s	3.0 ± 2.0 meq/h
Maximal (after SC histamine acid phosphate, 0.004 mg/kg body weight, and preceded by 50 mg promethazine, or after betazole, 1.7 mg/kg body weight, or pentagastrin, 6 µg/kg body weight)		
Females (mean ± 1 SD)	4.4 ± 1.4 µmol/s	16 ± 5 meq/h
Males (mean ± 1 SD)	6.4 ± 1.4 µmol/s	23 ± 5 meq/h
Basal acid output/maximal acid output ratio	≤0.6	≤0.6
Gastrin, serum	0–200 µg/L	0–200 pg/mL
Secretin test (pancreatic exocrine function): 1 unit/kg body weight, IV		
Volume (pancreatic juice) in 80 min	>2.0 mL/kg	>2.0 mL/kg
Bicarbonate concentration	>80 mmol/L	>80 meq/L
Bicarbonate output in 30 min	>10 mmol	>10 meq

TABLE 15

BODY FLUIDS AND OTHER MASS DATA

	REFERENCE RANGE	
	SI UNITS	CONVENTIONAL UNITS
Ascitic fluid: Body fluid		
Total volume (lean) of body weight	50% (in obese) to 70%	
Intracellular	30–40% of body weight	
Extracellular	20–30% of body weight	
Blood		
Total volume		
Males	69 mL/kg body weight	
Females	65 mL/kg body weight	
Plasma volume		
Males	39 mL/kg body weight	
Females	40 mL/kg body weight	
Red blood cell volume		
Males	30 mL/kg body weight	1.15–1.21 L/m^2 of body surface area
Females	25 mL/kg body weight	0.95–1.00 L/m^2 of body surface area
Body mass index	18.5–24.9 kg/m^2	18.5–24.9 kg/m^2

TABLE 16

RADIATION-DERIVED UNITS

QUANTITY	MEASURES	OLD UNIT	SI UNIT	SPECIAL NAME FOR SI UNIT (ABBREVIATION)	CONVERSION
Activity	Rate of radioactive decay	curie (Ci)	Disintegrations per second (dps)	becquerel (Bq)	1 Ci = 3.7 × 10^{10} Bq 1 mCi = 37 MBq 1 Bq = 2.703 × 10^{-11} Ci
Exposure	Amount of ionizations produced in dry air by x-rays or gamma rays, per unit of mass	roentgen (R)	Coulomb per kilogram (C/kg)	none	1 C/kg = 3876 R 1 R = 2.58 × 10^{-4} C/kg 1 mR = 258 pC/kg
Air kerma	Sum of initial energies of charged particles liberated by ionizing radiation in air, per unit of mass	rad	Joule per kilogram (J/kg)	gray (Gy)	1 Gy = 100 rad 1 rad = 0.01 Gy 1 mrad = 10 µGy
Absorbed dose	Energy deposited per unit of mass in a medium, e.g., an organ/tissue	rad	Joule per kilogram (J/kg)	gray (Gy)	1 Gy = 100 rad 1 rad = 0.01 Gy 1 mrad = 10 µGy
Equivalent dose	Energy deposited per unit of mass in a medium, e.g., an organ/tissue, weighted to reflect type(s) of radiation	rem	Joule per kilogram (J/kg)	sievert (Sv)	1 Sv = 100 rem 1 rem = 0.01 Sv 1 mrem = 10 µSv
Effective dose	Energy deposited per unit of mass in a reference individual, doubly weighted to reflect type(s) of radiation and organ(s) irradiated	rem	Joule per kilogram (J/kg)	sievert (Sv)	1 Sv = 100 rem 1 rem = 0.01 Sv 1 mrem = 10 µSv

ᴀᴄᴋɴᴏᴡʟᴇᴅɢᴍᴇɴᴛs

The contributions of Drs. Daniel J. Fink, Patrick M. Sluss, James L. Januzzi, and Kent B. Lewandrowski to this chapter in previous editions of Harrison's Principles of Internal Medicine are gratefully acknowledged. We also express our gratitude to Drs. Amudha Palanisamy and Scott Fink for careful review of tables and helpful suggestions.

APPENDIX

Laboratory Values of Clinical Importance

REVIEW AND SELF-ASSESSMENT[a]

Charles Wiener ■ **Cynthia D. Brown** ■ **Anna R. Hemnes**

QUESTIONS

DIRECTIONS: Choose the **one best** response to each question.

1. A 62-year-old man presents to his physician complaining of shortness of breath. All of the following findings are consistent with left ventricular dysfunction as a cause of the patient's dyspnea EXCEPT:

A. Feeling of chest tightness
B. Nocturnal dyspnea
C. Orthopnea
D. Pulsus paradoxus greater than 10 mmHg
E. Sensation of air hunger

2. A 48-year-old man is evaluated for hypoxia of unknown etiology. He recently has noticed shortness of breath that is worse with exertion and in the upright position. It is relieved with lying down. On physical examination, he is visibly dyspneic with minimal exertion. He is noted to have a resting oxygen saturation of 89% on room air. When lying down, his oxygen saturation increases to 93%. His pulmonary examination shows no wheezes or crackles. His cardiac examination findings are normal without murmur. His chest radiograph reports a possible 1-cm lung nodule in the right lower lobe. On 100% oxygen and in the upright position, the patient has an oxygen saturation of 90%. What is the most likely cause of the patient's hypoxia?

A. Circulatory hypoxia
B. Hypoventilation
C. Intracardiac right-to-left shunting
D. Intrapulmonary right-to-left shunting
E. Ventilation–perfusion mismatch

3. A patient is evaluated in the emergency department for peripheral cyanosis. All of the following are potential etiologies EXCEPT:

A. Cold exposure
B. Deep venous thrombosis

3. (*Continued*)
C. Methemoglobinemia
D. Peripheral vascular disease
E. Raynaud's phenomenon

4. A 35-year-old woman is seen in clinic for evaluation of dyspnea. Which of the following physical findings would fit the diagnosis of idiopathic pulmonary arterial hypertension?

A. Elevated neck veins, normal S_1 and S_2, II/VI diastolic blowing murmur heard at the right upper sternal border
B. Elevated neck veins; singular, loud S_2; II/VI systolic murmur left lower sternal border
C. Elevated neck veins; loud, fixed, split S_2; III/VI systolic murmur left lower sternal border
D. Elevated neck veins, expiratory splitting of S_2, II/VI harsh systolic murmur left upper sternal border
E. Elevated neck veins, barrel chest, prolonged expiratory phase

5. A 75-year-old woman with widely metastatic non–small cell lung cancer is admitted to the intensive care unit with a systolic blood pressure of 73/25 mmHg. She presented complaining of fatigue and worsening dyspnea over the last 3–5 days. Her physical examination shows elevated neck veins. Chest radiograph shows a massive, water bottle–shaped heart shadow and no new pulmonary infiltrates. Which of the following additional findings is most likely present on physical examination?

A. Fall in systolic blood pressure greater than 10 mmHg with inspiration
B. Lack of fall of the jugular venous pressure with inspiration
C. Late diastolic murmur with opening snap
D. Pulsus parvus et tardus
E. Slow y-descent of jugular venous pressure tracing

---

[a]Questions and answers were taken from Wiener C et al (eds): *Harrison's Principles of Internal Medicine Self-Assessment and Board Review*, 18th ed. New York: McGraw-Hill, 2012.

6. A 78-year-old man is admitted to the intensive care unit with decompensated heart failure. He has long-standing ischemic cardiomyopathy. Electrocardiogram (ECG) shows atrial fibrillation and left bundle branch block. Chest radiograph shows cardiomegaly and bilateral alveolar infiltrates with Kerley's B-lines. Which of the following is least likely to be present on physical examination?

A. Fourth heart sound
B. Irregular heart rate
C. Pulsus alternans
D. Reversed splitting of the second heart sound
E. Third heart sound

7. A 45-year-old man is admitted to the intensive care unit with symptoms of congestive heart failure. He is addicted to heroin and cocaine and uses both drugs daily via injection. His blood cultures have yielded methicillin-sensitive *Staphylococcus aureus* in four of four bottles within 12 hours. His vital signs show a blood pressure of 110/40 mmHg and a heart rate of 132 beats/min. There is a IV/VI diastolic murmur heard along the left sternal border. A schematic representation of the carotid pulsation is shown in **Figure 7**. What is the most likely cause of the patient's murmur?

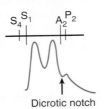

$S_4 \, S_1$ $A_2 \, P_2$

Dicrotic notch

FIGURE 7

A. Aortic regurgitation
B. Aortic stenosis
C. Mitral stenosis
D. Mitral regurgitation
E. Tricuspid regurgitation

8. A 72-year-old man seeks evaluation for leg pain with ambulation. He describes the pain as an aching to crampy pain in the muscles of his thighs. The pain subsides within minutes of resting. On rare occasions, he has noted numbness of his right foot at rest, and pain in his right leg has woken him at night. He has a history of hypertension and cerebrovascular disease. Four years previously, he had a transient ischemic attack and underwent right carotid endarterectomy. He currently takes aspirin, irbesartan, hydrochlorothiazide, and atenolol on a daily basis. On examination, he is noted to have diminished dorsalis pedis

8. (*Continued*)
and posterior tibial pulses bilaterally. The right dorsal pedis pulse is faint. There is loss of hair in the distal extremities. Capillary refill is approximately 5 seconds in the right foot and 3 seconds in the left foot. Which of the following findings would be suggestive of critical ischemia of the right foot?

A. Ankle-brachial index less than 0.3
B. Ankle-brachial index less than 0.9
C. Ankle-brachial index greater than 1.2
D. Lack of palpable dorsalis pedis pulse
E. Presence of pitting edema of the extremities

9. A 24-year-old man is referred to cardiology after an episode of syncope while playing basketball. He has no recollection of the event, but he was told that he collapsed while running. He awakened lying on the ground and suffered multiple contusions as a result of the fall. He has always been an active individual but recently has developed some chest pain with exertion that has caused him to restrict his activity. His father died at age 44 while rock climbing. He believes his father's cause of death was sudden cardiac death and recalls being told his father had an enlarged heart. On examination, the patient has a III/VI mid-systolic crescendo-decrescendo murmur. His electrocardiogram shows evidence of left ventricular hypertrophy. You suspect hypertrophic cardiomyopathy as the cause of the patient's heart disease. Which of the following maneuvers would be expected to cause an increase in the loudness of the murmur?

A. Hand-grip exercise
B. Squatting
C. Standing
D. Valsalva maneuver
E. A and B
F. C and D

10. An 18-year-old college freshman is being evaluated for a heart murmur heard at health screening. She reports an active lifestyle, no past medical history, and no cardiac symptoms. She has a mid-systolic murmur that follows a nonejection sound and crescendos with S_2. The murmur duration is greater when going from supine to standing and decreases when squatting. The murmur is heard best along the lower left sternal border and apex. Her electrocardiogram is normal. Which of the following is the most likely condition causing the murmur?

A. Aortic stenosis
B. Hypertrophic obstructive cardiomyopathy

10. (*Continued*)
    C. Mitral valve prolapse
    D. Pulmonic stenosis
    E. Tricuspid regurgitation

11. Which of the following characteristics makes a heart murmur more likely to be caused by tricuspid regurgitation than mitral regurgitation?

    A. Decreased intensity with amyl nitrate
    B. Inaudible A_2 at the apex
    C. Prominent c-v wave in jugular pulse
    D. Onset signaled by a mid-systolic click
    E. Wide splitting of S_2

12. You are examining a 25-year-old patient in clinic who came in for a routine examination. Cardiac auscultation reveals a second heart sound that is split and does not vary with respiration. There is also a grade 2–3 mid-systolic murmur at the midsternal border. Which of the following is most likely?

    A. Atrial septal defect
    B. Hypertrophic obstructive cardiomyopathy
    C. Left bundle branch block
    D. Normal physiology
    E. Pulmonary hypertension

13. Left bundle branch block is indicative of which of the following sets of conditions?

    A. Atrial septal defect, coronary heart disease, aortic valve disease
    B. Coronary heart disease, aortic valve disease, hypertensive heart disease
    C. Coronary heart disease, aortic valve disease, pulmonary hypertension
    D. Pulmonary embolism, cardiomyopathy, hypertensive heart disease
    E. Pulmonary hypertension, pulmonary embolism, mitral stenosis

14. A 57-year-old man with long-standing ischemic cardiomyopathy is seen in the clinic for a routine visit. He reports good compliance with his diuretic regimen, but has seen his weight fall about 2 kg since his last visit. Routine chemistries are drawn and show a potassium value of 2.0 meq/L. The patient is referred to the emergency department for repletion of potassium. Which of the following is likely to be found on ECG before administration of potassium?

    A. Diminution of P wave amplitude
    B. Osborne waves

14. (*Continued*)
    C. Prolongation of QT interval
    D. Prominent U waves
    E. Scooped ST segments

15. A 55-year-old woman from El Salvador is seen in the emergency department because of gradual onset of dyspnea on exertion. She denies chest pain, cough, wheezing, sputum, or fever. Her chest radiograph is notable for large pulmonary arteries and left atrial enlargement, but no parenchymal infiltrate. ECG shows a tall R in lead V_1 and right axis deviation. Which of the following is most likely to be found on her echocardiography?

    A. Aortic regurgitation
    B. Aortic stenosis
    C. Low left ventricular ejection fraction
    D. Mitral stenosis
    E. Tricuspid stenosis

16. A 29-year-old woman is in the intensive care unit with rhabdomyolysis due to compartment syndrome of the lower extremities after a car accident. Her clinical course has been complicated by acute renal failure and severe pain. She has undergone fasciotomies and is admitted to the intensive care unit. An ECG is obtained (shown in **Figure 16**). What is the most appropriate course of action at this point?

    A. 18-lead ECG
    B. Coronary catheterization
    C. Hemodialysis
    D. Intravenous fluids and a loop diuretic
    E. Ventilation/perfusion imaging

17. Acute hyperkalemia is associated with which of the following electrocardiographic changes?

    A. Decrease in the PR interval
    B. Prolongation of the ST segment
    C. Prominent U waves
    D. QRS widening
    E. T-wave flattening

18. The ECG shown below (**Figure 18**) was most likely obtained from which of the following patients?

    A. A 33-year-old female with acute-onset severe headache, disorientation, and intraventricular blood on head CT scan
    B. A 42-year-old male with sudden-onset chest pain while playing tennis

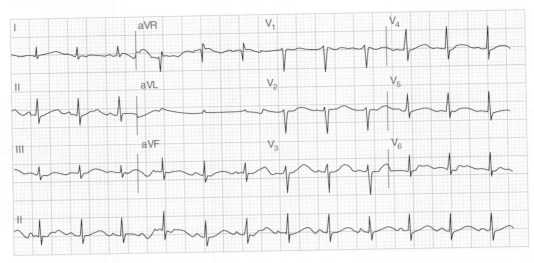

FIGURE 16

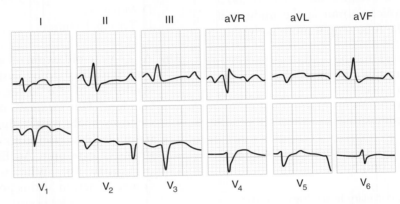

FIGURE 18

18. (*Continued*)
   C. A 54-year-old female with a long history of smoking and 2 days of increasing shortness of breath and wheezing
   D. A 64-year-old female with end-stage renal insufficiency who missed dialysis for the last 4 days
   E. A 78-year-old male with syncope, delayed carotid upstrokes, and a harsh systolic murmur in the right second intercostal space

19. You are evaluating a new patient in your clinic who has brought in the ECG shown below (**Figure 19**) to the visit. The ECG was performed on the patient 2 weeks ago. What complaint do you expect to elicit from the patient?

   A. Angina
   B. Hemoptysis
   C. Paroxysmal nocturnal dyspnea
   D. Pleuritic chest pain
   E. Tachypalpitations

20. All the following ECG findings are suggestive of left ventricular hypertrophy EXCEPT:

   A. (S in V_1 + R in V_5 or V_6) greater than 35 mm
   B. R in aVL greater than 11 mm
   C. R in aVF greater than 20 mm
   D. (R in I + S in III) greater than 25 mm
   E. R in aVR greater than 8 mm

21. Based on the electrocardiogram below (**Figure 21**), treating which condition might specifically improve this patient's tachycardia?

   A. Anemia
   B. Chronic obstructive pulmonary disease (COPD)
   C. Myocardial ischemia
   D. Pain

22. A 75-year-old man is undergoing routine cardiac catheterization for evaluation of stable angina that has not responded to medical therapy. He is inquiring about the risks associated with the procedure. Which of

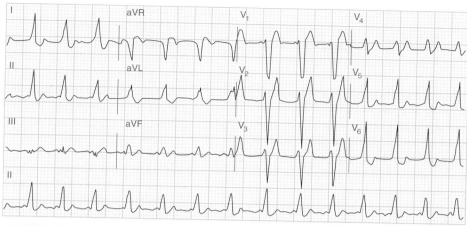

FIGURE 19

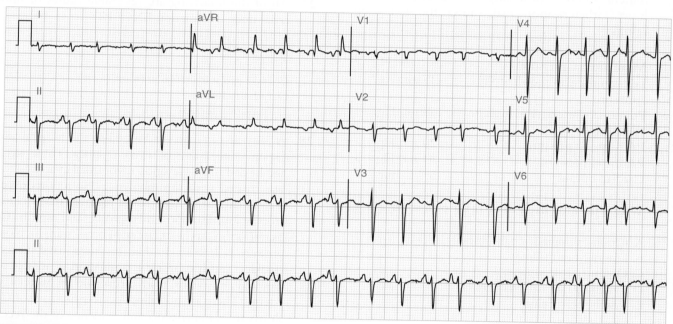

FIGURE 21

22. (*Continued*)

the following is the most common complication of cardiac catheterization and coronary angiography?

A. Acute renal failure
B. Bradyarrhythmias
C. Myocardial infarction
D. Tachyarrhythmias
E. Vascular access site bleeding

23. Which of the following patients is an appropriate candidate for right heart catheterization?

A. A 54-year-old woman with dyspnea of unclear etiology; a loud, fixed split second heart sound; normal chest radiograph; and evidence of bidirectional shunt across her interatrial septum

23. (*Continued*)

B. A 54-year-old man with an episode of sustained monomorphic ventricular tachycardia while at the casino terminated with bystander defibrillation. After arrival in the emergency department, the patient is hemodynamically stable.
C. A 63-year-old woman with a history of tobacco abuse, hypercholesterolemia, and type 2 diabetes mellitus with chest pain at rest, a normal ECG, and mild elevation in serum troponin value
D. A 66-year-old man with a history of diabetes and hypercholesterolemia brought to the emergency department with 1 hour of substernal chest pain and shortness of breath. His blood pressure is 95/60 mmHg with a heart rate of 115 beats/min. An ECG shows a new left bundle branch block since his prior ECG 1 month ago.

23. (*Continued*)

E. A 79-year-old man seen in the cardiology clinic for evaluation of severe aortic stenosis found on echocardiography performed for evaluation of dyspnea

24. A 55-year-old woman is undergoing evaluation of dyspnea on exertion. She has a history of hypertension since age 32 and is also obese with a body mass index (BMI) of 44 kg/m². Her pulmonary function tests show mild restrictive lung disease. An echocardiogram shows a thickened left-ventricular wall, left-ventricular ejection fraction of 70%, and findings suggestive of pulmonary hypertension with an estimated right-ventricular systolic pressure of 55 mmHg, but the echocardiogram is technically difficult and of poor quality. She undergoes a right heart catheterization that shows the following results:

Mean arterial pressure	110 mmHg
Left-ventricular end-diastolic pressure	25 mmHg
Pulmonary artery (PA) systolic pressure	48 mmHg
PA diastolic pressure	20 mmHg
PA mean pressure	34 mmHg
Cardiac output	5.9 L/min

What is the most likely cause of the patient's dyspnea?

A. Chronic thromboembolic disease
B. Diastolic heart failure
C. Obstructive sleep apnea
D. Pulmonary arterial hypertension
E. Systolic heart failure

25. Which of the following is a risk factor for the development of thromboembolism in patients with the tachycardia-bradycardia variant of sick sinus syndrome?

A. Age greater than 50 years
B. Atrial enlargement
C. Diabetes mellitus
D. Prothrombin 20210 mutation
E. None of the above; there is no increased risk of thromboembolism with the tachycardia-bradycardia variant of sick sinus syndrome.

26. A 38-year-old man is evaluated for the recent onset of feeling fatigued. He is a busy executive and active triathlete. He competed a challenging course 1 week earlier without difficulty but feels tired at other times. Laboratory examination, including hematocrit

26. (*Continued*)

and TSH, are unremarkable. Because his wife reports occasional snoring, a sleep study is recommended. There are no notable apneas, but ECG monitoring during the night shows sinus bradycardia. His heart rate varies between 42 and 56 while sleeping. His resting heart rate while awake is 65–72 beats/min. Which of the following is the most appropriate management for his bradycardia?

A. Carotid sinus massage
B. Intermittent nocturnal wakening
C. Measurement of free T_4
D. No specific therapy
E. Referral for pacemaker placement

27. All of the following are reversible causes of sinoatrial node dysfunction EXCEPT:

A. Hypothermia
B. Hypothyroidism
C. Increased intracranial pressure
D. Lithium toxicity
E. Radiation therapy

28. A 58-year-old man is admitted to the hospital after experiencing 2 days of severe dyspnea. Three weeks ago he had an ST elevation myocardial infarction that was treated with thrombolytics. He reports excellent adherence to his medical regimen that includes atorvastatin, lisinopril, metoprolol, and aspirin. On examination, his heart rate is 44 beats/min, his blood pressure is 100/45 mmHg, his lungs have bilateral crackles, and his cardiac examination is notable for elevated neck veins, bradycardia, and 2+ bilateral leg edema. There are no gallops or new murmurs. ECG shows sinus bradycardia and evidence of the recent infarct, but no acute changes. Which of the following is the most appropriate next management step?

A. Begin dopamine
B. Hold metoprolol
C. Measure TSH
D. Refer for pacemaker placement
E. Refer for urgent coronary angiography

29. A 23-year-old college student home for the summer is evaluated in the emergency department for dizziness that began within the last 3 days. He reports a rash on his right leg that looked like a target several days ago, but is otherwise healthy. Physical examination shows bradycardia at 40 beats/min and blood pressure of 88/42 mmHg; oxygen saturation is normal. His examination is otherwise unremarkable except for a bulls-eye rash over the right upper thigh.

29. (*Continued*)
ECG shows third-degree AV block. Which of the following laboratory studies is most likely to reveal the etiology of his signs and symptoms?

A. ANA
B. HLA B27 testing
C. *Borrelia burgdorferi* ELISA
D. RPR
E. SCL-70

30. In the tracing below (**Figure 30**), what type of conduction abnormality is present and where in the conduction pathway is the block usually found?

A. First-degree AV block; intranodal
B. Second-degree AV block type 1; intranodal
C. Second-degree AV block type 2; infranodal
D. Second-degree AV block type 2; intranodal

31. A 47-year-old woman with a history of tobacco abuse and ulcerative colitis is evaluated for intermittent palpitations. She reports that for the last 6 months every 2–4 days she notes a sensation of her heart "flip-flopping" in her chest for approximately 5 minutes. She has not noted any precipitating factors and has not felt lightheaded or had chest pains with these episodes. Her physical examination is normal. A resting ECG reveals sinus rhythm and no abnormalities. Aside from checking serum electrolytes, which of the following is the most appropriate testing?

A. Abdominal CT with oral and IV contrast
B. Event monitor
C. Holter monitor
D. Reassurance with no further testing needed
E. Referral for EP study

32. After further testing, the patient in question 31 is found to have several episodes of atrial premature contractions. Which of the following statements regarding the dysrhythmia in this patient is true?

A. Atrial premature contractions are less common than ventricular premature contractions on extended ECG monitoring.

32. (*Continued*)
B. Echocardiography is indicated to determine if structural heart disease is present.
C. Metoprolol should be initiated for symptom control.
D. The patient should be reassured that this is not a dangerous condition and does not require further evaluation.
E. The patient should undergo a stress test to determine if ischemia is present.

33. A 55-year-old man with end-stage COPD is admitted to the intensive care unit with an exacerbation of his obstructive lung disease. Because of hypercarbic respiratory failure, he is intubated and placed on assist-control mechanical ventilation. Despite aggressive sedation, his ventilator alarms several times that peak inspiratory pressures are high. The physician is called to the bedside to evaluate tachycardia. Examination is notable for a blood pressure of 112/68 mmHg and heart rate of 180 beats/min. Cardiac examination shows a regular rhythm, but no other abnormality. Breath sounds are decreased on the right. ECG shows narrow complex tachycardia. With carotid sinus massage, the heart rate transiently drops to 130 beats/min, but then returns to 180 beats/min. Which of the following is the most appropriate next step in management?

A. Adenosine 25-mg IV push
B. Amiodarone 200-mg IV push
C. Chest radiograph
D. Metoprolol 5-mg IV push
E. Sedation followed by cardioversion

34. All of the following are risk factors for stroke in a patient with atrial fibrillation EXCEPT:

A. Diabetes mellitus
B. History of congestive heart failure
C. History of stroke
D. Hypertension
E. Left atrial size greater than 4.0 cm

35. Which of the following statements regarding restoration of sinus rhythm after atrial fibrillation is true?

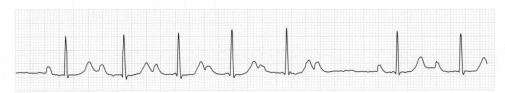

FIGURE 30

35. (*Continued*)

A. Dofetilide may be safely started on an outpatient basis.

B. In patients who are treated with pharmacotherapy and are found to be in sinus rhythm, a prolonged Holter monitor should be worn to determine if anticoagulation could be safely stopped.

C. Patients who have pharmacologically maintained sinus rhythm after atrial fibrillation have improved survival compared with patients who are treated with rate control and anticoagulation.

D. Recurrence of atrial fibrillation is uncommon when pharmacotherapy is used to maintain sinus rhythm.

36. A 57-year-old woman with a history of a surgically corrected atrial septal defect in childhood presents to the emergency department with palpitations for 3 days. She is found to have a heart rate of 153 beats/min and blood pressure of 128/75 mmHg, and an ECG shows atrial flutter. An echocardiogram demonstrates moderate right and left atrial dilation, postoperative changes from her surgery, and normal left and right ventricular function. Which of the following is true?

A. Anticoagulation with dabigatran should be initiated.

B. If a transesophageal echocardiogram does not demonstrate left atrial thrombus, she may be cardioverted without anticoagulation.

C. Intravenous heparin should be started immediately.

D. She should be immediately cardioverted.

E. Transthoracic echocardiogram is adequate to rule out the presence of left atrial thrombus.

37. A patient presents with palpitations and shortness of breath for 6 hours. In the emergency department waiting room an ECG is performed (shown in **Figure 37**). Which of the following is most likely to be found on physical examination?

A. Diffuse abdominal tenderness with guarding

B. Diffuse expiratory polyphonic wheezing with poor air movement and hyperinflation

C. Left ventricular heave and third heart sound

D. Supraclavicular lymphadenopathy

E. Vesicular rash over right T_5 dermatome

38. A 43-year-old woman is seen in the emergency department after sudden onset of palpitations 30 minutes prior to her visit. She was seated at her work computer when the symptoms began. Aside from low back pain, she is otherwise healthy. In triage, her heart rate is 178 beats/min, and blood pressure is 98/56 mmHg with normal oxygen saturation. On physical examination, she has a "frog sign" in her neck and tachycardia, but is otherwise normal. ECG shows a narrow complex tachycardia without identifiable P waves. Which of the following is the most appropriate first step to manage her tachycardia?

A. 5 mg metoprolol IV

B. 6 mg adenosine IV

C. 10 mg verapamil IV

D. Carotid sinus massage

E. DC cardioversion using 100 J

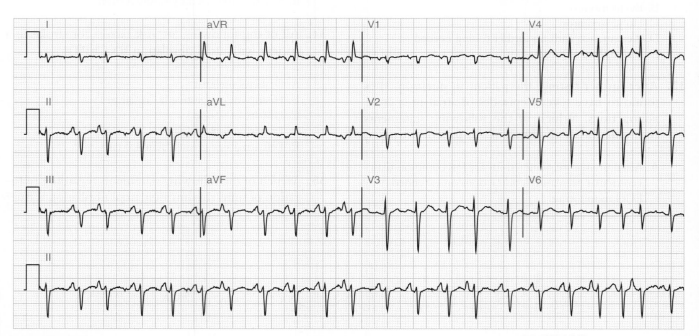

FIGURE 37

39. A 37-year-old man who is healthy aside from a prior knee surgery is evaluated in the emergency department for palpitations that developed suddenly while eating dinner. He is found to have a heart rate of 193 beats/min, blood pressure of 92/52 mmHg, and normal oxygen saturation. His physical examination is normal aside from tachycardia and mild diaphoresis. An ECG obtained before his knee surgery shows delta waves in the early precordial leads. His current ECG shows wide complex tachycardia. Which of the following therapies is contraindicated for treatment of his tachyarrhythmia?

   A. Adenosine
   B. Carotid sinus massage
   C. DC cardioversion
   D. Digoxin
   E. Metoprolol

40. In an ECG with wide complex tachycardia, which of the following clues most strongly supports the diagnosis of ventricular tachycardia?

   A. Atrial-ventricular dissociation
   B. Classic right bundle branch block pattern
   C. Irregularly irregular rhythm with changing QRS complexes
   D. QRS duration greater than 120 milliseconds
   E. Slowing of rate with carotid sinus massage

41. A 40-year-old male with diabetes and schizophrenia is started on antibiotic therapy for chronic osteomyelitis in the hospital. His osteomyelitis has developed just under an ulcer where he has been injecting heroin. He is found suddenly unresponsive by the nursing staff. His electrocardiogram is

41. (*Continued*)
   shown in **Figure 41**. The most likely cause of this rhythm is which of the following substances?

   A. Furosemide
   B. Metronidazole
   C. Droperidol
   D. Metformin
   E. Heroin

42. Normal sinus rhythm is restored with electrical cardioversion in the patient in question 41. A 12-lead electrocardiogram is notable for a prolonged QT interval. Besides stopping the offending drug, the most appropriate management for this rhythm disturbance should include intravenous administration of which of the following?

   A. Amiodarone
   B. Lidocaine
   C. Magnesium
   D. Metoprolol
   E. Potassium

43. You are caring for a patient with heart rate–related angina. With minor elevations in heart rate, the patient has anginal symptoms that impact his quality of life. On review of a 24-hour Holter monitor, it appears that the patient has sinus tachycardia at the time of his symptoms. What is the mechanism for this patient's arrhythmia?

   A. Delayed afterdepolarizations
   B. Early afterdepolarizations
   C. Increased automaticity
   D. Reentry pathway

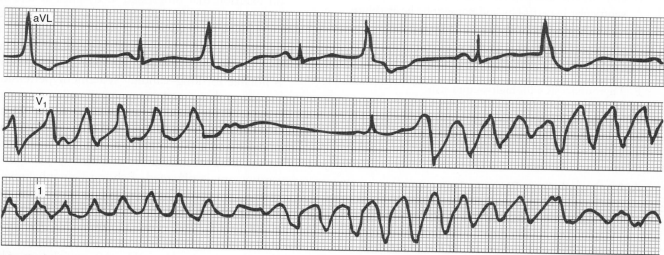

FIGURE 41

44. Where are the most common drivers of atrial fibrillation anatomically located?

A. Left atrial appendage
B. Mitral annulus
C. Pulmonary vein orifice
D. Sinus venosus
E. Sinus node

45. Symptoms of atrial fibrillation vary dramatically from patient to patient. A patient with which of the following clinical conditions will likely be the most symptomatic (e.g., short of breath) if the patient develops atrial fibrillation?

A. Acute alcohol intoxication
B. Hypertrophic cardiomyopathy
C. Hyperthyroidism
D. Hypothermia
E. Postoperative after thoracotomy

46. A 47-year-old postmenopausal woman is seen for onset of severe dyspnea over the last few weeks. She reports no preceding chest pain, cough, sputum, or fever, though she does report leg swelling. Physical examination is notable for a blood pressure of 145/78 mmHg and heart rate of 123 beats/min. Exophthalmos is present as well as bilateral inspiratory crackles occupying approximately one-third of the lower chest; neck vein distention; normal cardiac rhythm, though tachycardia is present; and a third heart sound with no murmur. Bilateral lower extremity edema and a fine hand tremor are also present. Which of the following is the most likely pathophysiologic explanation for her heart failure?

A. Anemia with high-output state
B. Chronic systemic hypertension with resultant left ventricular hypertrophy and nonsystolic heart failure
C. Hemochromatosis with subsequent restrictive cardiomyopathy
D. Myocardial infarction with depressed left ventricular systolic function
E. Thyrotoxicosis with high-output state

47. Which of the following statements is true regarding measurement of plasma BNP to diagnose heart failure?

A. An elevated plasma BNP in a dyspneic patient confirms the diagnosis of left heart failure.
B. In the presence of renal failure, BNP levels are suppressed even when heart failure is present.
C. Plasma BNP levels may be falsely low in patients with obesity and heart failure.

47. (*Continued*)
D. Serial measurement of BNP in the therapy of decompensated heart failure should be used to guide therapy.
E. All of the above are true.

48. A 64-year-old man with an ischemic cardiomyopathy, ejection fraction 35%, and stage C heart failure is seen in the cardiology clinic for evaluation of his disease status. The patient reports a regular exercise regimen of walking on the treadmill several times weekly and occasional exacerbations of his leg edema that he manages with an extra dose of furosemide. He has never been hospitalized for heart failure. His current medical regimen includes lisinopril, aspirin, furosemide, atorvastatin, digoxin, spironolactone, and metoprolol. He is interested in stopping medications because of their expense. Which of the following statements is true regarding his medical regimen?

A. ACE inhibition therapy has not been shown to improve heart failure symptoms.
B. Beta blocker therapy in this patient may be exacerbating his occasional need for extra furosemide and therefore should be stopped.
C. He should be switched from spironolactone to eplerenone for improved efficacy, as seen in patients with EF less than 35%.
D. If digoxin is withdrawn, he will likely have worsening symptoms.
E. If he is intolerant to lisinopril because of cough, it would be reasonable to switch him to an angiotensin-receptor blocker.

49. A 78-year-old slender woman is seen in the emergency department after several weeks of dyspnea on exertion that progressed to dyspnea at rest following a summer cookout where she consumed multiple pickled vegetables. She also complains of leg swelling, orthopnea, and occasionally awakening at night with dyspnea. Her past medical history is notable for long-standing systemic hypertension, uterine prolapse, and an anxiety disorder. Examination confirms the presence of heart failure with a laterally displaced and sustained point of maximum impulse and a fourth heart sound. She is admitted to the hospital and given diuretics, and an echocardiogram is obtained. Echocardiography reveals severe left ventricular hypertrophy with an ejection fraction of 70%, but there are no focal wall motion abnormalities, and aortic and mitral valvular function is intact. Her right ventricular systolic pressure is estimated to be 45 mmHg. After resolution of her

49. (*Continued*)

heart failure symptoms with diuresis, the patient is ready for discharge. Which of the following medications have been shown to improve mortality in patients with heart failure with preserved ejection fraction and should be included in this patient's regimen?

A. Digoxin
B. Lisinopril
C. Metoprolol
D. Sildenafil
E. None of the above

50. A 68-year-old man with a history of myocardial infarction and congestive heart failure is comfortable at rest. However, when walking to his car he develops dyspnea, fatigue, and sometimes palpitations. He must rest for several minutes before these symptoms resolve. His New York Heart Association classification is which of the following?

A. Class I
B. Class II
C. Class III
D. Class IV

51. The husband of a 68-year-old woman with congestive heart failure is concerned because his wife appears to stop breathing for periods of time when she sleeps. He has noticed that she stops breathing for approximately 10 seconds and then follows this with a similar period of hyperventilation. This does not wake her from sleep. She does not snore. She feels well rested in the morning but is very dyspneic with even mild activity. What is your next step in management?

A. Electroencephalography
B. Maximize heart failure management
C. Nasal continuous positive airway pressure (CPAP) during sleep
D. Obtain a sleep study
E. Prescribe bronchodilators

52. A 53-year-old man undergoes cardiac transplantation for end-stage ischemic cardiomyopathy due to an underlying familial hypercholesterolemic disorder. His donor was a 23-year-old motor vehicle accident victim. The patient does well for the first 3 years after transplantation with only a single episode of acute rejection. He shows good compliance with his immunosuppression regimen, which includes prednisone and sirolimus.

52. (*Continued*)

He is evaluated at a routine follow-up visit and reports that he has developed dyspnea on exertion. His pulmonary function tests are unchanged and a chest radiograph is normal. He undergoes right and left heart catheterization with biopsy of the transplanted heart. Severe, diffuse, concentric, and longitudinal coronary artery disease is found on coronary angiography, and histology shows no evidence of acute rejection. Which of the following statements is true regarding the coronary atherosclerosis found in this patient?

A. No immunosuppressive regimen has been shown to have a lower incidence of coronary atherosclerosis after cardiac transplantation.
B. The coronary atherosclerosis is most likely immunologic injury of the vascular endothelium in the transplanted organ.
C. The current coronary atherosclerosis after cardiac transplant is likely due to atherosclerosis present prior to transplantation.
D. The patient's underlying cholesterol disorder did not predispose him to recurrent coronary atherosclerosis after cardiac transplantation.
E. Therapy with statins has not been associated with a reduced incidence of this complication of transplantation.

53. Which of the following is a known complication of ventricular assist device placement in patients with end-stage heart failure?

A. Cerebrovascular accident
B. Infection of insertion site
C. Mechanical device failure
D. Thromboembolism
E. All of the above

54. All of the following are potential complications of an atrial septal defect in adults EXCEPT:

A. Air embolism from a central venous catheter
B. Arterial oxygen desaturation with exertion
C. Embolic cerebrovascular accident
D. Pulmonary arterial hypertension
E. Unstable angina

55. A 32-year-old woman is seen by her primary care physician clinic for routine follow-up of her hypothyroidism. She also has a history of complex congenital heart disease with a partially corrected VSD with predominantly right to left shunt across her patch. She is doing well and is able to work in janitorial services without severe dyspnea. She denies

55. (*Continued*)

any heart failure or neurologic symptoms, but does have a peripheral oxygen saturation of 78%. A routine CBC is drawn and shows a hematocrit of 65%. Which of the following is the most appropriate management of her elevated hematocrit?

A. Begin oxygen therapy
B. Check co-oximetry on arterial blood gas sample
C. Check serum erythropoietin level
D. Expectant waiting
E. Refer to hematology for phlebotomy

56. A 43-year-old man recently was found to have an asymptomatic atrial septal defect that was closed using a percutaneous patch 1 month ago without complication. He is undergoing a root canal at the dentist next week and calls his primary care office to determine if antibiotic prophylaxis is indicated. Which of the following statements is true regarding antibiotic prophylaxis in this patient?

A. Because he had only simple congenital heart disease, no prophylaxis is indicated.
B. Because the lesion is corrected, no prophylaxis is indicated.
C. He should avoid potentially bacteremic dental procedures unless no other alternative is available.
D. Routine antibiotic prophylaxis is indicated for bacteremic dental procedures, particularly if the patch is less than 6 months old.
E. Routine antibiotic prophylaxis is indicated for bacteremic dental procedures whenever foreign material is present.

57. A 20-year-old man undergoes a physical examination with chest radiograph for enrollment in the military. He has had a normal childhood without any major illness. There is no history of sinusitis, pneumonia, or chronic respiratory disease. Chest radiograph shows dextrocardia. On closer physical examination, a spleen tip is palpable on the right of the abdomen and the liver can be percussed on the left. Which of the following is true regarding his condition?

A. He is likely to have aortic stenosis.
B. He is likely to have aspermia.
C. He is likely to have an atrial septal defect.
D. He is likely to have a ventriculoseptal defect.
E. He is likely to otherwise be normal.

58. A 24-year-old male seeks medical attention for the recent onset of headaches. The headaches are described as "pounding" and occur during the day and night. He has had minimal relief with acetaminophen.

58. (*Continued*)

Physical examination is notable for a blood pressure of 185/115 mmHg in the right arm, a heart rate of 70 beats/min, arterioventricular (AV) nicking on funduscopic examination, normal jugular veins and carotid arteries, a pressure-loaded PMI with an apical S_4, no abdominal bruits, and reduced pulses in both lower extremities. Review of symptoms is positive only for leg fatigue with exertion. Additional measurement of blood pressure reveals the following:

Right arm	185/115
Left arm	188/113
Right thigh	100/60
Left thigh	102/58

Which of the following diagnostic studies is most likely to demonstrate the cause of the headaches?

A. MRI of the head
B. MRI of the kidney
C. MRI of the thorax
D. 24-hour urinary 5-HIAA
E. 24-hour urinary free cortisol

59. The patient described in question 58 is most likely to have which of the following associated cardiac abnormalities?

A. Bicuspid aortic valve
B. Mitral stenosis
C. Preexcitation syndrome
D. Right bundle branch block
E. Tricuspid atresia

60. Mitral stenosis is frequently complicated by pulmonary hypertension. Which of the following is a cause of pulmonary hypertension in mitral stenosis?

A. Interstitial edema in the walls of small pulmonary vessels
B. Passive transmission of elevated left atrial pressure
C. Obliterative changes in the pulmonary vascular bed
D. Pulmonary arteriolar constriction
E. All of the above

61. A 58-year-old man with a history of systemic hypertension, hyperlipidemia, and tobacco abuse is admitted to the intensive care unit with crushing chest pain associated with ST-segment elevation and small precordial Q waves. Because his symptoms have been present for 36 hours, he is not a candidate for thrombolytics. On admission to the ICU, his systemic blood pressure is 123/67 mmHg, heart rate is 67 beats/min after beta blockade, and

61. (*Continued*)

his oxygenation saturation is 93% on 2L nasal cannula. The remainder of the physical examination is normal. He is treated with lisinopril, aspirin, heparin, and metoprolol. Before transfer can be arranged to a tertiary center, the patient reports extreme dyspnea. He is found to be diaphoretic and to have a heart rate of 80 beats/min, blood pressure of 84/56 mmHg, and oxygen saturation of 93% on 100% non-rebreather. His lungs have bilateral crackles throughout, and neck veins are moderately elevated. ECG is unchanged. Chest radiograph shows new alveolar infiltrates in the right lung greater than the left. Which of the following is a likely finding on physical examination?

A. A fourth heart sound, III/VI systolic murmur heard best at the apex with a "cooing" quality that radiates to the axilla

B. A right ventricular heave, loud second heart sound, III/VI murmur increasing with inspiration at the right lower sternal border

C. A third heart sound, III/VI crescendo-decrescendo murmur heard best at the right upper sternal border

D. Diffuse urticarial reaction, wheezing on pulmonary examination

E. Mucosal edema, finger swelling, stridor

62. Which of the following is the most appropriate next step in therapy for the patient in question 61?

A. Aerosolized albuterol

B. Initiation of norepinephrine infusion

C. Intravenous infusion of nitroprusside

D. Intravenous methylprednisolone

E. Placement of intraaortic balloon pump

63. A 26-year-old healthy woman is seen for a pap smear at a routine office visit. She feels well and has no complaints and no significant past medical history. Her internist performs a full physical examination and a mid-systolic click is heard. No murmur or gallop is present. She is concerned about this finding. Which of the following statements is true regarding her examination finding?

A. In most patients with this disorder, an underlying cause such as a heritable disorder of connective tissue is found.

B. Infective endocarditis prophylaxis is indicated for dental procedures potentially associated with bacteremia.

C. Most patients are asymptomatic from this lesion and will remain so their entire life.

D. She should begin therapy with aspirin 325 mg po daily.

E. This disorder cannot be visualized on echocardiography.

64. A 78-year-old man is evaluated for the onset of dyspnea on exertion. He has a long history of tobacco abuse, obesity, and diabetes mellitus. His current medications include metformin, aspirin, and occasional ibuprofen. On physical examination his peripheral pulses show a delayed peak and he has a prominent left ventricular heave. He is in a regular rhythm with a IV/VI mid-systolic murmur that is loudest at the base of the heart and radiates to the carotid arteries. A fourth heart sound is present. Echocardiography confirms severe aortic stenosis without other valvular lesions. Which of the following most likely contributed to the development of his cardiac lesion?

A. Congenital bicuspid aortic valve

B. Diabetes mellitus

C. Occult rheumatic heart disease

D. Underlying connective tissue disease

E. None of the above

65. A 63-year-old man presents with new-onset exertional syncope and is found to have aortic stenosis. In counseling the patient, you tell him that your therapeutic recommendation is based on the observation that untreated patients with his presentation have a predicted average life span of:

A. 5 years

B. 4 years

C. 3 years

D. 2 years

E. 1 year

66. Which of the following physical examination findings suggests severe aortic regurgitation?

A. Corrigan's pulse

B. Pulsus alternans

C. Pulsus bigeminus

D. Pulsus paradoxus

E. Pulsus parvus et tardus

67. A 41-year-old Somali woman is seen in clinic for onset of hemoptysis in the sixth month of her pregnancy. This is her fourth pregnancy and the others were uncomplicated, though she was 35 years old at the birth of her last child. Prior to this, she had been healthy. She reports mild dyspnea beginning at the fourth month of her pregnancy with onset of mild leg swelling shortly thereafter that she attributed to her pregnancy. The dyspnea has become severe, and she is now limited to walking around her house. She began to cough small amounts of bloody sputum 5 days ago. She had neither fever

67. (*Continued*)

nor purulent sputum and has not responded to a course of antibiotics prescribed by her obstetrician. Physical examination is notable for a normal temperature, heart rate of 110 beats/min, blood pressure of 108/60 mmHg, and oxygen saturation of 91% on room air. No source of bleeding is seen in her nares or oropharynx. Her lungs have diffuse crackles, and cardiac examination shows moderately elevated neck veins, a regular heart rhythm, a loud second heart sound, and a low-pitched diastolic rumble heard best at the apex. The abdomen has a gravid uterus, and 1+ lower extremity edema is present. Which of the following is most likely to demonstrate the cause of her symptoms?

A. Bronchoscopy
B. Chest CT with contrast
C. Echocardiogram
D. Right heart catheterization
E. Upper airway inspection by an otolaryngologist

68. In the patient described in question 67, which of the following should be prescribed at her visit to alleviate her symptoms?

A. Benazepril
B. Digoxin
C. Furosemide
D. Heparin
E. Levofloxacin

69. Which of the following patients with echocardiographic evidence of significant mitral regurgitation has the best indication for surgery with the most favorable likelihood of a positive outcome?

A. A 52-year-old man with an ejection fraction of 25%, NYHA class III symptoms, and a left-ventricular end-systolic dimension of 60 mm
B. A 54-year-old man with an ejection fraction of 30%, NYHA class II symptoms, and pulmonary hypertension
C. A 63-year-old man in sinus rhythm without symptoms, an ejection fraction of 65%, and a normal right heart catheterization
D. A 66-year-old man without symptoms, an ejection fraction of 50%, and left-ventricular end-systolic dimension of 45 mm
E. A 72-year-old asymptomatic woman with newly discovered atrial fibrillation, ejection fraction of 60%, and end-systolic dimension of 35 mm

70. All of the following are potential causes of tricuspid regurgitation EXCEPT:

A. Congenital heart disease
B. Infective endocarditis
C. Inferior wall myocardial infarction
D. Pulmonary arterial hypertension
E. Rheumatic heart disease
F. All of the above will cause tricuspid regurgitation

71. All the following are true about cardiac valve replacement EXCEPT:

A. Bioprosthetic valve replacement is preferred to mechanical valve replacement in younger patients because of the superior durability of the valve.
B. Bioprosthetic valves have a low incidence of thromboembolic complications.
C. The risk of thrombosis with mechanical valve replacement is higher in the mitral position than in the aortic position.
D. Mechanical valves are relatively contraindicated in patients who wish to become pregnant.
E. Double-disk tilting mechanical prosthetic valves offer superior hemodynamic characteristics over single-disk tilting valves.

72. Which of the following infectious agents have been associated with the development of inflammatory myocarditis?

A. Coxsackievirus
B. Diphtheria
C. Q fever
D. *Trypanosoma cruzi*
E. All of the above

73. All of the following are risk factors for the development of peripartum cardiomyopathy EXCEPT:

A. Advanced maternal age
B. Malnutrition
C. Primiparity
D. Twin pregnancy
E. Use of tocolytics

74. A 67-year-old man with a long history of alcohol abuse presents with findings consistent with left ventricular failure including pulmonary edema and congestion. He undergoes right heart catheterization and left heart catheterization. No significant coronary artery disease is found. Which of the following right heart catheterization numbers (see **Table 74**) would support a diagnosis of beriberi heart disease?

74. (*Continued*)

TABLE 74					
	RIGHT ATRIAL PRESSURE (mmHg)	**MEAN PULMONARY ARTERIAL PRESSURE (mmHg)**	**PULMONARY CAPILLARY WEDGE PRESSURE (mmHg)**	**CARDIAC OUTPUT (L/min)**	**SYSTEMIC VASCULAR RESISTANCE (dyn • s/cm^5)**
A.	18	30	24	12	610
B.	4	15	12	6	1050
C.	24	35	28	3	2140
D.	24	48	8	5	2140
E.	2	10	2	4	2140

75. A 20-year-old basketball player is seen for evaluation prior to beginning another season of competitive sports. A harsh systolic murmur is heard at the left lower sternal border. Which of the following maneuvers will enhance this murmur if hypertrophic cardiomyopathy is the underlying cause?

A. Hand grip
B. Leaning forward while sitting
C. Lying left side down
D. Squatting
E. Valsalva maneuver

76. A 62-year-old woman presents to your office with dyspnea of 4 months duration. She has a history of monoclonal gammopathy of unclear significance (MGUS) and has been lost to follow-up for the past 5 years. She is able to do only minimal activity before she has to rest but has no symptoms at rest. She has developed orthopnea but denies paroxysmal nocturnal dyspnea. She complains of fatigue, lightheadedness, and lower extremity swelling. On examination, blood pressure is 110/90 mmHg and heart rate is 94 beats/min. Jugular venous pressure is elevated, and the jugular venous wave does not fall with inspiration. An S_3 and S_4 are present, as well as a mitral regurgitation murmur. The point of maximal impulse is not displaced. Abdominal examination is significant for ascites and a large, tender, pulsatile liver. Chest radiograph shows bilateral pulmonary edema. An electrocardiogram shows an old left bundle branch block. Which clinical features differentiate constrictive pericarditis from restrictive cardiomyopathy?

A. Elevated jugular venous pressure
B. Kussmaul's sign
C. Narrow pulse pressure
D. Pulsatile liver
E. None of the above

77. You are evaluating a new patient in the clinic. The 25-year-old patient was diagnosed with "heart failure" in another state and has since relocated. He has New York Heart Association class II symptoms and denies angina. He presents for evaluation and management. The patient has been wheelchair bound for many years and has severe scoliosis. He has no family history of hyperlipidemia. His physical examination is notable for bilateral lung crackles, an S_3, and no cyanosis. An electrocardiogram (ECG) is obtained in the clinic and shows tall R waves in V_1 and V_2 with deep Qs in V_5 and V_6. An echocardiogram reports severe global left ventricular dysfunction with reduced ejection fraction. What is the most likely diagnosis?

A. Amyotrophic lateral sclerosis
B. Atrial septal defect
C. Chronic thromboembolic disease
D. Duchenne's muscular dystrophy
E. Ischemic cardiomyopathy

78. A 35-year-old woman with a history of tobacco abuse presents to the emergency department because of severe chest pain radiating to both arms. The pain began 8 hours ago and is worse with inspiration. She has been unable to lie down as this markedly exacerbates the pain, but she feels better with sitting forward. Examination is notable for a heart rate of 96 beats/min, blood pressure of 145/78 mmHg, and oxygen saturation of 98%. Lungs are clear and a friction rub with three components is audible and is best heard at the left lower sternal border. Which of the following are most likely to be found on her ECG?

A. Diffusely inverted T waves in the precordial leads
B. PR elevation in leads II, III, and aVF
C. Sinus tachycardia

78. (*Continued*)

    D. ST-segment elevation in I, aVL, and V_2–V_6 with upward concavity and reciprocal depressions in aVR

    E. ST-segment elevation V_1–V_6 with convex curvature and reciprocal depressions in aVR

79. Which of the following statements is true regarding pulsus paradoxus?

    A. It consists of a greater than 15 mmHg increase in systolic arterial pressure with inspiration.

    B. It may be found in patients with severe obstructive lung disease.

    C. It is the reversal of a normal phenomenon during inspiration.

    D. It results from right ventricular distention during expiration resulting in compression of the left ventricular volume and subsequent reduction in systolic pulse pressure.

    E. All of the above are true.

80. Which of the following are features of Beck's triad in cardiac tamponade?

    A. Hypotension, electrical alternans, prominent x-descent in neck veins

    B. Hypotension, muffled heart sounds, electrical alternans

    C. Hypotension, muffled heart sounds, jugular venous distention

    D. Kussmaul's sign, hypotension, muffled heart sounds

    E. Muffled heart sounds, hypotension, friction rub

81. A 35-year-old woman is admitted to the hospital with malaise, weight gain, increasing abdominal girth, and edema. The symptoms began about 3 months ago and gradually progressed. The patient reports an increase in waist size of approximately 15 cm. The swelling in her legs has gotten increasingly worse such that she now feels her thighs are swollen as well. She has dyspnea on exertion and two-pillow orthopnea. She has a past history of Hodgkin's disease diagnosed at age 18. She was treated at that time with chemotherapy and mediastinal irradiation. On physical examination, she has temporal wasting and appears chronically ill. Her current weight is 96 kg, which reflects an increase of 11 kg over the past 3 months. Her vital signs are normal. Her jugular venous pressure is approximately 16 cm, and the neck veins do not collapse on inspiration. Heart sounds are distant. There is a third heart sound heard shortly after aortic valve closure. The sound is short and abrupt and is heard best at the apex. The liver is enlarged and pulsatile. Ascites is present.

81. (*Continued*)

There is pitting edema extending throughout the lower extremities and onto the abdominal wall. Echocardiogram shows pericardial thickening, dilatation of the inferior vena cava and hepatic veins, and abrupt cessation of ventricular filling in early diastole. Ejection fraction is 65%. What is the best approach for treatment of this patient?

    A. Aggressive diuresis only

    B. Cardiac transplantation

    C. Mitral valve replacement

    D. Pericardial resection

    E. Pericardiocentesis

82. A 19-year-old previously healthy hockey player is defending the goal when he is hit in the left chest with a hockey puck. He immediately collapses to the ice. His coach runs to his side and finds him unresponsive and without a pulse. Which of the following is most likely responsible for this syndrome?

    A. Aortic rupture

    B. Cardiac tamponade

    C. Commotio cordis

    D. Hypertrophic cardiomyopathy

    E. Tension pneumothorax

83. Which of the following is the most common cause of native valve infective endocarditis in the community?

    A. Coagulase-negative staphylococci

    B. Coagulase-positive staphylococci

    C. Enterococci

    D. Fastidious gram-negative coccobacilli

    E. Non-enterococcal streptococci

84. All of the following are minor criteria in the Duke criteria for the clinical diagnosis of infective endocarditis EXCEPT:

    A. Immunologic phenomena (glomerulonephritis, Osler nodes, Roth spots)

    B. New valvular regurgitation on transthoracic echocardiogram

    C. Predisposing condition (heart condition, intravenous drug use)

    D. Temperature >38.0°C

    E. Vascular phenomena (arterial emboli, septic pulmonary emboli, Janeway lesions, and so on)

85. Which of the following patients should receive antibiotic prophylaxis to prevent infective endocarditis?

85. (*Continued*)

A. A 23-year-old woman with known mitral valve prolapse undergoing a gingival surgery

B. A 24-year-old woman who had an atrial septal defect completely corrected 22 years ago who is undergoing elective cystoscopy for painless hematuria

C. A 30-year-old man with a history of intravenous drug use and prior endocarditis undergoing operative drainage of a prostatic abscess

D. A 45-year-old man who received a prosthetic mitral valve 5 years ago undergoing routine dental cleaning

E. A 63-year-old woman who received a prosthetic aortic valve 2 years ago undergoing screening colonoscopy

86. A 38-year-old homeless man presents to the emergency department with a transient ischemic attack characterized by a facial droop and left arm weakness lasting 20 minutes and left upper quadrant pain. He reports intermittent subjective fevers, diaphoresis, and chills for the past 2 weeks. He has had no recent travel or contact with animals. He has taken no recent antibiotics. Physical examination reveals a slightly distressed man with disheveled appearance. His temperature is 38.2°C, heart rate is 90 beats/min, and blood pressure is 127/74 mmHg. He has poor dentition. Cardiac examination reveals an early diastolic murmur over the left third intercostal space. His spleen is tender and 2 cm descended below the costal margin. He has tender painful red nodules on the tips of the third finger of his right hand and on the fourth finger of his left hand that are new. He has nits evident on his clothes consistent with body louse infection. His white blood cell count is 14,500/μL with 5% band forms and 93% polymorphonuclear cells. Blood cultures are drawn followed by empirical vancomycin therapy. These cultures remain negative for growth 5 days later. He remains febrile but hemodynamically stable but does develop a new lesion on his toe similar to those on his fingers on hospital day 3. A transthoracic echocardiogram reveals a 1-cm mobile vegetation on the cusp of his aortic valve and moderate aortic regurgitation. A CT scan of the abdomen shows an enlarged spleen with wedge-shaped splenic and renal infarctions. What test should be sent to confirm the most likely diagnosis?

A. *Bartonella* serology

B. Epstein-Barr virus (EBV) heterophile antibody

C. HIV polymerase chain reaction (PCR)

D. Peripheral blood smear

E. Q fever serology

87. In a patient with bacterial endocarditis, which of the following echocardiographic lesions is most likely to lead to embolization?

A. 5-mm mitral valve vegetation

B. 5-mm tricuspid valve vegetation

C. 11-mm aortic valve vegetation

D. 11-mm mitral valve vegetation

E. 11-mm tricuspid valve vegetation

88. A patient is admitted with fevers, malaise, and diffuse joint pains. His initial blood cultures reveal methicillin-resistant *Staphylococcus aureus* (MRSA) in all culture bottles. He has no arthritis on examination, and his renal function is normal. Echocardiogram shows a 5-mm vegetation on the aortic valve. He is initiated on IV vancomycin at 15 mg/kg every 12 hours. Four days later, the patient remains febrile, and cultures remain positive for MRSA. In addition to a search for embolic foci of infection, which of the following changes would you make to his treatment regimen?

A. No change

B. Add gentamicin

C. Add rifampin

D. Check the vancomycin serum peak and trough levels and consider tid dosing

E. Discontinue vancomycin, start daptomycin

89. Which of the following is the most common clinical presentation of acute rheumatic fever (ARF)?

A. Carditis

B. Chorea

C. Erythema marginatum

D. Polyarthritis

E. Subcutaneous nodules

90. A 19-year-old recent immigrant from Ethiopia comes to your clinic to establish primary care. She currently feels well. Her past medical history is notable for a recent admission to the hospital for new-onset atrial fibrillation. As a child in Ethiopia, she developed an illness that caused uncontrolled flailing of her limbs and tongue lasting approximately 1 month. She also has had three episodes of migratory large-joint arthritis during her adolescence that resolved with pills that she received from the pharmacy. She is currently taking metoprolol and warfarin and has no known drug allergies. Physical examination reveals an irregularly irregular heartbeat with normal blood pressure. Her point of maximal impulse (PMI) is most prominent at the

90. (*Continued*)

midclavicular line and is normal in size. An early diastolic rumble and a 3/6 holosystolic murmur are heard at the apex. A soft early diastolic murmur is also heard at the left third intercostal space. You refer her to a cardiologist for evaluation of valve replacement and echocardiography. What other intervention might you consider at this time?

A. Glucocorticoids
B. Daily aspirin
C. Daily doxycycline
D. Monthly penicillin G injections
E. Penicillin G injections as needed for all sore throats

91. All of the following statements regarding cardiogenic shock are true EXCEPT:

A. Approximately 80% of cases of cardiogenic shock complicating acute myocardial infarction are attributable to acute severe mitral regurgitation.
B. Cardiogenic shock is more common in ST-segment elevation than non–ST-segment elevation myocardial infarction.
C. Cardiogenic shock is uncommon in inferior wall myocardial infarction.
D. Cardiogenic shock may occur in the absence of significant coronary stenosis.
E. Pulmonary capillary wedge pressure is elevated in cardiogenic shock.

92. Aortic counterpulsation with an intraaortic balloon pump has which of the following as an advantage over therapy with infused vasopressors or inotropes in a patient with acute ST-segment elevation myocardial infarction and cardiogenic shock?

A. Increased heart rate
B. Increased left ventricular afterload
C. Lower diastolic blood pressure
D. Not contraindicated in acute aortic regurgitation
E. Reduced myocardial oxygen consumption

93. Which of the following is the most common electrical mechanism to explain sudden cardiac death?

A. Asystole
B. Bradycardia
C. Pulseless electrical activity (PEA)
D. Pulseless ventricular tachycardia (PVT)
E. Ventricular fibrillation

94. All of the following statements regarding successful resuscitation from sudden cardiac death are true EXCEPT:

94. (*Continued*)

A. Advanced age does not affect the likelihood of immediate resuscitation, only the probability of hospital discharge.
B. After out-of-hospital cardiac arrest, survival rates are approximately 25% if defibrillation is administered after 5 minutes.
C. If the initial rhythm in an out-of-hospital cardiac arrest is pulseless ventricular tachycardia, the patient has a higher probability of survival than asystole.
D. Prompt CPR followed by prompt defibrillation improves outcomes in all settings.
E. The probability of survival from cardiac arrest is higher if the event takes place in a public setting than at home.

95. A 32-year-old man is evaluated at a routine clinic visit for coronary risk factors. He is healthy and reports no tobacco use, his systemic blood pressure is normal, and he does not have diabetes. His family history is notable for high cholesterol in his mother and maternal grandparents. Physical examination shows tendon xanthomas. A fasting cholesterol is notable for a low-density lipoprotein cholesterol (LDL-C) of 387 mg/dL. Which of the following is the most likely genetic disorder affecting this individual?

A. Autosomal dominant hypercholesterolemia
B. Familial defective apoB-100
C. Familial hepatic lipase deficiency
D. Familial hypercholesterolemia
E. Lipoprotein lipase deficiency

96. All of the following are potential causes of elevated LDL EXCEPT:

A. Anorexia nervosa
B. Cirrhosis
C. Hypothyroidism
D. Nephrotic syndrome
E. Thiazide diuretics

97. A 16-year-old male is brought to your clinic by his parents due to concern about his weight. He has not seen a physician for many years. He states that he has gained weight due to inactivity and that he is less active because of exertional chest pain. He takes no medications. He was adopted and his parents do not know the medical history of his biological parents. Physical examination is notable for stage 1 hypertension and body mass index of 30 kg/m². He has xanthomas on his hands, heels, and buttocks. Laboratory testing shows a low-density

97. (*Continued*)

lipoprotein (LDL) of 210 mg/dL, creatinine of 0.7 mg/dL, total bilirubin of 3.1 mg/dL, haptoglobin below 6 mg/dL, and a glycosylated hemoglobin of 6.7%. You suspect a hereditary lipoproteinemia due to the clinical and laboratory findings. Which test would be diagnostic of the primary lipoprotein disorder in this patient?

A. Congo red staining of xanthoma biopsy
B. CT scan of the liver
C. Family pedigree analysis
D. Gas chromatography
E. LDL receptor function in skin biopsy

98. Your 60-year-old patient with a monoclonal gammopathy of unclear significance presents for a follow-up visit and to review recent laboratory data. His creatinine is newly elevated to 2.0 mg/dL, potassium is 3.7 mg/dL, calcium is 12.2 mg/dL, low-density lipoprotein (LDL) is 202 mg/dL, and triglycerides are 209 mg/dL. On further questioning he reports 3 months of swelling around the eyes and "foamy" urine. On examination, he has anasarca. Concerned for multiple myeloma and nephrotic syndrome, you order a urine protein/creatinine ratio, which returns at 14:1. Which treatment option would be most appropriate to treat his lipid abnormalities?

A. Cholesterol ester transfer protein inhibitor
B. Dietary management
C. HMG-CoA reductase inhibitors
D. Lipid apheresis
E. Niacin and fibrates

99. A 48-year-old white man is seen in the clinic for a routine physical examination. He reports no complaints. Examination shows a blood pressure of 134/82 mmHg with a normal heart rate. BMI is 31 kg/m². The remainder of his physical examination is normal. Which of the following is true regarding lifestyle modification?

A. Brisk walking for as little as 10 minutes, 4 days per week will lower his blood pressure to within the normal range.
B. Dietary NaCl restriction of less than 6 g per day will reduce his blood pressure.
C. Lifestyle modification will have no effect on his blood pressure.
D. Reduction of alcohol consumption to three or fewer drinks per day will decrease his blood pressure.
E. Weight loss of approximately 9 kg can be expected to bring his blood pressure to within the normal limit.

100. A 46-year-old white female presents to your office with concerns about her diagnosis of hypertension 1 month previously. She asks you about her likelihood of developing complications of hypertension, including renal failure and stroke. She denies any past medical history other than hypertension and has no symptoms that suggest secondary causes. She currently is taking hydrochlorothiazide 25 mg/d. She smokes half a pack of cigarettes daily and drinks alcohol no more than once per week. Her family history is significant for hypertension in both parents. Her mother died of a cerebrovascular accident. Her father is alive but has coronary artery disease and is on hemodialysis. Her blood pressure is 138/90 mmHg. Body mass index is 23. She has no retinal exudates or other signs of hypertensive retinopathy. Her point of maximal cardiac impulse is not displaced but is sustained. Her rate and rhythm are regular and without gallops. She has good peripheral pulses. An electrocardiogram reveals an axis of −30 degrees with borderline voltage criteria for left ventricular hypertrophy. Creatinine is 1.0 mg/dL. Which of the following items in her history and physical examination is a risk factor for a poor prognosis in a patient with hypertension?

A. Family history of renal failure and cerebrovascular disease
B. Persistent elevation in blood pressure after the initiation of therapy
C. Ongoing tobacco use
D. Ongoing use of alcohol
E. Presence of left ventricular hypertrophy on ECG

101. A 28-year-old female has hypertension that is difficult to control. She was diagnosed at age 26. Since that time she has been on increasing amounts of medication. Her current regimen consists of labetalol 1000 mg bid, lisinopril 40 mg qd, clonidine 0.1 mg bid, and amlodipine 5 mg qd. On physical examination she appears to be without distress. Blood pressure is 168/100 mmHg, and heart rate is 84 beats/min. Cardiac examination is unremarkable, without rubs, gallops, or murmurs. She has good peripheral pulses and has no edema. Her physical appearance does not reveal any hirsutism, fat maldistribution, or abnormalities of genitalia. Laboratory studies reveal a potassium of 2.8 meq/dL and a serum bicarbonate of 32 meq/dL. Fasting blood glucose is 114 mg/dL. What is the likely diagnosis?

A. Congenital adrenal hyperplasia
B. Fibromuscular dysplasia
C. Cushing's syndrome

101. (*Continued*)

    D. Conn's syndrome

    E. Pheochromocytoma

102. What is the best way to diagnose this disease in question 101?

    A. Renal vein renin levels

    B. 24-hour urine collection for metanephrines

    C. Magnetic resonance imaging of the renal arteries

    D. 24-hour urine collection for cortisol

    E. Plasma aldosterone/renin ratio

103. Which of the following patients with aortic dissection or hematoma is best managed *without* surgical therapy?

    A. A 74-year-old male with a dissection involving the root of the aorta.

    B. A 45-year-old female with a dissection involving the aorta distal to the great vessel origin but cephalad to the renal arteries.

    C. A 58-year-old male with aortic dissection involving the distal aorta and the bilateral renal arteries.

    D. A 69-year-old male with an intramural hematoma within the aortic root.

    E. All of the above patients require surgical management of their aortic disease.

104. A 68-year-old male presents to your office for routine follow-up care. He reports that he is feeling well and has no complaints. His past medical history is significant for hypertension and hypercholesterolemia. He continues to smoke a pack of cigarettes daily. He is taking chlorthalidone 25 mg daily, atenolol 25 mg daily, and pravastatin 40 mg nightly. Blood pressure is 133/85 mmHg, and heart rate is 66 beats/min. Cardiac and pulmonary examinations are unremarkable. A pulsatile abdominal mass is felt just to the left of the umbilicus and measures approximately 4 cm. You confirm the diagnosis of abdominal aortic aneurysm by CT imaging. It is located infrarenally and measures 4.5 cm. All the following are true about the patient's diagnosis EXCEPT:

    A. The 5-year risk of rupture of an aneurysm of this size is 1–2%.

    B. Surgical or endovascular intervention is warranted because of the size of the aneurysm.

    C. Infrarenal endovascular stent placement is an option if the aneurysm experiences continued growth in light of the location of the aneurysm infrarenally.

104. (*Continued*)

    D. Surgical or endovascular intervention is warranted if the patient develops symptoms of recurrent abdominal or back pain.

    E. Surgical or endovascular intervention is warranted if the aneurysm expands beyond 5.5 cm.

105. A 32-year-old female is seen in the emergency department for acute shortness of breath. A helical CT shows no evidence of pulmonary embolus, but incidental note is made of dilatation of the ascending aorta to 4.3 cm. All the following are associated with this finding EXCEPT:

    A. Syphilis

    B. Takayasu's arteritis

    C. Giant cell arteritis

    D. Rheumatoid arthritis

    E. Systemic lupus erythematosus

106. A 68-year-old man with a history of coronary artery disease is seen in his primary care clinic for complaint of cough with sputum production. His care provider is concerned about pneumonia, so a chest radiograph is ordered. On the chest radiograph, the aorta appears tortuous with a widened mediastinum. A contrast-enhanced CT of the chest confirms the presence of a descending thoracic aortic aneurysm measuring 4 cm with no evidence of dissection. What is the most appropriate management of this patient?

    A. Consult interventional radiology for placement of an endovascular stent.

    B. Consult thoracic surgery for repair.

    C. No further evaluation is needed.

    D. Perform yearly contrast-enhanced chest CT and refer for surgical repair when the aneurysm size is greater than 4.5 cm.

    E. Treat with beta blockers, perform yearly contrast-enhanced chest CT, and refer for surgical repair if the aneurysm grows more than 1 cm/year.

107. A 37-year-old woman with no significant past medical history except for a childhood murmur is evaluated for severe pain of sudden onset in her right lower extremity. Examination is notable for a young, uncomfortable woman with normal vital signs except for a heart rate of 110 beats/min. Right leg has pallor distal to the right knee and is cold to the touch, and the dorsalis pedis pulse is absent. Which of the following studies is likely to diagnose the underlying reason for the patient's presentation?

    A. Angiography of right lower extremity

    B. Blood cultures

107. (*Continued*)

    C. Echocardiogram with bubble study

    D. Serum c-ANCA

    E. Venous ultrasound of right upper extremity

108. Doppler echocardiography is most useful for diagnosis of which of the following cardiac lesions?

    A. Determination of cardiac mass in a patient with an audible "plop" on examination

108. (*Continued*)

    B. Determination of left ventricular ejection fraction in a patient with a history of myocardial infarction

    C. Diagnosis of myocardial ischemia in a patient with atypical chest pain

    D. Diagnosis of pericardial effusion

    E. Diastolic filling assessment in a patient with suspected heart failure with preserved ejection fraction

ANSWERS

1. The answer is D.

(*Chap. 5*) Shortness of breath, or dyspnea, is a common presenting complaint in primary care. However, dyspnea is a complex symptom and is defined as the subjective experience of breathing discomfort that includes components of physical as well as psychosocial factors. A significant body of research has been developed regarding the language by which a patient describes dyspnea with certain factors being more common in specific diseases. Individuals with airways diseases (asthma, chronic obstructive pulmonary disease [COPD]) often describe air hunger, increased work of breathing, and the sensation of being unable to get a deep breath because of hyperinflation. In addition, individuals with asthma often complain of a tightness in the chest. Individuals with cardiac causes of dyspnea also describe chest tightness and air hunger but do not have the same sensation of being unable to draw a deep breath or have increased work of breathing. A careful history will also lead to further clues regarding the cause of dyspnea. Nocturnal dyspnea is seen in congestive heart failure or asthma, and orthopnea is reported in heart failure, diaphragmatic weakness, and asthma that is triggered by esophageal reflux. When discussing exertional dyspnea, it is important to assess if the dyspnea is chronic and progressive or episodic. Whereas episodic dyspnea is more common in myocardial ischemia and asthma, COPD and interstitial lung diseases present with a persistent dyspnea. Platypnea is a rare presentation of dyspnea in which a patient is dyspneic in the upright position and feels improved with lying flat. On physical examination of a patient with dyspnea, the physician should observe the patient's ability to speak and the use of accessory muscle or preference of the tripod position. As part of vital signs, a pulsus paradoxus may be measured with a value of greater than 10 mmHg common in asthma and COPD. Pulsus paradoxus greater than 10 mmHg may also occur in pericardial tamponade. Lung examination may demonstrate decreased diaphragmatic excursion, crackles, or wheezes that allow one to determine the cause of dyspnea. Further workup may include pulmonary function testing, chest radiography, chest CT, electrocardiography, echocardiography, or exercise testing, among others, to ascertain the cause of dyspnea.

2. The answer is D.

(*Chap. 6*) When a patient presents for evaluation of hypoxia, it is important to consider the underlying mechanism of hypoxia in order to determine the etiology. The primary causes of hypoxia are related to respiratory disease and include ventilation/perfusion (V/Q) mismatch, hypoventilation, and intrapulmonary right-to-left shunting. Causes of hypoxia outside of the respiratory system include intracardiac right-to-left shunting, high-altitude hypoxia, anemic hypoxia, circulatory hypoxia, and carbon monoxide poisoning. In this patient, the mechanism of hypoxia can be narrowed to two possibilities—intracardiac versus intrapulmonary right-to-left shunting—quite easily because the patient failed to correct his hypoxia in response to 100% oxygen. The history of platypnea and orthodeoxia is suggestive that the likely cause is intrapulmonary rather than intracardiac shunting. The finding of a possible lung nodule on chest radiographs in the lower lung fields also is supportive of a pulmonary cause of shunting through an arteriovenous malformation, which can appear as a lung nodule on chest x-ray. An intracardiac right-to-left shunt is caused by congenital cardiac malformations and Eisenmenger syndrome. If there was an intracardiac cause of shunt, the cardiac examination would be expected to demonstrate a murmur and/or evidence of pulmonary hypertension.

    V/Q mismatch is the most common cause of hypoxia and results from perfusion of areas of the lung that receive limited ventilation. Examples of V/Q mismatch include asthma, chronic obstructive pulmonary disease, and pulmonary embolus. Hypoxia caused by V/Q mismatch can be corrected with supplemental oxygen. Hypoventilation can be caused by multiple causes, including acute respiratory depression or chronic respiratory failure with elevations in $PaCO_2$. Hypoxia caused by hypoventilation is also correctable with oxygen but frequently has a normal alveolar–arterial oxygen gradient.

    Causes of hypoxia outside the respiratory system are less common. High-altitude hypoxia becomes apparent when individuals travel to elevations greater than 3000 m. Anemic hypoxia is not associated with a decrease in PaO_2, but a decrease in hemoglobin does cause decreased oxygen-carrying capacity in the blood and relative tissue hypoxia if severe. Circulatory hypoxia refers to tissue hypoxia that occurs because of a decrease cardiac output that leads to greater tissue extraction of oxygen. As a result, the venous partial pressure of oxygen is reduced, and there is an increased arterial-mixed venous oxygen gradient.

3. The answer is C.

(Chap. 6) In the evaluation of cyanosis, the first step is to differentiate central from peripheral cyanosis. In central cyanosis, because the etiology is either reduced oxygen saturation or abnormal hemoglobin, the physical findings include bluish discoloration of both mucous membranes and skin. In contrast, peripheral cyanosis is associated with normal oxygen saturation but slowing of blood flow and an increased fraction of oxygen extraction from blood; subsequently, the physical findings are present only in the skin and extremities. Mucous membranes are spared. Peripheral cyanosis is commonly caused by cold exposure with vasoconstriction in the digits. Similar physiology is found in Raynaud's phenomenon. Peripheral vascular disease and deep venous thrombosis result in slowed blood flow and increased oxygen extraction with subsequent cyanosis. Methemoglobinemia causes abnormal hemoglobin that circulates systemically. Consequently, the cyanosis associated with this disorder is systemic. Other common causes of central cyanosis include severe lung disease with hypoxemia, right-to-left intracardiac shunting, and pulmonary arteriovenous malformations.

4. The answer is B.

(Chaps. 9, 40) Pulmonary hypertension is associated with a loud second heart sound that is heard to be louder than the first heart sound at the cardiac base. In idiopathic pulmonary arterial hypertension, there is no associated congenital lesion, such as atrial septal defect (ASD). In ASD, the components of the second heart sound, aortic and pulmonic valve closure, do not alter their timing with respect to respiratory cycle and are always widely split, and thus are described as "fixed split." In idiopathic pulmonary arterial hypertension, the components of the second heart sound are nearly superimposed and loud; often there is little respiratory variation. The soft systolic murmur at the left lower sternal border of tricuspid regurgitation is nearly always present in pulmonary hypertension of all etiologies. Idiopathic pulmonary arterial hypertension, by definition, is not associated with a parenchymal lung disease such as emphysema. Patients with idiopathic pulmonary arterial hypertension should not have physical findings associated with chronic airways disease.

5. The answer is A.

(Chap. 9) The patient is very likely to have pericardial tamponade from metastatic cancer as suggested by her elevated neck veins, heart shadow shape and size, and predisposing condition. Because of the exaggerated interventricular dependence, the normal (<10 mmHg) fall in systemic blood pressure with inspiration is exaggerated (often >15 mmHg) with cardiac tamponade. This is referred to as pulsus paradoxus, though it is in fact an augmentation of a normal finding. Kussmaul's sign, or a lack of fall of the jugular venous pressure with inspiration, usually denotes a lack of compliance in the right ventricle, as seen most frequently in constrictive pericarditis, though it may be found in restrictive cardiomyopathy or massive pulmonary embolism. A rapid y-descent, which follows the peak of the v wave, of jugular venous pressure tracing is indicative of cardiac tamponade. Pulsus parvus et tardus, or small and slow arterial pulsation, is a late finding in aortic stenosis. Late diastolic murmur and opening snap is found in mitral stenosis.

6. The answer is A.

(Chap. 9) A fourth heart sound indicates left ventricular presystolic expansion and is common among patients in whom active atrial contraction is important for ventricular filling. A fourth heart sound is not found in atrial fibrillation. An irregular heart rate is characteristic of atrial fibrillation. The irregular rate is often characterized as "irregularly irregular." A third heart sound occurs during the rapid filling phase of ventricular diastole and indicates heart failure. Reversed splitting of the second heart sound occurs with left bundle branch block, as this patient has. Finally, pulsus alternans is beat-to-beat variability in pulse amplitude. It is present when only every other Korotkoff sound is audible as the cuff pressure is lowered slowly. It is thought to be due to cyclic changes in intracellular calcium and action potential duration and is associated with severe left ventricular failure.

7. The answer is A.

(Chap. 9) The presentation of this patient is consistent with the diagnosis of acute valvular dysfunction due to infective endocarditis. The presence of a widened pulse pressure and diastolic murmur heard best along the lower sternal border suggests aortic regurgitation. Panel C of Figure 9-2 shows a typical bisferiens pulse that is characteristic of aortic regurgitation. With a bisferiens pulse, there are two distinct pulsations that can be palpated with systole. The initial pulse represents an exaggerated percussion wave reflecting the increased stroke volume that occurs in aortic regurgitation, with the second peak reflecting the tidal, or anacrotic, wave.

Infective endocarditis causes loss of valvular integrity and acutely causes valvular regurgitation. Of the other options, both mitral regurgitation and tricuspid regurgitation (choice E) would cause systolic and not diastolic murmurs. A hyperkinetic pulse may occur in these conditions, particularly if associated with fever or sepsis.

With a hyperkinetic pulse the usual dichrotic notch is more pronounced, as seen in panel E of the figure. Mitral stenosis causes a diastolic murmur but is not a common lesion associated with infective endocarditis, unless underlying valvular stenosis was present prior to acquiring the infection. It is not associated with a bisferiens pulse. Aortic stenosis is associated with pulsus parvus et tardus, with a delayed and prolonged carotid upstroke as shown in panel B of the figure. Aortic stenosis has an associated harsh crescendo-decrescendo systolic murmur.

8.   The answer is A.

(Chap. 9) Peripheral arterial disease (PAD) affects 5–8% of Americans, with increasing incidence with age. Over the age of 65, the incidence of PAD rises to between 12% and 20%. The primary symptom of PAD is claudication. As this patient describes, claudication occurs with ambulation and is often described as a crampy to aching pain that is relieved with rest. On physical examination, those with PAD often have diminished peripheral pulses, delayed capillary refill, and hair loss in the distal extremities. The skin is often cool to the touch with a thin, shiny appearance. In severe PAD, pain in the extremities occurs at rest. Diagnosis of PAD can be suggested by these findings and should be documented by determination of the ankle-brachial index (ABI), as physical examination alone is insufficient to diagnose PAD. Although lack of a palpable pulse suggests critical ischemia, it is not diagnostic. To perform an ABI, blood pressures are determined in the arm and the lower extremities. Either the dorsalis pedis or posterior tibial pulses can be used. The ABI is calculated by dividing the ankle systolic pressure by the brachial systolic pressure. A resting ABI less than 0.9 is abnormal, but critical ischemia with rest pain does not occur until the ABI is less than 0.3. In individuals with heavily calcified blood vessels, the ABI can be abnormally elevated (ABI >1.2) when PAD is present. In this situation, toe pressures to determine ABI or employing imaging techniques such as MRI or arteriography should be considered. Lower extremity edema is suggestive of congestive heart failure, not PAD.

9.   The answer is F.

(Chap. 9) When a murmur of uncertain cause is identified on physical examination, a variety of physiologic maneuvers can be used to assist in the elucidation of the cause. Commonly used physiologic maneuvers include change with respiration, Valsalva maneuver, position, and exercise. In hypertrophic cardiomyopathy, there is asymmetric hypertrophy of the interventricular septum, which creates a dynamic outflow obstruction. Maneuvers that decrease left-ventricular filling will cause an increase in the intensity of the murmur, whereas those that increase left-ventricular filling will cause a decrease in the murmur. Of the interventions listed, both standing and a

Valsalva maneuver will decrease venous return and subsequently decrease left ventricular filling, resulting in an increase in the loudness of the murmur of hypertrophic cardiomyopathy. Alternatively, squatting will increase venous return and thus decrease the murmur. Maximum hand-grip exercise also will result in a decreased loudness of the murmur.

10.   The answer is C.

(Chap. 10) Mitral valve prolapse is characterized by a mid-systolic nonejection sound (click) followed by a late systolic murmur that crescendos and terminates with S_2. A decrease in venous return induced by standing will move the click closer to S_1 and increase the duration of the murmur. Squatting will increase venous return and shorten the duration of the murmur. The murmur of hypertrophic cardiomyopathy behaves in a similar fashion, but there would be no nonejection click, and left ventricular hypertrophy would be expected on electrocardiography (ECG). Aortic stenosis is best heard at the right second intercostal space radiating to the carotid and is crescendo-decrescendo in character. Congenital pulmonic stenosis is crescendo-decrescendo in character and is heard best in the second to third left intercostal space. If severe, there is a parasternal lift right ventricular overload on ECG. Tricuspid regurgitation causes a holosystolic, not mid-systolic, murmur that increases with inspiration.

11.   The answer is C.

(Chap. 10) Tricuspid regurgitation and mitral regurgitation (along with ventricular septal defect) cause holosystolic murmurs. These murmurs have their onset with S_1 and terminate at or with S_2. Whereas tricuspid regurgitation is heard best over the left sternal border, mitral regurgitation is heard best at the apex with radiation to the base or axilla. The onset of a murmur after S_1 with a nonejection sound (click) is characteristic of mitral valve prolapse. Amyl nitrate decreases the intensity of mitral regurgitation and ventricular septal defect murmurs. Tricuspid regurgitation increases with inspiration. Wide splitting of S_2 is characteristic of ventricular septal defects. Inaudible A_2 at the ventricular apex is characteristic of mitral regurgitation. Because of the incompetent tricuspid valve, the murmur of tricuspid regurgitation is associated with prominent c-v waves and a sharp y-descent in the jugular venous pulse.

12.   The answer is A.

(Chap. 10) Evaluating the splitting of the aortic (A_2) and pulmonic (P_2) components of the second heart sound (S_2) during auscultation can be diagnostically useful. In normal conditions, P_2 follows A_2, and the splitting increases during inspiration. Reversed (or paradoxical) splitting of S_2, when P_2 precedes A_2 during expiration (and they come closer together during inspiration),

is attributable to a delay in A_2 and is characteristic of severe aortic stenosis, hypertrophic obstructive cardiomyopathy, left bundle branch block, right ventricular pacing, or acute myocardial ischemia. Wide splitting of S_2 is an accentuation of the physiologic pattern usually caused by delayed pulmonic valve closing (right bundle branch block, pulmonary stenosis, pulmonary hypertension) or early aortic valve closure (severe mitral regurgitation). Fixed splitting (no respiratory variation) with the murmur described is characteristic of an atrial septal defect. This is an important finding because it may be asymptomatic until the third or fourth decade of life and, if undiagnosed, may lead to severe pulmonary hypertension and Eisenmenger syndrome.

13. The answer is B.

(Chap. 11) Left bundle branch, defined by QRS interval greater than 120 milliseconds with typical pattern in V_1 and V_6, is associated with four conditions: coronary heart disease, hypertensive heart disease, aortic valve disease, and cardiomyopathy. In all cases, the left bundle branch block is associated with increased risk of cardiovascular morbidity and mortality. These conditions share left ventricular pathology. In contrast, right bundle branch block is associated with congenital heart disease, pulmonary vascular disease, and less frequently valvular heart disease.

14. The answer is D.

(Chap. 11) The classic findings of hypokalemia are prominent U waves due to prolonged ventricular repolarization. Scooped ST segments are commonly seen with digoxin toxicity. Low P wave amplitude is found in early hyperkalemia. Prolonged QT intervals are often due to drug toxicity such as tricyclic antidepressant overdose, procainamide, quinidine disopyramide, and phenothiazines. Finally, Osborne waves, or convex elevation of the J point, are found in severe hypothermia and are due to repolarization prolongation.

15. The answer is D.

(Chaps. 11, 20, and 40) The patient presents from a country with likely low rates of treatment for childhood streptococcal infection and was subsequently at high risk for rheumatic heart disease. Her large pulmonary arteries in the absence of parenchymal infiltrates suggests pulmonary hypertension and her ECG shows right ventricular hypertrophy, characterized by a relatively tall R wave in lead V_1, or R greater than or equal to S wave. This is highly likely to be due to mitral stenosis. While aortic stenosis and regurgitation are possible causes, these are less likely. Tricuspid stenosis is not associated with right ventricular hypertrophy. Left ventricular systolic failure may cause pulmonary venous hypertension, but more commonly is associated with evidence of left heart failure on examination.

16. The answer is D.

(Chaps. 11 and 41) This ECG shows a short ST segment that is most prominent in V_2, V_3, V_4, and V_5. Hypercalcemia, by shortening the duration of repolarization, abbreviates the total time from depolarization through repolarization. This is manifested on the surface ECG by a short QT interval. In this scenario, the hypercalcemia is due to the rhabdomyolysis and renal failure. Fluids and a loop diuretic are an appropriate therapy for hypercalcemia. Hemodialysis is seldom indicated. Hemodialysis is indicated for significant hyperkalemia, which may also develop after rhabdomyolysis, manifest by "tenting" of the T waves or widening of the QRS. Classic ECG manifestations of a pulmonary embolus (S_1, Q_3, T_3 pattern) are infrequent in patients with pulmonary embolism (PE), though the changes may be seen with massive PE. There are no signs of myocardial ischemia on this ECG, which would make coronary catheterization and 18-lead ECG interpretation of low yield.

17. The answer is D.

(Chap. 11) Hyperkalemia leads to partial depolarization of cardiac cells. As a result, there is slowing of the upstroke of the action potential as well as reduced duration of repolarization. The T wave becomes peaked, the RS complex widens and may merge with the T wave (giving a sine-wave appearance), and the P wave becomes shallow or disappears. Prominent U waves are associated with hypokalemia; ST-segment prolongation is associated with hypocalcemia.

18. The answer is C.

(Chaps. 11 and 21) The ECG shows slight right axis deviation and low voltage. These changes are typical of emphysema when the thorax is hyperinflated with air and the flattened diaphragm pulls the heart inferiorly and vertically. An acute central nervous system (CNS) event such as a subarachnoid hemorrhage may cause QT prolongation with deep, wide inverted T waves. Hyperkalemia will cause peaked narrowed T waves or a wide QRS complex. Patients with hypertrophic cardiomyopathy will have left ventricular hypertrophy and widespread deep, broad Q waves.

19. The answer is E.

(Chaps. 11 and 43) This ECG tracing shows the triad of a short PR interval, wide QRS, and delta waves (seen best in leads I, II, and V_5) consistent with Wolff-Parkinson-White (WPW) syndrome. Patients with WPW syndrome are commonly diagnosed asymptomatically when an ECG is performed showing the classic findings. Symptoms are due to conduction via an accessory pathway and include tachypalpitations, lightheadedness, syncope, cardiopulmonary collapse, and sudden cardiac death. Life-threatening presentations are usually due to the development of atrial fibrillation or atrial flutter with

1:1 conduction, both of which can precipitate ventricular fibrillation. Unstable angina is mainly associated with ST-segment abnormalities, although conduction abnormalities may be seen. Pulmonary embolism, which may cause hemoptysis and pleuritic chest pain, has nonspecific ECG findings including $S_1Q_3T_3$ (acute right ventricular failure) or T-wave abnormalities.

20. The answer is E.

(Chap. 11) The limb lead aVR generally has a negative deflection, as the primary vector for ventricular depolarization is directed down and away from this lead. Therefore, in the case of left ventricular hypertrophy the negative deflection, or S wave, would be expected to be larger without an effect on the R wave. There are multiple criteria for diagnosing left ventricular hypertrophy on ECG.

21. The answer is B.

(Chaps. 11 and 43) This ECG tracing shows multifocal atrial tachycardia (MAT), right atrial overload, a superior axis, and poor R-wave progression in the precordial leads. There are varying P-wave morphologies (more than three morphologies) and P-P intervals. MAT is most commonly caused by COPD, but other conditions associated with this arrhythmia include coronary artery disease, congestive heart failure, valvular heart disease, diabetes mellitus, hypokalemia, hypomagnesemia, azotemia, postoperative state, and pulmonary embolism. Anemia, pain, and myocardial ischemia are also causes of tachycardia that should be considered when managing a new tachycardia. These states are usually associated with sinus tachycardia.

22. The answer is E.

(Chap. 13) Although myocardial infarction, stroke, and death are complications that have been reported with cardiac catheterization (all with a frequency of <0.1%), the more common complications are tachy- or bradyarrhythmias, acute renal failure, and vascular complications. Vascular access site bleeding is the most common complication of cardiac catheterization, occurring in 1.5–2% of patients. When catheterization is performed in an emergent fashion for acute myocardial infarction or for hemodynamically unstable patients, the complication rate may rise substantially.

23. The answer is A.

(Chap. 13) Although right heart catheterization is no longer routinely performed at the time of left heart catheterization, there remain important indications for this procedure. These include evaluation of unexplained dyspnea, especially when there is a suspicion of pulmonary hypertension; diagnosis of valvular heart disease such as mitral regurgitation; pericardial disease; right and/or left ventricular dysfunction, particularly for

determination of severity; diagnosis of congenital heart disease; and suspected intracardiac shunts. In this case, the patient likely has an atrial septal defect with physical examination findings of a loud, fixed split second heart sound and perhaps associated dyspnea. During right heart catheterization, the pulmonary arterial pressures will be measured to assess for pulmonary hypertension, and venous saturation will be measured at the inferior vena cava, right atrium, right ventricle, and pulmonary artery to assess for evidence of an increase in saturation suggestive of intracardiac shunt. All the other patients described would be more appropriately served with a left heart catheterization and coronary angiogram.

24. The answer is B.

(Chaps. 13 and 40) In the diagnostic algorithm for pulmonary hypertension, the right heart catheterization is important to document the presence and degree of pulmonary hypertension. The right-ventricular systolic pressure (RVSP) on echocardiography provides an estimate of pulmonary arterial pressures, but accurate determination of the RVSP relies on the presence of tricuspid regurgitation and good quality echocardiography. This patient's body habitus is prohibitive in obtaining good windows for echocardiography. Thus, a right heart catheterization is imperative for documenting pulmonary hypertension, as well as for determining the cause. The right heart catheterization demonstrates an elevated mean arterial pressure, elevated left-ventricular end-diastolic pressure (pulmonary capillary wedge pressure), and elevated mean pulmonary artery pressure. In the presence of a normal cardiac output and an elevated left-ventricular ejection fraction, this is consistent with the diagnosis of diastolic heart failure. Systolic heart failure is associated with similar indices on right heart catheterization, but left-ventricular function is depressed in systolic heart failure. The other causes listed as options are known causes of pulmonary hypertension but would not be expected to cause an increase in the left-ventricular end-diastolic pressure. Obstructive sleep apnea is usually associated only with mild elevations in pulmonary artery pressure. This patient's BMI puts her at risk for obstructive sleep apnea but would not be responsible for these right heart catheterization values. Both chronic thromboembolic disease and pulmonary arterial hypertension can cause severe elevations in the pulmonary arterial pressure but have a normal left atrial pressure.

25. The answer is B.

(Chap. 15) The tachycardia-bradycardia variant of sick sinus syndrome is associated with an increased risk of thromboembolism, particularly when similar risk factors are present that increase the risk of thromboembolism in patients with atrial fibrillation. Specific risk factors associated with highest risk include age greater than 65 years and prior history of stroke, valvular heart

disease, left ventricular dysfunction, or atrial enlargement. Patients with these risk factors should be treated with anticoagulation.

26. The answer is D.
(*Chap. 15*) Bradycardia is frequently present in trained athletes, particularly at night, where heart rates are usually between 40 and 60 beats/min. While sleep apnea can be associated with bradycardia, no apnea was found in this patient on overnight polysomnography. Other possible causes of bradycardia in this patient such as hypothyroidism have been ruled out. Measurement of free T_4 is not indicated with a normal TSH. Pacemaker insertion is not indicated for his normal physiology. Carotid sinus massage is likely to cause further bradycardia. Fatigue is likely due to his stressful job.

27. The answer is E.
(*Chap. 15*) Sinoatrial dysfunction is often divided into intrinsic disease and extrinsic disease of the node. This is a critical distinction, as extrinsic causes are often reversible and pacemaker placement is not required. Drug toxicity is a common cause of extrinsic, reversible sinoatrial dysfunction, with common culprits including beta blockers, calcium channel blockers, lithium toxicity, narcotics, pentamidine, and clonidine. Hypothyroidism, sleep apnea, hypoxia, hypothermia, and increased intracranial pressure are all reversible forms of extrinsic dysfunction. Radiation therapy can result in permanent dysfunction of the node and therefore is an irreversible, or intrinsic, cause of sinoatrial node dysfunction. In symptomatic patients, pacemaker insertion may be indicated.

28. The answer is B.
(*Chap. 15*) When there is evidence of sinoatrial node dysfunction, as manifest in this patient with sinus bradycardia, the first approach is to search for reversible causes. In this case, excessive beta blockade is the most likely explanation for his bradycardia and symptoms. Stopping the metoprolol at least temporarily is in order. There are no urgent indications for temporary or permanent pacemaker placement, as he does not have a high-level AV block, syncope, or shock. His heart failure should reverse when his heart rate increases. Although pharmacologic chronotropic stimulation can increase heart rate temporarily, his moderate symptoms suggest that simply waiting for the beta blocker to be metabolized will be adequate. There is no evidence of new infarction or post-infarct angina; thus the patient does not require urgent revascularization. Once the patient is stabilized, the risks and benefits of restarting the beta blocker at a lower dosage may be considered.

29. The answer is C.
(*Chap. 15*) The patient presents with a classic bulls-eye lesion, or erythema migrans, consistent with Lyme disease.

Cardiac conduction abnormalities are common in Lyme disease, often involving the AV node. Temporary pacing may be necessary, but the conduction abnormalities usually resolve. The most common test to diagnose this condition is an ELISA with confirmatory Western blot. Other infectious etiologies can present with heart block such as syphilis and Chagas' disease, but these would not be associated with the characteristic Lyme rash. Autoimmune and infiltrative diseases may also present with conduction system disease such as ankylosing spondylitis, rheumatoid arthritis, scleroderma, and systemic lupus erythematosus.

30. The answer is B.
(*Chap. 15*) Second-degree AV block type 1 (Mobitz type 1) is characterized by a progressive lengthening of the PR interval preceding a pause. The pause in this tracing is between the third and fourth QRS complex. First-degree AV block is a slowing of conduction through the AV junction and is diagnosed when the PR interval is greater than 200 milliseconds. Type 2 second-degree AV block is characterized by intermittent failure of conduction of the P wave without changes in the preceding PR or RR intervals. Second-degree AV block type 2 usually occurs in the distal or infra-His conduction systems.

31 and 32.   The answers are B and D, respectively.
(*Chap. 16*) The patient has persistent, non–life-threatening palpitations that distress her enough to seek medical attention. A continuous Holter monitor for 24 hours is appropriate for patients in whom the symptoms happen several times a day in which an event monitor is triggered by the patient when symptoms occur and thus can be worn for a longer period of time. There is no indication of gastrointestinal triggers, so abdominal CT would not be helpful. The atrial premature contractions are uncomplicated, do not require additional diagnostic evaluation at this time, and pose no additional health risk. EP referral is indicated for patients with life-threatening or severe symptoms such as syncope.

33. The answer is C.
(*Chap. 16*) The patient has physiologic sinus tachycardia related to a pneumothorax, for which he was at risk from his obstructive lung disease and volume-cycled mechanical ventilation. The increased peak inspiratory pressure on the mechanical ventilator is due to the reduced respiratory system compliance from the pneumothorax. Physiologic sinus tachycardia often comes on slowly and responds poorly to carotid sinus massage with gradual return to original rate. Pharmacologic interventions are usually unsuccessful with correction of the underlying cause required for resolution of the tachycardia. In this case, a tension pneumothorax is confirmed by chest radiograph and, with placement of a chest tube, the tachycardia resolves. Other causes of physiologic sinus

tachycardia include pain, hyperthyroidism, anxiety, anemia, hypotension, fever, and exercise.

34. The answer is E.

(Chap. 16) Patients at the highest risk for stroke associated with atrial fibrillation include those with a prior history of stroke, TIA, or embolism, and patients with hypertension, diabetes mellitus, congestive heart failure, rheumatic heart disease, LV dysfunction, and marked left atrial dilation of greater than 5.0 cm or age greater than 65 years. Anticoagulation should be strongly considered in these patients. Increased left atrial size is a risk factor for chronic atrial fibrillation.

35. The answer is B.

(Chap. 16) The AFFIRM and RACE trials compared outcomes in survival and thromboembolic events in patients with atrial fibrillation using two treatment strategies: rate control and anticoagulation versus pharmacotherapy to maintain sinus rhythm. There was no difference in events in the two groups, which is thought to be due to the inefficiencies of pharmacotherapy, with over half of patients failing drug therapy, and also the high rates of asymptomatic atrial fibrillation in the sinus rhythm group. Thus, when considering discontinuation of anticoagulation in patients who have maintained sinus rhythm, placing a prolonged ECG monitor is recommended to ensure that asymptomatic atrial fibrillation is not present. Because of the risk of QT prolongation and polymorphic ventricular tachycardia, initiation of dofetilide and sotalol in the hospital is recommended.

36. The answer is C.

(Chap. 16) The patient has atrial flutter, which has a high risk of thromboembolic events and should be treated the same as atrial fibrillation. If atrial flutter has been present for more than 24–48 hours without anticoagulation, a transesophageal echocardiogram may be performed to rule out left atrial thrombus. If this is not present, cardioversion may be attempted, with anticoagulation continued for 1 month if successful. Transthoracic echocardiography is inadequate to rule out left atrial thrombus. The patient is hemodynamically stable and has no indications for acute cardioversion. Dabigatran is not currently FDA approved for atrial flutter. Intravenous heparin should be started immediately if there are no contraindications, given the greater than 12-hour duration of symptoms.

37. The answer is B.

(Chap. 16) The ECG shows at least three different P-wave morphologies with three different PR intervals, which is the hallmark of multifocal atrial tachycardia. This is the signature tachycardia of patients with significant pulmonary disease and is commonly seen in patients with chronic obstructive pulmonary disease, as suggested by diffuse polyphonic expiratory wheezing and hyperinflation.

38. The answer is D.

(Chap. 16) The patient has classic symptoms for an AV nodal reentrant tachycardia. The so-called frog sign (prominent venous pulsations in the neck due to cannon A waves seen in AV dissociation) on physical examination is frequently present and suggests simultaneous atrial and ventricular contraction. First-line therapy for these reentrant narrow complex tachyarrhythmias is carotid sinus massage to increase vagal tone. Often this is all that is required to return the patient to sinus rhythm. If that is not successful, IV adenosine 6–12 mg may be attempted. If adenosine fails, intravenous beta blockers or calcium channel blockers may be used (diltiazem or verapamil). Finally, in hemodynamically compromised patients or those who have failed to respond to previous measures, DC cardioversion with 100–200 J is indicated.

39. The answer is D.

(Chap. 16) The patient has an accessory conduction pathway, as evidenced by the delta waves on his baseline ECG. He now presents with atrial fibrillation through the accessory pathway. The wide complex is not due to ventricular arrhythmia but rather the aberrant accessory conduction through the accessory pathway. In general, this reentrant tachycardia may be treated as all others, with the exception of avoiding digoxin and verapamil, both of which may cause deterioration to ventricular fibrillation. Digoxin is thought to shorten the refractory period of the accessory pathway and thus can precipitate degeneration to ventricular fibrillation. Verapamil is thought to cause systemic vasodilation, with a resultant increase in sympathetic tone, and thus may precipitate ventricular fibrillation as well.

40. The answer is A.

(Chap. 16) Atrial-ventricular dissociation is a classic finding in ventricular tachycardia. Physical examination may show jugular vein cannon A waves when the atria contracts against a closed tricuspid valve and the ECG will manifest this with atrial capture and/or fusion beats. Other findings on ECG of ventricular tachycardia include QRS duration greater than 140 milliseconds for right bundle branch pattern in V_1 or greater than 160 milliseconds for left bundle morphology in lead V_1, frontal plane axis of -90 to $180°$, delayed activation during initial phase of the QRS complex, or bizarre QRS pattern that does not mimic typical right or left bundle branch block QRS complex patterns. An irregularly irregular rhythm with changing QRS complexes suggests atrial fibrillation with ventricular preexcitation. Carotid sinus massage, aimed at increasing vagal tone and slowing AV node conduction, is not effective at slowing ventricular tachycardia because the reentrant focus is below the AV node.

41 and 42.   The answers are C and C, respectively.

(Chap. 16) The patient's rhythm is torsade de pointes, with polymorphic ventricular tachycardia and QRS complexes with variations in amplitude and cycle length, giving the appearance of oscillation about an axis. Torsades de pointes are associated with a prolonged QT interval; thus, anything that is associated with a prolonged QT can potentially cause torsade. Most commonly, electrolyte disturbances such as hypokalemia and hypomagnesemia, phenothiazines, fluoroquinolones, antiarrhythmic drugs, tricyclic antidepressants, intracranial events, and bradyarrhythmias are associated with this malignant arrhythmia. Management, besides stabilization, which may require electrical cardioversion, consists of removing the offending agent. In addition, success in rhythm termination or prevention has been reported with the administration of magnesium as well as overdrive atrial or ventricular pacing, which will shorten the QT interval. Beta blockers are indicated for patients with congenital long QT syndrome, but are not indicated in this patient.

43.   The answer is C.

(Chap. 16) There are three main mechanisms by which arrhythmias are initiated and maintained: automaticity, afterdepolarizations, and reentry. Automaticity, such as that seen with sinus tachycardia, atrial premature complexes, and some atrial tachycardias, is due to an increase in the slope of phase 4 of the action potential. The depolarization threshold is reached more quickly and repeatedly. Afterdepolarizations are associated with an increase in cellular calcium accumulation, leading to repeated myocardial depolarization during phase 3 (early) and phase 4 (delayed) of the action potential. Early afterdepolarizations may be related to the initiation of torsades de pointes. Delayed afterdepolarizations are responsible for arrhythmias related to digoxin toxicity and for catecholamine-induced ventricular tachycardia. Reentry is due to inhomogeneities in myocardial conduction and refractory periods. With reentry, conduction is blocked in one pathway, allowing slow conduction in the other. This allows for sufficient delay so that the blocked site has time for reentry and propagation of the tachycardia within the two pathways. Reentry appears to be the mechanism for most supraventricular and ventricular tachycardias.

44.   The answer is C.

(Chap. 16) The mechanisms for atrial fibrillation initiation and maintenance are still debated; however, there are anatomic structures that play a role in both of these processes. Muscularized tissue at the orifices of the pulmonary vein inlets are the predominant anatomic drivers of atrial fibrillation, although metabolic disturbances (e.g., hyperthyroidism, inflammation, infection) are also very common. Radio-frequency ablation of the tissue in the area of the pulmonary vein inlets can terminate atrial fibrillation; however, recurrences are not uncommon and other anatomic drivers may be present. The left atrial appendage is an important site of thrombus formation in patients with atrial fibrillation. Any focus within the left or right atrium can be a focus of reentry of focal atrial tachycardia, including the mitral annulus or sinus venosus. Increased automaticity of the sinus node is the mechanism for sinus tachycardia.

45.   The answer is B.

(Chap. 16) Symptoms of atrial fibrillation vary dramatically. The most common symptom is tachypalpitations; however, the hemodynamic effects account for symptoms of impaired left ventricular filling. In atrial fibrillation, there is not an effective atrial contraction to augment late-diastolic left ventricular filling. In patients with impaired ventricular diastolic function, this loss of effective atrial contraction causes impaired left ventricular filling, increased left atrial filling pressures, and pulmonary congestion. These hemodynamic effects are more common in the elderly and in patients with long-standing hypertension, hypertrophic cardiomyopathy, and obstructive aortic valve disease. The tachycardia of atrial fibrillation further compromises left ventricular filling and increases atrial filling pressures. Atrial fibrillation may occur with acute alcohol intoxication, with warming of hypothermic patients, and postoperatively after thoracic surgery. The magnitude of the hemodynamic effect and symptoms will be related to ventricular rate (a slower rate allows more time for left ventricular filling) and underlying cardiac function.

46.   The answer is E.

(Chap. 17) The patient presents with evidence of heart failure by history, and physical examination confirms this diagnosis. Physical examination also shows exophthalmos and a fine tremor, which are suggestive of hyperthyroidism. Thyrotoxicosis, along with anemia, nutritional disorders, and systemic arteriovenous shunting, can all cause high-output heart failure. Although systolic and diastolic dysfunction are more common causes of heart failure, disorders associated with a high-output state are often reversible, and therefore a diagnosis should be pursued when clinical clues suggest this may be present.

47.   The answer is C.

(Chap. 17) Circulating levels of natriuretic peptides may be a useful adjunctive tool in the diagnosis of heart failure, but they cannot replace clinical judgment. BNP or N-terminal BNP are most commonly used and are released from the failing heart, though their release is not specific to left or right heart failure; thus, elevations are commonly seen in cor pulmonale associated with pulmonary vascular disease as well as in patients with left heart failure. Additionally, there are a number of factors that may affect the level of BNP that is normally released from the failing heart. Age and renal dysfunction increase plasma BNP levels. Obesity is associated with falsely low BNP levels. Although BNP levels may normalize after therapy, serial monitoring of this peptide is not presently recommended as a guide for heart failure therapy.

48. The answer is E.

(Chap. 17) Several drugs have been shown to prevent disease progression in heart failure including ACE inhibitors, angiotensin receptor blockers, beta blockers, and aldosterone antagonists. ACE inhibition has been shown to improve symptoms and survival, reduce cardiac hypertrophy, and reduce hospitalizations. Its use is often complicated by cough related to kinin potentiation, which is an acceptable reason to switch to an angiotensin receptor blocker. Digoxin therapy has not been shown to improve survival, may be associated with dose toxicity, and in patients with stable disease who are not frequently hospitalized, can usually be withdrawn. Beta blocker therapy may occasionally be associated with worsening heart failure symptoms at the time of initiation, but this can usually be managed with increased diuretics. The benefits of beta blockers would far outweigh the nuisance of occasional extra diuretics in this patient. Aldosterone antagonists such as spironolactone and eplerenone are recommended for patients with EF less than 35% who are receiving standard therapy as above. There is no known benefit to one member of this class of drugs over another.

49. The answer is E.

(Chap. 17) Although there is a wealth of information on which drugs will improve symptoms and survival in heart failure with reduced ejection fraction, little is known about heart failure with preserved ejection fraction. In fact, there are no proven or approved pharmacologic therapies for patients with heart failure and preserved ejection fraction. Therapy should be aimed at treating the predisposing factors for development of this condition, i.e., treat systemic hypertension if present, reverse ischemia if appropriate, etc. Precipitating factors, such as dietary indiscretion in this patient, atrial fibrillation, or infection, may be addressed to improve symptoms. Sildenafil is currently only approved for therapy of pulmonary arterial hypertension and is not proven to be useful for pulmonary hypertension associated with heart failure with preserved ejection fraction.

50. The answer is C.

(Chap. 17) The New York Heart Association (NYHA) classification is a tool to define criteria that describe the functional ability and clinical manifestations of patients in heart failure. It is also used in patients with pulmonary

hypertension. These criteria have been shown to have prognostic value with worsening survival as class increases. They are also useful to clinicians when reading studies to understand the entry and exclusion criteria of large clinical trials. Class I is used for patients with no limiting symptoms; class II for patients with slight or mild limitation; class III implies no symptoms at rest but dyspnea or angina or palpitations with little exertion—patients are moderately limited; class IV is used for severely limited patients in whom even minimal activity causes symptoms. Treatment guidelines also frequently base recommendations on these clinical stages. This patient has symptoms with mild exertion but is comfortable at rest; therefore, he is NYHA class III.

51. The answer is B.

(Chap. 17) Patients with severe congestive heart failure often exhibit Cheyne-Stokes breathing, defined as intercurrent short periods of hypoventilation and hyperventilation. The mechanism is thought to relate to the prolonged circulation time between the lungs and the respiratory control centers in the brain, leading to poor respiratory control of $PaCO_2$. The degree of Cheyne-Stokes breathing is related to the severity of heart failure. This pattern of breathing is different from obstructive sleep apnea, which is notable for loud snoring, periods of apnea, and sudden waking. Patients are also often hypersomnolent during the day. While sleep apnea is managed with weight loss and overnight CPAP, Cheyne-Stokes breathing is difficult to address as it is often a sign of advanced systolic dysfunction and implies a poor prognosis. All efforts to further maximize heart failure management are indicated. A sleep study would demonstrate this pattern of breathing, but this history and clinical presentation is typical. There is no role for bronchodilators or an electroencephalogram.

52. The answer is B.

(Chap. 18) Coronary artery disease is a common late complication after cardiac transplantation and is thought to be due to a primary immunologic injury of the vascular endothelium, though it is influenced by nonimmunologic factors such as dyslipidemia, diabetes mellitus, and cytomegalovirus infection. Use of mycophenolate, mofetil, and the mammalian target of rapamycin sirolimus have been associated with a lower short-term incidence of coronary intimal thickening. Similarly, statin use has been shown to reduce the incidence of this complication. Because donors are generally young, the coronary artery disease after transplantation is not thought to be due to coronary lesions present pretransplantation.

53. The answer is E.

(Chap. 17) Ventricular assist device therapy can be used either as a "bridge" to transplantation in eligible candidates or as a final destination in patients with end-stage heart failure who are not transplant candidates. There are four FDA-approved devices, all of which share common complications including thromboembolism, cerebrovascular accident, device failure, and infection.

54. The answer is E.

(Chap. 19) Atrial septal defect (ASD) is a not uncommon simple congenital heart disease lesion that is often diagnosed in adults. Because of chronic left-to-right shunting of intracardiac blood, pulmonary arterial hypertension is a well-recognized common complication. With the development of pulmonary arterial hypertension, the potential for paradoxical embolization of either air or thrombotic material from the right atrium to the systemic circulation is increased. Similarly, with exertion in the context of pulmonary arterial hypertension and ASD, blood may shunt right to left, leading to systemic arterial oxygen desaturation. Atrial fibrillation or other supraventricular arrhythmias may occur, also as a result of atrial stretching with the lesion. While atherosclerosis and unstable angina may certainly occur in adults, is not a reported complication of ASD.

55. The answer is D.

(Chap. 19) The patient has secondary erythrocytosis due to Eisenmenger's syndrome and chronic arterial hypoxemia. Her partially corrected left-to-right shunt resulted in chronic pulmonary circulation overflow and the subsequent development of pulmonary arterial hypertension. With a rise in pulmonary vascular pressure, the shunt reverses to become predominantly right to left, which causes systemic oxygen desaturation. Because hypoxemia is caused by shunt and not ventilation/perfusion mismatch (as in typical COPD), it is not responsive to oxygen therapy. Peripheral desaturation results in decreased oxygen delivery to the kidneys, increased erythropoietin secretion, and resultant erythrocytosis. Erythropoietin levels would be expected to be elevated in this case (in contrast to polycythemia vera rubra). Phlebotomy is only used for patients with symptomatic erythrocytosis; hyperviscosity symptoms, including neurologic symptoms such as transient ischemic attack; epistaxis or bleeding symptoms; or visual changes. Because iron depletion may worsen viscosity even at a lower hematocrit, it is considered as only a temporary therapy for management of erythrocytosis in Eisenmenger's syndrome. This patient had no symptoms referable to erythrocytosis; therefore, expectant management is most appropriate.

56. The answer is D.

(Chap. 19) Routine antibiotic prophylaxis is indicated for bacteremic dental procedures or instrumentation through an infected site in most patients with operated congenital heart disease, particularly whenever foreign material is present. The one exception is patches that don't have

a post-placement high-grade leak, where prophylaxis is only required for 6 months until endothelialization.

57. The answer is E.

(Chap. 19) The patient presents with dextrocardia on his chest radiograph and situs inversus, or complete mirror image situs inversus on examination. When dextrocardia occurs in isolation without situs inversus, multiple cardiac abnormalities are frequently present. Alternatively, when dextrocardia occurs with situs inversus, other cardiac defects are unlikely. Kartagener's syndrome with mucociliary dysfunction may underlie situs inversus, but it is associated with sinusitis and chronic bronchitis, which this patient did not have.

58 and 59. The answers are C and A, respectively.

(Chap. 19) This patient has a coarctation of the aorta presenting with marked hypertension proximal to the lesion. The narrowing most commonly occurs distal to the origin of the left subclavian artery, explaining the equal pressure in the arms and reduced pressure in the legs. Coarctations account for approximately 7% of congenital cardiac abnormalities, occur more frequently (2×) in men than in women, and are associated with gonadal dysgenesis and bicuspid aortic valves. Adults will present with hypertension, manifestations of hypertension in the upper body (headache, epistaxis), or leg claudication. Physical examination reveals diminished and/or delayed lower extremity pulses, enlarged collateral vessels in the upper body, or reduced development of the lower extremities. Cardiac examination may reveal findings consistent with left ventricular (LV) hypertrophy. There may be no murmur, a mid-systolic murmur over the anterior chest and back, or an aortic murmur with a bicuspid valve. Transthoracic (suprasternal/parasternal) or transesophageal echocardiography, contrast CT or MRI of the thorax, or cardiac catheterization can be diagnostic. MRI of the head would not be useful diagnostically. The clinical picture is not consistent with renal artery stenosis, pheochromocytoma, carcinoid, or Cushing's syndrome.

60. The answer is E.

(Chap. 20) Mitral stenosis is one of the leading causes of pulmonary hypertension worldwide, particularly in developing countries where the treatment of streptococcal disease is less available. The primary determinants of pulmonary artery pressure are left atrial pressure, pulmonary vascular resistance, and flow. Mitral stenosis may restrict flow from the left atrium to the left ventricle, and thus is associated with left atrial hypertension and passive pulmonary hypertension (due to back pressure). Additionally, the pulmonary vascular bed may actively vasoconstrict in response to left atrial hypertension. Additional contributors to pulmonary hypertension in mitral stenosis include interstitial edema in the walls of

small pulmonary vessels and, in end-stage disease, obliterative changes in the pulmonary vascular bed as may be seen in some forms of pulmonary arterial hypertension. Pulmonary hypertension related to mitral stenosis is generally reversible with correction of the valvular lesion.

61 and 62.   The answers are A and E, respectively.

(Chap. 20) The patient presents with a relatively stable ST elevation myocardial infarction. He likely has extensive necrosis given the duration of symptoms and ECG findings, and thus is at risk for complication of myocardial infarction. In this case, his acute dyspnea, worsening oxygenation, and asymmetric edema on chest radiograph all point to acute mitral regurgitation from papillary muscle rupture. An allergic reaction to a medication should not cause severe hypoxemia. It may cause rather mild reversible hypoxemia, and should not cause an abnormal chest radiograph. The classic finding of acute mitral regurgitation is a relatively loud systolic murmur heard best at the apex and radiating to the axilla. The murmur is described as having a "cooing" or "seagull-like" quality. A fourth heart sound is also common. Management of acute mitral regurgitation includes afterload and preload reduction, if possible, often with intravenous nitroprusside. If patients are unable to tolerate medical interventions to achieve this because of systemic hypotension, as in this patient, an intraaortic balloon pump is indicated. Albuterol and methylprednisolone are indicated for acute bronchospasm due to primary airways disease, but would not be helpful for the management of cardiogenic shock.

63.   The answer is C.

(Chap. 20) The patient has classic physical examination findings for mitral valve prolapse with a mid-systolic click that may or may not be associated with a systolic murmur. Mitral valve prolapse is generally thought to be a benign lesion, with most patients never developing symptoms during their lifetimes. While many patients with heritable connective tissue disorders such as Marfan's syndrome have mitral valve prolapse, in the majority of cases, a cause is not identified. Mitral valve prolapse may be seen on echocardiography by systolic displacement of the mitral valve leaflets by at least 2 mm into the left atrium. Doppler imaging may also be helpful to define the condition. Because the lesion is generally benign, endocarditis prophylaxis is generally not indicated unless the patient has a prior history of endocarditis. Although some patients develop atrial arrhythmias in conjunction with mitral valve prolapse, prophylactic antiplatelet agents or warfarin are not recommended, as most patients do not have complications.

64.   The answer is B.

(Chap. 20) The patient has aortic stenosis that presented late in life. While bicuspid aortic valve underlies nearly half of all aortic stenosis cases, this lesion typically presents earlier in life, and only 40% of patients greater than 70 years old with aortic stenosis who undergo surgery have a bicuspid valve. Rheumatic heart disease may cause aortic stenosis, but almost invariably mitral stenosis is also present. Underlying connective tissue disease is not known to be associated. Modern research on the development of aortic stenosis has shown that several traditional atherosclerotic risk factors are present such as diabetes mellitus, smoking, chronic kidney disease, and the metabolic syndrome. Polymorphisms of the vitamin D receptor have also been demonstrated in patients with symptomatic aortic stenosis.

65.   The answer is C.

(Chap. 20) Exertional syncope is a late finding in aortic stenosis (AS) and portends a poor prognosis. Patients with this symptom or with angina pectoris have an average time to death of 3 years. Patients with dyspnea have 2 years, and patients with heart failure have an average time to death of 1.5–2 years. Because of these data, patients with severe AS and symptoms should be strongly considered for surgical therapy.

66.   The answer is A.

(Chap. 20) Patients with severe aortic regurgitation will have a "water-hammer" pulse that collapses suddenly as arterial pressure rapidly falls during late systole and diastole, a so-called Corrigan's pulse. Capillary pulsations seen in the nail bed in severe aortic regurgitation are named Quincke's pulse. Traube's sign, or a pistol shot sound, may be heard over the femoral arteries and Duroziez's sign, with a to-and-fro murmur over the femoral artery, have also been described. Pulsus parvus et tardus is found in severe aortic stenosis. Pulsus bigeminus occurs when there is a shorter interval after a normal beat with a following low volume pulse, often with a premature ventricular beat. Pulsus paradoxus has been described with pericardial tamponade or severe obstructive lung disease. Pulsus alternans is alternating large and small volume pulses seen in severe heart failure.

67 and 68.   The answers are C and C, respectively.

(Chap. 20) The patient presents with heart failure during her second trimester from a region with high rates of rheumatic fever. She is therefore at risk for rheumatic mitral stenosis, which often presents during the second trimester of pregnancy as the cardiac output must rise to accommodate the fetus and intravascular volume expands substantially. The stenotic valve cannot accommodate the increased flow demands of pregnancy, and congestive heart failure ensues with secondary pulmonary venous hypertension. The patient has evidence of heart failure on examination with pulmonary hypertension. Her diastolic rumble is characteristic of mitral stenosis. Finally, hemoptysis is not an infrequent finding in severe mitral stenosis and may be due to the rupture of pulmonary-bronchial venous connections secondary to pulmonary venous hypertension. Occasionally, pink frothy sputum can be found in patients with frank alveolar hemorrhage related to elevated pulmonary capillary pressure. Mitral stenosis is readily demonstrated by echocardiography. While right heart catheterization may demonstrate pulmonary hypertension and an elevated pulmonary capillary wedge pressure, the etiology of these findings will remain unknown without imaging of the left heart. Short-term management of mitral stenosis with heart failure should include diuretics. As the patient does not have left ventricular failure, ACE inhibition and digoxin are not likely to alleviate her symptoms. Occasionally, beta blockade may improve symptoms, particularly in patients with symptomatic atrial arrhythmias. Anticoagulation is not indicated in mitral stenosis alone unless atrial arrhythmias or pulmonary embolism is present. As infection does not underlie the patient's hemoptysis, further antibiotics will not be helpful.

69. The answer is D.
(*Chap. 20*) Indications for surgical repair of mitral regurgitation are dependent on left-ventricular function, ventricular size, and the presence of sequelae of chronic mitral regurgitation. The experience of the surgeon and the likelihood of successful mitral valve repair are also important considerations. The management strategy for chronic severe mitral regurgitation depends on the presence of symptoms, left-ventricular function, left-ventricular dimensions, and the presence of complicating factors such as pulmonary hypertension and atrial fibrillation. With very depressed left-ventricular function (<30% or end-systolic dimension >55 mm), the risk of surgery increases, left-ventricular recovery is often incomplete, and long-term survival is reduced. However, since medical therapy offers little for these patients, surgical repair should be considered if there is a high likelihood of success (>90%). When ejection fraction is between 30% and 60%, and end-systolic dimension rises above 40 mm, surgical repair is indicated even in the absence of symptoms, owing to the excellent long-term results achieved in this group. Waiting for worsening left-ventricular function leads to irreversible left-ventricular remodeling. Pulmonary hypertension and atrial fibrillation are important to consider as markers for worsening regurgitation. For asymptomatic patients with normal left-ventricular function and dimensions, the presence of new pulmonary hypertension or atrial fibrillation in patients with normal ejection fraction and end-systolic dimensions are class IIa indications for mitral valve repair.

70. The answer is F.
(*Chap. 20*) Tricuspid regurgitation is most commonly caused by dilation of the tricuspid annulus due to right-ventricular enlargement of any cause. Any cause of left-ventricular failure that results in right-ventricular

failure may lead to tricuspid regurgitation. Congenital heart diseases or pulmonary arterial hypertension leading to right-ventricular failure will dilate the tricuspid annulus. Inferior wall infarction may involve the right ventricle. Rheumatic heart disease may involve the tricuspid valve, although less commonly than the mitral valve. Infective endocarditis, particularly in IV drug users, will infect the tricuspid valve, causing vegetations and regurgitation. Other causes of tricuspid regurgitation include carcinoid heart disease, endomyocardial fibrosis, congenital defects of the atrioventricular canal, and right-ventricular pacemakers.

71. The answer is A.
(*Chap. 20*) Bioprosthetic valves are made from human, porcine, or bovine tissue. The major advantage of a bioprosthetic valve is the low incidence of thromboembolic phenomena, particularly 3 months after implantation. Although in the immediate postoperative period some anticoagulation may occur, after 3 months there is no further need for anticoagulation or monitoring. The downside is the natural history and longevity of the bioprosthetic valve. Bioprosthetic valves tend to degenerate mechanically. Approximately 50% will need replacement at 15 years. Therefore, these valves are useful in patients with contraindications to anticoagulation, such as elderly patients with comorbidities and younger patients who desire to become pregnant. Elderly people may also be spared the need for repeat surgery, as their life span may be shorter than the natural history of the bioprosthesis. Mechanical valves offer superior durability. Hemodynamic parameters are improved with double-disk valves compared with single-disk or ball-and-chain valves. However, thrombogenicity is high and chronic anticoagulation is mandatory. Younger patients with no contraindications to anticoagulation may be better served by mechanical valve replacement.

72. The answer is E.
(*Chap. 21*) Many infectious etiologies have been associated with the development of inflammatory myocarditis including viral agents (coxsackie, adenovirus, HIV, hepatitis C) and parasitic agents, with Chagas disease or *T. cruzi* being most prominent, but also toxoplasmosis. Additionally, bacterial etiologies like diphtheria, spirochetal disease like *Borrelia burgdorferi*, rickettsial disease, and fungal infections have been associated.

73. The answer is C.
(*Chap. 21*) Peripartum cardiomyopathy is a rare complication of pregnancy and can occur during the last trimester or within the first 6 months postpartum. Risk factors include advanced age, increased parity, twin pregnancy, malnutrition, use of tocolytic therapy for premature labor, and preeclampsia.

74. The answer is A.

(Chap. 21) Beriberi heart disease is a dilated cardiomyopathy due to thiamine deficiency. While uncommon in developed countries, this condition still occurs in patients who derive most of their calories from alcohol and has been reported in teenagers who eat only highly processed foods. This condition involves systemic vasodilation with a very high cardiac output in its early stages. In advanced disease, a low-output state can occur. Thiamine repletion can lead to a complete recovery. Patient A has evidence of heart failure with systemic vasodilation and elevated cardiac output, as would be found in beriberi. Alternatively, patient B has normal hemodynamics. Patient C has evidence of low-output heart failure with systemic vasoconstriction. Patient D has elevated pulmonary arterial pressures with right heart failure in conjunction with normal pulmonary capillary wedge pressure, consistent with primary pulmonary vascular disease, e.g., pulmonary arterial hypertension. Patient E has low right heart filling pressures, with somewhat low cardiac output and elevated systemic vascular resistance, as might be found in hypovolemic shock.

75. The answer is E.

(Chap. 21) Hypertrophic cardiomyopathy usually presents between age 20 and 40 years, with the most common symptom being dyspnea. Many patients are, however, asymptomatic and the only clue to the presence of this potentially deadly disease is physical examination. Physical examination will show a harsh systolic murmur heard best at the left lower sternal border arising from both the outflow tract turbulence during ventricular ejection and the often concomitant mitral regurgitation. Maneuvers that decrease ventricular volume such as Valsalva or moving from squatting to standing will enhance the murmur. Conversely, maneuvers that increase left ventricular volume will decrease the murmur's intensity. These include hand grip and squatting. Having the patient lie with the left side down and leaning forward may make the friction rub of pericarditis more audible.

76. The answer is E.

(Chap. 21) A common diagnostic dilemma is differentiating constrictive pericarditis from a restrictive cardiomyopathy. Elevated jugular venous pressure is almost universally present in both. Kussmaul's sign (increase or no change in jugular venous pressure with inspiration) can be seen in both conditions. Other signs of heart failure do not reliably distinguish the two conditions. In restrictive cardiomyopathy, the apical impulse is usually easier to palpate than in constrictive pericarditis, and mitral regurgitation is more common. These clinical signs, however, are not reliable to differentiate the two entities. In conjunction with clinical information and additional imaging studies of the left ventricle and pericardium, certain pathognomic findings increase

diagnostic certainty. A thickened or calcified pericardium increases the likelihood of constrictive pericarditis. Conduction abnormalities are more common in infiltrating diseases of the myocardium. In constrictive pericarditis, measurements of diastolic pressures will show equilibrium between the ventricles, while unequal pressures and/or isolated elevated left ventricular pressures are more consistent with restrictive cardiomyopathy. The classic "square root sign" during right heart catheterization (deep, sharp drop in right ventricular pressure in early diastole, followed by a plateau during which there is no further increase in right ventricular pressure) can be seen in both restrictive cardiomyopathy and constrictive pericarditis. The presence of a paraprotein abnormality (MGUS, myeloma, amyloid) makes restrictive cardiomyopathy more common.

77. The answer is D.

(Chap. 21) Cardiac involvement is common in many of the neuromuscular diseases. The ECG pattern of Duchenne's muscular dystrophy is unique and consists of tall R waves in the right precordial leads with an R/S ratio greater than 1.0, often with deep Q waves in the limb and precordial leads. These patients often have a variety of supraventricular and ventricular arrhythmias, and are at risk for sudden death due to the intrinsic cardiomyopathy as well as the low ejection fraction. Implantable cardioverter defibrillators should be considered in the appropriate patient. Global left ventricular dysfunction is a common finding in dilated cardiomyopathies, whereas focal wall motion abnormalities and angina are more common if there is ischemic myocardium. This patient is at risk for venous thromboembolism; however, chronic thromboembolism would not account for the severity of the left heart failure and would present with findings consistent with pulmonary hypertension. Amyotrophic lateral sclerosis is a disease of motor neurons and does not involve the heart. This patient would be young for that diagnosis. An advanced atrial septal defect would present with cyanosis and heart failure (Eisenmenger's physiology).

78. The answer is D.

(Chap. 22) The patient has a classic presentation for acute pericarditis with constant or pleuritic chest pain, exacerbated by lying flat and alleviated by sitting forward. Serum biomarkers may show mild evidence of myocardial injury from myocardial inflammation, but are generally not substantially elevated. Friction rub is frequently present, has three components, and is best heard while the patient is upright and leaning forward. In the acute stages, ECG classically shows ST-segment elevation with upward concavity in two or three standard limb leads and V_2 through V_6 with reciprocal changes in aVR. Convex curvature is more commonly found in acute myocardial infarction. PR depression may be

found. After several days, the ST changes resolve and T waves become inverted. After weeks to months, the ECG returns to normal.

79. The answer is B.

(Chap. 22) Pulsus paradoxus is an exaggeration of the normal phenomenon in which systolic blood pressure declines 10 mmHg or less with inspiration. Pulsus paradoxus is typically seen in patients with pericardial tamponade and in patients with severe obstructive lung disease (COPD, asthma). In pulsus paradoxus due to pericardial tamponade, the inspiratory systolic blood pressure decline is greater due to the tight incompressible pericardial sac. The right ventricle distends with inspiration, compressing the left ventricle and resulting in decreased systolic pulse pressure in the systemic circulation. In severe obstructive lung disease, the inspiratory decline of systolic blood pressure may be due to the markedly negative pleural pressure either causing left ventricular compression (due to increased RV venous return) or increased LV impedance to ejection (increased afterload).

80. The answer is C.

(Chap. 22) Beck's triad can be used to alert clinicians to the potential presence of cardiac tamponade. The principal features are hypotension, muffled or absent heart sounds, and elevated neck veins, often with prominent x-descent and absent y-descent. These are due to the failure of ventricular filling and limited cardiac output. Kussmaul's sign is seen in restrictive cardiomyopathy and pericardial constriction, not tamponade. Friction rub may be seen in any condition associated with pericardial inflammation.

81. The answer is D.

(Chap. 22) This patient's presentation and physical examination are most consistent with the diagnosis of constrictive pericarditis. The most common cause of constrictive pericarditis worldwide is tuberculosis, but given the low incidence of tuberculosis in the United States, constrictive pericarditis is a rare condition in this country. With the increasing ability to cure Hodgkin's disease with mediastinal irradiation, many cases of constrictive pericarditis in the United States involve patients who received curative radiation therapy 10–20 years prior. These patients are also at risk for premature coronary artery disease. Risks for these complications include dose of radiation and radiation windows that include the heart. Other rare causes of constrictive pericarditis are recurrent acute pericarditis, hemorrhagic pericarditis, prior cardiac surgery, mediastinal irradiation, chronic infection, and neoplastic disease. Physiologically, constrictive pericarditis is characterized by the inability of the ventricles to fill because of the noncompliant pericardium. In early diastole, the ventricles fill rapidly, but filling stops abruptly when the elastic limit of the

pericardium is reached. Clinically, patients present with generalized malaise, cachexia, and anasarca. Exertional dyspnea is common, and orthopnea is generally mild. Ascites and hepatomegaly occur because of increased venous pressure. In rare cases, cirrhosis may develop from chronic congestive hepatopathy. The jugular venous pressure is elevated, and the neck veins fail to collapse on inspiration (Kussmaul's sign). Heart sounds may be muffled. A pericardial knock is frequently heard. This is a third heart sound that occurs 0.09–0.12 seconds after aortic valve closure at the cardiac apex. Right heart catheterization would show the "square root sign" characterized by an abrupt y-descent followed by a gradual rise in ventricular pressure. This finding, however, is not pathognomonic of constrictive pericarditis and can be seen in restrictive cardiomyopathy of any cause. Echocardiogram shows a thickened pericardium, dilatation of the inferior vena cava and hepatic veins, and an abrupt cessation of ventricular filling in early diastole. Pericardial resection is the only definitive treatment of constrictive pericarditis. Diuresis and sodium restriction are useful in managing volume status preoperatively, and paracentesis may be necessary. Operative mortality ranges from 5–10%. Underlying cardiac function is normal; thus, cardiac transplantation is not indicated. Pericardiocentesis is indicated for the diagnostic removal of pericardial fluid and cardiac tamponade, which is not present on the patient's echocardiogram. Mitral valve stenosis may present similarly with anasarca, congestive hepatic failure, and ascites. However, pulmonary edema and pleural effusions are also common. Examination would be expected to demonstrate a diastolic murmur, and echocardiogram should show a normal pericardium and a thickened immobile mitral valve. Mitral valve replacement would be indicated if mitral stenosis were the cause of the patient's symptoms.

82. The answer is C.

(Chap. 23) Blunt, nonpenetrating trauma such as that described here can result in commotio cordis, which occurs when the trauma impacts the heart during the susceptible phase of repolarization just before the peak of the T wave and results in ventricular fibrillation. This syndrome is most common in young athletes who are playing hockey, football, baseball, or lacrosse, for example. Treatment is prompt defibrillation. While aortic rupture, myocardial rupture with cardiac tamponade, and tension pneumothorax may occur with chest wall trauma, their presentation should be less immediate after the trauma. Hypertrophic cardiomyopathy may present with sudden cardiac death, as in this case, but the preceding chest trauma makes commotio cordis more likely.

83. The answer is E.

(Chap. 25) The etiologic agents of infective endocarditis vary by host (see Figure 25-1). Community-acquired native valve endocarditis remains an important clinical problem, particularly in elderly people. In those patients, streptococci (*Viridans* spp., *S. gallolyticus*, other nongroup A and other group streptococci, and *Abiotrophia* spp.) account for approximately 40% of cases. *Staphylococcus aureus* (30%) is next most common. Enterococci, HACEK group, coagulase-negative, and culture-negative cases each account for less than 10% of community-acquired native valve cases. In health care–associated, injection drug use–associated, and greater than 12-month-old prosthetic valve endocarditis, *S. aureus* is most common. Coagulase-negative staphylococcus is the most common organism in prosthetic valve endocarditis less than 12 months. Enterococci cause endocarditis in approximately 10% to 15% of cases in health care–associated, 2- to 12-month prosthetic valve, and injection drug use cases. Culture-negative endocarditis accounts for 5% to 10% of cases in all of the aforementioned clinical scenarios.

84. The answer is B.

(*Chap. 25*) The Duke criteria for diagnosis of infective endocarditis are a set of major and minor clinical, laboratory, and echocardiographic criteria that are highly sensitive and specific. The presence of two major criteria, one major criterion and three minor criteria, or five minor criteria allows a clinical diagnosis of definite endocarditis (see Table 25-3). Evidence of echocardiographic involvement as evidenced by an oscillating mass (vegetation) on a valve, supporting structure, or implanted material; an intracardiac abscess or partial dehiscence of a prosthetic valve; or a new valvular regurgitation are major criteria in the Duke classification. An increase or change in preexisting murmur by clinical examination is not sufficient. Transthoracic echocardiography is specific for infective endocarditis but only finds vegetations in about 65% of patients with definite endocarditis. It is not adequate for evaluation of prosthetic valves or for intracardiac complications. Transesophageal echocardiography is more sensitive, detecting abnormalities in more than 90% of cases of definite endocarditis.

85. The answer is C.

(*Chap. 25*) The recommendations for prophylaxis to prevent infective endocarditis have undergone change recently with a change to recommending it for fewer patients. The most recent American Heart Association guidelines (*Circulation* 116:1736, 2007) reverse many of the former recommendations based on indirect evidence suggesting that benefit is minimal and is not supported by cost-benefit or cost-effectiveness studies. Current recommendations advise prophylactic antibiotics only for those at highest risk for severe morbidity or mortality from endocarditis undergoing manipulation of gingival tissue or periapical region of the teeth, perforation of the oral mucosa, or a procedure on an infected site. Prophylaxis is not advised for routine gastrointestinal or genitourinary

procedures. High-risk patients include those with prior endocarditis, prosthetic heart valves, unrepaired cyanotic congenital heart disease lesions, recently (<6 months) repaired congenital heart lesions, incompletely repaired congenital heart disease lesions, and valvulopathy after cardiac transplant. The British Society for Antimicrobial Chemotherapy does recommend prophylaxis for at-risk patients undergoing selected gastrointestinal or genitourinary procedures; however, the National Institute for Health and Clinical Excellence in the United Kingdom advised discontinuation of the practice (*http://www.nice.org.uk/guidance/cg64*).

86. The answer is A.

(*Chap. 25*) This patient has culture-negative endocarditis, a rare entity defined as clinical evidence of infectious endocarditis in the absence of positive blood cultures. In this case, evidence for subacute bacterial endocarditis includes valvular regurgitation; an aortic valve vegetation; and embolic phenomena on the extremities, spleen, and kidneys. A common reason for negative blood cultures is prior antibiotics. In the absence of this, the two most common pathogens (both of which are technically difficult to isolate in blood culture bottles) are Q fever, *Coxiella burnetii* (typically associated with close contact with livestock), and *Bartonella* spp. In this case, the patient's homelessness and body louse infestation are clues for *Bartonella quintana* infection. Diagnosis is made by blood culture about 25% of the time. Otherwise, direct polymerase chain reaction of valvular tissue, if available, or acute and convalescent serologies are diagnostic options. Empirical therapy for culture-negative endocarditis usually includes ceftriaxone and gentamicin with or without doxycycline. For confirmed *Bartonella* endocarditis, optimal therapy is gentamicin plus doxycycline. EBV and HIV do not cause endocarditis. A peripheral blood smear would not be diagnostic.

87. The answer is D.

(*Chap. 25*) Although any valvular vegetation can embolize, vegetations located on the mitral valve and vegetations larger than 10 mm are greatest risk of embolizing. Of the answer choices, C, D, and E are large enough to increase the risk of embolization. However, only choice D demonstrates the risks of both size and location. Hematogenously seeded infection from an embolized vegetation may involve any organ but particularly affects those organs with the highest blood flow. They are seen in up to 50% of patients with endocarditis. Tricuspid lesions lead to pulmonary septic emboli, which are common in injection drug users. Mitral and aortic lesions can lead to embolic infections in the skin, spleen, kidneys, meninges, and skeletal system. A dreaded neurologic complication is mycotic aneurysm, focal dilations of arteries at points in the arterial wall that have been weakened by infection in the vasa vasorum or septic emboli, leading to hemorrhage.

88. The answer is A.

(*Chap. 25*) Patients with infective endocarditis on antibiotic therapy can be expected to demonstrate clinical improvement within 5 to 7 days. Blood cultures frequently remain positive for 3 to 5 days for *Staphylococcus aureus* treated with β–lactam antibiotics and 7 to 9 days with vancomycin. Neither rifampin nor gentamicin has been shown to provide clinical benefit in the scenario described in this question. Vancomycin peak and trough levels have not been shown to improve drug efficacy in infective endocarditis. It is too early in therapy to consider this case representative of vancomycin failure. The efficacy of daptomycin or linezolid because an alternative to vancomycin for left-sided MRSA endocarditis has not been established.

89. The answer is D.

(*Chap. 26*) Acute rheumatic fever (ARF) is almost universally due to group A streptococcal disease at the present time, though virtually all streptococcal disease may be capable of precipitating rheumatic fever. Although skin infections may be associated with rheumatic fever, far and away the most common presentation is with preceding pharyngitis. There is a latent period of approximately 3 weeks from an episode of sore throat to presentation of ARF. The most common manifestations are fever and polyarthritis, with polyarthritis being present in 60–75% of cases. Carditis may also be present, though somewhat less frequently in 50–60% of cases. Chorea and indolent carditis may have a subacute presentation. Chorea is present in 2–30% of affected individuals, while erythema marginatum and subcutaneous nodules are rare. Sixty percent of patients with ARF progress to rheumatic heart disease, with the endocardium, pericardium, and myocardium all potentially involved. All patients with ARF should receive antibiotics sufficient to treat the precipitating group A streptococcal infection.

90. The answer is D.

(*Chap. 26*) This patient has a history very suggestive of recurrent bouts of ARF with evidence of mitral regurgitation, mitral stenosis, and aortic regurgitation on physical examination. This and the presence of atrial fibrillation imply severe rheumatic heart disease. Risk factors for this condition include poverty and crowded living conditions. As a result, ARF is considerably more common in the developing world. Daily aspirin is the treatment of choice for the migratory large-joint arthritis and fever that are common manifestations of ARF. Practitioners sometimes use steroids during acute bouts of carditis to quell inflammation, though this remains a controversial practice and has no role between flares of ARF. Secondary prophylaxis with either daily oral penicillin or, preferably, monthly IM injections is considered the best method to prevent further episodes of ARF, and therefore prevent further valvular damage. Primary prophylaxis with penicillin on an as-needed basis is equally effective for preventing further bouts of carditis. However, most episodes of sore throat are too minor for patients to present to a physician. Therefore, secondary prophylaxis is considered preferable in patients who already have severe valvular disease. Doxycycline is not a first-line agent for group A *Streptococcus*, the pathogen that incites ARF.

91. The answer is A.

(*Chap. 28*) Cardiogenic shock (CS) is characterized by systemic hypoperfusion caused by severe depression of the cardiac index (<2.2 L/min/m^2) and sustained systolic arterial hypotension (<90 mmHg) despite an elevated filling pressure (pulmonary capillary wedge pressure >18 mmHg). It is associated with in-hospital mortality rates above 50%. Acute myocardial infarction (MI) with left ventricular dysfunction is the most common cause of cardiogenic shock. Other complications of acute MI such as mitral regurgitation or free wall rupture are far less common. CS is the leading cause of death of patients hospitalized with MI. Early reperfusion therapy for acute MI decreases the incidence of CS. Shock typically is associated with ST-segment elevation MI and is less common with non–ST-segment elevation MI. In patients with acute MI, older age, female sex, prior MI, diabetes, and anterior MI location are all associated with an increased risk of CS. Shock associated with a first inferior MI should prompt a search for a mechanical cause. Reinfarction soon after MI increases the risk of CS. Two-thirds of patients with CS have flow-limiting stenoses in all three major coronary arteries, and 20% have stenosis of the left main coronary artery. CS may rarely occur in the absence of significant stenosis, as seen in LV apical ballooning/Takotsubo's cardiomyopathy.

92. The answer is E.

(*Chap. 28*) In patients with acute myocardial infarction and cardiogenic shock, percutaneous coronary intervention can improve mortality rate and outcomes. Stabilizing the patient in cardiogenic shock is an important first maneuver. Initial therapy is aimed at maintaining adequate systemic and coronary perfusion by raising systemic blood pressure with vasopressors and adjusting volume status to a level that ensures optimum left ventricular filling pressure. Decreased diastolic blood pressure is detrimental because it reduces coronary blood flow. However, vasopressor and inotropic agents have the potential to exacerbate the ischemic process by raising myocardial oxygen consumption, increasing heart rate, or increasing left ventricular afterload. Norepinephrine is associated with fewer adverse events, including arrhythmias, compared with dopamine. Dobutamine has greater inotropic than chronotropic action but may cause a reduction in blood pressure due to vasodilation. Aortic counterpulsation with an intraaortic balloon pump (IABP) is helpful in rapidly stabilizing patients because it is capable of augmenting both arterial diastolic pressure and cardiac output. The balloon is automatically inflated during early diastole, augmenting coronary blood flow, and it collapses in early systole, reducing the left ventricular afterload. IABP improves hemodynamic status temporarily in most patients with cardiogenic shock. In contrast to vasopressors and inotropic agents, myocardial O_2 consumption is reduced, ameliorating ischemia. IABP is contraindicated if aortic regurgitation is present or aortic dissection is suspected.

93. The answer is E.

(Chap. 29) The most common electrical mechanism for cardiac arrest is ventricular fibrillation, which is responsible for 50–80% of cardiac arrests. Severe persistent bradyarrhythmias, asystole, and pulseless electrical activity (PEA: organized electrical activity, unusually slow, without mechanical response, formerly called electromechanical dissociation) cause another 20–30%. Pulseless sustained ventricular tachycardia (a rapid arrhythmia distinct from PEA) is a less common mechanism. Acute low cardiac output states, having a precipitous onset also may present clinically as a cardiac arrest. These hemodynamic causes include massive acute pulmonary emboli, internal blood loss from a ruptured aortic aneurysm, intense anaphylaxis, and cardiac rupture with tamponade after myocardial infarction. Sudden deaths from these causes are not typically included in the category of sudden cardiac death.

94. The answer is A.

(Chap. 29) The probability of achieving successful resuscitation from cardiac arrest is related to the interval from onset of loss of circulation to institution of resuscitative efforts, the setting in which the event occurs, the mechanism (ventricular fibrillation, ventricular tachycardia, PEA, asystole), and the clinical status of the patient before the cardiac arrest. Return of circulation and survival rates as a result of defibrillation decrease almost linearly from the first minute to 10 minutes. After 5 minutes, survival rates are no better than 25–30% in out-of-hospital settings. Settings in which it is possible to institute prompt cardiopulmonary resuscitation (CPR) followed by prompt defibrillation provide a better chance of a successful outcome. However, the outcome in intensive care units (ICUs) and other in-hospital environments is heavily influenced by the patient's preceding clinical status. The immediate outcome is good for cardiac arrest occurring in ICUs in the presence of an acute cardiac event or transient metabolic disturbance, but survival among patients with far-advanced chronic cardiac disease or advanced noncardiac diseases (e.g., renal failure, pneumonia, sepsis, diabetes, cancer) is low and not much better in the in-hospital than in the out-of-hospital setting. Survival from unexpected cardiac arrest in unmonitored areas in a hospital is not much better than that it is for witnessed out-of-hospital arrests. Because implementation of community response systems, survival from out-of-hospital cardiac arrest has improved, although it still remains low under most circumstances. Survival probabilities in public sites exceed those in the home environment. This may be because many patients with at home cardiac arrest have severe underlying cardiac disease. The success rate for initial resuscitation and survival to hospital discharge after an out-of-hospital cardiac arrest depends heavily on the mechanism of the event. Most cardiac arrests that are caused by ventricular fibrillation (VF) begin with a run of nonsustained or sustained ventricular tachycardia (VT), which then degenerates into VF. When the mechanism is pulseless VT, the outcome is best, VF is the next most successful, and asystole and PEA generate dismal outcome statistics. Advanced age also adversely influences the chances of successful resuscitation as well as outcomes after resuscitation.

95. The answer is D.

(Chap. 31) Mutation of the LDL receptor results in hypercholesterolemia. This mutation may be homozygous or heterozygous and occurs in approximately 1/500 people in its heterozygous form. Homozygous disease is more severe, with the development of symptomatic coronary atherosclerosis in childhood, while heterozygous patients have hypercholesterolemia from birth, and disease recognition is usually not until adulthood when patients are found to have tendon xanthomas or coronary artery disease. In patients with heterozygous disease, there is generally a family history on at least one side of the family. In familial hypercholesterolemia, there is an elevation of LDL-C between 200 and 400 mg/dL without alterations in chylomicrons or VLDL. Familial defective apoB-100 has a similar presentation but is less common (1/1000). Autosomal dominant history may be present in this family to suggest autosomal dominant hypercholesterolemia; however, this condition is quite rare (<1/1,000,000) and therefore much less likely. Familial hepatic lipase deficiency and lipoprotein lipase deficiency are associated with increased chylomicrons, not LDL-C, and present with eruptive xanthomas, hepatosplenomegaly, and pancreatitis. These conditions occur rarely (<1/1,000,000).

96. The answer is B.

(Chap. 31) There are many secondary forms of elevated LDL that warrant consideration in a patient found to have abnormal LDL. These include hypothyroidism, nephritic syndrome, cholestasis, acute intermittent porphyria, anorexia nervosa, hepatoma, and drugs such as thiazides, cyclosporine, and Tegretol. Cirrhosis is associated with reduced LDL because of inadequate production. Malabsorption, malnutrition, Gaucher's disease, chronic infectious disease, hyperthyroidism, and niacin toxicity are all similarly associated with reduced LDL.

97. The answer is D.

(Chap. 31) This patient has signs and symptoms of familial hypercholesterolemia (FH) with elevated plasma LDL, normal triglycerides, tendon xanthomas, and premature coronary artery disease. FH is an autosomal codominant lipoprotein disorder that is the most common of these syndromes caused by a single gene disorder. It has a higher prevalence in Afrikaners, Christian Lebanese, and French Canadians. There is no definitive diagnostic test for FH. It may be diagnosed with a skin biopsy that shows reduced LDL receptor activity in cultured fibroblasts (although there is considerable overlap with normals). FH is predominantly a clinical diagnosis, although molecular diagnostics are being developed. Hemolysis is not a feature of FH. Sitosterolemia is distinguished from FH by episodes of hemolysis. It is a rare autosomal recessive disorder that causes a marked increase in the dietary absorption of plant sterols. Hemolysis is due to incorporation of plant sterols into the red blood cell membrane. Sitosterolemia is confirmed by demonstrating an increase in the plasma levels of sitosterol using gas chromatography. CT scanning of the liver does not sufficiently differentiate between the hyperlipoproteinemias. Many of the primary lipoproteinemias, including sitosterolemia, are inherited in an autosomal recessive pattern, and thus a pedigree analysis would not be likely to isolate the disorder.

98. The answer is C.

(Chap. 31) This patient has nephrotic syndrome, which is likely a result of multiple myeloma. The hyperlipidemia of nephrotic syndrome appears to be due to a combination of increased hepatic production and decreased clearance of very low-density lipoproteins, with increased LDL production. It is usually mixed but can manifest as hypercholesterolemia or hypertriglyceridemia. Effective treatment of the underlying renal disease normalizes the lipid profile. Of the choices presented, HMG-CoA reductase inhibitors would be the most effective to reduce this patient's LDL. Dietary management is an important component of lifestyle modification but seldom results in a greater than 10% fall in LDL. Niacin and fibrates would be indicated if the triglycerides were higher, but the LDL is the more important lipid abnormality to address at this time. Lipid apheresis is reserved for patients who cannot tolerate the lipid-lowering drugs or who have a genetic lipid disorder refractory to medication. Cholesterol ester transfer protein inhibitors have been shown to raise high-density lipoprotein levels, and their role in the treatment of lipoproteinemias is still under investigation.

99. The answer is E.

(Chap. 37) The patient presents with prehypertension, as evidenced by systolic blood pressure of 120–139 mmHg or diastolic blood pressure of 80–89 mmHg. Although at this blood pressure medication therapy is not indicated, the MRFIT trial clearly showed a graded influence of both systolic and diastolic blood pressure on cardiovascular mortality including down to within normal range at 120 mmHg systolic. Thus, lifestyle modification is in order for the patient described here. Alcohol consumption is recommended to be two or fewer drinks per day for men and one drink or less per day for women. NaCl consumption of less than 6 g per day has been shown to reduce blood pressure in patients with established hypertension and in certain ethnic groups. To reduce blood pressure, regular moderate to intense aerobic activity for 30 minutes 6–7 days per week is recommended. Finally, a weight loss of 9.2 kg has been shown to drop blood on average 6/3 mmHg.

100. The answer is C.

(Chap. 37) Several factors have been shown to confer an increased risk of complications from hypertension. In the patient described here there is only one: ongoing tobacco use. Epidemiologic factors that have poorer prognosis include African-American race, male sex, and onset of hypertension in youth. In addition, comorbid factors that independently increase the risk of atherosclerosis worsen the prognosis in patients with hypertension. These factors include hypercholesterolemia, obesity, diabetes mellitus, and tobacco use. Physical and laboratory examination showing evidence of end-organ damage also may portend a poorer prognosis. This includes evidence of retinal damage or hypertensive heart disease with cardiac enlargement or congestive heart failure. Furthermore, electrocardiographic evidence of ischemia or left ventricular strain but not left ventricular hypertrophy alone may predict worse outcomes. A family history of hypertensive complications does not worsen the prognosis if diastolic blood pressure is maintained at less than 110 mmHg.

101 and 102.   The answers are D and E, respectively.

(Chap. 37) This patient presents at a young age with hypertension that is difficult to control, raising the question of secondary causes of hypertension. The most likely diagnosis in this patient is primary hyperaldosteronism, also known as Conn's syndrome. The patient has no physical features that suggest congenital adrenal hyperplasia or Cushing's syndrome. In addition, there is no glucose intolerance, as is commonly seen in Cushing's syndrome. The lack of episodic symptoms and the labile hypertension make pheochromocytoma unlikely. The findings of hypokalemia and metabolic alkalosis in the presence of difficult to control hypertension yield the likely diagnosis of Conn's syndrome. Diagnosis of the disease can be difficult, but the preferred test is the plasma aldosterone/renin ratio. This test should be performed at 8 A.M., and a ratio above 30 to 50 is diagnostic of primary hyperaldosteronism. Caution should be taken in interpreting this test while the patient is on ACE inhibitor therapy, as ACE inhibitors can falsely elevate plasma renin activity. However, a plasma renin level that is undetectable or an elevated aldosterone/renin ratio in the presence of ACE inhibitor therapy is highly suggestive of primary hyperaldosteronism. Selective adrenal vein renin sampling may be performed after the diagnosis to help determine if the process is unilateral or bilateral. Although fibromuscular dysplasia is a common secondary cause of hypertension in young females, the presence of hypokalemia and metabolic alkalosis should suggest Conn's syndrome. Thus, magnetic resonance imaging of the renal arteries is unnecessary in this case. Measurement of 24-hour urine collection for potassium wasting and aldosterone secretion can be useful in the diagnosis of Conn's syndrome. The measurement of metanephrines or cortisol is not indicated.

103. The answer is B.

(Chap. 38) For all patients with aortic dissection or hematoma, appropriate management includes reduction of shear stress with beta blockade and management of systemic hypertension to reduce tension on the dissection. However, emergent or urgent surgical therapy is indicated to patients with ascending aortic dissection and intramural hematomas (type A), and for complicated type B dissections (distal aorta). Complications that would warrant surgical intervention include propagation despite medical therapy, compromise of major branches, impending rupture, or continued pain. Thus, patient B has a distal dissection without evidence of complications and is the best candidate for medical therapy.

104. The answer is B.

(Chap. 38) Abdominal aortic aneurysms (AAAs) affect 1–2% of men older than age 50. Most AAAs are asymptomatic and are found incidentally on physical examination. The predisposing factors for AAA are the same as those for other cardiovascular disease, with over 90% being associated with atherosclerotic disease. Most AAAs are located infrarenally, and recent data suggest that an uncomplicated infrarenal AAA may be treated with endovascular stenting instead of the usual surgical grafting. Indications for proceeding to surgery include any patient with symptoms or an aneurysm that is growing rapidly. Serial ultrasonography or CT imaging is imperative, and all aneurysms larger than 5.5 cm warrant intervention because of the high mortality associated with repair of ruptured aortic aneurysms. The rupture rate of an AAA is directly related to size, with the 5-year risk of rupture being 1–2% with aneurysms less than 5 cm and 20–40% with aneurysms greater than 5 cm.

The mortality of patients undergoing elective repair is 1–2% and is greater than 50% for the emergent treatment of a ruptured AAA. Preoperative cardiac evaluation before elective repair is imperative, as coexisting coronary artery disease is common.

105. The answer is E.

(Chap. 38) Aortitis and ascending aortic aneurysms are commonly caused by cystic medial necrosis and mesoaortitis that result in damage to the elastic fibers of the aortic wall with thinning and weakening. Many infectious, inflammatory, and inherited conditions have been associated with this finding, including syphilis, tuberculosis, mycotic aneurysm, Takayasu's arteritis, giant cell arteritis, rheumatoid arthritis, and the spondyloarthropathies (ankylosing spondylitis, psoriatic arthritis, Reiter's syndrome, Behçet's disease). In addition, it can be seen with the genetic disorders Marfan's syndrome and Ehlers-Danlos syndrome.

106. The answer is E.

(Chap. 38) Descending aortic aneurysms are most commonly associated with atherosclerosis. The average growth rate is approximately 0.1–0.2 cm yearly. The risk of rupture and subsequent management are related to the size of the aneurysm as well as symptoms related to the aneurysm. However, most thoracic aortic aneurysms are asymptomatic. When symptoms do occur, they are frequently related to mechanical complications of the aneurysm causing compression of adjacent structures. This includes the trachea and esophagus, and symptoms can include cough, chest pain, hoarseness, and dysphagia. The risk of rupture is approximately 2–3% yearly for aneurysms less than 4 cm and increases to 7% per year once the size is greater than 6 cm. Management of descending aortic aneurysms includes blood pressure control. Beta blockers are recommended because they decrease the contractility of the heart and thus decrease aortic wall stress, potentially slowing aneurysmal growth. Individuals with thoracic aortic aneurysms should be monitored with chest imaging at least yearly, or more frequently if new symptoms develop. This can include CT angiography, MRI, or transesophageal echocardiography. Operative repair is indicated if the aneurysm expands by more than 1 cm in a year or reaches a diameter of more than 5.5–6.0 cm. Endovascular stenting for the treatment of thoracic aortic aneurysms is a relatively new procedure with limited long-term results available. The largest study to date included more than 400 patients with a variety of indications for thoracic endovascular stents. In 249 patients, the indication for stent was thoracic aortic aneurysm. This study showed an initial success rate of 87.1%, with a 30-day mortality rate of 10%. However, if the procedure was done emergently, the mortality rate at 30 days was 28%. At 1 year, data were available on only 96 of the original 249 patients with

degenerative thoracic aneurysms. In these individuals, 80% continued to have satisfactory outcomes with stenting and 14% showed growth of the aneurysm (LJ Leurs, *J Vasc Surg* 40:670, 2004). Ongoing studies with long-term follow-up are needed before endovascular stenting can be recommended for the treatment of thoracic aortic aneurysms, although in individuals who are not candidates for surgery, stenting should be considered.

107. The answer is C.

(Chap. 39) The patient presents with classic signs of arterial occlusion with limb pain, physical examination showing pallor, and a pulseless, cold leg. She has no risk factors for central or peripheral atherosclerotic disease; thus angiogram would simply confirm the diagnosis of arterial occlusion, not demonstrate her predisposing condition. In the absence of fever or systemic symptoms, vasculitis and endocarditis are unlikely sources of arterial embolization. She likely had a paradoxical embolism in the context of an atrial septal defect, which was the source of her childhood murmur. Because many of these patients develop pulmonary hypertension with time, she is now at risk for a paradoxical embolism. Although in this context, arterial emboli frequently originate from venous thrombus, the thrombi cannot produce a paradoxical embolism in the absence of right-to-left shunt, such as in a large patent foramen ovale or an atrial septal defect.

108. The answer is E.

(Chap. 42) Doppler echocardiography uses ultrasound reflecting off moving red blood cells to determine flow velocity within a structure, in this case the heart or great vessels. Thus, it is most useful for determining abnormal flow or flow limitation. Specifically, it is useful in defining valvular regurgitation or stenosis, cardiac output when combined with the cross-sectional area, and diastolic filling of the ventricle. Heart failure with preserved ejection fraction is associated with impaired left ventricle relaxation in early diastole and subsequently there is reduced early transmitral flow compared to normal individuals. Although Doppler might be helpful to determine the physiologic consequence of pericardial effusion, i.e., tamponade, two-dimensional (2D) echocardiography is the preferred mode for effusion diagnosis. Similarly, 2D echocardiography is used to calculate ejection fraction and diagnose cardiac masses. Diagnosis of ischemia can be made with the addition of physiologic or pharmacologic stress to echocardiography, but not with Doppler echocardiography.

INDEX

Bold page number indicates the start of the main discussion of the topic. Page numbers with "f" or "t" refer to figures and tables, respectively. Pages numbers with "V" refer to pages that describe the videos on the website.